MENTAL AND NEUROLOGICAL PUBLIC HEALTH:

A GLOBAL PERSPECTIVE

MENTAL AND NEUROLOGICAL PUBLIC HEALTH:

A GLOBAL PERSPECTIVE

EDITOR-IN-CHIEF

Vikram Patel
London School of Hygiene & Tropical Medicine and Sangath, Goa, India

ASSOCIATE EDITORS

Alistair Woodward
University of Auckland, Auckland, New Zealand

Valery L. Feigin
Auckland University of Technology, AUT North Shore Campus, Auckland,
New Zealand

H.K. Heggenhougen
Centre for International Health, University of Bergen, Bergen, Norway, Department of
International Health, Boston University School of Public Health and Department of Global Health
and Social Medicine, Harvard Medical School

Stella R. Quah
Duke-NUS Graduate Medical School Singapore, Singapore

AMSTERDAM • BOSTON • HEIDELBERG • LONDON • NEW YORK • OXFORD
PARIS • SAN DIEGO • SAN FRANCISCO • SINGAPORE • SYDNEY • TOKYO
Academic Press is an imprint of Elsevier

ACADEMIC
PRESS

Academic Press is an imprint of Elsevier
525 B Street, Suite 1900, San Diego, CA 92101-4495, USA
30 Corporate Drive, Suite 400, Burlington, MA 01803, USA
32 Jamestown Road, London NW1 7BY, UK
Radarweg 29, PO Box 211, 1000 AE Amsterdam, The Netherlands

First edition 2010

British Library Cataloguing in Publication Data
A catalogue record for this book is available from the British Library

Library of Congress Cataloging-in-Publication Data
Mental and neurological public health : a global perspective / editor-in-chief Vikram Patel ... [et al.]. – 1st ed.
    p. ; cm.
ISBN 978-0-12-810202-2
1. Mental health planning. 2. Mental health services. 3. Nervous system–Diseases–Treatment. I. Patel, Vikram.
[DNLM: 1. Mental Disorders–epidemiology. 2. Mental Health. 3. Nervous System Diseases–epidemiology. 4. Public Health. 5. World Health.
WM 140 M5482 2010]
RA790.5.M416 2010
362.196'89–dc22

                                                                                    2010001076

For information on all Academic Press publications
visit our website at elsevierdirect.com

PRINTED AND BOUND IN USA
10 11 12 13 10 9 8 7 6 5 4 3 2 1

CONTENTS

SECTION 3   PUBLIC HEALTH POLICY AND PRACTICE

CONTRIBUTORS

M Astejada
National Center of Neurology and Psychiatry, Tokyo, Japan

T F Babor
University of Connecticut School of Medicine, Farmington, CT, USA

D Baliunas
Centre for Addiction and Mental Health, Toronto, Canada

R L Barrett
Stanford University, Stanford, CA, USA

A E Becker
Massachusetts General Hospital, Boston, MA, USA

E D Belay
Centers for Disease Control and Prevention, Atlanta, GA, USA

J Bradshaw
Monash University, Clayton, VIC, Australia

T S Brugha
University of Leicester, Leicester, UK

R A Bryant
University of New South Wales, Sydney, NSW, Australia

R Burkard
University at Buffalo, Buffalo, NY, USA

J A Buxton
University of British Columbia, Vancouver, BC, Canada

S Casswell
Massey University, Auckland, New Zealand

P S Chandra
National Institute of Mental Health and Neuro Sciences, Bangalore, India

S H Cho
Columbia University, New York, NY, USA

A Cohen
Harvard Medical School, Boston, MA, USA

M J Crawford
Imperial College London, London, UK

A Culebras
Upstate Medical University, Syracuse, NY, USA

S Cvetkovski
Turning Point Alcohol and Drug Centre Inc., Fitzroy, VIC, Australia

J de Gans
University of Amsterdam, Amsterdam, The Netherlands

D De Leo
Griffith University, Brisbane, Queensland, Australia

L Degenhardt
University of New South Wales, Sydney, Australia

S S Delinsky
Massachusetts General Hospital, Boston, MA, USA

J Derenne
Massachusetts General Hospital, Boston, MA, USA

Y Dhansay
University of Cape Town, Cape Town, South Africa

G Donnan
University of Melbourne, Melbourne, VIC, Australia

B Easton
Centre for Social and Health Outcomes Research and Evaluation (SHORE) Massey University, Wellington, New Zealand

F Faggiano
Avogadro University, Novara, Italy

S V Faraone
SUNY Upstate Medical University, Syracuse, NY, USA

V Feigin
The University of Auckland, Auckland, New Zealand

A J Flisher
University of Cape Town, Cape Town, South Africa

M Freeman
Human Sciences Research Council, Pretoria, South Africa

C L Fry
Monash University, Frankston, VIC, Australia

M Funk
World Health Organization, Geneva, Switzerland

A P Giardino
Texas Children's Health Plan, Houston, TX, USA

K Glanz
Rollins School of Public Health, Emory University, Atlanta, GA, USA

S J Glatt
SUNY Upstate Medical University, Syracuse, NY, USA

P Griffiths
EMCDDA, Lisbon, Portugal

O Gureje
University of Ibadan, Ibadan, Nigeria

M Haden
Vancouver Coastal Health, Vancouver, BC, Canada

W Hall
University of Queensland, Herston, Australia

S Hatherill
University of Cape Town, Cape Town, South Africa

R Härtl
New York-Presbyterian Hospital, New York, NY, USA

D B Heath
Brown University, Providence, RI, USA

T Hemachudha
King Chulalongkorn Memorial Hospital, Bangkok, Thailand

H Herrman
University of Melbourne, Melbourne, VIC, Australia

I B Hickie
The University of Sydney, Sydney, NSW, Australia

L Hill
The Centre for Social and Health Outcomes Research and Evaluation (SHORE), Massey University, Auckland, New Zealand

H D Holder
Prevention Research Center, Pacific Institute for Research and Evaluation, Berkeley, CA, USA

R Jenkins
Institute of Psychiatry, London, UK

T J John
Christian Medical College, Vellore, India

A Kagee
Stellenbosch University, Matieland, South Africa

A Kleinman
Harvard University, Cambridge, MA, USA

E Klimkeit
Monash University, Clayton, VIC, Australia

J Knopman
New York-Presbyterian Hospital, New York, NY, USA

A D Korczyn
Tel-Aviv University, Ramat-Aviv, Israel

V A S Krishna
Washington University School of Medicine, St. Louis, MO, USA

K Krysinska
Griffith University, Brisbane, Queensland, Australia

U Lundberg
Stockholm University, Stockholm, Sweden

K Magruder
Medical University of South Carolina, Charleston, SC, USA

M C Malicdan
National Center of Neurology and Psychiatry, Tokyo, Japan

R G Mathias
University of British Columbia, Vancouver, BC, Canada

A May
University of Hamburg, Hamburg, Germany

R McKean-Cowdin
Keck School of Medicine of the University of Southern California, Los Angeles, CA, USA

R McKetin
University of New South Wales, Sydney, Australia

M Meacham
EMCDDA, Lisbon, Portugal

H Meltzer
University of Leicester, Leicester, UK

H Minas
University of Melbourne, Melbourne, Australia

M G Monteiro
Pan American Health Organization/World Health Organization, Washington, DC, USA

R Moodie
University of Melbourne, Melbourne, VIC, Australia

A Nickerson
University of New South Wales, Sydney, NSW, Australia

I Nishino
National Center of Neurology and Psychiatry, Tokyo, Japan

G S Norquist
University of Mississippi Medical Center, Jackson, MS, USA

B Oladeji
University of Ibadan, Ibadan, Nigeria

R Pararajasegaram
World Health Organization, Geneva, Switzerland

J Patra
Centre for Addiction and Mental Health, Toronto, Canada

D Pilgrim
University of Central Lancashire, Preston, Lancashire, UK

S Popova
Centre for Addiction and Mental Health, Toronto, Canada

C M Poser
Harvard Medical School, Boston, MA, USA

S G Post
Case Western Reserve University, Cleveland, OH, USA

V Poznyak
World Health Organization, Geneva, Switzerland

S Preston-Martin
Keck School of Medicine of the University of Southern California, Los Angeles, CA, USA

V N G P Raghunandan
National Institute of Mental Health and Neuro Sciences, Bangalore, India

L D Ravdin
Weill Medical College of Cornell University, New York, NY, USA

P Razavi
Keck School of Medicine of the University of Southern California, Los Angeles, CA, USA

J Rehm
Centre for Addiction and Mental Health, Toronto, Canada

S Resnikoff
World Health Organization, Geneva, Switzerland

N Rinehart
Monash University, Clayton, VIC, Australia

M Roerecke
Centre for Addiction and Mental Health, Toronto, Canada

B Saraceno
World Health Organization, Geneva, Switzerland

S Saxena
World Health Organization, Geneva, Switzerland

S C Schachter
Harvard Medical School, Boston, MA, USA

P Sharan
All India Institute of Medical Sciences, New Delhi, India

D Silove
University of New South Wales, Sydney, NSW, Australia

N Sindicich
University of New South Wales, Sydney, Australia

I Skoog
The Sahlgrenska Academy at the University of Göteborg, Göteborg, Sweden

S S Spudich
University of California at San Francisco, San Francisco, CA, USA

T Stockwell
Centre for Addictions Research of British Columbia, Victoria, Canada

J E Stryker
Rollins School of Public Health, Emory University, Atlanta, GA, USA

M Taj
Schizophrenia Research Foundation, Chennai, India

M Tarnopolsky
McMaster University, Hamilton, ON, Canada

B Taylor
Centre for Addiction and Mental Health, Toronto, Canada

V Tepsumethanon
King Chulalongkorn Memorial Hospital, Bangkok, Thailand

R Thara
Schizophrenia Research Foundation, Chennai, India

S Tirupati
The University of Newcastle, Newcastle, NSW, Australia

M T Tsuang
University of California, San Diego, La Jolla, CA, USA; Harvard Institute of Psychiatric Epidemiology and Genetics, Boston, MA, USA; Veterans Affairs San Diego Healthcare System, San Diego, CA, USA

T B Üstün
World Health Organization, Geneva, Switzerland

D van de Beek
University of Amsterdam, Amsterdam, The Netherlands

F Vigna-Taglianti
Piedmont Centre for Drug Addiction Epidemiology, Grugliasco, Italy

S Wacharapluesadee
King Chulalongkorn Memorial Hospital, Bangkok, Thailand

H Wilde
King Chulalongkorn Memorial Hospital, Bangkok, Thailand

L H Yang
Columbia University, New York, NY, USA

PREFACE

Health problems related to disorders affecting the nervous system may manifest in a variety of ways, affect people across the life course, and present themselves to health practitioners working in very diverse settings. While, in the context of clinical care, there may appear to be little in common between autism and epilepsy in childhood, depression and substance abuse in adulthood, and dementia in the elderly, they do in fact share a number of features: they are mostly mediated through brain dysfunction or abnormalities, are often chronic in course, typically benefit from multi-component interventions, and are among the most neglected conditions in global health. One of the most common trends worldwide is the low proportion of people affected by brain dysfunction or abnormalities who receive adequate medical care. This 'treatment gap' is estimated to be acutely serious in low income countries where only about one of every ten persons affected might actually receive treatment. Many of these conditions are associated with high levels of stigma and discrimination and frank human rights violations. Prevention of these conditions and closing the treatment gap for those who are already affected, are among the current global health priorities. It is in this context that this volume on the international public health analysis of mental and neurological disorders is particularly relevant.

Although the acknowledgement of the global health significance of mental, substance use, and neurological disorders is relatively recent, there have been significant advances in our knowledge base which can inform public health policy, programs, and practice. The time is ripe to take stock of what we know and to synthesize the evidence and opportunities to fill gaps in the evidence. Thus, for example, questions regarding the relative role of 'up-stream' versus proximal determinants and the roles of social and biological factors in determining risk for these conditions, the methods for detection and measurement, the individual and population level interventions for prevention, treatment and rehabilitation, and the public health policies which enable these are critical issues for the future growth of the disciplines of mental and neurological public health.

This volume brings together 59 chapters from the Psychiatry, Neurology, Substance Abuse, and Child Development sections of the *International Encyclopedia of Public Health*. These chapters address the public health implications of 'brain disorders' in a comprehensive manner and from a global perspective. The volume is divided into three sections. The first section 'Epidemiology' comprises chapters on the epidemiology and research methods of mental and neurological disorders. Section 2 'Clinical Syndromes' addresses specific clinical syndromes reviewing the evidence on these syndromes, key clinical features, epidemiology, treatment and prevention, and related public health policy and practices. Section 3 deals with broader principles of public health practice and policy relevant to mental and neurological disorders. The sheer diversity of subjects and authors in this volume is a testimony to the rich variety and depth that this discipline has to offer. We anticipate the volume will become the standard reference for students and practitioners of public health aspects of mental and neurological disorders.

Vikram Patel
Alistair Woodward
Valery L. Feigin
H.K. Heggenhougen
and
Stella R. Quah

SECTION 1
EPIDEMIOLOGY

Alcohol Consumption: Overview of International Trends

M G Monteiro, Pan American Health Organization/World Health Organization, Washington, DC, USA
J Rehm and B Taylor, Centre for Addiction and Mental Health, Toronto, Canada
T Stockwell, Centre for Addictions Research of British Columbia, Victoria, Canada

Introduction

Alcohol consumption is linked to over 60 health conditions and the related burden of disease is high; it ranks as the fifth most important risk factor for the burden of disease worldwide (Rehm *et al.*, 2003b); (WHO, 2002) and ranked first in the region of the Americas for the year 2000 (Rehm and Monteiro, 2005). There is ample evidence that the overall consumption of alcohol in a population is a good proxy for the percentage of heavy drinkers in that population. Overall consumption is related to all-cause mortality and alcohol-specific mortality and disability (Edwards *et al.*, 1994); therefore, changes in consumption lead to changes in the overall as well as the alcohol-specific disease burden in a population. As a result, national and international trends in alcohol consumption are related to disease outcomes and serve as monitoring tools of policy changes at country, regional, and global levels.

Two Dimensions of Alcohol Consumption

There are two dimensions of alcohol consumption: average volume of consumption and patterns of drinking, both of which are related to disease burden (Rehm *et al.*, 2003). Average volume, or per capita consumption, is related mostly to long-term health consequences, including alcohol dependence. Although average volume is also related to acute consequences, such as injuries, several studies indicate that the ability to predict such injuries is increased by taking patterns of drinking into account (Rehm *et al.*, 1996). For example, the same average volume of consumption (1 drink per day) can be consumed in one day of the week (7 drinks on one occasion) or through daily drinking (1 drink per day over 7 days), and the expected outcomes are different. In other words, how an individual drinks, which is influenced by cultural context, can moderate the impact of average volume of consumption on mortality and morbidity.

The pattern of drinking (how, when, and how much is consumed) has been related to acute health outcomes such as injuries and also to chronic diseases such as coronary heart disease and sudden cardiac death (Rehm *et al.*, 2006).

As part of the World Health Organization (WHO) Comparative Assessment of Risk Factors for the Global Burden of Disease study (2000), both dimensions of alcohol consumption for different regions of the world were quantified. It is beyond the scope of this article to cover details of such study, which can be found in other publications (Rehm *et al.*, 2003a, b). This article provides an overview of some methodological issues regarding these two dimensions relevant for comparative studies at the national level, and presents an international trend analysis as well.

Methodological Issues

The WHO has recently updated international guidelines for monitoring alcohol consumption and related harm (WHO, 2000). This guide provides details on how to calculate per capita consumption and related harms, including limitations and problems in interpreting the data. It should be consulted when planning to collect and use national and international estimates.

Estimating Per Capita Consumption by Country

Estimating the average volume of alcohol consumption in a country is best made using national sales and production and/or taxation data, as population surveys invariably underestimate total alcohol consumption. Retail sales data are the most accurate means of estimating how alcohol is consumed in a population, as governments often monitor sales data for tax collection purposes. Although there are some limitations to this type of data (e.g., beverages can be purchased yet not consumed in the same year, stockpiling can occur before a tax increase, neither home production nor smuggling is accounted for), it is still a relatively reliable source.

When gathering these data, the three major categories of alcoholic beverages (beer, wine, and distilled spirits) available within a country should be included in the estimates. In many developing countries, however, local beverages are as important as the three major categories (e.g., cider, fruit wines, *shochu, aguardiente, cachaca, samsu*) but often do not fall into the other categories or are sold in informal markets or are not taxed. Therefore, additional survey data can provide information on who drinks what type of beverages (at least by gender and age groups), which can then be useful in monitoring trends in consumption and relating specific beverages to specific harms.

Per capita consumption figures are given in liters of pure alcohol, which require estimates and/or assumptions about alcohol content of different beverages. Beer, for example, is usually estimated at 5% pure alcohol, but it can vary from 0.9 to 12%. As there is no international standard, countries should make periodic efforts to estimate median alcohol content of each beverage category as they can vary widely from country to country as well as within regions of the same country.

According to WHO recommendations, the total estimated adult alcohol consumption for a country is equal to the total alcohol production plus alcohol imports minus alcohol exports (in the same year) divided by the total population of 15 years of age and over. However, in calculating the average consumption of the total population there may be an underestimate of consumption, particularly in developing countries in which a large proportion of the population is under 15 years of age.

Market research firms serving the alcoholic beverage industry, or industry associations are a good source of data (e.g., *Impact Databank*, *World Drink Trends*, *Statistical Handbook*); however, these data are expensive to obtain and therefore of limited use by governments or researchers. These publications do not cover all countries, especially developing countries, and the information is often not reliable. However, in the absence of any other more reliable source of information, they can be used to supplement data at country and international levels.

The impact of tourism can also be substantial, and some estimate of the size of the tourist population in a given year (15 years of age and older) can be used for estimating adult per capita consumption for a country. If there are special sales taxes or measures for alcoholic beverages sold to tourists that can distinguish them from local consumption, the estimates can be done more adequately.

The United Nations Food and Agriculture Organization (FAO) publishes the most complete set of statistics available on the production and trade of beer, wine, and distilled spirits, and this set can be used in the absence of sales data. These statistics are collected from annual questionnaires sent to ministries of agriculture and trade (they are also available to the public on the FAO's website, see under 'Relevant Websites' section). The data consist of estimates of production and trade in metric tons for wine; vermouth; must of grape; fermented beverages; spirits; sorghum, millet, maize, and barley beer; and wheat-fermented and rice-fermented beverages. Beverage data are converted into metric tons of pure alcohol and then all beers are combined into a single beer category, all wines into a wine category, and all spirits into a 'beverages, alcoholic' or distilled spirits category (WHO, 2000). However, the data rely on national reporting (and not all countries are included) and do not include estimates of unrecorded consumption (e.g., home production, duty-free alcohol, smuggling). Nonetheless, the FAO remains the most comprehensive international data source on production of alcoholic beverages. Caution needs to be taken, however, in interpreting the data. Because only large-scale industrial production is quantified, data for countries with substantial informal, low-technology, or home production will be underestimated, as is the case with several African countries. In addition, when data are missing, the gaps are filled with repeated information of the last year reported. As the country population grows, per capita consumption may artificially decline, thus providing a false trend (WHO, 2000).

Estimating Levels of Consumption and Patterns of Drinking

General population surveys can provide a wide range of information on where drinking takes place, patterns of consumption, sociodemographic correlates, and alcohol-related harms. At the simplest level of analysis, they can provide information regarding, for example, the number of abstainers in the population in the last 12 months, lifetime abstainers, and consumption of alcohol by gender. There is variation worldwide on the rates of abstinence for men and women. There are countries in which the rate of abstinence is very high for both genders (e.g., where drinking is prohibited for religious reasons), and countries in which most of the drinking is done by males, with females drinking relatively less. Some European countries present no differences between genders. When rates of abstinence are considered, the average amount of alcohol consumption per drinker can be much greater than expected.

Population-level data cannot, however, identify different drinking patterns in a population, who does the drinking (e.g., which age groups), how patterns relate to socioeconomic characteristics of the population or to gender, where the drinking takes place, when and how it is consumed, if it is concentrated into special occasions of high consumption, such as in festivals or holidays, or is more evenly distributed throughout the year.

Surveys can also indicate the prevalence of high-, moderate-, and low-risk drinkers, according to clearly defined criteria. Patterns of drinking are not uniform across different studies thus, for the global burden of disease study, patterns of drinking have to be defined and estimated. A key informant questionnaire was sent to countries and, after two surveys, data were obtained from 63 countries in all regions but the Eastern Mediterranean. Four different aspects of drinking were covered by the survey: heavy drinking occasions (e.g., festive drinking at fiestas or community celebrations, the proportion of drinking occasions in which drinkers get drunk, the proportion of drinkers who drink daily or nearly daily, drinking with meals, and drinking in public places.

The results of this and other such surveys were combined with available national or regional survey results (unpublished information or publications in peer-review journals). They were then analyzed using optimal scaling analysis, which is similar to factor analysis but permits the simultaneous inclusion of ordinal and categorical data, to determine the number of underlying dimensions and the relations of items to each dimension. The analysis identified one dimension called a detrimental impact that leads to increased mortality and morbidity.

The countries were then classified into four categories and assigned values from 1 (least risky drinking pattern) to 4 (most risky drinking pattern). Rates of abstention were taken into account separately in the final comparative risk analysis (for the final algorithms for calculating pattern scores, see Rehm *et al.*, 2003b).

Rates of a variety of alcohol-related problems can be explored by surveys and linked to patterns of drinking and amount or frequency of drinking. Information on alcohol use disorders, using validated instruments such as AUDIT (Babor *et al.*, 2001) and CAGE (Ewing, 1984), and diagnostic criteria such as those found in the ICD-10 or DSM-IV, can be of value. This information is important when assessing coverage of treatment services in a particular country and then planning the organization of health treatment systems to respond to the range of alcohol-related problems.

On surveys, the most used and recommended questions regarding alcohol consumption are quantity-frequency, graduated frequency, and recent recall (WHO, in press). Even though there is still little agreement in the literature on which questions to include in surveys, and how to ask them, international collaborative studies have tried to increase comparability of data by agreeing on common indicators on a core number of areas, thus some progress has been made. Two studies are the GEN-ACIS study (Gender, Alcohol, Culture: An International Study), which included 35 countries from most regions of the world and assessed alcohol consumption and related problems from the adult general population, and the ESPAD (European School Survey Project on Alcohol and Drugs), which collected information from school students 13–15 years of age in European countries in 1995, 1999, and 2003, using the same basic questionnaire.

There are numerous methodological issues to be considered when planning, undertaking, and interpreting data from surveys. These include reference period, beverage-specific or overall questions on consumption, quantity per drinking day versus quantity per drinking occasion, drink size and alcohol content of alcoholic beverages (and mixed drinks), criteria for defining a drinker or non-drinker, validity and reliability of the survey instrument in the absence of international standardization, criteria for risk drinking (on a single occasion and average daily consumption, for acute or chronic problems), sample selection, and sample size, among others. The WHO guide (2000) is a good source of information on these methodological issues and how to address them.

WHO Alcohol Database

Although several attempts have been made in the past at summarizing world and regional drinking trends from a public health perspective, a key initiative from the WHO has become the most comprehensive source of data on alcohol in the world. In 1996, the WHO organized the Global Alcohol Database, bringing together the most reliable and updated information on alcohol consumption and related harm by country. It was created by the Marin Institute for the Prevention of Alcohol and Other Drug Problems, and maintained for some time by the Swiss Institute for the Prevention of Alcohol Problems. It is currently hosted and maintained by the Centre for Addiction and Mental Health in Toronto, Canada. Data from recorded production are included as well as data from national surveys and estimations of unrecorded consumption, health effects, national alcohol policies, and interventions. The database has information from the majority of countries in the world, although there are many gaps in the validity and reliability of the information.

In 1999 the WHO published the first *Global Status Report on Alcohol*, which included estimates of adult per capita consumption for most countries, relying on a combination of national and regional estimates, industry data, and data from the FAO and the UN Statistical Office (WHO, 1999). In 2001, it published the *Global Status Report: Alcohol and Young People* (WHO, 2001). In 2004, WHO (2004a) published the *Global Status Report: Alcohol Policy* and the *Global Status Report on Alcohol 2004* (2004b). The latter publication provided time-series analysis from 1961 to 2001 for all beverages, and also for beer, spirits, and wine separately, in liters of pure alcohol per adult per year in each country. Data regarding alcohol consumption from cross-border shopping, smuggling, legal or illegal home production (unless included in FAO estimates), or tourists were not included, however, estimates were given for recent years for many countries. The adult per capita consumption estimates were based on either FAO or World Drink Trends data, except for a few countries in which data were available directly from governments. The WHO estimates of adult per capita consumption are regularly updated, in support of WHO initiatives and global burden of disease calculations.

The following section illustrates some examples of uses of the WHO database for analyzing international trends in alcohol consumption, globally and regionally.

Data available up to 2003, in most cases, were used for all analysis. Even though there are methodological limitations inherent in the data, the results still provide interesting and useful information.

Results of Data Collection

Table 1 summarizes the characteristics of adult alcohol consumption in different regions of the world for the year 2002; **Figure 1** represents the global trend by beverage type (beer, wine, spirits) with time-series analysis from 1961–2003.

In most regions, spirits represent the main source of pure alcohol in total consumption, with the most growth during the last 30 years. Beer consumption, however, is also growing. Global wine production and consumption has decreased, mainly due to decreases in consumption in Southern Europe, a leading area of production and consumption in the world (one should bear in mind that regional differences can cancel each other out therefore looking only at the data at global levels might be misleading). **Figures 2, 3,** and **4** are regional analyses of trends; **Figure 5** shows that the two regions showing recent and continuing increases in consumption are South-East Asia and the Western Pacific.

The average adult per capita consumption, including unrecorded consumption, for 2002 is compared by country in **Figure 6**, indicating how countries and regions differ in their overall consumption levels. **Figure 7** illustrates the WHO subregions that show the typical pattern of alcohol consumption around the world for the year 2002. As can be seen, detrimental patterns of consumption are the norm in the vast majority of the developing world, which means that in those countries, there is no evidence that the population drinks at low-risk levels. Not surprisingly, there were no protective effects of low levels of alcohol consumption found for these countries.

Age and gender

Information by age and gender is insufficient for international comparisons across time on volume or patterns of alcohol consumption. Only recently, internationally comparable data have been collected in different countries. The ESPAD surveys in European countries, for example, which collected data in 1995, 1999, and 2003 among 13- to 15-year-old school children, indicated that lifetime use of alcohol (i.e., 40 times or more) has increased in several countries, as well as in the proportion of people who had been drunk 20 times or more in their lifetime (trends were not uniform across all participating countries).

Table 1   Characteristics of alcohol consumption in the world in 2002

WHO region	Adult population (1000's)[a]	Percent of abstainers		Adult total per capita alcohol consumption (in liters of pure alcohol)	Unrecorded consumption	Pattern value[b]	Recorded beverage most consumed
		M	W				
Africa D	180 316	59.3	69.3	7.2	2.2	2.8	Other fermented beverages
Africa E	208 662	55.4	73.3	6.9	2.7	3.1	Other fermented beverages and beer
America A	262 651	32.0	52.0	9.4	1.1	2.0	Beer
America B	311 514	18.0	39.1	8.4	2.6	3.1	Beer
America D	46 049	32.1	51.0	7.4	4.0	3.1	Spirits and beer
Eastern Mediterranean B	94 901	86.9	95.0	1.0	0.7	2.6	Spirits
Eastern Mediterranean D	219 457	90.8	98.9	0.6	0.4	2.6	Beer
Europe A	347 001	11.4	23.0	12.1	1.3	1.5	Beer and wine
Europe B	155 544	38.6	62.4	7.5	2.8	2.9	Spirits and beer
Europe C	197 891	13.0	26.9	14.9	6.1	3.9	Spirits
South East Asia B	215 853	77.6	96.9	2.3	0.9	3.0	Spirits
South East Asia D	854 450	79.0	98.0	1.9	1.6	3.0	Spirits
Western Pacific A	131 308	13.0	29.0	9.4	1.7	2.0	Spirits
Western Pacific B	1 164 701	26.3	62.5	6.0	1.1	2.2	Spirits
World	4 388 297	44.8	65.6	6.2	1.7	2.6	Spirits (53%)

[a]The adult per capita consumption is an average of the available data from 2001 to 2003 (usually the arithmetic mean of the 3 years).
[b]This 4-point scale reflects how people drink instead of how much, and is very important in determining alcohol-attributable harms. A score of 1 characterizes a less detrimental drinking behavior (moderate consumption with meals, no irregular heavy drinking), whereas a score of 4 (highest level of irregular, heavy drinking) characterizes alcohol consumption in the most detrimental way for health. Source: WHO Expert Committee on Problems Related to Alcohol Consumption (2007) Second Report, WHO Technical Report Series 944, World Health Organization Geneva, Switzerland. WHO.

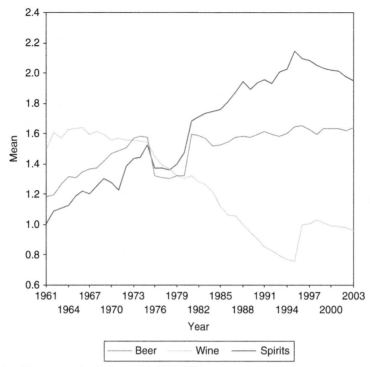

Figure 1   Beer, wine, and spirit consumption in the world, 1961–2003.

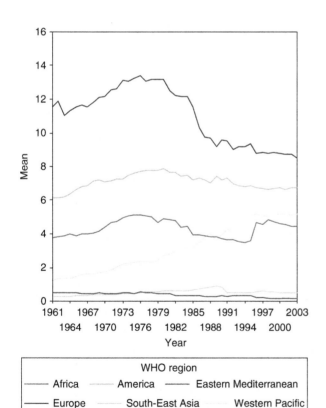

Figure 2   Adult per capita consumption in six WHO Regions: Africa, Americas, Eastern Mediterranean, Europe, South-East Asia, and Western Pacific, 1961–2003.

Mortality data

Analysis of mortality data from alcohol-related causes indicated that alcohol is responsible for most deaths among young people aged 15–29 years (WHO, 2002), but it is unknown if this has increased over the years, is a new phenomenon, or has been happening for decades because the data have not been analyzed in such a way that would show alcohol as a key risk factor.

Alcohol Consumption in Various Regions of the World

Both overall volume of alcohol consumption and patterns of drinking have considerable measurement error but remain the best indicators against which alcohol-related health burden is calculated. Adult per capita consumption should include, in many countries, an estimate of unrecorded consumption (even though that estimate will have limitations). In addition, systematic collection of data at country level is needed for trend analysis, but given the low priority given to alcohol (despite its importance as a risk factor for disease burden), and the limited resources in middle- and low-income countries, it remains a challenge to promote alcohol policies in the absence of reliable data.

Alcohol consumption has decreased or stabilized in developed countries overall, although averages are still considered high, with a pattern of use that is not as

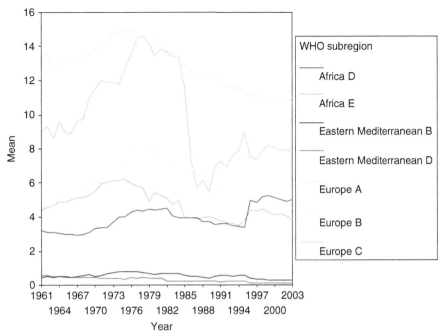

Figure 3 Adult per capita consumption in seven WHO subregions: Africa D and E, Eastern Mediterranean B and D, and Europe A, B, and C, 1961–2003.

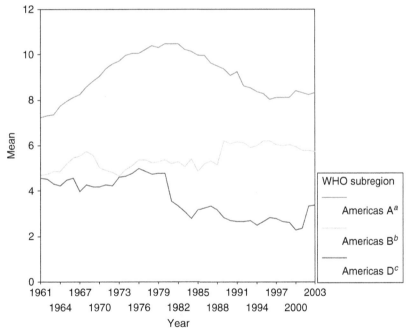

Figure 4 Adult per capita consumption in three WHO subregions: Americas A, B, and D, 1961–2003.
[a]Canada, Cuba, United States of America.
[b]Antigua and Barbuda, Argentina, Bahamas, Barbados, Belize, Brazil, Chile, Colombia, Costa Rica, Dominica, Dominican Republic, El Salvador, Grenada, Guyana, Honduras, Jamaica, Mexico, Panama, Paraguay, Saint Kitts and Nevis, Saint Lucia, Saint Vincent and the Grenadines, Suriname, Trinidad and Tobago, Uruguay, Venezuela.
[c]Bolivia, Ecuador, Guatemala, Haiti, Nicaragua, Peru.

detrimental as seen in other countries. Several European countries, aware of their high per capita consumption of alcohol, have enacted the best examples of alcohol control policies over the years based on high prices and taxation, low allowance for duty-free imports, and limits on the hours of sale of alcohol. These have led to measurable decreases in consumption and related harm. More recently, as a result of policy changes, new increases in alcohol consumption and

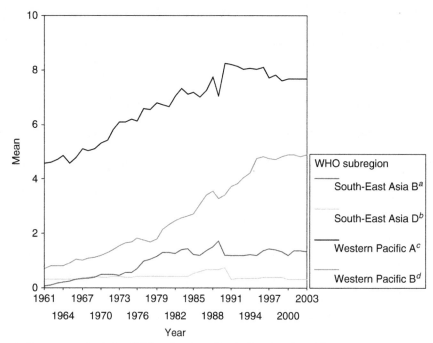

Figure 5 Adult per capita consumption in four WHO subregions: South-East Asia B and D, and Western Pacific A and B, 1961–2003.
[a]Indonesia, Sri Lanka, Thailand.
[b]Bangladesh, Bhutan, Democratic People's Republic of Korea, India, Maldives, Myanmar, Nepal.
[c]Australia, Brunei Darussalam, Japan, New Zealand, Singapore.
[d]Cambodia, China, Cook Islands, Fiji, Kiribati, Lao People's Democratic Republic, Malaysia, Marshall Islands, Micronesia
(Federated States of), Mongolia, Nauru, Niue, Palau, Papua New Guinea, Phillipines, Republic of Korea, Samoa, Solomon Islands,
Tonga, Tuvalu, Vanuatu, Vietnam.

related harm have been reported, such as in Sweden, Finland, Canada, and the UK, among others. Given that in many countries, unrecorded alcohol consumption is significant but difficult to estimate, these trends can be seen as an underestimation of the real situation, for example, upward trends are informally reported in Latin America.

In contrast, other regions of the world have shown less concern about the drinking habits of their residents. These regions risk further escalation of the problem. European markets are considered saturated, as the levels of consumption have stabilized (although the pattern of drinking might change, e.g., more binge drinking). As a result, alcohol marketing strategies have focused on new markets, including Asia and Latin America.

The Americas

Whereas the United States and Canada have population characteristics similar to Western Europe, in the other regions of the Americas countries are at different stages of development, some with relatively higher child and adult mortality rates, and an age structure different from that in developed countries. Latin America and the Caribbean have large proportions of young people, the age group that drinks the most (Levy, 1999). The problem is compounded because alcohol policies are absent or nearly so in these countries, thus creating a fertile ground

for the growth of alcohol-related problems. Informal and/ or illicit production and smuggling are known to be widespread in several countries in the Americas e.g., Brazil, Mexico, Nicaragua, and Bolivia, with little or no government control over them.

It is useful to look at the situation in the Americas as an example of international trends. Despite great subregional variations in per capita alcohol consumption, the population-weighted average value in the Americas is about 9 liters per person, well above the global average of 5.8 liters of per capita consumption (Rehm and Monteiro, 2005). In addition, irregular, heavy drinking occasions are very common, leading to a drinking pattern that is harmful to health. This translates into acute health problems, such as intentional and nonintentional injuries, including homicides, traffic crashes, violence, drowning, and suicides. At the same time, a significant proportion of the population with alcohol use disorders, particularly dependence, develop chronic health problems resulting in many years of life lost to disabilities and accounting for over 50% of all alcohol-related disease burden. It is estimated that there are over 30 million people that meet diagnostic criteria for alcohol use disorders in Latin America and the Caribbean, and over 75% did not receive any care (Kohn et al., 2005).

Most of the alcohol-related disease burden in the Americas (77.4%) occurs in the population aged 15–44,

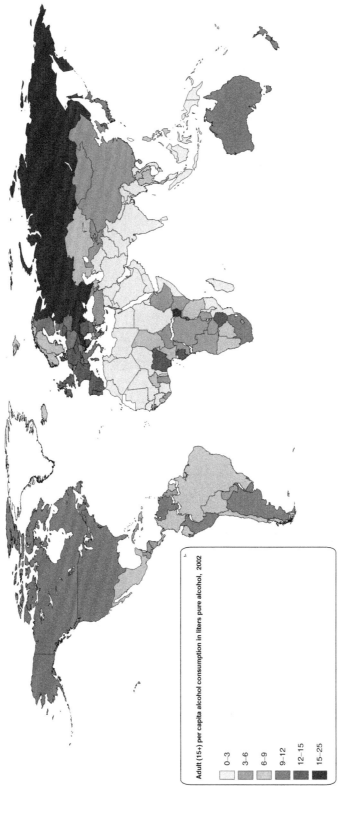

Figure 6 Adult per capita consumption including unrecorded consumption in 2002 (based on average 2001–03).

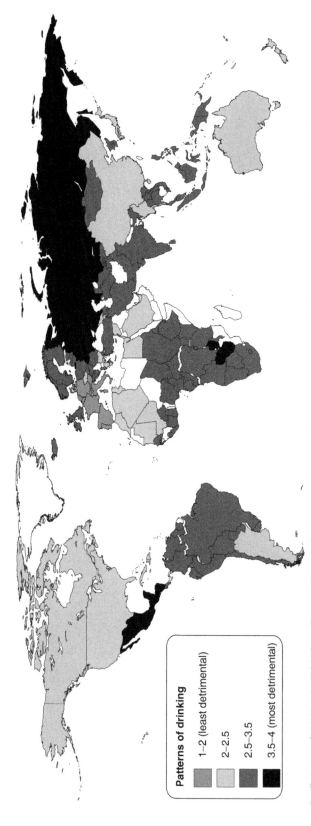

Figure 7   Patterns of drinking in 2002. From Rehm J, Patra J, Baliunas D, Popova S, Roerecke M, and Taylor B (2006) Alcohol consumption and global burden of disease 2002. Report to WHO. Geneva: World Health Organization.

Patterns of drinking

- 1–2 (least detrimental)
- 2–2.5
- 2.5–3.5
- 3.5–4 (most detrimental)

indicating that the most active and productive life years are being lost by a preventable factor, that is, alcohol consumption (Rehm and Monteiro, 2005). Socioeconomic development tends to be associated with higher levels of alcohol consumption, as people with more disposable income will spend more on alcoholic beverages (as they become more accessible and available). Concomitantly, for those living in poverty, expenditures on alcohol consumption can ruin family finances and their chances to attain better education, shelter, nutrition, health, and access to other goods and services (Room *et al.*, 2002).

Conclusion

The absence of effective national policies renders untenable the current situation. The public is largely uninformed about how alcohol consumption is related to harms, and what works to reduce public health problems from such consumption. They often believe their personal freedoms are at stake when alcohol controls are proposed. International and national trends can be critical information for advocacy groups, policy makers, and the public in the promotion of effective strategies. There is a need to continue to improve the knowledge base about alcohol consumption and patterns of drinking, using standardized indicators and collecting systematic information by age and gender, and both developed and developing countries.

See also: Alcohol: The Burden of Disease; Alcohol—Socio-Economic Impacts (Including Externalities); Alcoholism Treatment; Alcohol Industry.

Citations

Babor T, Higgins-Biddle JC, Saunders JB, and Monteiro MG (2001) AUDIT: Alcohol Use Disorders Identification Test: Guidelines for use in primary care. WHO/MSD/MSB/01.6a. Geneva, Switzerland: World Health Organization.
Edwards G, Anderson P, Babor TF, *et al.* (1994) *Alcohol Policy and the Public Good.* Oxford, UK: Oxford University Press.
Ewing JA (1984) Detecting Alcoholism: The CAGE questionnaire. *Journal of the American Medical Association* 252: 1905–1907
Kohn R, Levav I, Caldas de Almeida JM, *et al.* (2005) Los trastornos mentales en América Latina y el Caribe: Asunto prioritario para la salud publica. *Revista panamericana de salud pública* 18(4/5): 229–240.
Levy DT (1999) *Costs of Underage Drinking.* Washington, DC: Pacific Institute for Research and Evaluation.
Rehm J, Ashley MJ, Room R, *et al.* (1996) Drinking patterns and their consequences: Report from an international meeting. *Addiction* 91: 1615–1621.
Rehm J, Rehn N, Room R, *et al.* (2003a) The global distribution of average volume of alcohol consumption and patterns of drinking. *European Addiction Research* 9: 147–156.
Rehm J, Room R, Monteiro M, *et al.* (2003b) Alcohol as a risk factor for global burden of disease. *European Addiction Research* 9: 157–164.
Rehm J and Monteiro M (2005) Alcohol consumption and burden of disease in the Americas – implications for alcohol policy. *Pan American Journal of Public Health* 18(4/5): 241–248.
Rehm J, Patra J, Baliunas D, Popova S, Roerecke M, and Taylor B (2006) Alcohol consumption and global burden of disease 2002. Report to WHO. Geneva, Switzerland: World Health Organization.
Room R, Jernigan D, Carlini-Marlatt B, *et al.* (2002) Alcohol in developing societies: A public health approach vol. 46). Geneva, Switzerland: Finnish Foundation for Alcohol Studies.
World Health Organization (WHO) (1999) *Global Status Report on Alcohol.* Geneva, Switzerland: WHO, Substance Abuse Department.
World Health Organization (WHO) (2000) *International Guide for Monitoring Alcohol Consumption and Related Harm.* Geneva, Switzerland: WHO, http://whqlibdocowho.int/hq/2000/WHO_MSD_MSB_00.4.pdf.
World Health Organization (WHO) (2001) *Global Status Report: Alcohol and Young People.* Geneva, Switzerland: WHO, Substance Abuse Department.
World Health Organization (WHO) (2002) *World Health Report 2002: Reducing Risks, Promoting Healthy Life.* Geneva, Switzerland: WHO.
World Health Organization (WHO) (2004) *Global Status Report: Alcohol Policy.* Geneva, Switzerland: WHO, Department of Mental Health and Substance Abuse.
WHO Expert Committee on Problems Related to Alcohol Consumption (2007) Second Report, WHO Technical Report Series 944, World Health Organization Geneva, Switzerland. WHO.

Further Reading

Babor T, Caetano R, Edwards G, *et al.* (2003) Alcohol: no ordinary commodity. *Research and Public Policy.* Oxford, UK: Oxford University Press.
Chisholm D, *et al.* (2004) Reducing the global burden of hazardous alcohol use: a comparative cost-effectiveness analysis. *Journal of Studies on Alcohol* 65: 782–793.
International Agency for Research on Cancer (1998) Alcohol drinking. (*IARC Monographs on the Evaluation of Carcinogenic Risks to Humans* vol 44; http://monographs.iarc.fr/ENG/vol44.pdf).

Relevant Websites

http://www.espad.org – The European School Survey Project on Alcohol and Other Drugs.
http://www.fao.org – Food and Agriculture Organization of the United Nations.
http://www.who.int/alcohol – WHO Statistical Information System (WHOSIS).

Alcohol: The Burden of Disease

J Rehm, J Patra, D Baliunas, S Popova, M Roerecke, and B Taylor, Centre for Addiction and Mental Health, Toronto, Canada

Introduction

In the World Health Organization (WHO) Comparative Risk Assessment (CRA) study (Ezzati *et al.*, 2004; Lopez *et al.*, 2006; for details on alcohol, see Rehm *et al.*, 2004), alcohol proved to be one of the most important risk factors for global burden of disease (GBD), ranking fifth, just behind tobacco (alcohol attributable burden in 2000: 4.0% of global burden compared to 4.1% of tobacco). Only being under weight, resulting mainly from malnutrition and underfeeding, unsafe sex, and high blood pressure, had more impact on burden of disease than these two substances (WHO, 2002).

This article outlines the comprehensive background of and updates the comparative risk analyses and their calculations on alcohol-attributable burden of disease. It is based on:

- A review of evidence on developments of alcohol exposure in different parts of the world between 2001 and 2003 based on the WHO Global Alcohol Database (GAD);
- An update of current knowledge on the relationships between consumption of alcohol and disease and injury outcomes; and
- New calculations on burden of disease for the year 2002 undertaken by Colin Mathers and his team at the WHO (Mathers *et al.*, 2003).

Establishing Alcohol as a Risk Factor for Burden of Disease

Dimensions of Alcohol Relevant for Burden of Disease and Social Harm

The relationship between alcohol consumption and health and social outcomes is complex and multidimensional. **Figure 1** gives an overview. Alcohol consumption is linked to health and social consequences through three intermediate outcomes: direct biochemical effects, intoxication, and dependence (Rehm *et al.*, 2003a). An example of such direct biochemical effects is the promotion of blood clot dissolution or direct toxic effects on acinar cells triggering pancreatic damage. **Figure 1** shows only the main causal pathways thus indirect consequences were not included. For example, the model does not explicitly cover the situation in which a drunk driver kills somebody and, due to the emotional impact of this event on the drunk driver, he or she loses employment and becomes socially marginalized. In this example, the model covers the effects of alcohol on acute consequences (i.e., the driving accident), but does not explicitly cover the subsequent job loss and social marginalization.

Intoxication and dependence are, of course, also influenced by biochemistry. However, since these two intermediate outcomes are central in shaping the effect of alcohol on many health and social outcomes, they are discussed separately. The other pathways are often specific for one disease or a limited group of diseases. Both intoxication and dependence are defined as health outcomes in the *International Classification of Diseases* (ICD-10).

Direct biochemical effects, intoxication, and alcohol dependence

Direct biochemical effects of alcohol may influence chronic disease either in a beneficial or harmful way. Beneficial effects include the influence of moderate drinking on coronary heart disease by way of effects on reduction of plaque deposits in arteries, on protection against blood clot formation, and on promotion of blood clot dissolution. Examples of harmful effects include increasing the risk for high blood pressure and direct toxic effects on acinar cells triggering pancreatic damage or hormonal disturbances. The label of direct toxic and beneficial effects is used to summarize all the biochemical effects of alcohol on body functions, which are independent of intoxication and dependence. In terms of the level of burden, special emphasis should be given to the hepatotoxic properties of some forms of alcohol, such as surrogate alcohol in Russia and other countries in Central and Eastern Europe (McKee *et al.*, 2005).

Intoxication is a powerful mediator mainly for acute outcomes, such as accidents, intentional injuries or deaths, and domestic conflict and violence, although intoxication episodes can also be implicated in chronic health and social problems. The effects of alcohol on the central nervous system mainly determine the subjective feeling of intoxication. These effects are felt and can be measured even at consumption levels that are light to moderate (Eckhardt *et al.*, 1998).

Alcohol dependence is a disorder in itself, but is also a powerful mechanism sustaining alcohol consumption and mediating its impact on both chronic and acute physiological and social consequences of alcohol (Rehm *et al.*, 2004).

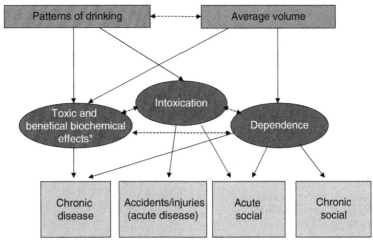

Figure 1 Model of alcohol consumption, intermediate outcomes, and long-term consequences. Asterisk indicates independent of intoxication or dependence. Reproduced from Rehm J, Room R, Graham K, *et al.* (2003a) The relationship of average volume of alcohol consumption and patterns of drinking to burden of disease – an overview. *Addiction* 98: 1209–1228, with permission of Blackwell Publishing.

This article is restricted to health consequences only. However, when analyzing the burden of disease linked to alcohol one should not overlook that in some regions and countries, the social harm related to alcohol is more important or costly than the health consequences.

To Which Disease and Injury Conditions is Alcohol Causally Relevant?

Two general types of disease and injury conditions causally impacted by alcohol can be distinguished (Rehm *et al.*, 2003a): (1) disease and injury conditions that are caused by alcohol by definition (e.g., alcohol dependence or alcohol intoxication), and (2) disease and injury conditions in which alcohol is a contributory cause. In identifying the latter (current burden of disease study), the usual epidemiological standards were applied. Thus, to establish sufficient evidence of causality there had to be: (1) consistent evidence of an association (positive or negative) between alcohol consumption and the disease or injury; (2) chance, confounding variables, and other bias could be ruled out with reasonable confidence as factors in this association; and (3) evidence of a plausible mediating process (English *et al.*, 1995). These judgments were made using the usual criteria for establishing causality in epidemiology, with the most weight placed on the following four criteria:

1. Consistency across studies;
2. Established experimental biological evidence of mediating processes or at least physiological plausibility (biological mechanisms);
3. Strength of the association (effect size); and
4. Temporality (i.e., cause before effect).

Disease and injury conditions wholly attributable to alcohol

With regard to the attribution of alcohol-relatedness, the conditions shown in **Table 1** are, by definition, wholly attributable to alcohol and thus have an alcohol-attributable fraction of 100% (AAF; see under 'Risk relations' for equation). In other words, in a counterfactual scenario of no presence of alcohol, these disease conditions would not exist. For these conditions, no statistical procedures are necessary to estimate risk relationships. This does not mean that the underlying data are always free of measurement error, that is, that all diagnoses of 'alcoholic cirrhosis of liver' are caused by alcohol. Measurement error may also work in the opposite direction, for example, alcoholic liver cirrhoses are not identified as such and erroneously classified as other forms of liver cirrhosis.

Chronic disease conditions and injuries in which alcohol is a contributory cause

Table 2 gives an overview of chronic conditions that are not wholly attributable to alcohol, but in which alcohol has been identified as causally relevant, based on the previously mentioned four criteria. Two examples of the considerations undertaken with regard to somewhat controversial outcomes illustrate this process. For lung cancer, after adjusting for smoking, meta-analyses showed a clear relationship. However, since evidence for the possible biological mechanism was not conclusive and residual confounding from smoking could not be excluded, English and colleagues (1995), in their first seminal assessment, decided to exclude lung cancer from the list of diseases causally influenced by alcohol. A decade later, we still believe this judgment is correct, although some tentative pathways have meanwhile been established.

Table 1   Disease and injury conditions that are by definition alcohol related (AAF = 1 or 100%)

ICD 10 code	Disease or injury condition
E24.4	Alcohol-induced pseudo-Cushing's syndrome
F10.0, F10.3-F10.9	Alcoholic psychoses and other alcohol-related mental and behavioral disorders
F10.1	Alcohol abuse
F10.2	Alcohol dependence syndrome
G31.2	Degeneration of nervous system due to alcohol
G62.1	Alcoholic polyneuropathy
G72.1	Alcoholic myopathy
I42.6	Alcoholic cardiomyopathy
K29.2	Alcoholic gastritis
K70.0	Alcoholic fatty liver
K70.1	Alcoholic hepatitis
K70.2	Alcoholic fibrosis and sclerosis of liver
K70.3	Alcoholic cirrhosis of the liver
K70.4	Alcoholic hepatic failure
K70.9	Alcoholic liver disease, unspecified
K86.0	Alcohol-induced chronic pancreatitis
O35.4	Maternal care of (suspected) damage to fetus from alcohol
P04.3	Fetus and newborn affected by maternal use of alcohol
Q86.0	Fetal alcohol syndrome (dysmorphic)
R78.0	Finding of alcohol in blood
T51	Toxic effect of alcohol
X45	Accidental poisoning by and exposure to alcohol
X65	Intentional self-poisoning by and exposure to alcohol
Y15	Poisoning by and exposure to alcohol, undetermined intent. Supplementary factors related to causes of morbidity and mortality classified elsewhere
Y90	Evidence of alcohol involvement determined by blood alcohol level
Y91	Evidence of alcohol involvement determined by level of intoxication
Z72.1	Problems related to lifestyle: alcohol use

In contrast, although English *et al.* (1995) concluded there was not sufficient evidence linking alcohol consumption and breast cancer, recent advances both in biological and epidemiological research have changed this evaluation, so that breast cancer was included in this article as an alcohol-related outcome. Similar scientific advances hold true for colorectal cancer. These two conditions were the only two that had been added to the list in the last decade.

Measuring Alcohol Exposure: Key Indicators of Alcohol Consumption at Country and Regional Levels

The following key indicators of exposure are involved in estimating alcohol-attributable burden of disease (Rehm *et al.*, 2004):

- Adult per capita consumption of recorded alcohol;
- Adult per capita consumption of unrecorded alcohol;
- Prevalence of abstention by age and sex;
- Prevalence of different categories of average volume of alcohol consumption by age and sex; and
- Score for patterns of drinking.

We first discuss each of the indicators separately and then the overall procedure to estimate exposure for alcohol-attributable burden of disease.

Adult per capita consumption of recorded alcohol

Per capita data on alcohol consumption denote the consumption in liters of pure alcohol per inhabitant in a given year. These data are available for the majority of countries, often in time series, and avoid the underestimation of total volume of consumption commonly seen in survey data. Adult per capita consumption, that is, consumption by everyone aged 15 and above, is regarded as preferable to per capita consumption *per se* as the overwhelming proportion of alcohol is consumed in adulthood. The age pyramid varies in different countries, therefore per capita consumption figures based on the total population tend to relatively underestimate consumption among drinkers in countries in which the larger proportion of the population is below age 15, as is the case in many developing countries. (For more information and guidance on estimating per capita consumption, see WHO, 2000.)

There are three principal sources of data for per capita estimates: national government data, data from the Food and Agriculture Organization of the United Nations (FAO), and data from the alcohol industry (Rehm *et al.*, 2003b).

Where available, the best and most reliable data generally stem from national governments, usually based on sales figures, tax revenue, and/or production data. Generally, sales data are considered the most accurate,

Table 2 Disease and injury conditions that are not by definition wholly attributable to alcohol (AAF < 1)

ICD 10 code	Disease or injury condition
C00–C14	Mouth and oropharynx cancers
C15	Esophagus cancer
C18–C21	Colon and rectum cancers
C22	Liver cancer
C32	Laryngeal cancer
C50	Breast cancer
D00–D48	Other neoplasms
	Diabetes
E10–E14	Diabetes mellitus
	Neuropsychiatric conditions
F32–F33	Unipolar major depression
G40–G41	Epilepsy
	Cardiovascular diseases
I10–I13	Hypertensive heart disease
I20–I25	Ischemic heart disease
I47–I49	Cardiac arrhythmias
150–I52, I23, I25.0, I97.0, I97.1, I98.1	Heart failure and ill-defined complications of heart disease
I60–I69	Cerebrovascular disease
I60–I62	Ischemic stroke
I63–I66	Hemorrhagic stroke
I85	Esophageal varices
	Digestive diseases
K74	Fibrosis and cirrhosis of liver, without mention of alcohol
K80	Cholelithiasis
K85, K86.1	Acute and chronic pancreatitis (not alcohol induced)
	Skin diseases
L40	Psoriasis
	Conditions arising during the perinatal period
P05–P07	Low birth weight and short gestation
	Unintentional injuries
a	Road traffic accidents
X40–X49	Poisonings (except X45 – Accidental poisoning by and exposure to alcohol)
W00–W19	Falls
X00–X09	Fires
W65–W74	Drownings
bRest of V and W20–W64, W75–W99, X10–X39, X50–X59, Y40–Y86, Y88, Y89	Other unintentional injuries
	Intentional injuries
X60–X84, Y87.0	Self-inflicted injuries
X85–Y09, Y87.1	Violence and homicide
Y35	Other intentional injuries

aV01.1–V01.9, V02.1–V02.9, V03.1–V03.9, V04.1–V04.9, V06.1–V06.9, V09.2, V09.3, V10.4–V10.9, V11.4–V11.9, V12.3–V12.9, V13.3–V13.9, V14.3–V14.9, V15.4–V15.9, V16.4–V16.9, V17.4–V17.9, V18.4–V18.9, V19.4–V19.6, V20.3–V20.9, V21.3–V21.9, V22.3–V22.9, V23.3–V23.9, V24.3–V24.9, V25.3–V25.9, V26.3–V26.9, V27.3–V27.9, V28.3–V28.9, V29.4–V29.9, V30.4–V30.9, V31.4–V31.9, V32.4–V32.9, V33.4–V33.9, V34.4–V34.9, V35.4–V35.9, V36.4–V36.9, V37.4–V37.9, V38.4–V38.9, V39.4–V39.9, V40.4–V40.9, V41.4–V41.9, V42.4–V42.9, V43.4–V43.9, V44.4–V44.9, V45.4–V45.9, V46.4–V46.9, V47.4–V47.9, V48.4–V48.9, V49.4–V49.9, V50.4–V50.9, V51.4–V51.9, V52.4–V52.9, V53.4– V53.9, V54.4–V54.9, V55.4–V55.9, V56.4–V56.9, V57.4–V57.9, V58.4–V58.9, V59.4–V59.9, V60.4–V60.9, V61.4–V61.9, V62.4– V62.9, V63.4–V63.9, V64.4–V64.9, V65.4–V65.9, V66.4–V66.9, V67.4–V67.9, V68.4–V68.9, V69.4–V69.9, V70.4–V70.9, V71.4– V71.9, V72.4–V72.9, V73.4–V73.9, V74.4–V74.9, V75.4–V75.9, V76.4–V76.9, V77.4–V77.9, V78.4–V78.9, V79.4–V79.9, V80.3–V80.5, V81.1, V82.1, V83.0–V83.3, V84.0–V84.3, V85.0–V85.3, V86.0–V86.3, V87.0–V87.8, V89.2, V89.9, V99, Y850.
bRest of V = V-series – a.

provided that sales of alcoholic beverages are separated from sales of any other possible items sold at a given location, and that sales data are beverage specific. One of the drawbacks of production data is that they are always dependent on accurate export and import data, as otherwise the production figures will yield an under- or an overestimation.

The most complete and comprehensive international data set on per capita consumption is published by FAO. FAOSTAT, the database of the FAO, publishes production and trade data for almost 200 countries for different types of alcoholic beverages. The estimates are based on official reports of production by national governments, mainly as replies by the ministries of agriculture to an annual FAO questionnaire. The statistics on imports and exports derive mainly from customs departments. If these sources are not available, other government data such as statistical yearbooks are consulted. The accuracy of the FAO data relies on member nations reporting the data. It is likely that the data underestimate informal, home, and illegal production.

The third main source of data comes from the alcohol industry. In this category the most widely used source is World Drink Trends (WDT). WDT estimates are based on total sales in liters divided by the total mid-year population and use conversion rates that are not published. WDT also tries to calculate the consumption of both incoming and outgoing tourists. Currently, at least partial data are available for 58 countries. There are other alcohol industry sources, as well as market research companies, which are less systematic, contain fewer countries, and are more limited in time scope.

The WHO GAD also systematically collects and compares per capita data from different sources on a regular basis using United Nations (UN) data for population estimates (for procedures and further information, see WHO, 2004; Rehm et al., 2003b).

The main limitations of adult per capita estimates are twofold: (1) they do not incorporate most of unrecorded consumption (see the following section), and (2) they are only aggregate statistics that cannot easily be disaggregated into sex and age groups. Thus, surveys have to play a crucial role in any analysis of risk of alcohol for burden of disease.

Adult per capita consumption of unrecorded alcohol

Unrecorded consumption stems from a variety of sources:

- Home production of alcoholic beverages;
- Illegal production and sale of alcoholic beverages;
- Illegal and legal import of alcoholic beverages; and
- Other production and use of alcoholic beverages, not taxed and/or part of the official production and sales statistics.

Most of these categories are self-explanatory. However, the relation between legal import of alcoholic beverages and unrecorded consumption deserves further exploration. Consider Sweden as an example. Alcohol has been traditionally sold in monopoly stores. After joining the European Union (EU) and after a grace period, the very generous travel allowances of the EU became law, which allowed anybody to import several hundred bottles of beer or wine providing that they claimed these imports exclusively for personal use. As a result, recorded sales went down in parts of the country with borders nearby, and this kind of unrecorded consumption went up. For the year 2002 for Sweden, it is thus estimated that about 3 liters of the overall adult per capita consumption of approximately 9 liters was unrecorded.

How is unrecorded consumption estimated? The preceding Swedish data given stem from survey information. Currently, survey data are probably the most widely used source for estimating unrecorded consumption but there are other methods, such as indirect calculations based on use of raw materials for alcohol production (e.g., sugar or fruits), or based on indicators strongly related to overall alcohol consumption such as alcohol poisoning. Of course, the latter methodology is not possible as part of a study trying to estimate alcohol-attributable burden of disease, as it would lead to circular reasoning.

Prevalence of abstention by age and sex

Prevalence of abstention was assessed by surveys. Abstention information is part of many surveys, not necessarily restricted to health or alcohol surveys. Last-year abstention is usually measured, however, there is an error introduced using this measurement, as former drinkers who stopped drinking for health reasons have a higher risk for mortality and morbidity compared to lifetime abstainers, in most cases exceeding the risk of moderate drinkers. However, this error will result in an underestimation of alcohol-attributable burden when risk relations are applied, which are based on lifetime abstention, and will result in correct estimation if risk relations used are based on all kinds of abstention. Thus, this decision will never

result in an overestimation of alcohol-attributable burden, and is therefore acceptable. Moreover, it can be suspected that former drinkers quitting for health reasons are mainly to be found in developed countries, and to a lesser degree in developing countries and emerging economies.

For the current estimate of alcohol-attributable burden for the year 2002 discussed in this article, large representative surveys were used, which are in closest proximity to the year 2002. Data on abstention from these surveys is available from 118 out of 184 countries included (64.1% of the countries), representing 92.8% of the adult population in all the countries.

Prevalence of different categories of average volume of alcohol consumption by age and sex

Prevalence of different categories of average volume of alcohol consumption by age and sex was also assessed by survey. The same criteria for survey selection as specified previously applied. The categories of drinking as defined in **Table 3** were used, constructed in a way that the risk of many chronic diseases such as alcohol-related cancers were about the same for both men and women in the same category (Rehm et al., 2004). These categories were first used as the basis to derive attributable fractions in the first Australian study on the costs of substance abuse (English et al., 1995) and have been used in many epidemiological and cost-of-illness studies.

The results of the surveys constitute only the raw input into the exposure calculations. They have to be made comparable to be used in a risk assessment by adjusting them to per capita consumption (Rehm et al., 2004, 2006).

Score for patterns of drinking

Patterns of drinking impact certain disease categories such as ischemic heart disease or injuries independently of volume consumed. To quantify the impact of patterns of drinking, a score has been constructed and validated for the CRA of the year 2000. The score and its underlying algorithms have been described in detail elsewhere (Rehm et al., 2003b, 2004). It comprises four different aspects of heavy drinking: high usual quantity of alcohol per occasion, frequency of festive drinking at fiestas or community

Table 3   Definition of drinking categories[a]

Drinking categories	Men	Women
Abstainer or very light drinker	0 – <0.25 g/day	0 – <0.25 g/day
Drinking category I	0.25 – <40 g/day	0.25 – <20 g/day
Drinking category II	40 – <60 g/day	20 – <40 g/day
Drinking category III	60 + g/day	40 + g/day

[a]The limits of these categories are stated in grams of pure alcohol per day. For reference, a bottle of table wine contains about 70 g of ethanol; 0.25 g/day corresponds to somewhat less than one glass of wine per month.

celebrations, proportion of drinking occasions when drinkers get drunk, and distribution of the same amount of drinking over several occasions, as well as no drinking with meals and drinking in public places. These aspects were found to be related to one underlying dimension in an optimal scaling analysis. In several analyses with different methodology, they were found to be related to ischemic heart disease and to different forms of injury.

Patterns scores have been assessed by a mixed methodology of key expert interviews and surveys. They are part of the GAD, and currently only one score per country has been calculated. There are efforts to apply this methodology sex-specifically.

Data Indicating Burden of Disease

Both event-based and time-based measures indicating population health status are used in the usual analyses on burden of disease. We will present the burden of alcohol for the year 2002. Mortality, as measured in number of deaths, was the event measure. Years of life lost due to premature mortality (YLL) and burden of disease, as measured in disability-adjusted life years (DALYs), constituted the time-based gap measures (Murray *et al.*, 2002; Rehm *et al.*, 2004). The DALY measure combines YLL with years of life lost to living with a disability. Estimates for mortality and DALYs for the years 2002 and 2005 were

directly obtained by the WHO (Mathers *et al.*, 2003). YLL and DALYs were 3% age-discounted and age-weighted to be comparable with the GBD study. Population data were obtained from UN population division. Age groups used were: 0–4 years, 5–14 years, 15–29 years, 30–44 years, 45–59 years, 60–69 years, and 70+ years.

Definition of Regions

The regional classification used in this article was defined by the WHO on the basis of levels of adult and infant mortality. The regional groups are organized as follows: A stands for very low child and low adult mortality, B for low child and low adult mortality, C for low child and high adult mortality, D for high child and high adult mortality, and E for high child and very high adult mortality. There were 14 subregions defined in total. The allocation of countries into different subregions can be found in **Table 4**.

Relating Alcohol Exposure to Disease and Injury Outcomes

Defining alcohol-attributable diseases

Alcohol consumption was found to be related to the following GBD categories: conditions arising during the perinatal period: low birth weight; cancers: mouth and oropharynx cancers, esophageal cancer, colon and rectal cancers, liver cancer, breast cancer and

Table 4 Classification of countries into WHO subregions

Africa D	Algeria, Angola, Benin, Burkina Faso, Cameroon, Cape Verde, Chad, Comoros, Equatorial Guinea, Gabon, Gambia, Ghana, Guinea, Guinea-Bissau, Liberia, Madagascar, Mali, Mauritania, Mauritius, Niger, Nigeria, Sao Tome and Principe, Senegal, Seychelles, Sierra Leone, Togo
Africa E	Botswana, Burundi, Central African Republic, Congo, Côte d'Ivoire, Democratic Republic of the Congo, Eritrea, Ethiopia, Kenya, Lesotho, Malawi, Mozambique, Namibia, Rwanda, South Africa, Swaziland, Uganda, United Republic of Tanzania, Zambia, Zimbabwe
Americas A	Canada, Cuba, United States of America
Americas B	Antigua and Barbuda, Argentina, Bahamas, Barbados, Belize, Brazil, Chile, Colombia, Costa Rica, Dominica, Dominican Republic, El Salvador, Grenada, Guyana, Honduras, Jamaica, Mexico, Panama, Paraguay, Saint Kitts and Nevis, Saint Lucia, Saint Vincent and the Grenadines, Suriname, Trinidad and Tobago, Uruguay, Venezuela
Americas D	Bolivia, Ecuador, Guatemala, Haiti, Nicaragua, Peru
Eastern Mediterranean B	Bahrain, Iran (Islamic Republic of), Jordan, Kuwait, Lebanon, Libyan Arab Jamahiriya, Oman, Qatar, Saudi Arabia, Syrian Arab Republic, Tunisia, United Arab Emirates
Eastern Mediterranean D	Afghanistan, Djibouti, Egypt, Iraq, Morocco, Pakistan, Somalia, Sudan, Yemen
Europe A	Andorra, Austria, Belgium, Croatia, Cyprus, Czech Republic, Denmark, Finland, France, Germany, Greece, Iceland, Ireland, Israel, Italy, Luxembourg, Malta, Monaco, Netherlands, Norway, Portugal, San Marino, Slovenia, Spain, Sweden, Switzerland, United Kingdom
Europe B	Albania, Armenia, Azerbaijan, Bosnia and Herzegovina, Bulgaria, Georgia, Kyrgyzstan, Poland, Romania, Slovakia, The Former Yugoslav Republic Of Macedonia, Tajikistan, Turkmenistan, Turkey, Uzbekistan, Yugoslavia
Europe C	Belarus, Estonia, Hungary, Kazakhstan, Latvia, Lithuania, Republic of Moldova, Russian Federation, Ukraine
South East Asia B	Indonesia, Sri Lanka, Thailand
South East Asia D	Bangladesh, Bhutan, Democratic People's Republic of Korea, India, Maldives, Myanmar, Nepal
Western Pacific A	Australia, Brunei Darussalam, Japan, New Zealand, Singapore
Western Pacific B	Cambodia, China, Cook Islands, Fiji, Kiribati, Lao People's Democratic Republic, Malaysia, Marshall Islands, Micronesia (Federated States of), Mongolia, Nauru, Niue, Palau, Papua New Guinea, Philippines, Republic of Korea, Samoa, Solomon Islands, Tonga, Tuvalu, Vanuatu, Vietnam

other neoplasms; diabetes mellitus; neuropsychiatric conditions: alcohol-use disorders, epilepsy; cardiovascular diseases: hypertensive heart disease, ischemic heart disease; cerebrovascular diseases: hemorrhagic stroke, ischemic stroke; cirrhosis of the liver; unintentional injuries: road traffic accidents, poisonings, falls, drownings, and other unintentional injuries; intentional injuries: self-inflicted injuries, violence, and other intentional injuries.

These disease categories are the same as for the CRA 2000 with one exception: colorectal cancer has been added. In other words, all of the major review studies in the 1990s and in the early part of this decade concluded a causal relationship between alcohol and the respective disease or injury category selected, except for colorectal cancer, for which some of the evidence is newer.

Risk relations

Table 5 gives an overview on relative risks (RR) for different diseases by drinking categories. For most chronic disease categories, AAFs of disease were derived from combining prevalence of exposure and RR estimates based on meta-analyses using the following formula:

$$AF = \left[\sum\nolimits_{i=1}^{k} P_i (RR_i - 1) \right] / \left[\sum\nolimits_{i=0}^{k} P_i (RR_i - 1) + 1 \right]$$

in which $_i$ is exposure category with baseline exposure or no exposure ($i = 0$), RR_i is RR at exposure level $_i$ compared to no consumption, and P_i is prevalence of the $_i$th category of exposure.

AAFs, as derived from the preceding formula, can be interpreted as reflecting the proportion of disease that would not exist if there had been no alcohol consumption. For depression and injuries, AAFs were taken from the CRA study (see Rehm *et al.*, 2004, for a detailed description of underlying assumptions and calculations). Protective effects of alcohol consumption on ischemic heart disease, strokes, and diabetes were not estimated in all non-A regions due to the evidence that the pattern of drinking for most alcohol consumption is not protective in these regions (for physiological mechanisms, see Puddey *et al.*, 1999). Thus, where in A regions a RR of less than 1 would represent the protective effect for strokes and diabetes, in non-A regions a RR of 1 was used. For ischemic heart disease, the results of pooled, cross-sectional time-series analyses were used (Rehm *et al.*, 2004).

Consumption and Alcohol-Attributable Burden: A Global Overview

Global Patterns of Drinking and Burden of Disease

Figure 2 gives an overview of adult per capita consumption in different countries. Overall, there is wide variation around the global average of 6.2 liters of pure alcohol consumed per adult per year. The countries with highest overall consumption are in Eastern Europe around the Russian Federation, but other areas of Europe also have high overall consumption. The Americas are the region with the next highest overall consumption. Except for some individual countries, alcohol consumption is lower in other parts of the world. In interpreting these numbers one should keep in mind that the majority of the adult population around the world actually abstain from drinking alcohol. **Table 6** gives further details on consumption.

Deaths attributable to alcohol consumption for all age groups are shown in **Table 7**. Both those deaths caused and prevented by alcohol consumption are shown, but for both sexes the number of deaths caused by alcohol consumption far exceeds the number prevented. Among men the number of deaths caused is approximately 20 times greater than the number prevented, among women the comparable figure is approximately three times greater. Alcohol consumption was responsible for approximately 1.8 million net deaths among men and close to 300 000 net deaths among women. Overall, in 2002, 6.1% of all deaths among men and 1.1% of all deaths among women were attributable to alcohol consumption. Among men, the single largest category of alcohol-attributable deaths was unintentional injuries, which accounted for 25.9% of deaths caused by alcohol consumption.

The second largest category of deaths caused by alcohol among men was cardiovascular disease deaths, which accounted for 23.3% of alcohol-attributable deaths. The burden of alcohol-attributable cardiovascular disease deaths, however, was offset somewhat by those deaths that were prevented by alcohol consumption: about 20% as many deaths were prevented by alcohol consumption as were caused by alcohol consumption. Cancer deaths make up the third largest category of deaths caused by alcohol consumption, accounting for 18.7% of alcohol-attributable deaths among men. Among women, the single largest category of alcohol-attributable deaths was cancer deaths, which accounted for 25.0% of deaths caused by alcohol consumption; deaths due to cirrhosis of the liver account for 18.2% of alcohol-attributable deaths among women.

The second largest category of deaths among women caused by alcohol consumption was unintentional injuries, which accounted for 22.7% of alcohol-attributable deaths. Cardiovascular disease deaths and liver cirrhosis deaths accounted for 18.2% of the total each. In contrast to the situation observed among men, cardiovascular disease deaths prevented by alcohol consumption among women exceeded those caused by alcohol consumption by approximately 70%.

Overall, deaths relatively increased in comparison to the CRA analyses for 2000 (Rehm *et al.*, 2004), both for men and women (see **Table 7**). This increase is mainly

Table 5 Relative risks for alcohol-attributable diseases and injuries by consumption stratum (reference group is 'current abstainers') for globally available disease categories

Disease condition	ICD-10	GBD code	Drinking category IRR	Drinking category IIRR	Drinking category IIIRR	Sources and comments
Conditions arising during the perinatal period: Low birth weight and short gestation	P05–P07	U050	M/W 1.00	M/W 1.40	M/W 1.40	Gutjahr et al., 2001; Rehm et al., 2004
Mouth and oropharynx cancers	C00–C14	U061	M/W 1.45	M/W 1.85	M/W 5.39	Gutjahr et al., 2001
Esophagus cancer	C15	U062	M/W 1.80	M/W 2.38	M/W 4.36	Gutjahr et al., 2001
Colon and rectum cancers	C18–C21	U064	M/W 1.00	M 1.16 W 1.01	M/W 1.41	Cho et al., 2004
Liver cancer	C22	U065	M/W 1.45	M/W 3.03	M/W 3.60	Gutjahr et al., 2001
Breast cancer	C50	U069	<45 yrs W 1.15 45+ yrs W 1.14	<45 yrs W 1.41 45+ yrs W 1.38	<45 yrs W 1.46 45+ yrs W 1.62	Ridolfo and Stevenson, 2001
Other neoplasms	D00–D48	U078	M/W 1.10	M/W 1.30	M/W 1.70	Rehm et al., 2004
Diabetes mellitus (A regions)	E10–E14	U079	M 0.99 W 0.92	M 0.57 W 0.87	M 0.73 W 1.13	Gutjahr et al., 2001
Diabetes mellitus (non-A regions)	E10–E14	U079	M/W 1.00	M/W 1.00	M 1.00 W 1.13	Gutjahr et al., 2001
Mental and behavioral disorders due to use of alcohol	F10	U086	n/a	n/a	n/a	AF 100%
Unipolar major depression[a]	F32–F33	U082				Rehm et al., 2004
Epilepsy	G40, G41	U085	M 1.23 W 1.34	M 7.52 W 7.22	M 6.83 W 7.52	Gutjahr et al., 2001
Hypertensive heart disease	I10–I13	U106	M 1.33 W 1.15	M 2.04 W 1.53	M 2.91 W 2.19	Corrao et al., 1999
Ischemic heart disease[a]	I20–I25	U107	M/W 0.82	M/W 0.83	M 1.00 W 1.12	Corrao et al., 2000; Rehm et al., 2004
Hemorrhagic stroke (A regions)	I60–I62	U108	M 1.12 W 0.74	M 1.40 W 1.04	M 1.54 W 1.94	Reynolds et al., 2003
Hemorrhagic stroke (non-A regions)	I60–I62	U108	M 1.12 W 1.00	M 1.40 W 1.04	M 1.54 W 1.94	Reynolds et al., 2003
Ischemic stroke (A regions)	I63	U108	M 0.94 W 0.66	M 1.13 W 0.84	M 1.19 W 1.53	Reynolds et al., 2003
Ischemic stroke (non-A regions)	I63	U108	M/W 1.00	M 1.13 W 1.00	M 1.19 W 1.53	Reynolds et al., 2003
Cirrhosis of the liver[a]	K74	U117	M/W 1.26	M/W 9.54	M/W 13.0	Rehm et al., 2004
Road traffic accidents[a]	[b]	U150				Rehm et al., 2004
Poisonings[a]	X40–X49	U151				Rehm et al., 2004
Falls[a]	W00–W19	U152				Rehm et al., 2004
Drownings[a]	W65–W74	U154				Rehm et al., 2004

Continued

Table 5 Continued

Other unintentional injuries[a]	[c]Rest of V, W20–W64, W75–W99, X10–X39, X50–X59, Y40–Y86, Y88, Y89	U155	Rehm et al., 2004
Self-inflicted injuries[a]	X60–X84, Y870	U157	Rehm et al., 2004
Violence and homicide[a]	X85–Y09, Y871	U158	Rehm et al., 2004
Other intentional injuries[a]	Y35	U160	Rehm et al., 2004

For all injury categories (shaded areas), the approach assuming that consumption strata specific RRs are generalizable across countries was only used as a sensitivity analysis. The main analyses used region-specific alcohol-attributable fractions, based on both the level of consumption and drinking pattern (for derivation see Rehm et al., 2004)

[a]AAFs are taken from CRA for non-A regions (based on pooled cross-sectional time-series analyses).
[b]V01.1–V01.9, V02.1–V02.9, V03.1–V03.9, V04.1–V04.9, V06.1–V06.9, V09.2, V09.3, V10.4–V10.9, V11.4–V11.9, V12.3–V12.9, V13.3–V13.9, V14.3–V14.9, V15.4–V15.9, V16.4–V16.9, V17.4–V17.9, V18.4–V18.9, V19.4–V19.6, V20.3–V20.9, V21.3–V21.9, V22.9, V23.3–V24.9, V25.3–V25.9, V26.3–V26.9, V27.3–V27.9, V28.3–V28.9, V29.4–V29.9, V30.4–V30.9, V31.4–V31.9, V32.4–V32.9, V33.4–V33.9, V34.4–V34.9, V35.4–V35.9, V36.4–V36.9, V37.4–V37.9, V38.4–V38.9, V39.4–V39.9, V40.4–V40.9, V41.4–V41.9, V42.4–V42.9, V43.4–V43.9, V44.4–V44.9, V45.4–V45.9, V46.4–V46.9, V47.4–V47.9, V48.4–V48.9, V49.4–V49.9, V50.4–V50.9, V51.4–V51.9, V52.4–V52.9, V53.4–V53.9, V54.4–V54.9, V55.4–V55.9, V56.4–V56.9, V57.4–V57.9, V58.4–V58.9, V59.4–V59.9, V60.4–V60.9, V61.4–V61.9, V62.4–V62.9, V63.4–V63.9, V64.4–V64.9, V65.4–V65.9, V66.4–V66.9, V67.4–V67.9, V68.4–V68.9, V69.4–V69.9, V70.4–V70.9, V71.4–V71.9, V72.4–V72.9, V73.4–V73.9, V74.4–V74.9, V75.4–V75.9, V76.4–V76.9, V77.4–V77.9, V78.4–V78.9, V79.4–V79.9, V80.3–V80.5, V81.1, V82.1, V83.0–V83.3, V84.0–V84.3, V85.0–V85.3, V86.0–V86.3, V87.0–V87.8, V89.2, V89.9, V99, Y850.
[c]Rest of V = V-series —[b].
RR, relative risk; n/a, not applicable.

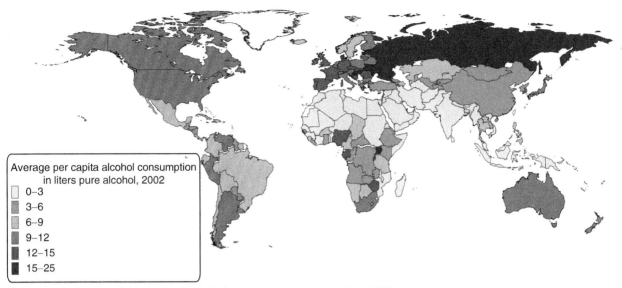

Figure 2 Adult per capita consumption including unrecorded consumption in 2002.

Table 6 Characteristics of alcohol consumption in the world in 2002

WHO Region	Adult population[a]	Percent of abstainers M[b]	Percent of abstainers W[b]	Total alcohol consumption[c]	Unrecorded consumption	Pattern value	Recorded beverage most consumed
Africa D	180 316	59.3	69.3	7.2	2.2	2.8	Other fermented beverages
Africa E	208 662	55.4	73.3	6.9	2.7	3.1	Other fermented beverages and beer
America A	262 651	32.0	52.0	9.4	1.1	2.0	Beer
America B	311 514	18.0	39.1	8.4	2.6	3.1	Beer
America D	46 049	32.1	51.0	7.4	4.0	3.1	Spirits and beer
Eastern Mediterranean B	94 901	86.9	95.0	1.0	0.7	2.6	Spirits
Eastern Mediterranean D	219 457	90.8	98.9	0.6	0.4	2.6	Beer
Europe A	347 001	11.4	23.0	12.1	1.3	1.5	Beer and wine
Europe B	155 544	38.6	62.4	7.5	2.8	2.9	Spirits and beer
Europe C	197 891	13.0	26.9	14.9	6.1	3.9	Spirits
South East Asia B	215 853	77.6	96.9	2.3	0.9	3.0	Spirits
South East Asia D	854 450	79.0	98.0	1.9	1.6	3.0	Spirits
Western Pacific A	131 308	13.0	29.0	9.4	1.7	2.0	Spirits
Western Pacific B	1 164 701	26.2	62.5	6.0	1.1	2.2	Spirits
World	4 388 297	44.8	65.6	6.2	1.7	2.6	Spirits (53%)

[a]Numbers in thousands.
[b]M = Men, W = Women.
[c]Adult per capita (age 15+) consumption for 2002 in liters of pure alcohol, derived as average of yearly consumptions from 2001 to 2003, including unrecorded consumption.

due to chronic disease deaths, whereas the relative impact of alcohol-attributable injuries decreased.

The net impact of alcohol on mortality was relatively larger in younger age groups, again for both sexes. Whereas 3.7% of all deaths were attributable to alcohol in all age groups (6.1% in men; 1.1% in women), 5% of the deaths under the age of 60 were attributable to this risk factor (7.5% in men; 1.7% in women; **Table 8**). Injury deaths especially occurred relatively early in life.

More details on premature deaths attributable to alcohol consumption (i.e., for those 0–59 years of age) are shown in **Table 8**. Both those premature deaths caused and prevented by alcohol consumption are shown, and, as was the case for deaths for all ages, the number of premature deaths caused by alcohol consumption far exceeds the number prevented. In fact, this pattern is greater for those in the younger age group: among men the number of premature deaths caused is approximately 80 times greater than the number prevented, and among women

Table 7   Deaths (in 1000s) attributable to alcohol consumption in the world in 2002

Disease category	M^a	W^a	Total M and W	% M	% W	Total % M and W
Maternal and perinatal conditions (low birth weight)	1	1	3	0.1	0.3	0.1
Cancer	361	105	466	18.7	25.0	19.8
Diabetes mellitus	0	1	1	0.0	0.2	0.0
Neuropsychiatric disorders	106	25	130	5.5	5.9	5.5
Cardiovascular diseases	452	77	528	23.3	18.2	22.4
Cirrhosis of the liver	293	77	370	15.2	18.2	15.7
Unintentional injuries	501	96	597	25.9	22.7	25.3
Intentional injuries	220	40	260	11.4	9.6	11.1
Total alcohol-attributable deaths 'caused'	1934	421	2355	100.0	100.0	100.0
Diabetes mellitus	−8	−5	−12	7.7	3.5	5.3
Cardiovascular diseases	−90	−130	−220	92.3	96.5	94.7
Total alcohol-attributable deaths 'prevented'	−98	−135	−232	100.0	100.0	100.0
All alcohol-attributable net deaths	1836	287	2123	100.0	100.0	100.0
All deaths	29 891	27 138	57 029			
Percentage of all net deaths attributable to alcohol	6.1%	1.1%	3.7%			

^{a}M = Men, W = Women.

Table 8   Premature deaths (in 1000s; 0–59 years of age) attributable to alcohol consumption in the world in 2002

Disease category	M^a	W^a	Total M and W	% M	% W	Total % M and W
Maternal and perinatal conditions (low birth weight)	1	1	3	0.1	0.5	0.2
Cancer	159	45	204	13.3	20.6	14.5
Diabetes mellitus	0	0	0	0.0	0.0	0.0
Neuropsychiatric disorders	80	18	98	6.7	8.3	7.0
Cardiovascular diseases	149	16	165	12.5	7.2	11.7
Cirrhosis of the liver	180	41	221	15.1	18.6	15.6
Unintentional injuries	424	65	489	35.6	29.8	34.7
Intentional injuries	198	33	231	16.6	15.0	16.4
Total alcohol-attributable deaths 'caused'	1191	218	1409	100.0	100.0	100.0
Diabetes mellitus	−3	0	−3	16.9	8.7	14.9
Cardiovascular diseases	−12	−4	−17	83.1	91.3	85.1
Total alcohol-attributable deaths 'prevented'	−15	−5	−20	100.0	100.0	100.0
All alcohol-attributable net deaths	1177	213	1390	100.0	100.0	100.0
All deaths	15 664	12 371	28 035			
Percentage of all net deaths attributable to alcohol	7.5%	1.7%	5.0%			

^{a}M = Men, W = Women.

the comparable figure is approximately 40 times greater. Alcohol consumption was responsible for close to 1.2 million net premature deaths among men and approximately 200 000 net premature deaths among women. Overall, in 2002, 7.5% of all premature deaths among men and 1.7% of all premature deaths among women were attributable to alcohol consumption. Among men, injuries alone make up more than half of the alcohol-attributable premature deaths.

The single largest category of alcohol-attributable premature deaths, which was more than twice as large as the next largest category, was unintentional injuries, and accounted for 35.6% of premature deaths caused by alcohol consumption among men. The next largest category of premature deaths caused by alcohol was intentional injuries, which accounted for 16.6% of

alcohol-attributable premature deaths. The third largest category of premature deaths caused by alcohol was cirrhosis of the liver, which accounted for 15.1% of alcohol-attributable premature deaths. Cardiovascular disease deaths encompassed only 12.5% of premature deaths among men. Alcohol consumption prevented a relatively smaller number of deaths in this disease category as compared to the overall as well: in contrast to a figure of 20% for all ages, only about 8% as many premature deaths were prevented as were caused by alcohol consumption among men.

As was the case among men, among women the single largest category of alcohol-attributable premature deaths was unintentional injuries, which accounted for 29.8% of premature deaths caused by alcohol consumption. The next largest category of premature deaths caused by alcohol consumption was cancer deaths, which accounted for 20.6% of alcohol-attributable premature deaths among women. Deaths due to cirrhosis of the liver make up the third largest category of premature deaths caused by alcohol consumption, accounting for 18.6% of alcohol-attributable premature deaths among women.

Alcohol-attributable YLLs are shown in **Table 9**. YLLs are a summary measure that take the age at which death occurs into account, thereby giving higher weight to deaths that occur among younger-aged populations (i.e., higher number of years of life lost). As usual, the proportion of alcohol-attributable YLLs among all YLLs exceeds the proportion of alcohol-attributable deaths among all deaths. This is another indication that alcohol kills relatively early in life, thus time-based gap measures such as YLLs indicate proportionally higher burden of

disease than event-based measures (i.e., 3.7% of global mortality was attributable to alcohol [cf. **Table 7**] vs. 4.1% of YLL [cf. **Table 9**]).

Table 9 illustrates these data, in which over half of all the alcohol-attributable YLLs are accounted for by intentional and unintentional injury categories combined, which tend to affect younger populations. In contrast, lower relative percentages of YLLs due to diseases are more associated with older-aged populations (e.g., cancers and cardiovascular diseases). Over three times as many YLLs occur among men compared to women worldwide, for the simple reason that men tend to drink more than women, both in number of occasions and in quantity of alcohol consumed per occasion. In addition, across all disease categories caused by alcohol consumption, raw numbers of YLLs among men are four to five times higher than those seen for women.

Table 9 Years of life lost (YLLs in 1000s) attributable to alcohol consumption in the world in 2002

Disease category	M[a]	M[a]	Total M and W	% M	% W	Total % M and W
Maternal and perinatal conditions (low birth weight)	47	37	83	0.1	0.5	0.2
Cancer	4510	1368	5878	13.5	20.4	14.7
Diabetes mellitus	0	12	12	0.0	0.2	0.0
Neuropsychiatric disorders	2005	484	2489	6.0	7.2	6.2
Cardiovascular diseases	5003	791	5794	15.0	11.8	14.4
Cirrhosis of the liver	4403	1118	5521	13.2	16.7	13.8
Unintentional injuries	11910	1963	13873	35.6	29.3	34.6
Intentional injuries	5540	934	6475	16.6	13.9	16.1
Total alcohol-attributable burden 'caused' in YLLs	33417	6707	40124	100.0	100.0	100.0
Diabetes mellitus	−85	−41	−126	9.8	3.8	6.5
Cardiovascular diseases	−779	−1041	−1820	90.2	96.2	93.5
Total alcohol-attributable burden 'prevented' in YLLs	−864	−1082	−1946	100.0	100.0	100.0
All alcohol-attributable net YLLs	32553	5625	38177	100.0	100.0	100.0
All YLLS	496059	426418	922476			
Percentage of all net YLLs attributable to alcohol	6.6%	1.3%	4.1%			

[a]M = Men, W = Women

Table 10 Disability-adjusted life years (DALYs) (in 1000s) attributable to alcohol consumption in the world in 2002.

Disease category	M[a]	W[a]	Total M and W	% M	% W	Total % M and W
Maternal and perinatal conditions (low birth weight)	52	42	94	0.1	0.4	0.1
Cancer	4593	1460	6054	8.2	12.9	9.0
Diabetes mellitus	0	20	20	0.0	0.2	0.0
Neuropsychiatric disorders	19393	3722	23115	34.6	32.9	34.3
Cardiovascular diseases	5711	887	6598	10.2	7.8	9.8
Cirrhosis of the liver	5415	1468	6883	9.7	13.0	10.2
Unintentional injuries	14499	2647	17146	25.9	23.4	25.5
Intentional injuries	6366	1051	7417	11.4	9.3	11.0
Total alcohol-attributable burden 'caused' in DALYs	56029	11297	67326	100.0	100.0	100.0
Diabetes mellitus	−225	−86	−312	21.3	6.7	13.3
Cardiovascular diseases.	−834	−1205	−2039	78.7	93.3	86.7
Total alcohol-attributable burden 'prevented' in DALYs	−1059	−1291	−2351	100.0	100.0	100.0
All alcohol-attributable net DALYs	54970	10006	64975	100.0	100.0	100.0
All DALYs	772912	717213	1490126			
Percentage of all net DALYs attributable to alcohol	7.1%	1.4%	4.4%			

[a]M = Men, W = Women.

Table 11   Average age at death and alcohol attributable fractions by age and sex in world, 2002

	Men Avg age	Women Avg age	Men 0–4	Men 5–14	Men 15–29	Men 30–44	Men 45–59	Men 60–69	Men 70 plus	Women 0–4	Women 5–14	Women 15–29	Women 30–44	Women 45–59	Women 60–69	Women 70 plus
Low birth weight and short gestation	0.0	0.0	0.2%	–	–	–	–	–	–	0.2%	–	–	–	–	–	–
Mouth and oropharynx cancers	60.3	64.1	–	–	19.9%	34.3%	37.5%	26.3%	20.9%	–	–	10.5%	14.3%	13.2%	11.4%	7.3%
Esophagus cancer	65.4	66.6	–	–	31.8%	44.6%	46.5%	39.7%	36.4%	–	–	10.7%	19.0%	20.8%	14.8%	12.1%
Colon and rectum cancers	63.9	63.6	–	–	3.9%	6.6%	7.6%	5.7%	2.9%	–	–	1.3%	1.5%	2.0%	1.2%	0.5%
Liver cancer	60.8	63.7	–	–	32.0%	43.0%	43.2%	36.4%	31.8%	–	–	13.9%	21.3%	20.0%	16.0%	12.7%
Breast cancer	–	61.4	–	–	–	–	–	–	–	–	–	6.1%	8.2%	8.9%	7.1%	5.9%
Other neoplasms	63.9	66.8	–	–	7.1%	10.5%	12.3%	10.0%	7.8%	–	–	4.8%	5.6%	5.7%	5.1%	4.7%
Diabetes mellitus	66.1	81.8	–	–	–1.0%	–2.0%	–2.2%	–2.0%	–1.3%	–	–	0.2%	–0.1%	0.0%	–0.3%	–1.2%
Unipolar depressive disorders	61.4	76.7	–	–	0.0%	2.0%	2.0%	2.3%	7.5%	–	–	0.5%	0.1%	0.1%	0.2%	1.7%
Epilepsy	41.7	42.5	–	–	51.4%	63.5%	63.0%	46.2%	30.5%	–	–	29.2%	36.5%	35.4%	28.1%	18.6%
Mental and behavioral disorders due to use of alcohol	51.1	54.9	100.0%	100.0%	100.0%	100.0%	100.0%	100.0%	100.0%	100.0%	100.0%	100.0%	100.0%	100.0%	100.0%	100.0%

Hypertensive heart disease	68.4	72.2	–	–	17.8%	28.6%	28.0%	22.5%	19.3%	–	–	6.1%	9.3%	8.3%	6.0%	5.0%
Ischemic heart disease	57.7	81.8	–	–	4.6%	7.0%	7.6%	3.9%	0.7%	–	–	0.0%	–0.2%	–0.3%	–0.2%	–1.4%
Cerebrovascular disease	68.4	89.7	–	–	6.7%	10.9%	9.1%	6.6%	4.6%	–	–	1.9%	2.2%	1.9%	0.6%	–2.6%
Cirrhosis of the liver	56.4	59.3	–	–	47.7%	71.2%	67.4%	56.8%	43.9%	–	–	13.7%	38.3%	37.9%	31.9%	20.4%
Road traffic accidents	35.2	39.6	9.3%	10.1%	32.0%	34.4%	17.8%	14.8%	14.1%	5.4%	6.6%	9.3%	12.8%	9.6%	7.6%	8.1%
Poisonings	43.7	46.7	0.0%	0.0%	31.7%	26.5%	25.6%	24.0%	9.2%	0.0%	0.0%	16.2%	13.5%	14.4%	10.3%	5.2%
Falls	53.3	63.3	0.0%	0.0%	18.4%	21.2%	22.1%	16.5%	11.0%	0.0%	0.0%	7.6%	9.1%	8.8%	6.0%	3.5%
Drownings	40.0	47.7	0.0%	0.0%	23.3%	32.9%	33.1%	27.1%	21.5%	0.0%	0.0%	14.3%	19.2%	20.6%	15.8%	16.2%
Other	42.2	52.9	10.5%	8.6%	27.2%	30.3%	29.6%	28.8%	24.5%	2.7%	2.3%	11.2%	14.6%	13.3%	13.8%	15.0%
Self-inflicted injuries	40.6	43.5	0.0%	0.0%	15.4%	17.3%	14.2%	13.2%	5.9%	0.0%	0.0%	4.9%	6.3%	5.5%	6.3%	4.1%
Violence and homicide	35.4	41.1	9.0%	9.4%	32.5%	32.6%	34.1%	33.6%	26.3%	8.0%	8.7%	20.8%	21.9%	22.0%	21.0%	23.6%
Other intentional injuries	36.3	44.5	0.0%	0.0%	14.9%	13.6%	13.1%	10.5%	5.1%	0.0%	0.0%	7.2%	11.1%	10.8%	7.0%	2.8%
Total	51.9	47.0														

(Row label "Other" under Poisonings/Falls/Drownings group refers to "Other unintentional injuries".)

Table 12 Alcohol attributable fractions of DALY by age and sex in world, 2002

	Men							Women						
	0–4	5–14	15–29	30–44	45–59	60–69	70 plus	0–4	5–14	15–29	30–44	45–59	60–69	70 plus
Low birth weight and short gestation	0.2%	–	–	–	–	–	–	0.2%	–	–	–	–	–	–
Mouth and oropharynx cancers	–	–	20.9%	35.6%	38.9%	27.2%	32.4%	–	–	11.0%	15.1%	13.9%	12.1%	13.4%
Esophagus cancer	–	–	34.0%	47.6%	49.7%	41.2%	55.5%	–	–	10.9%	20.4%	21.8%	15.3%	20.9%
Colon and rectum cancers	–	–	4.2%	6.9%	8.2%	6.0%	4.7%	–	–	1.4%	1.6%	2.1%	1.3%	0.9%
Liver cancer	–	–	32.8%	45.4%	44.3%	37.6%	48.1%	–	–	14.2%	22.0%	20.8%	16.4%	21.4%
Breast cancer	–	–	–	–	–	–	–	–	–	7.0%	9.0%	9.5%	7.4%	10.5%
Other neoplasms	–	–	7.4%	10.7%	12.8%	10.5%	14.5%	–	–	4.9%	5.7%	5.8%	5.3%	10.1%
Diabetes mellitus	–	–	–1.3%	–2.8%	–3.9%	–2.9%	–2.3%	–	–	0.0%	–0.5%	–0.5%	–0.6%	–2.0%
Unipolar depressive disorders	–	–	3.4%	3.6%	3.7%	4.0%	4.7%	–	–	0.6%	0.6%	0.6%	0.6%	0.9%
Epilepsy	–	–	46.9%	60.3%	59.5%	47.7%	45.0%	–	–	28.5%	34.3%	34.7%	28.8%	28.2%
Mental and behavioral disorders due to use of alcohol	100.0%	100.0%	100.0%	100.0%	100.0%	100.0%	100.0%	100.0%	100.0%	100.0%	100.0%	100.0%	100.0%	100.0%
Hypertensive heart disease	–	–	18.4%	30.0%	29.4%	23.1%	32.0%	–	–	6.3%	9.7%	8.6%	6.1%	9.5%
Ischemic heart disease	–	–	4.6%	7.2%	7.8%	3.9%	1.1%	–	–	–0.1%	–0.4%	–0.4%	–0.3%	–2.9%
Cerebrovascular disease	–	–	6.9%	11.3%	9.6%	6.9%	7.5%	–	–	2.0%	1.7%	1.5%	0.2%	–5.1%
Cirrhosis of the liver	–	–	50.9%	73.8%	68.6%	57.4%	65.0%	–	–	16.7%	40.1%	38.6%	32.2%	30.8%
Road traffic accidents	1.5%	11.3%	29.7%	31.9%	16.8%	14.5%	21.5%	1.3%	6.8%	8.1%	11.5%	8.9%	7.5%	12.4%
Poisonings	0.0%	0.0%	32.2%	26.7%	25.1%	23.6%	14.2%	0.0%	0.0%	15.9%	13.5%	14.6%	10.5%	8.7%
Falls	0.0%	0.0%	11.9%	15.6%	18.4%	14.6%	17.0%	0.0%	0.0%	4.3%	5.6%	6.8%	4.7%	5.5%
Drownings	0.0%	0.0%	23.2%	32.7%	33.2%	27.6%	35.9%	0.0%	0.0%	14.1%	18.9%	20.5%	16.2%	29.2%
Other unintentional injuries	2.2%	8.5%	18.6%	21.6%	22.1%	22.4%	34.4%	0.4%	2.8%	7.1%	8.8%	9.1%	9.9%	24.8%
Self-inflicted injuries	0.0%	0.0%	15.2%	17.1%	14.0%	13.4%	9.2%	0.0%	0.0%	4.4%	6.1%	5.4%	6.4%	6.5%
Violence and homicide	0.7%	8.3%	26.6%	27.3%	30.4%	31.6%	39.7%	0.3%	10.0%	17.1%	18.9%	20.3%	20.8%	33.5%
Other intentional injuries	0.0%	0.0%	14.0%	12.8%	12.8%	10.7%	7.5%	0.0%	0.0%	7.2%	11.1%	10.5%	7.0%	5.0%

However, there are some proportional variations within disease categories that deviate from this overall trend. For example, among alcohol-attributable YLL caused, the proportion of alcohol-attributable YLLs among women is proportionally higher for cancers, neuropsychiatric disorders, and liver cirrhosis. Among burden prevented, however, women have higher raw numbers and relative proportions of YLLs prevented due to their more moderate use of alcohol generally. Among men, however, the lower proportion of cardiovascular disease YLLs prevented is due to the higher alcohol consumption and more hazardous drinking pattern.

Alcohol-attributable YLLs and DALYs were also slightly higher in 2002 compared to 2000 (Rehm *et al.*, 2004). **Table 10** shows global alcohol-attributable DALYs for 2002. DALYs are proportionally higher overall than both deaths or YLLs because this summary measure of burden of disease additionally accounts for years lived with a disability prior to death, and many alcohol-attributable diseases are not fatal.

For this reason, the most striking difference between alcohol-attributable deaths and YLLs and this table is the high contribution of neuropsychiatric disorders to the overall alcohol-attributable burden for both men and women (proportionally, between three- and fivefold higher for DALYs than for the other burden measures). For DALYs, the burden of alcohol-attributable neuropsychiatric disorders now approximately equals that of injury categories combined. Many of the same trends exist in alcohol-attributable DALYs as were seen in alcohol-attributable YLLs, such as the disparity among men and women with respect to prevented deaths, especially in cardiovascular diseases, and the gender-based disease distribution among alcohol-attributable DALYs caused (among women, cancer and cirrhosis of the liver are proportionally higher; among men, injury categories and cardiovascular diseases are higher).

Table 11 shows the AAFs and average age of death for each alcohol-attributable disease category examined in this report. One will notice that for acute outcomes such as injury categories, the average age for alcohol-attributable outcome is lower. In addition, the ages for these outcomes are usually a number of years older for women than for men, indicating that these alcohol-attributable disease deaths occur in men at a younger age. With respect to the AAFs, one can see that they are universally higher for men than women in the same age group, and, in most cases, decrease as age increases. This is because in most countries volume of drinking decreases with age.

Table 12 shows the AAFs used for DALY calculations. Note the overall increased proportion for men compared to women and increased fractions for some chronic conditions such as unipolar.

Conclusions and Implications

Alcohol is one of the most important risk factors for burden of disease globally. Given the current trends both in exposure, with expected increases in alcohol consumption in the most populous countries India and China, and in outcomes, with an overall relative increase in alcohol-attributable causes of death, the detrimental impact of alcohol is expected to increase in the future if no additional interventions are introduced.

A large part of alcohol-attributable burden is avoidable, however, and some of it in the short term (WHO, 2002). It is beyond the scope of this article to detail potential interventions to achieve this goal. However, such interventions exist (e.g., Babor *et al.*, 2003), not only for the developed world, but also for developing countries, and they are cost-effective in comparison to other public health measures. Thus, it is up to public health policy to set priorities establishing such interventions.

See also: Alcohol Consumption: Overview of International Trends; Alcohol Industry; Alcoholism Treatment; Alcohol—Socio-Economic Impacts (Including Externalities).

Citations

Babor T, Caetano R, Casswell S, *et al.* (2003) *Alcohol: No Ordinary Commodity. Research and Public Policy.* Oxford and London: Oxford University Press.

Cho E, Smith WSA, Ritz J, *et al.* (2004) Alcohol intake and colorectal cancer: A pooled analysis of 8 cohort studies. *Annals of Internal Medicine* 140(8): 603–613.

Corrao G, Bagnardi V, Zambon A, *et al.* (1999) Exploring the dose-response relationship between alcohol consumption and the risk of several alcohol-related conditions: A meta-analysis. *Addiction* 94: 1551–1573.

Corrao G, Rubbiati L, Bagnardi V, *et al.* (2000) Alcohol and coronary heart disease: A meta analysis. *Addiction* 95(10): 1505–1523.

English D, Holman C, Milne E, *et al.* (1995) *The Quantification of Drug-caused Morbidity and Mortality in Australia 1995.* Canberra, Australia: Commonwealth Department of Human Services and Health.

Eckardt M, File S, Gessa G, *et al.* (1988) Effects of moderate alcohol consumption on the central nervous system. *Alcoholism, Clinical and Experimental Research* 22: 998–1040.

Ezzati M, Lopez AD, Rodgers A, *et al.* (2004) *Comparative Quantification of Health Risks. Global and Regional Burden of Disease Attributable to Selected Major Risk Factors.* Geneva, Switzerland: WHO.

Gutjahr E, Gmel G, and Rehm J (2001) Relation between average alcohol consumption and disease: An overview. *European Addiction Research* 7(3): 117–127.

Lopez AD, Mathers CD, Ezzati M, *et al.* (2006) *Global Burden of Disease and Risk Factors.* New York and Washington: Oxford University Press and The World Bank.

Mathers CD, Bernard C, Iburg K, *et al.* (2003) *The Global Burden of Disease in 2002: Data Sources, Methods and Results. GPE Discussion Paper No. 54.* Geneva, Switzerland: WHO.

McKee M, Suzcs S, Sarvary A, et al. (2005) The composition of surrogate alcohols consumed in Russia. *Alcoholism: Clinical and Experimental Research* 29(10): 1884–1888.

Murray CJL, Salomon JA, Mathers CD, et al. (2002) *Summary Measures of Population Health: Concepts, Ethics, Measurement and Applications.* Geneva, Switzerland: WHO.

Puddey IB, Rakic V, Dimmitt SB, et al. (1999) Influence of pattern of drinking on cardiovascular disease and cardiovascular risk factors – A review. *Addiction* 94: 649–663.

Rehm J, Patra J, Baliunas D, et al. (2006) Alcohol consumption and global burden of disease 2002. *Report to WHO.* Geneva, Switzerland: WHO.

Rehm J, Rehn N, Room R, et al. (2003b) The global distribution of average volume of alcohol consumption and patterns of drinking. *European Addiction Research* 9: 147–156.

Rehm J, Room R, Graham K, et al. (2003a) The relationship of average volume of alcohol consumption and patterns of drinking to burden of disease – an overview. *Addiction* 98: 1209–1228.

Rehm J, Room R, Monteiro M, et al. (2004) Alcohol use. In: Ezzati M, Lopez A, Rodgers A and Murray C (eds.) *Comparative Quantification of Health Risks. Global and Regional Burden of Disease Attributable to Selected Major Risk Factors,* vol. 1, pp. 959–1108. Geneva, Switzerland: WHO.

Reynolds K, Lewis B, Nolen JD, et al. (2003) Alcohol consumption and risk of stroke: A meta-analysis. *Journal of the American Medical Association* 289(5): 579–588.

Ridolfo B and Stevenson C (2001) The quantification of drug-caused mortality and morbidity in Australia 1998. Canberra, Australia: Australian Institute of Health and Welfare.

World Health Organization (WHO) (2000) *International Guide for Monitoring Alcohol Consumption and Related Harm.* Geneva, Switzerland: WHO Department of Mental Health and Substance Dependence.

World Health Organization (WHO) (2002) *World Health Report: Reducing Risks, Promoting Health Life.* Geneva, Switzerland: WHO.

World Health Organization (WHO) (2004) *Global Status Report on Alcohol 2004.* Geneva, Switzerland: WHO.

Further Reading

Jamison DT, Breman JG, Measham AR, et al. (eds.) *Disease Control Priorities in Developing Countries*, 2nd edn. Washington: Oxford University Press and World Bank.

Rehm J, Klotsche J, and Patra J (2007) Comparative quantification of alcohol exposure as risk factor for global burden of disease. *International Journal of Methods in Psychiatric Research* 16(2): 66–76.

Rehm J, Sulkowska U, Manczuk M, et al. (2007) Alcohol accounts for a high proportion of premature mortality in central and eastern Europe. *International Journal of Epidemiology* 36: 458–467.

Room R, Babor T, and Rehm J (2005) Alcohol and public health: a review. *Lancet* 365: 519–530.

Relevant Website

http://www3.who.int/whosis – WHO Global Alcohol Database.

Alcohol—Socio-Economic Impacts (Including Externalities)

B Easton, Centre for Social and Health Outcomes Research and Evaluation (SHORE) Massey University, Wellington, New Zealand

Depending on the cultural context and particular circumstances, the same drink of alcohol can generate a feeling of benign content, or moroseness, or stupor. The immediate health benefits for the individual may also be benign (or even beneficial), or the drink may result in injury or death – in the short run from accident or in the long run from one of the diseases alcohol can precipitate. The consequences for others may also be benign or beneficial, or damaging or mortal from violence or collateral accident. Someone may be born as the result of intentional or unintentional impregnation. The loss of production due to lower workplace productivity or non-attendance from drinking alcohol may cause financial loss to the drinker and possibly to others. Alcohol may, or may not, generate additional costs in many sectors of the economy, especially in the criminal system, in the health system, and in the transport system. The national budget probably gains from the specific tax it levies on alcoholic beverages, but this levy may, or may not, cover its costs from the consumption of alcohol.

The impact of alcohol consumption is so multifarious that it is not easy to track all its social and economic impacts. This review confines itself to those to which social costs of alcohol misuse studies have paid most attention, excluding the burden of disease caused by alcohol which is covered in this encyclopedia by Rehm. The framework used is that of the WHO report, *International Guidelines for Estimating the Costs of Substance Abuse* (Single *et al.*, 2003), and related and subsequent studies, although some of the technical issues, such as the valuation of life, counterfactual hypotheses, and discounting, are not considered here.

As the opening sentence reminds us, the social and economic impact of alcohol is affected by the cultural context, even though the physiological impact may not be. This means that each country, or culture within a country, has its own quantitative and qualitative particularities. This entry deals with the heterogeneity by including in its bibliography recent country-specific studies (especially cost studies, because they look at most dimensions of the impact).

Following brief discussions on externalities and irrationality, the main areas of impact are dealt with in alphabetical order, because their relative significance will vary from country to country.

Externalities

The social cost of an activity is the total of all the costs associated with it, including both the costs borne by the economic agent involved and all costs borne by society at large. This includes the costs reflected in the organization's charge (price), which covers the use of the various resources (including labor capital and risk as well as natural resources) excluding taxation, together with the costs external to the firm's private costs. If social costs are greater than private costs – the costs of purchase – then a negative externality is present.

When the market economy is working effectively, and there are no external social costs, rational consumers will purchase and consume the product only if it is more valuable to them than the price paid for it. In this case, society is better off since the consumers deem themselves better off from the transaction, and society is no worse off, since it has traded off the social costs of the consumption for the payment, which embodies the ability to purchase other products with equivalent social costs.

There are all sorts of subtle assumptions embodied in this analysis: Public health analysis often worries about the equity in the distribution of income – the power to purchase. But even if those assumptions hold (near enough), alcoholic beverages are one of a number of products for which the purchase price cannot generally equal social costs because the social cost of each unit of consumption varies greatly. Thus the social cost of the first drink in a session may reflect the private cost, but later drinks may generate additional social costs in poor health, material damage, public and private outlays that were ignored when the drinking decision was made, violence to others, and even death to the drinker or, in the case of motor vehicle accidents and the like, to innocent bystanders.

As a later section discusses, taxation and other public policy measures aim to reconcile in one way or another the inconsistency between the purchase price and social costs. However, there is still likely to be a substantial difference for at least a number of significant ingestions.

A useful term is misuse for occasions where the consumption generates outcomes that were unintended by the consumer and not taken into account when the purchase or drinking decision was made. It is sometimes preferred to abuse in order to emphasize that much alcohol consumption is useful, in the sense of its social impact being benign or even (mildly) beneficial.

Irrationality

The previous discussion has assumed that consumers are acting rationally, taking into consideration all the costs of the consumption that affect them (although they may discount costs in the more distant future).

However, it is not immediately obvious that rationality applies when there is drunkenness or addiction. Economists explore this by using a theoretical definition of irrationality where consumers show time inconsistency between decisions, as for example when they go into a bar to have three drinks, change their minds in consequence of the resulting euphoria and drink more, and the following day regret the change of mind (Ainslie, 1992; Frederick et al., 2002; O'Donoghue and Rabin, 2003).

It is unclear how to define externalities in such circumstances. The tendency has been to ignore such irrationality, but increasingly cost of alcohol studies need to address it, incorporating it in a rigorous way consistent with the theory.

Crime

Pernanem et al. (2000, 2002), based on Goldstein (1985), propose four models (modes might be a better word) to account for alcohol-associated crime.

1. The pharmacological model, in which intoxication encourages the commission of crimes which otherwise would not have been committed.
2. The economic means model, in which crimes are committed to fund alcohol consumption.
3. The systemic model, involving the illegal economy, as in unlawful brewing or distilling or sale of liquor.
4. The substance-defined model, where actions are defined as being criminal by laws which regulate drug use, such as drunkenness in a public place, supplying underage or drunk people (if that be illegal) and drunk-driving.

Note these apply also to illicit drugs, for which modes 3 and 4 are more important than for alcohol.

This crime causes social costs, both directly via damage to property and individuals but also with consequent costs to the public purse for policing, justice and corrections, transport management, and indirectly when it adds to concerns about community safety and security.

Estimating the attributable fractions (the proportions which alcohol causes) for criminal activity is much less advanced than for disease. Because law, practices of enforcement, and culture vary by country, fractions cannot be easily borrowed from other jurisdictions. (Indeed care is also required in generalizing research findings on the relationship between crime and alcohol.)

Harm to Others

As well as affecting the health of its drinkers, alcohol can affect the health of others. These effects include:

1. Children born as the result of an unplanned conception as a result of intoxication (it is not obvious how to deal with this);
2. Fetal alcohol syndrome and fetal alcohol effects, said to be the major source of mental illness and behavioral disorders, and generating on average a large public cost during their lifetime (Harwood, 2000);
3. Pain and suffering, abuse, violence, injury, and death experienced by those close to the drinker;
4. Pain and suffering, violence, and death including from motor vehicle accidents, experienced by the wider public.

There are rarely good estimates of these phenomena, and the incidence and costs vary from country to country.

Motor Vehicle Accidents

As well as injury and death from motor vehicle accidents caused by alcohol consumption, there is damage to cars and property, the costs of law enforcement and prevention (which may include road design), and the costs of administrating the insurance system. (There are also costs in the resulting travel delays.)

Motor vehicle accidents are particularly onerous, but there are other types of accidents. Industrial accidents caused by alcohol are covered in the next section.

Production Losses

Drinking alcohol may result in production losses from the following:

1. Reduced workforce size as a consequence of death or premature retirement;
2. Absenteeism from sickness or injury;
3. Reduced on-the-job productivity from sickness or injury and accidents.

Alcohol misuse may also cause loss of production in the unpaid household sector and in other non-market activities. Although the informal economy is not included in the standard measures of market output (such as GDP or GNP), the losses or production in it caused by alcohol misuse may be significant.

Public Spending

Most of the above-mentioned events impact to some extent on public spending (or, for those countries that depend more upon private provision, on the private insurance system). Such an impact is a classic externality, because it is unlikely to be taken into account by the drinker.

Among the most significant sectors affected by additional spending are costs to the health system (at every level from prevention to advanced tertiary specialties, but also for nursing care later in life), social security or other forms of public income maintenance, traffic management, and also to policing, justice, and corrections.

Taxation and Public Policy

Historically, specific taxes on alcohol were imposed because they could be readily collected at brewery, distillery, or port. (There are greater difficulties collecting excise from small vineyards.) Later in some but not all jurisdictions, the justification for special duties shifted from convenience to a notion of the propriety of taxing sinful activities.

More recently, in some jurisdictions, alcohol taxes have been justified by the arguments that raising the cost of alcohol better reconciles the private cost and social cost of alcohol consumption. If so, pure logic might conclude that the level of taxation should be related to the quantity of absolute alcohol rather than the value of the drink, imposing more heavily on low-value drinks. An extension would be to focus on the minimum cost of alcohol, structuring the excise to maintain a minimum cost of absolute alcohol, where some of the worse social costs occur (Easton, 2002).

However, no country has an economically rational alcohol taxation regime, and revenue considerations still remain as important in its design as political and cultural considerations.

Moreover, as previously mentioned, the divergence between private and social cost varies from drink to drink, so a taxation regime cannot be perfect. Therefore, other public policy measures have to be implemented. Insofar as such policy measures are effective, there would be a reduction in the divergence between private and social cost, and the optimal excise duty would be lower than if the policies are ineffective.

Table 1   The (tangible) social costs of alcohol as a proportion of GDP

	Australia 1998–99	Canada 1992
Costs of crime, law and order	0.42%	0.20%
Health-care costs	0.03%	0.19%
Loss of production	0.23%	0.60%
Motor vehicle accidents	0.24%	0.07%
Other government resource costs	NA	0.03%
Total	0.92%	1.09%

Source: Collins DJ and Lapsley HM (2002) *Counting the Cost: Estimates of the Social Costs of Drug Abuse in Australia in 1998–9*. Canberra, Australia: National Drug Strategy Monograph Series No. 49; Single E, Robson L, Xie X, and Rehm J (1998) The economic costs of alcohol, tobacco and illicit drugs in Canada, 1992. *Addiction* 93(7): 983–998.

Conclusion

The impacts of alcohol consumption are manifold, and it is not practical to list them all. The ones discussed here are generally those which are known to be largest in quantifiable terms, as measured by their impact on GDP (or GNP) the standard measure of the aggregate output produced in the formal economy (generally valued at market prices). This approach asks what of the available production had to be diverted to deal with the costs of alcohol misuse. (Technically it is an estimate based on supposing that if alcohol misuse had not occurred, what additional resources would have been available for consumption and other purposes.)

Table 1 provides estimates for two countries of this (tangible) social cost of alcohol, as a proportion of GDP. The estimates come from studies that broadly conform to the *International Guidelines* (Single *et al.*, 2003). They do not include estimates of the intangible costs, arising from death, injury, and poor-quality life that alcohol misuse generates (avoiding, among other things, the problem of valuing life). Nor do they include the impact on the informal economy, because there is no measure of the aggregate value of its output (the equivalent of GDP).

In each case the costs are estimated to be near 1% of GDP, the implication being that without alcohol misuse effective GDP would be 1% greater. However, the increase in GDP per capita would be lower, depending on the mortality impact on the population.

Note that despite using the same international guidelines, there are considerable differences between the subtotals, only some of which may be explained by classification differences or by the different cultures and institutional arrangements of Australia and Canada. Nevertheless, while other countries may have different social costs of alcohol misuse, representing the waste from drinkers not taking into consideration the social consequences of their decisions, the magnitude as a proportion of total output is likely to be significant. The quantification reinforces the common sense conclusion of a need for behavior change and public policies in regard to alcohol consumption in order to reduce its misuse.

See also: Alcohol Consumption: Overview of International Trends; Alcohol: The Burden of Disease; Alcohol Industry; Alcoholism Treatment.

Citations

Ainslie G (1992) *Picoeconomics*. Cambridge, UK: Cambridge University Press.

Collins DJ and Lapsley HM (2002) *Counting the Cost: Estimates of the Social Costs of Drug Abuse in Australia in 1998–9*. Canberra, Australia: National Drug Strategy Monograph Series No. 49.

Easton B (2002) *Taxing Harm: Modernising Alcohol Excise Duties*. Wellington Alcohol Advisory Council of New Zealand. http://www.eastonbh.ac.nz/?p=272.

Frederick S, Loewenstein G, and O'Donoghue T (2002) Time discounting and time preference: A critical review. *Journal of Economic Literature* XL: 351–401.

Goldstein PJ (1985) The drugs/violence nexus: A tripartite conceptual framework. *Journal of Drug Issues* 14: 493–506.

Harwood H (2000) *Updating Estimates of the Economic Costs of Alcohol Abuse in the United States: Estimates, Update Methods, and Data*. Report prepared by the Lewin Group for the National Institutes on Alcohol Abuse and Alcoholism. Washington, DC.

O'Donoghue T and Rabin M (2003) Studying optimal paternalism illustrated with a model of sin taxes. *American Economic Review Papers and Proceedings* 93(2): 186–191.

Pernanen K, Brochu S, Cousineau M-M, Cournoyer LG, and Fu Sun (2000) Attributable fractions for alcohol and illicit drugs in relation to crime in Canada: Conceptualization, methods and internal consistency of estimates. *Bulletin on Narcotics* LII (1, 2). United Nations Drug Control Programme.

Pernanen K, Cousineau M-M, Brochu S, and Fu Sun (2002) *Proportions of Crimes Associated with Alcohol and Other Drugs in Canada*. Ottawa: Canadian Centre on Substance Abuse.

Single E, Robson L, Xie X, and Rehm J (1998) The economic costs of alcohol, tobacco and illicit drugs in Canada, 1992. *Addiction* 93(7): 983–998.

Single E, Collins D, Easton B, *et al.* (2003) *International Guidelines for Estimating the Costs of Substance Abuse,* 2nd edn. Geneva, Switzerland: World Health Organisation.

Further Reading

Andlin-Sobocki P and Rehm J (2005) Cost of addiction in Europe. *European Journal of Neurology* 12(supplement 1): 28–33.

Babor T, Caetano R, Casswell S, *et al.* (2003) *Alcohol: No Ordinary Commodity. Research and Public Policy*. Oxford, UK: Oxford University Press.

Collins D, Lapsley H, Brochu S, *et al.* (2006) *International Guidelines for the Estimation of the Avoidable Costs of Substance Abuse*. Ottawa, Canada: Canadian Centre on Substance Abuse.

Easton B (1997) *The Social Costs of Tobacco Use and Alcohol Misuse*. Public Health Monograph No. 2. Wellington, New Zealand: Department of Public Health Wellington School of Medicine.

Elster J (ed.) (1999) *Addiction: Entries and Exits*. New York: Russell Sage Foundation.

Gmel G, Rehm J, Room R, and Greenfield T (2000) Dimensions of alcohol-related social and health consequences in survey research. *Journal of Substance Abuse* 12: 113–138.

Haworth A and Simpson R (2004) *Moonshine Markets*. New York: Brunner Routledge.

Heather N, Peters T and Stockwell T (eds.) (2001) *International Handbook of Alcohol Dependence and Problems*. Chichester, UK: John Wiley & Sons.

Huakau J, Asiasiga L, Ford M, *et al.* (2005) New Zealand Pacific peoples' drinking style: too much or nothing at all? *New Zealand Medical Journal* 118: 1491.

Klingemann H and Gmel G (eds.) (2001) *Mapping the Social Consequences of Alcohol Consumption*. Dordrecht, the Netherlands: Kluwer Academic Publishers.

Mathers C, Bernard C, Iburg K, *et al.* (2003) *Global Burden of Disease in 2002: Data Sources, Methods and Results*. Global Programme on Evidence for Health Policy Discussion Paper No. 54. Geneva, Switzerland: World Health Organization.

Österberg E and Karlsson T (eds.) (2002) *Alcohol Policies in EU Member States and Norway: A Collection of Country Reports*. Helsinki, Finland: STAKES.

Rice D, Kelman S, Miller L, and Dunmeyer S (1990) *The Economic Cost of Alcohol and Drug Abuse and Mental Illness, 1985*. DHHS Publication No. ADM90–1694. San Francisco, CA: Institute for Health and Aging, University of California.

Room R, Babor T, and Rehm J (2005) Alcohol and public health. *Lancet* 365(9458): 519–530.

Single E and Easton B (2001) *Estimating the Economic Costs of Alcohol Misuse: Why We Should Do It Even Though We Shouldn't Pay Too Much Attention to the Bottom Line Results*. Paper presented at the annual meeting of the Kettil Bruun society for Social and Epidemiological research on Alcohol Toronto, May 2001.

Skog OJ (1985) The collectivity of drinking cultures: A theory of the distribution of alcohol consumption. *British Journal of Addiction* 80(1): 83–99.

Child Abuse/Treatment

A P Giardino, Texas Children's Health Plan, Houston, TX, USA

Introduction

Child abuse and neglect, synonymous with the more current term 'child maltreatment,' is a multifactorial problem affecting the health and well-being of large numbers of children worldwide. Ever-increasing amounts of research into the cause and effects of child abuse, what treatments are most effective in ameliorating its consequences, and how best to prevent it from occurring in the first place are being conducted and reported upon. One research team has commented that studying child maltreatment is akin to climbing a mountain: The further you ascend, the more you see that you have to climb (Gough and Lynch, 2000). Because of the multifaceted causes of child abuse and neglect and owing to the wide range of observed responses by children exposed to abuse and neglect, this mountain-climbing analogy rings true to professionals and advocates interested in understanding the child maltreatment problem.

Approximately a decade and a half ago, in a commentary about the public health implications for violence published in the prestigious *Journal of the American Medical Association*, Rosenberg, O'Carroll, and Powell (1992) from the U.S. Centers for Disease Control defined child abuse as a component of interpersonal violence and made clear that both public health as a field and public health-minded professionals as a group ought to rightly address violence including child abuse because:

> Violence is a major cause of injuries and deaths . . . probably has no simple solution, but the public health method

of health-event surveillance, epidemiologic analysis, and intervention design and evaluation can undoubtedly make important contributions to the solution.

> (p. 3072)

Dr. James Gilligan (2000), writing in the equally prestigious *Lancet*, draws an insightful comparison of the public health approach to preventing epidemics to the necessary approach to addressing the public health aspects of violence including child maltreatment:

> A century and a half ago, public health and preventive medicine discovered that cleaning up the water supply and the sewer system was more effective in preventing epidemics of illness and death than all the doctors, medicines, and hospitals in the world. When those same medical specialties are applied to the study of violence, we discover that cleaning up the social and economic system, by reducing the huge inequities in income and wealth between the rich and the poor, are more effective in preventing epidemics of violence and death than all the police, prisons, and punishments in the world.

> (p. 1803)

The United Nations Office of the High Commissioner for Human Rights (1996), in discussing the ratification of the Convention on the Rights of the Child, calls for attention to the health, safety, and development of children throughout the world, including "children who have suffered mistreatment, neglect or exploitation" who need appropriate services in order to recover from this trauma (p. 5). In August 2006, the UN Secretary General received an in-depth study from an appointed independent expert that presented a global study of the problem of violence against children and presented a sobering picture of the magnitude of the problem of abuse and mistreatment of our planet's children. The independent expert, Paolo Sergio Pinheiro, began the report with the observation that no violence against children can be justified and that all violence is preventable. Specifically, Mr. Pinheiro, in describing the intended result of sharing the report's results with the Secretary General, stated:

> The Study should mark a turning point – an end to adult justification of violence against children, whether accepted as 'tradition' or disguised as 'discipline.' There can be no compromise in challenging violence against children. Children's uniqueness – their potential and vulnerability, their dependence on adults – makes it imperative that they have more, not less, protection from violence.

Much of the violence described in this UN report would be seen as child abuse and neglect, so this call to action includes a call to stop child abuse and neglect perpetrated against the world's children. Finally, the World Health Organization (WHO) in collaboration with the International Society for the Prevention of Child Abuse and Neglect (ISPCAN) in 2006 issued a worldwide guide on preventing child maltreatment, in the hopes of generating action to protect children and also to systematize the collection of evidence in the study of child maltreatment such that the impact of such prevention efforts can be quantified and assessed.

This article will briefly summarize what is known about the problem of child abuse and neglect from a public health perspective, focusing on the size of the problem worldwide and looking at the risk factors for being maltreated, what the known consequences are of being exposed to this form of violence, and, finally, what is proposed as being effective at preventing this form of violence that threatens the health and well being of children throughout the globe.

Definitions and Typologies

Child abuse and neglect can be broadly defined as occurring when harm to a child happens by the actions or omissions of someone in a caregiving role for the child. The harm can be an actual injury or a significant risk to the health and safety of a child. The WHO defines child abuse as including all forms of physical and/or emotional ill treatment, sexual abuse, neglect or negligent treatment, or commercial or other exploitation that results in actual or potential harm to the child's health, survival, development, or dignity in the context of a relationship of responsibility, trust, or power (WHO, 1999). Child abuse and neglect is then further categorized into five different subtypes, namely, physical abuse, sexual abuse, neglect and negligent treatment, emotional abuse, and exploitation. See **Table 1** for WHO definitions of each child maltreatment subtype.

Physical abuse typically refers to bodily injuries that are observable on physical examination, via diagnostic testing, or through various imaging techniques and include bruising, cuts and/or abrasions of the skin, various degrees of burns, and broken bones. Head and brain injuries are particularly concerning in infants because of the risk for severe injury to the developing child that often results in disability or even death.

Child sexual abuse (CSA) is a form of child maltreatment in which a child or adolescent is engaged in sexual activities to which they can not developmentally consent by an older, more dominant person. These imposed sexual activities may include exhibitionism, inappropriate viewing of the child, allowing the child to view inappropriate sexual material, taking sexually related photographs of the child, sexualized kissing, fondling, masturbation, digital or object penetration of the vagina or anus, and oral–genital, genital–genital, and anal–genital contact (Sgroi, 1982).

Neglect occurs when a child's caregivers fail to provide for the child's basic needs. These basic needs are wide-ranging and are described by the United Kingdom's Hobbs, Hanks, and Wynne (1993) as typically including such things as food, warmth, clothing, shelter and protection, grooming and hygiene, fresh air and sunlight, activity and rest, prevention from illness and accidents, affection, continuity of care, security of belonging, nurture, and opportunity to learn.

Emotional or psychological abuse refers to styles of child rearing that are injurious to the child's sense of self-worth and well-being. Its forms are listed in **Table 1**.

Finally, commercial exploitation, often involving the commercial sexual exploitation of children (CSEC), is being increasingly identified. In this, children and adolescents are involved in the production of pornographic materials, prostitution, and human trafficking across national borders for the sexual pleasure of people willing to pay for the material produced or for sexual access to the children themselves.

Child maltreatment may be seen as part of the continuum of family violence, and increasing attention is being paid to the relationship of child abuse, specifically physical abuse, to the well-recognized problem of domestic violence or its synonym, interpersonal violence. In 2006, the United Nations International Children's Emergency Fund (UNICEF) in conjunction with The Body Shop International through the Stop Violence in the Home campaign issued a report entitled "Behind closed doors: The impact of domestic violence on children," which reported the following findings:

Table 1   WHO definitions of child abuse and neglect sub-types

Sub-type	Definition
Physical abuse	Actual or potential physical harm from an interaction or lack of interaction, which is reasonably within the control of a parent or person in a position of responsibility, power, or trust. There may be single or repeated incidents (WHO, 1999)
Child sexual abuse	The involvement of a child in sexual activity that he or she does not fully comprehend, is unable to give informed consent to, or for which the child is not developmentally prepared and cannot give consent, or that violates the laws or social taboos of society. Child sexual abuse is evidenced by an activity between a child and an adult or another child who by age or development is in a relationship of responsibility, trust or power, the activity being intended to gratify or satisfy the needs of the other person. This may include but is not limited to the inducement or coercion of a child to engage in any unlawful sexual activity; the exploitative use of a child in prostitution or other unlawful sexual practices; the exploitative use of children in pornographic performances and materials (WHO, 1999)
Neglect and negligent treatment	The inattention or omission on the part of the caregiver to provide for the development of the child in all spheres: health, education, emotional development, nutrition, shelter, and safe living conditions, in the context of resources reasonably available to the family or caretakers and causes, or has a high probability of causing harm to the child's health or physical, mental, spiritual, moral, or social development. This includes the failure to properly supervise and protect children from harm as much as is feasible (WHO, 1999)
Emotional abuse	The failure to provide a developmentally appropriate, supportive environment, including the availability of a primary attachment figure, so that the child can develop a stable and full range of emotional and social competencies commensurate with her or his personal potential, and in the context of the society in which the child dwells. There may also be acts toward the child that cause or have a high probability of causing harm to the child's health or physical, mental, spiritual, moral, or social development. These acts must be reasonably within the control of the parent or person in a relationship of responsibility, trust, or power. Acts include restriction of movement, patterns of belittling, denigrating, scape-goating, threatening, scaring, discriminating, ridiculing, or other non-physical forms of hostile or rejecting treatment (WHO, 1999)
Exploitation, commercial or other forms	Refers to use of the child in work or other activities for the benefit of others. This includes, but is not limited to, child labor and child prostitution. These activities are to the detriment of the child's physical or mental health, education, moral, or social-emotional development (WHO, 1999)

Adapted from: http://www.who.int/violence_injury_prevention/violence/neglect/en/

- Children who live with and are aware of violence in the home face many challenges and risks that can last throughout their lives.
- There is an increased risk of children in domestic violence situations becoming victims of abuse themselves.
- There is a significant risk of ever-increasing harm to children's physical, emotional, and social development when they find themselves in living situations affected by domestic violence.
- There is a strong likelihood that behaviors and attitudes that underlie domestic violence may become a continuing cycle of violence that impacts the following generation.

The year prior to the report, the Stop Violence in the Home campaign was launched in 35 countries throughout Africa, the Americas, Asia, Australia, Europe, and the Middle East.

In a landmark study, researchers Tjaden and Theonnes discussed a range of issues related to violence against women in various settings and they (Tjaden and Theonnes, 1998), identified the overlap of child abuse and domestic violence. They refer to children often being in "harm's way" when there is intimate partner violence in the home or

family setting. **Figure 1** demonstrates this overlapping, often coexistent relationship.

Finally, regretfully, noncaregivers also harm children. This type of violence and injury is seen as a different type of problem and is defined as physical or sexual assault rather than as child abuse or child maltreatment, since abuse occurs in the context of a caregiving relationship that fails to protect the child, whereas assault is violence perpetrated against a child from someone not in a caregiving role.

Epidemiology

A caregiving context underlies child abuse and neglect. Thus, gaining accurate incidence and prevalence statistics on child maltreatment is notoriously difficult for public health officials owing to the shrouding of problems that occur primarily in the private, potentially isolated familial context as well as to the stigma attached to harming children in one's care. On a global basis, with the wide range of cultural norms surrounding privacy in the home, parental rights, and the rights of children, this problem is magnified. According to the report of the independent expert for the UN study on violence against children, the

Multilevel risk factor

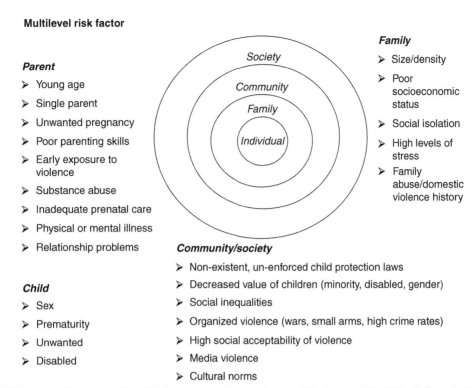

Parent

➢ Young age
➢ Single parent
➢ Unwanted pregnancy
➢ Poor parenting skills
➢ Early exposure to violence
➢ Substance abuse
➢ Inadequate prenatal care
➢ Physical or mental illness
➢ Relationship problems

Child

➢ Sex
➢ Prematurity
➢ Unwanted
➢ Disabled

Family

➢ Size/density
➢ Poor socioeconomic status
➢ Social isolation
➢ High levels of stress
➢ Family abuse/domestic violence history

Community/society

➢ Non-existent, un-enforced child protection laws
➢ Decreased value of children (minority, disabled, gender)
➢ Social inequalities
➢ Organized violence (wars, small arms, high crime rates)
➢ High social acceptability of violence
➢ Media violence
➢ Cultural norms

Figure 1   WHO human ecology model for child abuse and neglect risk factors. Adapted from World Health Organization (2006) *Injuries and Prevention: Child Abuse & Neglect*. http://www.who.int/violence_injury_prevention/violence/neglect/en/ accessed 7/18/06).

global scope of the maltreatment of children is estimated as follows:

- Approximately 53 000 children died worldwide as a result of homicide in 2002.
- Up to 80–98% of children suffer physical punishment in their homes, with at least one-third experiencing severe physical punishment from the use of an implement (e.g., belt, stick, whip).
- Between 20–65% of school-aged children have been verbally or physically bullied in the past 30 days.
- Approximately 150 million girls and 73 million boys under 18 experienced forced sexual intercourse or other forms of sexual violence during 2002.
- Between 100–140 million girls and women have undergone some form of genital cutting or mutilation.
- At least 218 million children were involved in child labor practices, with at least 126 million of these being engaged in hazardous work in 2004 (this is an 11% decrease from the child labor observed in 2002 and a 25% decrease in the number of children in hazardous work).
- In 2000, at least 5.7 million children were in forced or bonded labor, at least 1.8 million were in prostitution and pornography, and 1.2 million were victims of trafficking.

The numbers above are believed to be underestimates because of the illegal, illicit, and stigmatized nature of child maltreatment as well as the well-established underreporting of this problem.

The U.S. Example

An illustrative example of the public health challenges to measuring the national scope of the child maltreatment problem via epidemiologic efforts is the data from the United States regarding the incidence and prevalence of child sexual abuse. Historically, professional attention to the problem of child abuse and neglect is entering its fifth decade in the United States, after the landmark *JAMA* publication of C. Henry Kempe and colleagues' article (1962) detailing the injury of children at the hands of caregivers entitled "The battered child syndrome." Nearly 15 years later, C. Henry Kempe challenged his colleagues again with the publication of an address entitled "The hidden epidemic" that chronicled the existence of child sexual abuse in our midst.

Incidence

Incidence studies look at the number of new cases of abuse and neglect that occur in a given time period, typically one year's time frame. Recent national compilations of U.S. data consistently find that approximately 3 million reports of suspected child maltreatment are being made to child protective services (CPS) agencies for investigation. Of these, ultimately, after processing and investigation, anywhere from 900 000 to about 1 million children are found to have been maltreated; thus, about 1 million cases are substantiated each year in the United States. Specifically, in 2005 there were approximately 3.3 million reports made to CPS involving alleged maltreatment of nearly 6 million children and, after processing and investigation, approximately 899 000 children were determined to have been victims of maltreatment (referred to as being substantiated) (U.S. Dept. of Health and Human Services, 2007). Approximately 60% of the cases are substantiated for child neglect in which a basic need is not met; 15% of cases are substantiated for physical abuse in which a child sustains an injury at the hands of his or her caregivers; approximately 10% are substantiated for CSA; and the remainder are cases of emotional abuse, educational neglect, and combinations of the different forms of child abuse and neglect.

In addition to the annual compilations of individual state data discussed above, the U.S. Congress mandated a series of national incidence studies to determine the national incidence of child abuse and neglect from representative samples of the population. These national incidence studies were viewed as necessary to overcome the well-recognized underreporting to official agencies for all forms of child abuse and neglect, especially of CSA. The Third National Incidence Study on Child Abuse and Neglect (NIS-3), conducted in 1993 and published in 1996, captured data on possible cases of sexual abuse, as inclusively as possible, by using data collection techniques that did not rely solely on state child protective services reports (Sedlak and Broadhurst, 1996). The NIS-3 included

a number of methodological enhancements beyond what was employed in the first and second national incidence studies (NIS-1 and NIS-2) and was able to more completely characterize the full continuum of cases that were known to professionals, not just those known to CPS. Even this approach, however, may underestimate the true number of cases of maltreatment and particularly CSA because it does not capture cases known to nonsampled types of agencies and, of course, does not capture those cases not known to anyone other than the child victim and perpetrator. The NIS approach is frequently displayed as an 'iceberg,' with the visible portion of the iceberg being the cases known to CPS, the portions of the iceberg below the surface being those cases known to other professionals but not known by CPS, and the deepest portion being those cases not known to anyone except the victim and perpetrator (Sedlak, 2001). **Figure 2** displays the NIS iceberg approach to conceptualizing the awareness that professionals have about the numbers of cases of abuse, known and unknown, with those known being visible 'above the water line' and those unknown (unreported) being 'below the water line' and potentially being quite large.

The NIS-3 estimated an overall rate of child maltreatment in the U.S. in 1993 of 23.1 per 1000 children (representing 1 553 8000 children) if stringent rules were used (called the harm standard) and 41.9 per 1000 (representing 2 815 600) if less stringent rules were used (called the endangerment standard). Over half the cases were for neglect, followed sequentially by physical abuse, sexual abuse, emotional abuse, and various forms of educational

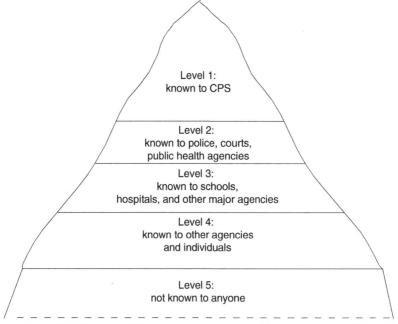

Figure 2 Levels of recognition of Child Abuse and Neglect Children's Bureau, Administration for Children, Youth and Families, Administration for Children and Families. U.S. Department of Health and Human Services. A History of the National Incidence Study of Child Abuse and Neglect. 2001. https://www.nis4.org/NIS_History.pdf (accessed Fubruary 14, 2008).

maltreatment. The Fourth National Incidence Study (NIS-4) is currently underway and will provide the most up-to-date epidemiologic incidence data once completed. The NIS methodology views maltreated children who are investigated by CPS agencies as representing only the 'tip of the iceberg,' so children investigated by CPS are included, along with maltreated children who are identified by professionals in a wide range of agencies in representative communities. The NIS-4, underway at the time of this printing, uses data gathered from a nationally representative sample of 122 counties, and the final report for the NIS-4 is expected to be available by February 2008. CPS agencies in these counties provide data about all children in cases they accept for investigation during one of two reference periods (September 4–December 3, 2005 or February 4–May 3, 2006). Additionally, professionals in these same counties serve as NIS-4 sentinels and will report data about maltreated children identified from the following organizations: elementary and secondary public schools; public health departments; public housing authorities; short-stay general and children's hospitals; state, county, and municipal police/sheriff departments; licensed day care centers; juvenile probation departments; voluntary social services and mental health agencies; and shelters for runaway and homeless youth or victims of domestic violence.

In the mid-1980s, Finkelhor and colleagues (1986) noted that yearly occurrence rates for CSA substantially underestimated its incidence, primarily because the identification and reporting of sexual abuse is discouraged because of the nature of sexual abuse, the secrecy and shame associated with it, the criminal sanctions against it, and the young age of its victims. In addition, varying levels of professional education and public awareness affect the frequency of case detection and make it difficult to judge the true scope of the problem accurately. Most authorities agree that published incidence figures dealing with the occurrence of child sexual abuse are in reality underestimates of the actual incidence of sexual maltreatment.

The specific rate for CSA appeared to decrease throughout the 1990s, with a decrease in the rate from 2.3 per 1000 in 1990 to 1.6 per 1000 in 1998. As more data became available, Finkelhor and Jones (2004) were able to provide a national estimate of the number of sexual abuse cases substantiated by CPS from 1992 to 2000; the number of substantiated sexual abuse cases peaked at 149 800 in 1992, followed by annual declines through 2000, reaching a low of 89 355 in 2000.

Prevalence

As an alternative to examining incidence of sexual abuse, there has been a great deal of interest in the prevalence of sexual abuse. Prevalence looks at the proportion of the population who have been sexually abused during their childhood. Incidence studies rely on data reported to county, state, and national authorities such as seen with the state compilations and NIS-3 data reported above and are recognized as deficient because of the suspected large amount of underreporting that Finkelhor has observed. Prevalence studies, on the other hand, rely on victim and offender self-reports. Because it is believed that most sexual abuse goes unreported, studies that rely on large survey data from a variety of potential victim populations may more accurately reflect the scope of the problem. Prevalence studies, however, may suffer from several problems:

- differences in definition of sexual abuse (e.g., inclusion of noncontact sexual abuse such as exposure, inappropriate comments or requests for sex; inclusion of incidents involving peers as perpetrators; and use of specific age differences between participants, such as age difference greater than 5 years);
- differences in sample characteristics (e.g., age of subject, education level of subject, ethnicity of subject, and region of country surveyed);
- differences in methodological characteristics of studies (e.g., sampling techniques, specifically around populations selected to sample; random vs. nonrandom techniques (e.g., random dialing telephone surveys vs. nonrandom surveys of undergraduates taking an introductory psychology course); and questioning techniques, specifically around face-to-face interviews, self-administered questionnaires, and phone call surveys).

In a comprehensive review of 16 survey-type prevalence studies of nonclinical, North American samples that were performed over three decades, Gorey and Leslie (1997) attempted to adjust or correct the reported prevalence figures for females and males who had experienced sexual abuse in their childhood. The adjustments were done to account for as much variation as possible that might be attributed to differences in each study's response rate and the definitions of abuse used. The authors explained that these corrections were necessary because adults who are aware that they have experienced sexual abuse in their childhood are more likely to respond to surveys addressing this issue, so a high response rate is necessary to balance this out. Additionally, the definition adjustment was necessary because how the survey questions are phrased is central to how the respondents answer the questions. The unadjusted prevalence rates for having experienced childhood sexual abuse was 22.3% for women and 8.5% for men. When adjustments were made in the calculation for a survey response rate of 60% or more (considered a good survey), the prevalence rates became 16.8% for women and 7.9% for men. Additionally, when the calculations were done excluding the broadest, noncontact form of sexual abuse (exhibitionism) from the comparisons, the prevalence figures were 14.5%

for women and 7.2% for men. Using these adjustments, the authors argued that the prevalence rates during the three decades in which the studies were done had not changed significantly.

Professionals in the child abuse field have conservatively used Finkelhor's (1994) U.S. prevalence estimates of 20% for women and 5–10% for men. The careful analysis by Gorey and Leslie (1997) suggest that prevalence figures should at their upper end be set at about 17% for women and 8% for men (Leventhal, 1998). Finally, both Runyan (1998) and Leventhal (1998) individually call for rigorous, epidemiologically sound future studies that limit bias and that are longitudinal in design and focused on the clinically relevant areas of risk and prognosis. This call for increased rigor is echoed in the jointly sponsored WHO and ISPCAN report on preventing child maltreatment (2006).

Consequences: Physical and Psychological Effects

Child maltreatment may have physical, psychological, and emotional effects. The immediate physical consequences vary depending on the type and severity of the injury; depending on the structures and organ systems involved, child maltreatment may have long-term consequences as well. The immediate and long-term physical consequences are often visible and obvious. The psychological and developmental aspects may be less obvious and may be more complex to understand. The anticipated negative impact of child maltreatment on a child's psychological functioning and developmental trajectory may be lessened by 'mediating' factors that include the child's coping strategies and personality characteristics, supportive people in the child's environment, and perceived level of response to the identification of the abuse and neglect once it comes to light. Certainly, children do best when in an environment that provides positive, nurturing interactions that promote psychomotor, cognitive, psychosocial, and emotional well-being. If these aspects are absent, as is the case in an abusive or neglectful situation, then the child's development can be impaired. For example, if the abusive environment interferes with the achievement of an internal sense of safety and trust, the child may as a result have difficulty attaining developmental tasks related to cooperation and interactive play. The extent of the negative impact on the child's psychological and developmental progress could be modified, however, by the various mitigating factors mentioned above. Typical negative consequences that may be seen in cases of physical abuse and neglect include behavioral difficulties related to self-control such as aggression, violence, and juvenile delinquency; psychosocial and cognitive problems such as decreased academic and vocational achievement; and psychological disorders such as poor attachment formation, low levels of empathy, and low self-esteem (Silverman, 1996).

Physical Consequences

Child abuse and neglect can have a wide range of both immediate and long-term consequences on nearly every dimension of a child's physical, emotional, cognitive, developmental, and social health and well-being. Perhaps the easiest to understand are the potential physical health consequences from physical abuse. Injury types vary, and children may experience skin and soft-tissue injuries such as bruises, abrasions, lacerations, and burns. Skeletal injuries include fractures and sprains, as well as abdominal and chest injuries to major organs and structures. Central nervous system injuries may occur to the brain and spinal cord. A variety of other types of injuries to the eyes, face, and teeth are possible, as well as injuries resulting from poisoning. Depending on the severity of the injury, the number of injuries, and the duration of abusive caregiving, children may recover fully or may suffer long-term consequences. Some children are so injured that they have long-term disfigurement, as from severe burns from an immersion-type injury in hot liquid; some may have long-term neurological disabilities, as might be seen from a shaking-impact injury to an infant's fragile skull and brain. Other children may experience a level of violence so severe that their life is violently ended.

Physical injuries to the genitalia from CSA are increasingly understood to be relatively uncommon, primarily due to the perpetrator's desire to elude being detected and as a result engaging in activities with the child that are unlikely to cause physical signs and symptoms that would prompt a medical evaluation and hence detection. Heger and colleagues (2002) have identified a number of possible reasons for a general paucity in genital findings on physical examination, which include the perspective that the perpetrator does not want to be detected, as well as specific anatomic and physiologic characteristics of the child victim and also specific psychological and social factors that seem to promote underreporting or late reporting of the abuse, which permits time for minor injuries to heal.

In addition to the injuries that might be seen to the genitalia, CSA has been associated with a number of 'functional' physical complaints, which are so called because extensive medical diagnostic workups do not reveal obvious physical etiologies to the symptoms described. Specifically, Berkowitz (1998) discusses a number of medical effects from child maltreatment that impact on the child's physical health and well-being, including most notably abdominal or gastrointestinal disorders, genital and anal disorders, and various forms of somatization, including headaches and pain syndromes.

Neglect may lead to poor growth, injury, and death. Perhaps the most commonly recognized physical manifestation of neglect is seen in cases in which the child's basic need for food and nutrition is not met. In these cases, which are frequently referred to as psychosocial failure to thrive (FTT), the child receives inadequate nutrition to sustain his or her anticipated growth potential. The child's growth parameters fall below the expected percentile and demonstrate a pattern of growth retardation. **Figure 3**(**a** and **b**) demonstrates the types of growth curves that might be seen in typical cases of FTT.

Other physical symptoms that might be seen in neglect cases are a lack of hygiene and appropriate cleanliness. In cases in which the child is not provided with adequate clothing or shelter for the climate, one might see frostbite injuries, heat prostration, or even death from exposure to the elements.

Of particular note when discussing potential long-term physical health consequences of child abuse and neglect on children as they grown into adulthood are a set of well-designed epidemiologic studies by Felitti and Anda referred to collectively as the Adverse Childhood Experience (ACE) studies. In these epidemiologic studies, over 17 000 health records were analyzed – and the findings were astounding, in that children who had experienced a variety of adverse experiences in childhood, including child abuse and neglect, were found to be at higher risk for a number of health problems in adulthood, including cardiovascular disease, diabetes, and clinical depression. **Figure 4** illustrates the ACE

pyramid, which graphically represents the ACE studies' conceptual model of how these adverse childhood exposures work in the aging adult's life to lead to poor health outcomes.

Psychological Consequences

Suffering injury or neglect at the hands of a caregiver is a negative event and typically characterizes a negative caregiving environment that may predispose children who have been abused or neglected to a wide range of potential mental health problems. The child's response to the abusive events and abusive environment varies widely, however. Depending on a number of mitigating or protective factors, a child's acute and long-term consequences may vary from mild to severe. These include individual characteristics such as sense of self-esteem, autonomy, and inherent intelligence; family characteristics such as the availability of a caring, nonabusing caregiver; and social characteristics such as access to health-care services within one's community.

Mental health professionals have characterized the mental health consequences of child maltreatment along several continua including:

1. a severity range going from mild to severe symptoms and conditions;
2. a time course range going from relatively short-term effects to those that are long term, sometimes even lifelong; and

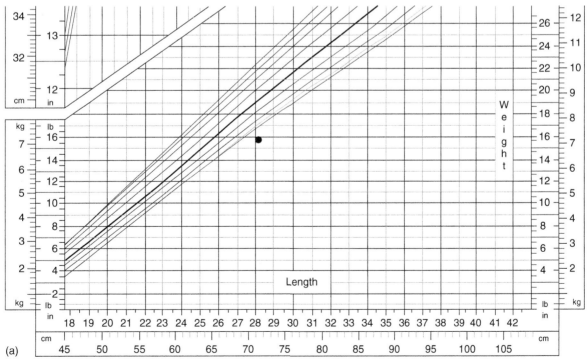

Figure 3 Continued

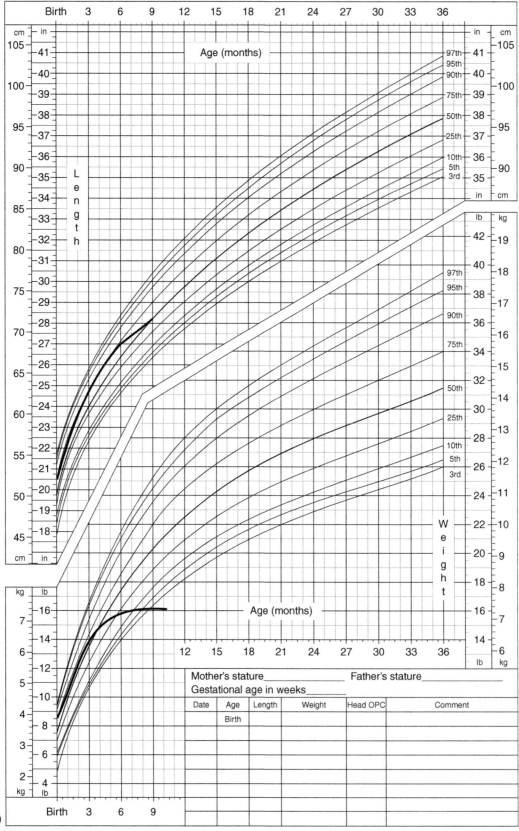

Figure 3 (a) Typical growth chart showing weight crossing several percentiles and reaching a level below the fifth percentile. curve and length dropping, but not as prominently; and (b) Weight for length curve also below the fifth percentile. Graphs courtesy of Dr. Hans Kersten, St. Christopher's Hospital for Children Grow Clinic, Philadelphia, PA.

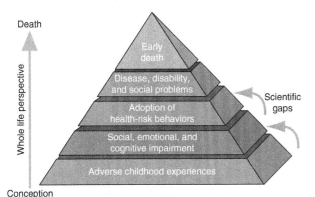

Figure 4 Conception: The Ace Pyramid represents the conceptual framework for the study and graphically represents how adverse experiences in childhood may lead to circumstances that promote poor health outcomes in adulthood. Adopted from Felitti VJ, Anda RF, Nordenberg D, *et al.* (1998) Relationship of childhood abuse and household dysfunction to many of the leading causes of death in adults: The adverse childhood experiences (ACE) study. *American Journal of Preventive Medicine* 14(4): 245–258.

3. an internalizing versus externalizing type of symptom pattern, ranging from children who internalize and respond to the stress by withdrawing and becoming depressed to those children who externalize and become aggressive and disruptive in response to the trauma.

In looking at acute and long-term mental health consequences, both Kendall-Tackett and colleagues (1993) and Paolucci and colleagues (2001) have concluded that no universal response pattern and psychological consequence can be found in all cases of child abuse and child sexual abuse. Paolucci and her colleagues (2001) conducted a meta-analysis of published research on the effects of child sexual abuse and identified 37 English-language studies published between 1981 and 1995 that collectively contained 25 367 people. Despite not finding conclusive evidence to support a specific or universal child sexual abuse syndrome, they found clear evidence of a link between experiencing child sexual abuse and a set of multifaceted negative short-term and long-term consequences impacting the child's development and emotional well-being. These negative consequences included posttraumatic stress disorder, depression, suicide, sexual promiscuity, poor academic performance, and risk for the victim to adopt perpetrator-like behavior toward others.

Intervening on Behalf of the Children and Family

Effective public health intervention begins with case identification. Reporting of suspected cases of abuse and neglect has wide variation throughout the world. In the United States, there are mandatory reporting requirements in all 50 states that require professionals to alert authorities about suspicions of potential child abuse and neglect. Mandated reporters include professionals who by virtue of their work with children are obligated to make reports to the child protective services agency and in some cases to law enforcement. Physicians, nurses, and teachers are consistently included in the list of mandated reporters. The UN, WHO, and ISPCAN support the notion of mandated reporting as a means to ensure the identification of children who are being harmed by abusive caregivers.

Health-Care Evaluation

The medical evaluation of suspected abuse and neglect is fairly standardized and follows the typical health-care evaluation format, namely, history or interview from child and caregiver, complete head-to-toe physical examination of the child, appropriate laboratory/diagnostic studies, consideration of diagnostic possibilities consistent with the findings in the case (the differential diagnosis), and the formulation of a diagnostic impression and treatment plan. The health-care evaluation forms an important component of the overall investigation of a case of suspected child maltreatment. A comprehensive investigation also requires the input of the child welfare agency, which should focus on the safety and custody issues of the affected child, as well as the input of law enforcement, which should be responsible for criminal investigation and for protection of the child from further violence from the alleged perpetrator.

Investigation and Service Delivery

Psychosocial management that requires a significant amount of coordination among various service providers, including the physician and other health-care providers, complements the medical management.

The child welfare agency, frequently referred to as child protective services, in each community should be responsible for performing investigations of suspicion of child maltreatment. CPS will assess the caregivers' background, caregiving abilities and potential, environmental safety, risk for repeat abuse, and risk to other siblings. A variety of treatment options are available, ranging from periodic contact with the child and family to removal of the child from the home, either temporarily or permanently, with termination of parental rights. The CPS process for child maltreatment cases in the United States, for example, typically involves the following steps (DePanfilis and Salus, 1992):

- Intake – Screening of reports and acceptance of case;
- Initial risk assessment – Caregiver interviews, medical information gathering, home evaluation, and possibility of contact with law enforcement;

- Case planning – Determination of safety for the child with essentially three options:
    1. The child goes home with the caregiver with or without services, depending on the circumstances.
    2. The child is removed from home and family with caregivers' consent, and caregivers are offered services to assist them in working toward reunifying with the child.
    3. The child is removed from the home and family without caregivers' consent, involving court action and incorporation of legal steps and processes to determine the ultimate plan for the child.

In the United States, once a report of possible abuse or neglect is made by someone who is concerned, usually in the form of a call to the state or county hotline followed by some form of written documentation, the state laws outline a timeline for the subsequent evaluation. CPS will screen the information, conduct an investigation, and provide supportive services for the child and family. Law enforcement may become involved, depending on the locality and the circumstances of the case. Under state statute, the people making the report in good faith will be able to claim immunity from criminal and civil liability should an angry caregiver file a lawsuit against them for making the report even if it ultimately is determined that no maltreatment has occurred. Certain professionals, such as physicians, who fail to make a report of suspected abuse may be held liable for failing to report the case under the state's statues.

Prevention

Preventing child maltreatment before it occurs and exposes the child to its potential negative physical and psychological consequences remains the ultimate goal of the public health professional, regardless of level of activity, including international, national, regional, or local/ institutional. The collaborative WHO and ISPCAN report on prevention begins with seeking a sound scientific public health approach and promotes more accurate identification and reporting, and more effective intervention on behalf of children who are at risk or who have already been harmed as a result of child abuse and neglect. Additionally, a special focus on childhood fatalities resulting from preventable causes and prevention strategies for all potentially fatal childhood events can be developed, including those from abusive and nonabusive causes. Using the public health model, strategies dealing with preventable causes of death, in particular those related to child maltreatment, can be thought of as being primary, secondary, or tertiary.

Primary (or universal) prevention deals with broad, relatively untargeted initiatives aimed at reaching all of a community's members. Secondary (or selected) prevention efforts are more focused initiatives aimed at individuals or groups who are deemed at higher risk for the exposure to the problem – those children and families who have indicators that suggest a higher risk for child maltreatment. For example, a secondary child maltreatment prevention effort might be targeted to first-time teen mothers, who may have fewer parenting skills when compared to an older mother with several children. Tertiary (or intervention) prevention are efforts directed at providing treatment-oriented services to those children already victims of abuse. The WHO/ISPCAN guide for prevention concludes with a call for (1) information for effective action, (2) prevention of child maltreatment, and (3) care services for victims and families, which includes child protection as well. The prevention strategy called for in this guide describes a comprehensive plan that includes interventions at all levels of the human ecology model and that addresses an array of risk including, among others, cultural norms conducive to child maltreatment and to unwanted pregnancies.

Conclusion

Child abuse and neglect is increasingly recognized as a significant risk to the health and well-being of children in every nation in our world. From a public health perspective, the ever-increasingly accurate epidemiologic statistics that are being collected, analyzed, and publicly shared serve a number of purposes beyond simply being an academic exercise. First, by looking at accurate numbers that have solid academic foundations, victims, the public, and all concerned professionals and organizations can begin to see the magnitude of the problem requiring focused attention and action. This is important with regard to developing interventions, treatment services, and prevention efforts, and informs training efforts as well. In addition, having accurate measures of the problem allows for a baseline in which there is some degree of confidence from which to measure the problem's worsening or improvement. Several reports from international organizations were released in 2006 and, in the words of the UN's independent expert, Paolo Sergio Pinheiro, it is time to move beyond any excuses that might distract our united, international resolve to make the protection of children from the risks posed by exposure to abuse and neglect a high priority that is firmly committed to success – in short, let us commit to making these reports a true turning point, and let us all redouble our efforts to implement the calls toward effective action to protect children.

Citations

Berkowitz CD (1998) Medical consequences of child sexual abuse. *Child Abuse and Neglect* 22(6): 541–550.
DePanfilis D and Salus MK (1992) *Child Protective Services: A Guide for Caseworkers*. Washington, DC: Department of Health and Human Services, National Center on Child Abuse and Neglect.

Felitti VJ (2002) The relationship of adverse childhood experiences to adult health: Turning gold into lead. *Permanente Journal* 6(1). http://xnet.kp.org/permanentejournal/winter02/goldtolead.html (accessed January 2008).

Felitti VJ, Anda RF, Nordenberg D, *et al.* (1998) Relationship of childhood abuse and household dysfunction to many of the leading causes of death in adults: The adverse childhood experiences (ACE) study. *American Journal of Preventive Medicine* 14(4): 245–258.

Finkelhor D (ed.) (1986) *A Sourcebook on Child Sexual Abuse.* Beverly Hills, CA: Sage.

Finkelhor D (1994) Current information on the scope and nature of child sexual abuse. *Future of Children* 4: 31–53.

Finkelhor D and Jones LM (2004) *Explanations for the Decline in Child Sexual Abuse Cases.* Washington DC: United States Department of Justice, Office of Justice Programs, office of Juvenille Justice and Delinquency Prevention.

Gilligan J (2000) Violence in public health and preventive medicine. *Lancet* 355: 1802–1804.

Gorey KM and Leslie DR (1997) The prevalence of child sexual abuse: Integrative review adjustment for potential response and measurement biases. *Child Abuse and Neglect* 21: 391–398.

Gough D and Lynch MA (2000) Taking child abuse research seriously. *Child Abuse Review* 9: 1–5.

Heger A, Ticson L, Velasquez O, and Bernier R (2002) Children referred for possible sexual abuse: Medical findings in 2384 children. *Child Abuse and Neglect* 26: 645–659.

Hobbs CJ, Hanks GI, and Wynne JM (1999) *Child Abuse and Neglect: A Clinician's Handbook,* 2nd edn. London: Churchill Livingston.

International Child Abuse Network (1999) *The World Health Report on the Consultation on Child Abuse Prevention.* Geneva, Switzerland: The World Health Organization.

Kempe C, Silverman F, Steele B, Droegemueller W, and Silver H (1962) The battered-child syndrome. *Journal of the American Medical Association* 181: 17–24.

Kempe CH (1978) Sexual abuse, another hidden pediatric problem: The 1977 C. Anderson Aldrich Lecture. *Pediatrics* 62: 383–389.

Kendall-Tackett K, Williams L, and Finkelhor D (1993) Impact of sexual abuse on children: A review and synthesis of recent empirical studies. *Psychological Bulletin* 113: 164–180.

Leventhal JM (1998) Epidemiology of sexual abuse of children: Old problems, new directions. *Child Abuse and Neglect* 22(6): 481–491.

Paolucci EO, Genuis ML, and Violato C (2001) A meta-analysis of the published research on the effects of child sexual abuse. *Journal of Psychology* 135(1): 17–36.

Rosenberg ML, O'Carroll PW, and Powell KE (1992) Let's be clear: Violence is a public health problem. *Journal of the American Medical Association* 267(22): 3071–3072.

Runyan DK (1998) Prevalence, risk, sensitivity, and specificity: a commentary on the epidemiology of child sexual abuse and the development of a research agenda. *Child Abuse & Neglect* 22(6): 493–498.

Sedlak AJ and Broadhurst DD (1996) *Third National Incidence Study of Child Abuse and Neglect (NIS-3 Final Report).* Washington, D.C.: U. S. Department of Health and Human Services (Contract #105–94–1840).

Sedlak AJ (2001) *A History of the National Incidence Study of Child Abuse and Neglect.* Rockville, MD: Westat, Inc. https://www.nis4.org/NIS_History.pdf (accessed January 2008).

Sgroi SM (ed.) (1982) *Handbook of Clinical Intervention in Child Sexual Abuse.* Lexington, MA: Lexington.

Silverman AB, Reinherz HZ, and Giaconia RM (1996) The long-term sequelae of child and adolescent abuse: A longitudinal community study. *Child Abuse and Neglect* 20(8): 709–723.

Tjaden P and Theonnes N (1998) Prevalence, incidence, and consequences of violence against women: findings from the national violence against women survey. *Research in Brief,* pp. 1–16.

United Nations Office of the High Commissioner for Human Rights (1996) Fact Sheet No. 10 (Rev. 1), The *Rights of the Child.* (http://www.unhchr.ch/html/menu6/2/fs10.htm, accessed 7/12/2006).

United Nations, General Assembly (29 August 2006) *Rights of the Child*: Note by the Secretary –General. 61st Session, Item 62(a) provisional agenda, Promotion and protection of the rights of children, A/61/299. http://www.violencestudy.org/IMG/pdf/English.pdf (accessed 14 February 2008).

UNICEF/Body, Shop (2006) http://www.unicef.org/protection/files/BehindclosedDoors.pdf (accessed 11 February 2008).

U.S. Department of Health and Human Services (USDHHS) (2007) *Child Maltreatment 2005: Summary of Key Findings.* Washington, DC: Government Printing Office.

World Health Organization (2006) *Injuries and prevention: Child Abuse & Neglect.* (http://www.who.int/violence_injury_prevention/violence/neglect/en/ accessed 7/18/06).

Further Reading

Alexander R and Giardino AP (eds.) (2005) *Child Maltreatment: A Photographic Atlas* 3rd edn, vol. 2. St. Louis, MO: GW Medical Publications.

Cooper S, Estes R, Giardino AP, Kellog N, and Vieth V (eds.) (2003) *The Sexual Exploitation of Children.* St. Louis, MO: GW Medical Publications.

Giardino AP and Alexander R (eds.) (2005) *Child Maltreatment: A Clinical Guide and Reference* 3rd edn, vol. 1. St. Louis, MO: GW Medical Publications.

Kendall-Tackett KA and Giacomoni SM (2005) *Child Victimization: Maltreatment, Bullying, and Dating Violence: Prevention and Intervention.* Kingston, NJ: Civic Research Institute.

Relevant Websites

https://www.nis4.org/nis4.asp – U.S. Dept. of Health and Human Services, NIS-4 Description.

http://whqlibdoc.who.int/publications/2006/9241594365_eng.pdf – WHO, Preventing Child Maltreatment: A Guide to Taking Action and Generating Evidence.

Classification of Mental Disorders: Principles and Concepts

T B Üstün, World Health Organization, Geneva, Switzerland

Introduction

The diagnosis and classification of mental disorders has been a controversial issue throughout history. Multiple philosophical and theoretical approaches have been put forward to understand the nature of mental disorders in their various forms and types. Only in the last half of the twentieth century have systematic efforts toward an operational classification enabled scientific studies regarding the description, possible causes, and treatment responses to mental disorders. A common way of defining, describing, naming, and classifying mental disorders was made possible by the International Classification of Diseases (ICD) Mental Disorders (World Health Organization, 1992, 1993) developed by the World Health Organization and also the Diagnostic and Statistical Manual (DSM) of Mental Disorders (American Psychiatric Association, 1994). General acceptance of the ICD and DSM rests on the merits of their descriptive and operational approach toward diagnosis (Stengel, 1959). Operational criteria are logical descriptive statements about the clinical features of the disorders, which can be observed or measured if possible, and as a whole identify similar groups of disorders. These classifications have greatly facilitated practice, teaching, and research by distinguishing the mental illnesses from each other. The absence of etiological information linked to brain physiology, however, has limited the understanding of mental illness.

Classification of mental disorders creates great interest because it offers a synthesis of our current knowledge of mental disorders. A classification represents a way of seeing the whole spectrum of mental disorders and hence provides a general overview. As an accepted standard of theory and knowledge, a classification reflects both the nature of mental disorders and our approach to knowing them. The classification of mental disorders may thus yield some knowledge about the essence of the underlying mechanisms of mental disorders and it may offer some clues toward an understanding of how the brain works. At the same time, the organization of the classification may reflect the conceptual path of how we know and group various mental disorders. Having all this knowledge organized in a classification presents a challenge in terms of consistency and coherence. It also helps us to identify the limits of our knowledge and leads to further research on unresolved issues.

Uses of Mental Health Classifications

Classification of mental disorders has traditionally started from practical efforts to seek similarities and differences among patient groups. Today its greatest use is for administrative and reimbursement purposes. In addition, researchers use mental disorder classifications to identify homogeneous groups of patient populations so as to explore their characteristics and possible determinants of mental illness such as the cause, treatment response, and outcome. Use of mental disorder classifications has also gained importance as a guide in teaching and clinical practice. Earlier practice of psychiatry and behavioral medicine was mainly based on clinical judgment and speculative theories about etiology; the introduction of operational diagnostics has demystified aspects of various practices: Identification of a clinical feature should be defined, observed, and if possible measured in a similar way independent of the assessor. One of the greatest achievements of mental disorder classifications so far has been understanding that mental illnesses could be explained as brain dysfunctions. For example, schizophrenia, which was seen as a myth or a societal label, was defined as an integration of mental functions originating in the brain: Errors in thought processing, for example, result in this mental disorder.

Epistemological State of Mental Health Classifications

The current classifications of mental disorders have largely been built on observation of so-called pathological human behaviors or deviant mental states. They identify patterns of signs or symptoms that are observable and relatively stable over time, across different cultural settings, that can be informed by new knowledge of the way the mind and brain work. Such a classification is a reflection of (a) natural observable phenomena; (b) cultural ways of understanding these; and (c) the social context in which these experiences occur. Since one of the major purposes of a diagnostic classification is to help clinicians communicate with each other by identifying patterns linked to disability, interventions, and outcomes, these classifications have often evolved based on the sorting techniques that clinicians use. All psychiatric classifications are therefore human tools intended for use within a social system. Therefore in thinking about the

Table 1   Timeline of landmark events in psychiatric classification in the twentieth century

Late nineteenth century	Human-rights-based treatment of mentally ill (Pinel, Tuke, Rush and others)
1895	Freud asserts mental disorders are caused by the unconscious mechanisms and uses the psychoanalytic method for assessment and therapy
1910	Watson and Skinner founded behaviorism, which advocates the use of experimental procedures to study observable behavior in relation to the environment
1917	Precursor of DSM: the American Medico-Psychological Association and the United States Bureau of the Census produced the statistical manual including 59 mental illnesses to classify mental inpatients
1922	Krapelin stressed the likely physiological causes of mental disorders and their study through well-defined tests and measurements
1930	ECT was introduced as a reliable method to treat depression
1948	ICD-6 and DSM-I (1952) listing 106 mental illnesses
1955	Major psychotropic drugs introduced to alleviate symptoms of mental illness
1959	Stengel: quest for operational criteria
1960	Deinstitutionalization of mental patients started in Italy, United States, UK
1967	Lin *et al.*: WHO Programme on Diagnosis of Mental Disorders
1968	ICD-8 and DSM-II
1970	Robins and Guze criteria for validity of mental disorders, including clinical description (symptom clusters); laboratory studies; treatment response; family studies and long-term follow-up
1980	DSM-III: fulfilling Stengel's operational criteria quest and paralleling ICD-9 from 1975
1994	ICD-10 and DSM-IV: following a 5-year global collaborative effort

classification of mental disorders, multiple factors need to be taken into account, simply because our understanding of genetics, physiology, individual development, behavioral patterns, interpersonal relations, family structures, social changes, and cultural factors all affect how we think about a classification. The twentieth century was marked by several distinct phases in the way mental phenomena and disorders have come to be understood (see **Table 1**). The determinism of psychoanalysis and early behaviorism has been superseded by the logical empiricism of biological psychiatry that is searching for the underpinnings of human behavior in the brain in particular and in human biology in general.

Our current knowledge of psychiatric disorders remains limited because of the lack of disease-specific markers and is largely based on observation of concurrent behavioral and psychological phenomena, on response to pharmacological and other treatments, and on data on the familial aggregation of these elements. The task of creating a universal classification of mental disorders is, therefore, a very challenging one that seeks to integrate a variety of findings within a unifying conceptual framework.

ICD-10 System of Classification of Mental Disorders

The International Classification of Diseases (ICD) is the result of an effort to create a universal diagnostic system that began at an international statistical congress in 1853 with an agreement to prepare the causes of death for common international use. Subsequently, periodic revisions

were made and, in 1948, when the World Health Organization was formed, the 6th revision of the ICD was produced. Since this date, Member States have decided to use the ICD in their national health statistics. The 6th revision of the ICD for the first time contained a separate section on mental disorders. Since then, extensive efforts have been undertaken to better define mental disorders. Work on the ICD Chapter V for mental disorders has been significantly supported by international work, mainly by the development of the Diagnostic and Statistical Manual (DSM) of Mental Disorders (American Psychiatric Association, 1994). There has been a synchrony between ICD 6 and DSM I, ICD 8 and DSM II, ICD-9 and DSM III, and ICD-10 and DSM IV, with increasing harmony and consistency between the two thanks to the international collaboration between WHO, APA, WPA, and a large network of international collaborative centers. Similarly, work on national classificatory systems, such as the Chinese Classification of Mental Disorders (CCMD) in China, The Latin American Guide for Psychiatric Diagnosis, and the Cuban Glossary of Psychiatry have been standardized with ICD-10 Chapter V, forming a useful internationally comparable yet culturally adapted system.

In the most recent 10th revision of the International Classification of Diseases (ICD-10), the mental disorders chapter has been considerably expanded and several different descriptions are available for the diagnostic categories: The clinical description and diagnostic guidelines (CDDG) (World Health Organization, 1992), a set of diagnostic criteria for research (DCR) (World Health Organization, 1993), diagnostic and management guidelines for mental disorders in primary care (PC) (World Health Organization, 1996), a pocket guide (Cooper, 1994), a multiaxial version (World Health Organization, 1997), and a lexicon (World Health Organization, 1989). These interrelated components all share a common foundation of ICD grouping and definitions yet differentiate to meet the needs of different users.

In the ICD-10, explicit diagnostic criteria and rule-based classification have replaced the art of diagnosis with a reliable and replicable descriptive scheme that has considerable predictive validity in terms of effective interventions. Its development has relied on international consultation and has been linked to the development of assessment instruments. The mental disorders chapter of the ICD-10 has undergone extensive testing in two phases to evaluate the CDDG (Sartorius et al., 1993) as well as the DCR (Sartorius et al., 1995) and agreement between different assessors as measured by the kappa statistic for most categories was over 0.70, indicating very good agreement. Low agreement categories were later revised so as to improve the reliable use of the classification.

Main Principles and Concepts for Classification of Mental Disorders

The new classification systems have generally greatly facilitated teaching, clinical practice, scientific research, and communication. These improvements depend on better definition of concepts and application of certain principles such as definition of the unit of classification; identification of thresholds between wellness and illness; clinical significance and utility; classification style and other factors. These concepts and principles are briefly described below.

Unit of Classification: Definition of Mental Disorder

While ICD is a classification of diseases (or disorders in the context of mental illness), there is no explicit agreement on the definition of a mental disorder (or disease). Disease in general is now proposed by the WHO to be defined as a set of dysfunction(s) in any of the body systems defined by:

- Symptomatology and manifestations: Known pattern of signs, symptoms, and related findings;
- Etiology: An underlying explanatory mechanism;
- Course and outcome: A distinct pattern of development over time;
- Treatment response: A known pattern of response to interventions;
- Linkage to genetic factors, e.g., genotypes, patterns of gene expression;
- Linkage to interacting environmental factors.

The status of disorder is less well defined and it refers to a similar group of syndromes that share similar features usually without having a clear-cut etiological explanation.

This ambiguity creates a fuzzy boundary between wellness and arbitrarily defined disorder. At the lowest level, a mental disorder is an identifiable and distinct set of signs and symptoms that commonly produce disability, and that the healers in the society claim to be able to ameliorate through various interventions. While practical, such a definition can lead to error; for example, homosexuality was once defined as a mental disorder.

The answer to the question 'What is a disorder?' needs to be evaluated against rigorous scientific standards rather than just from societal or personal points of view. Robins and Guze (1970) in their classic paper proposed five phases for establishing the validity of psychiatric diagnosis: Clinical description, laboratory studies, delimitation from other disorders, follow-up study to show diagnostic homogeneity over time, and family study to demonstrate the familial aggregation of the syndrome. Experience gathered since then shows that some of these criteria lead to contradictory conclusions. For example, if one wants to define schizophrenia by its diagnostic stability over time, the best approach is to define the illness at the very outset by a duration criterion of 6 months of continuous illness, which tends to select for subjects with a poor outcome. In contrast, the familial aggregation of schizophrenia is best demonstrated when the notion of the disorder is broadened to include the notion of schizotaxia – a broad-spectrum notion that views the predisposition to schizophrenia to be characterized by negative symptoms (such as withdrawal, motivation loss, disorganized speech, and blunted effect, etc.) – neuropsychological impairment, and neurobiological abnormalities, and schizophrenia to be a psychotic neurotoxic endpoint in the process. The latter approach suggests that narrowing the definition of schizophrenia using the former strategy may in fact hinder progress in identifying the genetic causes of the disorder (Tsuang et al., 2000).

Threshold for Illness

The lack of a definition of what is a disorder also creates an ambiguity. In many instances, for example, depressive disorders, the distribution of mental disorder symptoms forms a continuum in a population without a distinct threshold. This raises questions on where to set the threshold. Even when clinicians have agreed on an arbitrary expert consensus on the placement of a threshold, there remains a large proportion of so-called subthreshold cases that do not fulfill the criteria for a disorder but suffer from signs of mental disorders and display significant disability (e.g., inability to perform daily activities) (Hasin and Paykin, 1999). A good illustration is subthreshold depression. Perhaps the most common of psychiatric presentations in primary care, subjects with this diagnosis do not meet the diagnostic criteria for any depressive disorder in the classification systems and yet are associated with sufficient distress to lead to a consultation and have an impact on the person's functioning (Pincus *et al.*, 1999). There is a need to understand what establishes normal mood fluctuations in response to life events: Every person may react with sadness to the loss of a loved one, but may come out of grief in time by a homeostatic regulation of the mood. In some people, however, this homeostatic regulation fails and a disorder takes place. It is therefore necessary to know the exact nature and determinants of these events so as to clearly identify the disorder (Kendler *et al.*, 1992).

Clinical Significance

Use of operational descriptions has resulted in augmented numbers of cases identified in the community surveys. Similarly, the numbers of cases in clinical studies identified through research criteria but somehow not diagnosed by clinicians were also increased (Regier *et al.*, 1998; Spitzer and Wakefield, 1999). It has therefore been suggested that the criterion of clinical significance be used to define mental disorders. Clinical significance has two main components: (a) Distress; (b) disability. Distress is expressed by the subjects or their significant relatives in terms of worry, concern, suffering, and pain about the condition. There are many clinical cases, however, in which distress may not be expressed or be explicitly denied. The second component, disability, may usually be associated with diseases (as people who are ill cannot function properly in their daily functions), but not always need to be there (Ustun *et al.*, 1998). For example, a person may have tuberculosis with bacillus-positive status but may not exhibit any functional limitations. Similar examples could be given for HIV infection and other infections, noncommunicable diseases such as diabetes and hypertension, or any type of cancer. In all these conditions, diagnosis is conditional on the presence of a physiological disturbance and does not require any disability to be present. Hence, calling for the existence of disability (i.e., functional impairment in DSM parlance) is controversial because it creates an unequal theoretical position between so-called physical and mental illnesses. This issue remains a key target for further revision of current diagnostic classifications, ICD, and ICF.

The development of the International Classification of functioning, disability, and health (ICF) (World Health Organization, 2001) is an important landmark in this regard. The distinct assessment and classification of disability is a strong theoretical and practical requirement to refine the definition of mental disorders. The separate classification of disease and disability phenomena in ICD and ICF is likely to lead to better understanding the underlying body function impairments for mental disorders and associated disability. In this way, we would be able to describe and delineate the features of mental illness more clearly.

Classification by Syndrome Similarity

In the current mental disorder classifications, disorders are grouped by similarity of their clinical features. All substance-related disorders are grouped together, similarly as psychotic disorders, mood disorders, or anxiety disorders. An important grouping issue is about lumping and splitting. Different users have different needs and views regarding the level of detail of a classification. Usually, for primary care and initial clinical care uses, one needs broad categories of classification that lump relatively similar cases. On the other hand, some users search for even minor differences that may identify different aspects such as response to treatment. Current classification systems are debated in terms of whether the level of detail and the number of diagnostic categories are justified. Also, as scientific knowledge advances, we become aware that the current grouping of classifications may not fully fit neurobiology. For example, obsessive compulsive disorder has been grouped with anxiety disorders even though it has been shown to have a totally different neural circuit (Montgomery, 1993; Lucey *et al.*, 1997; Liebowitz, 1998). Similarly, despite the hair-splitting categorizations of anxiety and depressive disorders with complex exclusion rules, clinical and epidemiological studies indicate high rates of comorbidity and similar psychopharmacological agents prove efficacious in their treatment (Mineka *et al.*, 1998; Boerner and Moller, 1999; Kaufman and Charney, 2000; Kessler *et al.*, 2001). Despite the belief in distinct genetic mechanisms between schizophrenia and bipolar disorders, family studies have shown the concurrent heritability (Kendler *et al.*, 1998). Such examples will inevitably accumulate to identify paradoxes in grouping depending on the appearance or the essence (i.e., the underlying mechanisms).

Atheoretical Approach

The separation of the diagnostic criteria from etiological theories (i.e., what causes mental disorder) was an explicit approach undertaken to avoid being speculative, since these theories about causation had not been empirically tested. However this atheoretical approach has also been severely criticized because if one takes a totally atheoretical and solely operational approach, it may be possible to classify normal but statistically uncommon phenomena as psychiatric disorders, for example, one can propose to classify happiness as a disorder (Kendler *et al.*, 1992).

Diagnostic categories have been proposed and accepted merely because of recognizable patterns of co-occurring symptoms rather than because of a true understanding of their distinctive nature that would make them discrete categories within a classification.

Classification Approach: Mind, Brain, or Context?

Recent progress in the cognitive sciences, developmental neurobiology, and real-time *in vivo* imaging of the intact human brain has provided us with new insights into the basic correlates of emotions and cognitions that should inform a new psychopathology. A better understanding of the neural circuitry involved in complex emotional and cognitive functions will accelerate the development of testable hypotheses about the exact pathophysiological basis of mental disorders.

Genetic sciences emphasize the interaction between the genome and the environment. This approach is important in understanding the plasticity of the human brain and how it malfunctions in mental disorders. There is not necessarily a molecular pathology for every mental sign, and there may be multiple paths that may explain the progress of gene expression through central nervous system function to emotional and cognitive constructs.

Progress in the neural sciences is already blurring the boundaries of the brain and mind, yet such a mind–body dualism as expressed in the organic versus nonorganic distinction in the ICD (but not in DSM) does have a utility. It directs the clinician to pay special attention to an underlying physical state as the cause of the mental disturbance. However, the term organic implies an outmoded functional versus structural and mind versus body dualism. Similarly, at the other end of the spectrum, cultural relativism can undermine efforts toward the meaningful diagnosis of mental disorders. The view that stigma and labeling can wrongly define a person as ill implies that mental illnesses are myths created by society. This has resulted in a devaluation of insights that are inherent in a cultural perspective. A similar danger of further dismissing the role of cultural factors in the causation, maintenance, and outcome of mental disorders exists when culture is seen as antithetical to neurobiology.

International Use: Need for Universalism and Diversity

Although some cultural elements have been included in the ICD and DSM, such as culture-bound syndromes, much remains to be done. There is a need to move beyond this because of the role that culture plays in the manifestation of mental disorders. Culture-bound syndromes reflect an extreme view and represent generally rare exotic cases, and provide little if any understanding of the complex interaction between culture and mental phenomena. There is a need for a better cultural formulation of diagnosis and for informed research to address the impact of culture on the explanatory, pathoplastic, and therapeutic processes. Unless typologies are formulated on the basis of careful research, sound theory, and clinical relevance, they are likely to be relegated to the status of historical artifacts.

Etic versus emic approaches

There is a fundamental dilemma with all international crosscultural comparisons: The need to provide an international common language without losing sight of the unique experiences that occur as a feature of living in different social and cultural contexts. There is a need to look for global, universal features of mental conditions, an approach that is driven by analysis and emphasizes similarities rather than differences. This etic approach relies on multigroup comparisons and is often carried out from a viewpoint that is located outside of the system. On the other hand, an emic approach emphasizes the local and specific interpretation that is more bound within culture interpretation. Although the etic and emic approaches are usually presented as opposites, perhaps a balance between the two approaches is in the interest of an international classification. The cultural applicability of international classification warrants careful consideration in future comparative research. For example, WHO's research on drinking norms definitely show differences in terms of thresholds of problem drinking and dependence in wet and dry cultures (Room *et al.*, 1996). Cultural differences in the meaning of mental distress may vary in different ways:

1. In terms of threshold, the point at which respondents from different societies recognize a disorder as something serious;
2. Whether the entities described in international classifications count as problems in all cultures;
3. In causal assumptions about how mental problems arise;
4. In the extent to which there exist culture-specific manifestations of symptoms not adequately captured by official disease nomenclature.

Categorical and Dimensional Models

There are two quite different ways of conceptualizing mental disorders: As dimensions of symptoms or as categories, often by identifying a threshold on the dimension. Clinicians are usually obliged to use categorical concepts, as they must decide who is sufficiently ill to justify treatment. But in our efforts to understand the relationships between social and biological variables, dimensional models are more appropriate (Goldberg,

2000). Dimensional models are more consistent with the polygenic models of inheritance favored for most mental disorders. These models assume that a number of genes combine with one another and interact with the environmental factors to cause the disorder. Persons can thus have various doses of the risk factors that predispose to the illness and depending on the dose, the severity of the manifest condition may vary along a continuum. Such approaches have been shown to provide important clinical advantages with psychotic illnesses (Ustun *et al.*, 1997) and personality disorders.

The Concept of Comorbidity

The concept of comorbidity becomes important when the classification logic posits discrete categories. Comorbidity, the concurrence of more than one diagnosis, does occur in real life and it is more the norm rather than the exception. The phenomenon of comorbidity poses a great challenge to the classification because it can be an artefact of hierarchical rules used in classification systems. Excessive splitting of classical syndromes into subtypes of disorders with overlapping boundaries and indefinite thresholds adds to the confusion. Though the co-occurrence of pathology in different subsystems of the body is indeed possible, it can either be attributed to the same underlying etiological cause affecting different body systems (as is the case, for example, with diabetes causing hyperglycemia, peripheral neuropathy, and nephropathy) or to distinct causes that just happen to co-occur (as is the case with diabetes and a lacerated wound following an injury). Further, the notion of comorbidity can only be accepted when the categories are not mutually exclusive, in order to avoid category errors.

Future of Mental Health Classifications

WHO's network on the family of international classifications has planned for an overall revision of the classification of diseases before 2015. Similarly, DSM has announced a revision by 2012. This period will allow for a more extensive knowledge base to develop and build up mechanisms so that such a knowledge base informs the mental health classifications. In particular, new information on genetics, neurobiology, and epidemiology can be used in an iterative process to update the categories, criteria, and grouping of disorders. A sound epistemological approach could be used to identify the disorder, disease, and disability. It is expected that future classifications should go beyond an expert consensus and reliability. Operationalization and reliability are indeed useful guides for classifications; however, they are not sufficient for validity. An evidence-based review mechanism and focused empirical testing for specific categorizations should be started. Underlying physiological mechanisms should be preferred for disease grouping instead of traditional conventions. Applicability and reliability of the new proposals for classification should be tested in field trials.

The ICD and DSM in their current forms are both descriptive classifications with operationally defined criteria and rule-based approaches to generating diagnoses. The efforts to harmonize the two classifications have left minor differences between the two systems. Currently, both systems are not entirely homologous, but in a large majority of criteria they are identical or differ in a insignificant ways in terms of diagnostic categories and criteria. Differences are most marked in the case of near-threshold, mild, or moderate conditions. Discordance is particularly high with categories such as posttraumatic stress disorder and harmful use or abuse of substances (Andrews *et al.*, 1999; Farmer and McGuffin, 1999; First and Pincus, 1999; van Os *et al.*, 2000). Substantive differences between the ICD and DSM also exist; for example, the ICD separates disability from diagnosis, and the ICD does not put personality disorders or physical disorders in a different axis.

Future classifications will be more than a common language between clinicians. First, the use of computerization in health records will require linkages between clinical symptoms, laboratory findings, and other features of diseases. A number of various domains will have to come together to build classification systems. Such a comprehensive integrated system will require identification of each entity and relations between them as a sound ontology-based system. Different use cases on clinical utility, quality of care, research, administrative reimbursement uses can be defined with different levels of granularity based on such a flexible system. Second, the health information should be shared by all parties, including consumers and providers, which will require more elaborate systems. Consumers and various care providers sharing the same classification system will require different levels of complexity, which is based on the same groupings expressed in different terms. In terms of comparison of views between different users, countries and across-time use of a common international classification is essential. The closer this system comes to the scientific evidence, the more reliable and valid its use between different agents will become.

See also: Measurement of Psychiatric and Psychological Disorders and Outcomes in Populations; Mental Health: Morbidity and Impact; Women's Mental Health.

Citations

American Psychiatric Association (1994) *Diagnostic and Statistical Manual of Mental Disorders*, 4th edn. (DSM-IV). Washington, DC: American Psychiatric Association.

Andrews G, Slade T, and Peters L (1999) Classification in psychiatry: ICD-10 versus DSM-IV. Editorial. *British Journal of Psychiatry* 174: 3–5.

Bentall RPA (1992) Proposal to classify happiness as a psychiatric disorder. *Journal of Medical Ethics* 18: 94–98.

Boerner RJ and Moller HJ (1999) The importance of new antidepressants in the treatment of anxiety/depressive disorders. *Pharmacopsychiatry* 32: 119–126.

Cooper JE (1994) *Pocket Guide to the ICD-10 Classification of Mental and Behavioural Disorders, with Glossary and Diagnostic Criteria for Research*. Edinburgh: Churchill Livingstone.

Farmer A and McGuffin A (1999) Comparing ICD-10 and DSM-IV. *British Journal of Psychiatry* 175: 587–588.

First MB (2004) Clinical utility. *American Journal of Psychiatry* 161(6): 946–954.

First MB and Pincus HA (1999) Classification in psychiatry: ICD-10 v. DSM-IV. A response [editorial]. *British Journal of Psychiatry* 175: 205–209.

Goldberg D (2000) Plato versus Aristotle. Categorical and dimensional models for common mental disorders. *Comprehensive Psychiatry* 41(2 supplement 1): 8–13.

Hasin D and Paykin A (1999) Dependence symptoms but no diagnosis: Diagnostic 'orphans' in a 1992 national sample. *Drug and Alcohol Dependence* 53(3): 215–222.

Kaufman J and Charney D (2000) Comorbidity of mood and anxiety disorders. *Depression and Anxiety* 12(supplement 1): 69–76.

Kendler KS, Neale MC, Kessler RC, Heath AC, and Eaves LJ (1992) A population based study of major depression in women – The impact of varying definitions of illness. *Archives of General Psychiatry* 49: 257–265.

Kendler KS, Karkowski LM, and Walsh D (1998) The structure of psychosis: Latent class analysis of probands from the Roscommon Family Study. *Archives of General Psychiatry* 55: 492–499.

Kessler RC, Keller MB, and Wittchen HU (2001) The epidemiology of generalized anxiety disorder. *Psychiatric Clinics of North America* 24: 19–39.

Liebowitz MR (1998) Anxiety disorders and obsessive compulsive disorder. *Neuropsychobiology* 37: 69–71.

Lucey JV, Costa DC, Busatto GP, *et al.* (1997) Caudate regional cerebral blood flow in obsessive-compulsive disorder, panic disorder and healthy controls on single photon emission computerised tomography. *Psychiatry Research* 74: 25–33.

Mineka S, Watson D, and Clark LA (1998) Comorbidity of anxiety and unipolar mood disorders. *Annual Review of Psychology* 49: 377–412.

Montgomery SA (1993) Obsessive compulsive disorder is not an anxiety disorder. *International Clinical Psychopharmacology* 8(supplement 1): 57–62.

Pincus HA, Davis WW, and McQueen LE (1999) 'Subthreshold' mental disorders. A review and synthesis of studies on minor depression and other 'brand names'. *British Journal of Psychiatry* 174: 288–296.

Regier DA, Kaelber CT, Rae DS, *et al.* (1998) Limitations of diagnostic criteria and assessment instruments for mental disorders: Implications for research and policy. *Archives of General Psychiatry* 55: 109–115.

Robins E and Guze SB (1970) Establishment of diagnostic validity in psychiatric illness: Its application to schizophrenia. *American Journal of Psychiatry* 126: 983–987.

Room R, Janca A, Bennett LA, Schmidt L, and Sartorius N (1996) WHO cross-cultural applicability research on diagnosis and assessment of substance use disorders: An overview of methods and selected results. *Addiction* 91: 199–220.

Sartorius N, Kaelber CT, Cooper JE, *et al.* (1993) Progress toward achieving a common language in psychiatry. Results from the field trial of the clinical guidelines accompanying the WHO classification of mental and behavioral disorders in ICD-10. *Archives of General Psychiatry* 50: 115–124.

Sartorius N, Ustun TB, Korten A, Cooper JE, and van Drimmelen J (1995) Progress toward achieving a common language in psychiatry, II: Results from the international field trials of the ICD-10 diagnostic criteria for research for mental and behavioral disorders. *American Journal of Psychiatry* 152: 1427–1437.

Spitzer RL and Wakefield JC (1999) DSM-IV criteria for clinical significance. Does it help solve the false positive problem? *American Journal of Psychiatry* 156: 1856–1864.

Stengel E (1959) Classification of mental disorders. *Bulletin of the World Health Organization* 21: 601–603.

Tsuang MT, Stone WS, and Faraone SV (2000) Toward reformulating the diagnosis of schizophrenia. *American Journal of Psychiatry* 157: 1041–1050.

Ustun B, Compton W, Mager D, *et al.* (1997) WHO Study on the reliability and validity of the alcohol and drug use disorder instruments: Overview of methods and results. *Drug and Alcohol Dependence* 47: 161–169.

Ustun TB, Chatterji S, and Rehm J (1998) Limitations of diagnostic paradigm: It doesn't explain "need". *Archives of General Psychiatry* 55: 1145–1146.

van Os J, Gilvarry C, Bale R, *et al.* (2000) Diagnostic value of the DSM and ICD categories of psychosis: An evidence-based approach. UK700 Group. *Social Psychiatry and Psychiatric Epidemiology* 35: 305–311.

World Health Organization (1989) *Lexicon of Psychiatric and Mental Health Terms*. Geneva, Switzerland: World Health Organization.

World Health Organization (1992) *The ICD-10 Classification of Mental and Behavioural Disorders: Clinical Descriptions and Diagnostic Guidelines*. Geneva, Switzerland: World Health Organization.

World Health Organization (1993) *The ICD-10 Classification of Mental and Behavioural Disorders: Diagnostic Criteria for Research*. Geneva, Switzerland: World Health Organization.

World Health Organization (1996) *Diagnostic and Management Guidelines for Mental Disorders in Primary Care: ICD-10 Primary Care Version*. Bern, Switzerland: Hogrefe and Huber.

World Health Organization (1997) *Multiaxial Presentation of the ICD-10 for Use in Adult Psychiatry*. Cambridge, UK: Cambridge University Press.

World Health Organization (2001) *International Classification of Functioning, Disability and Health (ICF)*. Geneva, Switzerland: World Health Organization.

Relevant Website

http://www.who.int/classifications/icd/ICDRevision/en/index.html – WHO.

Health Behavior and Risk Factors

K Glanz and J E Stryker, Rollins School of Public Health, Emory University, Atlanta, GA, USA

Why Health Behavior Is Important

Health-related behavior is one of the most vital elements to the public's health and well-being. Its importance has grown during the past century, as sanitation has improved and medicine has advanced so that once deadly or incurable diseases can be prevented or successfully treated. Thus, health-related behavior is an increasing focus of attention in public health and improving health-related behavior is central to public health activities.

The major causes of death in the United States and other developed countries are chronic diseases such as heart disease, cancer, and stroke. The causes of each of these diseases include health risk behaviors. Behavioral factors are thought to contribute to almost half of the deaths in the United States. The most common behavioral contributors to mortality, or death, in 2000 were tobacco, poor diet and physical inactivity, and alcohol use; other significant causes of death include firearms, sexual behavior, motor vehicle crashes, and illicit use of drugs. These behaviors were responsible for nearly one million deaths in just a single year (Mokdad *et al.*, 2004). The resurgence of infectious diseases, including foodborne illness and tuberculosis, and the emergence of new infectious diseases such as antibiotic-resistant infections, HIV/AIDS, hepatitis C, and human papillomavirus (HPV) are also influenced by human behaviors. Of the 12 leading causes of death, behavioral factors are related to all of them. The social and economic costs related to these behaviors can all be greatly reduced by changes in individuals' behaviors.

Over the past 20 years, there has been a dramatic increase in public, private, and professional interest in preventing disability and death through changes in lifestyle behaviors and participation in screening programs. Much of this interest has been stimulated by changes in disease patterns from infectious to chronic diseases as leading causes of death, the aging of the population, rapidly escalating health-care costs, and data linking individual health risk behaviors to increased rates of morbidity and mortality.

Although there is more information about what constitutes healthy behavior and risk factors than ever before, this has not always led people to practice healthier behaviors. There have been some positive changes: In the United States in the late 1980s and 1990s, average daily intake of dietary fat dropped from 36% to 34% of total energy, seat belt use increased from 42% to 67%, and the number of women over the age of 40 who had breast exams and mammograms doubled. However, not all the news is favorable. More adults and children are overweight. Diabetes is increasing in near-epidemic proportions. More adolescents are sexually active. After major increases in seat belt use in the early 1990s, rates declined slightly and remain at 67%, well below the target rate of 85% (NCHS, 2001). One-fifth of children under three years old have not received a basic series of vaccinations for polio, measles, diphtheria, and other diseases. Ethnic minorities and those in poverty experience a disproportionate burden of preventable disease and disability, and for many conditions the gap between disadvantaged and affluent groups is widening (House and Williams, 2000).

Patterns of risk factors and their impact on the burden of disease vary across regions of the world, with the most striking differences found between developing and developed regions. In the poorest regions, behaviors associated with childhood and maternal malnutrition, unsafe sex, tobacco and alcohol use, and personal and household hygiene are leading causes of disease burden (Ezzati *et al.*, 2002). In both developing and developed regions, behavioral risk factors of alcohol use, tobacco, and cardiovascular risks strongly influenced by dietary and physical activity behaviors – high blood pressure and high cholesterol – are major causes of disease burden (Ezzati *et al.*, 2002). Updated projections of global mortality and the burden of disease suggest that noncommunicable diseases will increase in the next two decades, and that tobacco-attributable deaths in particular will continue to rise. Global HIV/AIDS deaths are projected to more than double and to become the leading cause of disease burden in middle- and low-income countries by 2015 (Mathers and Loncar, 2006). Both health behavior and medical care will influence emerging disease patterns: for example, the reach of effective antiretroviral drugs and increased prevention activity have the potential to affect these projections from the World Health Organization between now and 2030 (Mathers and Loncar, 2006).

Definitions of Health Behavior

Health behavior encompasses a large field of study that cuts across various disciplines, including psychology, education, sociology, public health, epidemiology, and anthropology. In the broadest sense, 'health behavior' refers to the actions of individuals, groups, and organizations as well as their determinants, correlates, and consequences, including social change, policy development and implementation, improved coping skills, and enhanced quality of life. Health behavior includes not only observable, overt actions but also the mental events and feeling states that can be reported and measured. Health behavior has been defined as "those personal attributes such as beliefs, expectations, motives, values, perceptions, and other cognitive elements; personality characteristics, including affective and emotional states and traits; and overt behavior patterns, actions, and habits that relate to health maintenance, to health restoration, and to health improvement" (Gochman, 1982).

Gochman's definition is consistent with the definitions of specific categories of overt health behavior proposed by Kasl and Cobb in their seminal articles (1966a, b). They define three categories of health behavior as follows:

Preventive health behavior. Any activity undertaken by an individual who believes him- or herself to be healthy, for the purpose of preventing or detecting illness in an asymptomatic state, is defined as preventive health behavior. This can include self-protective behavior, such as wearing a helmet when riding a bicycle, using seat belts, or wearing a condom during sexual activity.

Illness behavior. Illness behavior is any activity undertaken by an individual (who believes she or he is ill) to define his or her state of health and discover a suitable remedy (Kasl and Cobb, 1966a).

Sick-role behavior. Any activity undertaken by an individual who considers her- or himself to be ill, for the purpose of getting well, is defined as sick-role behavior. It includes receiving treatment from medical providers, which generally involves a whole range of dependent behaviors, and leads to some degree of exemption from one's usual responsibilities (Kasl and Cobb, 1966b).

These classic definitions have stood the test of time, and continue to be used by students and public health workers alike. However, the lines between these three categories have blurred somewhat over time. For example, the period of survival after a major illness event such as a heart attack or a cancer diagnosis has become longer as treatments and disease management have improved. Cancer survivors can benefit from increased physical activity after initial treatment, both to improve quality of life and to prevent recurrence of the cancer. Diabetes self-management involves a complex set of behaviors that help to reduce health risks and prolong healthy functioning. So, a person who has been diagnosed with a serious disease may practice preventive health behavior for both disease management and prevention of further health risks.

As well, classic definitions of health behavior emphasize the actions of individuals, in contrast to a public health perspective, which is concerned with individuals as part of a larger community. Also, individuals' actions (behaviors)

are what determine many of the social conditions that affect people's health. For example, people act collectively to make laws and policies and to implement and enforce them.

Additional useful distinctions can be made between 'episodic' and 'lifestyle' behaviors, or habits. Episodic health behavior can be something that is done once, or periodically, like getting immunizations or a flu shot. It can also be something that one does only to oneself, such as putting on sunscreen, or a behavior that affects others, like putting up a shade cover so children at the playground are protected from the sun.

Lifestyle behaviors, or health habits, are actions that are performed over a long period of time, such as eating a healthful (or unhealthy) diet, getting regular physical activity, and avoiding tobacco use. A composite of various healthful behaviors is often referred to as a 'healthy lifestyle.' However, most people do not practice all healthful or risky behaviors consistently, for instance, someone might get regular, health-promoting exercise several times a week but be a cigarette smoker who seldom brushes his or her teeth. Or someone might quit smoking, only to begin overeating as a substitute. In the ideal, the person who practices a variety of behaviors in a health-enhancing manner can be described as having a healthy lifestyle. More realistically, though, many people practice *some*, but not all, lifestyle behaviors in a healthy manner.

At-Risk Populations as Defined by Their Health Behaviors

The idea of 'risk factors' or 'at-risk populations' is complex and involves many dimensions of risk.

Biological risk

Biological risk involves risks that are part of one's physical make-up, and may involve hereditary disorders or genetic predisposition to certain diseases. For example, some of the better-known hereditary diseases such as Tay-Sachs disease, Huntington's disease, and cystic fibrosis are primarily biologically determined and, to date, there are no known behaviors to recommend for preventing them. Other biological risks can be addressed, at least partly, by preventive health behavior: fair-skinned people are at greater risk for skin cancer, and someone whose parent died of a heart attack in their 40s is likely to have an increased risk for heart disease. Fair-skinned people can make strong efforts to avoid exposure to ultraviolet radiation (UVR) or sunlight, and those with a family history of heart disease can avoid tobacco, maintain a healthy weight, and manage risk factors such as high blood pressure and high cholesterol. There are other biological predispositions that confer increased risk to people in combination with certain exposures – often behavioral – that are increasingly being uncovered through scientific research in molecular epidemiology, also often known as genetic epidemiology. For example, a man with a family history of colon cancer who eats a lot of red meat might be increasing his risk more than would a woman with no relatives who have had the disease.

Environmental risk

Another category of risk is environmental risk, which may or may not be within the control of individuals' behavior. Examples include air pollution, water pollution, congested traffic, and characteristics of the 'built environment' such as urban sprawl. These risks may affect people's health directly – such as when high levels of particles in the air cause asthma or allergies to flair up, or indirectly through health behavior – such as when people spend a lot of time in their cars, being sedentary, because of lengthy commuting distances to work.

Social risk factors

Social risk factors have been increasingly recognized by social scientists and epidemiologists over the past 30 years (Berkman and Kawachi, 2000). Social isolation is thought to increase the risk of both physical and psychological health problems. Again, this can be considered a direct social risk or one that operates through behaviors such as poor self-care, and increased use of alcohol and drugs. In contrast, social support systems are believed to be protective to individuals and 'social capital' is a construct that describes communities that are more likely to be cohesive, trusting, and to have better health.

Behavioral risk factors

Finally, behavioral risk factors are risks identified specifically with the practice, or failure to practice, an action or series of actions that are associated with health outcomes. These include tobacco use, poor diet, physical inactivity, risky sexual behavior, poor dental hygiene, drinking and driving, and many others that are important contributing causes to illness or inadequate disease management.

Determinants of Health Behavior

There are many questions about how health behavior develops and is sustained. Therefore, both public health workers and scientific researchers continue to attempt to understand the nature and causes of many different health behaviors that lead to varying levels of risk for disease. An understanding of the determinants of health behavior is critical for developing effective interventions that may reinforce or change behavior. Numerous theories and models have been developed to understand health behavior and its determinants. The determinants of health behavior are complex and multifaceted, so one single theory rarely can explain a health behavior (Glanz et al., 2002). Because of this, some models have been developed that use multiple theories to help understand a specific problem in a particular setting or context.

Behavioral Theories

Broadly speaking, these theories and models can be broken down into two categories: (1) theories of behavioral prediction or explanation; and (2) theories of behavior change or action. Explanatory or predictive theories help to identify factors that may influence a health behavior; if properly specified, explanatory theories should be able to predict reasonably well who will be more or less likely to perform a given behavior. In contrast, theories and models of behavior change focus on the change process; these theories tend to detail stages through which individuals progress before achieving lasting health behavior change. Though these two types of theories often have different emphases, they are complementary. For example, knowing the reasons why someone smokes is important for the development of effective smoking cessation materials, but equally important is an understanding of how someone who has made several unsuccessful quit attempts in the past can progress to becoming a nonsmoker.

The major theories can be classified into roughly three categories: (1) individual level, focusing on constructs such as knowledge and attitudes; (2) interpersonal level, emphasizing social factors such as social norms or social support; and (3) structural or environmental, emphasizing multiple levels of influence, including access to resources, laws, and policies. The most commonly used theories cut across these levels. Glanz et al. (2002, 2005) have conducted several reviews of health behavior theories presented in major health education, health behavior, and preventive medicine journals. The most common health behavior theories used in research published in health education, health behavior, and preventive medicine journals are briefly described here.

The health belief model (Rosenstock, 1974) was originally developed to explain why people took or did not take advantage of preventive services such as disease screening and immunizations. The model suggests that when a person perceives a threat that has severe consequences, and believes she or he is likely to take action. To take action against that threat (i.e., change their behavior), the individual must also perceive that the benefits outweigh the costs of the preventive action.

The theory of reasoned action (Ajzen and Fishbein, 1980) proposes that the most proximal indicator of actual behavior is behavioral intention. Behavioral intentions, in turn, are a function of (1) attitudes toward the behavior, and (2) subjective norms regarding the behavior. Attitudes are made up of beliefs about the positive and negative consequences associated with performing the behavior, as well as an individual's evaluation of those consequences. Subjective norms are a function of normative beliefs that people who are important to the individual think they should or should not perform the behavior, as well as that individual's general motivation to comply with a particular person's wishes.

An extension of the theory of reasoned action, the theory of planned behavior (Ajzen, 1985) includes the idea of perceived behavioral control. Perceived behavioral control depends on specific beliefs about the likelihood that certain conditions might affect the ability to control the behavior, and whether those conditions would encourage or constrain behavioral performance. Perceived behavioral control is similar to self-efficacy, found in social cognitive theory.

Social cognitive theory (SCT) (Bandura, 1986) purports that people and their environments are thought to interact continuously. A basic premise of SCT is that people learn not only through their experiences, but also by watching the way other people act and the results they achieve. According to SCT, three primary factors affect behavior. First, individuals must have self-efficacy, or the confidence in their ability to perform particular behaviors (akin to perceived behavioral control above). Second, individuals must have personal goals that provide them with meaningful incentives for change. Third, the perceived advantages of practicing the behavior must outweigh the obstacles that hinder behavior change.

Like SCT, social ecological models of behavior change emphasize the importance of the interplay between individuals and their environments. Sallis and Owen (2002) suggest the following with respect to health behavior determinants: (1) individual, social, and environmental forces determine health behavior; (2) both natural and built environments influence health behavior, including actual and perceived influence; (3) different levels of aggregation (including individuals, families, organizations, communities, and populations) need to be considered, both to understand and to change health behavior; and (4) behavior-specific ecological models may improve behavioral prediction and change.

The stages of change model – or the transtheoretical model – addresses individuals' readiness to change their behaviors from unhealthy to healthy (DiClemente *et al.*, 1991). Its basic premise is that behavior change is a process and not an event, and that individuals are at varying levels of readiness to change. This means that people at different points in the process of change can benefit from different programs for change. In developing successful behavior change intervention, the programs work best if matched to the person's stage at that time. For example, a smoker who has never thought about quitting will need different messages (to motivate the smoker to think

about quitting) than a smoker who has made repeated unsuccessful attempts (to build self-efficacy to quit).

It is useful to consider these various theories in context, relative to the level of analysis (individual, social, environmental) and to determine whether they focus primarily on explaining or changing behavior. The health belief model, the theory of reasoned action, and the theory of planned behavior can all be considered explanatory theories of individual health behavior, in that they all have a clearly defined set of constructs, specify the relationships between constructs, and focus on individual explanations for health behavior. SCT, which contains a larger number of constructs, and a more dynamic relationship between individuals and their environments, shares some features with the aforementioned theories, as well as similarities with social ecological models of behavior. By viewing behavior as a dynamic process, and highlighting the importance of social and environmental determinants, SCT and social ecological models are more complex, and provide a more holistic approach to behavior change. Finally, the stages of change model focuses on the behavior change process, and are best used in conjunction with other behavioral theories.

Overlap of Behavioral Theories

Various theories of health-related behavior often overlap. Not surprisingly, these explanations for behavior and models for change share several important cross-cutting issues and constructs. This section highlights a few of the most important of these.

Behavior change as a process

One central idea that has gained wide acceptance in recent years is the simple notion that behavior change is a process, not an event. Rather, it is important to think of the change process as one that occurs in stages. It may involve more than someone deciding one day to stop smoking and the next day becoming a nonsmoker for life. Also, most people won't be able to dramatically change their eating pattern all at once. The idea that behavior change occurs gradually is not new, but it has gained wider acceptance in the past few years. Indeed, some multistage theories of behavior change date back more than 50 years (Lewin, 1935; Weinstein, 1993).

Changing behaviors versus maintaining behavior change

Even when there is good initial compliance to a health-related behavior using change advice or attempts (e.g., applying sunscreen or changing diet), relapse is very common. Thus undertaking initial behavior changes and maintaining behavior change are very different and require different types of programs and/or self-management strategies. For example, someone could quit smoking by going 'cold turkey,' but they will probably be tempted again, perhaps at a party where their friends are smoking. To maintain cessation behavior requires developing self-management and coping strategies, and establishing new behavior patterns that emphasize perceived control, environmental management, and improved confidence in one's ability to avoid temptation.

Barriers to actions, pros and cons, and decisional balance

The concept of barriers to action, or perceived obstacles, is often mentioned in theories of health behavior. An extension of the concept of barriers to action involves the net benefits of action, also referred to as 'benefits minus barriers' in the health belief model (Glanz and Rimer, 2005). In the stages of change model, there are parallel constructs labeled as the pros (the benefits of change) and cons (the costs of change) (Prochaska et al., 1992). Taken together, these are known as decisional balance, or the pros minus cons, similar to the net benefits of action in the health belief model. In the theory of reasoned action and theory of planned behavior, attitudes, norms, and perceived behavioral control each consists of the sum of different positive and negative beliefs. The idea that individuals engage in relative weighing of the pros and cons has its origins in models of decision making, and has been considered important for many years (Lewin, 1935; Janis and Mann, 1977). Indeed, this notion is basic to models of rational decision making, in which people intellectually think about the advantages and disadvantages, obstacles and facilitators, barriers and benefits, or pros and cons, of engaging in a particular action.

Behavior-Change Strategies for At-Risk Populations

Why Focus on High-Risk Populations?

From a public health perspective, it may be prudent to focus on high-risk populations and especially those who are at risk because of their health behaviors. There are limited resources to encourage and support risk reduction efforts, and focusing those resources (time, money, programs) on those at high risk may be more efficient. People have variable levels of need as defined by the chances that they will get sick or die prematurely, and it makes sense to concentrate efforts on those with greatest need. Intervention strategies may have a larger effect on people who are at risk, and further, the risk (and association perceptions of risk) may increase the salience of the issue and the motivation to change.

Health Risk Communication

A decision to focus behavioral interventions on high-risk populations must be accompanied by an understanding of how best to reach and communicate with these vulnerable populations. Principles of effective health and risk communication should guide the development of strategies and materials for behavior change among at-risk populations. Two key issues to focus on are (1) determining how to reach the desired audience, and (2) specific 'message' considerations for at-risk populations.

There are two primary options for reaching an at-risk population: through targeting (or audience segmentation) or tailoring. Targeting at-risk populations is most effective when there is a channel to effectively reach those populations; that is, there is a preferred medium that is shared among the population. Many demographic variables, such as age, gender, or race/ethnicity, can be predictors both of high-risk behaviors and of channel preferences. For example, adolescents are at greater risk for smoking initiation, and there are various ways to reach this population almost exclusively, such as through teen magazines.

There are also 'psychographic' variables that can be used for targeting at-risk populations. An example of psychographic targeting of these populations is the SENTAR, or sensation-seeking targeting approach (Palmgreen et al., 2001), which has been a successful targeting strategy to reach adolescents at greatest risk for drug use. Researchers found that sensation seeking, or the need for novel, complex, and emotionally intense stimuli, is a personality trait that can predict: (a) adolescents at greatest risk for drug use; and (b) the types of messages that are most appealing to those adolescents. With this information, messages that appeal to at-risk adolescents can be developed and then can be inserted into programming preferred by the high-sensation seekers, thereby ensuring that messages will reach the desired population.

In contrast to targeting, which focuses on delivering the same set of messages to a homogeneous group, tailoring involves delivering messages that are individualized, and based on personal assessments. Tailoring acknowledges that even among a relatively homogeneous at-risk population, there may be differences in the underlying beliefs, values, or norms that are associated with a given health behavior. After identifying these salient beliefs through an initial assessment, a computerized algorithm can be used to create individually tailored materials. Researchers have found that people may pay more attention, process more deeply, and make greater behavioral changes when messages are tailored rather than generic (Kreuter et al., 1999; Skinner et al., 1999). The disadvantage of using a tailored approach is that the messages can only be generated for those who have provided information about themselves – usually by completing a questionnaire – so tailored materials are usually more expensive to produce and typically have a smaller reach than targeted approaches.

When designing messages for at-risk individuals, special attention should be paid to the way that risk is discussed. Dual processing theories (Leventhal, 1971; Witte, 1992) suggest that when individuals are faced with risky or 'threatening' information, they may react in one of two ways: (1) they can become fearful, which can trigger avoidance and denial; or (2) they can become alert to the danger, vigilant, and motivated to do whatever is necessary to alleviate the threat.

Messages that inform people that they have an elevated risk for developing a negative health outcome, or for performing an unhealthy behavior, tend to heighten fear. If that fear is elevated, and people are not also told how they can reduce their risk, then any other messages will likely not be processed. In contrast, if fear is elevated and is coupled with efficacy messages (e.g., there is an effective response to reduce risk, and the individual is able to make the recommended changes), then individuals will be more likely to be motivated to reduce the threat.

Conclusion

Understanding and improving health-related behavior is key to improving public health and individual well-being. Focusing on at-risk populations is one strategy for maximizing public health impact. In general, behavioral interventions will be more effective if they are theoretically based. Communication strategies targeting high-risk individuals should be carefully crafted and properly pretested to ensure that the messages do not trigger denial or avoidance. Whereas policies, laws, and regulations can affect health behaviors, individual beliefs and motivations must also be considered in public health efforts. Behavior change is incremental. Many people who are at greatest risk for negative health outcomes have practiced a lifetime of less than optimal health behaviors of one sort or another. It is unreasonable to expect that significant and lasting changes will occur during a short period of time. Public health programs need to identify and maximize the benefits or advantages of positive change, push or pull participants along the continuum of change, and consider changes in educational programs and environmental supports to help people who have made changes maintain them over the long term.

Citations

Ajzen I (1985) Intention, perceived control, and weight loss: An application of the theory of planned behavior. *Journal of Personality and Social Psychology* 49(3): 843–851.

Ajzen I and Fishbein M (1980) *Understanding Attitudes and Predicting Social Behavior.* Englewood Cliffs, NJ: Prentice-Hall.

Bandura A (1986) *Social Foundations of Thought and Action: A Social Cognitive Theory.* Englewood Cliffs, NJ: Prentice-Hall.

Berkman LF and Kawachi I (2000) *Social Epidemiology.* New York: Oxford University Press.

DiClemente CC, Fairhurst SK, Velasquez MM, Prochaska JO, Velicer WF, and Rossi JS (1991) The process of smoking cessation – an analysis of precontemplation, contemplation, and preparation stages of change. *Journal of Consulting and Clinical Psychology* 59(2): 295–304.

Ezzati M, Lopez AD, Rodgers A, Vander Hoorn S, and Murray CJ (2002) Comparative Risk Assessment Collaborating Group. Selected major risk factors and global regional burden of disease. *Lancet* 360(9343): 1347–1360.

Glanz K and Rimer BK (2005) *Theory at a Glance: A Guide for Health Promotion Practice,* 2nd edn. NIH Publication No. 05–3896. Bethesda, MD: National Cancer Institute. http://www.nci.nih.gov/PDF/481f5d53-63df-41bc-bfaf-5aa48ee1da4d/TAAG3.pdf (accessed August 2007).

Glanz K, Rimer BK, and Lewis FM (2002) *Health Behavior and Health Education: Theory, Research and Practice,* 3rd edn. San Francisco, CA: Jossey-Bass.

Gochman DS (1982) Labels, systems, and motives: Some perspectives on future research. *Health Education Quarterly* 9: 167–174.

House JS and Williams DR (2000) Understanding and reducing socioeconomic and racial/ethnic disparities in health. In: Smedley BD and Syme SL (eds.) *Promoting Health: Intervention Strategies from Social and Behavioral Research*, pp. 81–124. Washington, DC: National Academy Press

Janis I and Mann L (1977) *Decision Making: A Psychological Analysis of Conflict.* New York: Free Press.

Kasl SV and Cobb S (1966a) Health behavior, illness behavior, and sick-role behavior: I. Health and illness behavior. *Archives of Environmental Health* 12: 246–266.

Kasl SV and Cobb S (1966b) Health behavior, illness behavior, and sick-role behavior: II. Sick-role behavior. *Archives of Environmental Health* 12: 531–541.

Kreuter MW, Strecher VJ, and Glassman B (1999) One size does not fit all: The case for tailoring print materials. *Annals of Behavioral Medicine* 21(4): 276–283.

Leventhal H (1971) Fear appeals and persuasion: The differentiation of a motivational construct. *American Journal of Public Health* 61: 1205–1224.

Lewin K (1935) *A Dynamic Theory of Personality.* New York: McGraw Hill.

Mathers CD and Loncar D (2006) Projections of global mortality and burden of disease from 2002 to 2030. *PLoS Medicine* 3(11): 2011–2030, e442.

Mokdad AH, Marks JS, Stroup DF, and Gerberding JL (2004) Actual causes of death in the United States, 2000. *Journal of the American Medical Association (JAMA)* 291: 1239–1245. Correction published in (2005). *Journal of the American Medical Association* 293: 298.

National Center for Health Statistics (NCHS) (2001) *Healthy People 2000: Final Review.* DHHS Publication No. 01–0256. Hyattsville, MD: Public Health Service.

Palmgreen P, Donohew L, Lorch EP, Hoyle RH, and Stephenson MT (2001) Television campaigns and adolescent marijuana use: Tests of sensation seeking targeting. *American Journal of Public Health* 91(2): 292–296.

Prochaska JO, DiClemente CC, and Norcross JC (1992) In search of how people change: Applications to addictive behaviors. *American Psychologist* 47: 1102–1114.

Rosenstock IM (1974) Historical origins of the Health Belief Model. *Health Education Monographs* 2: 328–335.

Sallis JF and Owen N (2002) Ecological models of behavior. In: Glanz K, Rimer BK, and Lewis FM (eds.) *Health Education and Health Behavior: Theory, Research and Practice.* 3rd edn. pp. 462–484. San Francisco, CA: Jossey-Bass.

Skinner CS, Campbell MK, Rimer BK, Curry S, and Prochaska JO (1999) How effective is tailored print communication? *Annals of Behavioral Medicine* 21(4): 290–298.

Weinstein ND (1993) Testing four competing theories of health-protective behavior. *Health Psychology* 12: 324–333.

Witte K (1992) Putting the fear back into fear appeals: The extended parallel process model. *Communication Monographs* 59(4): 329–349.

Further Reading

Committee on Communication for Behavior Change in the 21st Century (2002) Speaking of health: Assessing health communication strategies for diverse populations. Washington, DC: Institute of Medicine.

Kreuter MW, Farrell D, Olevitch L, and Brennan L (2000) *Tailoring Health Messages: Customizing Communication with Computer Technology.* Mahwah, NJ: Lawrence Erlbaum.

Relevant Websites

http://www.josseybass.com/WileyCDA/WileyTitle/producted–078796149.html – Health Behavior and Health Education: Theory, Research, and Practice, 4th Edition.

http://www.1000.nih.gov/behaviorchange/overview.htm – Innovative Approches to Disease Prevention through Behavior Change.

http://www.cancercontrol.cancer.gov/brp/constructs – National Cancer Institute.

Illicit Drug Use and the Burden of Disease

W Hall, University of Queensland, Herston, Australia

L Degenhardt and N Sindicich, University of New South Wales, Sydney, Australia

Introduction

Illicit drugs are those whose nonmedical use is prohibited by international law, namely: amfetamine-type stimulants (ATS), one of a class of sympathomimetic amines with powerful stimulant action on the central nervous system (CNS); cannabis, a generic term for psychoactive preparations (e.g., marijuana, hashish, and hash oil) derived from the *cannabis sativa* plant; cocaine, an alkaloid CNS stimulant drug that is derived from the coca plant; heroin, an opioid drug derived from the opium poppy; other opioids, derivatives from the opium poppy, and their synthetic analogues, which act on the opioid receptors in the brain (they have the capacity to relieve pain and produce a sense of euphoria, as well as cause stupor, coma, and respiratory depression); and ecstasy (3,4 methylene-dioxymethamfetamine, or MDMA), a synthetic drug that is used as a stimulant.

This article focuses on the burden of disease (BOD) attributable to the use of cannabis, amfetamines, cocaine, and opioids. Other substances that are illegal in most countries, such as MDMA and solvents, are not included because there is insufficient research to quantify their health risks.

Global Prevalence of Illicit Drug Use

The first challenge in quantifying the burden of disease attributable to illicit drugs is estimating the prevalence of their use. The illegality of illicit drug use makes this difficult to quantify because illicit drug users are 'hidden' and are thus difficult to identify, and even when they can be located and interviewed, they may attempt to conceal their drug use.

The United Nations Drug Control Programme (UNDCP) provides a convenient tabulation of the most recent estimates of the global prevalence of illicit drug use (**Table 1**). The quality of the data collected and reported by the UNDCP varies across countries and regions from high-quality national survey data to key informant and indicator data of uncertain validity. The prevalence estimates for each type of illicit drug cannot be added together because many individuals use more than one.

Cannabis is the most widely used illicit drug with 162.4 million persons over the age of 15 estimated to have used cannabis in the past year during the early 2000s. Patterns of cannabis use have been most extensively studied in the United States, Canada, Australia, and Europe. Europe generally has lower rates of use than Australia, Canada, and the United States. The limited data from developing countries suggest that with exceptions (e.g., Jamaica, South Africa) rates of cannabis use are much lower in Africa, Asia, and South America than in Europe and English-speaking countries.

The ATS are the next most widely used illicit drugs, with 24.9 million people estimated to have used these drugs globally in 2006. The highest rates of per capita use were in Oceania, North America, and Europe.

Table 1   Annual prevalence (%) of illicit drug use among 15–64-year-olds (UNODC-World Drug Report 2006)

Region	Opioids	No. of opioid users	Cocaine	No. of cocaine users	ATS[b]	No. of ATS users	Cannabis	No. of cannabis users
Europe	0.7	4 030 000	0.7	3 524 000	0.5	2 700 000	5.6	30 800 000
West & Central Europe	0.5	1 565 000	1.1	3 333 000	0.7	2 185 000	7.4	23 400 000
South-East Europe	0.2	180 000	0.1	64 000	0.2	180 000	2.3	1 900 000
Eastern Europe	1.6	2 285 000	0.1	127 000	0.2	335 000	3.8	5 500 000
Americas	0.4	2 280 000	1.5	8 440 000	0.8	4 320 000	6.4	36 700 000
North America	0.5	1 300 000	2.3	6 459 000	1.1	3 190 000	10.3	29 400 000
South America	0.3	980 000	0.7	1 981 000	0.4	1 130 000	2.6	7 300 000
Asia	0.3	8 530 000	0.1	260 000	0.6	15 250 000	2.1	52 100 000
Oceania[a]	0.4	890 000	0.9	175 000	3.0	610 000	15.3	3 200 000
Africa	0.2	910 000	0.2	959 000	0.4	2 000 000	8.1	39 600 000
Global	0.4	15 840 000	0.3	13 358 000	0.6	24 880 000	3.9	162 400 000

[a]Refers to Australia and New Zealand and the islands that comprise Polynesia, Melanesia, and Micronesia.
[b]Amfetamine-type stimulants.

The illicit opioids were the third most common form of illicit drug use. Globally, illicit opioids were estimated to have been used by 15.8 million people. The highest rates of opioid use appear to be in the developed world, where estimates of use in the past year are around 0.4–0.5% of adults aged 15 or more.

Cocaine was the least widely used of the major illicit drugs, with its global use declining from third place in 1997. A total of 13.3 million adults were estimated to have used cocaine globally in 2006. The highest prevalence of use was in the United States, with lower reported rates of use in other developed societies (see **Table 1**).

Defining Problem Illicit Drug Use

We follow the *International Classification of Diseases* (ICD-10) in distinguishing between 'harmful drug use' and 'drug dependence.' Harmful drug use is defined by evidence of substance-related physical (e.g., organ damage) and psychological harm (e.g., drug-induced psychosis). In the ICD-10 drug dependence requires the presence of three or more of the following indicators: a strong desire to take the substance; impaired control over its use; a withdrawal syndrome on ceasing or reducing use; tolerance to the effects of the drug; requiring larger doses to achieve the desired psychological effect; a disproportionate amount of the user's time is spent obtaining, using, and recovering from drug use; and the user continues to take drugs despite associated problems. These problems should have occurred at some time during the previous year for at least a month.

There are no widely accepted gold standard methods for producing credible estimates of the number of people who make up the hidden population of problem drug users. The preferred strategy is to look for convergence in estimates produced by a variety of different methods of direct and indirect estimation. Direct estimation methods attempt to estimate the number of illicit drug users in representative samples of the population by way of surveys. Indirect estimation methods use information from known populations of illicit drug users (such as those who have died of opioid overdoses or have been treated) to estimate the size of the total hidden population of illicit drug users.

Adverse Health Effects of Illicit Drug Use

Cannabis

Effects on mortality

A Swedish study of mortality over 15 years among male military conscripts found an increased risk of premature death from violence and accidents among men who had smoked cannabis 50 or more times by age 18. However, the association between mortality and cannabis use disappeared after statistical adjustment for alcohol and other drug use. Sidney *et al.* (1997) reported a 10-year study of mortality in cannabis users among 65 171 members of the Kaiser Permanente medical care program aged between 15 and 49. The sample comprised 38% who had never used cannabis, 20% who had used less than six times, 20% who were former users, and 22% who were current cannabis users. Regular cannabis use had a small association with premature mortality that was explained by increased AIDS deaths in men, probably because cannabis use was a correlate of male homosexual behavior in this cohort.

Cannabis produces dose-related impairments in cognitive and behavioral functions that may potentially impair driving an automobile or operating machinery. The effects of recreational doses of cannabis on driving performance in laboratory simulators and standardized driving courses have been reported as similar to blood alcohol concentrations between 0.07% and 0.10%. However, studies of the effects of cannabis on driving under more realistic conditions on roads have found much more modest impairments. Epidemiological studies of motor vehicle accidents have produced equivocal results because most drivers who have cannabinoids in their blood also have high blood alcohol levels.

Morbidity

A cannabis dependence syndrome occurs in heavy chronic users of cannabis. Regular cannabis users develop tolerance to THC, some experience withdrawal symptoms on cessation of use, and some report problems controlling their cannabis use. The risk of dependence is about one in ten among those who ever use the drug.

Cognitive effects: Long-term daily cannabis use does not severely impair cognitive function but it may more subtly impair memory, attention, and the integration of complex information. It remains unclear whether these effects are due to the cumulative effect of regular cannabis use on cannabinoid receptors in the brain or are the residual effects of THC that will disappear after an extended period of abstinence.

Psychotic disorders: There is now reasonable evidence that chronic cannabis use may precipitate a psychosis in vulnerable individuals.

The gateway hypothesis: Among adolescents in developed societies alcohol and tobacco have typically been used before cannabis, which in turn, has been used before hallucinogens, amfetamine, heroin, and cocaine. Generally, the earlier the age of first use, and the greater the involvement with cannabis, the more likely a young person is to use other illicit drugs. The role played by cannabis in this sequence remains controversial. The hypothesis that cannabis use has a pharmacological effect that increases the risk of using other illicit drugs is not strongly supported. More plausible hypotheses are that the relationship is explained by a combination of: (1) early recruitment into cannabis use of nonconforming adolescents who are more likely to use other illicit drugs; (2) a shared genetic vulnerability to dependence on cannabis and other illicit drugs; and (3) socialization of cannabis users within a drug-using subculture that increases the opportunity and encourages the use of other illicit drugs.

Adolescent psychosocial outcomes: Cannabis use is associated with failure to complete high school, early family formation, poor mental health, and involvement in drug-related crime. In the case of each of these outcomes the strong associations in cross-sectional data are more modest when one takes into account that cannabis users often

show characteristics before they use cannabis that predict these outcomes, for example, have lower academic aspirations and poorer school performance than peers who do not use.

Amfetamine-Type Stimulants

Amfetamine users who inject the drug are at high risk of blood-borne infections through needle sharing. Amfetamine users are as likely as opioid users to share injection equipment. Primary amfetamine users are also a sexually active group, small proportions of whom engage in paid sex to support drug use.

High-dose amfetamine use, especially by injection, can result in a schizophreniform paranoid psychosis, associated with loosening of associations, delusions, and hallucinations. The psychosis could be reproduced by the injection of large doses in addicts and by the repeated administration of large doses to normal volunteers. High proportions of regular amfetamine users report symptoms such as anxiety, panic attacks, paranoia, and depression. The emergence of such symptoms is associated with injecting the drugs, greater frequency of use, and dependence on amfetamines.

In high doses, amfetamines can be lethal but the risk is low compared to the risks of overdose from heroin. Amfetamine-related deaths are due to the effects of amfetamines on the cardiovascular system, for example, cardiac failure and cerebral vascular accidents. Amfetamines appear to be neurotoxic with animal studies indicating that heavy amfetamine use results in dopaminergic depletion. More recently, deficits in performance on neuropsychological tests have been demonstrated in human users.

Illicit Opioids

Mortality

Four main causes of premature death are elevated in illicit opioid users compared with peers who do not use these drugs: drug overdose, HIV/AIDS, suicide, and trauma. In the ICD-10, drug overdose refers to deaths caused by: (a) accidental or intentional fatal poisoning caused by specific drugs, and (b) poisoning deaths among dependent drug users that are attributed to drug dependence. Despite the conceptual simplicity of drug overdose deaths it has been difficult to precisely quantify the number of such deaths in developed countries with well-developed vital statistics. The connection between illicit opioid use and HIV/AIDS arises from injectors sharing contaminated injecting equipment.

Illicit opioid users report high rates of suicide attempts and show elevated rates of suicide mortality. These deaths are probably underreported because cultural variations in attitudes toward suicide may influence coroners' and mortality registrars' willingness to classify deaths among young adults as intentional.

Rates of death from motor vehicle accidents, other forms of accidental death, and homicide have all been found to be elevated in cohort studies of illicit opioid users. It is likely that these causes of death are underestimated among illicit opioid users because they may not be recognized as drug-related.

Morbidity

Each of the major causes of premature mortality in illicit opioid users (overdose, HIV, attempted suicide, and accidents) causes substantial morbidity. So too does chronic infection with hepatitis B (HBV) and hepatitis C (HCV) viruses. Opioid-dependent persons have a high prevalence of major depression and anxiety disorders. It is unclear what proportion of these disorders preceded and contributed to the development of problem drug use or vice versa. Nor is it clear to what extent preexisting psychiatric disorders have been exacerbated by problem illicit drug use.

Cocaine

Regular cocaine users who inject cocaine or smoke crack cocaine are likely to develop dependence and problems related to their cocaine use. In the United States it has been estimated that one in six cocaine users becomes dependent on the drug. High rates of cocaine dependence are found among persons treated for alcohol and drug problems and among arrestees in the United States.

In large doses cocaine is cardiotoxic in cocaine-naïve and -tolerant individuals. The vasoconstrictor effects of cocaine in large doses place great strain on the cardiovascular system that can cause fatal cardiac arrests, cerebral vascular accidents, seizures, and hyperthermia in healthy young adults.

In the United States, regular cocaine users report high rates of anxiety and affective disorders. The repeated use of large doses of cocaine can also produce a paranoid psychosis. Persons who are acutely intoxicated by cocaine can become violent, especially those who develop a paranoid psychosis. Animal studies suggest that cocaine use may be neurotoxic in large doses but it is unclear whether it is also neurotoxic in humans.

Cocaine injecting, either on its own or in combination with heroin (known as speedballs), is associated with more frequent injection, needle sharing, increased sexual risk-taking, and HIV infection. An association between cocaine use and HIV risk-taking has been reported in Europe, Australia, and the United States. Crack cocaine smoking has also been linked to higher levels of needle risk, sexual risk-taking, and HIV infection. Two mechanisms probably underlie the relationship between cocaine use and HIV infection. First, the short half-life of cocaine promotes a much higher frequency of injecting than that seen in heroin injectors. Second, cocaine itself disinhibits and stimulates users, encouraging them to take greater risks with sexual activity and needle use.

Quantifying Mortality and Morbidity Attributable to Illicit Drug Use

The best evidence that illicit drug use is a cause of premature death comes from cohort studies of illicit drug users (for a detailed review, see Degenhardt et al., 2004). The available cohort studies have a number of major limitations; we consider the following four.

First, the majority of cohort studies of illicit drug users have included people seeking treatment for problem drug use. A small number of studies have compared mortality of drug users while in and out of treatment (Degenhardt et al., 2004).

Second, injecting opioid users are overrepresented in these cohort studies by comparison with cocaine, other stimulant, and cannabis users. The few studies that report mortality in problem illicit opioid and stimulant use suggest that it is higher among opioid users because of the higher rate of fatal overdose. Stimulant users appear to have higher rates of blood-borne virus infections such as HBV and HCV from sharing injection equipment and exchanging sex for drugs.

Third, the cohort studies have predominantly been done in developed countries. Extrapolating from these to drug users in developing countries is problematic because the latter generally have all-cause mortality rates that are significantly higher than the developed countries.

Fourth, the majority of the cohort studies were conducted before the HIV/AIDS epidemic began to affect mortality among injecting drug users. There have been changes in the epidemiology of HIV and other drug-related conditions since these studies were conducted, which reduces their value in predicting contemporary illicit drug-related mortality.

Despite these limitations, the cohort studies have identified causes of mortality that are more prevalent among problem illicit drug users than their age peers. There are good reasons for believing that the relationships are causal for deaths caused by drug overdose and blood-borne virus infection. Opioids cause respiratory depression that can cause death, especially when used in combination with other CNS depressants such as alcohol and benzodiazepines. Cocaine and amfetamines can cause fatal cardiac arrhythmias and strokes that are very rare causes of death in young adults who do not use these drugs. The viruses that cause HIV/AIDS, and HBV and HCV infections, are efficiently spread by contaminated blood in shared injection equipment.

The case for illicit drug use being a contributory cause of suicide is indirect. Depression is a risk factor for suicide and it occurs at higher rates among illicit drug users. Alcohol and opioids use and dependence have been shown in case-control and prospective studies to increase suicide risk in persons with depression. Opioid-dependent persons in treatment also report very high rates of attempted suicide.

The case for a causal connection between illicit drug use and trauma deaths is also indirect. Driving while intoxicated by alcohol is a well-known risk factor for fatal motor vehicle crashes and heavy alcohol use is common among illicit drug users. Opioids are also intoxicating substances that adversely affect driving, although they are less commonly found in persons killed in fatal car crashes.

Estimates of the Global Burden of Disease Attributable to Illicit Drug Use

The global burden of death and disability attributable to illicit drugs was first estimated by Donoghoe as part of the Global Burden of Disease project. Donoghoe (Murray and Lopez, 1997) estimated that illicit drug use was responsible for 100 000 deaths globally in 1990; 62% of these deaths occurred in developing countries. Donoghoe's estimate was based on the attributable fractions of various causes of mortality and morbidity attributable to illicit drug use.

Murray and Lopez (1997) estimated the contribution that illicit drugs made to the global burden of disease (GBD) by combining Donoghoe's mortality estimate with an estimate of disability attributable to illicit drug dependence. The burden of disease was assessed by the number of disability-adjusted life years (DALYs) accounted for by each risk factor. This was the sum of years of life lost from premature mortality due to the risk factor and the number of years lived with disability (adjusted for the severity of the disability). The contribution that illicit drug use made to global burden of disease was assessed along with tobacco and alcohol and a list of other risk factors.

Comparative estimates of contributions made by alcohol, tobacco, and illicit drugs to the GBD are shown in **Table 2** for established market economies (EME), formerly socialist economies (FSE), China (CHN), Latin America and the Caribbean (LAC), other Asia and Islands (OAI), Middle Eastern crescent (MEC), India (IND), and sub-Saharan Africa (SSA). Overall, 0.5% of GBD in 1990 was attributed to illicit drug use compared with 2.6% for tobacco and 3.5% for alcohol. Illicit drug use accounted for nearly 20% of the disease burden of tobacco even though this legal drug was used by a much larger proportion of the world's population. The contribution of illicit drugs to GBD was higher for males in all regions and highest in developed countries (1.5%), as were the contributions of tobacco (12.1%) and alcohol (9.6%).

Degenhardt and colleagues (2004) updated Donoghoe's estimates for illicit drug use in 2000 in the Comparative Risk Assessment project. This project updated and improved on the Murray and Lopez (1997) estimates

Table 2   Percentage of DALYs attributable to tobacco, alcohol and illicit drugs in various global regions in 1990

Subregion	Tobacco	Alcohol	Illicit drugs
EME	11.7	10.3	2.3
FSE	12.5	8.3	1.3
IND	0.6	1.6	0.1
CHN	3.9	2.3	0.3
OAI	1.5	2.8	0.4
SSA	0.4	2.6	0.2
LAC	1.4	9.7	1.6
MEC	1.2	0.4	0.7
Developed	12.1	9.6	1.9
Developing	1.4	2.7	0.4
World	2.6	3.5	0.6

Source: Murray CJL and Lopez AD (1997) Global mortality, disability, and the contribution of risk factors: Global Burden of Disease study. *The Lancet* 349: 1436–1442.

of GBD that was attributable to alcohol, tobacco, illicit drugs, and many of the same risk factors assessed in 1990. Illicit drug use was defined as the use by injection or the long duration use of amfetamines, cocaine, or opioids. UNDCP data were used to estimate the prevalence of use of these illicit drugs in different world regions. Data from the United States and Australia were used to estimate the proportion of people that had used these drugs in the past year who were problem users. Cohort studies of mortality in illicit drug users provided estimates of the annual mortality among illicit drug users that could be attributed to AIDS, overdose, suicide, and trauma. Degenhardt *et al.* (2004) also used an estimate of overall excess mortality among illicit drug users (SMR) that was derived from all causes of death in the cohort studies.

Degenhardt *et al.* (2004) used direct methods to estimate the number of deaths attributed to illicit drug use in each country by applying attributable fractions to each of the relevant ICD-classified causes of death in national mortality statistics. They also used indirect methods to estimate the excess mortality attributable to problem illicit drug use by using overall mortality risk among illicit drug users and the estimated prevalence of problem illicit drug use in each population.

A major difficulty in applying the direct method was the poor quality of mortality data in many countries. This was exemplified by deaths by overdose, the only cause of death wholly attributable to illicit drug use. Overdose deaths should be the most easily quantified but major difficulties have been identified in many developed countries in assigning deaths to this cause.

Degenhardt *et al.* (2004) estimated that the median number of global deaths attributable to illicit drugs in 2000 produced by summing the deaths due to overdose, AIDS, trauma, and suicide was 240 483. The median estimate obtained by applying the all-cause mortality to the estimated prevalence of illicit drug use was 197 383.

Table 3   Median estimates of mortality attributable to illicit drug use in 14 WHO subregions (Degenhardt et al., 2004)

Subregion	AIDS	Opioid overdose	Suicide	Trauma
AFR-D	4 003	1 891	1 191	2 768
AFR-E	1 334	407	64	922
AMR-A	10 698	6 397	2 034	4 057
AMR-B	5 349	1 845	922	2 342
AMR-D	1 035	498	78	716
EMR B	962	3 881	673	813
EMR D	4 273	12 852	2 015	2 954
EUR-A	6 236	5 527	2 355	3 387
EUR-B	733	1 281	1 465	651
EUR-C	773	6 895	4 156	830
SEAR-B	1 586	955	576	797
SEAR-D	57 011	22 989	14 982	3 128
WPR-A	1 310	825	1 251	1 028
WPR-B	10 122	2 909	456	9 295
Total (median)	105 425	69 152	32 216	33 689

AFR-D, Africa D; AFR-E, Africa E; AMR-A, Americas A; AMR-B, Americas B; AMR-D, Americas D; EMR-B, Eastern Mediterranean B; EMR-D, Eastern Mediterranean D; EUR-A, Europe A; EUR-B, Europe B; EUR-C, Europe C; SEAR-B, South East Asia B; SEAR-D, South East Asia D; WPR-A, Western Pacific A; WPR-B, Western Pacific B
A: very low child and very low adult mortality
B: low child and low adult mortality
C: low child and high adult mortality
D: high child and high adult mortality
E: very high child and very high adult mortality

Both estimates had wide uncertainty intervals around them. The estimated numbers of deaths for each method also varied between subregions, reflecting considerable uncertainty about the prevalence of drug use and the poor quality of mortality data in many developing countries (**Tables 3** and **4**).

Degenhardt et al.'s (2004) estimates nonetheless suggested that illicit drug use was a significant global cause of premature mortality among young adults. As they stressed, they probably underestimated the total disease burden attributable to illicit drugs because of: (a) a lack of data on mortality attributable to the use of cannabis and newer synthetic ATS stimulants; (b) differences between World Health Organization (WHO) subregions in the quality of mortality data; and (c) an absence of data on mortality attributable to HBV and HCV and violence.

The estimated contribution of illicit drug use to GBD was higher in 2000 than in 1990 (0.8% vs. 0.5%). This was largely because the estimated number of deaths attributed to illicit drug use in 2000 was approximately twice that estimated by Donoghoe in 1990. Comparison of the contributions of tobacco, alcohol, and illicit drug use to GBD in various world regions produced similar results to the 1990 comparison. The contribution of illicit drugs to GBD was less than tobacco and alcohol but disproportionately high when compared to its much lower prevalence of use than the legal drugs. All drugs

Table 4   Estimates of total mortality attributed to illicit drug use in 14 subregions (using the sum of four main causes, and estimates of all-cause mortality) (Degenhardt et al., 2004)

Subregion	Population (000s) >15 years	Sum of four causes of mortality[a]	Population mortality rate (per 1000)	All-cause mortality[b]	Population mortality rate (per 1000)
AFR-D	159 577	9 853	0.06	19 046	0.12
AFR-E	190 152	2 727	0.01	8 286	0.04
AMR-A	255 420	23 186	0.09	40 356	0.16
AMR-B	297 625	10 458	0.04	18 425	0.06
AMR-D	44 658	2 327	0.05	2 522	0.06
EMR-B	86 853	6 329	0.07	5 012	0.06
EMR-D	204 039	22 094	0.11	10 411	0.05
EUR-A	339 446	17 505	0.05	16 453	0.05
EUR-B	161 213	4 130	0.03	5 794	0.04
EUR-C	152 432	12 654	0.08	10 709	0.07
SEAR-B	206 870	3 914	0.02	5 688	0.03
SEAR-D	818 521	98 110	0.12	11 024	0.01
WPR-A	129 888	4 414	0.03	9 916	0.08
WPR-B	1 131 503	22 782	0.02	33 741	0.03
Global	4 178 197	240 483	0.06	197 383	0.05

[a]Sum of the median estimates of the following four causes: AIDS, opioid overdose, suicide via opioids, and trauma.
[b]Median estimates of all-cause mortality derived from SMR analyses and pooled CMRs.
AFR-D, Africa D; AFR-E, Africa E; AMR-A, Americas A; AMR-B, Americas B; AMR-D, Americas D; EMR-B, Eastern Mediterranean B; EMR-D, Eastern Mediterranean D; EUR-A, Europe A; EUR-B, Europe B; EUR-C, Europe C; SEAR-B, South East Asia B; SEAR-D, South East Asia D; WPR-A, Western Pacific A; WPR-B, Western Pacific B
A: very low child and very low adult mortality
B: low child and low adult mortality
C: low child and high adult mortality
D: high child and high adult mortality
E: very high child and very high adult mortality

Table 5   Percentage contribution to burden of disease for tobacco, alcohol, and illicit drugs in selected world regions 2000

Subregion	Tobacco		Alcohol		Illicit drugs	
	Males	Females	Males	Females	Males	Females
High-mortality developing countries AFR-D, AFR-E, AMR-D, EMR-D, SEAR-D	3.4	0.6	2.6	0.5	0.8	0.2
Low-mortality developing regions – emerging economies AMR-B, EMR-B, SEAR-B, WPR-B	6.2	1.3	9.8	2.0	1.2	0.3
Developed regions AMR-A, EUR-A, EUR-B, EUR-C, WPR-A	17.1	6.3	14.0	3.3	2.3	1.2
World	6.3	5402	6.5	1477	1.1	0.4

Source: Rehm J, Taylor B, and Room R (2006) Global burden of disease from alcohol, illicit drugs and tobacco. *Drug and Alcohol Review* 25: 503–513.
AFR-D, Africa D; AFR-E, Africa E; AMR-A, Americas A; AMR-B, Americas B; AMR-D, Americas D; EMR-B, Eastern Mediterranean B; EMR-D, Eastern Mediterranean D; EUR-A, Europe A; EUR-B, Europe B; EUR-C, Europe C; SEAR-B, South East Asia B; SEAR-D, South East Asia D; WPR-A, Western Pacific A; WPR-B, Western Pacific B
A: very low child and very low adult mortality
B: low child and low adult mortality
C: low child and high adult mortality
D: high child and high adult mortality
E: very high child and very high adult mortality

made a larger contribution in disease burden in men than in women in all regions and their contribution to GBD was largest in developed regions (**Table 5**).

Australian Studies of the Burden of Disease Attributable to Illicit Drugs

Two studies have been conducted in Australia of the major determinants of disease burden using similar methods to those of the GBD. Mathers *et al.* (2000) estimated the contribution that tobacco, alcohol, and illicit drugs (primarily heroin use) made to the burden of disease in Australia in 1996. The results were broadly consistent with those of the original GBD estimate and the 2000 update in that tobacco use accounted for the largest proportion of disease burden (**Table 6**). Alcohol and illicit drugs contributed similarly to disease burden because the authors included an estimate of the benefits of moderate alcohol consumption which offset some of the harm that its use caused (Mathers *et al.*, 2000).

Begg *et al.* (2007) estimated the major contributors to burden of disease in Australia in 2003 using updated methods and mortality data. Their results (**Table 7**) indicated that the contribution of illicit drug use to BOD in Australia had doubled between 1996 and 2003. This increase was partly due to a heroin epidemic in Australia in the mid to late 1990s that produced a steep increase in overdose deaths. It also increased because of the inclusion of higher morbidity estimates for each drug type. The latter were derived by applying disability weights to estimates of the population prevalence of different types of illicit drug dependence obtained in the National Survey of Mental Health and Well-Being conducted in 1997. The

Table 6   Contribution of tobacco, alcohol, and illicit drugs to burden of disease in Australia in 1996

Drug	Males	Females	Persons
Tobacco	12.1	6.8	9.7
Alcohol (net)	4.2	−0.1	2.1
Illicit drugs	2.2	1.3	0.9

Source: Mathers CD, Vos ET, Stevenson CE (1999) *The Burden of Disease and Injury in Australia.* Canberra, Australia: Australian Institute of Health and Welfare.

Table 7   Contribution of tobacco, alcohol, and illicit drugs to burden of disease in Australia in 2003

Drug	Males	Females	Persons
Tobacco	9.6	5.8	7.7
Alcohol (net)	3.8	0.07	2.3
Illicit drugs	2.6	1.2	2.0

Source: Begg S, Vos T, Barker B, et al. (2007) *The Burden of Disease and Injury in Australia 2003.* Canberra: Australian Institute of Health and Welfare. http://www.aihw.gov.au/publications/hwe/bodaiia03/bodaiia03.pdf (accessed October 2007).

burden attributable to tobacco use declined between 1996 and 2003 in line with a decline in the population prevalence of tobacco smoking since 1996. The contribution of alcohol changed marginally, despite different methods of estimating its health benefits.

Research Priorities

The quantification of disease burden attributable to illicit drug use is in its infancy even in developed countries with good mortality and morbidity data collection systems. The following are research priorities to improve the quality of future estimates.

First, we need better estimates of the prevalence of problem illicit drug use in developed and developing countries. Second, in developed countries we need cohort studies of injecting and other problem illicit drug users who are *not* in treatment. Third, we need better studies of morbidity in illicit drug users attributable to nonfatal overdoses, HBV and HCV, suicide attempts, and trauma in developed and developing countries. Fourth, we need better-designed prospective studies of mortality and morbidity among more representative samples of problem illicit drug users in developing countries, especially those with high rates of injecting drug users (IDU) and high rates of HIV/AIDS infection.

Conclusions

Notwithstanding the limitations of existing methods of estimation, illicit drug use makes a substantial contribution to GBD that is disproportionate to the low prevalence of this form of drug use.

The contribution to disease burden is clearest for illicit opioid injecting in developed countries where it produces a high rate of premature mortality from drug overdose, trauma, and suicide, and in some settings, HIV/AIDS.

Illicit use of ATS stimulants and cocaine probably also contributes to increased disease burden by way of increased mortality from overdose and HIV/AIDS. The contributions of these types of illicit drug use have been less extensively studied even in developed countries with high rates of use.

Cannabis is probably not a major contributor to premature mortality apart possibly from some deaths from motor vehicle accidents and suicide. Its contribution to morbidity has probably been underestimated because of a lack of population estimates of cannabis dependence and uncertainty about the contributions of cannabis use to psychosis, poor mental health, and poor psychosocial outcomes in adolescence.

Existing estimates almost certainly underestimate the contribution of illicit drug use to burden of disease for a number of reasons. First, the coverage of illicit drug types has been limited. Second, considerable uncertainty remains about the contribution that different types of illicit drug use make to premature mortality. Third, there is a dearth of data on the contribution that all illicit drug use makes to morbidity.

See also: Control and Regulation of Currently Illegal Drugs; Illicit Drug Trends Globally.

Citations

Begg S, Vos T, Barker B, *et al.* (2007) *The burden of disease and injury in Australia 2003.* Canberra: Australian Institute of Health and Welfare. http://www.aihw.gov.au/publications/hwe/bodaiia03/bodaiia03.pdf (accessed October 2007).

Degenhardt LD, Hall WD, Warner-Smith M, *et al.* (2004) Illicit drug use. In: Ezzati M, Lopez AD, Rodgers A, *et al.* (eds.) *Comparative Quantification of Health Risks: Global and Regional Burden of Disease Attributable to Selected Major Risk Factors* vol. 1, pp. 1109–1176. Geneva, Switzerland: World Health Organization.

Mathers CD, Vos ET, Stevenson CE (1999) *The Burden of Disease and Injury in Australia.* Canberra, Australia: Australian Institute of Health and Welfare.

Mathers CD, Vos ET, Stevenson CE, *et al.* (2000) The Australian Burden of Disease study: Measuring the loss of health from diseases, injuries and risk factors. *Medical Journal of Australia* 172: 592–596.

Murray CJL and Lopez AD (1997) Global mortality, disability, and the contribution of risk factors: Global Burden of Disease study. *The Lancet* 349: 1436–1442.

Rehm J, Taylor B, and Room R (2006) Global burden of disease from alcohol, illicit drugs and tobacco. *Drug and Alcohol Review* 25: 503–513.

Sidney S, Beck JE, Tekawa IS, *et al.* (1997) Marijuana use and mortality. *American Journal of Public Health* 87: 585–590.

Further Reading

Andreasson S and Allebeck P (1990) Cannabis and mortality among young men: A longitudinal study of Swedish conscripts. *Scandinavian Journal of Social Medicine* 18: 9–15.

Darke S, Degenhardt LD, and Mattick RP (eds.) (2007) *Mortality among Illicit Drug Users: Epidemiology, Causes and Intervention.* Cambridge, UK: Cambridge University Press.

Ezzati M, Lopez AD, Rodgers A, *et al.* (2002) Selected major risk factors and global and regional burden of disease. *The Lancet* 360: 1347–1360.

Hall WD and Pacula RL (2003) *Cannabis Use and Dependence: Public Health and Public Policy.* Cambridge, UK: Cambridge University Press.

Hall WD, Ross JE, Lynskey MT, *et al.* (2000) How many dependent heroin users are there in Australia? *Medical Journal of Australia* 173: 528–531.

MacDonald M, Wodak A, Dolan K, *et al.* (2000) Hepatitis C virus antibody prevalence among injecting drug users at selected needle and syringe programs in Australia, 1995–1997. *Medical Journal of Australia* 172: 57–61.

Macleod J, Oakes R, Copello A, *et al.* (2004) Psychological and social sequelae of cannabis and other illicit drug use by young people: A systematic review of longitudinal, general population studies. *The Lancet* 363: 1579–1588.

Platt JJ (1997) *Cocaine Addiction: Theory, Research, and Treatment.* Cambridge, MA: Harvard University Press.

United Nations Office on Drugs and Crime (2006) *World Drug Report 2006. Volume 2: Statistics.* Vienna: UNODC.

Measurement of Psychiatric and Psychological Disorders and Outcomes in Populations

T S Brugha and H Meltzer, University of Leicester, Leicester, UK

The measurement of mental and behavioral disorders poses three particular challenges. First, there are no laboratory or similar independent confirmatory diagnostic technologies; instead, the nature of these disorders requires the collection of subjective psychological information on inner states of feeling, thinking, and perceiving, together with, sometimes, reliable information on behavior over time. Second, nearly all measures involve a retrospective element that relies on recall, whereas ideally information should be collected prospectively, requiring a more costly longitudinal element. Third, there is the challenge of achieving external or criterion validity.

This article covers the principles of measurement in psychiatric epidemiology, including discussions around international aspects (e.g., cross-population issues, including excluded groups, and issues of culture), measurement of specific disorders, and application of measurement methods in public health contexts (e.g., surveillance and screening in health settings). Enormous progress has been made in developing and applying such methods, including their use in very large-scale international surveys in recent years. Policy and decision makers can now readily access the information they need but must first understand the potential and limitations of current measurement methods.

It is assumed that the reader of this article is already familiar with basic clinical measurement, epidemiological, and public health concepts. This article points selectively to the ways in which such concepts have been developed in relation to measurement and public mental health. In order to illustrate this with the most up-to-date examples, we refer to survey methods used in Great Britain to collect information for policy on children (Green *et al.*, 2005), adults, and older people (Singleton *et al.*, 2001), but we also refer to more widely known, similar methods used elsewhere in relation to studies of the adult population, including high-quality national surveys in low-income countries. Such surveys have generated not only official government and policy reports but also numerous articles in academic journals. The article begins with a discussion of the nature of mental disorder, study design and measurement issues, procedures and techniques, and the interpretation of findings.

Nature of Mental Disorder

For further reading please see Farmer *et al.* (2002).

Psychopathology

Concepts of psychopathology were first described in the clinical literature on severe mental disorders such as psychosis in the nineteenth century (Farmer *et al.*, 2002). Attempts to define these with a view to their reliable measurement developed in the following century (Wing *et al.*, 1974). Soon after this, work was extended to a wide range of mental and behavioral disorders to support the emergence of detailed mental disorder classification systems (World Health Organization Division of Mental Health, 1992; World Health Organization, 1992, 1993; American Psychiatric Association, 1994).

The psychopathology of mental disorders can be considered in terms of specific mental functions. Emotion in the form of mood and anxiety is given prominence in such systems with relatively little attention given to other emotions such as anger or happiness (except in the form of inappropriate elation in mania or bipolar disorder). Abnormalities of the experience and perception of reality in the form of psychotic hallucinations is given prominence, together with beliefs that are clearly false and not shared with another person (in contrast to subculturally approved beliefs). Cognitive impairment as seen in mental retardation (also known as learning disability or as intellectual disability) and dementia also receive prominence. Problems due to misuse of psychoactive drugs and their effects on mental functioning have taken greater prominence in recent years. New areas hardly touched on in surveys include developmental, behavioral, and personality abnormalities.

Definition and Classification of Disorders

Until now the official classification systems (American Psychiatric Association, 1994; World Health Organization Division of Mental Health, 1990) have relied exclusively on binary definitions of disorders (Brugha, 2002): either the person has or does not have the disorder. This has been an enormously important and successful development in helping mental disorders to be considered and included in general health policy debates. However, critics have questioned the large number of categories of mental disorder, most of which would not register in surveys of public mental health in the general population anyway. Furthermore, the underlying nature of common mental disorder is likely to be dimensional without obvious cut points representing a diagnostic threshold (**Figure 1**). Dimensional

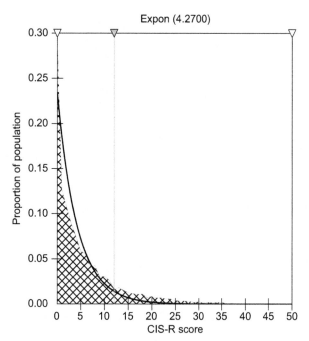

Figure 1   Proportion of population by full range of common mental disorder (CIS-R) scores, and fitted exponential curve. (Goodness of fit (RMS error) test statistic = 0.029E-04.) From Melzer D, Tom B, Brugha T, Fryers T, and Meltzer H (2002) Common mental disorder symptom counts in populations: Are there distinct case groups above epidemiological cutoffs? *Psychological Medicine* 32: 1195–1201.

approaches are, however, promised in future revisions of the classification system. Even within the ICD-10 system, depression is described in terms of levels of severity. Subthreshold levels are likely to be given greater prominence in the future in much the same way that clinical medicine increasingly recognizes the significance of lower levels of blood pressure or of serum lipids in terms of prediction of future morbidity. A stepped-care approach to the management of depression that uses these different levels of severity is already officially recommended in Great Britain by the National Institute for Health and Clinical Excellence. This is important for policymakers to consider because it implies that most (but not all) published prevalence tables for depressive disorder do not take into account such clinically significant distinctions.

Purposes of epidemiological methods (epidemiological estimates, modeling determinants, treatment planning, and needs assessment)

It makes sense that any data collection using epidemiological methods should be preceded by a careful consideration of the purposes for which they will be used. Yet convention often seems to overtake such considerations.

A key question should be whether the purpose is research, audit, or surveillance. Research should aim to

answer a key question and related subsidiary questions and should be designed and planned as such. The purpose of audit is to improve a process or service by examining its functioning against defined objectives and standards; audit should not be carried out without inclusion of a process for correcting flaws in the process or service being audited. Surveillance is similar to audit but is designed to monitor trends in populations over time and to alert decision makers to any changes that require early or urgent action.

A further difficulty may lie in a misunderstanding of the differences between clinical and epidemiological assessment. The measurement of psychiatric disorders in national surveys, which aim to provide population estimates, differs substantially from methods used in judicial and clinical decisions, for example, for benefits, compensation, and need for services. Methods used for assessing individuals, say, for a treatment program, are rarely the same as those required in epidemiology for classifying populations. In the case of the former, detailed and time-consuming assessments by a range of professionals of contexts such as family situations are justified because such methods are sensitive to individual circumstances and produce results that are equitable between individuals. In surveys, provided that the methods used deal adequately with the majority of people and can be done within a relatively short time, it matters little if a small minority have been classified differently than they would had more detailed procedures been used.

Quality of data

Conclusions regarding epidemiological estimates, the modeling of possible determinants, service planning, and needs assessment all require the use of comparisons. Comparisons have little value or legitimacy if the data employed are not collected reliably. The types of measures available are discussed later in this article. Because it is essential that epidemiological methods are reproducible (reliable), comparison may be either too costly or impractical when purely clinical measures are used. However, it is also important in developing either a new measure or in using an existing measure in a population with different language or culture, that it is generally accepted as representing descriptions used in clinical settings. Small-scale comparisons of epidemiological questionnaires and systematic clinical evaluations have been carried out occasionally in general population samples. At first sight the level of agreement between these appears to be poor and likely to be limited by the uncertain consistency with which clinical assessments can be used outside in the general population where most conditions are less severe and more fluctuant over time. It is reassuring therefore that clinical and epidemiological measures, when compared in clinical settings, can show high levels of agreement.

Design Issues

Study designs can be divided into the experimental and nonexperimental; the former are infrequently used in the collection of information on psychiatric and psychological disorders in the general population. New mental health policies are seldom subjected to the rigors of experimental evaluation in the general population, although where feasible this can be particularly informative. One experimental design variant that may be particularly feasible in practice is the cluster randomized evaluation. Examples are beginning to appear in the mental health field in which the cluster is an organizational unit, for example, a primary care practice, a specialist team: existing and new policies can be compared between randomly allocated cluster units (MacArthur et al., 2002). Another example makes use of the classroom or work team unit, which could be used in prevention policy trials. As in any experiment involving human subjects, ethical considerations arise: interventions can have wanted and unwanted effects, and those participating should be informed. Careful consideration should be given to anticipating possible harm and minimizing its likelihood; experiments are only justifiable when there is genuine uncertainty about the outcome.

A detailed discussion of the use of different designs in psychiatric epidemiology can by found in a chapter by Zahner and colleagues (1995). Here we focus selectively on the factors that are sometimes neglected in the design of studies in the general population. Most first-generation mental health surveys were typically small, based in a local community, and carried out by a small academic team. The past two decades have seen the emergence of adequately powered, large sample size surveys using complex, often clustered sampling methods, systematically developed and tested structured instruments, and specialized 'survey' methods of analysis, carried out by collaborations between professional survey organizations and academic researchers, which are referred to in examples that follow.

Cross-sectional Surveys

This article refers mainly to the use of cross-sectional and longitudinal designs. Great attention is paid in such surveys to ensuring the representativeness of subjects so that inferences are generalizable and can be used, for example, at a national level and sometimes in small area statistics. Because we regard this as a fundamental issue, which is often inadequately handled in surveys other than those carried out by large (generic) survey organizations, we give this particular emphasis here.

The approach taken by one of us to the challenge of sampling children nationally illustrates some of the factors that can and need to be considered. Several methods of obtaining a representative sample of children in Great Britain were considered: carrying out a postal sift of the general population to identify households with children, sampling through schools, using administrative databases, and piggybacking on other surveys. It was decided to draw the sample from administrative records, specifically, the Child Benefit Records held by the Child Benefit Centre (CBC). Parents of each child under 16 living in the United Kingdom are entitled to receive child benefits unless the child is under the care of social services. Using these centralized records as a sampling frame was preferred to carrying out a postal sift of over 100 000 addresses or sampling through schools. The postal sift would have been time consuming and expensive. The designers did not want to sample through schools because they wanted the initial contact to be with parents who then would give signed consent to approach the child's teacher. A two-hour survey was regarded as too long for piggybacking on other surveys.

Use of centralized records (see later also) does have some disadvantages; access to the records can be problematic and the frame may not be accurate or comprehensive. It was realized that some child benefit records did not have postal codes attributed to addresses: 10% in a first survey and 5% in the repeat. The Child Benefit Centre had no evidence that records with postal codes were different from those without. The addresses with missing postal codes probably represent a mixture of people who did not know their postal code at the time of applying for child benefits and those who simply forgot to enter the details on the form. If there are other factors which differentiate between households with and without postal-coded addresses, the key question is to what extent these factors are related to the mental health of children. Because these factors are unknown, one does not know what biases may have been introduced into the survey by omitting the addresses without postal codes.

The survey design dealt with the problem of omission of children in the care of social services by carrying out a separate survey of this vulnerable group even though such children represent only 0.5% of the population in England. Previous research had indicated high rates of mental disorders among this group. Also excluded from the original sample were cases in which 'action' was being invoked, such as occur with the death of the child or a change of address. These are administrative actions as distinct from some legal process concerning the child and hence should not bias the sample in any way.

Small-area statistical estimates are population approximations developed by specialized statistical procedures such as spatial interpolation. They allow policymakers, local planners, and individual users of services to extrapolate census and survey data to specific local areas. Very large survey sample sizes may be used in conjunction with census data allowing linkages between different information sources on economics, health, crime, quality of the environment, and so forth. The estimates obtained may be subject to census (or survey) or modeling error. Trend estimates may not be directly comparable from year to year because of changes in boundaries, data, and methodology. Estimates can be improved by the use of spatially more precise, geographically coded, building identifiers. Alternatively postal code data or an equivalent coding system are essential but will not be available in all parts of the world.

Screening and full assessment

Although in the children survey example all respondents were administered the same set of questions, many surveys employed two-stage or multiphase survey designs. The first stage consists of a self-report questionnaire administered to the full sample by lay interviewers who do not need to have any clinical training. In a second stage, a randomly selected subsample will undergo a more complex and detailed assessment, possibly involving some degree of clinical expertise. The second phase might involve a full clinical assessment of one or more forms of mental disorder, analogous to a second stage of a population dietary survey in which a random subsample of first-stage respondents undergoes a more detailed inventory of all food kept in a household, and of food purchases within a past number of days, which may be carried out by a smaller team of research dieticians.

There are considerable advantages and also disadvantages to both the single and two-phase designs; these are well discussed in the literature (Newman *et al.*, 1990; Shrout and Newman, 1989). The advantages of the single stage approach are as follows:

- Detailed information is collected on all respondents. A sample distribution can be produced on all subscales even though only those with an above-threshold score will have psychopathology.
- With the possibility of a longitudinal element in the survey, there is a large pool of respondents from which to select controls who could be matched on several characteristics to the children who exhibit significant psychiatric symptoms during the first-stage interview.
- A one-phase design is likely to increase the overall response rate compared with a two-phase (screening plus clinical assessment) design.
- A one-stage design reduces the burden put on respondents. Ideally, a two-phase design would require a screening questionnaire to be followed up with an assessment interview administered to the selected respondent. A one-stage design only requires one interview.

One of the advantages of a one-phase over a two-phase design is that it can be carried out in a far shorter time scale.

The main disadvantage of a one-stage design is cost. The administration is far cheaper in two-stage designs, although they are likely to have more biases and less precision.

Cohort and Longitudinal Surveys

Cross sectional surveys explore associations between two variables (x and y) whereas prospective surveys allow the researcher to investigate the problem of unknown direction of causality ($x \rightarrow y$, $x \leftarrow y$, $x \leftrightarrow y$). In relation to mental disorder they can also provide invaluable information on the persistence and duration of mental disorder over time in the population (in general the commoner and less severe forms of disorder in adulthood tend to be of short duration rather than long lasting). However, they are not appropriate for examining treatment and service effectiveness prospectively because, if anything, at a given time, those having treatment are likely to be more severely ill and to have a poorer subsequent health outcome.

In our experience the more common obstacle to successfully carrying out a longitudinal study is a failure to include this element in the design from the beginning of the study, a 'keeping in touch component.' This is essential if the number followed up successfully is to be maximized. In an adequately funded 'keeping in touch' program, respondents are regularly sent reminders and updates, often including personal birthday greetings, on the progress and successful achievement of the study, thus sustaining what can be a considerable commitment on the part of respondents. This of course requires sustained funding over much longer periods some of which could be used to provide incentives.

Informed Consent

According to Martin (2000), the validity of survey research depends crucially on obtaining as high response rates as possible from the sample selected for a survey. However, individuals selected have a right to make an informed decision about whether or not to participate. Martin argues that without personal contact with an interviewer, the conditions needed to obtain informed consent cannot be achieved. Use of opt-out procedures based on a letter (and opt-in procedures to an even great extent) guarantees neither that the information needed to ensure that consent is informed reaches the right person nor that the person has read and fully understood what participation entails. Martin has concluded that truly informed consent can be obtained only if it is sought by an interviewer trained to explain the survey fully and answer all questions. This is analogous to a personal approach to take part in a clinical trial in which informed consent must also be obtained.

The survey research literature and standard survey practice both emphasize the importance of motivating people to agree to take part in surveys by stressing the importance of the survey and of their personal contribution. There is no evidence that such motivation is seen as exerting undue pressure. The voluntary nature of surveys is always explained, and respondents are free to refuse to answer particular questions or to terminate their participation at any stage. Additional safeguards in the case of the longitudinal and panel surveys are that explicit permission is sought to continue at each stage of the survey, so initial consent does not imply consent to every part of the survey process (Martin, 2000).

Case Control Studies

Measures of exposure status can be compared in which disease status is determined at the time of subject selection. This design may be useful in studying rare conditions, events, or exposures. However, unless these are obtained in the same population setting from which controls are drawn, comparisons and resulting estimates may be biased. This design is rarely used in this field.

Information Sources

Types of information sources can be divided into administrative and survey or census. Some very useful studies can be performed by means of existing well-collected administrative data, thus avoiding the high cost of new data collection and using those resources instead for the important tasks of analysis and dissemination.

Administrative Sources

For cultural and legal reasons, administrative authorities will probably have the best data on causes of death such as suicide and homicide. Data can exist in registers of independent organizations, provider services, or of the authority organization itself.

Censuses

Censuses are a similar source of data; the main advantage is that they collect whole-population data. But census sources are limited by the fact that questions on health are rare and virtually unheard of in relation to psychological and mental health. Other disadvantages are that they are carried out relatively infrequently, rely on proxy information (provided by one household member), and rely on another service such as the postal service to convey data.

Surveys

Surveys can be an efficient and relatively low-cost method for obtaining large numbers of observations in a systematic, reliable way and provide powerful methods for addressing questions on health. Such survey data sets are increasingly archived after a period of time and therefore remain available to the wider research community and to policy advisers (see the Relevant Websites section at the end of this article). This is good in that better use is made of such data at little extra cost, but it can have bad effects also, particularly in a complex area such as mental health, unless the original survey designers can contribute the analysis and interpretation of the data in order to obviate serious misunderstandings.

Mental health surveys

Early mental health surveys tended to be carried out on small samples obtained in single communities and were typically conducted by an individual or small academic team. Estimates from these studies carried little precision, and only substantial effects were demonstrable. Large-scale, statistically more powerful, survey methodologies began to impinge on the field of psychiatric surveys with the Epidemiologic Catchment Area Survey of Mental Disorders (ECA) (Robins et al., 1984), British National Psychiatric Morbidity Surveys (Jenkins et al., 1997) (see Relevant Websites), the National Comorbidity Survey (NCS) (Kessler et al., 1994), and now the WHO World Mental Health Survey (Demyttenaere et al., 2004), all of which have served to transform the field. Not only did this development herald the introduction of new instruments for assessing mental disorders (see below) but it also served to refine sampling and statistical methods used to generate scientific and policy information. Such surveys have probably been more successful in answering questions about effects within subgroups of the population such as those who are economically disadvantaged. They have also been effective in collecting representative data from difficult-to-reach populations, including low-income populations in less economically developed parts of the world. General health surveys and social and economic surveys have also made increased use of measures of mental and physical health and functioning, thus bringing evidence to a much wider community of policymakers and decision makers.

Registers

Disease and service registers have also played a key part, although few countries have been willing to or capable of operating these over sustained periods. Scandinavian countries, most notably Denmark, have made a contribution in this regard to studying, for example, rarer conditions such as bipolar disorder and other specific forms of psychosis within a whole population context. External researchers have also been able to work collaboratively with those responsible for maintaining such registers. The use of such sources must include a careful consideration of the quality of the register's coding of data.

Services

Although services ought to be able to provide information on rarer events and conditions in practice, for example, we have found such sources to be unable to furnish reliable information except, of course, when they are linked to a register that is managed to high scientific standards. A key issue that may underlie this situation is that the purposes for which data are collected and used by a service are likely to be very different from those of scientific or policy researchers. Services may be able to supply information on the use of such services, providing diagnostic coded data (sometimes in close accord with an accepted set of definitions).

Record Linkage

Linking data on respondents or service users across population care sectors and agencies can be of value in ensuring continuity of care, evaluation, and planning of mental health services, depending of course on the aforementioned issue of data quality. Notable research examples have involved linking data on suicide with data on previous service usage. Useful recent examples of the use of record linkage to support services are the Ontario Data Linkage System (Squire *et al.*, 2002) and the Western Australia Linked Database system (Holman *et al.*, 1999).

Measurement Methods

As discussed earlier, we make a distinction in this section between measures suitable for clinical settings and requiring some clinical experience and measures that can be either self-completed or administered by a lay interviewer that are not only less costly to use but are also more feasible to use in the kinds of large-scale general population surveys needed to obtain information that is useful in planning and policy development. Further background reading about these kinds of measures can also be obtained elsewhere (Thompson, 1988; Biemer *et al.*, 1991; Farmer *et al.*, 2002).

Unstructured Methods

When an investigator is beginning to study a new area of research or is beginning to study an understood construct but in a new population or cultural context or setting, it may be prudent to start with qualitative assessments as a first stage in identifying key themes and concepts and in particular the language in which they are expressed.

Once a structured (or semistructured) instrument has been drafted, testing can be enhanced by means of cognitive interviewing (Biemer *et al.*, 1991). After the test respondent answers each question, an interviewer then asks the respondent questions such as: What do you think was meant by that question? What were you thinking when you answered that question? Why did you answer it that way?

Qualitative analytical methods are used to summarize key points emerging from such interviews; questions are revised and further testing is carried out, and so on.

The more structured methods of measurement described further on were developed because of concerns about the use of unstructured measures such as the clinician mental state assessment. Given the all-important consideration of instrument reliability, mentioned previously, we do not propose to give further consideration to unstructured approaches to the assessment of mental health functioning.

Structured Measures

Fully structured measures are completed by study respondents. They can be either directly completed in the form of self-completion, 'paper and pencil' questionnaires although such methods are increasingly computer assisted; (see the Procedures section) or they can be administered face-to-face by a lay interviewer. When an interviewer administers a questionnaire, the interviewer must not impose her or his judgment on the responses to the questionnaire, which must be chosen by the respondent or left blank, unfilled. Considerable ingenuity has gone into the development of such questionnaires in order to gather information on the criteria needed to determine the presence of specified types of psychiatric disorder. Such techniques were first developed within the social survey field in order to collect information on complex social and economic issues. The principles involved began to be used in the field of mental disorders in the 1970s and 1980s. A strength but also a limitation of such interviewer-administered questionnaires is the use of branching rules: when a respondent states that they do not have a particular characteristic (e.g., symptoms of depression in general, being currently unemployed) further questions about depression or about the effects of being unemployed need not be asked. Such methods allow a great deal of information to be collected selectively but are limited by the sensitivity and specificity and positive and negative predictive value of the initial 'screening' or 'sifting' questions.

Self-report questionnaires

Self-report questionnaire can be used at little cost because interviewers need not be directly involved in their administration. A comprehensive listing of such questionnaires can be found in Farmer *et al.* (2002), where rating scales are also described. The best-known examples of such self-report measures for adults are the General Health Questionnaire (Goldberg, 1972), the Short-Form Questionnaire (Ware, 1993), which also assesses physical aspects of health and functioning, and the Strengths and Difficulties Questionnaire for children (Goodman *et al.*, 2000b). These measures have been used in a considerable number of large-scale surveys (including prospective or panel studies), which mainly focus on general health rather than specifically on mental disorder. Also widely used is the Edinburgh Postnatal Depression Scale to screen for perinatal maternal depression (Cox *et al.*, 1987). A promising new measure recommended for identifying more severe forms of mental disorder are the new K6 and K10 Scales (Kessler *et al.*, 2003). A great deal of attention has focused on the psychometric properties of these measures. Unfortunately, their deceptively simple appearance may disguise the enormous work that goes into their development. Therefore, researchers should be very cautious in trying to develop measures of their own, because questionnaire design and development is a highly specialized undertaking.

Structured diagnostic interviews

As already explained, diagnostic interviews extend the concept of self-report further; they either require an interviewer or, in some studies, a computer to administer the interview directly (interviewers will typically also use a computer rather than printed paper to help them correctly follow branching rules). Comprehensive listings are provided by Farmer *et al.* (2002). The limitations of these useful and efficient interview branching techniques need to be considered. For example, a respondent, perhaps for reasons of social desirability, may deny having symptoms of depression based on stem questions, which might otherwise have been picked up if nonstem questions (for example, about the physical effects of depression and accompanying thoughts) were asked in a nonbranching questionnaire. Therefore, some researchers prefer to use the self-report questionnaire formats that do not include any branching structure.

The first widely used such interview was the Diagnostic Interview Schedule, which later evolved into a series of interviews that carry the common title Composite International Diagnostic Interview (CIDI) (Robins *et al.*, 1988). Although lengthy and highly detailed, this quality has not been detrimental to their widespread use, including in the collection of survey data in low-income countries. However, they are not suitable for measuring severe mental disorders, and there are many different versions of the CIDI, thus limiting comparison between different studies. Less known are similar diagnostic interviews used in the British National Survey Programme (see Relevant Websites). For the child surveys, worth mentioning is a particularly novel solution to the challenge to combine fully structured questions and the use of clinical ratings in the Development and Well-Being Assessment (DAWBA) (Goodman *et al.*, 2000a). The questionnaire used structured interviewing supplemented by open-ended questions. When definite symptoms were identified by the structured questions, interviewers used open-ended questions and supplementary prompts to get parents to describe the child's' problems in their own words. The wording of the prompts was specified. Answers to the open-ended questions and any other respondent comments were transcribed verbatim by the interviewers but were not rated by them. Interviewers were also given the opportunity to make additional comments, where appropriate, on the respondents' understanding and motivation.

A small team of experienced clinicians reviewed the transcripts and interviewers' comments to ensure that the answers to structured questions were not misleading. The same clinical reviewers could also consider clashes of information between different informants, deciding which account to prioritize. Furthermore, children with clinically relevant problems that did not quite meet the operationalized diagnostic criteria could be assigned suitable diagnoses by the clinical raters. There are no other existing diagnostic tools that combine the advantages of structured and semistructured assessments in this way, which is why a new set of measures were specifically designed for this survey. The new measures and their validity are described in more detail elsewhere (Goodman *et al.*, 2000a).

Semistructured

The term 'semistructured' is used to refer to measures that could be considered as lying in between the pre-worded, fully structured measures and largely unstructured qualitative interviews just described. In the sense that it is used here, 'semistructured' refers to a style of interviewing that is flexible and more conversational but critically different in that the interviewer (either the interviewer or others on the research team) has two additional responsibilities: first, the selective framing of supplementary questions in order to add clarification and to respond to the way subjects at first answer and appear to understand questions; and second, sifting through the interview content and deciding on the final ratings. Issues of feasibility, cost, and complexity of the phenomena to be measured will bear on the choice of which approach to use in a study, as discussed earlier.

Diagnostic interviews

Diagnostic interviews are discussed in detail elsewhere (Farmer *et al.*, 2002; Thompson, 1988). As for fully structured diagnostic interviews, all the information needed for the mental disorder classification system is sought (and these interviews also use branching techniques). Because the interviewer is required to provide the judgment of each rating in a semistructured interview as compared to the respondent in a fully structured interview, great care is needed to ensure the consistency of such ratings between interviewers and across time within one study not to mention between studies. Little is known about how successful such efforts are. There is little doubt that such approaches will be very costly in most settings. However, in low-income populations the cost of interviews also may be lower; there may also be advantages arising from the flexible 'clinical' conversational style of such interviews that could serve to minimize misunderstanding among respondents who are perhaps less well acquainted with Western psychological terms. However, these are all conjectural matters for further investigation. Some of the issues are also discussed elsewhere in the wider context of survey measures in general (Biemer *et al.*, 1991).

In a previous section we discussed the DAWBA (Goodman *et al.*, 2000a), which combines a fully structured and a partial semistructured element that has been shown to be reliable in generating DSM-IV and ICD-10 categories. The most widely used such measure in adult mental health surveys is the Structured Clinical Interview for DSM (SCID) (Spitzer *et al.*, 1992). Also used, particularly to elucidate psychotic forms of disorder, is the Schedules for Clinical Assessment in Neuropsychiatry (SCAN) (World Health Organization Division of Mental Health, 1992). Both should be administered by clinically experienced, specifically trained clinicians or by interviewers with greatly extended training that provides such experience (Brugha *et al.*, 1999). The SCAN provides dimensional and ICD-10 and DSM-IV diagnostic outputs and has been translated extensively; the SCID-I provides DSM-IV outputs only and also exists in a number of translated forms.

Rating Scales

Rating scales are similar to semistructured interviews in that the person administering the scale judges the ratings. However, far less guidance is provided on how to collect the data. Such measures were developed in order to efficiently make use of the observations of a clinician, who presumably would already have conducted a mental state assessment, in treating a patient. These approaches have for many years been in widespread use in clinical treatment trials but are rarely used in surveys. Examples can be found in Farmer *et al.* (2002) and Thompson (1988).

Cross-Population Issues

A number of references have been made to considerations that are of importance when measuring mental health in different cultures and language settings. This principle should be extended to consideration of any subpopulation that could be marginalized or excluded, such as prisoners (Brugha *et al.*, 2004) and those with sensory impairment. For example, a version of the DIS interview has been developed for deaf people (Montoya *et al.*, 2004).

Culture and ethnicity

There is a large body of evidence suggesting that the idioms for mental distress vary across different ethnic groups (Sproston and Nazroo, 2002). The implication of possible cultural differences in symptomatic experience is that standardized research instruments will perform inconsistently across different ethnic groups, greatly restricting the validity of conclusions based on their use in surveys. Although there is some evidence of the universality of the major forms of clinical psychopathology (Cheng *et al.*, 2000), this is not universally accepted. Fundamental issues about the transferability of Western psychological and psychopathological concepts continue to be debated. Invaluable experience of the practicalities and scope for addressing such challenges has come from the International Pilot Studies of Schizophrenia and subsequent research under WHO auspices (Jablensky *et al.*, 1992) and from recent work within the general population survey paradigm of the diverse cultures and languages found in urban Britain (Sproston and Nazroo, 2002), which included detailed qualitative, unstructured assessments carried out in the first language of respondents.

Translation methods and protocols

A great deal of experience has been built up in translating (Sartorius, 1998) and testing instruments in different population and cultural settings. Great emphasis has been placed on the use of both forward- and back-translation. Recent developments emphasize that it is the concepts rather than the words that need to be translated, thus preserving meaning as far as possible. In order for questions to be understood in a way that is comparable within and across populations that rely on different languages and dialects, it is necessary to have a translation procedure that yields equivalent versions of the questions across a variety of settings and cultures.

There are three main problems that occur when trying to standardize the translation process across countries:

- linguistic differences caused by changes in the meaning of words between dialects;
- translation difficulties; and
- differences that arise when applying a concept across cultures.

The conceptual translational method relies on detailed explanations of the terms used in each survey question, as well as the underlying concepts that the questions were intended to measure. This approach differs from the forward-backward method in the 'backward' step, during which rather than translating the question back into the original language, a checker determines whether each question was properly translated such that the intended concepts were actually captured (Robine and Jagger, 2002; Robine and Jagger, 2003).

Measurement of Specific Disorders

As mentioned earlier, mental health survey approaches and programs in a given geographic setting sometimes begin by assessing an overall or 'common mental disorder' outcome that may be dimensional (see **Figure 1**) or based on a categorical case definition. This approach can also be embedded into surveys that assess other aspects of health, economic and social functioning. The influence of clinical psychiatry has led to an expectation of data on specific categories of mental disorder. Most surveys have focused on more common internalizing disorders: anxiety and depression in adults, conduct and emotional disorders in children and young people. Many surveys also attempt to measure rarer and more complex disorders (in terms of diagnostic criteria and their measurement), such as obsessive compulsive disorder and psychosis in adults and attention deficit disorder and developmental disorders in children (e.g., tick disorder and autism). Externalizing disorders involving the use of substances and alcohol are also often assessed; other disorders of behavior, such as personality disorder, are rarely assessed. These expectations are likely to be increasingly questioned in favor of the more practical and parsimonious value of information on severity, complexity *per se*, and persistence over time.

Procedures (Surveys Mainly)

The procedures used in surveys also determine quality, cost, and acceptability. Quality (or accuracy) is the most difficult of these to evaluate. A notable example is that it has been shown that audio computer-assisted self-interviewing (ACASI) administration can yield more information on mental health than that obtained from an interviewer-administered, paper-and-pencil (I-PAPI) mental health module of the CIDI (Epstein *et al.*, 2001).

Face to Face

In face-to-face procedures the respondent is administered the questions by an interviewer who will typically visit the person's home or other agreed-upon place. Although costly, such methods are regarded as of high quality. The researcher has control over the quality of the training and procedures used by interviewers.

Postal

Respondents complete and return a questionnaire by post, usually using a prepaid cover or envelope. Unless additional steps are taken to ensure cooperation, response rates tend to be so low as to make the information provided of limited value, but methods for increasing response rates have been developed. Costs are understandably very low. It may come as a surprise, however, to find that quality can be high, possibly because respondents have time to think more carefully about questions and also because social desirability factors play less of a part (Bushery *et al.*, 1996) than in face-to-face interviews. However, self-completion methods that are fully anonymous are now often included within a face-to-face interview procedure.

Electronic and Digital

Various electronic methods have gradually been introduced; some of these are under active development and likely to become either more sophisticated or drop out of use. In most contexts and cases, costs are lower than for the equivalent interviewer-based approach, although start-up costs may be very high.

Procedures include computer-assisted telephone interviewing, the Internet, interactive voice response over telephone (IVR), and so forth. IVR is a more automated version of telephone interviewing but may be limited by the proportion of the population who subscribe. Telephone interviewing is used widely by commercial organizations in some populations, and this may lead to resistance among some of the public and thus compromise the representativeness of survey findings.

Start-up costs for Internet surveys, although dropping, are still high but then fall to almost zero per unit cost. They may share some of the advantages of accuracy of postal methods. Data can be collected from all over the world (which may be either an advantage or a disadvantage) and is immediately available for analysis. Other computer-administered methods include audio-computer-assisted interviewing (ACASI), in which the respondent may wear ear phones; text to speech (TTS), which may use 'talking heads' (Avatars) that can be specifically gender and culture matched to the respondent; digital recording; and touch screen responses to questions.

Computer adaptive testing (CAT), in which the software calculates and determines the next question to ask in an interview, is probably limited to assessing fairly simple concepts and facts rather than attitudes; when we evaluated such a system in a comparison with a clinical evaluation of neurotic symptoms we found poor agreement (Brugha *et al.*, 1996).

Application of Measurement Methods in Public Health Contexts (e.g. Surveillance and Screening in Health Settings)

Government policy documents are beginning to suggest the use of surveillance methods such as repeat surveys over time in order to evaluate policies and success in implementing health objectives (e.g., England; Department of Health, 1999). National mental health strategies should set realistic targets for improvements in the mental health of the population (Jenkins *et al.*, 2002). The example of a common mental disorder for which there is a range of effective treatments deserves mention. Despite the high prevalence rates of common mental disorders, they have traditionally been underdetected and undertreated. In recent years changes in services should have improved this situation in Great Britain. A campaign by the Royal Colleges of General Practitioners and of Psychiatrists to increase awareness and the effective treatment of depression led to over half of general practitioners (GPs) taking part in teaching sessions on depression. The pharmaceutical industry successfully encouraged increased prescription of newer antidepressants. The effectiveness of such innovations may be evaluated by monitoring the mental health and treatment of representative samples of the whole population surveyed in 1993 and 2000. However, a recent examination of rates of such disorders in 1993 and 2000, during which rates of treatment increased dramatically, concluded that treatment with psychotropic medication alone is unlikely to improve the overall mental health of the population nationally (Brugha *et al.*, 2005). Similar conclusions have emerged since from the USA (Kessler *et al.*, 2005). Such evidence can be interpreted as pointing to the need to develop effective prevention policies for which surveillance methods would also be essential.

Policy Information and Decision Making

Little is known or understood about how policymakers use information from mental health surveys. Expectations are likely to be shaped by the nature and value of information used in physical health and evidence-based treatments and services, including prevention policies. This may be why information on the prevalence of mental disorders is often sought and provided, although the concept may have little meaning. A surprisingly large number of systematic reviews, often including the use of synthetic methods such as meta-analysis, have appeared in the psychiatric epidemiology literature in the past decade. Policymakers require guidance on the value of such reviews, given the technical difficulties faced in carrying out good-quality studies in this field.

Conclusions

Methods for measuring psychiatric and related psychological disorders and outcomes in populations have advanced considerably, particularly in the past two decades. Some long-standing assumptions have been tested, sometimes with surprising conclusions. Contemporary researchers pay particular attention to consistency and reproducibility of findings, in contrast to an earlier era in which clinical applicability often dominated the choice of the method used. Studies have become much larger and require the input of many more and different disciplines than in the past; this is probably to the good, as it may help render the topic of mental disorder more acceptable and less stigmatizing. Although the field seems new and technologically exciting, old principles are still important: simplicity and clarity of purpose, an appropriate design, the use of well-tested measures, and the interpretation of findings with a clear understanding of the limitations of the methods used. The measurement of mental disorder now stands equal in importance, in methodological rigor and usefulness, to other major public health topics.

Citations

American Psychiatric Association (1994) *Diagnostic and Statistical Manual of Mental Disorders, Fourth Edition.* Washington, DC: American Psychiatric Association.

Biemer P, Groves RM, Lyberg LE, Mathiowetz NA, and Sudman S (1991) *Measurement Errors in Surveys.* New York: John Wiley & Sons.

Brugha TS (2002) The end of the beginning: A requiem for the categorisation of mental disorder? *Psychological Medicine* 32(7): 1149–1154.

Brugha TS, Teather D, Wills KM, Kaul A, and Dignon A (1996) Present state examination by microcomputer: Objectives and experience of preliminary steps. *International Journal of Methods in Psychiatric Research* 6: 143–151.

Brugha TS, Nienhuis FJ, Bagchi D, Smith J, and Meltzer H (1999) The survey form of SCAN: The feasibility of using experienced lay survey interviewers to administer a semi-structured systematic clinical assessment of psychotic and non psychotic disorders. *Psychological Medicine* 29(3): 703–712.

Brugha TS, Bebbington PE, Singleton N, *et al.* (2004) Trends in service use and treatment for mental disorders in adults throughout Great Britain. *The British Journal of Psychiatry* 185: 378–384.

Brugha T, Singleton N, Meltzer H, *et al.* (2005) Psychosis in the community and in prisons: A report from the British National Survey of Psychiatric Morbidity. *American Journal of Psychiatry* 162(4): 774–780.

Cheng ATA, Tien AY, Brugha TS, *et al.* (2000) Cross-cultural implementation of a Chinese version of the Schedules for Clinical Assessment in Neuropsychiatry (SCAN) in Taiwan. *British Journal of Psychiatry* 178: 567–572.

Cox JL, Holden JM, and Sagovsky R (1987) Detection of postnatal depression. Development of the 10 item Edinburgh Postnatal Depression Scale. *British Journal of Psychiatry* 150: 782–786.

Demyttenaere K, Bruffaerts R, Posada-Villa J, *et al.* (2004) Prevalence, severity, and unmet need for treatment of mental disorders in the World Health Organization World Mental Health Surveys. *Journal of the American Medical Association* 291(21): 2581–2590.

Department of Health (1999) *National Service Frameworks for Mental Health. Modern Standards and Service Models*, pp. 149. London: Department of Health.

Epstein JF, Barker PR, and Kroutil LA (2001) Mode Effects in Self-Reported Mental Health Data. *Public Opinion Quarterly* 65(4): 529–549.

Farmer A, McGuffin P, and Williams J (2002) *Measuring Psychopathology.* Oxford, UK: Oxford University Press.

Goldberg DP (1972) *The Detection of Psychiatric Illness by Questionnaire.* Oxford, UK: Oxford University Press.

Goodman R, Ford T, Richards H, Gatward R, and Meltzer H (2000a) The Development and Well-Being Assessment: Description and initial validation of an integrated assessment of child and adolescent psychopathology. *Journal of Child Psychology and Psychiatry*, JID 0375361, 41(5): 645–655.

Goodman R, Ford T, Simmons H, Gatward R, and Meltzer H (2000b) Using the Strengths and Difficulties Questionnaire (SDQ) to screen for child psychiatric disorders in a community sample. *British Journal of Psychiatry*, JID 0342367, 177: 534–539.

Green H, McGinnity A, Meltzer H, Ford T, and Goodman R (2005) *Mental Health of Children and Young People in Great Britain, 2004.* Hampshire, UK: Palgrave McMillan.

Holman CD, Bass AJ, Rouse IL, and Hobbs MS (1999) Population-based linkage of health records in Western Australia: Development of a health services research linked database. *Australia and New Zealand Journal of Public Health* 23(5): 453–459.

Jablensky A, Sartorius N, Ernberg G, *et al.* (1992) Schizophrenia: Manifestations, incidence and course in different cultures. A World Health Organization ten-country study [published erratum appears in Psychological Medicine Monograph Suppl. 1992, Nov. 22(4): following 1092]. *Psychological Medicine Monograph Supplement* 20: 1–97.

Jenkins R, Bebbington P, Brugha T, *et al.* (1997) The national psychiatric morbidity surveys of Great Britain – Strategy and methods. *Psychological Medicine* 27(4): 765–774.

Kessler RC, McGonagle KA, Zhao S, *et al.* (1994) Lifetime and 12-month prevalence of DSM-III-R psychiatric disorders in the United States. Results from the National Comorbidity Survey. *Archives of General Psychiatry* 51(1): 8–19.

Kessler RC, Barker PR, Colpe LJ, *et al.* (2003) Screening for serious mental illness in the general population. *Archives of General Psychiatry* 60(2): 184–189.

Kessler RC, Demler O, Frank RG, *et al.* (2005) Prevalence and treatment of mental disorders, 1990 to 2003. *The New England Journal of Medicine* 352(24): 2515–2523.

MacArthur C, Winter HR, Bick DE, *et al.* (2002) Effects of redesigned community postnatal care on women's' health 4 months after birth: A cluster randomised controlled trial. *Lancet* 359(9304): 378–385.

Martin J, Social Survey Division, ONF (ed.) (2000) *Informed Consent in the Context of Survey Research.* London: Office for National Statistics.

Montoya LA, Egnatovich R, Eckhardt E, *et al.* (2004) Translation Challenges and Strategies: The ASL Translation of a Computer-Based Psychiatric Diagnostic Interview 4(4): 314–344.

Newman SC, Shrout PE, and Bland RC (1990) The efficiency of two-phase designs in prevalence surveys of mental disorders [published erratum appears in *Psychological Medicine* 1990, Aug. 20(3): following 745]. *Psychological Medicine* 20(1): 183–193.

Robine JM and Jagger C (2003) Creating a coherent set of indicators to monitor health across Europe: The Euro-REVES 2 project. *European Journal of Public Health* 13(3 Suppl): 6–14.

Robine JM and Jagger C (eds.) Euro-REVES (2002) *Report to Eurostat on European Health Status Module.* Geneva, Switzerland: EUROSTAT.

Robins LE, Helzer JE, Weissman MM, *et al.* (1984) Lifetime prevalence of specific psychiatric disorders in three sites. *Archives of General Psychiatry* 41: 949–957.

Robins LN, Wing J, Wittchen HU, *et al.* (1988) The Composite International Diagnostic Interview. An epidemiologic instrument suitable for use in conjunction with different diagnostic systems and in different cultures. *Archives of General Psychiatry* 45(12): 1069–1077.

Sartorius N (1998) SCAN translation. In: Wing JK and Ustün TB (eds.) *Diagnosis and Clinical Measurement in Psychiatry. A Reference Manual for SCAN/PSE-10*, pp. 44–57. Cambridge, UK: Cambridge University Press.

Shrout PE and Newman SC (1989) Design of two-phase prevalence surveys of rare disorders. *Biometrics* 45(2): 549–555.

Singleton N, Bumpstead R, O'Brien M, Lee A and Meltzer H, National Statistics (eds.) (2001) *Psychiatric Morbidity among Adults Living in Private Households*, pp. 154. London: The Stationary Office.

Spitzer RL, Williams JB, Gibbon M, and First MB (1992) The Structured Clinical Interview for DSM-III-R (SCID). I: History, rationale, and description. *Archives of General Psychiatry* 49(8): 624–629.

Sproston K and Nazroo JY (eds.) (2002) *Ethnic Minority Psychiatric Illness Rates in the Community (EMPIRIC) – Quantitative Report*, pp. 210. London: The Stationary Office.

Squire L, Bedard M, Hegge L, and Polischuk V (2002) Current evaluation and future needs of a mental health data linkage system in a remote region: A Canadian experience. *Journal of Behavioral Health Services Research* 29(4): 476–480.

Thompson C (1988) *The Instruments of Psychiatric Research,* 1st edn. Chichester, UK: Wiley.

Ware JE (1993) *SF-36 Health Survey.* Boston, MA: Medical Outcomes Trust.

Wing JK, Cooper J, and Sartorius N (1974) *Measurement and Classification of Psychiatric Symptoms.* Cambridge, UK: Cambridge University Press.

World Health Organization (1992) *ICD-10 Classification of Mental and Behavioural Disorders: Clinical Descriptions and Diagnostic Guidelines.* Geneva, Switzerland: World Health Organization.

World Health Organization (1993) *The ICD-10 Classification of Mental and Behavioural Disorders: Diagnostic Criteria for Research.* Geneva, Switzerland: WHO.

World Health Organization Division of Mental Health (1990) *ICD-10, chapter 5, Mental and Behavioural Disorders (Including Disorders of Psychological Development): Diagnostic Criteria for Research (May 1990 Draft for Field Trials).* Geneva, Switzerland: World Health Organization. (Distribution: limited).

World Health Organization Division of Mental Health WHO SCAN Advisory Committee (ed.) (1992) *SCAN Schedules for Clinical Assessment in Neuropsychiatry,* Version 1.0, pp. 242. Geneva, Switzerland: World Health Organization.

Zahner GE, Chung-Cheng H, and Fleming JA (1995) Introduction to epidemiological research methods. In: Tsuang M, Tohen M and Zahner GE (eds.) *Textbook in Psychiatric Epidemiology*, pp. 23–54. New York: Wiley.

Further Reading

American Statistical Association (1996) How interview mode affects data reliability. *Proceedings of the Survey Research Methods Section, American Statistical Association.* Alexandria, VA: American Statistical Association.

Biemer P, Groves RM, Lyberg LE, Mathiowetz NA, and Sudman S (1991) *Measurement Errors in Surveys.* New York: John Wiley & Sons.

Farmer A, McGuffin P, and Williams J (2002) *Measuring Psychopathology.* Oxford, UK: Oxford University Press.

Green H, McGinnity A, Meltzer H, Ford T, and Goodman R (2005) *Mental Health of Children and Young People in Great Britain, 2004.* Hampshire, UK: Palgrave McMillan.

Shrout PE and Newman SC (1989) Design of two-phase prevalence surveys of rare disorders. *Biometrics* 45(2): 549–555.

Singleton N, Bumpstead R, O'Brien M, Lee A and Meltzer H (eds.) (2001) *Psychiatric Morbidity Among Adults Living in Private Households*, pp. 154. London: The Stationary Office National Statistics.

Sproston K and Nazroo JY (2002) *Ethnic Minority Psychiatric Illness Rates in the Community (EMPIRIC) – Quantitative Report*, pp. 210. London: The Stationary Office.

Thompson C (1988) *The Instruments of Psychiatric Research*, 1st edn. Chichester, UK: John Wiley & Sons.

Wing JK, Cooper J, and Sartorius N (1974) *Measurement and Classification of Psychiatric Symptoms.* Cambridge, UK: Cambridge University Press.

World Health Organization (1993) *The ICD-10 Classification of Mental and Behavioural Disorders: Diagnostic Criteria for Research.* Geneva, Switzerland: WHO.

Zahner GE, Chung-Cheng H, and Fleming JA (1995) Introduction to epidemiological research methods. In: Tsuang M, Tohen M and Zahner GE (eds.) *Textbook in Psychiatric Epidemiology*, pp. 23–54. New York: John Wiley & Sons.

Relevant Websites

http://www.hcp.med.harvard.edu/wmh/ – Department of Health Care Policy, Harvard Medical School.

http://www.nice.org.uk/page.aspx?o=235213 – National Institute for Clinical Excellence, Depression Treatment Guideline.

http://www.dh.gov.uk/PublicationsAndStatistics/Published/Survey/ListOfSurveySince1990/SurveyListMentalHealth/fs/en – Reports of National Surveys of Psychiatric Morbidity, England.

http://www.data-archive.ac.uk – UK Data Archive.

Mental Health and Physical Health (Including HIV/AIDS)

A Kagee, Stellenbosch University, Matieland, South Africa
M Freeman, Human Sciences Research Council, Pretoria, South Africa

Introduction

According to the World Health Report 2001, over the past 20 years a fundamental and inseparable connection between mental and physical health has been convincingly established (WHO, 2001). Both mental and physical health are influenced by a combination of biological, psychological, and social factors. Thoughts, feelings, and behavior have a major impact on physical health. Conversely, physical health has an important influence on mental health and well-being. The report notes two critical pathways through which this occurs: Physiological systems such as neuroendocrine and immune functioning and health behavior. These pathways are not independent: Behavior may affect physiology, while physiological functioning may in turn affect health behavior. In this article, we examine the historical shift that has occurred from a dualistic conception of health and illness to the biopsychosocial model that emphasizes an integration of mind and body. We explore this interrelationship using the examples of somatoform disorder, chronic pain, HIV/AIDS, cardiovascular disease, cancer, and diabetes. Finally, we focus on some of the somatic manifestations of mental illness.

Historical Development of an Integrated Model

The Biomedical Model

In the seventeenth century, the mind and body were considered to be two separate entities, largely unrelated to each other and influenced by discrete sets of factors. René Descartes, a major proponent of a dualistic conceptualization of mind and body, considered it appropriate that the functioning of the body should fall in the realm of science, while the workings of the mind and soul should be the concern of philosophy and, subsequently psychology. In the strongly religious atmosphere of this era, Cartesian dualism provided an important restraint on the influential Christian church from interfering in scientific activities that were considered previously taboo, such as the dissection of corpses, which was considered sinful and was forbidden by the European church. However, if it could be agreed that scientists would be concerned with the body and nothing else, it would no longer be the prerogative of the church to interfere in scientific affairs. In return, the soul and mind would remain the domain of the clergy and outside of the realm of science. In this context, mind and body were separate and the boundary between the two was seen as impermeable.

Dualism became highly influential in informing the biomedical model of health care. The medical model, whose hegemony went largely unchallenged for more than two centuries, embraces the view that illness is caused by internal or external agents that arrest or alter the normal functioning of the body. Such agents include bacteria, viruses, toxins, carcinogens, or genes. In the medical model, the objective is to identify the etiological factors associated with poor health and rectify these so as to restore the body to optimal functioning. Accordingly, humans are chiefly biological organisms who can be understood by examining their constituent parts. In its extreme form, the only conceptual apparatuses required by the biomedical model to understand human functioning are physical and chemical in nature. This emphasis has led to the ascendance of disciplines such as anatomy, physiology, and biochemistry in traditional biomedicine. Disease in the biomedical paradigm occurs when there is disruption in normal biological functioning, usually caused by an identifiable event of a physical or chemical nature. Medical treatment from this perspective involves physical or chemical agents to correct the disruption and restore the body to health.

The Biopsychosocial Model

With further discoveries in the health sciences in the nineteenth and twentieth centuries, it became apparent that a dualistic conceptualization of health and illness was an inadequate explanatory model. It was instead recognized that the physiological regulation of the body's various systems (e.g., the digestive and respiratory systems) entailed a series of complex interactions and feedback loops involving a variety of variables. The utility of linear and mechanistic causal models of illness thus diminished and a greater emphasis was placed on a systemic understanding of human functioning. Thus, viruses and bacteria remained necessary conditions for the occurrence of illness but were no longer considered sufficient. Instead, disease is thought to occur as a result of the interaction between host systems and disease agents. This interaction is characterized by complexity and nonlinearity, with an emphasis on systemic rather than mechanistic functioning. It has become accepted that human health and well-being are shaped by a multitude of factors that include behavior, personality, cognitive style, and social, economic and political relationships.

The biopsychosocial model emphasizes the interaction of psychological, social, economic, behavioral, biological, and physical factors in influencing the functioning of human beings. As such, it invokes a systemic understanding in which elements are arranged hierarchically so that change in one element of a system affects other parts. Human beings are highly complex systems that consist of organ systems, organs, tissue, cells, and chemical elements located in a historical, social, and economic context. Yet, while this context influences individuals, the environment is similarly affected by human interpretation, action, interaction, and social change. Thus, environment influences human behavior and is also simultaneously influenced by it. Similarly, behavior may influence biological processes but may also be influenced by such processes. The biopsychosocial model considers the boundary between the psychological and physical dimensions of human functioning to be a highly permeable mediator of reciprocal influences. The emphasis on multiple elements and their

dynamic interplay provides a complex and nuanced understanding of the factors that influence health.

The biopsychosocial model defines health and illness as 'the product of a combination of factors that include biological characteristics (e.g. genetic predisposition), behavioral factors (e.g. lifestyle, stress, health beliefs), and social conditions (e.g. cultural influences, family relationships, and social support)' (American Psychological Association, 2001). Political and economic structures and systems as well as (their associated) health systems and approaches to financing of health care have also been found to directly affect health.

Mental and physical health intersect in various ways. While in reality it is often not possible to separate out these relationships, the following are important identifiable junctures between mental and physical health.

- Mental health status may impact on health risk behaviors;
- Mental problems may manifest as or impact on physical health problems;
- Diseases may attack both the brain and other organs or functions of the body;
- Physical ailments may affect mental functioning;
- A mental disorder may influence the course of physical disease;
- Medication given for the treatment of both mental and physical health problems may affect the other.

Having addressed some of the paradigmatic and theoretical considerations regarding mental and physical health, we now focus on specific conditions such as somatization, chronic pain, HIV and AIDS, cardiovascular disease, cancer, and diabetes. Our analysis is in keeping with the biopsychosocial model to the extent that we de-emphasize rigid divisions between the two dimensions of health.

Health Conditions

Somatoform Disorders

When physical symptoms occur in patients that are not fully explained by a general medical condition, these are usually referred to as somatoform disorders. In the category of somatoform disorders, the DSM-IV-TR includes somatization disorder (characterized by pain, gastrointestinal, and sexual problems), conversion disorder (involving unexplained symptoms that affect motor or sensory function), and hypochondriasis (characterized by the idea that one may have a serious disease, based on misinterpretation of bodily symptoms). Complaints about pain, nausea, erectile dysfunction, paralysis, and excessive concerns about illness in the absence of objective evidence to support such concerns may fall into the category of somatization disorder. The features of this condition that differentiate it from a general medical condition are the involvement of more than one unrelated organ system, chronicity of complaints without the development of structural abnormalities, and the absence of laboratory evidence that suggests a medical condition. Somatization has been shown to pose serious medical, social, and economic problems and may be difficult to manage clinically.

Various theories have been postulated to explain somatoform disorders. We review the psychoanalytic and the communicative perspectives. The idea that physical symptoms could be removed by influencing the mind rose to prominence in the nineteenth century and formed the foundation of the work of psychologists such as Jean Charcot, Pierre Janet, Josef Breuer, and Sigmund Freud. The psychoanalytic perspective advanced by Freud suggests that an unexplained physical symptom is a defense in response to anxiety from unacceptable unconscious conflict. The theory holds that the individual experiences anxiety because of an unacceptable idea or experience, against which the conversion is a defense. Psychic energy is then converted into a somatic symptom, which debilitates the physical organ. By this process, the somatic loss symbolizes the underlying psychic conflict.

The communicative perspective holds that somatizing patients may be defending against a variety of feelings such as depression, guilt, or anger. The patient then uses the problem of somatization to cope with these emotions and negotiate personal interactions that may be considered stressful. In the communicative perspective, the condition of alexithymia has been associated with somatization. This term has been used to refer to persons who have difficulty in expressing their feelings. Thus when asked to express feelings in response to loss, a typical response may be a report about physical symptoms such as headaches. There appears to be some evidence suggesting a relationship between somatization and alexithymia. Alexithymic persons have been shown to be particularly susceptible to somatoform disorders and psychosomatic problems. Somatization has often been viewed as a defense against awareness of emotional distress or as a masked version of depression. In a population-based epidemiologic survey, among respondents with five or more somatic symptoms, 63% reported psychological problems and 50% met criteria for a psychiatric diagnosis. Among persons without somatic symptoms on the other hand, these figures were 7% and 6%, respectively (Simon and VonKorf, 1991).

Common diagnostic conditions associated with somatization include chronic fatigue syndrome (CFS) and fibromyalgia. CFS is considered a revision of a condition that first occurred in the nineteenth century named neurasthenia, which referred to undue exhaustion in the context of minimal physical effort. It has been demonstrated that CFS is often comorbid with psychiatric illness. Fibromyalgia is related to chronic fatigue and is characterized by muscle pain and tenderness. This condition is also often accompanied by depression and sleep disturbance.

In keeping with the biopsychosocial paradigm, it is postulated that if the mind and brain transact, then, being regulated by the brain, organ systems are subject to influence by the mind and, in turn, anything that affects the mind (e.g., society and culture). As an example of the nonlinearity of the mind–body interaction, we examine the question of chronic pain and its association with psychological disturbance.

Chronic Pain

The traditional biomedical model of chronic pain is that it is caused by an identifiable disease state or tissue damage. Medical interventions are aimed at correcting the physical pathology with the intention of removing the experience of pain. While there have been considerable advances in fields such as anatomy and neurophysiology, much of patients' reported experiences of pain cannot be accounted for only by physical factors. For example, there are many instances when patients have reported dissimilar subjective experiences of pain despite identical physical stimuli to produce them; the association between the extent of injury and the intensity of reported pain has been shown to be modest; it has been suggested that between 30% and 50% of patients seeking medical treatment may not have a specific diagnosable condition (Dworkin and Massoth, 1994); and the majority of patients who present with chronic back pain do not have a physical basis for their condition.

Many chronic pain researchers place a strong emphasis on the distinction between disease and illness. Disease refers to the objective biological event such as trauma or physiological changes to body tissue. Illness, on the other hand, refers to the patient's subjective appraisal of the biological event and is associated with the experience of physical discomfort, emotional distress, behavioral limitations, and psychosocial disruption. While the biomedical model has traditionally focused on disease, the emphasis of the biopsychosocial model is primarily on illness.

Chronic pain in terms of the biopsychosocial model is best understood as the result of ongoing and multifactorial processes in which there is a dynamic and reciprocal relationship between the biological, psychological, and social factors shaping patients' experiences. The dynamics of these reciprocal relationships may occur in at least three ways. First, biological factors initiate and maintain physical sensations, psychological factors may influence the manner in which a person appraises and perceives physiological signs and social factors may influence how patients respond behaviorally to these perceptions. Second, psychological and mood-related factors affect biological processes by having an effect on hormone production and the autonomic nervous system. Behavioral responses may also have an effect on biological factors, as in the case of a patient who refrains from strenuous activities in order to reduce symptoms of pain. Third, biological factors and pharmaceutical treatment can cause fatigue, influence a patient's ability to concentrate, and affect their ability to engage in certain activities. Various examples demonstrate the interrelationship between these factors. For example, soldiers who sustain injuries on a battlefield report feeling considerably less pain than they would if the same injury had occurred elsewhere; athletes typically report feeling pain after a sports injury only once they are off the sports field; and patients who have the same degree of physical deterioration as measured by objective tests may have very different subjective perceptions of pain. Patients may also report pain in the absence of any objective evidence of tissue damage. These examples provide an indication of the complexity of the pain experience.

Gate Control Theory

Probably the most successful attempt at understanding perception of pain is gate control theory (Melzack and Wall, 1982). In his original work, Melzack noted that pain is an adaptive response to ensure the survival of the species as it ensures that a person avoids a stimulus in order to avoid injury, for example a hot plate that causes tissue damage. Gate control theory suggests that there are three systems that converge to affect the way in which pain is perceived, namely, sensory-discriminative, motivational-affective, and cognitive-evaluative. The model thus rejects the dichotomous view that pain is either physiological or psychological and suggests an integration of peripheral stimuli with psychological variables such as mood and anxiety in the experience of pain. The pain experience involves an ongoing set of activities that is reflexive at the beginning and may be modified by excitatory and inhibitory influences and the level of activity in the CNS. GCT proposes that there is a series of neurophysiological mechanisms located in the dorsal horn of each segment of the spinal cord. The activity of these mechanisms mediates the experience of pain and depends in part on both sensory information from the external environment (e.g., temperature and touch) and brain processes related to emotional state, past learning, and expectations. The meaning attributed to the stimulation is then transmitted back to the gate via nerve fibres that go from the brain to the spinal cord. In this way, the experience of pain is related to a combination of sensory input (tissue damage) and the psychological and behavioral state of the person.

Chronic Pain and Psychopathology

Emotional distress is common among persons experiencing chronic pain (Gatchel, 1996). Gatchel proposes a three-stage model to account for the relationship between chronic pain and distress. In Stage 1, the individual experiences emotional distress as a consequence of experiencing pain when it is acute, as pain is most commonly associated with physical harm. In Stage 2 when the pain does not remit and becomes chronic, psychological reactions may include learned helplessness, depression, emotional distress, anger, and somatization. While the model does not suppose a personality type that predisposes an individual to experiencing pain, it presumes that the nature and extent of these problems depend on the preexisting psychological characteristics and social context of the person. There appears to be mixed evidence concerning whether depression is a consequence of chronic pain or whether chronic pain is part of a symptom cluster of depression. In Stage 3 of the model, as the behavioral or psychological problems persist, the person may adopt a sick role, which permits him or her to be excused from responsibilities and obligations. Physical deconditioning may also occur alongside the progression of patients along the trajectory of this model, as a lack of physical activity may result in muscular atrophy and in turn in a decrease in physical capacity. Physical deconditioning may have a deleterious effect on emotional well-being and self-esteem, which may lead to additional psychological difficulties. Those chronic pain patients who experience depression may, as part of the symptom picture of this condition, experience a decrease in their level of motivation to engage in work, social, or recreational activities, which may in turn further contribute to physical deconditioning.

Chronic Pain and Depression

There is considerable evidence of a close relationship between chronic pain and symptoms of depression. However, this relationship is complex and possibly overlapping as the diagnostic criteria for mild depressive disorder also include some physical problems that could be attributed to chronic pain, such as sleep disturbance, energy loss, change in appetite, and weight gain or loss. Criterion contamination of this nature makes the process of accurate diagnosis of depression difficult. The various efforts to determine the causal direction between pain and depression may be organized in the following manner (Dersh et al., 2002):

- the antecedent hypothesis, which holds that depression precedes the onset of chronic pain;
- the consequence hypothesis, which states that depression follows the onset of pain;
- the scar hypothesis, which speculates that prior episodes of depression predispose pain patients to further episodes of depression;
- the cognitive behavioral mediation hypothesis, which states that cognitions mediate the relationship between chronic pain and the development of depression;

- the common pathogenic mechanisms hypothesis, which states that both pain and depression have a common etiological factor.

In a review of several studies addressing these various hypotheses, little support was found for the antecedent hypothesis, but robust support was found for the consequence hypothesis and the cognitive behavioral mediation hypothesis, which are in many ways compatible with each other (Fishbain *et al.*, 1997). Some support was also found for the scar and common mechanisms hypotheses. The scar hypothesis assumes a genetic predisposition to depression and is supported by findings that suggest that a higher proportion of patients with chronic pain have family members with depression than those in the general population. There is also evidence that common processes are involved in the mechanisms of pain and mood disturbance. For example, nociceptive (pain-related) and affective pathways are thought to coincide anatomically; the neurotransmitters associated with mood disorders, namely norepinephrine and serotonin, have some involvement in the gate control mechanism described above; and antidepressant medication has been shown to relieve chronic pain (Dersh *et al.*, 2002). It is apparent therefore that the relationship between chronic pain and depression is complex and dynamic, rather than linear and mechanistic.

Chronic Pain and Other Mental Disorders

Depression is by far the most common psychological association with chronic pain. Yet, it is evident that conditions such as substance abuse, anxiety, somatoform disorders, and personality disorders may be common among patients suffering chronic pain. The association between these disorders and chronic pain have received much less empirical scrutiny than mood disorders and the trajectory of their causal pathways awaits investigation.

HIV/AIDS and Mental Health

The complex interrelationship between mental and physical health is starkly exemplified with respect to HIV/AIDS. Five key mechanisms through which this occurs are presented.

Mental Health Status as a Precursor to HIV/AIDS

In the United States, people with severe mental illness are nearly 20 times more likely to be infected with HIV than the general population. Lack of appreciation of risk, impaired social interactions, low levels of assertiveness, low use of condoms, injecting drug use, multiple partners,

and homelessness appear to be some of the reasons for the higher infection rates.

Higher rates of infection have not been reported in the few studies that have been conducted in developing countries, where the prevalence of HIV in people with mental illness has usually mirrored population prevalence. It is possible that because studies have primarily been done in closed systems of in-patient psychiatric institutions that people have been somewhat protected from the infection. However, once infection does take root within a closed system, the chances of widespread infection are increased. Given high-risk sexual behaviors in people with mental illness globally, higher rates in this grouping should be anticipated.

HIV Infection Affects the Central Nervous System

Infiltration of HIV into the CNS is common, often resulting in HIV dementia and minor cognitive disorder. HIV can be detected in the cerebrospinal fluid of over 90% of asymptomatic patients while 75% of AIDS patients have been found to have brain pathology at autopsy. Between 30% and 50% of HIV-seropositive individuals are estimated to experience some cognitive–motor problems (Grant *et al.*, 1999). HIV invades the brain early in the infection process and in a certain proportion of people psychotic symptoms manifest, especially in late-stage AIDS. Manic episodes are above the population norm in people with HIV (around 5%), especially at more advanced stages of the disease, and are the most common reason for psychiatric hospitalization in the HIV seropositive population in the United Kingdom.

Mental Disorders and HIV/AIDS

Studies of the mental health status of people infected with HIV have consistently found a higher prevalence of mental health problems than is found in community or clinical samples, ranging from relatively mild distress to a full mental disorder.

Mood disorder is the most frequent psychiatric complication associated with people with HIV/AIDS. High levels of major depression, mild depressive disorder and dysthymia have been found in seropositive individuals. Bing *et al.* (2001) found a 36% 1-year prevalence of depression among a large national sample of HIV-positive men and women in the US. In a meta-analysis of studies comparing HIV-positive and HIV-negative samples, Ciesla and Roberts (2001) showed that major depressive disorder occurred nearly twice as often among HIV-positive than HIV-negative patients. In a review of studies of mental health problems of HIV-infected people in developing countries, Collins *et al.* (2006) also found a significantly higher prevalence of depressive symptoms among HIV-positive people compared with controls.

Feelings of anxiety and distress are a normal and arguably even a healthy response to a diagnosis of HIV. However anxiety may reach clinical levels and impair overall functioning and people's capacity for adequate self-care. The prevalence of anxiety disorders in studies in the US range from negligible to around 40%. Anxiety can be provoked by the unpredictability of the virus and by certain milestones such as initial diagnosis, first opportunistic infection, declining CD4 count, or the onset or progression of an AIDS-defining illness.

Since the introduction of antiretroviral therapy (ART) in developed countries, the mental health and quality of life of people living with HIV/AIDS has improved considerably. Firstly, the progressive neuropsychiatric progression of HIV is diminished. Secondly people's psychological responses to living with HIV/AIDS are deeply affected by treatment. A number of cross-sectional as well as longitudinal studies have shown decreased depression for people on ART. However, there is other evidence that suggests that ART does not itself alleviate depression and that a diagnosis of HIV remains profoundly distressing for most people. In London, even though there was a significant decrease in the number of referrals for adjustment disorder and organic brain syndromes from pre-ART to post-ART eras, there was an increase in the proportion of people experiencing depressive disorders. People tended to have new problems and anxieties around forming relationships, disclosure, and demoralization around the side effects of medication.

Mental Disorder May Influence Health Behaviors

An HIV-positive person needs to engage in a number of behaviors to maintain good health. For example, he or she must engage in protected sex to avoid reinfection, eat nutritious food, refrain from excessive use of alcohol, seek treatment for opportunistic infections when needed and, if antiretroviral treatment is required, adhere to the medication regimen (95% adherence is needed). The person's psychological state is likely to affect his or her ability to engage in these behaviors.

As part of the HIV/AIDS Treatment Adherence, Health Outcomes and Cost Study Group, Uldall *et al.* (2004) reviewed over 50 studies that examined mental illness and substance abuse and the impacts on adherence. Mental health problems were found to be barriers to adherence in a number of community samples, for example in a population-based cohort and in a national probability sample of people living with HIV/AIDS engaged in primary care. This association has been found to be particularly significant in women. While the introduction of HAART in the US has reduced HIV-associated dementia, two studies have shown that mental flexibility was strongly associated with poor adherence. The effect of depression on HIV medication has also been extensively studied. At least eight studies have shown that adherence to antiretroviral medication is adversely affected by mood disturbance. A number of studies have reported associations between adherence and generalized anxiety disorder, panic disorder, PTSD, recent trauma, and social phobia.

Initial studies in Africa have pointed to high levels of ART adherence. However, in a recent analysis of African adherence research Gill *et al.* (2005) caution against complacency and conclude that adherence rates in Africa are in fact quite variable and often poor. They suggest that additional research is urgently needed to determine patient-level barriers. They also suggest that ways of increasing adherence levels need to be found. In some pilot treatment sites, people with mental health and substance-abuse problems have been excluded from programs in order not to compromise the program. While it is not clear to what extent such exclusion corresponds with program success rates, given that mental health and substance abuse have been regularly found to be barriers to adherence in developed countries, this relationship seems possible and needs further exploration.

Does Treatment of Mental Disorder Improve Adherence?

The evidence that mental health problems impair HIV treatment is far more comprehensive than the evidence available on treating mental health problems and thereby improving ART adherence. Nonetheless, there is some research that indicates efficacy resulting from mental health and psychosocial interventions.

According to Uldall *et al.* (2004), most of the interventions that have been designed to improve adherence have focused on cognitive-behavioral skills, such as helping individuals with remembering to take their medication and improving medication-taking self-efficacy, rather than treating mental health problems in order to improve adherence and overall health. However, a retrospective study based on pharmaceutical records found that antiretroviral adherence was higher for depressed patients who received antidepressant medication than those who did not. It was also higher for those who adhered to their psychiatric medication.

In a study on the impacts of self-efficacy on HIV viral load and distress in women living with AIDS, Ironson *et al.* (2005) showed an improved course of illness linked to their SMART/EST intervention. They suggest that this may be the effect of improved adherence linked to their intervention. One US study on severely nonadherent patients showed that continuous and personalized counseling improved adherence and virologic outcomes. Motivational interviewing has also been utilized to improve adherence, although with mixed results.

Side Effects of Medication

In a minority of patients, mania and psychosis can occur due to the AIDS medication they receive such as AZT, 3TC, efavirenz, abacavir, and nevirapine. People taking efavirenz may experience nightmares and have other paranoid symptoms. These usually resolve within 2–3 weeks but may persist. Patients who have had multiple episodes of depression are at particular risk of having negative reactions to efavirenz.

Cardiovascular Disease

The most common psychological attributes associated with persons with cardiac disease are type A behavior pattern (TABP). TABP is a predisposition to think, feel, and act in a time-urgent, aggressive, and impatient manner. This constellation of behaviors first reached the attention of researchers in the 1950s when two cardiologists, Friedman and Rosenman, observed that their heart patients behaved similarly to one another during clinic visits. Patients sat on the edge of their seats while waiting for appointments, as if they were ready to bolt at any instant. In fact, the waiting room seats became worn in a rather unusual way: only in the front. The original work on TABP was conducted in the 1970s (Friedman and Rosenman, 1974), and it was consistently found that the combination of cognitive, emotional, and behavioral predispositions was predictive of coronary heart disease. These predispositions included time urgency, impatience, aggression toward others, and a propensity toward hostility. In accounting for the relationship between TABP and CHD, it is thought that appraising the world in a time-urgent and hostile manner can lead to chronic psychosocial stress via a mechanism involving excessive sympathetic nervous system activation, which in turn leads to an exacerbation of coronary artery atherosclerosis.

While TABP is a well-documented antecedent of CHD, there have also been psychological effects of heart disease. Clinical depression is a prominent psychological feature of CHD patients and may be a strong predictor of death. In a large-scale national community survey, 52.1% of heart patients displayed symptoms of depression, and of these 30.1% met the criteria for clinical depression (Purebl *et al.*, 2006). However, other estimates have been somewhat lower. CHD patients who experience depression are considered to be at greater risk of dying of a subsequent heart attack than nondepressed patients. Various pathways between depression and CAD have been considered, including behavioral mechanisms that involve poor adherence to medical and behavioral recommendations, diminished heart rate variability, stress-induced ischemia, platelet activation, and immunological dysregulation (Faller, 2005). Studies of efficacy and effectiveness for depression have generally been conducted with non-CHD patients and have provided support for psychological treatments such as cognitive behavioral therapy and interpersonal therapy. In addition, aerobic exercise as a means to elevate mood may have additional benefits of addressing the cardiovascular condition from which patients suffer.

Cancer

While many of the psychosocial concerns of cancer are unique to the specific type of cancer, there are several common psychological and behavioral factors that define most oncology patients. Nezu and colleagues (1999) have systematically identified the psychological issues that patients may face when confronting cancer. When first detecting symptoms, the patient may experience anxiety and fear, which in some cases may lead to a delay in seeking a diagnosis. The task at hand in this early stage of illness is to seek the most appropriate and available medical attention. Upon diagnosis, many patients experience emotional distress, anxiety, anticipatory grief, and anger, have to engage with the stress of treatment decision making, and have to adjust to a new role and related responsibilities. The process of undergoing treatment may also in many cases present its own challenges.

Treatment requires the marshalling of effort, energy, and support in combating cancer, accompanied by anxiety and grief with the loss of well-being. Common treatments for cancer include chemotherapy, radiation therapy, and surgery. Chemotherapy is a systemic therapy that involves introducing medication into the body with the intention of destroying cancer cells. The side effects of chemotherapy occur because of the medication's inability to differentiate between cancerous cells and normal cells. Common side effects of chemotherapy include hair loss, mouth sores, diarrhea, nausea and emesis, loss of appetite, and fatigue. Radiation therapy is considered a local therapy in that it is directed at a specific area of the body that is affected by cancer. Similar to chemotherapy, radiation that destroys cancer cells may also harm noncancerous ones; thus side effects are usually related to the area of the body being treated. For example, radiation targeted at the abdomen may lead to diarrhea, while radiation directed at the mouth may lead to changes in taste and sensitivity. Surgery is a local treatment that usually involves the loss of body tissue that is affected by cancer, such as the breast, prostate, lung, or larynx. Many patients may experience anxiety prior to surgery and some may experience emotional difficulties related to their altered body image.

At posttreatment, many patients may be concerned with the fear of recurrence and anxiety as the health-care team may be less available to provide support.

Many patients who have been through treatment report re-evaluating their life priorities. Among patients who experience a recurrence of cancer, common emotional responses include disappointment, guilt, anxiety, anger, and grief. Treatment decision-making is accompanied by psychological adaptation to treatment and follow-up evaluation. When facing death from cancer that has metastasized to other parts of the body, common experiences among patients include fear of abandonment, suffering, and anxiety and sadness related to loss of control over their lives. Patients may engage in a re-evaluation of their lives and try to find meaning to their experience with cancer.

In general, emotional distress is commonly experienced by many cancer patients, especially when their diagnosis is unexpected. Specifically, symptoms of depression and anxiety are common, while psychiatric disorders such as major depression and posttraumatic stress disorder occur in a minority of patients. It has been argued that cancer patients are no more likely to experience major depression than general medical patients. In a study of psychiatric morbidity of breast cancer patients, the prevalence estimates of emotional distress, major depression, and generalized anxiety disorder were 29%, 9%, and 6%, respectively (Coyne et al., 2004). Distress among cancer patients may be most appropriately ameliorated with social and family support, information about treatment options, and psychological counseling. For the minority of patients who meet the criteria for a psychiatric disorder, psychotropic medication is likely to be appropriate.

Personality and Cancer

The question of whether personality factors play a role in precipitating the onset of cancer is controversial. The major proponent of the view that certain personality characteristics are associated with cancer is Hans Eysenck, who has conducted several studies on the so-called type C, or cancer-prone personality (Eysenck, 2000). According to Eysenck, persons at increased risk of developing cancer tend to be unassertive, harmony-seeking, unable to express emotions, and have difficulties in coping that may lead to helplessness and depression. There appear to be some data to support this contention. For example, in a prospective study in which a sample of 1353 healthy persons were followed for 10 years until death, personality traits that involved blocking of feelings and needs in important relationships appeared to be associated with certain cancers, most notably breast cancer (Grossarth-Maticek et al., 1997). Eysenck even went so far as to propose autonomy training to move personality characteristics away from type C tendencies (Eysenck, 2000).

On the other hand, results of other investigations have yielded null findings on the relationship of personality factors and carcinogenesis. In a prospective study

of 5133 adults, the incidence of cardiovascular disease was significantly predicted by emotional lability, behavioral control, and TABP, but the incidence of cancer was unrelated to these variables. In an examination of the relationship between personality factors and cancer, Amelang and Schmidt-Rathiens (2003) conclude that personality factors are of little importance and explain less than 2% of the health–disease variance. These authors have shown that the significance of these variables has decreased over the past several years, while the biomedical predictors of carcinogenesis have remained robust. The conclusion of this review is that 'hypotheses addressing the causal relationships between personality and disease are of little value' (Amelang and Schmidt-Rathiens, 2003: 22).

It may well be the case that certain personality factors predispose certain people to engaging in behaviors that place them at greater risk for developing certain kinds of cancer. For example, the relationship between smoking and lung cancer has been well documented. However, the case for personality characteristics as a carcinogenic or even constituting a risk factor for cancer remains unconvincing.

Diabetes

Psychological difficulties common among endocrine patients include poor adherence to medication and lifestyle regimens, poor adjustment to the illness, an exacerbation of medical symptoms by stress, and psychiatric problems such as depression and anxiety. Aikens and Wagner (2003) classified 65 consecutive referrals seen in a behavioral endocrinology service in terms of the primary presenting problem or the corresponding DSM-IV diagnosis: major depression (15%), adjustment disorder (8%), dysthymic disorder (8%), specific phobia (8%), regimen nonadherence (13%), and stress affecting diabetes mellitus (21%).

In most of the literature on the psychological and behavioral aspects of diabetes, treatment adherence is a salient theme. Medications that are prescribed following consultation with a medical professional are usually dispensed with an expectation of close to perfect adherence. Such expectations pertain to the dosage, timing, ingestion with specific foods, contraindications regarding ingestion with other medicines, and consistent adherence to the treatment regimen over time (World Health Organization, 2003). These details are of crucial importance in maximizing the health benefits from medical treatment. Patient nonadherence may therefore have severe implications for the control of symptoms, recovery time, quality of life, and mortality. Among the factors associated with adherence in diabetes patients are health literacy, social support, and emotional problems.

Health literacy implies an awareness of the importance of adherence even when actual symptoms are absent. Behavioral regimens such as restricted fat and sugar intake, exercise, and adherence to specific medications in many cases serve an important preventive function by controlling blood sugar and insulin levels. In the absence of overt symptoms, for many patients adherence may appear to be unimportant. Yet, the longer-term health consequences of nonadherence may be severe, as symptoms will inevitably develop.

Considerable research has demonstrated consistently that social support is a strong predictor of medical adherence. Social support for adherence is defined as encouragement from family and friends for the patient to cooperate with the recommendations and prescriptions of a health professional. The expression of concern and encouragement from others to engage in health-promoting behaviors, including medication adherence, combine with social desirability needs on the part of the patient to yield higher rates of medical cooperation. An issue related to social support, namely the relationship between the health-care worker and patient, has also been shown to be strongly associated with adherence. Data obtained by Roberts (2002) further suggest that medical providers viewed communicating with patients about adherence issues as an essential component of the health-care service. While the provider–patient relationship may ostensibly constitute an example of social support, it also extends beyond this. The health professional is often seen as a person of authority, in the possession of specific expertise that is unobtainable elsewhere, and as someone in whom the patient solely invests hope for assistance in the recovery process.

Emotional problems such as depression appear to be common among patients with diabetes. Depressive symptoms such as loss of interest in activities, decreased energy, fatigue, difficulties in concentrating, remembering and making decisions, and appetite disturbance may seriously affect the extent to which patients are adherent to their dietary and lifestyle regimens. Anxiety may be related to diabetes in at least three ways: Symptoms of anxiety may be produced by sympathetic nervous system responses to hyperglycemia; endocrine abnormalities may be exacerbated by normal physiological stress responses, and the psychological stress of living with a chronic illness and managing the challenging self-care tasks may have a general negative effect on mood. Hypoglycemic fear is also a concern for insulin-dependent diabetes patients as hypoglycemia is a highly distressing experience that can cause serious physical consequences that include unconsciousness, coma, and in extreme cases, death.

Somatic Symptoms Associated with Mental Illness

Somatic symptoms form part of the symptom picture of a number of psychiatric illnesses, most notably major depressive disorder. The symptoms of depression, for example, include weight loss or gain, sleep disturbance, and fatigue or loss of energy. When criterion contamination of this nature occurs, it may be suggested that physical symptoms are 'caused' by a mental condition. Such an appraisal may tend toward dualism and a distortion of a complex condition, which has both mental and physical features. Yet, from a treatment perspective it is essential to understand the etiological features of a disease.

In assessing patients for depression, the DSMIV-TR criteria stipulate that these symptoms should not be due to the direct effects of a medical condition, such as hypothyroidism. Hypothyroidism, a condition in which the body lacks sufficient thyroid hormone and is caused by the inflammation of the thyroid gland, is said to mimic the symptoms of major depressive disorder. The symptoms of hypothyroidism thus similarly include fatigue, weakness, weight gain or difficulty losing weight, depressed mood, irritability, memory impairment, and a decreased libido, which can cause difficulties for mental health professionals in distinguishing between the two conditions. There are clear implications for treatment if patients are misdiagnosed: Hypothyroidism is effectively treated with hormone therapy, while the most efficacious treatment for depression is a combination of antidepressant medication and psychological counseling. Among cancer patients as well, common somatic symptoms include pain, fatigue, weakness, and reduced energy. Symptoms such as these make the process of diagnosing depression and anxiety in cancer patients a complex process, again with important treatment implications.

On the other hand, there are somatic symptoms that are associated with a mental illness as well. In general, somatic symptoms of depression create diagnostic dilemmas in the assessment of patients with medical comorbidities because symptoms may be due to either the medical condition or depressive illness. In an effort to determine whether the etiology of somatic symptoms was due to an illness condition or mood disturbance among older patients, Drayer and colleagues (2005) showed that scores on measures of somatization, namely the Asberg Side Effects Rating Scale and the Utvalg for Kliniske Undersogelser (UKU), were significantly correlated with psychological symptoms of depression but not with medical comorbidities (Drayer et al., 2005). These authors recommended that when assessing medical disorders with multiple somatic complaints, clinicians should consider the possibility that such symptoms may be due to depressive illness rather than solely due to the medical disorder. Further, it may be necessary to assess the effects of antidepressant medication on somatic symptoms. For example, in a 32-week trial testing the effects of citalopram, a selective serotonin reuptake inhibitor, on somatic symptoms among patients with anxiety and anxious depression, it was concluded that somatic symptoms often improve with successful antidepressant medication management (Lenze *et al.*, 2005).

Health and Behavior Change

Health behavior is a key determinant of overall health, and a person's health behavior is in turn highly dependent on that person's mental health and psychological state. Many noncommunicable diseases such as cardiovascular disease and diabetes are linked to unhealthy behavior such as alcohol and tobacco use, poor diet, and a sedentary lifestyle. Health behavior is also an important determinant of communicable diseases through, for example, unsafe sex practices. Health-care-seeking behavior is similarly influenced by mental health. Three exemplars of theoretical models on health behavior change need mention.

Theory of Planned Behavior

The Theory of Planned Behavior (TPB) postulates that the likelihood of an individual engaging in a health behavior (for example, regular exercise) is correlated with the strength of his or her intention to engage in the behavior. A behavioral intention represents an individual's commitment to act and is itself the outcome of a combination of several variables. According to the TPB, the factors that directly influence intentions to engage in a health behavior include the person's attitudes toward the behavior, the person's perception of subjective group norms concerning the behavior, and the extent to which the person perceives him- or herself to have control concerning the behavior (Fishbein, 2002).

Health Belief Model

The Health Belief Model (HBM) hypothesizes that health-related behavior depends on the combination of several factors, namely, perceived susceptibility, perceived severity, perceived benefits, perceived barriers, cues to action, and self-efficacy. Perceived susceptibility refers to an individual's opinion of the chances of contracting the illness condition. Perceived severity refers to an individual's opinion of how serious a condition and its consequences are. Perceived benefits refer to one's belief in the efficacy of the recommended health behavior in reducing the risk or seriousness of the condition. Perceived barriers refer to the perception of cost associated with adhering to a recommended health behavior if it is likely to be beneficial in reducing or eliminating the perceived threat. Self-efficacy refers to the level of confidence in one's ability to perform the health behavior in question. Those persons who have low self-efficacy will have low confidence in their ability, which will have an effect on the likelihood of the behavior being performed. The HBM has been applied with considerable success to a range of health behaviors and populations, particularly preventive behaviors, such as diet, exercise, smoking cessation, vaccination, and contraception and sick role behaviors such as adherence to recommended medical treatments.

The Transtheoretical Model

This theory proposes that individuals progress through five interlocking stages in their effort to engage in health behaviors. Precontemplation is the time during which people are not seriously thinking about changing the behavior that will permit the attainment of better health. In this stage, individuals are either unaware or underaware of their health problems and the need to alter their behavior. During the stage of contemplation, people are aware that a health problem exists and have earnestly begun thinking about behavior change but have not yet committed themselves to taking action. The third stage of the model is preparation, in which the individual is preparing to enact the health behavior in question. The next stage is the action stage, when individuals are making unambiguous changes in their behavior, experiences, or environment in order to address health problems. The beginning of the maintenance stage is sometimes defined as 6 months following taking overt action to engage in the desired health behavior. Progression through the stages defined by the model is not necessarily linear since in many instances relapses occur and individuals return to either the precontemplation or contemplation stages before finally succeeding in maintenance.

Conclusion and Implications

In defining health as a state of complete physical, mental, and social well-being and not merely the absence of disease and infirmity, the countries involved in developing this World Health Organization definition of health in 1948 portrayed great insight and understanding of the components of health. It is unlikely, however, that at the time they realized just how interdependent all the elements in the definition in fact are to health and illness. These relationships are now becoming clearer. While much research is still needed to fully understand these relationships and mechanisms, conceptualizing the components as useful products of language that help explain different influences on health and well-being is an important step forward. Despite the evidence that the distinction between mental and physical health is permeable, in reality this distinction remains in the minds of many and in the health services of most countries. A number of shifts are needed to change this.

- Health worker education. The education of health workers rarely conceptualizes health as being a product of physical, mental, and social influences. Where this does happen, it is often in a linear manner. Even within many public health approaches where there is a growing emphasis on the social aspects of health, there is only minimal emphasis on the psychological or behavioral aspects. A comprehensive and integrated understanding of health needs to become the norm in order to change the way health workers think about and engage with their patients. Such an understanding should also result in health workers becoming more involved in prevention of health problems.

- Integration of mental and physical health care. The integration of mental health into general health care, where this has occurred, has been an important step forward in health-care treatment. However, this approach is still in its infancy, especially in developing countries. Separating physical and mental health services reinforces difference and mitigates against treating a whole person. Moreover, separation often leads to poorer accessibility of mental health services when, for example, only physical health care is provided at local clinics or hospitals.

- Stigma and discrimination. Mental health problems as well as some physical health problems, such as HIV/AIDS, are highly stigmatized in most countries and people are often discriminated against both by members of the public and health workers. Redressing stigma and discrimination is essential for good health within a population, as health seeking behavior and health service provision may be adversely affected. Stigmatization also negatively influences the course of illness.

- Promoting health-related behavior. The relationships between lifestyle and treatment behaviors and health are being increasingly recognized as fundamental. Integrating more of the behavioral sciences with the health sciences is a crucial step that needs to be taken boldly.

See also: Happiness, Health & Altruism; Mental Health and Physical Health (Including HIV/AIDS); Mental Health and Substance abuse; Stress and (Public) Health.

Citations

Aikens JE and Wagner LI (2002) A review of empirically-based psychological assessment and intervention procedures for adults with diabetes mellitus. *Advances in Medical Psychotherapy and Psychodiagnosis* 11: 59–74.

Amelang M and Schmidt-Rathjens C (2003) Personality, cancer and coronary heart disease: Fictions and fact in the etiological research. *Psychologische-Rundschau* 54(1): 12–23.

American Psychological Association (2001) Health Psychology, Mission Statement. http://www.health-psych.org/mission.php (accessed October 2007).

Bing EG, Burnam MA, Longshore D, et al. (2001) Psychiatric disorders and drug use among human immunodeficiency virus-infected adults in the United States. *Archives of General Psychiatry* 58: 721–728.

Ciesla JA and Roberts JE (2001) Meta analysis of the relationship between HIV infection and risk for depressive disorders. *American Journal of Psychiatry* 158: 725–730.

Collins PY, Holman AR, Freeman M, and Patel V (2006) What is the relevance of mental health to HIV/AIDS care and treatment programs in developing countries? A systematic review. *AIDS* 20: 1571–1582.

Coyne JC, Palmer SC, Shapiro PJ, Thompson R, and DeMichele A (2004) Distress, psychiatric morbidity, and prescriptions for psychotropic medication in a breast cancer waiting room sample. *General Hospital Psychiatry* 26: 121–128.

Dersh J, Polatin PB, and Gatchel RJ (2002) Chronic pain and psychopathology: Research findings and theoretical considerations. *Psychosomatic Medicine* 64(5): 773–786.

Drayer RA, Mulsant BH, Lenze EJ, et al. (2005) Somatic symptoms of depression in elderly patients with medical comorbidities. *International Journal of Geriatric Psychiatry* 20: 973–982.

Dworkin SF and Massoth DL (1994) Temporomandibular disorders and chronic pain: Disease or illness? *Journal of Prosthetic Dentistry* 72(1): 29–38.

Eysenck HJ (2000) Personality as a risk factor in cancer and coronary heart disease. In: Kenny DT, Carlson JG, McGuigan FJ and Sheppard JL (eds.) *Stress and Health: Research and Clinical Applications*, pp. 291–318. Amsterdam the Netherlands: Harwood Academic Publishers.

Faller H (2005) Depression. A prognostic factor in coronary artery disease/depression. *Psychotherapeut* 50(4): 265–273.

Fishbain DA, Cutler RB, Rosomoff HL, and Rosomoff RS (1997) Chronic pain-associated depression: Antecedent or consequence of chronic pain? A review. *Clinical Journal of Pain* 13(2): 116–137.

Fishbein M (2002) The role of theory in HIV prevention. In: Marks DF (ed.) *The Health Psychology Reader*, pp. 120–126. London: Sage.

Gatchel RJ (1996) Psychological disorders and chronic pain: Cause and effect relationships. In: Gatchel RJ and Turk DC (eds.) *Psychological Approaches to Pain Management: A Practitioner's Handbook.* New York: Guilford Press.

Gill C, Hamer D, Simon J, et al. (2005) No room for complacency about adherence to antiretroviral therapy in Sub-Saharan Africa. *AIDS* 1243–1249.

Grant I, Marcotte TD, and Heaton RK (1999) Neurocognitive complications of HIV Disease. *Psychological Science* 10: 191–195.

Grossarth-Maticek R, Eysenck HJ, Pfeifer A, Schmidt P, and Koppel G (1997) The specific action of different personality risk factors on cancer of the breast, cervix, corpus uteri and other types of cancer: A prospective investigation. *Personality and Individual Differences* 23(6): 949–960.

Ironson G, Weiss S, Lydston D, et al. (2005) The impact of improved self-efficacy on HIV viral load and distress in culturally diverse women living with AIDS: The SMART/EST Women's project. *AIDS Care* 17(2): 222–236.

Lenze EJ, Karp JF, Mulsant BH, et al. (2005) Somatic symptoms in late-life anxiety: Treatment issues. *Journal of Geriatric Psychiatry and Neurology* 18(2): 89–96.

Melzack OR and Wall PD (1982) *The Challenge of Pain.* New York: Basic Books.

Nezu AM, Nezu CM, Friedman SH, Faddis S, and Houts PS (1999) *Helping Cancer Patients Cope.* Washington, DC: American Psychological Association.

Purebl G, Birkas E, Csoboth C, Szumska I, and Kopp MS (2006) The relationship of biological and psychological risk factors of cardiovascular disorder in a large-scale national representative community survey. *Behavioural Medicine* 31(4): 133–139.

Roberts KJ (2002) Physician–patient relationships, patient satisfaction, and antiretroviral medication adherence among HIV-infected adults attending a public health clinic. *AIDS Patient Care and STDS* 16(1): 43–50.

Simon GE and VonKorff M (1991) Somatization and psychiatric disorder in the NIMH Epidemiologic Catchment Area study. *American Journal of Psychiatry* 148(11): 1494–1500.

Uldall K, Palmer N, Whetten K, and Mellins C (2004) Adherence in people living with HIV/AIDS, mental illness, and chemical dependency: A review of the literature. *AIDS Care* 16(supplement 1): S71–S96.

World Health Organization (2001) *Mental Health: New Understanding, New Hope.* Geneva, Switzerland: World Health Organization.

World Health Organization (2003) *Adherence to Long Term Therapies: Evidence for Action.* Geneva, Switzerland: World Health Organization.

Further Reading

Conner M and Norman P (1996) *Predicting Health Behavior: Research and Practice with Social Cognition Models.* Buckingham, UK: Open University Press.

Cournos F and Forstein M (eds.) (2000) *What Mental Health Practitioners Need to Know About HIV and AIDS.* San Francisco, CA: Jossey-Bass.

Engel G (1977) The need for a new medical model: a challenge for biomedicine. *Science* 196: 128–136.

Lipowski ZJ (1988) Somatization: The concept and its clinical application. *American Journal of Psychiatry* 14: 1358–1368.

Rozanski A, Blumenthal JA, and Kaplan J (1999) Impact of psychological factors on the pathogenesis of cardiovascular disease and implications for therapy. *Circulation* 99: 2192–2217.

Simon GE and VonKorff M (1991) Somatization and psychiatric disorder in the NIMH Epidemiologic Catchment Area study. *American Journal of Psychiatry* 148(11): 1494–1500.

Trimble M (2004) *Somatoform Disorders: A Medicolegal Guide.* Cambridge, UK: Cambridge University University Press.

Von Bertalanffy L (1969) *General System Theory: Foundations, Development, Applications.* New York: George Brazillier.

World Health Organization (2001) *Mental Health: New Understanding, New Hope.* Geneva, Switzerland: World Health Organization.

Mental Health and Substance Abuse

B Saraceno, M Funk, and V Poznyak, World Health Organization, Geneva, Switzerland

Introduction

An Increasing Burden of Disease Requiring an Effective Service Response

Around the world, it is estimated that at least 450 million people experience mental, neurological, or substance use disorders, including about 76 million experiencing alcohol use disorders and approximately 15 million, drug use disorders. One person in every four has been affected by a mental disorder at some stage during their life.

The disease burden of these disorders is enormous (**Figure 1** and **Table 1**), thus creating a devastating social and economic impact for individuals, families, and governments. In the year 2002 mental and substance use disorders accounted for 13% of the global burden of disease (WHO, 2004).

Although the burden is high, only a small proportion of people receive effective treatment and care (**Table 2**). A recent WHO study in 14 countries (Kohn *et al.*, 2004) has shown just how extensive is the treatment gap for mental health and substance abuse disorders. In high-income countries 35.5% to 50.3% of people suffering from serious mental health and substance use disorders did not receive treatment within the prior year. The corresponding range for low-income countries was even higher with 76% to 85% not receiving treatment. To reduce this treatment gap and the overall health burden, it is essential that services for mental, neurological and substance abuse disorders are put in place.

Relationship between Mental and Physical Disorders

Mental health is as important as physical health to the overall well-being of individuals. The data to substantiate this important relationship are becoming increasingly evident from studies examining comorbidity between mental and physical health problems.

Mental health and substance use disorders are often comorbid with many physical health problems such as cancer, HIV/AIDS, diabetes, tuberculosis, hepatitis, liver cirrhosis, and heart disease among others. For example, a review of studies (**Figure 2**) reports that the 1-year prevalence of depression in people living with HIV/AIDS can be as high as 44%; and as high as 33% in those people who have cancer. This is compared with the estimated 10% prevalence rates in the general population (Saraceno *et al.*, 2003). In addition, injecting drug use is one of the leading modes of HIV in the world (UNAIDS, 2006). In the United States in 1999 injecting drug users accounted for 18% of the reported HIV cases classified by a specific risk and at least 36% of all reported AIDS cases (CDC, 2001). The disability of individual sufferers and the burden on families increase with the number of comorbid conditions experienced. In addition, the presence of comorbidity has implications for the identification, treatment, and rehabilitation of affected individuals. For example, knowing that someone has diabetes or another relevant condition should lead the health

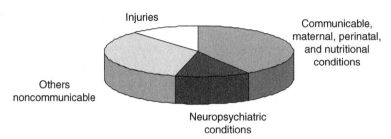

Figure 1 Distribution of disability-adjusted life years (DALYs) by causes (%). Changing history. *World Health Report 2004.* Geneva: World Health Organization.

Table 1   Distribution of disability-adjusted life years (DALYs) by causes (%)

Cause	Percentage
Communicable, maternal, perinatal, and nutritional conditions	41%
Neuropsychiatric conditions	13%
Others, noncommunicable diseases	34%
Injuries	12%

WHO (2004) *Changing History. World Health Report 2004.* Geneva, Switzerland: World Health Organization.

provider to conduct a mental health assessment to identify and treat any (previously unidentified) mental disorder. Finally, because mental disorders such as depression significantly reduce treatment compliance, treatment for the mental disorder can lead to greatly improved outcomes for the 'physical' health problem.

For overall health outcomes to be improved on the population level, interventions for mental health and substance use disorders must be accessible to those in need and have to be provided through services in general health care. Providers of these services should be able to identify mental and substance use disorders, understand the links between mental and physical disorders, and have the skills to address both dimensions for any one health problem.

Link between Poverty and Mental Health

Studies over the last 20 years indicate a close reciprocal association between poverty and mental ill-health (Patel, 2001). Not only can poverty increase the risk of developing a mental disorder but having a mental disorder can be an important factor leading people into poverty (**Figure 3**). Common mental disorders are about twice as frequent among the poor as among the rich (Patel *et al.*, 1999). In relation to severe mental disorders, and schizophrenia specifically, data from developed countries show that people with the lowest socioeconomic status (SES) have 8 times more relative risk for schizophrenia than those of the highest SES (Saraceno and Barbui, 1997).

It is therefore crucial that services are widely accessible to people with mental disorders including those living in poverty. The provision of effective treatment and care

can help people to recover and 'exit' the poverty in which they are living; however, this can only be achieved if services are accessible in terms of both physical reach and affordability. Providing ineffective treatment and care or services that go beyond the means of the individual concerned can act to drive them further into poverty. It is crucial that services are comprehensive and meet the variety of psychosocial needs of people with mental illness which are also required to bring them out of poverty (employment, education, social services).

Stigma and Human Rights Violations

People with mental and substance use disorders are stigmatized, excluded from society, and subject to human rights abuses. The stigma and misconceptions associated with mental disorders mean that people are marginalized and ostracized from society. People with mental disorders are often assumed to be lazy, weak, unintelligent, and incapable of making decisions, and these are common reasons why they are denied employment and education opportunities. In many countries people do not have access to the basic mental health care and treatment they require. Often the only care available is in psychiatric institutions which are themselves associated with gross human rights violations. People in these institutions are often exposed to inhuman and degrading living conditions, with little or no access to proper clothes, clean water, and food. They are also exposed to harmful practices such as the abusive use of seclusion and restraint.

Even when the physical environment of a mental health facility is adequate and clean with basic needs being provided for, neglect remains a key feature of institutional care. Many people receive no form of stimulation for months and even years. This aimlessness, inactivity, and social isolation is inhuman and degrading.

Services for mental health and substance abuse need to be respectful of human rights and the dignity of people with mental disorders and conducive to recovery. The treatment, care, and support provided must be comprehensive enough to meet the variety of psychosocial needs of those with mental illness that are required for re-integration into the community.

Table 2 Estimates of the median treatment gap (%) by mental health categories in each WHO region

Mental disorder	WHO region					
	Africa	Americas	Eastern Mediterranean	Europe	South-East Asia	Western Pacific
Schizophrenia	NA*	56.8	NA	17.8	28.7	35.9
Major depression	67.0	56.9	70.2	45.4	NA	48.1
Dysthymia	NA	48.6	NA	43.9	NA	50.0
Bipolar disorder	NA	60.2	NA	39.9	NA	52.6
Panic disorder	NA	55.4	NA	47.2	NA	66.7
Generalized anxiety	NA	49.6	NA	62.3	NA	55.6
Obsessive compulsive	NA	82.0	NA	24.6	NA	62.7
Alcohol abuse/dependence	NA	72.6	NA	92.4	NA	71.6

Kohn R, Saxena S, Levav I, and Saraceno B (2004) The treatment gap in mental health care. *Bulletin of World Health Organization* 82(11): 858–866.

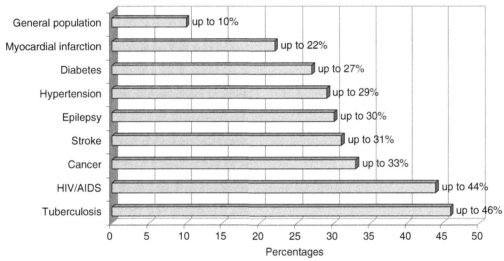

Figure 2 Major depression co-morbidity with physical illness. Saraceno B, Tarsitani L, and Fleischmann A (2003) *Public Health Implications of Depression* (WHO unpublished report).

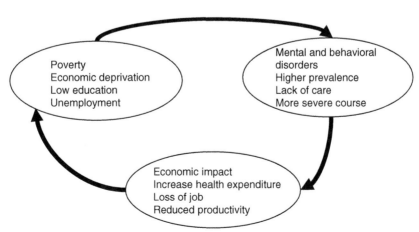

Figure 3 The vicious circle of poverty and mental disorders. Mental health: New understanding, new hope. *World Health Report 2001*. Geneva: World Health Organization.

Mental Health Service Organization

In many communities in countries all over the world, people are not able to access services and many of the available services are of poor quality. In low-income countries, the typical pattern of services is to have one or more psychiatric institutions based in urban areas and some informal community services provided by nongovernmental organizations (NGOs), traditional healers, spiritual healers, or religious groups. In middle- and high-income countries, it is not uncommon to find a predominance of institutional care services, although these countries have to varying degrees implemented a formal system of care involving community services, hospitals, and primary care.

WHO has developed a pyramid framework (**Figure 4**) which conceptualizes an *optimal mix of services for mental health*. It reinforces the idea that no single service will meet all needs, and that what is needed is an optimal mix of a range of services (Funk *et al.*, 2004).

According to this framework, and starting at the top of the pyramid, the least numerous services ought to be mental hospitals and specialist services, for example, psychiatric institutions and long-term residential treatment for alcohol and drug dependence. The second layer includes formal community mental health services (day care centers, outreach services, crisis services, and methadone clinics for opioid dependence patients) and general hospital-based services (psychiatric and substance abuse units in general hospitals). The third represents mental health services provided through primary health care. The fourth layer represents informal community mental health services, for example, traditional healers, village leaders, schoolteachers, and informal groups such as Alcoholics Anonymous or

Narcotics Anonymous. The fifth and final layer involves self-care management, that is, helping people to learn how to take care of themselves. Each of these levels is described in more detail in later sections of the article, including the strengths of and considerations for delivering care at that level.

Long-Stay Facilities

Psychiatric institutions and specialist services present the highest cost, yet are the least frequently needed service. Psychiatric institutions in both the developing and the developed world have a history of serious human rights violations. Clinical outcomes tend to be poor as a result of poor treatment and care practices and lack of rehabilitative activities in these hospitals. Where they exist, they consume most of the available specialist mental health resources and budget of the country, and this acts as a serious barrier to developing alternative or additional services.

Because of the high costs, often poor clinical outcomes, and human rights violations, mental hospitals represent the least desirable use of scarce financial resources available for mental health services (**Table 3**). Specialist residential services for alcohol and drug dependence may be needed for particular groups of clients and for most severe forms of substance use disorders, but their potential impact on population health is limited.

A very important recommendation of WHO is to replace psychiatric institutions by a network of services in the community. Essentially this means embarking on a process of deinstitutionalization – a planned and gradual transition from a predominantly institutionally based service model to a model that provides treatment and care

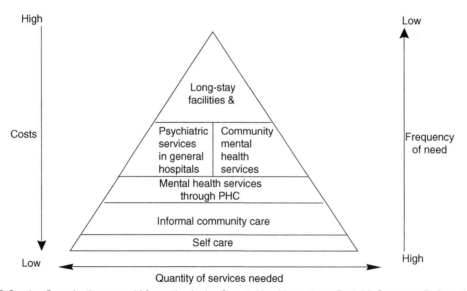

Figure 4   WHO Service Organization pyramid for optimal mix of mental health services. Funk M, Saraceno B, Drew N, Lund C, and Grigg M (2004) Mental health policy and plans: Promoting an optimal mix of services in developing countries. *International Journal of Mental Health* 33(2): 4–16.

Table 3 Approximate proportion of psychiatric beds in different settings in each WHO region and the world*

WHO regions	Mental hospitals (%)	General hospitals (%)
Africa	73.0	21.4
Americas	80.6	10.3
Eastern Mediterranean	83.0	8.8
Europe	63.5	21.8
South-East Asia	82.7	11.2
Western Pacific	60.1	34.5
World	68.6	19.8

*Other beds may be located in private and military hospitals, hospitals for special groups of population, long-term rehabilitation centers, etc.
WHO Mental Health Atlas 2005. Geneva: World Health Organization.

through community services, general hospitals, and primary health care.

The failure of many countries to make sure that these services are in place when psychiatric institutions close has led to problems of marginalization and homelessness.

Formal Community Mental Health Services

Within this category formal community mental health services refer to day centers, rehabilitation services, hospital diversion programs, mobile crisis teams, therapeutic and residential supervised services, and home help and support services that are based in the community.

Strengths

Providing community services has been shown to result in better physical health and mental health outcomes and better quality of life than treatment provided in institutions. In addition, shifting patients from mental hospitals to care in the community has been shown to be cost effective and ensures a better promotion and protection of the rights of people with mental and substance use disorders.

Considerations

First, the development of community services can require a vast and highly skilled group of professionals, thereby limiting the capacity of many countries to immediately put in place an extensive network of services. As a result, planners need to prioritize the development of some services, while developing others in a phased manner over time.

A second consideration in prioritizing the development of some community services over others is to identify the existing resources in the country. For example, in some countries fewer services such as halfway houses or group homes may be needed because of the availability of good family support. In situations like these planners need to acknowledge and actively support the efforts of families in caring for persons with mental disorders, rather than

working to build new group homes. Finally, community mental health services work best when they have strong links with general hospitals, primary health-care services, and informal community services.

Mental Health Services in General Hospitals

Another important WHO recommendation is to develop mental health services in general hospital settings. A common example of a service is a health unit within the general hospital itself, but this category also refers to other services such as consultation liaison services provided in the hospital. Specialist mental health professionals or general health workers with specialist training in psychiatry generally deliver these types of services.

Strengths

One of the most important advantages of this type of service is that it provides a setting to manage acute episodes of mental disorders. Second, there is the opportunity to simultaneously obtain medical treatment for comorbid physical illnesses, and it also allows access to specialist investigations and treatment. Third, the hospital can become a base for undergraduate and postgraduate teaching and training for many different types of health professionals, from physicians and nurses to psychiatrists, psychologists, and social workers.

Considerations

It is important to keep in mind some of the limitations of these services. Although general hospital services (short-stay wards and consultation-liaison services to other medical departments) can manage acute episodes of mental disorders quite well, they do not provide a solution for people with chronic disorders who end up in the admission–discharge–admission cycle (revolving door syndrome) unless backed up by comprehensive primary health-care services or community services. Second, their location generally, in district headquarters and big cities, can create access problems especially in developing countries which lack good, reliable, and cheap public transportation services.

Mental Health Services in Primary Health Care

Integration of mental health care into primary health care has been a fundamental WHO policy since the Alma Ata Declaration in 1978 and continues to be so. Services referred to in this category refer to mental health care and promotional and preventive activities conducted by health workers at the first level of formal health care; for example, general practitioners, nurses, and other staff providing assessment, treatment, and referral services for mental and substance use disorders. Early identification and management of hazardous and harmful drinking is a good example of an activity at the level of primary health care that, if widely implemented, can have a significant effect on population levels of alcohol-related problems (Whitlock *et al.*, 2004).

Strengths

As discussed in relation to general hospital care, providing treatment for mental and substance use disorders in primary health care improves access to mental health services and specialist services for substance use disorders as well as to treatment of comorbid physical conditions. Additionally, stigma is reduced – and acceptability for users improved – when seeking mental health care from a primary health-care provider. In terms of clinical outcomes it has been found that, for most common mental disorders, primary health care can deliver good care and certainly better care than that provided in psychiatric hospitals. From a management perspective, integrating health services for mental and substance use disorders into primary health care can be an important solution to addressing human resource shortages in the delivery of mental health interventions.

Considerations

Integration requires a lot of careful planning and there are likely to be several issues and challenges that will need to be addressed. For example, integration into primary health care requires investment in the training of staff to detect and treat mental and substance use disorders. Ongoing supervision is also of utmost importance, and mental health professionals should be available to primary care staff, as required, to give advice as well as guidance on management and treatment of people with mental and substance use disorders.

The issue of availability of time needs to be addressed. In many countries primary health-care staff are overburdened with work as they are expected to deliver multiple health-care programs. Governments cannot ignore the need to increase the numbers of primary health-care staff who are either partially or entirely devoted to mental health care.

Informal Community Mental Health Services

These refer to services provided in the community but that do not form part of the formal health and welfare system. These may include, but are not limited to, services delivered by traditional healers and professionals in other sectors (social and village/community workers, teachers, police) as well as services delivered by nonprofessional organizations or lay persons (such as consumer and family associations, advocacy groups, and NGOs).

Strengths

In many countries, informal community services are the first point of contact for a majority of persons with mental and substance use disorders and sometimes they represent the only service available to them. These services can play an important supportive role in improving outcomes for persons with mental disorders. They can help maintain community integration and provide a supportive network which reduces the risk of relapse. These services enjoy high acceptability and there are few barriers to access as they are nearly always based in the community. The high degree of community acceptability also reduces the likelihood of stigma associated with using these services.

Considerations

Informal community mental health services should not form the core of mental health service provision and countries would be ill-advised to depend solely on these services. Rather they form a useful complement to formal mental health services and can form useful alliances with such services.

There is also the issue of the quality of these services given that many currently fall out of the ambit of regulation in many countries. Indeed, it is not uncommon to find services providing either ineffective or inappropriate and harmful care. In many instances, human rights violations are committed.

Self-Care

The level of self-care refers to individuals' knowledge and skills to manage their mental health disorders on their own or with the help of family and friends.

Strengths

The service level of self-care acknowledges the role and autonomy of individuals (and families) to deal with their own psychological or mental health problems given access to the right information and guidance. Low-cost resources – for example, written materials or radio programs – can be used to promote self-care in the community.

Considerations

Problems related to mental health and substance use vary widely in complexity and severity, and medical and other professional expertise are essential for some of the more severe and complex cases. However, for all cases, the provision of information and support goes a long way in helping people take control of their illness and reduce their dependence on the health system.

Key Principles for Organizing Services

Even if the 'ideal' service organization model, as depicted in **Figure 4**, is adopted, it would not result in optimal treatment and care for persons with mental and substance use disorders unless a number of key 'principles' for organizing services are respected. These include the need to have services and care that promote accessibility, comprehensiveness, effectiveness, continuity and coordination, needs-led care, equity, and respect for human rights.

To deliver a high standard of mental health treatment and care, it is necessary to adopt an integrated system of service delivery that comprehensively addresses the full range of psychosocial needs of people with mental and substance use disorders (WHO, 2003).

Accessibility

Essential mental health care, including both outpatient and inpatient care, should be available locally so that people do not have to travel long distances. Accessibility also implies that services should be affordable and acceptable. Barriers to access include stigma and discrimination; low awareness of available services; a lack of well-organized primary mental health care; inadequate links between services; inadequate mental health training of primary health-care staff; and poor identification of cases in the community. Sometimes legislative barriers prevent development of effective services, such as substitution therapy programs for people with opioid dependence.

Comprehensiveness

Persons with mental and substance use disorders need and can benefit from a range of different coordinated services incorporating the use of case management, multidisciplinary teams, crisis intervention, assertive outreach, patient advocacy, and practical support as well as a range of treatment options. In addition to dealing with acute/chronic 'health' needs of persons, services need to address longer-term community integration needs, such as social services, housing, education, and employment. Collaboration with other sectors is essential in this regard.

Continuity and Coordination of Care

Health systems in most countries, and especially those in developing countries, are designed to provide health care on the basis of the throughput model. This emphasizes the importance of vigorous treatment of acute episodes in the expectation that most patients will make a reasonably complete recovery without a need for ongoing care until the next acute episode. Many mental and substance use disorders, especially those with a chronic course or with a relapsing–remitting pattern, are better managed by services that adopt a continuing care model. This emphasizes the long-term nature of the disorders and the need for a continuing therapeutic input.

A continuing care approach also emphasizes the need to address the totality of patients' needs, including their social, occupational, and psychological needs. Such approaches therefore require the coordination of patients' medical and social care needs in the community and collaboration between different care agencies.

Needs-led Care

To be effective, it is essential that mental health services be designed on a needs-led basis rather than on a service-led basis. This means adapting services to users' needs, and not the other way round. Too often, services are developed and run primarily from a managerial perspective and users have to adjust to the peculiar structures of the services they need to access.

Effectiveness

Service development should be guided by evidence of the effectiveness of particular interventions and models of service provision. For example, there is a growing evidence base of effective interventions for many mental disorders, among them depression, schizophrenia, and alcohol and opioid dependence. In addition, there is growing evidence of the effectiveness of treatment and care based on the community and the general hospital.

Equity

People's access to services of good quality should be based on need. Equity means that all segments of the population are able to access services and that possible inequities are taken into account. For most policy makers, the improvement of equity involves working toward greater equality in outcomes or status among individuals, regardless of the income group to which they belong or the region in which they reside.

Respect for Human Rights

International human rights norms and standards should be respected when providing services for people with mental disorders. People with mental and substance use disorders have the same civil, economic, political, social, and cultural rights as everyone else in the community and these rights should be upheld.

Variables Influencing Service Organization and Provision

The exact form of service organization ultimately depends on a number of wider contextual variables related to the country's social, cultural, political, and economic contexts.

In this section we define a 'model' in which different, but sometimes interrelated, wider societal variables interplay to influence service organization for mental health. The model has a number of implications, one of which is that changing the mental health system toward that described in the WHO service organization pyramid will require a number of paradigm shifts. These paradigm shifts and interventions to support them are discussed in the next section.

Essentially the model defines four important groupings of variables. The first grouping refers to the level of *resources* of a country at large and the resources specifically devoted to the mental health system. In this context it is important to note that resources and economic development can differ considerably throughout the country, leading to vast differences in service systems, for example, between different states and between urban and rural areas.

We know that a minimal level of resources is required to provide an effective mental health system. Low-income countries, sometimes, just do not have the required resources to build effective and responsive mental health systems. Having said that, a country can be a middle- or even a high-income country but still have a poorly functioning mental health system because mental health is not considered a priority for investment. Furthermore, although low economic development is a barrier to a well-functioning mental health system, some poor countries or poor areas within countries have been able to develop some innovative services. Often these make use of 'freely' available resources in the community as opposed to 'more costly' services available in the formal health system.

What is also interesting is that the more resources a country has to invest in their mental health system the more influential other variables, such as the prevailing paradigm for mental health, become in shaping that system.

Essentially, the prevailing *paradigm* for mental health, the second grouping of variables in this model, will greatly influence the formation of mental health service providers and clinical practice in countries. To date, there have been two distinct approaches: the biomedical approach and the psychosocial approach. The biomedical approach has been the most predominant, and continues to influence service delivery structures in most parts of the world. Its limitations are that it focuses exclusively on the physical aspects of mental disorders and not enough on psychosocial dimensions. Its influences are seen in the mental health system in terms of an over-reliance on hospital care at secondary and tertiary levels.

The psychosocial approach, in contrast, recognizes that successful treatment requires attention to biologically based treatments within the context of a broader approach to ensure that people with mental disorders are integrated into the community and leading as normal lives as possible. Where a psychosocial orientation or model operates in countries, the mental health system tends to be better geared toward the lower end of the WHO pyramid, that is, community mental health services, primary health care, and informal community services.

The third grouping refers to the *value system* of countries, for example, the relative importance given to individual rights and collective norms and the degree to which value systems are directed toward human rights, equality, equity, and so on.

Countries in which social control is an important feature and in which individual needs are seen as insignificant in comparison are more likely to provide a mental health system reliant purely on institutional care. In these scenarios, services as well as clinical practice are based more on ideology than evidence. Here the problem is not necessarily that there is an absence of care – in fact, in some of these countries mental health-care facilities and providers can be numerous – but that the care provided is limited to institutions emphasizing control and containment rather than rehabilitation. This is the type of care that WHO actively discourages.

Countries in which value systems emphasize human rights as well as equality and equity tend to provide mental health systems that are more (1) protective of individuals and their rights, (2) responsive to individual needs, and (3) likely to have structures in place to offer some degree of protection against violations and discrimination.

The fourth grouping of variables refers to the *environment*, for example, the degree to which both the political and economic environments provide long-term *stability or instability*. Countries undergoing rapid change, economic and political crisis, and civil war are likely to experience ongoing disruptions to any existing mental health system, and in serious conflict situations a total destruction of the existing system of care, at the very time when mental health needs are likely to be greatest. The end result of these influences is chaos, lack of coordination, and unregulated care, paralleled by greater emphasis on informal community services, a greater reliance on the private sector, NGOs, and aid programs. On a more positive note, in the rebuilding of systems following crises, the classic inhibiting factors for change, such as historical patterns of funding, no longer prevail, and so open up new opportunities to leave behind the negative and inefficient aspects of old systems in order to move toward more efficient mental health system models.

Changing the Paradigm – Important Roles of Training, Policy, and Legislation

The knowledge base for putting in place a comprehensive mental health system is now available. Systems limited to a few large mental asylums in the main urban areas, disconnecting hospitalized people with mental disorders from their family and community, and run by a small number of overburdened health workers, are no longer acceptable. However, whereas mental health care has undergone major changes toward community-based care in some countries during the past 50 years, the majority have not been able to achieve this.

Worldwide, there remains a widespread need in many countries to radically shift models of mental health care, not only in terms of the practical organization of services but in terms of the mental health-care paradigm itself. Radically reforming or introducing new models of training and policy and legislation can help promote the required paradigm shift.

Shift from a Biomedical to a Biopsychosocial Approach

An important shift is required to move from a biomedical model to a biopsychosocial model. The evidence indicates that mental and substance use disorders result from a complex interaction of biological, psychological, and social factors and that treatment options based solely on a biomedical approach are failing because they have not addressed the psychological and social dimensions. Health-care providers need to adopt treatment approaches that (1) actively involve the patient in his or her treatment and care plan, (2) educate the main care provider or family on how to support the patient, and (3) provide for rehabilitation support, vocational support, social support, and any other intervention that may be required to help persons reintegrate into their community.

Shift to Multidisciplinary Teams

In order to take into account the many dimensions of mental health, treatment and care should no longer be delivered by any one mental health professional alone but by a multidisciplinary team, which, depending on the country, might include psychiatrists, psychologists, nurses, general practitioners, occupational therapists, and community/social workers sharing their expertise and working in collaboration, each with their own roles and responsibilities. There also needs to be collaboration between mental health teams and other non-health providers in health, welfare, employment, criminal justice, and education sectors in order to meet the range of needs that people with mental disorders might have.

Reforming Education and Training Models

Radically reforming or introducing new models of training can help promote the required paradigm shift. In many developed and developing countries, the education curriculum for health and allied health professionals contains limited content in mental health. Much of what is provided is focused on institutional models of care, the diagnosis of disorders, and administration of medication, while essentially ignoring other important mental health issues and aspects of treatment. Outdated curricula act to reinforce existing and outdated mental health paradigms.

Essential to building a qualified workforce for mental health is the incorporation of mental health into the education of a wide spectrum of health workers and professionals, with mental health concepts introduced early, reinforced and expanded throughout the curricula, and developed through experiential learning opportunities. Education and training should be informed by evidence for the mental health and service requirements of the country. In most countries this requires the reorientation of the treatment framework from custodial institutional models of mental health care to community-based treatment, emphasizing the integration of mental health into general health care and the development of community care alternatives. In addition to building knowledge and skills, for example, communication and interpersonal skills training also needs to promote fundamental changes in the attitudes and beliefs of those being trained and the promotion of a human rights approach to treatment and care.

Changes to Policy and Legislative Framework

The necessary reform of services and the required paradigm shift in the attitudes, beliefs, and values of policy makers and planners can be promoted by the introduction of modern national policies and legislation in line with best practice and international human rights standards. The mental health policy of a government is the official guideline for a number of interrelated strategic directions for improving the mental health of a population, including an important focus on service delivery. A policy provides the overall direction for mental health in a country by defining the vision for the future, and the values and principles on which the vision is based, and by establishing objectives and a model for action (WHO, 2005a). A mental health plan is the operational arm of the policy and details the strategies and activities that will be implemented to achieve the objectives of the policy.

Both strategies and activities are complementary and useful tools to (1) promote development of mental health services or their reform, such as the integration of mental health into primary health care, development of community mental health services, and deinstitutionalization; (2) promote access to services in urban, rural, and poor areas and to underserved populations in a way that is affordable; and (3) improve the overall functioning of services – by, for example, committing to put in place a well-equipped workforce, good-quality treatment practices, and mental health and substance abuse information systems.

Mental health policies and plans should promote effective preventive and treatment interventions for substance use disorders within the health system; however, in addition, public health policies aimed at controlling alcohol and other substances are also required.

Mental health legislation is also a very powerful tool in that it can be used to legally reinforce these policy objectives. In addition, because it is legally enforceable and penalties can be applied it can be an effective mechanism to reduce human rights violations and discrimination, promote human rights in services and the community, and encourage autonomy and liberty of people with mental disorders (WHO, 2005b).

Despite the important role that policy and plans can have, we know that 38% of countries do not have a mental health policy, and even more countries have policies that are not implemented or that do not reflect best practice. In addition, 22% of countries do not have any mental health legislation, 57% have legislation that is more than 10 years old, and 15% have legislation dating to the pre-1960s, before most of the currently used treatment methods became available (WHO, 2005c).

The combined effects of outdated policy and legislation are to preserve outdated thinking about people with mental disorders as incapable and 'crazy,' unable to make decisions for themselves, or as 'criminals' when related to people with drug dependence. It reinforces the use of outmoded treatment methods and institutional services and actively denies people their human rights. Modernizing policy and legislation is therefore of utmost importance to establish and enforce the basic requirements for service development, quality of care, and respect of human rights, and can as a consequence lead to changes in fundamental attitudes and beliefs and the required paradigm shift.

Citations

CDC (2001) *HIV Prevention Strategic Plan Through 2005.* Atlanta, GA: Centers for Disease Control and Prevention (CDC).

Funk M, Saraceno B, Drew N, Lund C, and Grigg M (2004) Mental health policy and plans: Promoting an optimal mix of services in developing countries. *International Journal of Mental Health* 33(2): 4–16.

Kohn R, Saxena S, Levav I, and Saraceno B (2004) The treatment gap in mental health care. *Bulletin of World Health Organization* 82(11): 858–866.

Patel V (2001) Poverty, inequality and mental health in developing countries. In: Leon D and Walt G (eds.) *Poverty, Inequality and Health*, pp. 247–262. Oxford, UK: Oxford University Press.

Patel V, Araya R, De Lima M, Ludermir A, and Todd C (1999) Women, poverty and common mental disorders in four restructuring societies. *Social Science and Medicine* 49(11): 1461–1471.

Saraceno B and Barbui C (1997) Poverty and mental illness. *Canadian Journal of Psychiatry* 42(3): 285–290.

Saraceno B, Tarsitani L, and Fleischmann A (2003) *Public health implications of depression.* (WHO unpublished report).

UNAIDS (2006) *Report on the Global AIDS Epidemic.* A UNAIDS 10th anniversary special edition. Geneva, Switzerland: UNAIDS.

Whitlock EP, Polen MR, Grenn CA, Orleans T, and Klein J (2004) Behavioural counseling interventions in primary care to reduce risky/harmful alcohol use by adults: A summary of the evidence for the U.S. preventive services task force. *Annals of Internal Medicine* 140: 557–568.

WHO (2001) *Mental Health: New Understanding, New Hope.* World Health Report 2001. Geneva, Switzerland: World Health Organization.

WHO (2003) *Organization of Services for Mental Health.* Mental Health Policy and Service Guidance Package. Geneva, Switzerland: World Health Organization.

WHO (2004) *Changing History.* World Health Report 2004. Geneva, Switzerland: World Health Organization.

WHO (2005a) *Mental Health Policy, Plans and Programmes* (updated version). Mental Health Policy and Service Guidance Package. Geneva, Switzerland: World Health Organization.

WHO (2005b) *Stop Exclusion, Dare to Care: WHO Resource Book on Mental Health, Human Rights and Legislation.* Geneva, Switzerland: World Health Organization.

WHO (2005c) *WHO Mental Health Atlas 2005.* Geneva, Switzerland: World Health Organization.

Further Reading

Cohen A (2001) *The Effectiveness of Mental Health Services in Primary Care: The View from the Developing World.* World Health Organization. Geneva, Switzerland: Nations for Mental Health.

WHO (1990) *The Introduction of a Mental Health Component into Primary Health Care.* Geneva, Switzerland: World Health Organization.

WHO (2002) *Mental Health Global Action Programme (mhGAP): Close the Gap, Dare to Care.* Geneva, Switzerland: World Health Organization.

WHO (2003) *Investing in Mental Health.* Geneva, Switzerland: World Health Organization.

WHO (2003) *Planning and Budgeting to Deliver Services for Mental Health.* Mental Health Policy and Service Guidance Package. Geneva, Switzerland: World Health Organization.

WHO (2004) *Neuroscience of Psychoactive Substance Use and Dependence.* Geneva, Switzerland: World Health Organization.

WHO (2005) *Human Resources and Training in Mental Health.* Geneva, Switzerland: World Health OrganizationMental Health Policy and Service Guidance Package.

WHO (2007) *Research and Evaluation.* Mental Health Policy and Service Guidance Package. Geneva, Switzerland: World Health Organization.

Relevant Websites

http://www.cdc.gov/hiv/pubs/prev-strat-plan.pdf – Centers for Disease Control and Prevention (CDC).

http://www.unaids.org/en/HIV_data/2006Global Report – UNAIDS.

http://www.who.int/mental_health – World Health Organization (WHO).

http://www.who.int/substance_abuse/publications/en/Neuroscience.pdf – World Health Organization (WHO).

http://www.who.int/whr – World Health Organization (WHO).

Mental Health Epidemiology (Psychiatric Epidemiology)

G S Norquist, University of Mississippi Medical Center, Jackson, MS, USA
K Magruder, Medical University of South Carolina, Charleston, SC, USA

Overview

Background

Epidemiology (derived from the Greek *epi* meaning upon, *demos* meaning people, and *logos* meaning study) is the study of factors that influence the occurrence, distribution, prevention, and control of diseases and other health-related events in human populations. It provides a framework that helps public health officials identify important health problems, their magnitude and causative factors.

Epidemiology has been traditionally an observational science of populations but more recently newer areas in the field (e.g., clinical epidemiology) have initiated interventions in populations. By determining the personal characteristics and environmental exposures that increase risk for disease, epidemiologists identify individual risks and assist in the development of public health policy to alleviate personal and environmental exposures. They have helped to understand the factors that influence the risk of developing chronic diseases such as schizophrenia.

A variety of types of studies are used in epidemiology. The most common found in mental health are cross-sectional (prevalence) studies. Data from such studies have been used to determine levels of need, to identify groups that are at highest risk for disease, and to determine changes over time in the occurrence of disorders. Such data are particularly informative in public policy for allocating resources and developing public health prevention strategies. More recently, psychiatric epidemiology has focused on determining better ways to classify people into more homogeneous disease groups to focus interventions into populations in which they will be most successful. In addition, the field has sought to determine risk factors (including biological and social) for the development of disorders to promote future efforts at prevention. One of the key issues is identification of the factors that are responsible for the occurrence of a particular mental health problem.

The purpose of this article is to provide a general overview of epidemiology in the mental health area. The term mental health in this article refers to conditions defined in the *Diagnostic and Statistical Manual of Mental Disorders* (DSM) and the *International Statistical Classification of Diseases and Related Health Problems* (ICD) *Classification of Mental and Behavioral Disorders*. Thus, it will refer to disorders that are sometimes called psychiatric or neuropsychiatric (including substance use disorders).

The article presents key examples of methods and assessment instruments used in mental health epidemiology. However, a detailed review and discussion of epidemiologic methods and instruments is beyond the scope of this article. For such details, the reader is referred to several textbooks on mental health epidemiology listed in the 'Further reading' section.

History

The early period of epidemiology is marked by a focus on health issues related to the growing industrial revolution in Europe. Public health officials were concerned with general social reform and the effects of overcrowding in urban industrial areas, with an emphasis on sanitary conditions. In the mental health area, there was concern that environmental toxins were the cause of disorders. For example, mercury was considered a cause of psychosis and lead exposure was suspected as a contributor to mental disorders. One of the early founders of epidemiology, William Farr, was among the first to study mental illnesses. He studied the physical condition of inmates in English asylums in the early part of the nineteenth century. During this time, many thought there was a virtual epidemic of mental illness but another important figure in epidemiology, John Snow, insisted the increase was more likely the result of an increase in detection rather than a true increase in incidence.

The second period in the development of epidemiology began around the start of the twentieth century and focused on germs as a cause of disease. Epidemiology became virtually synonymous with the study of infectious diseases. One of the causes of insanity identified during this time was the late effects of syphilis. Discovery of the spirochete that causes this illness led to the development of the first medication to stop this infectious agent (Salvarsan 606). Although emphasis was placed on finding infectious agents, there were some epidemiologists at this time who studied other causes of disease. One notable finding during this time was the association of nutritional deficiency with the occurrence of pellagra. Initially it was thought to be due to an infectious agent but studies in institutionalized populations (including those in mental institutions) led to the association with nutritional deficiency.

After the Second World War, infectious diseases started to decline in the higher-income countries. However, those countries realized the increasing importance of non-communicable diseases such as cardiovascular disease. This led to a move away from consideration of single etiologic factors and to the consideration of various risk factors that could lead to disease development. New methods such as cohort and case-control designs were developed to identify these risk factors. Mental illnesses were also considered to be chronic noncommunicable disorders, but initial epidemiological work in psychiatry focused more on counting disease in community surveys rather than the study of risk factors. Thus, there were very few cohort or case-control studies in the early part of this era that focused on mental illnesses. Most of the studies in mental health during the initial years of this period were unstructured face-to-face field surveys with poor reliability.

In the late 1970s during the Carter administration in the United States, a special commission on mental health called for a study to obtain information on mental illness across the United States. Around the same time, the third edition of the *Diagnostic and Statistical Manual* (DSM-III) was published in the United States. It moved toward use of explicit criteria to make a diagnosis and increased the reliability of making such diagnoses. This standard nomenclature made it possible to develop measures that could be used in large community surveys.

Substance abuse had for some time not been considered a true disorder but rather a weakness of character or a personality disorder. However, after the Second World War it was recognized as a major public health problem, and the field sought to quantify it through assessments that focused on alcohol and drug use disorders. As a result of this effort, the significant impact of such disorders has now been recognized as well as the frequent comorbidity with other psychiatric disorders.

In recent years, mental health epidemiology has expanded to include attention to genetics and the molecular basis of disease. This has brought more attention to determination of biological risk factors through the field of genetic epidemiology. Attention has also been focused on social processes that can affect exposure to risk factors. This field of social epidemiology seeks to understand how social factors might influence differences in health status across populations.

Methods

Issues for Mental Health

One of the major problems in psychiatric epidemiology has been the difficulty in measuring mental and substance abuse disorders reliably and validly. Determination of a case is made on the basis of symptoms and not clear objective signs like a biopsy result. Because diagnosis is dependent on symptom reports from individuals there can be significant problems with biased reporting (both over- and underreporting). A key concern is the lack of objective, well-defined biological markers of mental illness.

There are continuing debates in the field about how to define the presence of an illness and whether there should be categorical definitions or use of a dimensional model. A dimensional approach focuses on a collection of symptoms and involves a quantitative assessment of the number of symptoms a person has from a few to many. Another approach is to define pathology in terms of a syndrome. In this scheme, a pattern of symptoms may include essential symptoms and others associated with the syndrome. This type of scheme takes the duration of symptoms into consideration and may include severity of the symptoms and resulting disability. Depending on the types of symptoms present, the duration and disability, a syndrome may be considered to be present or absent. Thus, this becomes a dichotomous measure (present or absent) and the resulting conditions are placed into categories of disorders.

Other problems in making diagnoses in mental health are the changes in symptoms over time, even without treatment, and the potential for recall bias (i.e., failure to remember past symptoms). The latter is a particular problem when trying to assess lifetime diagnoses. Stigma may also affect what a person reports about his/her behavior. Some people may not want to report symptoms due to embarrassment and may not come forward for treatment.

Terms

Below are listed some common terms used in psychiatric epidemiological studies. Familiarity with these will aid the reader in understanding such studies. A more detailed description of the various epidemiologic terms can be found in resources listed in the section titled 'Further Reading.'

- Case: This represents the presence of a mental or substance abuse disorder in a person.
- Case registry: A database of people with a defined mental and/or substance use disorder. It may include other data such as demographic and clinical treatment information.
- Comorbidity: This is the presence in a person of at least two different disorders. It may be used to represent the occurrence of somatic or psychiatric disorders and simultaneous or lifetime occurrence.
- Control group: This is a group of people who are used as a basis for comparison to another group. Depending on the study design, control subjects do not receive the experimental intervention or are healthy and do not possess the disorder or risk factor in question.
- Incidence: This represents the number of new cases or events that occur during a particular period of time.

- Odds ratio (OR): A measure of the odds of an event/disorder occurring in one group compared to the odds of the event/disorder occurring in another group. Thus, an odds ratio of one (1) means that the event/disorder is equally likely to occur in both groups. If the odds ratio is greater than one (>1), then the event/disorder is more likely to occur in the first group. If less than one (<1), then the event/disorder is less likely to occur in the first group.
- Predictive value of a test: The positive predictive value of a test or screen is the proportion of all people who test positive on a screen who actually have the disorder being screened. The negative predictive value is the proportion of all people who test negative on a screen who do not have the disorder being screened.
- Prevalence: This represents the number of cases/events that exist during a particular period of time. This figure would include both new cases (incidence) and those that were already present but still existed during the defined period of time. It is expressed in terms of the period of time defined to contain the cases or events. Thus, point prevalence would be the prevalence at a specific point in time. Period prevalence would expand the time over which cases or events could be present. For example, one might have one month, 6 months, 12 months (1 year), or lifetime prevalence. Period prevalence is used more often these days in mental health epidemiology because the diagnosis of mental disorders requires the occurrence of symptoms over periods of time.
- Risk factor: This is something that increases the chance for development of a disorder or the occurrence of an event. It is important to note that it is not necessarily causal but rather associated with the disorder or event. There may also be more than one risk factor for a given disorder and a particular combination of such factors may be necessary before a disorder develops. Risk factors can be inherent in the individual (e.g., age and gender) or they may represent an exposure (e.g., substance abuse, economic status).
- Reliability: This is the degree to which any particular measure produces consistent results even among different raters of the measure. Reliability is often a problem in making diagnoses of mental and substance abuse disorders.
- Sensitivity: This represents the proportion of people with a disorder in a population who are identified correctly by a screen or test as having a disorder.
- Specificity: This represents the proportion of people without a disorder in a population who are identified correctly by a screen or test as not having a disorder.
- Validity: This is the extent to which any given indicator of a disease actually represents the presence of that disease. In psychiatry, the gold standard against which validity is most often measured is the diagnosis made by a clinician.

Assessment

Background

The field of psychiatric epidemiology has developed various ways to assess and diagnose mental disorders. Some early studies used direct observation and assessment by clinicians. However, with the growing need for larger community surveys, it became too expensive to use clinicians to make every assessment. As a result, survey instruments were developed that could be used by either clinicians or trained lay interviewers to provide reliable diagnoses of mental illnesses.

Before considering the specific instruments used to measure mental disorders, it is important to understand how such disorders are determined. In psychiatric epidemiological studies, disorders are assessed usually through a set of defined questions. The set of questions is known as an instrument or test and can be divided into two types: A scale or schedule. An instrument can be administered through direct observation by a clinician, through trained lay interviewers, or self-report by the subject.

A scale is sometimes called a screen and usually focuses on the dimensional aspect of pathology. Responses to items or questions on a scale are given individual values and when added provide a score. The presence of pathology is determined by this overall score.

A schedule is more comprehensive and complex than a scale and determines various diagnoses through a structured set of questions. Some instruments have been designed to be administered by trained lay people (i.e., nonclinicians) in community settings. In addition, schedules determine if the symptoms are present at the time of the interview or occurred at some other point in time. They are designed to contain a variety of disease modules so one can opt to assess a selected number of diagnoses. Some are designed so a respondent who answers negatively to certain stem questions for a particular disease can skip the rest of the module.

Concern has been raised about the validity of schedules used in epidemiological studies. They may overestimate the prevalence of disorders, especially if compared to assessments made by clinicians. However, some recent studies seem to indicate clinician assessments may actually result in a larger number of identified cases (i.e., a higher prevalence) unless one looks only at recent symptoms when clinician assessments may have lower estimates of pathology. In addition to concerns about reliability and validity, a major issue is whether dimensional or categorical measurement is better. The concern is that categorical measurement is too restrictive and human behavior is not so easily divided into strict categories. Yet, dimensional measures such as scales often use cut points and thus create categories, while categorical measures involve some dimensional qualities.

Most branches of medicine use categorical diagnoses; thus such approaches are compatible with general medical diagnostic practice.

Instrument development

During the Second World War, several scales were developed to assess psychopathology such as the Maudsley Personality Inventory in the United Kingdom. The first structured interviews were conducted in two community surveys shortly after the Second World War. These were the Stirling County Study and the Midtown Manhattan Study. They used the Health Opinion Survey and the Twenty-Two Item Scale, respectively. Yet, the studies did not rely on the instruments for final diagnoses. Instead, they had psychiatrists review the results from the instruments. In spite of some differences in the way the two studies assessed psychiatric conditions, they both reported that about 20% of people had a mental disorder.

President Carter's Commission on Mental Health called for national information on psychiatric disorders and use of mental health services in the United States at the start of the 1980s. This led to the development of the Epidemiologic Catchment Area (ECA) study, the first national epidemiologic survey for psychiatric conditions in the United States. The Diagnostic Interview Schedule (DIS) was developed for use in the ECA. It was the first complex diagnostic schedule designed to be used in a community study and set the stage for future epidemiologic surveys around the world.

Around the time of the ECA study, the WHO collaborated with the U.S. Alcohol, Drug Abuse and Mental Health Administration to assess the state of international diagnosis and classification. A product of this collaboration was the development of a new instrument, the Composite International Diagnostic Interview (CIDI). This instrument is highly structured and does not allow interviewers to interpret responses, as was allowed in some early international studies that used the Present State Examination (PSE) developed in the United Kingdom. One version of the CIDI, the UM-CIDI, was used in the U.S. National Comorbidity Survey (NCS). The CIDI has been used in a variety of international epidemiologic surveys, including national surveys in Australia and Norway. The latest version is being used in the World Mental Health Project, which is attempting to provide an international estimate of mental disorders and the disability associated with them.

Instruments have also been developed for use in various clinical settings (e.g., primary care settings). The most prominent of these is the General Health Questionnaire (GHQ). Other instruments designed for this setting are the Personal Health Questionnaire, the Patient Health Questionnaire, the Medical Outcomes Study 36-Item Short Form Health Survey (SF-36), and the Primary Care Evaluation of Mental Disorder (PRIME-MD).

Other instruments have been designed to allow clinicians to make reliable assessments of patients in clinical settings. Among the most prominent of these is the Hamilton Rating Scale for assessment of depressive symptoms. Others include the Schedule for Affective Disorders and Schizophrenia (SADS) and the Structured Clinical Interview for DSM-III-R (SCID).

The selection of an instrument depends on what one wants to do with it. For example, if one wants to compare community data to those being collected around the world the choice at this time is the CIDI as it is being used in the largest international study to date.

Study Designs

Here are described the common study designs and examples of each related to mental health and substance abuse. The most common design used in traditional mental health epidemiological studies is the cross-sectional (prevalence) survey.

Nonexperimental or observational

In these types of studies, an investigator does not have control over exposure to an intervention or risk factor in any particular group. There are three basic types summarized here.

Cross-sectional (prevalence) surveys

In this type of study, one selects a population and determines the presence or absence of a disease or exposure to a risk factor by assessing the subject at a single point in time. The subject may be asked about past events but is not followed for any period of time. The classic epidemiological surveys in psychiatry have been cross-sectional in design (e.g., the ECA study). These studies are useful in determining the mental health status and service needs of community populations. A variety of techniques are used to sample community populations for such studies (e.g., stratified random sampling). A few of these cross-sectional studies have had additional follow-up interviews with subjects (e.g., the Stirling County Study). Such studies with a repeated assessment could be considered a hybrid design.

In addition, the type of instrument used in a cross-sectional survey can vary. One might create a case registry such as that used by the National Health Insurance in the United Kingdom. These could use assessments by both clinicians and individually administered instruments. However, a typical design is to administer an instrument to every subject from a survey population. A less expensive option is a two-stage design in which people are first given a short instrument (e.g., a scale) and those who test positive are then given a more thorough instrument to assess psychopathology.

Case-control study

In this type of study, one selects two different groups to compare. One is a group of people with the condition one wants to study (cases) and the other is a group of people who are as similar as possible to those people with the condition, except they do not have the condition (controls). One looks back in time to determine whether the two groups had different exposure to risk factors of interest. Although these types of studies are subject to potential biases (e.g., selection bias), they are relatively inexpensive and can be conducted quickly. For rare disorders, it is an efficient study design. If a case-control study indicates a finding of interest it can be tested through more rigorous methods such as a cohort study.

Cohort study

In this type of study, people are selected to be observed over time. These are usually conducted in a prospective (forward) fashion with disease-free subjects but can be done in a retrospective (backward) time fashion as long as the temporal sequence of exposure predating disease onset can be established. In contrast to case-control studies, groups are not defined by the presence of a disease, but rather by the presence of a risk factor or exposure and subjects are followed over a period of time. During the time of study, one looks for the development of new cases (incidence) and attempts to connect exposure to certain risk factors with the development of the disorder. These studies require large numbers of people since only a small number are likely to develop the condition of interest and thus can be quite costly and take long periods of time. Nevertheless, cohort studies can establish without question that risk factors predated disease onset and are an important strategy in epidemiology.

Experimental

Clinical trials

These types of studies are also known as randomized controlled clinical trials (RCTs). In this type of study, people are allocated randomly to either a group that receives an experimental intervention or a group that does not receive the intervention. Thus, the investigator can control both the distribution of subjects into comparison groups and the experimental condition for a group. By using random assignment, one can reduce greatly or eliminate the potential for selection bias. In addition, raters are usually blinded to the experimental intervention and in many studies placebos are used. Some recent clinical trials have utilized hybrid designs in which subjects are given some choice of the intervention and no placebo is used.

Studies and Results

Listed below are the designs of some of the most influential recent epidemiological studies in mental health. This is followed by a summary of results from these and some other studies. The reader is referred to the published full reports of the studies for comprehensive details and results.

Recent Studies

Epidemiologic Catchment Area Study

The Epidemiological Catchment Area (ECA) Study, funded by the U.S. National Institute of Mental Health, was launched in the early 1980s to assess the prevalence of mental and substance use disorders in the United States and the use of mental health services. Instead of a national probability sample, the ECA used five specific geographic regions in the U.S. to select population samples. Two waves of data were collected from subjects. The first wave started around 1980 and the second wave was collected 1 year later, with the last site finishing in the mid-1980s. The first wave had a combined sample size of a little over 20 000 people and the second wave was not able to assess about 21% of the first sample. It used the Diagnostic Interview Schedule (DIS) to obtain diagnoses for the major DSM-III diagnoses through trained lay interviewers in face-to-face community interviews. This was a ground-breaking study in that it was the first to use structured complex diagnostic interview schedules to obtain estimates of community mental health.

National Co-Morbidity Survey-Replication

This study is a replication of a similar study (National Co-Morbidity Survey) conducted in the early 1990s on a national sample in the United States. The National Co-Morbidity Survey-Replication (NCSR) is part of the World Mental Health Surveys described in the next section and was funded by the U.S. National Institute of Mental Health. It is a nationally representative (United States), cross-sectional household survey of people aged 18 and older. Interviews were conducted in person from 2001 to 2003 by trained lay interviewers using the WMH-CIDI. The response rate was approximately 71%, and the sample size was a little over 9200 people.

National Epidemiologic Survey on Alcohol and Related Conditions

The U.S. National Institute of Alcohol Abuse and Alcoholism launched a nationally representative survey of people 18 years and older in 2001. The National Epidemiologic Survey on Alcohol and Related Conditions (NESARC) study has two waves of data collection with the first wave completed in 2001–02. Although the survey is of noninstitutionalized populations, it did make an effort to include people who live in housing units more likely to have higher substance use patterns (e.g., shelters and group homes). The response rate for the first wave (81%) was much higher than previous surveys.

The survey used the Alcohol Use Disorder and Associated Disability Interview Schedule-DSM-IV version (AUDADIS-IV). This is a state of the art structured diagnostic interview that is designed to be used by lay interviewers. This instrument was designed to be more accurate than previous instruments in assessing alcohol and substance use disorders. The survey conducted face-to-face interviews with over 43 000 people across the United States.

WHO World Mental Health Surveys
In 1998 the WHO established the World Mental Health Survey (WMH) Consortium to address the limitations of previous surveys of mental health disorders around the world. Prior surveys were unable to adequately assess severity of disorders, interviews used in the surveys were not standardized to allow cross-national comparisons, and the majority of surveys were in high-income countries, thus limiting their generalizability to other areas of the world. The Consortium expanded the CIDI (WMH-CIDI) to include questions that would assess severity, impairment, and treatment. Surveys were then launched in 28 countries in each region of the world, including low-income countries.

Each area is using the WMH-CIDI, a fully structured diagnostic interview that uses trained lay interviewers to obtain information. Age of subjects varies by country, but the most common range is 18 and older. Sample sizes vary by country but all used multistage household probability sampling. Response rates have varied so far from lows around 45% to highs of about 88%. There are differences in the demographics, with some sites having young and less educated populations.

Global Burden of Disease
In the early 1990s, the WHO supported a study that was the first to use epidemiologic data and projections of disability from various disorders to estimate the public health burden of various medical disorders. The purpose of the study was to quantify the years of healthy life lost as a result of disease in the various countries of the world. The identified measure for this is known as DALYs (disability-adjusted life years) and incorporates death and disability from a disorder. This study, known as the Global Burden of Disease (GBD) study, had a significant influence on the perception of the impact of various disorders. Prior estimates had indicated infectious diseases were the most important causes of public health problems. However, this study, which considered not only mortality from a disease but the burden imposed by living with disability from the disease, changed the perception of which diseases were the most important in terms of impact on public health. Chronic diseases with significant effects on long-term disability (e.g., major

depression) now were considered more important from a public health perspective than had previously been projected. There were a number of criticisms about the methodology of the study and concerns about miscalculations of the impact of certain diseases (e.g., HIV/AIDS).

These projections were updated recently by the WHO to consider more current epidemiological data on burden of disease and mortality. In addition, the update moved from considering projections by only the eight regions of the world to project at the country level and then aggregated the results into regional and income-level groups. The various diseases and injury causes were grouped into three levels: Group I (communicable, maternal, nutritional causes), Group II (noncommunicable diseases), and Group III (injuries).

Data on Mental Illness and Substance Use Disorders

Table 1 shows a comparison of data from the three most prominent studies in the United States and a meta-analysis of studies conducted in Europe and the initial findings of the European component of the WHO World Mental Health Surveys. It is important to note that one cannot make clear comparisons across these studies as the time of data collection was different, the samples are obviously different, and the methods varied. However, despite these differences, it is remarkable that estimates are very close in some diseases. The obvious exception is the report from the ESMeD study, which has lower 12-month prevalence estimates. It is not clear why this would be the case, but it represents a summary of data from several European countries and if one looks at the range for those countries (**Table 2**) there is significant variation. In addition, there were some initial problems in the survey implementation in these countries that could have resulted in lower estimates. The meta-analysis represented in the column labeled Europe presents median estimates and the range is variable for these, especially alcohol dependence, depression, and specific phobia. For substance abuse, the figures from the NCS-R study are probably low because the module used to obtain these diagnoses did not consider responses to questions about dependence in those who did not respond positively to abuse questions.

Table 2 shows the first data from the WHO-Mental Health Survey (WMH). The estimates vary across countries despite similar methodology. However, there are likely to be cultural differences in the interpretation of the questions and the concept of mental illness. In addition, the stigma attached to mental illness and substance abuse may be greater in some areas and impede responses to such questions. An issue that often arises in any mental health survey is a concern that the disorders reported do not represent significant clinical problems. Thus, recent surveys such as the WMH have attempted to measure severity and

Table 1   Twelve-month prevalence of mental and substance use disorders (percent of study population)

	ECA	NCS-R	NESARC	Europe[e]	ESMeD[g]
Any mood disorders	9.5	9.5	9.3	9.1	4.5
Major depression	5.0	6.7	7.2	6.9	4.1
Dysthymia	[a]	1.5	1.8		1.1
Mania	1.2	0.6	1.7	0.9	
Any anxiety disorders	12.6	18.1	11.1	12.0	8.4
Panic disorder	1.3	2.7	2.1	1.8	0.7
Social phobia	2.1	6.8	2.8	2.3	1.6
Specific phobia	10.9	8.7	7.1	6.4	5.4
Generalized anxiety disorder	[b]	3.1	2.1	1.7	0.9
Any substance use disorder	9.5	3.8	9.3	3.4[f]	
Any alcohol use disorder	7.4	3.1[c]	8.5		1.0
Any drug use disorder	3.1	1.4[d]	2.0		
Any disorder	28.1	26.2		27.4	11.5

[a]All sites did not assess 12-month prevalence for dysthymia.
[b]All sites did not assess generalized anxiety disorder.
[c]Alcohol abuse only; see text.
[d]Drug abuse only; see text.
[e]Figures are median values from meta-analysis of multiple studies.
[f]Dependence only (excludes abuse).
[g]Figures are from recent update analysis except dysthymia and alcohol use which are from original analysis.
Data from: Regier DA, Narrow WE, Rae DS, *et al.* (1993) The de facto US mental and addictive disorders service system: Epidemiologic catchment area prospective 1-year prevalence rates of disorders and services. *Archives of General Psychiatry* 50: 85–94 (ECA); Kessler RC, Chiu WT, Demler O, *et al.* (2005) Prevalence, severity, and comorbidity of 12-month DSM-IV disorders in the national comorbidity survey replication. *Archives of General Psychiatry* 62: 617–627 (NCS-R); Grant BF, Stinson FS, Dawson DA, *et al.* (2004) Prevalence and co-occurrence of substance use disorders and independent mood and anxiety disorders. *Archives of General Psychiatry* 61: 807–816 (NESARC); Wittchen HU and Jacobi F (2005) Size and burden of mental disorders in Europe – A critical review and appraisal of 27 studies. *European Neuropsychopharmacology* 15: 357–376 (Europe); Alonso J and Lepine J (2007) Overview of key data from the European study of the epidemiology of mental disorders (ESEMeD). *Journal of Clinical Psychiatry* 68: 2, 3–9 (ESMeD).

disability. The WMH initial reports show variation in severity and disability but in some settings more than 50% of the cases are of serious or moderate severity. Days out of work are much higher for those with serious disorders than those classified as having mild severity.

Data on Comorbidities

Among the interesting findings from recent studies is the recognition that mental disorders and substance use disorder are comorbid at higher levels than was previously expected. The NESARC study found that 20% of people with a current substance use disorder also had a mood disorder. These disorders appear to be independent and not substance induced. Such findings on co-morbidity are important as they point to the need to assess and provide services for both mental and substance abuse disorders when a person is seen initially for one or the other disorder. There are no current data to clarify this increased co-morbidity among mental and substance abuse disorders. One may lead to the onset of the other type of disorder, there may be common genetic or environmental causes or the methods used to assess these disorders may overestimate co-morbidity. An understanding of these linkages could aid in development of preventive and treatment interventions for co-morbidity.

Burden of Disease Data

One can see in **Table 3** that noncommunicable diseases (Group II) are the most important causes of disease burden. By the year 2030, Group II causes are expected to have a greater impact on overall burden of disease around the world than Group I (communicable) causes. **Table 4** shows that major depression becomes a significant factor in the overall burden of disease regardless of a country's income level.

Although these updated projections address some of the criticism of the original Global Burden of Disease Study, there are still limitations to the study. Recent epidemiological studies such as the WHO-WMH study have improved what data are available for mental health, but there are still problems in the quality of such epidemiological data across regions. In addition, measures of disability are not ideal and projections are based on present data and various assumptions about future disease that could change with time. Thus, although data such as these are helpful for planning distribution of future health services, they must be interpreted with caution.

Service Use Data

Many of the epidemiological studies have assessed use of mental health services. As can be seen in **Table 5**, large

Table 2   Twelve-month prevalence of World Mental Health Composite International Diagnostic Interview/*Diagnostic and Statistical Manual of Mental Disorders*, 4th edn.[a]

Country anxiety mood impulse-control substance any (95% confidence interval)

Country	Anxiety	Mood	Impulse control	Substance	Any
Americas					
Columbia	10.0 (8.4–11.7)	6.8 (6.0–7.7)	3.9 (3.2–4.7)	2.8 (2.0–3.7)	17.8 (16.1–19.5)
Mexico	6.8 (5.6–7.9)[b]	4.8 (4.0–5.6)	1.3 (0.9–1.8)[e]	2.5 (1.8–3.3)	12.2 (10.5–13.80)
United States	18.2 (16.9–19.5)	9.6 (8.8–10.4)	6.8 (5.9–7.8)	3.8 (3.2–4.5)	26.4 (24.7–28.0)
Europe					
Belgium	6.9 (4.5–9.4)	6.2 (4.8–7.6)[d]	1.0 (0.3–1.8)[e]	1.2 (0.6–1.9)[j]	12.0 (9.6–14.3)
France	12.0 (9.8–14.2)	8.5 (6.4–10.6)[d]	1.4 (0.7–2.0)[e]	0.7 (0.3–1.2)[j]	18.4 (15.3–21.5)
Germany	6.2 (4.7–7.6)	3.6 (2.8–4.3)[d]	0.3 (0.1–0.6)[e]	1.1 (0.4–1.7)[j]	9.1 (7.3–10.8)
Italy	5.8 (4.5–7.1)	3.8 (3.1–4.5)[d]	0.3 (0.1–0.5)[e]	0.1 (0.0–0.2)[j]	8.2 (6.7–9.7)
Netherlands	8.8 (6.6–11.0)	6.9 (4.1–9.7)[d]	1.3 (0.4–2.2)[e]	3.0 (0.7–5.2)[j]	14.9 (12.2–17.6)
Spain	5.9 (4.5–7.3)	4.9 (4.0–5.8)[d]	0.5 (0.2–0.8)[e]	0.3 (0.0–0.5)[j]	9.2 (7.8–10.6)
Ukraine	7.1 (5.6–8.6)[b,c]	9.1 (7.3–10.9)[d]	3.2 (2.4–4.0)[f,g,h]	6.4 (4.8–8.1)[j]	20.5 (17.7–23.2)
Middle East/Africa					
Lebanon	11.2 (8.9–13.5)	6.6 (4.9–8.2)	1.7 (0.8–2.6)[f,h]	1.3 (0.0–2.8)	16.9 (13.6–20.2)
Nigeria	3.3 (2.4–4.2)	0.8 (0.5–1.0)	0.0 (0.0–0.1)[f,g,h]	0.8 (0.3–1.2)[j]	4.7 (3.6–5.8)
Asia					
Japan	5.3 (3.5–7.0)[b]	3.1 (2.2–4.1)[d]	1.0 (0.4–1.5)[f,g,h,i]	1.7 (0.3–3.0)	8.8 (6.4–11.2)
People's Republic of China					
Beijing	3.2 (1.8–4.6)[b]	2.5 (1.5–3.4)	2.6 (1.3–3.9)[f,g,h]	2.6 (1.2–3.9)	9.1 (6.0–12.1)
Shanghai	2.4 (0.9–3.9)[b]	1.7 (0.6–2.9)	0.7 (0.4–1.1)[f,g,h]	0.5 (0.3–0.6)	4.3 (2.7–5.9)

[a]Anxiety disorders include agoraphobia, generalized anxiety disorder, obsessive-compulsive disorder, panic disorder, posttraumatic stress disorder, social phobia, and specific phobia. Mood disorders include bipolar I and II disorders, dysthymia, and major depressive disorder. Impulse-control disorders include bulimia, intermittent explosive disorder, and reported persistence in the past 12 months of symptoms of three child-adolescent disorders (attention-deficit hyperactivity disorder, conduct disorder, and oppositional-defiant disorders). Substance disorders include alcohol or drug abuse or dependence, respondents who met full criteria at some time in their life and who continue to have any symptoms are considered to have 12-month dependence even if they currently do not meet full criteria for the disorder. Organic exclusions were made as specified in the *Diagnostic and Statistical Manual of Mental Health Disorders*, 4th edn., but diagnostic hierarchy rules were not used.
[b]Obsessive-compulsive disorder was not assessed.
[c]Specific phobia was not assessed.
[d]Bipolar disorders were not assessed.
[e]Intermittent explosive disorder was not assessed.
[f]Bulimia was not assessed.
[g]Attention-deficit hyperactivity disorder was not assessed.
[h]Oppositional-defiant disorder was not assessed.
[i]Conduct disorder was not assessed.
[j]Only alcohol abuse and dependence were assessed. No assessment was made of other drug abuse or dependence.
From WHO World Health Survey Consortium (2004) Prevalence, severity and unmet need for treatment of mental disorders in the World Health Organization world mental health surveys. *Journal of the American Medical Association* 291: 2581–2590. Copyright (2004) American Medical Association. All rights reserved.

numbers of people with a mental disorder during a 1-year period do not seek medical care for such services. Obviously, such data will differ according to the ability to access such services and the stigma attached to using them. However, it is interesting to note that even within countries that provide universal coverage there is still a large amount of unmet need (low use in those with disorders). The studies also looked at the use of a variety of other service sectors (including nontraditional providers). Such data show that even though significant numbers of people use other service sectors for mental health care there are still large numbers of people with a disorder who do not seek care anywhere. Those least likely to use services are the elderly, men, people without resources such as insurance, and those living in rural areas where care is not readily available.

Future Needs

Assessments and Methods

The field of mental health epidemiology has come a long way in the past 100 years, with tremendous growth since the end of the Second World War. Key to this expansion has been the development of explicit criteria for diagnostic assessment. These have increased reliability in making diagnoses and facilitated the development of instruments that can be used in large-scale community surveys. However, a number of issues still confront the field. Among the most prominent is the issue of diagnostic validity. Efforts are underway currently to update the DSM and ICD classification systems. That process has initiated discussions about the best ways to classify mental and substance abuse disorders and whether a more dimensional approach should be considered. Given the growing findings from basic neuroscience and genetics about potential biological causes of mental disorders, there is a need to connect this information with future diagnostic classifications. Collection of biological data in epidemiological studies could help to further this connection.

In addition to classification by symptoms, more attention should be focused on other aspects of disorder such as disability. A number of efforts are already underway in this area, but better assessments of severity, disability, and quality of life are needed. For many people with mental and substance abuse disorders, the most important end points in treatment are improvement in functional status and quality of life, not just a reduction in symptoms.

Table 3 Leading causes of DALYs (world)

2002	2030
1. Perinatal conditions	1. HIV/AIDS
2. Lower respiratory tract infections	2. Unipolar depressive disorders
3. HIV/AIDS	3. Ischemic heart disease
4. Unipolar depressive disorders	4. Road traffic accidents
5. Diarrheal disease	5. Perinatal conditions
6. Ischemic heart disease	6. Cerebrovascular disease
7. Cerebrovascular disease	7. COPD
8. Road traffic accidents	8. Lower respiratory tract infections
9. Malaria	9. Hearing loss, adult onset
10. Tuberculosis	10. Cataracts

From Mathers CD and Loncar D (2006) Projections of global mortality and burden of disease from 2002 to 2030. *PLoS Medicine* 3: 11: e442.

Previous studies have focused on cross-sectional looks at populations with very few cohort studies. Although they are less costly and perhaps easier to conduct, these prevalence studies have major limitation when trying to determine risk factors for development of disorders. Thus, the field needs to launch large cohort studies that would help delineate the various risk factors (biological, individual, environmental, and social) and the interplay among them. Only more comprehensive information is likely to lead us to a better understanding of the natural history of mental disorders and the various etiological factors that are involved in their development.

More international collaboration would be helpful. Previous studies have shown the importance of mental and substance abuse disorders as public health problems throughout the world. There is much to learn from different regions and standardization of assessments and classification systems together with collaborative large multinational studies would move the field much further.

Topics

A number of recent studies have looked at the interface between mental disorders and other medical disorders such as cardiovascular disease. More work in this area would help to delineate the impact of mental health on other medical disorders and vice versa. This could lead to new interventions for the prevention and early intervention of medical disorders that are co-morbid with mental health disorders.

Given the increasing attention to genetic factors in disease, genetic epidemiological studies in mental health offer an opportunity to understand the complex linkage between genes and environment. Recent work has shown that the presence of certain genes together with certain environmental exposures increases the risk for development of depression. Studies that address the impact of genes on response to pharmacological or psychotherapeutic interventions in the presence of particular environmental exposure would help to revolutionize treatments in mental health.

Table 4 Leading causes of DALYs (2030) by country income ranking

High income	Middle income	Low income
1. Unipolar depressive disorders	1. HIV/AIDS	1. HIV/AIDS
2. Ischemic heart disease	2. Unipolar depressive disorders	2. Perinatal conditions
3. Alzheimer and other dementias	3. Cerebrovascular disease	3. Unipolar depressive disorders
4. Alcohol use disorders	4. Ischemic heart disease	4. Road traffic accidents
5. Diabetes mellitus	5. COPD	5. Ischemic heart disease
6. Cerebrovascular disease	6. Road traffic accidents	6. Lower respiratory tract infections
7. Hearing loss, adult onset	7. Violence	7. Diarrheal diseases
8. Trachea, bronchus, lung cancers	8. Vision disorders, age-related	8. Cerebrovascular disease
9. Osteoarthritis	9. Hearing loss, adult onset	9. Cataracts
10. COPD	10. Diabetes mellitus	10. Malaria

From Mathers CD and Loncar D (2006) Projections of global mortality and burden of disease from 2002 to 2030. *PLoS Med* 3: 11: e442.

Table 5 Prevalence of 12-month use of mental health services (percent of those with mental disorder)

Sector	ESMeD	ECA	NCS-R
Mental health specialist	31.4	12.7	21.7
General medical physician	34.1	12.7	22.8

Data from Alonso J and Lepine J (2007) Overview of key data from the European study of the epidemiology of mental disorders (ESEMeD). *Journal Clinical Psychiatry* 68: 2, 3–9 (ESMeD); Regier DA, Narrow WE, Rae DS, *et al.* (1993) The de facto US mental and addictive disorders service system: Epidemiologic catchment area prospective 1-year prevalence rates of disorders and services. *Archives of General Psychiatry* 50: 85–94. (ECA); Wang PS, Lane M, Olfson M, *et al.* (2005) Twelve-month use of mental health services in the United States. *Archives of General Psychiatry* 62: 629–640 (NCS-R).

Epidemiological studies have tremendous potential to inform the allocation of public health resources. However, previous studies have tended to focus on specific individual factors that affect use of resources (e.g., insurance status, availability of services). Studies that address both individual factors and macro-level environmental factors (e.g., organization of services, public mental health policies) at the same time would strengthen the ability to make more informed public policy decisions for the provision of health-care services. This could lead to better systems of care, ensuring that limited services reach those most in need of them.

See also: Mental Health Etiology: Social Determinants; Mental Health: Morbidity and Impact; Mental Health Policy; Mental Health Promotion; Specific Mental Health Disorders: Eating Disorders; Specific Mental Health Disorders: Personality Disorders; Specific Mental Health Disorders: Psychotic Disorders; Specific Mental Health Disorders: Trauma and Mental Disorders; Women's Mental Health.

Citations

Alonso J and Lepine J (2007) Overview of key data from the European study of the epidemiology of mental disorders (ESEMeD). *Journal Clinical Psychiatry* 68: 2–9.

ESEMeD/MHEDEA 2000 Investigators (2004) Prevalence of mental disorders in Europe: Results from the European Study of the Epidemiology of Mental Disorders (ESEMeD) project. *Acta Psychiatrica Scandinavica Supplementum* 109 (supplement 420): 21–27.

Grant BF, Stinson FS, Dawson DA, *et al.* (2004) Prevalence and co-occurrence of substance use disorders and independent mood and anxiety disorders. *Archives of General Psychiatry* 61: 807–816.

Hughes CC, Tremblay MA, Rapoport RN, and Leighton AH (1960) *People of Cove and Woodlot: Communities from the Viewpoint of Social Psychiatry. Vol. 2, Stirling County Study of Psychiatric Disorder and Sociocultural Environment.* New York: Basic Books.

Kessler RC, Chiu WT, Demler O, *et al.* (2005) Prevalence, severity, and comorbidity of 12-month DSM-IV disorders in the national comorbidity survey replication. *Archives of General Psychiatry* 62: 617–627.

Mathers CD and Loncar D (2006) Projections of global mortality and burden of disease from 2002 to 2030. *PLoS Med* 3(11): e442.

Regier DA, Narrow WE, Rae DS, *et al.* (1993) The de facto US mental and addictive disorders service system: Epidemiologic catchment area prospective 1-year prevalence rates of disorders and services. *Archives of General Psychiatry* 50: 85–94.

Wang PS, Lane M, Olfson M, *et al.* (2005) Twelve-month use of mental health services in the United States. *Archives of General Psychiatry* 62: 629–640.

WHO World Health Survey Consortium (2004) Prevalence, severity and unmet need for treatment of mental disorders in the World Health Organization world mental health surveys. *Journal of the American Medical Association* 291: 2581–2590.

Wittchen HU and Jacobi F (2005) Size and burden of mental disorders in Europe – A critical review and appraisal of 27 studies. *European Neuropsychopharmacology* 15: 357–376.

Further Reading

Kessler RC, Demler O, Frank RG, *et al.* (2005) Prevalence and treatment of mental disorders, 1990 to 2003. *New England Journal of Medicine* 352(24): 2515–2522.

McDowell I (ed.) (2006) *Measuring Health: A Guide to Rating Scales and Questionnaires.* Oxford, UK: Oxford University Press.

Mezzich JE, Jorge MR, and Salloum IM (1994) *Psychiatric Epidemiology: Assessment of Concepts and Methods.* Baltimore, MD: Johns Hopkins University Press.

Murphy JM, Laird NM, Monson RR, *et al.* (2000) A 40-year perspective on the prevalence of depression. *Archives of General Psychiatry* 57: 209–215.

Murray CJL and Lopez AD (eds.) (1996) *The Global Burden of Disease: A Comprehensive Assessment of Mortality and Disability from Diseases Injuries and Risk Factors in 1990 and Projected to 2020.* Cambridge, MA: Harvard University Press.

Prince M, Stewart R, Ford T and Hotopf M (eds.) (2003) *Practical Psychiatric Epidemiology.* Oxford, UK: Oxford University Press.

Regier DA, Kaelber CT, Rae DS, *et al.* (1998) Limitations of diagnostic criteria and assessment instruments for mental disorders. *Archives of General Psychiatry* 55: 109–115.

Robins LN and Regier DA (eds.) (1991) *Psychiatric Disorders in America: The Epidemiological Catchment Area Study.* New York: Free Press.

Susser E, Schwartz S, Morabia A and Bromet EJ (eds.) (2006) *Psychiatric Epidemiology.* Oxford, UK: Oxford University Press.

Tsuang MT and Tohen M (eds.) (2002) *Textbook in Psychiatric Epidemiology.* New York: A John Wiley & Sons Inc.

US Department of Health, Human Services (1999) *Mental Health: A Report of the Surgeon General.* Rockville MD: US Department of Health and Human Services.

US Department of Health and Human Services (2001) *Mental Health: Culture Race, and Ethnicity: A Supplement to Mental Health: A Report of the Surgeon General.* Rockville MD: US Department of Health and Human Services.

World Health Organization (2001) *Mental Health: New Understanding New Hope.* Geneva, Switzerland: World Health Organization.

Relevant Websites

http://www.cdc.gov – Centers for Disease Control and Prevention.

http://www.hcp.med.harvard.edu/icpe – International Consortium in Psychiatric Epidemiology.

http://www.sinica.edu.tw/~ifpe – International Federation of Psychiatric Epidemiology.

http://www.niaaa.nih.gov – National Institute on Alcohol Abuse and Alcoholism.

http://www.nida.nih.gov – National Institute on Drug Abuse.

http://www.nimh.nih.gov – National Institute of Mental Health.

http://www.who.int – World Health Organization.

http://www.wparet.org – World Psychiatric Association.

Mental Health Etiology: Biological and Genetic Determinants

S J Glatt and S V Faraone, SUNY Upstate Medical University, Syracuse, NY, USA
M T Tsuang, University of California, San Diego, La Jolla, CA, USA; Harvard Institute of Psychiatric Epidemiology and Genetics, Boston, MA, USA; Veterans Affairs San Diego Healthcare System, San Diego, CA, USA

Introduction

The purpose of this article is to provide a broad overview of what we know about the genetic epidemiology of psychological and psychiatric ailments. As the title suggests, we provide a brief review of the genetic epidemiologic methods and principles that guide the search for genes influencing these conditions. We also evaluate the evidence implicating familial and genetic factors in general, and specific genes and alleles in particular. As one of the most heritable – and most often studied – psychiatric disorders, we will focus our review on schizophrenia; however, general principles will be emphasized, and particularly successful efforts directed at other mental disorders will also be highlighted where appropriate. The article concludes with a series of recommendations to hasten the discovery of risk genes for psychiatric disorders. Most psychiatric disorders exhibit complex, non-Mendelian inheritance patterns, and thus are thought to result from the joint effects of multiple genes and environmental factors. As such, we refer to the genes for psychiatric disorders as risk genes rather than disease genes, since none may be either necessary or sufficient to elicit illness.

Behavioral Genetic Methods and Principles

Family Studies

The first question that must be asked and answered when attempting to delineate the genetic and environmental components of a complex psychiatric disorder is: Does the phenotype run in families?, or, Is this phenotype familial? This question can be answered through the use of family studies. The basic design of the family study begins with the ascertainment of a group of subjects who are affected by the disorder (cases) and a comparable group of control subjects who do not have the disorder. Next, the biological relatives of these index subjects, or probands, are ascertained and evaluated for the presence of the illness, or in some cases, subthreshold forms of the illness. The rate of the disorder among family members of affected probands is then compared to the rate of the disorder among family members of control probands to determine the familial risk or relative risk.

If a psychiatric disorder has a genetic etiology, then biological relatives of cases should have a higher likelihood than relatives of controls of carrying the gene or genes that influenced illness in their relative, and thus they should be at greater risk for the illness themselves. In addition, the risk to relatives of cases should be correlated with their degree of relationship to the proband, or the amount of genes they share in common. First-degree relatives such as parents, siblings, and children, share 50% of their genes, on average, with the proband. Thus, first-degree relatives of cases should be at greater risk for the disorder than second-degree relatives (grandparents, uncles, aunts, nephews, nieces, and half-siblings), who share only 25% of their genes with the proband.

Twin Studies

Once a disorder has been established as familial, it becomes necessary to determine if that pattern is attributable to the inheritance of genes or to shared familial and other environmental factors. It is also important to quantify the contribution that genes make relative to that made by environmental factors, as this may encourage or discourage future molecular genetic studies; it may also influence the decisions made by individuals seeking genetic counseling and the usefulness of family information in identifying high-risk individuals to target for early intervention and prevention protocols. These questions can be answered by both twin studies and adoption studies but, mostly because of their relative ease to conduct and thus, their popularity, we focus on twin studies in this article.

In twin study designs, identical (monozygotic (MZ)), and fraternal (dizygotic (DZ)) twin-pairs are ascertained if at least one member of the pair is affected with a disorder. Twin-pairs are deemed concordant if both members of the pair have the illness, and are deemed discordant if only one member of the pair is affected. The ratio of concordant:discordant MZ twin-pairs is then compared to the ratio of concordant:discordant DZ twin-pairs.

MZ twins are derived from the same zygote and thus share 100% of their genetic material. In contrast, DZ twins result from separate fertilizations and thus share, on average, 50% of their genes – no more or less than any other pair of siblings. Thus, a typical MZ twin-pair will have 50% more genes in common than a typical DZ twin-pair. However, the degree of similarity in environmental exposures between members of a MZ twin-pair should be no different than that between members of a DZ twin-pair. Thus, any difference in concordance for a mental illness between the two types of twin-pairs can be attributed to the effects of the additional gene-sharing in the MZ twins.

If the concordance for a mental illness is higher among MZ twin-pairs than DZ twin-pairs, this is a good indication that there is a genetic contribution to the disorder; if MZ and DZ twin-pairs have approximately equal concordance rates, environmental factors are more strongly implicated. Frequently, concordance rates among twin-pairs are used to estimate the heritability of a disorder. Heritability measures the degree to which genetic factors influence variability in the manifestation of the phenotype. Heritability in the broad sense is the ratio of genetic to phenotypic variances, or the proportion of variance in schizophrenia risk that is accounted for by variability in genetic factors. A heritability of 1.0 indicates that all variability in the phenotype is due to genetic factors alone. In contrast, a heritability of zero attributes all phenotypic variation to environmental factors. Two points need to be carefully considered when interpreting heritability estimates, however. The first is that the heritability estimate is a maximum value, but the true heritability may be lower than its estimate in any given sample. The second is that heritability estimates are often context-dependent, and this is reflected by the fact that the heritability estimate accounts for the main effects of genetic factors but also gene-by-environment interactions. Thus, the entire heritability of a trait may be accounted for by the presence or absence of a necessary environmental cofactor. This is easiest to understand in the context of nonpsychiatric disorders, such as lung cancer. In the absence of important environmental cofactors such as exposure to cigarette smoke, the heritability would be much lower; in the case of phenylketonuria, lack of exposure to phenylalanine would reduce the heritability estimate to zero, since the condition would not occur at all. Recently, evidence of gene-by-environment interactions in psychiatry have been discovered and, in some cases, replicated. One such example of this is a commonly observed interaction of stress and a polymorphism in the serotonin transporter gene, which combine to increase the risk for major depression beyond the main effect of either risk factor.

General Familial and Genetic Factors Implicated in Mental Disorders

Family Studies

As shown in **Table 1**, many disorders identified in the *Diagnostic and Statistical Manual of Mental Disorder,* Fourth Edition (DSM-IV) (American Psychiatric Association, 1994) have been evaluated within the framework of a family study and have yielded an estimate of the risk of illness to a sibling of an affected person (λ_s). For the most part, familial risk estimates for psychiatric conditions have been found to range from 4 to 12, indicating that, depending on the disorder, a sibling of an affected individual is four to 12 times more likely to develop the disorder himself as compared to an individual from the general population.

It is noteworthy, however, that most family studies of psychiatric disorders that have included second- and third-degree relatives of the proband have observed a nonlinear relationship between relative risk for illness and degree of relationship to the proband (i.e., expected proportion of shared genes). Thus, for example, the consensus from studies of schizophrenia is that second-degree relatives of schizophrenia patients are at an approximately two- to threefold increased risk of illness, but first-degree relatives are at a tenfold increased risk despite a mere doubling of expected alleles shared with the proband. Furthermore, the risk to offspring of two schizophrenic parents, from whom the affected offspring received all of their genes, is not absolute ($\sim$46%); this pattern is also observed in studies of most other psychiatric disorders. These results underscore the complexity of the genetic bases for psychiatric disorders and imply that gene–gene interactions (epistasis) as well as environmental factors must contribute to their etiologies.

Collectively, the evidence from family studies suggests that psychiatric conditions do aggregate in families, that multiple genes and environmental factors may be involved in these illnesses, and that these disorders can present (even within families) with different degrees of severity. Despite this powerful evidence, it is important to recognize that familiality does not necessarily establish heritability. For example, religion and language are familial traits, as all members of the same family often practice the same religion and speak the same language. These facts do not reflect the transmission of religion genes or language genes through the family, but rather the common environment and upbringing that those family members share.

Twin Studies

The suggestions raised by these family studies can be formally evaluated through the use of twin studies, and as can be seen in **Table 1**, the heritability of many psychiatric disorders has already been examined. Of those psychiatric disorders described in the DSM-IV that have been the subject of a twin study, all but one was found to be significantly heritable. Estimates of the heritability of these disorders vary widely, from a high of more than 90% for autism (Bailey *et al.*, 1995) to a low of 0% for

Table 1　Results of family, twin, linkage, and association studies of psychiatric disorders[a]

Psychiatric disorder	Relative risk (λ_s)	Heritability (h^2)	Linked loci	Associated genes
Autism	22	93	7q	GABRAB3, SLC6A4
Tourette's syndrome	12	90	11q	SLITRK1, TBCD
Schizoaffective disorder	11	85	1q	DISC1
Bipolar disorder	8	84	6q, 8q	BDNF, DRD4, MAOA, SLC6A4
Schizophrenia	12	84	1q, 2q, 8p, 22q	DRD2, DTNBP1, HTR2A, NRG1, RGS4
Narcissistic personality disorder	–	79	–	–
Obsessive-compulsive personality disorder	–	78	–	–
Cannabis abuse	6	76	–	–
Attention-deficit/hyperactivity disorder	4	75	4p, 5p, 6q, 16p, 17p	DRD4, DRD5, SLC6A3, DBH, SLC6A4, HTR1B, SNAP25
Conduct disorder	–	74	9q, 17q	DRD4, SLC6A4
Anorexia nervosa	11	71	13q	BDNF, HTR2A, SLC6A2
Stuttering	5	70	12q, 18p	SOX3
Antisocial personality disorder	–	69	–	MAOA
Borderline personality disorder	–	69	–	–
Obsessive-compulsive disorder	4	68	17q, 13q, 11p	HTR2A, SLC6A4
Histrionic personality disorder	–	67	–	–
Stimulant abuse	–	66	–	–
Hallucinogen abuse	–	65	–	–
Gender identity disorder	–	62	–	–
Oppositional defiant disorder	–	61	–	–
Nicotine dependence	–	60	5q, 9q, 20q	CYP2A6, GABRAB2
Sleepwalking	–	60	–	–
Sedative abuse	–	59	–	–
Alzheimer's disease	2	58	4p, 7q, 10q, 12p, 12q, 17q, 19p, 20p	A2M, ACE, APOE, APP, BCHE, LRP1, MAPT, NOS3
Dependent personality disorder	–	57	–	–
Bulimia nervosa	4	55	10p	BDNF
Dyslexia	–	53	1p, 2p, 3p, 6p, 15q, 18p, Xq	DCDC2
Dissociative identity disorder	–	48	–	–
Pathological gambling	4	46	–	–
Panic disorder	5	43	9q, 13q, 22q	ADORA2A
Suicide	10	43	–	SLC6A4, TPH
Nightmare disorder	–	41	–	–
Agoraphobia	4	38	3q	–
Opiate abuse	10	38	17q	DRD4, OPRM1
Postpartum psychosis	11	38	–	TNFA, TPH
Posttraumatic stress disorder	–	38	–	–
Major depression	4	37	13q, 12q, 12q, 15q	DRD4, SLC6A3, TH
Narcolepsy	–	37	4p, 17q, 21q	HLA-DBQ1
Alcohol abuse	2	36	13q, 4q, 4p	ALDH2, ADH2, ADH3
Cocaine abuse	4	32	9q	–
Generalized anxiety disorder	6	32	–	–
Insomnia	–	32	12q, 14q, 20p	–
Schizoid personality disorder	4	29	–	–
Seasonal affective disorder	–	29	–	HTR2A
Simple phobia	4	29	14q	–
Avoidant personality disorder	4	28	–	–
Paranoid personality disorder	4	28	–	–
Schizotypal personality disorder	5	28	–	–
Social phobia	4	25	16q	–
Enuresis	–	24	12q, 13q	–
Dysthymia	–	20	–	–

[a]All values denote representative, replicated, or consensus estimates, but all available data relevant to each parameter may not be reflected in this table. Reprinted with permission from Recognition and Prevention of Major Mental and Substance Abuse Disorders, © 2007. American Psychiatric Publishing, Inc.

dysthymia (Lyons *et al.*, 1998). Thus, while some psychiatric disorders may have no genetic basis, most have a genetic component and several are predominantly attributable to genes.

Analogous to the results of family studies, MZ twins often have a rate of concordance for a psychiatric illness that is greater than twice that observed among DZ twins, even though their expected proportion of shared genes is only double that of DZ twins. For example, the best evidence from twin studies of schizophrenia suggests a rate of concordance of approximately 46–53% for MZ twins and 14–15% for DZ twins. These data further support the possibility of epistasis in the etiology of the disorder, and similar results have been observed in twin studies of other psychiatric conditions. Furthermore, MZ twins are not 100% concordant for any psychiatric disorder, confirming that environmental factors make a strong contribution to the overall risk, even for the most heritable mental disorders.

Molecular Genetic Methods and Principles

Linkage Studies

Knowing that genetic factors are involved in the etiology of a psychiatric disorder – and to what degree – is essential for designing optimal molecular genetic studies to reveal the chromosomal location of the responsible risk genes. To identify regions of chromosomes that have a high likelihood of harboring risk genes for an illness, linkage analysis is a highly appropriate strategy. Families are ascertained for linkage analysis through a proband affected with the disorder of interest. Each individual in the family is then genotyped at a series of DNA markers (not necessarily in genes) spaced evenly throughout the genome, and the cosegregation of these DNA markers with the illness is tracked in each pedigree. Evidence for cosegregation at each marker locus is summed across pedigrees to derive an index of the likelihood of the obtained patterns of marker-phenotype cosegregation given the sampled pedigree structures.

Although the DNA markers used for linkage analysis are not presumed to be actual risk genes for the disorder, they are numerous and dense enough to ensure that their coinheritance with a nearby (but unobserved) risk gene could be inferred with reasonable certainty based on the coinheritance of the marker with the phenotype that is influenced by that risk gene. In this design, the disorder serves as a proxy for the risk gene; thus DNA markers that cosegregate commonly with the disorder are presumed to cosegregate commonly with its underlying risk gene. Because the probability of cosegregation of two pieces of DNA is inversely proportional to the distance between them, the regularity of the cosegregation of the

DNA marker and the disorder gives an indirect indication of the genetic distance between the DNA marker and the unobserved risk gene.

The possible outcomes of a linkage analysis will vary based on the structure of families ascertained for analysis. For example, linkage analysis can be performed with affected sibling-pairs, or with other affected relative-pairs, or with small nuclear families, or with large extended pedigrees. Regardless of what family structure is the principal unit of analysis, the common output across methods is some index of the degree of phenotypic similarity of family members and the degree of genotypic similarity between those individuals at each DNA marker. These indices are summed across families to determine the overall evidence for linkage at a given locus in the full sample. If a given DNA marker cosegregates with illness through families more often than would be expected by chance, this indicates that the marker is linked (i.e., is in relatively close physical proximity) to a risk gene that influences expression of the disorder.

Association Studies

Once regions of certain chromosomes have been implicated from linkage analysis as harboring a risk gene for a disorder, the next step is to identify what specific gene is segregating through families to give rise to that linkage signal. A gene can be selected for such analysis subsequent to linkage analysis as a means to follow up on evidence for increased genetic similarity at a locus among affected individuals in a family (i.e., a positional candidate gene approach). Alternatively, specific genes can be examined in the absence of linkage information if there is some compelling physiological reason to suspect that the gene influences risk for a given disorder (i.e., a functional candidate gene approach). For example, dopamine-system genes, such as receptors and transporters, are commonly examined as functional candidates for schizophrenia, mood disorders, substance use disorders, and ADHD. In contrast to linkage analysis, which uses random DNA markers as proxies for nearby risk genes, genetic association analysis is an appropriate method for determining if a particular gene variant has a direct effect on risk for an illness, or is in tight linkage disequilibrium with such a gene. Recent developments in whole-genome association scan methods will marry the unbiased genomic survey approach of linkage analysis with the power and precision of association analysis and may shed new insights on previously unsuspected candidate genes for psychiatric disorders.

If a gene influences risk for a mental illness, this should be detectable as an increased frequency of the risk allele of the gene in cases compared to controls. Within the context of the family, this would be detectable as an increased likelihood of an affected patient receiving the risk allele of the gene from his parent, even when both the risk and normal forms of the gene were present in the parent and should have been transmitted to offspring with equal frequency and likelihood.

Specific Chromosomal Loci and Genes Implicated in Psychiatric Disorders

Linkage Studies

For the most heritable psychiatric disorders, including schizophrenia, bipolar disorder, and autism, numerous independent genome-wide linkage analyses have been performed (**Table 1**). In fact, each of these three disorders has been studied often enough by linkage analysis to allow for the quantitative combination of evidence across studies by meta-analysis. For autism, two meta-analyses have confirmed linkage to chromosome 7q, which was observed in several individual studies (Badner and Gershon, 2002a, 2002b; Trikalinos *et al.* 2006). Schizophrenia and bipolar disorder have also been subjected to more than one independent meta-analysis each, but with less agreement between the methods than has been observed for autism.

For schizophrenia, no less than 18 independent genome-wide linkage analyses have been published to date. Each of these studies has identified at least one chromosomal region in which either significant or suggestive evidence for linkage was observed. Unfortunately, the major findings from these genome-wide linkage scans do not, on first glance, appear to overlap to any great extent. Badner and Gershon (2002a) performed the first meta-analysis of these genome-wide linkage scans, and the results of their pooled analysis identified loci on chromosomes 8p, 13q, and 22q as the best candidates for harboring schizophrenia risk genes. Other promising regions included 1q, 2q, 6q, and 15q, but evidence for linkage at these loci was weaker, indicating a need for further replication. Subsequently, Lewis *et al.* (2003) conducted a meta-analysis of these and additional studies using an alternate methodology. Their results were somewhat different, identifying chromosome 2q as the prime candidate linked locus, and revealing somewhat weaker evidence for linkage on chromosomes 1q, 3p, 5q, 6p, 8p, 11q, 14p, 20q, and 22q. However, both meta-analyses were consistent in identifying chromosomes 1q, 2q, 8p, and 22q as the most reliably linked loci across individual studies.

For bipolar disorder, the first meta-analysis (that of Badner and Gershon, 2002a) found the strongest evidence for significant linkage on chromosomes 13q and 22q. (Of note, these were two of the three loci these authors also identified as linked to schizophrenia.) In stark contrast, the meta-analysis of Segurado *et al.* (2003) found the strongest evidence for linkage at loci on chromosomes 9p, 10q, and 14q. Most recently, a combined analysis of primary genotype data (rather than pooled study-level

results) from all 11 studies implicated chromosomes 6q and 8q as the strongest candidates for harboring risk genes for bipolar disorder, perhaps providing the best evidence to date on the topic.

Genome-wide linkage analyses have thus provided some strong leads (but some ambiguous ones as well) in the search for loci harboring risk genes for some mental illnesses; however, the method is certainly not optimal for detecting genes with small effects on risk. For example, Risch and Merikangas (1996) illustrated that a locus conferring four times greater risk for a disorder could be detected by linkage analysis in 200–4000 families; a reasonable number for today's large, multisite collaborative research studies. However, to detect a locus that increases risk by only 50%, a minimum of 18 000 families would be needed. This number of families is clearly unattainable by any single research group and, indeed, is beyond the reach of even the most effective research consortia. In fact, this number exceeds the total number of families studied to date in all published linkage analyses of schizophrenia, bipolar disorder, and autism combined. Therefore, for all practical purposes, we have reached an era where linkage analysis may no longer be a feasible strategy to detect genes that have a small but reliable influence on risk for complex mental disorders, especially those disorders with less of a heritable component to their etiologies.

Association Studies

When reviewing the status of behavioral genetic studies of psychiatric disorders, we saw that fewer conditions had been subjected to family studies than to twin studies, even though the former have traditionally preceded the latter in the chain of psychiatric genetic research (Faraone *et al.*, 1999). This may be due to the ease of ascertaining twins rather than entire families, as well as the enhanced inferential power afforded by the twin study method. Thus, while family studies give an indication of the familial aggregation of a disorder (which may or may not reflect genetic factors), a twin study can directly establish whether or not genes influence the disorder and to what degree. This same type of reversal is also true for molecular genetic studies, wherein linkage studies have recently become far outnumbered by association studies. Again, this may be due to the ease of ascertaining units of analysis for an association study (i.e., unrelated cases and controls or, at most, small nuclear families with one affected individual) relative to a linkage study (i.e., affected sibling-pairs or extended pedigrees). In addition, the information gleaned from an association study may be more direct than that from a linkage study, since the former can test for direct effects on risk for each studied polymorphism, while the latter only identifies linked loci that must then be subjected to further fine-mapping to identify risk-conferring genes. Furthermore, in contrast to linkage analysis, association analysis should be more effective at detecting genes with small effects on liability. For example, Risch and Merikangas (1996) showed that a locus increasing risk for a complex disorder by 50% could be detected in as few as 950 subjects. This number of samples is more feasible than that needed to detect the same effect by linkage analysis (i.e., 18 000 families). In fact, many of the pooled association studies conducted to date have attained such numbers of subjects.

Due to these favorable attributes of association methods, many studies (we estimate over 2700) of functional and positional candidate genes for psychiatric disorders have been conducted over the past two decades; however, only a handful of genes exhibit reasonably strong evidence for exerting reliable risk for one or more of these disorders (**Table 1**). The genes listed here are those that have been implicated by (1) strongly significant evidence from a very large primary study; (2) significant evidence from two or more independent research groups; or (3) significant pooled evidence from meta-analysis. Although the genes listed in this table represent relatively strong candidates for these disorders, we must reiterate at this point that none of these genes are proven risk factors for an illness, and none is either necessary or sufficient for producing any psychiatric disorder. In fact, most have been found to increase risk less than twofold and account for only a small portion of the aggregate risk for the given mental illness in the population. In addition, the risk alleles and haplotypes identified in one sample are often not the same as those implicated in other studies. Thus, more work is needed to definitively specify the nature and magnitude of the influences of these genes on risk for the various mental disorders to which they have been associated.

Despite these successes, association studies remain plagued by some limitations, including their propensity for producing false-positive results (Lohmueller *et al.*, 2003) and their limited breadth. Regarding the former, genes identified as associated with a mental illness in an initial study often overestimate the true effect size and subsequently fall victim to the winner's curse, wherein the same magnitude of an effect cannot be replicated (Ioannidis *et al.*, 2001; Glatt *et al.* 2003). As such, independent replication of genetic associations must be considered crucial for determining the role of a gene in a mental disorder. Regarding the latter, association methods have traditionally focused on one or at most a handful of genes at once, whereas linkage analysis constitutes a genome-wide survey of (relatively) unselected markers. Unfortunately, the prior probability of selecting the right candidate gene (out of ~25 000 human genes) and the right polymorphism (out of more than 10 000 000 in the human genome) for analysis is remote. Most candidate genes for mental disorders have been targeted based on their expression within systems widely implicated in the disorder (e.g., functional candidate genes in the dopamine neurotransmitter systems in schizophrenia). This approach has thus far proven essential for clarifying the nature of dysfunction within these recognized candidate pathways; however, it may not be optimal for identifying additional novel risk factors outside of these systems. The recent advancement of laboratory and statistical methods for genome-wide association analysis should allow for a more unbiased examination of association patterns throughout the genome and help resolve this dilemma in coming years (Thomas *et al.*, 2005).

Recommendations for Future Research

It is clear that the multifactorial polygenic etiologies and heterogeneity of psychiatric disorders obscure the discovery of their underlying genetic bases. The multifactorial polygenic nature of these diseases dictates that the signals obtained in linkage and association studies will be numerous and of very low intensity, while the heterogeneity of these disorders increases the noise against which these already-faint signals must be detected. Some of the most effective ways of combating these complexities are through the maximization of power, both by increasing sample size and by studying homogeneous groups of affected individuals. To identify the numerous genes with small effects on risk for psychiatric illness, various data-pooling strategies, such as direct combination of primary data or combination of study-level data by meta-analysis, can be particularly effective. However, to overcome the obstacles introduced by heterogeneity, delineating and studying smaller, more homogeneous subgroups of affected individuals may have the greatest beneficial effects on power. When used in tandem, the practices of pooling and splitting will yield maximal power for genetic studies, and hasten the discovery of the full compendium of risk genes for each heritable psychiatric condition. Other promising avenues for elucidating risk genes include the analysis of gene–gene and gene–environment interactions. An often overlooked potential benefit of genetic research on mental disorders is that, once risk genes are identified, environmental risk factors may become easier to detect within subgroups of subjects who do or do not possess those risk genes.

Since the first draft of the human genome was produced in 2001 (Lander *et al.*, 2001), scientists have been touting the promise of genetic analysis for identifying risk factors for common diseases and the development of personalized medicine. Yet, the vast potential of genetic studies to change the clinical practice of psychiatry remains almost entirely untapped. Presently, the results of behavior genetic analyses, such as the family and twin studies described in this article, can be useful in genetic counseling situations to inform individuals of their chances of becoming affected with a particular illness. In addition, this information can be used prospectively for family planning and to help parents understand the risks for mental illnesses that may be carried by their children. However, families still cannot be examined for linkage at a particular locus to determine if they exhibit a particular pattern of marker transmission that suggests who in the family is at risk. Similarly, individuals in the population cannot be tested for the possession of particular genotypes to determine their cumulative risk of developing a particular disorder. The leads that have been generated from molecular genetic studies are simply not yet understood well enough to allow such uses. However, with continued advancement of laboratory and analytic methods, reliable risk genes for some psychiatric disorders are sure to emerge in the coming years.

Once genetic risk factors for psychiatric conditions become established and widely recognized, they can serve many purposes for early intervention and prevention efforts. For example, an objective, gene-based laboratory test could facilitate the arrival at a primary or differential diagnosis much more quickly than is presently possible. This in turn could speed the initiation of appropriate treatments, which consequently may promote better prognoses (McGlashan, 1999). Ultimately, a panel of genetic markers for a mental illness might be administered to high-risk individuals from affected families or in the general population to determine their likelihood of progression toward illness even before any clinical symptoms are manifest, which would allow these individuals to be targeted for early intervention and prevention efforts as well. Ultimately, this line of investigation may foster medicinal chemistry applications and the development of novel therapeutics that more precisely target faulty DNA sequences in aberrant genes or active sites in its protein. While recent successes in identifying specific risk genes for mental disorders are encouraging, much more work is needed to replicate and refine these results, and translate them into meaningful clinical applications.

See also: Specific Mental Health Disorders: Child and Adolescent Mental Disorders; Specific Mental Health Disorders: Eating Disorders; Specific Mental Health Disorders: Mental Disorders Associated With Aging; Specific Mental Health Disorders: Psychotic Disorders.

Citations

American Psychiatric Association (1994) *Diagnostic and Statistical Manual of Mental Disorders (DSM-IV)*. Washington, DC: American Psychiatric Association.

Badner JA and Gershon ES (2002a) Meta-analysis of whole-genome linkage scans of bipolar disorder and schizophrenia. *Molecular Psychiatry* 7: 405–411.

Badner JA and Gershon ES (2002b) Regional meta-analysis of published data supports linkage of autism with markers on chromosome 7. *Molecular Psychiatry* 7: 56–66.

Bailey A, LeCouteur A, Gottesman I, *et al.* (1995) Autism as a strongly genetic disorder: Evidence from a British twin study. *Psychological Medicine* 25: 63–77.

Faraone SV, Tsuang D, and Tsuang MT (1999) *Genetics of Mental Disorders: A Guide for Students, Clinicians, and Researchers*. New York: Guilford.

Glatt SJ, Faraone SV, and Tsuang MT (2003) Meta-analysis identifies an association between the dopamine D2 receptor gene and schizophrenia. *Molecular Psychiatry* 8: 911–915.

Ioannidis JP, Ntzani EE, Trikalinos TA, and Contopoulos-Ioannidis DG (2001) Replication validity of genetic association studies. *Nature Genetics* 29: 306–309.

Lander ES, Linton LM, Birren B, *et al.* (2001) Initial sequencing and analysis of the human genome. *Nature* 409: 860–921.

Lewis CM, Levinson DF, Wise LH, *et al.* (2003) Genome scan meta-analysis of schizophrenia and bipolar disorder, part II: Schizophrenia. *American Journal of Human Genetics* 73: 34–48.

Lohmueller KE, Pearce CL, Pike M, Lander ES, and Hirschhorn JN (2003) Meta-analysis of genetic association studies supports a contribution of common variants to susceptibility to common disease. *Nature Genetics* 33: 177–182.

Lyons MJ, Eisen SA, Goldberg J, *et al.* (1998) A registry based twin study of depression in men. *Archives of General Psychiatry* 55: 468–472.

McGlashan TH (1999) Duration of untreated psychosis in first-episode schizophrenia: Marker or determinant of course? *Biological Psychiatry* 46: 899–907.

Risch N and Merikangas K (1996) The future of genetic studies of complex human diseases. *Science* 273: 1516–1517.

Segurado R, Detera-Wadleigh SD, Levinson DF, *et al.* (2003) Genome scan meta-analysis of schizophrenia and bipolar disorder, part III: Bipolar disorder. *American Journal of Human Genetics* 73: 49–62.

Thomas DC, Haile RW, and Duggan D (2005) Recent developments in genomewide association scans: A workshop summary and review. *American Journal of Human Genetics* 77: 337–345.

Trikalinos TA, Karvouni A, Zintzaras E, *et al.* (2006) A heterogeneity-based genome search meta-analysis for autism-spectrum disorders. *Molecular Psychiatry* 11: 29–36.

Further Reading

McGuffin P, Owen MJ, and Gottesman II (2002) *Psychiatric Genetics and Genomics*. New York: Oxford University Press.

Mental Health Etiology: Social Determinants

A Cohen, Harvard Medical School, Boston, MA, USA
H Minas, University of Melbourne, Melbourne, Australia

Historical Background

The origin of modern research on the social determinants of mental health and disorders is often traced to the work of Émile Durkheim, who demonstrated that cross-national variations in suicide rates reflected differences in social conditions rather than the characteristics of individuals. This line of reasoning – that social structures exert profound influence on the lives and well-being of individuals – has dominated thinking about the social determinants of mental disorders ever since. For example, the work of Robert Faris and H. Warren Dunham demonstrated that the prevalence of psychosis was higher in the poor and slum neighborhoods of Chicago than in wealthier districts of the city. Similarly, the research of Alexander Leighton and colleagues found that rates of mental disorder in Nigeria and Nova Scotia, Canada were highest in communities experiencing social disorganization. Durkheim's influence is apparent in more recent research on the characteristics of neighborhoods and variations in physical and mental health, a growing interest in the concept of social capital (see below), as well as, more generally, in research on the association of socioeconomic status and well-being.

Stress Models of Psychopathology

The 'stress-adversity' model of psychopathology, as formulated by Bruce Dohrenwend (2000), proposes that the degree to which environments present danger and hardship to individuals will be positively associated with risk for psychopathology. The association between environment and psychopathology will be reduced by the degree to which individuals have the ability to respond to and cope with the adversities.

How social groups come to be at increased risk of stress is central to considerations of the social determinants of mental health and disorders. As suggested by Leonard Pearlin (1989), relative well-being is associated with 'the structured arrangements of people's lives and by the repeated experiences that stem from these arrangements.' Thus, the social positions of particular populations put them at differential risk of stress. For example, the stress associated with becoming unemployed is different for a member of a poor family than it is for a member of a wealthy family. Further, being poor often means living in a crowded, polluted, and dangerous neighborhood, which is far more stressful, physically and psychologically, than being wealthy and able to afford living in a quiet suburb with tree-lined streets. Finally, differential access to effective medical care will have consequences for the relative well-being of social groups.

The 'stress-diathesis' model builds on the stress-adversity model by positing that risk for psychopathology is produced by an interaction between environmental stressors and individual vulnerability. One must not suppose, however, that individual vulnerability negates the notion of social determinants of well-being (Monroe and Simons, 1991). It is likely that individual vulnerability to common physical and mental disorders is evenly distributed in large populations. Therefore, exposure of subpopulations to different levels of stress will result in social differentials in the expression of those vulnerabilities. In view of this, one could say that the term 'social determinants' is an overly simplistic consideration of causality. It would be more accurate to refer to 'environment–gene interactions' as a primary source of social differentials in health and well-being. Even this is something of an oversimplification. Environments contain features that may mitigate or intensify the effects of social adversities. Thus, residents of a neighborhood with a relatively high degree of social capital (see below) may be less affected by an economic crisis; in contrast, residents of a neighborhood wracked by violence may be less capable of resilience in the face of a natural disaster.

Social Risk Factors for Mental Disorders

Gender

Gender, which may be thought of as the social roles designated for men and women in different sociocultural settings, carries with it differential risk for a range of mental disorders. For example, women are two to three times more likely than men to experience depression, and postnatal depression has been recognized as a significant problem worldwide. In most societies, completed suicide rates among men are much higher than among women, but rates of attempted suicide are much higher in women. Men are many times more likely to abuse substances, particularly alcohol. While it is likely that gender differences for common mental disorders are at least partially due to sociocultural factors, biological factors likely also play an important role.

Socioeconomic Status

Socioeconomic status (SES), which is variously measured by levels of income, educational attainment, occupation, and neighborhood characteristics (see below), exerts a profound influence on health status. On average, people of higher SES have rates of mortality and morbidity that are significantly lower than people of lower SES. The same relationship is true for mental disorders. For example, Ronald Kessler and colleagues (2003) have found that being unemployed, having less than 12 years of education, and having a low income are all associated with elevated prevalence of depression in a representative sample of adults in the United States. Findings from the Whitehall study (Stansfeld *et al.*, 2003), which examined the health of civil servants in the United Kingdom, also supports the notion of social inequalities in depression: Higher-grade civil servants had lower levels of depression than those in the lower grades. Other research demonstrates that the same relationship is true for psychosis: Low SES is associated with elevated rates of the disorder.

For a long time, there has been a debate over whether this pattern is the result of social drift or social causation. According to social drift theory, elevated rates of mental disorder are found among low SES groups because mental disorders impair the ability of individuals to raise themselves out of that status or limit the ability of individuals to maintain their higher status. Thus, mentally ill individuals drift into low SES. In contrast, the social causation theory suggests that risk for mental disorder is heightened for low SES individuals because of the stressful social environments in which they live.

Probably the best research to test the validity of these two competing theories was conducted by Bruce Dohrenwend and colleagues (1992). In an investigation of nearly 5000 Israeli-born adults, they found that (1) persons who had not graduated high school had rates of depression that were higher than persons who had graduated either high school or college; and, (2) educational status had no association with rates for schizophrenia. To further examine the relation between social status and mental disorder, Dohrenwend and colleagues also looked at rates of depression among adults of European (advantaged) and North African (disadvantaged) backgrounds. The results mirrored those for educational status: Those from disadvantaged backgrounds had elevated rates of depression, but rates of schizophrenia were the same for advantaged and disadvantaged groups. Thus, this research suggests that the social causation theory accounts for subpopulation inequalities in rates of depression, while the social drift theory accounts for subpopulation inequalities in rates of schizophrenia.

One must not assume that the various measures of SES, income and education in particular, are interchangeable. As demonstrated by Araya and colleagues (2003), the predictive power of these variables is very much context-dependent. They found an inverse relation between levels of education and the prevalence of common mental disorders in Chile, while in the United Kingdom level of income, but not education, was associated with prevalence, and in the United States both income and education were found to have significant associations with prevalence of common mental disorders.

Race/Ethnicity

Too often, social status as measured by membership in racial/ethnic groups is seen as a proxy for socioeconomic status. However, the relationship is much more complex. For example, although African-Americans in the United States are a socially disadvantaged group, their rates of depression and suicide are lower than the majority white population (in contrast to predictions based on SES). Other evidence suggests that African-Americans have higher rates of depressive symptoms and that their risk for persistent mood and anxiety disorders is higher (in keeping with predictions based on SES). The AESOP study (Fearon *et al.*, 2006) reports that incidence rates of psychosis among the African-Caribbean and black African populations in the United Kingdom are substantially higher than in white Britons, a finding that suggests that membership in a racial or ethnic minority may confer risk for mental disorder, independent of SES. In general, research from Australia, the United Kingdom, the Netherlands, Denmark, and Sweden support these findings in that immigrants, especially those from racial or ethnic backgrounds that are different from the host countries, are at increased risk for psychosis.

Psychosocial Environments

Social capital

The concept of social capital emerges from the work of Durkheim in that it looks to features of social environments to explain the collective behavior of individuals. Specifically, social capital may be defined as those properties of social units (e.g., neighborhoods, communities, cities, or provinces) that include, as defined by De Silva and colleagues (2005), 'the quantity and quality of formal and informal social interactions, civic participation, norms of reciprocity, and trust in others.' Research literature has demonstrated a strong and positive association between levels of social capital and the health status of communities, and there is growing evidence of an inverse association between social capital and risk for common mental disorders such as depression and anxiety. However, difficulties in precise definition and measurement of social capital must be overcome before it is possible to develop public mental health policies based on the concept of social capital.

Neighborhoods

There is now a large body of evidence demonstrating the association of neighborhood characteristics (e.g., proportion of households living in poverty) with physical health. There is also evidence that the collective level of depressive symptoms is influenced by the characteristics of neighborhoods. Indeed, a 2006 study by Cohen and colleagues shows that, compared to older residents of middle- and high-income neighborhoods, older residents of low-income neighborhoods are less likely to respond to even the best of antidepressant treatment. As noted above, Faris and Dunham found high rates of psychosis in the inner city of Chicago. Additionally, a recent meta-analysis by John McGrath and colleagues at the University of Queensland (2004) suggests that relatively high rates of schizophrenia are associated with urban residence.

Occupation and social status

There is increasing evidence that social inequalities in well-being are the consequence of psychological processes. For example, the Whitehall study (Stansfeld *et al.*, 2003) suggests that psychosocial work environments (e.g., the extent to which one may make decisions and use skills creatively) were more important than socioeconomic status in determining risk for depression. More generally, research by Michael Marmot (2004) suggests that subjective social status, that is, the perception of one's relative position in the social order, accounts for much of the social gradient in health and well-being.

Rapid Social Change and Social Disorganization

Durkheim associated rapid social change (e.g., political and economic upheavals) with what he termed as 'anomic' suicide – suicide caused by a collective experience of chaos and/or loss of meaning and purpose. The validity of the concept can be found in a number of examples. As a result of decades of political violence, suicide rates in Sri Lanka have gone from being among the lowest to among the highest in the world, particularly among young adults (Somasundaram, 2007). The startling increase of suicides in Japan since 1998 has been attributed to a range of economic factors, including unemployment, bankruptcy, and debt (Curtin, 2004). Gender inequities, as well as economic and social changes, are often cited to explain the high rates of suicide among young women in rural China. Perhaps the most dramatic example of anomic suicide is found among the indigenous peoples of the world, who have experienced massive social and cultural dislocations for hundreds of years. In Micronesia and Australia, for example, high rates of suicide and self-harm among young men are likely the result of social changes that have eroded traditional cultural activities and social structures that

helped to guide this age group through the difficult transition to adulthood.

Difficult and rapid social transformations are often associated with increased rates of substance abuse, alcohol-related problems, and suicide. Evidence of this is found, again, among the indigenous peoples of the world; high rates of alcoholism are found among indigenous groups in such disparate places as Australia, Taiwan, and North America.

Rates of mortality in Russia have gone through dramatic changes since the dissolution of the Soviet Union: a sharp increase immediately after 1991, substantial improvement between 1994 and 1998, and another decline after 1998. The result is that life expectancy in Russia (66 years) is alarmingly shorter than in the developed nations of the world ($\geq$78 years). To a large degree, the overall decline in the health status of the Russian population is due to alcohol abuse and related deaths, as well as violence. Since 1991, the rate of suicide in Russia has remained one of the highest in the world; it is also presumed that high levels of depression have contributed to high levels of alcohol abuse and suicide. Again, the indigenous peoples of the world provide a shocking example: Throughout the world, their life expectancies are much shorter – almost 20 years shorter in Australia, for example – than the general populations in which they live.

Globalization, specifically the spread of Western media and cultural values, has been associated with the appearance of anorexia nervosa in Hong Kong and other cities in China. Research in the late 1990s demonstrated an association between eating disorders among female Chinese high school students and their relative exposure to Western media and values. In Hong Kong, a highly Westernized city, the prevalence of eating disorders was high, while in the city of Shenzen and in rural Hunan the prevalence was moderate and low, respectively. Research from Fiji provides even stronger evidence of the causal relationship between the images portrayed in Western media and eating disorders. Just prior to the introduction of television (with programming primarily from the United States), a survey showed that female Fijian high school students had very low levels of eating disorders. Three years after the introduction of television, the same survey was administered among a comparable group of students. This time the respondents reported much higher levels of disordered eating behaviors. The change was attributed to the introduction of television and the pervasive images of women who were exceedingly thin (Becker, 2004).

Violence and Trauma

There is now a large body of evidence that links the experiences of violence and trauma to risk for depression and posttraumatic stress disorder (PTSD), in particular. The sociopolitical context of the refugee experience, predisplacement and postdisplacement, is associated with refugee mental health. Conflict, war, and disaster situations impact on fundamental family and community dynamics, resulting in profound negative changes at a collective level. Vietnamese and Cambodian victims of political violence and torture have been found to suffer from elevated rates of these disorders. Under the rule of the Taliban in Afghanistan, women suffered from high rates of depression and anxiety as a result of the extreme social restrictions under which they were forced to live. Indeed, there is extensive evidence from throughout the world about the mental health consequences of violence against women. The trauma of natural disasters – such as the tsunami that struck Aceh, Indonesia in 2004, earthquakes in China and India, or hurricanes in the southern United States – has been linked to increased rates of depression and PTSD. In sum, experiencing violence and/or trauma substantially increases the risk for mental distress.

Conclusion

There is strong evidence that links the social conditions in which people live and their psychological well-being. Socioeconomic status, characteristics of neighborhoods, exposure to violence, membership in racial or ethnic minorities, gender, and rapid social change all influence psychological well-being and confer differential risk for a range of mental disorders.

See also: Mental Health Epidemiology (Psychiatric Epidemiology); Historical Views of Mental Illness; Suicide and Self-Directed Violence.

Citations

Becker AE (2004) Television, disordered eating, and young women in Fiji: Negotiating body image and identity during rapid social change. *Culture, Medicine and Psychiatry* 28(4): 533–559.

Cohen A (1999) *The Mental Health of Indigenous People: An International Overview.* Geneva, Switzerland: World Health Organization.

Cohen A, Houck PR, Szanto K, *et al.* (2006) Social inequalities in response to antidepressant treatment in older adults. *Archives of General Psychiatry* 63(1): 50–56.

Curtin JS (2004) Suicide also rises in land of rising sun. *Asia Times Online* July 28. http://www.atimes.com/atimes/Japan/FG28Dh01. html (accessed October 2007).

De Silva MJ, McKenzie K, Harpham T, and Huttly SR (2005) Social capital and mental illness: A systematic review. *Journal of Epidemiology and Community Health* 59(8): 619–627.

Dohrenwend BP, Levav I, Shrout PE, *et al.* (1992) Socioeconomic status and psychiatric disorders: The causation-selection issue. *Science* 255: 946–952.

Durkheim E (1996) *Suicide.* New York: Free Press.

Fearon P, Kirkbride JB, Morgan C, *et al.* (2006) Incidence of schizophrenia and other psychoses in ethnic minority groups: Results from the MRC AESOP Study. *Psychological Medicine* 36(11): 1541–1550.

Kessler RC, Berglund P, Demler O, *et al.* (2003) The epidemiology of major depressive disorder: Results from the National Comorbidity Survey Replication (NCS-R). *Journal of the American Medical Association* 289(23): 3095–3105.

Lee S and Lee AM (2000) Disordered eating in three communities of China: a comparative study of female high school students in Hong Kong, Shenzhen, and rural Hunan. *International Journal of Eating Disorders* 27: 317–332.

Marmot M (2004) *The Status Syndrome: How Social Standing Affects Our Health and Longevity.* New York: Times Books.

McGrath J, Saha S, Welham J, *et al.* (2004) A systematic review of the incidence of schizophrenia: The distribution of rates and the influence of sex, urbanicity, migrant status, and methodology. *BMC Medicine* 2: 13.

Pearlin LI (1989) The sociological study of stress. *Journal of Health and Social Behavior* 30: 241–256.

Phillips MR, Li X, and Zhang Y (2002) Suicide rates in China, 1995–1999. *Lancet* 359: 835–840.

Pridemore WA and Spivak AL (2003) Patterns of suicide mortality in Russia. *Suicide and Life Threatening Behavior* 33(2): 132–150.

Shkolnikov V, McKee M, and Leon DA (2001) Changes in life expectancy in Russia in the mid-1990s. *Lancet* 357(9260): 917–921.

Somasundaram D (2007) Collective trauma in Northern Sri Lanka: A qualitative psychosocial-ecological study. *International Journal of Mental Health Systems* 1:5.

Stansfeld SA, Head J, Fuhrer R, Wardle J, and Cattell V (2003) Social inequalities in depressive symptoms and physical functioning in the Whitehall II study: Exploring a common cause explanation. *Journal of Epidemiology and Community Health* 57(5): 361–367.

Further Reading

Araya R, Lewis G, Rojas G, and Fritsch R (2003) Education and income: Which is more important for mental health? *Journal of Epidemiology and Community Health* 57(7): 501–505.

Berkman LF, Glass T, Brissette I, and Seeman TE (2000) From social integration to health: Durkheim in the new millennium. *Social Science and Medicine* 51(6): 843–857.

Cantor-Graae E (2005) Schizophrenia and migration: A meta-analysis and review. *American Journal of Psychiatry* 162(1): 12–24.

Faris RE and and Dunham HW (1939) *Mental Disorders in Urban Areas: an Ecological study of schizophrenia and other psychoses.* Chicago, IL: University of Chicago press.

Tsuang MT, Bar JL, Stone WS, and Faraone SV (2004) Gene-environment interactions in mental disorders. *World Psychiatry* 3(2): 73–83.

Mental Health: Morbidity and Impact

O Gureje and B Oladeji, University of Ibadan, Ibadan, Nigeria

Burden of Mental Disorders

The World Health Organization estimates that up to 450 million people are affected by mental, neurological and behavioral disorders worldwide. These disorders include unipolar depression, bipolar affective disorder, schizophrenia, alcohol and drug use disorders, posttraumatic disorder, panic disorder, Alzheimer's disease and other dementias, and primary insomnia. The prevalence of mental disorders is generally higher than that of any other class of chronic conditions and this is further reflected in the fact that four out of the six leading causes of years lived with disability are neurological or mental disorders. Even though estimates vary, depending on definition and ascertainment methods, in general approximately one in every four individuals will develop one or more mental disorders in their lifetime. Cross-national estimates of 12-month prevalence of between 4.3% and 26.4% have been reported in studies conducted among large community samples. In the community, the most common disorders are anxiety, mood, and substance use disorders. The burden attributable to mental disorders results not only from their high prevalence but also from the relatively early age of their onset as well as their tendency to be chronic or recurrent. For example, the median age of onset for anxiety disorders is early teenage and many affected individuals will go on to develop other types of mental disorder in adulthood.

Prevalence

Mental disorders are highly prevalent in the community. Large-scale community surveys, which have only become possible with the development in the last few decades of reliable lay-administered interviews, have shown that between 25% and 50% of adults will develop one mental disorder or the other in their lifetime. In a 12-month period, between one in ten and one in five adults will have significant levels of symptoms sufficient for a categorical diagnosis. Even though such estimates have generated controversy and concern about their reliability, their replication in several different settings has provided credibility. These estimates have varied depending on the mode of ascertainment, the diagnostic categories covered, and the age group studied. There is also variability between countries. For example, the largest mental health survey ever conducted, the World Mental Health Surveys,

reported rates of 12-month disorder that vary between 4.7% in Nigeria and 26.3% in the United States (**Table 1**). Whether this reflects the performance of the assessment tools, the reporting styles of people from different cultural backgrounds, or a true difference in propensity to develop mental disorders is still unknown. The likelihood is that some or all of these factors are involved. Irrespective of where they are conducted, it is a common observation that prevalence rates in the general adult population typically underestimate projected lifetime risk, so that more people are indeed likely to develop mental disorders in their lifetime than cross-sectional estimates suggest.

The most common group of mental disorders in the community is anxiety disorders. Lifetime estimates of anxiety disorders of up to 25% have been commonly reported. Among these, specific phobia is the most prevalent often followed by social phobia, posttraumatic disorder, and generalized anxiety disorder. Mood disorders, in particular major depressive disorder, are also highly prevalent, with some studies suggesting that up to one in five adults may experience at least one episode of depression in their lifetime. Substance use disorders may affect up to 10% of adults in their lifetime, with alcohol abuse the most prevalent condition reported. While anxiety and mood disorders tend to be more prevalent among females, males are commonly the more likely to report substance use disorders. Rates of substance use disorders, as a group, tend to vary considerably between cultural settings and age groups. However, there is now a common observation for a trend for a prominent cohort effect in which higher rates of these disorders are often to be found in the teens and young adults.

Nonaffective psychotic disorders and dementia are less common in the community. Schizophrenia has a lifetime risk of about 1%. There is evidence that males are more affected than females, with a male to female ratio of about 1.4, and that migrants, especially second-generation migrants, tend to have higher incidence than native-born individuals. Bipolar disorder also has a lifetime morbid risk of about 1%. However, recent studies suggest that subthreshold bipolar syndrome, which is also a disabling disorder, has a much higher prevalence in the community. In addition, several studies have now documented idespread experience of psychotic symptoms in the community, although the import for such experiences in regard to disability is not yet fully understood. About 1% of persons aged 65 years will have dementia. However, with the prevalence of the disorder doubling every 5 years, over 40% of elderly persons 90 years and above will have the disorder.

Table 1 Epidemiologic studies: Lifetime and 12-month rates of mental disorder

	US (NCS-R)	Europe (ESEMeD)	New Zealand (NZMHS)	Mexico (M-NCS)	Nigeria (NSMHWB)
Lifetime prevalence	46.4	25.0	39.5	26.1	12.0
12-month prevalence	26.3	9.6	20.7	12.2	4.7

NCS-R, National Comorbidity Survey-Reproduction; ESEMeD, European Study of the Epidemiology of Mental Disorders; NZMHS, New Zealand Mental Health Survey; M-NCS, Mexican National Comorbidity Survey; NSMHWB, Nigerian Survey of Mental Health and Well-Being.

Comorbidity

Mental disorders do not always occur in discrete forms. Many affected individuals will have more than one form of disorder, a phenomenon termed comorbidity. Defined as the presence, either simultaneously or in succession, of two or more specific disorders in an individual within a specified period of time, comorbidity has important implications for the level of impairment associated with mental disorders and for their prognosis. Persons with multiple disorders are commonly more disabled than those with single disorders but, in general, the implications of lifetime and 12-month comorbidity are somewhat different. Lifetime comorbidity rates can offer important opportunities for secondary prevention of mental disorders, as it has been shown that the experience of early-onset disorders confers a greater risk for the occurrence of another later-onset disorder; these later-onset disorders are frequently more persistent and severe. Twelve-month comorbidity, on the other hand, is often associated with symptom severity, with consequent increased burden on affected persons and increased demand for services. High rates of comorbidity have been reported in large community surveys. The Epidemiological Catchment Area study (ECA) and the National Comorbidity Survey in the United States reported 54% and 56%, respectively, of respondents with a lifetime history of at least one DSM III disorder met criteria for some other mental disorder. The Netherlands Mental Health Survey and Incidence study documented a 45% comorbidity rate, while the Australian National Mental Health Survey reported a 12-month comorbidity rate of 39%.

The most common comorbidity is between mood and anxiety disorders. More than 50% of patients with a mood disorder will meet diagnostic criteria for an anxiety disorder. Other conditions that may be comorbid with mood disorders include alcohol use disorders, personality disorders, dysthymia, somatoform disorders, drug abuse, and dependence and impulse control disorders. A substantial proportion of patients with schizophrenia have symptoms of obsessive-compulsive disorder (OCD) and schizophrenia patients with OCD may differ from those without OCD in severity of schizophrenia symptoms. Comorbidity also is common between mental disorders and substance-use disorders. Up to two-thirds of patients

attending alcohol and drug services have a comorbid mental disorder. Rates of alcohol-related problems are also high in patients attending mental health services.

The presence of multiple co-occurring disorders carries poor outcome. Comorbidity is associated with increased case severity, lower satisfaction with life, greater disability, longer illness course, and increased likelihood of attempting suicide. Furthermore, even though comorbidity increases the chance of seeking treatment and increases the chance of detection by primary care clinicians, it often complicates treatment and leads to poor response to treatment. In patients with major depressive disorders, comorbidity predicts longer duration of episode, recurrence of symptoms, and psychosocial impairment.

Child and Adolescent Mental Health

Two reasons make a consideration of child and adolescent mental health particularly important: Many mental disorders start during this period of life and childhood disorders often predict chronicity of adult disorders. A consequence of these factors is that the large percentage of the global burden of disease can be attributed to neuropsychiatric conditions in children and adolescents (World Health Organization, 2001). Indications are that about 10–20% of children and adolescents worldwide suffer from a serious mental illness.

Childhood psychiatric disorders can broadly be categorized into disorders that more typically affect children and adolescents and disorders that are more common in adulthood but with onset in childhood. Childhood and adolescent disorders include specific or pervasive developmental impairment or delay and behavioral disorders, such as attention deficit hyperactivity disorder (ADHD), conduct disorder, and emotional disorders.

Approximately 50% of adult mental disorders begin in childhood, with many starting before the age of 14 years. Anxiety and impulse control disorders often start in the early teens. The prevalence of major depressive disorder in preadolescent children may be up to 2%, with over a doubling of the rate occurring at the onset of puberty in adolescence. Major depressive disorder in adolescence is associated with a fourfold increased risk of depression in adulthood.

There is a high level of comorbidity in childhood and adolescent mental disorders. Depressed children and adolescents have higher rates of anxiety disorders, oppositional disorders, and ADHD. Childhood bipolar disorder is associated with high rates of alcohol and drug use, ADHD, and disruptive disorders. More than 50% of children with ADHD may have comorbid psychiatric disorders, with the most common conditions being oppositional defiant disorder, conduct disorder, and depression and anxiety disorders.

A diverse range of negative consequence is associated with childhood and adolescent mental disorders. Adolescents with anxiety disorders are at elevated risk for illicit drug dependence and failure to attend university. The presence of major depressive disorder (MDD) is related to poor outcome, high rates of suicide and suicide attempts, psychosocial impairments, and lower educational achievement. Conduct disorder tends to persist into adolescence and adulthood and is associated with juvenile delinquency, high school drop out rates, adult crime, antisocial behavior, unemployment, marital problems, poor parenting, and poor physical health. Suicide is the third leading cause of death in adolescents worldwide (World Health Organization, 2001). Depression and substance abuse are risk factors for adolescent suicidal behavior.

Child and adolescent mental disorders impose considerable costs on society. Direct medical costs may result from increased health-care utilization. For example, children with ADHD, depression, and conduct disorder are more likely to present with somatic complaints and have higher health-care utilization than children without such disorders. However, it has been estimated that the health sector cost resulting from child and adolescent mental health problems may be no more than 10% of the total costs to the society. More costs are incurred in the provision of foster and residential care and in the criminal, educational, and social welfare sectors.

Disability and Functional Limitation

Various concepts are still commonly employed in interchangeable and overlapping ways in the investigation of the impact of mental disorders on individuals. Thus, impairment, handicap, disability, and even quality of life and wellbeing are often used as if they denote similar sequelae of diseases. One example of the relative lack of specificity of current literature in the area is the diverse use to which common assessment tools in the field have been put. For example, the Medical Outcomes Study 36-Item Short-Form Health Survey (SF-36), has been used to assess activity limitation, disability, functional impairment, as well as quality of life. Recently, a heuristic organization of the consequences of disease has been provided by the World Health Organization in the International Classification of Impairment, Disabilities and Handicaps (ICIDH-2). The ICIDH-2 organizes the consequences of disease into three dimensions: (1) body functions and structure (symptoms and impairment), (2) activities, and (3) participation. This organization has yet to form the conceptual basis of existing research into the impact of mental disorders. Along with the World Health Organization Disability Assessment Scale second edition (WHO-DAS-II), which is conceptually linked to it, the ICIDH-2 will hopefully guide future work in this area.

An important metric that allows comparison of the societal impact of various health conditions was introduced in 1993 by the Harvard School of Public Health in collaboration with the World Bank and the World Health Organization. The metric, disability-adjusted life years (DALY), combines information on the impact of premature death and of disability and other nonfatal health outcomes. As described by the WHO (2001), DALY represents the sum of years of life lost due to premature mortality (YLL) in the population and the years lost due to disability for incident cases of the health condition. Using this metric, mental and neurological disorders have been shown to be among the most disabling health conditions. Cumulatively, these disorders accounted for 12.3% of the total DALYs lost due to all diseases and injuries in 2000. In 2005, neuropsychiatric disorders accounted for approximately 28% of total DALYs lost due to noncommunicable diseases (**Figure 1**).

One of the reasons why mental disorders rank so high among the most burdensome diseases in the world is that they are commonly associated with a significant degree of disability or inability to perform usual activities or roles. Disability refers to limitations in performing defined roles and tasks in the context of the individual's social and cultural environment. Thus, disability can be conceived as inability to fulfill socially or culturally sanctioned expectations within the domains of family, work, recreation, and self-care. Multiple domains of functioning may be affected. For example, focus is commonly directed at the impairment of occupational and physical functioning as well as at disability days. However, within the concept of psychosocial disability, functions relating to marriage, parenting, and social relationships are often studied. In recent years, studies have been extended to encompass disability in activities of daily living as well as instrumental activities of daily living. Thus, mental disorder may limit performance relating to mobility as well as cognition and may also reduce the capacity of affected individuals for personal self-care. The demonstration that mental disorders may affect not only psychosocial functioning, but also limit physical functioning has important implications for the understanding of the totality of the impact of mental disorders, especially in contrasting such disorders with common chronic physical conditions such as arthritis, heart diseases, and respiratory conditions. Using the Sheehan Disability Scale, a measure of functional

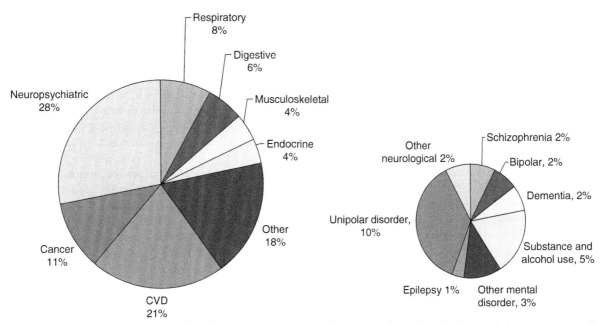

Figure 1   Disability adjusted life years (DALYs) due to non-communicable diseases in 2005; contributions of disease groups and of specific neuropsychiatric disorders. Adapted from Murray CJL and Lopez AD (1996) The Global Burden of Disease Volume 1: A comprehensive assessment of mortality and disability from diseases, injuries and risk factors in 1990 and projected to 2020. Cambridge, MA: Harvard University Press.

Table 2   Treatment and disability of 12-month cases of physical and mental disorders in developed and developing countries according to the World Mental Health Surveys

	Proportion treated		Proportion rated severely disabled[a]	
	Developed (%)	Developing (%)	Developed (%)	Developing (%)
Physical				
Arthritis	50.9	46.6	23.3	22.8
Cancer	51.8	59.6	16.6	23.9
Diabetes	94.4	76.6	13.6	23.7
High blood pressure	90.2	69.8	5.3	23.8
Mental				
Bipolar	29.1	13.4	68.3	52.1
Depression	29.3	8.1	65.8	52.0
Generalized anxiety disorder	31.6	7.2	56.3	42.0
Posttraumatic stress disorder	29.5	8.1	54.8	41.2

[a]Based on global ratings on the Sheehan Disability Scale. Adapted from Ormel J, Petukhova M, Chatterji S, et al. (in press). Disability and treatment of specific mental and physical disorders across the world: Results form the WHO World Mental Health Surveys. *British Journal of Psychiatry*.

impairment in the domains of work, home management, social life, and close relationships, data from the World Mental Health Surveys show that common mental disorders are more disabling than common chronic medical conditions, but, paradoxically, persons with mental disorders are much less likely to receive treatment (**Table 2**). The observations are true for both developed and developing countries, even though, as could be expected, cases of either physical or mental disorders are less likely to receive treatment if they reside in developing as compared to developed countries.

Schizophrenia and schizoaffective disorder constitute the fifth leading cause of disability and are responsible for more years of life lived with disability than all malignancies and HIV combined. Because the typical age of onset of schizophrenia is late adolescence or early adulthood, the illness often makes the achievement of a career or the establishment of a marital relationship impossible. The disability associated with schizophrenia often persists for the person's lifetime, with attendant cost to society in lost productivity. Persons with bipolar disorder also experience a significant level of disability and there is evidence that, even though the disorder is characterized by remissions and relapses, associated disability may persist even during periods of apparent remission.

Even though psychotic disorders are seriously disabling, they are not the only group of mental disorders with evidence of associated disability and functional impairment. Persons with common mental disorders also show significantly elevated levels of disability when compared with persons with no mental disorders. Also, common mental disorders are associated with levels of disability that are comparable or higher than those of chronic physical disorders such as arthritis and heart disease. A large body of evidence suggests that unipolar major depressive disorder is commonly associated with significant psychosocial disability. The Global Burden of Disease study found that depression was the fourth most burdensome of all medical conditions throughout the world in 1990, and predicted that it would become the second most burdensome by 2020. Unipolar depressive disorder accounts for so much disability globally because it is common, with a lifetime occurrence in the general population reaching nearly one in five, and often follows a chronic course. It is now known that even states of subthreshold depressive symptoms that do not attain diagnostic status are associated with considerable levels of disability and that significant increases in disability occur with each stepwise increment in depressive symptoms.

The evidence of significant level of disability in persons with other common mental disorders is now substantial. The widespread co-occurrence of common mental disorders often confounds the link between specific disorders and functional limitation. For example, comorbidity of anxiety disorders with depression may hide the unique contribution of the former to disability. However, several studies have now documented the association of individual mental disorders with disability both in primary care settings and in the community. Even though persons with comorbid generalized anxiety disorder (GAD) and depression are often more disabled than those with GAD or depression alone, it is now known that GAD is independently associated with significant disability. Analysis of large community surveys shows that persons with either GAD or major depression have comparable levels of impairment. Compared with persons without mental disorders, persons suffering from phobia report significantly poorer social, family, and work functioning. Panic disorder, posttraumatic stress disorder, as well as agoraphobia each make a specific and unique contribution to disability. When multiple disorders are examined, level of disability varies substantially with diagnosis, with particularly prominent levels of disability among individuals with affective disorder, panic disorder, posttraumatic stress disorder, and generalized anxiety disorder.

Determinants and Course of Disability in Mental Disorder

Longitudinal studies suggest that depression and disability often show synchrony of change, such that the remission of depression is associated with decrement in disability, while a worsening of depression is commonly accompanied by greater disability. However, symptomatic recovery does not always guarantee complete return to full functional capacity. Thus, even though there could be alleviation of disability when depressed patients become asymptomatic, there may continue to be persistence of disability even when full symptomatic remission has occurred. The question of whether psychopathology may cause residual debilitating functional impairment has important ramifications for rehabilitation and organization of postrecovery management of cases. As discussed by Ormel and colleagues (2004), postmorbid disability could be (1) the continuation of premorbid disability, predating the onset of any depressive episode (trait effect); (2) caused by ongoing postmorbid residual depressive symptoms (state effect); and (3) disability that emerged in the context of a depressive illness but has persisted in spite of the complete remission of the depression (scar effect). Their longitudinal study of a Dutch community cohort suggests that psychosocial disability in persons who have recovered from depression commonly reflects premorbid psychosocial disability and that scarring does not occur routinely in major depressive episodes. However, they also found the possibility of scarring in persons with severe recurrent major depression, an observation that may partly explain the apparent discordance of their findings from those of previous authors who have found evidence of scarring following mania and depression.

The emergence and persistence of disability in major depression may result from a variety of causes. Other than the severity of the depression, histories of previous episodes and of incomplete remission from them are important determinants of disability. Duration is often an important correlate of disability. However, it would seem that duration of depression may have a differential relationship with various aspects of disability, with impact on functioning in daily activities and none on social functioning. Also important are the presence of comorbidity of psychiatric disorders, personality traits of neuroticism, and perceived social support.

Even though most mental disorders are seriously disabling, the presence of disability does not always lead to seeking help. In some studies in the community, only about half of persons with mental illness who were rated as being disabled would have consulted a health provider. Persons who do not consult for medical intervention may feel that they do not need treatment. However, a finding that the presence of disability in the context of mental disorder does not lead to seeking help is curious and may result from perceived stigma or lack of knowledge of the availability of appropriate treatment on the part of affected individuals. Nevertheless, when affected persons do seek help, there is evidence that the presence of concomitant disability sensitizes the primary care physicians to the presence of psychological problems and thus aids detection and treatment.

Quality of Life

The term quality of life in the health-care field has become useful in integrating the patient's subjective experience of their life during illness into clinical care. This is done by relying on patient's subjective assessment of their quality of life. The importance of quality of life as an index of impact of mental illness lies in the need to capture indices of social and economic well-being and address the salience to those suffering from mental disorders of features such as autonomy, choice, life satisfaction, and self-actualization. Quality of life has become a valued assessment in those branches of medicine dealing with chronic suffering and disability. In mental health, it takes on an added importance: It embodies the regard accorded to patients as people with needs and concerns and not just as persons with illness. The assessment of quality of life in persons with mental illness is not without controversy (Katschnig *et al.*, 2006). Several dimensions of quality of life overlap considerably with psychopathological domains, thus raising the question about measurement redundancy. Also, there is some debate as to the validity of self-reported outcomes in the assessment of quality of life of persons with mental illness. This debate relates to the dissonance that may be observed between patients' subjective report and an objective evaluation of their position in life. In spite of these considerations, the assessment of the quality of life of persons affected by mental illness is now a central consideration in the evaluation of the totality of the impact of mental disorders.

There is considerable evidence that persons with mental disorders commonly rate their quality of life lower than those with no mental disorders. Multiple domains are often affected. Thus, poorer self-reported well-being in physical, social, environmental, as well as psychological domains may be reported. Persons with severe mental disorders, such as schizophrenia, bipolar disorder, dementia, and intellectual disabilities have lower scores on measures of quality of life than unaffected persons. There is also evidence that severe mental disorders are associated with more impairment in quality of life than common mental disorders such as mood and anxiety disorders, which themselves are associated with a substantial decrease in quality of life. Other than major depressive disorder

and generalized anxiety disorder, posttraumatic stress disorder, panic, social phobia, as well as primary insomnia and dependence states (including dependence on nicotine), are all associated with quality of life decrement.

Experience of stigma and discrimination is prevalent for people with mental illness and may be an important reason for impaired quality of life. Stigma can be defined as a social process with cognitive, attitudinal, behavioral, and structural elements that lead to social inequities, negative discriminatory treatment, and disadvantage to people with mental illness. Stigma can affect a variety of life situations of persons with mental illness, from befriending to neighborhood residence. It is a common source of disability for persons with mental health problems. A particularly important way in which stigma constitutes a burden for persons with mental illness is its potential to limit their opportunities for work. Work is important to mental health because it enhances a sense of self-worth and promotes social activity. When stigma and discrimination lead to exclusion from the workforce for people with mental illness, the result is not only material deprivation but a denial of the opportunity for full recovery and a perpetuation of disability.

Economic Cost

Studies of the economic costs of mental disorders are few and have been mainly conducted in the developed countries of North America and Europe. Estimates often include the costs of health service uptake, production losses, and patients' out-of-pocket costs. It may also include health benefit claim costs and salary-replacement payments for patients who are on sick leave or have short- or long-term disability. Most attention has been given to severe mental disorders such as Alzheimer's disease, schizophrenia, and bipolar disorder. Findings suggest that, not unexpectedly, economic costs vary by country. For example, the per capita resources spent on care for people with schizophrenia in the United States have been estimated to be twice that in Canada. Variation in the economic costs of mental disorders may reflect differences in the organization of service and per capita income, among other reasons.

Health benefit costs and health-related absences constitute a financial burden for employers. The average number of missed workdays by employees with bipolar disorder or schizophrenia may be two to three times more than for employees without such disorders. There is also substantial cost associated with informal caregiving. For Alzheimer's disease, the annual cost of caregiving time and caregiver's lost earnings may be up to US $18 000 per patient in some settings. The costs can add up to billions of dollars for countries. Community studies show common mental disorders to be associated with considerable economic cost. Depression imposes a much larger economic burden on the society than chronic conditions such as hypertension, rheumatoid arthritis, and asthma. Mood disorders tend to be associated with higher per capita cost than anxiety disorders and alcohol-related disorders. However, in view of their higher prevalence, anxiety disorders impose more economic costs on the society. In the productive age of 18–65 years, loss of productivity accounts for much of the economic cost of common mental disorders.

Impact on Caregivers

Persons suffering from illnesses such as dementia, intellectual disability, schizophrenia, and bipolar disorder commonly draw on informal family sources for their care. Indeed, families are important resources in the community care of people with a variety of mental illness. Parents, children, and spouses are the most common informal caregivers. There are more female than male carers across most cultures. Caring roles can be diverse, ranging from supervision, help with activities of daily living, to emotional support. Whatever the role, there is an extensive literature documenting the burden of caring for persons with mental illness on caregivers. The nature of the burden is often diverse. Psychological, physical, and social stresses are common. Among psychological distress, depression is the most extensively studied. For example, the prevalence of depression among carers of dementia sufferers may be up to 50%. Increased rates of anxiety and other psychiatric disorders are also found. Physical strain and physical health problems are frequent, especially when carers are themselves old. Compromised immune response has been reported and this is sometimes associated with increased susceptibility to physical illness, including infections. Economic loss is common, especially in lost earnings. Opportunities for social interactions and leisure are constrained and carers' quality of life is commonly lower than control groups with similar sociodemographic attributes but with no caring roles. Among patients' characteristics that increase burden on the carers are level of behavioral disturbance and severity of symptoms. Prolonged duration of contact between carer and patient is also a frequent factor.

Mortality

Excess mortality has been clearly documented in patients with mental disorders. This has been attributed to both natural and unnatural causes. Standardized mortality ratios (SMRs) for both natural (deaths resulting from somatic diseases) and unnatural (deaths due to accidents and suicide) causes of death in psychiatric patients are more than twice that of the general population. SMRs for unnatural causes of death are greater than that for natural causes. Neuropsychiatric disorders account for 1.4% of all years of life lost (YLL) and have been linked with significant reduction in life expectancy.

This excess mortality in patients with mental illness can be accounted for in part by the increased frequency of death from suicides and accidents. However, there is an excess mortality risk from all causes of death associated with mental disorders. Increased risk of death has been reported in patients with serious mental illness, particularly schizophrenia, dementia, major affective disorder, and substance use disorders. The leading causes of death include cardiovascular diseases, suicides, accidents, respiratory diseases, infections, and malignancies. Mortality rates are higher for men than women, but SMRs are higher for women. The highest mortality relative risk is observed between 20 and 40 years of age. There is increased risk of mortality in patients who had at least one episode of inpatient care compared with out-patients and more deaths occur in the first few years of follow-up after initial diagnosis and within a short time interval of last hospitalization.

The most commonly reported natural causes of death in psychiatric populations include cardiovascular disease, respiratory disease, infections, and metabolic disorders. The risk factors associated with this in patients with mental illness include higher rates of smoking and substance abuse, medication-induced weight gain, poor personal hygiene, and reduced physical activity. Another important factor is the health gap faced by people with mental illness; physical diseases are likely to go undetected or are inadequately treated. It has been suggested that up to one-third of psychiatric patients may harbor an undiagnosed medical condition. Some studies have also shown that patients with mental disorders may be less likely to receive appropriate medical or surgical intervention for physical illnesses than members of the general population with similar physical conditions.

Suicide and Accidental Deaths

Suicides and accidental deaths are a major cause of excess mortality in persons with mental disorders. Deaths from suicide and accidents are usually significantly higher than expected in patients than in other individuals. Accidental deaths have been linked to substance use disorders, especially alcohol use, depressive disorders, anxiety disorders, adjustment disorders, and personality disorders. Accidental deaths are more common in men than in women and are significantly increased in the presence of comorbidities. The risk of accidental death is increased in patients aged between 30 and 49 years.

Worldwide, suicide is estimated to represent 1.8% of the total global burden of disease in 1998. In 2000, approximately one million people died from suicide: a global mortality rate of 16 per 100 000. The majority of suicides occur in low- and middle-income countries. More than half of suicides occur in people aged 15–44 years; suicide is now ranked among the three leading causes of death in this age group for both sexes.

Mental disorders (particularly depression, substance abuse, schizophrenia, and other psychosis) are associated with more than 90% of all cases of suicide. Depression may account for up to 70% of all suicides. The lifetime risk of suicide in patients with mood disorders is about 30 times that of the general population. Higher rates of suicide are also found among unipolar depressed patients compared to those with bipolar affective disorders. The suicide risk in depressed patients is determined by the extent and severity of their symptoms. The severity of concurrent depressive symptoms rather than the presence of a depressive syndrome may determine suicidal behavior in patients with mixed affective or bipolar disorders. Schizophrenia is also associated with significant risk of suicide. The risk is increased, especially in young men, soon after diagnosis and in the presence of comorbid affective disorders.

High rates of psychiatric comorbidity have been reported in patients committing suicide. Comorbidity of psychiatric and personality disorder has been found to be an important risk factor for suicide. Personality traits that are thought to increase the risk of suicidal behavior include aggression and impulsivity. Mental illness necessitating admission has also been reported to be a strong risk factor for suicide. Suicidality is influenced by ethnic, sociodemographic, and psychological factors independent of diagnosis or diagnostic subgroup. Social and demographic factors associated with suicide include age, race, and marital status. Consistently lower rates of suicide have been reported in blacks compared to whites. On the other hand, higher mortality rates have been reported among separated, divorced, or widowed individuals than in those who were never married. Living alone has also been found to be a strong risk factor for suicide in psychiatric patients. With respect to gender, there are conflicting reports in the literature. Whereas some studies have found increased mortality in females, others report increased rates in men.

One of the strongest predictors of completed suicide is attempted suicide. Attempted suicide is also an indicator of extreme emotional distress (Kessler *et al.*, 2005). Epidemiologic surveys in the U.S. suggest that 1.1–4.6% of the general population attempt suicide at some time in their lifetime and that about 98% of those who make such an attempt may have a psychiatric diagnosis. The presence of any mental disorder is often a significant risk factor for suicidal attempt, but the odds for mood disorders are commonly higher than those for any other disorders. There is a significant link between suicidal attempts and comorbidity, with increased frequency of attempts with increasing number of psychiatric diagnoses. Adverse

experiences in childhood such as separation from parents, physical and sexual abuse, and maternal history of mental illness have been found to increase the likelihood of a history of lifetime suicidal attempt among adults (Gureje *et al.*, 2007). Given the relationship of such childhood adversities to mental disorders in adulthood, it is possible that they represent distal risk factors, while mental disorders represent more proximal vulnerabilities for suicidal behavior.

See also: Measurement of Psychiatric and Psychological Disorders and Outcomes in Populations; Mental Health Resources and Services; Stigma of Mental illness.

Citations

Gureje O, Kola L, Uwakwe R, et al. (2007) The profile and risks of suicidal behaviors in the Nigerian Survey of Mental Health and Well-Being. *Psychological Medicine* 37: 1–10.

Kessler RC, Berglund P, Borges G, Nock M, and Wang PS (2005) Trends in suicide ideation, plans, gestures and attempts in the United States 1990–1992 to 2001–2003. *Journal of the American Medical Association* 293: 2487–2495.

Ormel J, Oldenhinkel AJ, Nolen WA, and Vollebergh W (2004) Psychosocial disability before, during, and after a major depressive episode: A 3-wave population-based study of state, scar, and trait effects. *Archives of General Psychiatry* 61: 387–392.

Ormel J, Petukhova M, Chatterji S, et al. (in press). Disability and treatment of specific mental and physical disorders across the world: Results form the WHO World Mental Health Surveys. *British Journal of Psychiatry*.

World Health, Organization (2001) *The World Health Report 2001. Mental Health: New Understanding, New Hope.* Geneva, Switzerland: World Health Organization.

Further Reading

Belfer ML and Nurcombe B (2007) The epidemiology of child and adolescent mental disorder. In: Remschmidt H, Nurcombe B, Belfer ML, Sartorius N and Okasha A (eds.) *The Mental Health Needs of Children and Adolescents: An Area of Global Neglect*, pp. 1–11. Chichester, UK: John Wiley and Sons.

Bertelli M and Brown I (2006) Quality of life for people with intellectual disabilities. *Current Opinion in Psychiatry* 19: 508–513.

Buish-Bouwman MA, de Graaf R, Vollebergh WA, et al. (2006) Functional disability of mental disorders and comparison with physical disorders: A study among the general population of six European countries. *Acta Psychiatrica Scandinavica* 113(6): 492–500.

Cook JA (2006) Employment barriers for persons with psychiatric disabilities: Update of a report for the President's Commission. *Psychiatry Service* 57(10): 1391–1405.

Coryell W, Scheftner W, Keller M, Endicott J, Maser J, and Klerman GL (1993) The enduring psychosocial consequences of mania and depression. *American Journal of Psychiatry* 150: 720–727.

Evan S, Banerjee S, Leese M, and Huxley P (2007) The impact of mental illness on quality of life: A comparison of severe mental illness, common mental disorder and healthy population samples. *Quality of Life Resources* 16(1): 17–29.

Gardner HH, Kleinman NL, Brook RA, Rajagopalan K, Brizee TJ, and Smeeding JE (2006) The economic impact of bipolar disorder in an employed population from an employer perspective. *Journal of Clinical Psychiatry* 67(8): 1209–1218.

Harrington R, Fudge H, Rutter M, Pickles A, and Hill J (1990) Adult outcomes of childhood and adolescent depression: I. Psychiatric status. *Archives of General Psychiatry* 47: 465–473.

Katschnig H, Freeman H and Sartorius N (eds.) (2006) *Quality of Life in Mental Disorders.* 2nd edn. Chichester, UK: Wiley.

Keitner GI and Miller IW (1990) Family functioning and major depression: An overview. *American Journal of Psychiatry* 147: 1128–1137.

Knapp M, McCrone Fombonne E, Beecham J, and Wostear G (2002) The Maudsley long-term follow up of child and adolescent depression: 3. Impact of comorbid conduct disorder on service use and costs in adulthood. *British Journal of Psychiatry* 180: 19–23.

Kovess-Masfety V, Xavier M, Kustner BM, et al. (2006) Schizophrenia and quality of life: a one-year follow-up in four EU countries. *Biomedical Central Psychiatry* 6: 39.

Lopez-Bastida J, Serrano-Aguilar P, Perestelo-Perez L, and Oliva-Moreno J (2006) Social-economic costs and quality of life of Alzheimer disease in the Canary Islands, Spain. *Neurology* 67(12): 2186–2191.

Murray CJL and Lopez AD (1996) *The Global Burden of Disease: A Comprehensive Assessment of Mortality and Disability from Diseases, Injuries and Risk Factors in 1990 and Projected to 2020.* Cambridge, MA: Harvard University Press.

Schene AH, van Wijngaarden B, and Koeter MW (1998) Family caregiving in schizophrenia: Domains and distress. *Schizophrenic Bulletin* 24(4): 609–618.

Smit F, Cuijpers P, Oostenbrink J, et al. (2006) Costs of nine common mental disorders: Implications for curative and preventive psychiatry. *Journal of Mental Health Policy and Economics* 9(4): 193–200.

Stein MB, Roy-Byrne PP, Craske MG, et al. (2005) Functional impact and health utility of anxiety disorders in primary care outpatients. *Medical Care* 43(12): 1164–1170.

Stuart H (2006) Mental illness and employment discrimination. *Current Opinion in Psychiatry* 19: 522–526.

Trivedi MH, Rush AJ, Wisniewski SR, et al. (2006) Factors associated with healthy-related quality of life among outpatients with major depressive disorder: A STAR*D report. *Journal of Clinical Psychiatry* 67(2): 185–195.

WHO International Consortium in Psychiatric Epidemiology (2000) Cross-national comparisons of the prevalences and correlates of mental disorders. WHO International Consortium in Psychiatric Epidemiology. *Bulletin of the World Health Organization* 78: 413–426.

WHO World Mental Health Survey Consortium (2004) Prevalence, severity, and unmet need for treatment of mental disorders in the World Health Organization World Mental Health Surveys. *Journal of the American Medical Association* 291: 2581–2590.

Relevant Websites

http://www.nida.nih.gov/economiccosts – National Institute on Drug Abuse.

http://www.hcp.med.harvard.edu/wmh – The World Mental Health Survey Initiative.

http://www.who.int/healthinfo/bodproject/ – World Health Organization Burden of Disease.

Socio-Cultural Context of Substance Use/Abuse (Alcohol/Drugs/Tobacco)

D B Heath, Brown University, Providence, RI, USA

Glossary

Abuse As used in this article, excessive or problematic use.

Alcohol As used in this article, ethanol (C_2H_5OH), also called ethyl alcohol. Also any beverage that contains more than 1% ethanol by weight.

Drug As used in this article, any substance that changes behavior and/or consciousness when ingested.

Sociocultural Associated with the order of society and of the associated system of patterns of belief and behavior (i.e., culture).

The use of alcohol and drugs is an ancient and widespread custom among human beings throughout the world. Although some such usage is commonplace, specific beliefs and practices vary markedly from one population to another, and significant changes have occurred over time within many societies (Blum *et al.*, 1974). Far from being aberrant or isolated acts, alcohol and drug use are often highly valued and integrated with other aspects of the culture. This often involves important linkages between such use and religion, economics, diet, health beliefs and practices, social organization, literature and the arts, or other features of daily life, as well as with exceptional concerns. At the same time, it is important to acknowledge that alcohol and other drugs can be harmful to the user or others. They can be toxic, can greatly increase the risk of accidents, and can even cause physiological damage to various organs and social, psychological, and other disruptions. Dependence (often called addiction) is uncommon but is a major interference with a user's social obligations and expectations, which partly explains why abuse has been the subject of scientific study more than moderate use, which is much more common. In view of humankind's long ambivalence, a wide range of such sociocultural influences, in combination with the biophysiological impacts that alcohol and drugs have on the human organism, and a variety of psychological causes and effects, are all important for understanding the association between such usages and public health.

Alcohol/Drug Use in Evolutionary Perspective

There has been little systematic attention paid to alcohol or drug use by non-human animals, although Siegel (1989) reviewed the literature and described intoxication among various birds, fish, insects, mammals, and reptiles. Altered behavior after the ingestion of diverse substances was so commonplace that he characterized the quest for intoxication as a primary motivational force, the fourth drive (on a par with hunger, thirst, and sex).

As far as origins of alcohol/drug use are concerned, there is little in the way of empirical evidence, although myths, folktales, and popular beliefs abound, usually with respect to whatever substance is most favored locally. Given the present state of archaeological technology, there is little opportunity to know with confidence many details about alcohol/drug use by prehominid or ancient human beings. Speculation tends to emphasize either accidental discovery or imitation based on the observations of animals' reactions to naturally occurring substances.

In other instances, supernatural beings were said to have given alcohol or drugs to humankind. Dionysus was both the god and origin of wine for ancient Greeks; Bacchus was his counterpart for Romans. Similarly, Egyptians supposedly learned about beer (which they called liquid bread) from the god Osiris; in the Americas, Aztecs claimed to have got pulque from Mayahuel, a goddess with forty breasts.

Although alcohol/drug use are widespread phenomena in human cultures, they have not evolved in any discernible sequence overall, nor do they evidence similar or even analogous patterns over time in most parts of the world.

The earliest archaeological evidence of both beer and wine appears in the Near East about 7000 years ago. Beer rapidly diffused as a staple food, whereas wine was long a luxury product, although its popularity also spread both east and west. Drinking and drunkenness were both much appreciated, until Islam spread through much of the same area after 700 AD, and most interpreted Koranic injunctions as prohibiting the use of alcohol.

It remains a mystery why most of North America and the islands of the Pacific did not have alcoholic beverages until the arrival of Europeans. When such drinks were introduced, some peoples rejected them and others embraced them. The homebrewed beers of sub-Saharan Africa and what is now Latin America have tended to persist in both alimentary and ritual roles, even while industrial beers are gaining.

Distillation was probably invented by Arabs in North Africa and diffused to Western alchemists a couple of centuries before it became popular around 1200 AD. Opium, smoked or eaten, was highly esteemed as a tranquilizer throughout much of Asia, and derivatives of it served as such and as analgesics throughout Europe and North America in the nineteenth century. Heroin was originally hailed as a cure for opium addiction in much the same manner that cocaine was initially embraced as both mentally and physically therapeutic. Heroin and cocaine in various forms have enjoyed popularity in recent decades and are the basis of a vast international trade, much of which is illicit. Although caffeine is the active ingredient in coffee, tea, and chocolate, each of these beverages has its distinct history. Coffee spread from eastern Africa and the Near East, and, in the early years, was often suspected of eroding the moral values of those who drank it. Various governments banned it and closed coffeehouses as supposed hotbeds of immorality, sedition, and even revolution. But such prohibitions tended to be short-lived, and coffee is now extremely popular, with or without food, and is rarely even considered to be a drug. Although tea originated in Asia, it spread rapidly over the British Empire and is now a popular staple, similarly no longer viewed as a drug. Chocolate, having originated in pre-Columbian Mexico, underwent a similar dispersion linked with a similar trajectory from popularity to suspicion and on to acceptance as benign. Tobacco contains nicotine and other psychoactive substances; it similarly spread rapidly (from the Caribbean) to circle the globe in a few years, sometimes embraced and sometimes reviled, whether smoked, sniffed, or chewed. Recent health concerns have diminished its use in the developed world, although its popularity is still increasing in many poorer regions. Also during the past century, ether drinking has been replaced by solvent sniffing, and a variety of synthesized drugs now offer central nervous system (CNS) stimulation, relief from pain, or escape to bored or harried urbanites throughout the world system.

Alcohol/Drug Use among Humankind Today

There is so much variation among the substances that are used by human beings even now that it is not easy to provide just an illustrative sampling. More importantly, the social and cultural meanings, patterns of usage, values, and associated attitudes are yet more varied in ways that are important but rarely recognized. One convenient way of ordering such data is geographically, with a brief survey of influential drugs and outstanding uses as encountered in major world areas. This is not an arbitrary convention inasmuch as the natural environment comprises a complex interrelated system of soil, flora, fauna, climate, and other factors that can be viewed as the context for all human behaviors. With respect to alcohol, for example, the sugar content of plants affects their aptness for fermentation, and a shortage of fuel may preclude distillation. The molecular composition of a leaf or vine may harbor psychoactive potential, but it is moot unless ingested.

Biologists and ethnopharmacologists do not yet know why the Western Hemisphere is home to many times more psychoactive plants than the Eastern. Neither do historians or anthropologists understand how people came to use such plants, a tantalizing mystery in part because so many require elaborate processing and are highly toxic at various stages in their preparation.

Part of the ecological richness of what is now Latin America is a wealth of plants that have psychoactive properties and that have been used by native peoples in various ways. Coca grows throughout the area but is most potent at about 2000 m elevation in the Andes. The Incas and their descendants traded it far and wide; farmers still chronically chew it to relieve hunger, thirst, and cold, and shamans use it for divination, diagnosis, and other ritual purposes. Simple processing of it yields an addictive paste, and more sophisticated refinement yields powdered cocaine hydrochloride, which is widely used worldwide. Nowadays, it tends to be sniffed by wealthy users who find small quantities exciting but not interfering with the rest of their lives. The same drug tends to be taken by injection by a small group of poor and compulsive users who must often resort to crime or prostitution to feed their dependency.

Forested lowland areas of Latin America yield many snuffs, cactus fruits, and mushrooms that are still used by native peoples for myriad purposes. One of the most famous is ayahuasca, long a medication and inducer of visions that would be helpful to the community; it has recently become popular among outsiders who are seeking shortcuts to divine revelation or direct contact with what they interpret as primal forces of nature. Peyote, rich in LSD, was and is a sacrament to Huichol Indians in Mexico and to members of the Native American Church in North America. When chewed, it induces visual hallucinations that a believer interprets as directives for proper living, and it has diffused little beyond that religious context.

Snuffs and drinks made from a variety of plants are common throughout Latin America, but usually their magical powers are monopolized by a few specialists who provide services to the community. Drug-induced visions often allow practitioners to learn about enemies, the dead, or others, and have been reported in considerable detail. Ethnobotany and ethnopharmacology have become big business, and traditional native knowledge is being actively sought by international pharmaceutical companies. Drug tourism has recently become a small

source of income in some regions, as is the quest for shamanic and ecstatic experiences.

The islands of the Pacific generally lacked alcoholic beverages before the arrival of Europeans. Kava is a mild stimulant that was often mistaken for a fermented drink. Traditionally, it played an important ceremonial role in maintaining social hierarchy, but has gradually become secularized and popular. Its recent combination with alcohol often results in aggression, in contrast with its tranquilizing and sociable effects in traditional use. Although some populations in Oceania have not accepted alcohol, others have been transformed by it, especially as young men who lack meaningful social roles drink heavily and act out in boisterous ways. Similar problems often occur among aboriginal Australians, who are stereotyped as chronic drunkards although their average per capita consumption is lower than that of white Australians. The traditional native drug, pituri, is little used nowadays, but the sniffing of gasoline and other volatile substances is highly visible among the poorest of the aboriginal population.

Different drugs have long been favored in various parts of Asia. In the southeast, betel is still habitually chewed, even though many consider it unsightly. Opium derived from poppies is often smoked, eaten or sold to outsiders as a major commodity in trade. Those who become dependent in opium-producing regions tend to be the aged, for whom it serves as self-medication; despite easy availability, growers and traders rarely use it.

In northern Asia, the fly agaric mushroom is so esteemed as a hallucinogen that men drink urine to get a second-hand or prolonged dose of the active agent. China's many nationalities use alcohol in many different ways, often significantly embedded in social rituals, and the Russians' love of vodka is increasingly cited as a major cause of short life expectancy.

Across most of Europe, alcohol is widely known and enjoyed, although in very different ways. Cultures in the southern band of countries in Europe are often called 'wine cultures'; wine is common as an adjunct to meals, and average per capita alcohol consumption is exceptionally high. A middle band of so-called 'beer cultures' tend to favor beers and ales, whereas 'spirits cultures' line the north, with infrequent but heavy drinking of distillates. Recent decades have seen a remarkable trend toward homogeneity, with almost every country drinking less of its traditionally dominant beverage and more of others.

Throughout much of Africa, native beers are commonplace, often as the primary beverage and nutritionally important in the diet. The base varies, with barley, millet, honey, dates, maize, and palm nuts the most common. Apart from their value as food and refreshments, such beers have traditionally played important roles in gifting, purifying, signaling friendship, hospitality, or other symbolizing. Factory-made beer is gaining popularity in recent years, although many of the traditional uses continue. Drug use for psychoactive effects is relatively rare in most of Africa. In the sub-Saharan region, tobacco is commonly used as a relaxant but it lacks the special religious, judicial, and other symbolism that alcohol has. In the north, tea and coffee tend to be important as adjuncts to food and as hospitality, but few other drugs have much importance.

Sociocultural Influences in Alcohol/Drug Use

Anthropologists often define culture as the system of patterns of belief and behavior that shape the worldview of a given population, and society as the array of statuses and role relationships that describe the composition and organization of a population. By eliding the concepts, it is both convenient and revealing to attend to a variety of factors, social and cultural or sociocultural, that are important to human beings in their quotidian lives but that are rarely identified or measured in other terms or by other methods.

The conceptual linkage of 'alcohol and drugs' is also a fairly recent convention and one that has not yet gained general acceptance. In broad terms, it stands for a huge variety of substances that are psychoactive or mind altering when ingested. By changing the internal chemistry of the body, especially the transmission of messages across nerve cells in the brain, alcohol and drugs have various effects that are regulated in large part by their composition and dosage.

However, we have already seen that alcohol/drug use is far more complex than would be implied by the direct action of a chemical agent upon a host body; an enormous third class of variables is often referred to simply as the environment. For those reasons, alcohol/drug use is often characterized as a biopsychosocial phenomenon that cannot be understood unless all those several and diverse types of variables are taken into consideration.

In the simplest terms, there is no single meaning, use, or function that is assigned to alcohol or any drug in a universal manner. On the contrary, they are often evaluated in diametrically contrasting ways such that, for example, sometimes they are viewed as sacred and sometimes as sacrilegious, alternatively healthful and harmful, inspiring or repugnant, relaxing or stimulating, liberating or enslaving, and so forth. Because the scope of sociocultural influences on alcohol/drug use is so large, the following discussion is divided into sections that focus on patterns of use, associated attitudes, a variety of problems that are said to be linked with them, some benefits, and notes on prevention and treatment of problems.

Patterns of Alcohol/Drug Use

One need not seek out isolated or exotic populations in order to find significant differences in terms of alcohol/drug use. Within the United States, there are some Protestant groups for whom avoidance of coffee, tea, and alcohol are issues of faith, whereas others use wine in a key sacramental ritual. Switzerland and The Netherlands have become venues for drug tourism because their emphasis on harm-avoidance as crucial in public health policy is associated with more liberal treatment of drug selling and drug taking. So-called 'wet cultures' in southern Europe have relatively high rates of per capita alcohol consumption based on frequent drinking of small quantities, whereas so-called 'dry countries' in northern Europe have relatively low rates of consumption based on infrequent drinking but in large quantities.

Chinese and Arab attitudes about alcohol are of special interest because both groups long praised drinking and drunkenness as not only permissible and enjoyable, but even as desirable and commendable. Songs, poetry, paintings, and inscriptions on a variety of fine objects attest to these positive values in ancient times. Religious and political changes in both cultural systems have resulted in more negative views of alcohol, including episodic prohibition under various emperors of China and lasting prohibition under Shariah, the Islamic legal code enforced in some countries.

In the various areas where prohibition for secular reasons has been attempted, it has rarely endured long in the face of widespread criminality, corruption, and disregard for the law. Informal social controls often carry more weight than laws, however, so we often find that young people are not allowed to drink; females, if they drink, are often discouraged from having as much as males, and those in critical or liminal statuses (such as menstruation, initiation, pregnancy, devotion, to name a few) may find themselves hedged about with specific restrictions.

Cannabis nicely illustrates both cultural differences and rapid changes in drug use and associated symbols. There are communities in India where high-caste Hindus indulge in cannabis tea while low-caste members of the same village drink a locally made liqueur. Each group speaks lavishly about the benefits of its drink, and each deplores the other's. Closer to home, cannabis was long viewed in the United States as an unfortunate weakness of a few jazz musicians, blacks, or Hispanics, but not a threat to the white middle class. That abruptly changed when reefer madness was publicized as turning innocent young people into murderous or rapacious monsters after smoking a single cigarette. At the same time that laborers in Jamaica and Costa Rica were heavily smoking cannabis as an energizer, and finding that they could do more work, earn more, buy better houses, and educate their children, students there and elsewhere were finding relaxation and indifference in smaller doses of the same drug. Popular resentment against disproportionate punishment for cannabis use and in favor of the medical relief that it appears to provide for AIDS, glaucoma, chemotherapy, and other ills has resulted in a few states' recently opposing the federal ban on that drug in the United States.

Demography is far removed from pharmacology in anyone's view of the world, and yet it is a sociocultural influence that was crucial in shaping one form of drug use. Middle-aged men from several Levantine countries thoroughly enjoyed daily sessions in which they chewed qat leaves and quietly talked with male friends, but had to forgo such use when they went to work in Britain. When the expatriate colony there grew large enough to warrant it, an enterprising merchant was quick to fly in fresh qat so that stylized daily use could be resumed.

The imagery of opium as luxurious in oriental settings, nefarious when used to recruit Western women as sex slaves, inspiring for bohemian artists, analgesic in the hands of a physician, or addicting when offered by a pusher on the street all relate to the same substance and reflect changing ideological emphases and contexts.

Smoking tobacco was a concrete way of symbolizing the links between human beings and both natural and supernatural forces for many tribes of North American Indians. Cigarettes were thought feminine at the start of the twentieth century and masculine after World War I. Health warnings and the assertion of nonsmokers' rights have resulted in rapid reduction of smoking in many areas that are economically and politically dominant, while there has been a similarly abrupt rise in smoking in developing regions.

Modern technology and the global economy have facilitated the spread of alcohol and drugs, to the point where some would say that there is now a multisocietal and transcultural pattern. To the extent that such a pattern is meaningful, it could probably be described as consisting of name-branded beers, relatively expensive wines, and Scotch whisky as drinks that signal wealth and associated power or prestige. Industrially produced drugs tend to have a similar cachet, although cocaine, heroin, cannabis, and their derivatives have a truly global market, despite stringent legal and other restrictions. Such drugs are often used excessively by addicts for whom drug use has become a preoccupation that overwhelms concerns for health, family, or other workaday relationships. Although such usage is too often misinterpreted as typical and causes a variety of lamentable problems, it is rare in epidemiological terms.

In fact, there are few societies in which drugs are used more often than weekly, and fewer in which usage is casual and dissociated from connotations of the sacred or powerful. Tobacco, coffee, tea, and chocolate are rare exceptions to that generalization, although each of them also has its own kind of symbolic importance in various social and cultural contexts.

Special Attitudes about Alcohol/Drug Use

Alcohol and drug use are behaviors that are often the focus of considerable affect and emotion, whether in favor or in opposition. Different populations show a broad range of affect and emotion, from frequent and ostentatious use and praise to prohibition and vehement condemnation of the substances, their use, and the outcomes of such use. Popular attitudes are often significantly different with respect to different substances, or they may differ for different categories of users or different contexts and purposes of use. It is commonplace that popular attitudes differ from official attitudes as expressed by authorities and as codified in laws and regulations, which tend to be more restrictive although not always diligently enforced.

Many observers have remarked on the frequency with which such attitudes reflect a profound ambivalence, combining recognition of the inherent risk that excessive use may result in problems affecting not only the user but also others with appreciation of various short-term benefits that accrue to those who use such substances in moderate or sensible ways.

The crucial role of sociocultural influences on such use and special attitudes about use is evident in the fact that both use and attitudes have often varied significantly with respect to the same substance from time to time, often reversing within just a few years. A dramatic illustration is the United States, where the 1960s saw widespread alcohol/drug use as part of a movement toward greater independence and freedom from responsibility for individuals. In subsequent decades, an extreme negative connotation has been given to drugs, so strong that the very word is often interpreted as implying harm, risk, and illegality. Corporations that used to offer proudly a wide range of preventive or curative 'drugs' now deal in 'pharmaceuticals,' and some who favor abstinence from alcohol are quick to insist that it be treated like 'other drugs.' Such negative emotional loading is commonplace, regardless of legality or popularity of use. A fad for zero-tolerance has resulted in schools' disciplining students for sharing candies, individuals' having their vital medications taken from them, and so forth.

Problems Associated with Alcohol/Drug Use

A large part of what is written about alcohol/drug use in recent years has a distinctly negative bias, presuming that all use is abuse, so that vague but alarming statements are made about rapidly accelerating consumption around the world. Linked with consumption are a host of problems, some physical, others psychological, and still others social, that often affect nonusers as well as users. Such problems are quite variable, ranging from liver cirrhosis to absence from school or work, from spouse abuse to dependence or addiction, and from illegal trafficking to personal embarrassment. Those who have a primary concern with public health or law enforcement tend to emphasize different problems within their areas of responsibility, and the data are generally poor. Nevertheless, a closer look at their own numbers shows that fewer than 1 in 10 of those who admit to habitually using either drugs or alcohol experience any such problems in association with such use (Walton, 2002).

In most societies, about 90% of those who use alcohol do so without suffering any of the so-called alcohol-related problems that tend to be the focus of concern in public safety and health. It is generally estimated that roughly the same proportions hold among drug users. It is also common that those 10% of users who suffer various problems are responsible for at least 80% of overall consumption. With few exceptions, therefore, it can be said that alcohol/drug use is most often unproblematic except in the case of exceptionally heavy or excessive use, which is often referred to as abuse. Nevertheless, the reality and importance of alcohol/drug use and of related problems is such a preoccupation that it warrants our paying attention to at least five broad areas: economic, political, legal, health, and social welfare.

Economic

At the beginning of the twenty-first century, alcohol and drugs must be recognized as together comprising one of the major businesses in many parts of the world in terms of foreign currency although rarely in terms of employment. Statistics are lacking because most of the commerce is surreptitious and untaxed. Where governments actively try to control drug traffic, the direct costs are enormous and indirect costs are also substantial, including an illicit network of distribution, intense competition at every level of the market, and high costs to consumers, some of whom must rely on criminal activity to support their use of drugs.

Where alcohol/drugs are legal, they tend to provide at least some income from taxation; users are spared the extra burden of criminality for their habits, and the general crime rate tends to be lower. Where they are positively approved, few economic costs are evident.

In many frontier areas, alcohol was often used as a crucial commodity in trade. It combined high value in small volume and was produced by a technology that native people did not readily master. As such, it served as a tool of colonialism and even today is still used as part of wages in some developing regions. Growers, refiners, and major traffickers rarely use such products enough to become dependent on them, but it is not unusual to find that those who do the most lowly work in such a network receive partial payment in drugs and often become dependent.

Legality is not the only consideration, however; spouses or companions often complain that too much is spent on alcohol/drugs, leaving too little in the budget for other needs. In extreme cases, this can result in spouse or child abuse or neglect, although wealthy users can often spend huge amounts without suffering financially.

Compulsive use of alcohol/drugs can interfere with an individual's ability to take part in the labor market, as it does with other social relationships. In general, alcohol/drug use tends to occur in inverse proportion to income, education, and status, and the testimony of the heaviest users suggests that it is at least as often a symptom as it is a cause of their poverty. A quest for excitement, good feelings, or respites from daily tedium or frustrations has prompted many of those who could least afford it to turn to alcohol/drugs.

Political

As with any behavior, the degree of social acceptance, indifference, or rejection of alcohol/drug use is important in determining who does it, where, when, how, and with what consequences. Correlatively, alcohol/drug use is often cited as an important characteristic of particular individuals or categories of people, explaining or justifying their treatment by others in the society.

The significant profit margin that is involved in alcohol/drug traffic generates considerable wealth and correlatively, power and politics are involved even – or especially – in instances where the traffic is illegal. The problem of political influences associated with alcohol/drug use is aggravated where national boundaries are crossed and differing laws, policies, and groups of officials must be dealt with.

Where official policies fit well with popular beliefs and practices, alcohol/drug use tend to be unremarkable, often integrated with workaday activities and the pace of life. Where they are discrepant, alcohol/drug use can be a focus of social and cultural strains, defiance of the law, dissatisfaction, and prejudicial treatment of users.

One important political aspect of alcohol/drug use is the fiscal implications for the state. At various times, as much as 20% of Russia's income was derived from distilled spirits; more than half the retail price of beverage alcohol is taxed in several jurisdictions. A state monopoly can give money and power to the state; private enterprise in such commerce can bring significant pressures to bear on officials and legislators.

Even the predominant sociocultural view of morality is intertwined with politics and policies. Where drinkers and drug users are thought to be weak-willed, dissolute, frivolous, or irresponsible, they are often imprisoned or otherwise punished and rarely helped by public institutions. Where they are thought to suffer from a disease, a more philanthropic pattern of harm reduction, treatment, rehabilitation, or social support is often offered.

A striking contrast can be seen between the United States and The Netherlands. In the United States, sentencing for possession of certain drugs has resulted in the imprisonment of millions of individuals, with minorities disproportionately represented, even though studies consistently show those minority populations to be less involved in alcohol/drug use. An explicit emphasis on harm reduction rather than punishment in The Netherlands is reflected in the availability of cannabis in public tea shops, police permissiveness where drug users congregate at certain parks, and publicly sponsored needle exchange, drugs, and treatment for those who want them.

Just as some types of alcohol/drugs tend to be associated with disreputable persons and groups, others are thought to symbolize or demonstrate modernity, sophistication, wealth, or prestige. Those who have paid close attention to alcohol/drug policies cross-culturally and internationally are in broad agreement that scientific knowledge usually plays a smaller role than emotional appeals when it comes to shaping government policies. A costly U.S. war on drugs during recent decades has been declared effective by those who point to burgeoning prison populations and called ineffective by those who point to cheaper and more abundant drugs. Most activities of the war on drugs have been devoted to attempts at diminishing supply rather than reducing demand.

Legal

The majority of alcohol and drug use throughout the world is quite legal and by no means disapproved from the point of view of neighbors or public authorities. This is not to say that it has been ignored by the law.

A major part of the earliest known legal code (Hammurabi's) was devoted to beer and wine; the primary concern was not with restricting use but rather with protecting users from unscrupulous dealers. Because of its great popularity, alcohol has often been heavily taxed, with accompanying regulations to facilitate the monitoring of production and distribution.

Prohibition for secular purposes has been tried episodically in various areas, generally with mixed results. Sweden tried it for a time, switched to rationing, and settled on a system that combined state monopoly of production and distribution, which has subsequently been liberalized (at the behest of the European Union). Denmark banned beer for some years while allowing easy access to distilled spirits; the situation was reversed for another period of years, and now all alcohol beverages are readily available. Parts of Canada, Mexico, Finland, Honduras, and few other countries have briefly banned alcohol, but no such prohibition has lasted long. Smaller jurisdictions (states, provinces, counties, towns, reserves of Indians or native peoples, etc.) frequently ban sales but also frequently find it difficult to keep people from bringing in alcohol from outside, or producing it clandestinely.

Cycles of strong temperance ideology with associated restrictions have occurred with some regularity throughout the history of the United States, often in association with a bundle of attitudes favoring exercise, fresh air, wholesome foods, and clean living in general.

Many of the substances that are now not only legal but viewed as innocuous were viewed with suspicion earlier. For example, coffee and chocolate were often described in terms very similar to those that opponents now use for cannabis, and both sale and consumption of these items were outlawed in many jurisdictions.

A noteworthy example of rapid sociocultural change is the recent combination of popular concern and legal sanctions against driving while under the influence of alcohol. Within living memory, many countries have enacted laws that specify a certain blood-alcohol concentration as *prima facie* evidence of drunkenness and what used to be routinely treated as a joke has become a major offense.

The law is not color-blind, and some see racism in the fact that U.S. sanctions against possessing or selling crack (preferred by blacks) are ten times as severe as those for powdered cocaine (mostly used by whites). Many families and communities are deeply affected by alcohol/drug use, enforcement of laws against it, and by economic and other anomalies that are associated with alcohol and drugs.

Health

As with many of the other classes of problems, the most widely discussed negative outcomes for health are generally associated with frequent, heavy, and long-term use rather than with light or moderate use. Alcohol is a good example, about which many physicians approve two or three drinks a day, but warn against more than five or six within a few hours.

For many years, education about alcohol focused on major damage caused to various organ systems that was found only late in the careers of the heaviest drinkers, such as peripheral neuropathy, liver cirrhosis, or pancreatitis. Little recognition was given to the fact that fully 90% of those who drink never encountered any health problem as a result.

Ample publicity given to the link between tobacco use and cancer in recent decades has prompted nonsmokers to clamor for increasing smoke-free venues, to the point where a few entire cities have banned smoking in public places. Despite widespread health warnings, often mandated on each package, consumption is increasing among some populations so rapidly that it makes up for decreases among others.

Intravenous drugs are blamed, as is unprotected sex, for much of the rapid spread of hepatitis and HIV/AIDS in many parts of the world. The sharing of needles and other paraphernalia, together with frequent exchanges of sex for drugs, justify such concerns, especially among addicts who often spend considerable time together in crowded and unsanitary conditions.

The monstrous generation of crack babies that were predicted in the 1990s did not materialize, nor did that of fetal alcohol syndrome a decade earlier; evidently only long-term chronic use by the mother is harmful to the fetus. However, both the expense and the distractions of addiction often interfere with the complex sociocultural expectations of mothering in a broad sense, so that poor nutrition, lack of cleanliness, and associated health problems are common among addicts and their families.

For wealthy cosmopolitan individuals, misuse of prescription drugs, anxiolitics, and analgesics is a dangerous trend that is rapidly increasing. A rash of other synthesized drugs can be injurious if used in inappropriate combinations or by naive users. Examples are the so-called date-rape drug that has become a common adjunct to seduction and the drug Ecstasy (MMDA), which causes harmful hyperthermia and dehydration among young people at rave parties. The popular interest in sports is reflected in a preoccupation with steroids and other performance-enhancing drugs, even though their use is limited to a small segment of the population. The well-publicized epidemic of methamfetamine use is unusual for being more rural than urban and for having flourished especially in the midwestern United States, where other drugs have generally been less popular. Cheap and easy to produce, it is a stimulant and produces tolerance, which may be mistaken for instant addiction. Alarmist fears about meth-babies are reminiscent of similar fears about crack-babies a generation earlier.

Social Welfare

Sociocultural attitudes and values play a major role in shaping the nature and extent of problems that people associate with alcohol/drug use and with the public good. Negative labeling that brands a user as degenerate, irresponsible, or criminal carries stigma that sometimes discredits that person as undeserving of help from others. By contrast, identification of the compulsive user as suffering from an illness tends to be associated with a more supportive strategy of harm reduction.

In many urban or cosmopolitan areas, excessive alcohol/drug users constitute an underclass, marginal in economic, political, and other terms. Such marginality is sometimes a cause and sometimes an effect of alcohol/drug use, especially among minority populations who may simultaneously be suffering from cultural deprivation, ethnic prejudice, or related pressures in a society dominated by others with alien ways of thinking and acting.

Well-intentioned but misguided policies sometimes predominate in attempts to foster social welfare. One example is the presumption that using alcohol predisposes a person to use various drugs (the gateway or stepping-stone hypothesis), commonly cited as a threat to prevent young people from drinking, but with little evidence to support it.

Benefits Associated with Alcohol/Drug Use

There are many different kinds of benefits that people enjoy from alcohol/drug use, just as there are many different kinds of harm. Not all individuals experience the same benefits, just as not all suffer similar harms. Medicinal or therapeutic use to control or relieve symptoms is an important part of overall use; evidence is also rapidly accumulating about a number of long-term health benefits of moderate drinking, and the social and psychological benefits are so well known as to receive little scientific attention.

Many such benefits and harms have clear bases in physicochemical effects, but often they are also strongly influenced by sociocultural factors. For example, hallucinogens produce visual and other sensory stimuli that are exciting and inspiring for some who are artistically inclined. Drug-induced hallucinations often provide clues to the diagnosis of illness or to foretelling the future, but only among those who are culturally attuned to having such revelatory experiences and know how to interpret the cues.

Similarly, depressants and soporifics provide relaxation, which can be a boon for those for whom it is otherwise difficult to achieve. By contrast, stimulants can be useful to foster action and social interaction.

The symbolism of alcohol in terms of sociability and hospitality makes it sometimes an important part of business or a convenient way of signaling acceptance or approbation. Its widespread use as an adjunct to celebration lends special weight to certain events, and is linked to public demonstrations of approval. In general, those settings in which alcohol/drug use is a communal activity or a ceremonial one that has positive meaning for members of the group tend to be highly approved and rewarded in various sociocultural ways.

Prevention and Treatment of Alcohol/Drug Problems

Our historical and cross-cultural perspective has already shown that the very idea that certain problems are associated with alcohol/drug use is shaped by sociocultural influences and not merely by the effects that substances have on people. Different and changing views about what constitutes a problem, how alcohol/drug use relates to problems, and how such linkage can be broken are all important with respect to prevention and treatment.

Social and cultural variables have significance even at the level of identification and diagnosis of illnesses and disabilities.

In recent decades, WHO (the World Health Organization) has become increasingly aware of differences in the etiology, symptoms, meanings, and attitudes toward psychological states and syndromes. Successive efforts at specifying observable and objective diagnostic criteria and terminology, especially with reference to alcohol/drug use and abuse, have repeatedly and progressively been demonstrated to be widely misunderstood and misapplied, even by professional practitioners who had received advanced training at European or North American institutions and who appear to be skilled in the English language. This should not have surprised the WHO inasmuch as it is a quintessential demonstration of the important impact that sociocultural influences have on alcohol/drug use, not only as it is practiced by peoples throughout the world but even as it is conceived by scientists.

Despite such large and important differences, there is increasing recognition of the abundant evidence that patterns of use tend to be more important than simple quantity and frequency of consumption, which have been the most common measures of use. This accounts for the fact that groups with the highest per capita annual consumption of alcohol (based on frequent moderate ingestion) have fewer problems than groups with much lower consumption (based on episodic excessive drinking).

Risky or harmful levels of use are increasingly targeted for change by those concerned with public health. This involves gradual modification of policies that have emphasized reducing overall consumption (interdiction, taxation, labeling, restrictions of sales, and advertising, etc.) and development of approaches that focus on heavy users. Twelve-step or mutual help groups have enjoyed remarkable success in aiding those who independently choose to stop or lessen alcohol/drug use. A wide range of treatments, ranging from behavior modification to cue recognition and simple counseling have all been found helpful for certain abusers, and growing recognition that occasional relapse is normal rather than a signal of failure has helped even more clients to achieve sobriety. Occasional examples of culturally specific prevention and treatment have been successful. Sweat bath and Sun Dance for Native Americans or vows for Hispanic Catholics are examples, and receptiveness to the interests and attitudes of clients is important, although superficial gestures of supposed cultural appropriateness are not so important as was once believed.

It is crucial to keep in mind that few societies have ever been wholly free of alcohol/drug use and that the reduction of harm is a more realistic goal than universal abstinence.

See also: Alcohol: The Burden of Disease; Alcohol Consumption: Overview of International Trends; Alcohol Industry; Alcohol—Socio-Economic Impacts (Including Externalities); Alcoholism Treatment; Control and Regulation of Currently Illegal Drugs; Illicit Drug Trends Globally; Illicit Drug Use and the burden of Disease.

Citations

Blum RH and Associates (1974) *Society and Drugs: Social and Cultural Observations.* San Francisco, CA: Jossey Bass.
Siegel RK (1989) *Intoxication: Life in Pursuit of Artificial Paradise.* New York: Simon and Schuster.
Walton S (2002) *Out of It. A Cultural History of Intoxication.* New York: Harmony Books.

Further Reading

Coomber R and South N (eds.) (2004) *Drug Use and Cultural Context "Beyond the West": Tradition, Change and Post-Colonialism.* London: Free Association Books.
Davenport-Hines R (2002) *Pursuit of Oblivion: A Global History of Narcotics.* New York: Norton.
Grant M and Litvak J (eds.) (1998) *Drinking Patterns and their Consequences.* Washington, DC: Taylor and Francis.
Heath DB (2000) *Drinking Occasions: Comparative Perspectives on Alcohol and Culture.* Philadelphia, PA: Brunner/Mazell.
Heath DB (ed.) (1995) *International Handbook on Alcohol and Culture.* Westport, CT: Greenwood Press.
Jaffe JH (ed.) (1995) *Encyclopedia of Drugs and Alcohol,* 4 vols. New York: Macmillan Library Reference USA.
Knipe E (1995) *Culture, Society and Drugs: The Social Science Approach to Drug Use.* Prospect Heights, IL: Waveland Press.
MacCoun RJ and Reuter P (2001) *Drug War Heresies: Learning from Other Vices, Times and Places.* New York: Cambridge University Press.
McCarthy RG (ed.) (1959) *Drinking and Intoxication: Selected Readings in Social Attitudes and Controls.* Glencoe, IL: Free Press.
Musto DF (1987) *The American Disease: Origins of Narcotic Control,* rev. ed. New York: Oxford University Press.
Peele S and Grant M (eds.) (1999) *Alcohol and Pleasure: A Health Perspective.* Philadelphia, PA: Brunner/Mazell.
Pittman DJ and White HR (eds.) (1991) *Society, Culture and Drinking Patterns Reexamined.* New Brunswick, NJ: Rutgers Center of Alcohol Studies.
Rudgley R (1993) *Essential Substances: A Cultural History of Intoxicants in Society.* New York: Kodansha America.
Tracy SW and Acker CJ (eds.) (2004) *Altering American Consciousness: The History of Alcohol and Drug Use in the United States, 1800–2000.* Amherst, MA: University of Massachusetts Press.

SECTION 2
CLINICAL SYNDROMES

Alcoholism Treatment

T F Babor, University of Connecticut School of Medicine, Farmington, CT, USA

Introduction

Despite its positive role as a beverage, a mood enhancer, and a social lubricant, alcohol accounts for a significant portion of the global burden of disease and disability, primarily through its toxic effects on different organ systems in the body, its ability to cause psychomotor impairment through intoxication, and its dependence-producing properties that can impair the drinker's control over the frequency and amount of drinking. For these reasons, various interventions have been developed to help people who are experiencing medical and social problems associated with their misuse of beverage alcohol. This article reviews conceptual advances and scientific evidence within the framework of a public health approach to the management of alcohol-related problems through clinical interventions. Such an approach assumes that an organized response to alcohol use disorders requires a conceptual understanding of the medical condition, the availability of screening and diagnostic procedures to identify cases for treatment, and the existence of effective interventions that can be made available to people in need of treatment and early intervention.

Conceptual Overview: What Is Being Treated?

Alcohol consumption varies enormously in terms of the frequency and amount of drinking, not only among individuals, but also over time and between different population groups. Variations in drinking affect rates of alcohol-related problems and have implications for the organization of treatment interventions. There is no sharp demarcation between social or moderate drinking, on the one hand, and problem or harmful drinking, on the other. But as the average daily amount of alcohol consumed and frequency of intoxication increase, so does the incidence of medical and psychosocial problems in a society. As illustrated in **Figure 1**, three mechanisms have been identified to explain alcohol's ability to cause medical, psychological, and social harm (Babor *et al.*, 2003): (1) physical toxicity, (2) intoxication, and (3) dependence.

Alcohol is a toxic substance in terms of its direct and indirect effects on a wide range of body organs and organ systems. In addition, one of the main causes of alcohol-related harm in the general population is alcohol intoxication, which is strongly related to violence, traffic casualties, and other injuries. Alcohol dependence has many different contributory causes, including genetic vulnerability, but it is a condition that is often contracted by repeated exposure to alcohol. In general, the heavier the drinking, the greater the risk is of developing alcohol dependence.

As illustrated in **Figure 1**, the mechanisms of toxicity, intoxication, and dependence are closely related to the ways in which people consume alcohol, called patterns of drinking. Drinking patterns that lead to rapidly elevated blood alcohol levels result in problems associated with acute intoxication such as accidents, injuries, and violence. Similarly, drinking patterns that promote frequent and heavy alcohol consumption are associated with chronic health problems such as liver cirrhosis, cardiovascular disease, and depression. Sustained drinking may also result in alcohol dependence. Once dependence is present, it impairs a person's ability to control the frequency and amount of drinking. For these reasons, the public health response should be designed to address not only the treatment of alcohol dependence, but also the management of persons who are both harmful and hazardous drinkers. Harmful drinkers are people without serious alcohol dependence whose alcohol misuse is already causing problems to their health, whereas hazardous drinkers are people who drink in ways that increase the risk of experiencing health or social problems.

Alcohol dependence has long been recognized to run in families. There is an estimated sevenfold risk of alcohol dependence in first-degree relatives of alcohol-dependent individuals. But the majority of alcohol-dependent individuals do not have a first-degree relative who is alcohol dependent. This underscores the fact that the risk for alcohol dependence is also determined by environmental factors, which may interact in complex ways with genetics.

A variety of approaches have been proposed to describe the diverse types of alcohol dependence encountered in clinical settings (Hesselbrock and Hesselbrock, 2006), in the interest of developing specialized treatment interventions that would address the needs of different types of alcohol-dependent drinkers, commonly called alcoholics. These include diagnostic classifications based on single characteristics such as onset age of alcohol problems (early vs. later in life), drinking pattern (continuous vs. binge drinking), family history of alcoholism, personality style, and the presence or absence of psychopathology. Multidimensional approaches combine these characteristics into meaningful clusters. One of the best known of these typologies is the Type 1/Type 2 distinction developed by Cloninger and colleagues (1987). Type 1 alcoholics are characterized by the late onset of problem drinking, rapid development of behavioral tolerance to alcohol, prominent guilt and anxiety related to drinking, and infrequent fighting and arrests when drinking. Cloninger also termed this subtype milieu-limited, which emphasizes the etiologic role of environmental factors. In contrast, Type 2 alcoholics are characterized by early onset of an inability to abstain from alcohol, frequent fighting and arrests when drinking, and the absence of guilt and fear concerning drinking. Differences in the two subtypes are thought to result from differences in three basic personality (i.e., temperament) traits, each of which has a unique neurochemical and genetic substrate.

Babor and colleagues (1992) used statistical clustering techniques to derive a dichotomous typology (Type A vs. Type B) similar to that proposed earlier by Cloninger. The analysis identified two homogeneous subtypes that may have important implications for understanding the etiology of different forms of alcoholism. Type A alcoholics have a later onset of alcohol-related problems, few childhood psychological problems, a less severe drinking history, and a more benign course of the disorder. Type B alcoholics have an early onset of alcohol-related problems, childhood behavior problems, parental alcoholism, co-occurring psychopathology, a more problematic drinking history, severe alcohol dependence, and a worse prognosis.

In addition to these different types of alcoholics, there are also substantial differences in the manifestation of alcohol dependence among different gender, age, and racial/cultural groups, suggesting the need for different treatment approaches. Adolescents have comparatively short histories of heavy drinking, and physiological

dependence on alcohol and alcohol-related medical complications are rare. The manifestations of alcohol dependence in the elderly are often more subtle and nonspecific than those observed in younger individuals.

Detection, Diagnosis, and Assessment of Alcohol Use Disorders

Diagnosis is the first step in the selection of treatment for persons with alcohol use disorders. Diagnosis not only includes the core syndrome of alcohol dependence, but also related conditions such as alcohol withdrawal and comorbid medical and psychiatric disorders. Diagnostic criteria for alcohol use disorders are described in the *International Classification of Diseases*, 10th edition (ICD-10) (World Health Organization, 1992). These criteria were based upon the alcohol dependence syndrome (ADS) concept of Edwards and Gross (1976), a theoretical formulation of ADS that includes biological, cognitive, and behavioral elements. As illustrated in **Table 1**, the ICD-10 diagnosis of alcohol dependence is given when three or more of the six criteria are present. Because physiological dependence is associated with greater potential for medical problems (particularly acute alcohol withdrawal), the first two criteria to be considered are tolerance and withdrawal. The remaining criteria reflect the behavioral and cognitive dimensions of ADS: (a) impaired control (i.e., alcohol is consumed in larger amounts or over a longer period of time than was intended; there is a

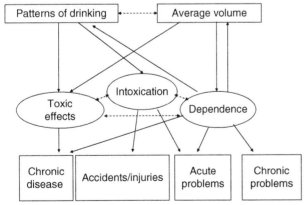

Figure 1 Schematic diagram illustrating how alcohol consumption is linked to alcohol-related problems through three mechanisms of action: Toxicity, intoxication, and dependence. Reproduced from Babor T, Caetano R, Casswell S, *et al.* (2003) *Alcohol: No Ordinary Commodity – Research and Public Policy.* Oxford, UK: Oxford University Press. By permission of Oxford University Press.

Table 1 Diagnostic guidelines for alcohol dependence syndrome according to the *International Classification of Diseases,* 10th edition

A definite diagnosis of dependence should usually be made only if three or more of the following have been experienced or exhibited at some time during the previous year:
 a. A strong desire or sense of compulsion to consume alcohol
 b. Difficulties in controlling alcohol consumption in terms of its onset, termination, or levels of use
 c. A physiological withdrawal state when alcohol use has ceased or been reduced
 d. Evidence of tolerance, such that increased doses of alcohol are required in order to achieve effects originally produced by lower doses
 e. Progressive neglect of alternative pleasures or interests because of alcohol use, increased amount of time necessary to consume alcohol or to recover from its effect
 f. Persisting with alcohol use despite clear evidence of overtly harmful consequences, such as harm to the liver through excessive drinking, depressive mood states consequent to periods of heavy use, or alcohol-related impairment of cognitive functioning

Adapted from World Health Organization (1992) *The ICD-10 Classification of Mental and Behavioural Disorders: Clinical Descriptions and Diagnostic Guidelines.* Geneva, Switzerland: World Health Organization.

persistent desire or unsuccessful efforts to cut down or control drinking; the individual continues to drink despite knowledge of a persistent or recurrent physical or psychological problem), and (b) increased salience of alcohol (i.e., a great deal of time spent drinking or recovering from its effects; important social, occupational, or recreational activities are given up or reduced due to drinking).

Alcohol withdrawal is a condition that follows a reduction in alcohol consumption or an abrupt cessation of drinking in alcohol-dependent individuals. Uncomplicated cases of alcohol withdrawal are characterized by increased heart rate, elevated blood pressure, hyperthermia, diaphoresis, tremor, nausea, vomiting, insomnia, and anxiety. Onset of withdrawal usually occurs between 4 and 12 h following the last drink. Symptom severity tends to peak around the second day, usually subsiding by the fourth or fifth day of abstinence. Alcohol withdrawal delirium (also known as delirium tremens) can occur in 5% of cases, usually between 36 and 72 h following alcohol cessation. This condition is characterized by autonomic hyperactivity as well as illusions, hallucinations, psychomotor agitation, cloudiness of consciousness, and disorientation. Prior history of delirium tremens, older age, poor nutritional status, comorbid medical conditions, and history of high tolerance to alcohol are predictors of increased severity of alcohol withdrawal.

In addition to alcohol dependence and alcohol withdrawal, chronic drinking is associated with disturbances in mood, sleep, and sexual function, which are typically included in the diagnostic evaluation. Alcohol-induced mood disorder is characterized by depressed mood and anhedonia, as well as expansive or irritable mood. Although mood disturbances are common among patients entering treatment, alcohol-induced mood symptoms tend to subside within 2–4 weeks following alcohol cessation. Heavy drinking can also induce generalized anxiety symptoms, panic attacks, and phobias. As with depression, a substantial improvement is often observed with abstinence with a full remission of taking as long as 3–4 weeks. Alcohol-induced psychotic disorder is another psychiatric syndrome observed in chronic alcoholics. This disorder is characterized by hallucinations or delusions that usually occur within a month of an alcohol intoxication or withdrawal episode. These psychotic symptoms tend to subside within a few weeks of abstinence, although some patients may require long-term treatment with antipsychotic medication.

Assessment of Alcohol Use Disorders

Improvements in the diagnosis of alcohol use disorders have been facilitated in part by the development of psychiatric and psychological tests. Comprehensive assessment provides the basis for accurate diagnosis and an individualized plan of treatment. Depending on the severity of alcohol dependence, the nature of comorbid medical

and psychiatric pathology, and the presence of family and other social supports, decisions can be made concerning the most appropriate intensity, setting, and modality of treatment. The optimal approach to the assessment of a drinking problem begins with the use of standardized measurement procedures, including screening tests and structured diagnostic interviews.

A number of self-report screening tests have been developed to identify alcoholics as well as persons at risk of alcohol problems. One of the most widely used screening tests is the CAGE (Ewing, 1984), which contains four questions: (1) Have you ever felt you ought to cut (the "C" in CAGE) down on your drinking? (2) Have people annoyed (A) you by criticizing your drinking? (3) Have you ever felt bad or guilty (G) about your drinking? (4) Have you ever had a drink first thing in the morning to steady your nerves or get rid of a hangover that is, an eye opener (E)? A score of 1 positive response suggests possible alcoholism and a score of two or more is interpreted as definite grounds for further diagnostic evaluation.

The Alcohol Use Disorders Identification Test (AUDIT) is a 10-item screening instrument developed by the World Health Organization for use in primary care settings (Saunders *et al.*, 1993). The AUDIT covers the domains of alcohol consumption, alcohol dependence, and alcohol-related consequences. It has been shown to be sensitive and specific in discriminating alcoholics from nonalcoholics and is superior to other tests in identifying hazardous drinkers. The AUDIT total score increases with the severity of alcohol dependence and related problems and can be used as part of a comprehensive approach to early identification and patient placement.

Following a positive screen or other indications of alcohol problems, diagnostic assessment should be conducted with a standard interview schedule. The alcohol sections of the Composite International Diagnostic Interview (CIDI) and the Structured Clinical Interview for DSM (SCID) provide accurate classification of alcohol use disorders according to both ICD criteria and the criteria contained in the *Diagnostic and Statistical Manual* of the American Psychiatric Association. An important purpose of clinical assessment is to obtain an estimate of illness severity. The number of ICD symptoms obtained using a structured interview or the total score on the AUDIT screening test can serve this purpose.

Several laboratory tests can be helpful in detecting heavy drinking and assessing its effects on liver function. Tests commonly used by clinicians include serum transaminases, bilirubin, gamma-glutamyl transpeptidase (GGTP), carbohydrate-deficient transferrin (CDT), and mean corpuscular volume (MCV) of erythrocytes.

Diagnostic assessment of people with alcohol dependence also includes measures of family alcohol history, psychopathology, social adjustment, personality disorder, and medical conditions.

Treatment, Early Intervention, and Long-Term Management

With progress in the understanding of how alcohol use disorders are manifested, whom they affect, and how they can be diagnosed, a broad range of interventions have been developed to manage people with alcohol dependence and harmful drinking. This section describes three types of intervention: (1) interventions designed for nondependent high-risk drinkers, (2) formal treatment for problem drinkers and alcoholics, and (3) mutual help organizations for alcoholics and their families.

Interventions Designed for Nondependent High-Risk Drinkers

Harmful drinking typically precedes the development of alcohol dependence, but it can also by definition cause serious medical and psychological problems in the absence of dependence. It is generally assumed that harmful drinking can be arrested before dependence develops if the drinker is motivated to reduce the quantity and frequency of alcohol consumption to amounts not exceeding moderation levels of no more than approximately one or two drinks a day (i.e., 20 g pure alcohol). With the increased interest in clinical preventive services in both developed and developing countries, early intervention programs have been developed by the World Health Organization to facilitate the management of harmful drinking in primary care and other health-care and social service settings. Following an initial assessment with a screening test such as the AUDIT, the patient is referred to either a diagnostic evaluation or a brief intervention with further monitoring. Brief interventions are characterized by their low intensity and short duration. They typically consist of one to three sessions of counseling and education and seek to motivate high-risk drinkers to moderate their alcohol consumption rather than promote total abstinence.

During the past two decades, more than 100 randomized controlled trials have been conducted to evaluate the efficacy of brief interventions. The results of these trials have been summarized in several integrative literature reviews and meta-analyses (for example, Whitlock et al., 2004). The cumulative evidence shows that clinically significant reductions in drinking and alcohol-related problems can follow from brief interventions. In general, nurses are as effective as doctors in producing behavior change. Regarding the nature of the intervention, drink resistance training, simple advice, and motivational enhancement approaches seem to be equally effective. In addition, brief interventions seem to be equally effective with adolescents, adults, older adults, and pregnant women. However, there is no evidence that these interventions are beneficial for alcohol-dependent individuals.

Specialized Treatment for Persons with Alcohol Dependence

In countries with well-developed health-care systems, the range of agencies and professional service providers involved in specialist treatment of alcohol-related problems is extensive. In addition to the medical sector, which encompasses psychiatric services and specialist treatment units, treatment is also delivered by social and welfare agencies, workplace programs, and court-mandated programs for persons convicted of drunk-driving. Some of the key issues that treatment research has addressed with increasing scientific rigor include the most effective detoxification measures, the impact of different treatment settings, whether some therapeutic modalities are better than others, the effects of treatment intensity, and factors that influence long-term outcomes.

Detoxification

As noted above, many patients with a history of chronic drinking (especially those with poor nutrition and prior experience of an abstinence syndrome) experience withdrawal symptoms, and for some patients alcohol withdrawal can be life-threatening. It is generally assumed that successful management of the alcohol withdrawal syndrome provides a basis for subsequent efforts at rehabilitation. Administration of thiamine and multivitamins is a low-cost, low-risk intervention that prevents alcohol-related neurological disturbances and is typically combined with supportive care and treatment of concurrent illness, including fluid and electrolyte repletion. Social detoxification, which involves the nonpharmacological treatment of alcohol withdrawal has been shown to be effective. It consists of frequent reassurance, monitoring of vital signs, personal attention, and general nursing care. Increasingly, detoxification is being done on an ambulatory basis, which is much less costly than hospital-based detoxification. A variety of medications have been used for the treatment of alcohol withdrawal, but the benzodiazepines, especially diazepam and chlordiazepoxide, have largely supplanted all other medications because of their favorable side-effect profiles.

Optimal Treatment Settings for Rehabilitation

Following detoxification, a variety of programmatic elements and therapeutic modalities have been incorporated into service settings designed to treat the patient's alcohol-related problems, promote abstinence from alcohol, and prevent relapse. Service settings are an important component of treatment for alcohol problems, not only because they control access to treatment, but also because the setting often determines the climate (sometimes called the milieu), the resources and the professional staff providing treatment. Alcohol treatment is typically provided in outpatient hospital settings, but it can also be delivered in psychiatric clinics, social service agencies, and health-care settings. Treatment is also delivered in residential settings, which include hospital-based rehabilitation programs, freestanding units, and psychiatric units.

In most comparative studies, outpatient programs have been found to produce outcomes comparable to those of residential programs. This conclusion, however, should be tempered by a consideration of the kinds of problem drinkers who are appropriate for each type of program (Finney *et al.*, 1996). Some studies comparing outpatient with residential treatment have not controlled for the possibility that patients who choose outpatient settings are less severely alcohol-dependent, less physically ill, or less psychiatrically impaired. Residential treatment may be indicated when motivation is weak to continue treatment, when patients are psychotic, depressed, or suicidal, and when there are medical complications. Other factors that affect the choice of treatment setting include patients' social stability, the severity of their symptoms, and the ability of a program to respond to individual needs. An obstacle to ambulatory treatment is the higher rate of attrition usually encountered among more severely impaired alcoholics. An obvious question is whether some treatment settings are more cost-effective than others. In general, the research evidence on the cost-effectiveness of different treatment modalities has consistently found that the more expensive modalities do not necessarily produce better treatment outcomes.

Therapeutic Modalities: Nonpharmacological

A variety of therapeutic modalities are used within the context of outpatient and residential treatment services, and many programs use a combination of these interventions. The approaches with the greatest amount of supporting evidence are behavior therapy, group therapy, family treatment, and motivational enhancement (Edwards *et al.*, 2003). Behavior therapists stress the importance of teaching new, adaptive skills designed to alter the conditions that precipitate and reinforce drinking. One example of this approach is relapse prevention, which focuses on coping with situations that represent high risk for heavy drinking. Research (Ouimette *et al.* 1999; Babor and Del Boca, 2003) also indicates that Twelve Step Facilitation, which is designed to introduce problem drinkers to the principles of Alcoholics Anonymous, is as effective as more theory-based therapies.

Therapeutic Modalities: Pharmacological

There are three kinds of pharmacotherapy for persons with alcohol dependence: Alcohol-sensitizing drugs,

medications to directly reduce drinking, and medications to treat comorbid psychopathology (Kranzler, 2000). Alcohol-sensitizing drugs such as disulfiram and calcium carbimide cause an unpleasant reaction when combined with alcohol. Although these drugs may help alcohol-dependent persons when special efforts are made to ensure compliance, their efficacy in the prevention or limitation of relapse has not been demonstrated. Several approaches to enhancing voluntary compliance with disulfiram therapy have been evaluated, such as the use of incentives, and enlisting the help of family members. Under these conditions, disulfiram can significantly increase the number of abstinent days and decrease total drinks consumed.

In contrast to drugs like disulfiram that precipitate an aversive reaction following drinking, another class of medications has been developed to reduce drinking and prevent relapse by operating on the specific brain neurotransmitter systems implicated in the control of alcohol consumption, including endogenous opioids, catecholamines (especially dopamine), and serotonin. Based on research suggesting that opioid antagonists, such as naltrexone, decrease ethanol consumption in laboratory animals and humans, a series of double-blind, placebo-controlled trials have been conducted with alcohol-dependent patients. In general, naltrexone has been found to be superior to placebo in delaying the time to relapse and reducing the rate of relapse to heavy drinking among patients (Kranzler and Van Kirk, 2001). The most comprehensive clinical trial of naltrexone therapy was conducted at 11 U.S. sites with nearly 1400 patients (Anton *et al.*, 2006). Naltrexone was associated with more abstinent days and reduced the risk of a heavy drinking day after a relapse. The effects, however, tended to be short-lived, with no advantage evident 1 year later after medication had been suspended. The findings open the possibility that naltrexone with medical management may be delivered by primary care clinicians as an alternative to traditional alcohol treatment programs. Another focus of medications research has been Acamprosate, an amino acid derivative. Multicenter studies conducted in a variety of countries have shown significant advantages for acamprosate over placebo, but other large-scale studies have been negative (Kranzler and Van Kirk 2001; Anton *et al.*, 2006). In summary, despite advances in the search for a pharmacological intervention that could reduce craving and other precipitants of relapse, the additive effects of pharmacotherapies have been marginal beyond standard counseling and behavior therapies.

Because psychiatric disorders may contribute to the development or maintenance of heavy drinking, it is generally believed that the treatment of psychiatric comorbidity may have beneficial effects on drinking outcomes. Subsequent to detoxification, many patients with alcohol dependence complain of persistent depression, anxiety, insomnia, and negative emotional states, including frustration and anger. These symptoms may last for weeks or months, and they may contribute to relapse. Although most instances of postwithdrawal depression and anxiety will spontaneously remit within a few days to several weeks, there are still substantial numbers of patients whose severe and persistent psychiatric symptoms may require treatment. In many cases antidepressants, such as the selective serotonin reuptake inhibitor fluoxetine, and nonbenzodiazepine anxiolytics, may treat the co-occurring disorder and also have a beneficial effect on treatment outcomes for alcohol use (Kranzler, 2000).

Treatment of Multiple Substance Use and Dependencies

Multiple substance use has become increasingly prevalent in many countries, and with it there has been an increase in the proportion of treatment-seeking alcoholics who have multiple dependencies. The pattern of multiple drug use depends on a variety of factors, including the cultural setting, the availability of different substances, and the age of the substance user. A pattern of tobacco and illicit drug use, for example, is common among young adult heavy drinkers. The drugs most frequently implicated with alcohol dependence are cocaine, opioids, cannabis, benzodiazepines, and nicotine. In general, the presence of multiple drug use in persons with alcohol dependence is associated with more severe dependence, worse retention in treatment, and poorer outcomes (Edwards *et al.*, 2003). Unfortunately, there has been little research on the treatment of multiple drug use, and virtually no attention to the sequencing of interventions in persons dependent on two or more substances. Is it better, for example, to treat multiple substance use simultaneously or should individual substances be addressed sequentially? In a study of cocaine- and alcohol-dependent patients (Carroll *et al.*, 2000), simultaneous treatment with disulfiram was associated with better treatment retention and abstinence from both substances, especially when combined with out-patient psychotherapy. But in the case of co-occurring dependence on alcohol and nicotine, research suggests that patients prefer sequential treatment and simultaneous cessation therapy can negatively impact alcohol use outcomes (Kodl *et al.*, 2006).

Treatment Matching and Patient Placement

In response to concerns about the inappropriate use of expensive residential treatment, patient placement criteria have been applied in some countries to standardize the way in which patients are assigned to different types and intensities of care. The *Patient Placement Criteria for the Treatment of Substance-Related Disorders*, of the American Society of Addiction Medicine (ASAM) provides detailed guidelines for different levels of care, including detoxification, outpatient, and residential care. The decision to refer the patient to a particular level of care is based on the following considerations: Acute intoxication and withdrawal, biomedical conditions, emotional/behavioral conditions, acceptance of treatment, relapse potential, and recovery environment.

Another approach to patient placement is based on the notion that patients should initially be matched to the least intensive level of care that is appropriate, and then stepped up to more intensive treatment settings if they do not respond. This approach is consistent with the ASAM criteria, which specify that residential treatment should not be recommended unless the patient has failed at outpatient treatment.

Another approach is called treatment matching, which relies on the cumulative evidence of research to suggest the treatment modalities most likely to produce favorable outcomes with different types of patients. In one large-scale study of treatment matching, patients with certain characteristics (e.g., severe dependence, high levels of anger, social networks that support drinking) responded marginally better to certain types of therapy (e.g., Twelve Step Facilitation, motivational enhancement, cognitive behavioral therapy, respectively) (Babor and Del Boca, 2003). Other research (McLellan *et al.*, 1993) suggests the importance of including psychological and social services within specialized treatment facilities in order to meet the diverse psychosocial needs of alcohol-dependent patients.

Long-Term Residential Care and Mutual Help Societies

Some people with alcohol dependence relapse repeatedly in spite of multiple treatment episodes. Long-term residential treatment is used in some countries for alcoholics who do not respond to more limited efforts at rehabilitation. Unfortunately, the effectiveness of these programs has not been evaluated systematically. In contrast, continuing care by means of aftercare groups and other mutual help organizations has received increased research attention. For example, a study of the long-term outcomes of treated and untreated alcoholics (Timko *et al.*, 2000) found that individuals who obtained help for a drinking problem, especially in a timely manner, had better outcomes over 8 years than those who did not receive help. The type of help they received (e.g., mutual help societies or specialized treatment) made little difference in long-term outcomes.

Although mutual help societies composed of recovering alcoholics are not considered a formal treatment, they are often used as a substitute, an alternative, and an adjunct to treatment. With an estimated 2.2 million members affiliated with more than 100 000 groups in

150 countries, Alcoholics Anonymous (AA) is by far the most widely utilized source of help for drinking problems in the world. Related organizations have been developed in a number of other countries, such as Danshukai in Japan, Krcuzbund in Germany, Croix d'Or and Vie Libre in France, Abstainers Clubs in Poland, Family Clubs in Italy, and Links in the Scandinavian countries.

Although it is regarded as one of the most useful resources for recovering alcoholics, the research literature supporting the efficacy of AA is limited. Attendance at AA tends to be correlated with long-term abstinence, but this may reflect motivation for recovery. Several large-scale, well-designed studies (Walsh *et al.*, 1991; Ouimette *et al.*, 1999) suggest that AA can have an incremental effect when combined with formal treatment, and AA attendance alone may be better than no intervention. When AA is combined with a 12-week individual therapy called Twelve Step Facilitation (TSF), one study (Babor and Del Boca, 2003) found that TSF not only increased affiliation with AA, it also had a demonstrable effect on clients whose social networks contained many drinking companions. This study suggested that AA is effective because it helps to change the drinker's social environment, rather than through some form of spiritual conversion.

Special Features Influencing Treatment

There is considerable evidence that links the outcome of alcohol dependence treatment to comorbid psychopathology. General measures of psychopathology, as well as the specific diagnoses of drug abuse, drug dependence, antisocial personality disorder, and major depressive disorder predict poorer outcomes in alcoholics (Edwards *et al.*, 2003). Demographic characteristics such as age, gender, and socioeconomic level also influence treatment outcomes.

A wide variety of treatment approaches have been adapted to suit the needs of women, adolescents, and the elderly, including multidisciplinary inpatient treatment programs, outpatient individual therapy, group therapy or day treatment, and outpatient recovery support groups. Although treatment programs with experience in treating these groups are better able to coordinate rehabilitation with medical and social services, there is little evidence that tailored treatment settings produce better outcomes than more generic programs.

Mediators and Moderators of Treatment Effectiveness

The investigation of mediators and moderators helps to answer questions about how and why treatment works (mediating effects) and for whom certain treatments work best (moderators). The search for mediators and moderators of treatment effects has taken place within the clinical technology model of treatment efficacy and treatment matching, which postulates that patient attributes and treatment process elements, respectively, constitute mediators and moderators of change in drinking following treatment. Studies show that matching to therapeutic orientation is not an essential ingredient to substantially enhanced outcomes, as previously believed (Babor and Del Boca, 2003). They also indicate that the mediational mechanisms underlying several of the most popular therapies are different than what is suggested by their proponents. In general, the Technology Model of (psychotherapy) treatment effectiveness may be flawed as it applies to alcohol dependence. Instead of distinct, non-overlapping elements, therapy may work through common mechanisms, such as empathy, an effective therapist–client alliance, a desire to change, inner resources, a supportive social network, and the provision of a culturally appropriate solution to a socially defined problem.

Aggregate Effects of Treatment

Given the scarcity of specialized treatment services in most countries, they are not likely to have an impact on aggregate rates of morbidity and mortality at the population level. Nevertheless, there is some evidence that treatment has the potential to produce an aggregate impact in countries where the treatment system is relatively well developed. For example, researchers have found an association between declining liver cirrhosis rates and the growth of specialized treatment (Smart and Mann, 2000).

Despite evidence of the effectiveness of treatment interventions, little attention has been paid to the mechanisms of action that would translate individual benefits to the population. Treatment interventions are primarily designed to serve the needs of individual patients and clients, but there are a number of ways that these interventions may have an impact at community and population levels: By raising public awareness of alcohol problems, influencing national and community agendas, involving health professionals in advocacy for prevention, and providing secondary benefits to families, employers, and automobile drivers. The effect of treatment interventions can also be manifested more directly by not only reducing the amount of alcohol consumed by the drinker (and his or her associated risks), but also influencing the social milieu of the drinker. By removing a source of reciprocal influence that is likely to contribute to the maintenance of heavy drinking subcultures, treatment may diminish the alcohol-related problem rates of an entire society.

Conclusion

This article has described a public health approach to the provision of services for people with alcohol use disorders. Such an approach is broadly conceived to include the consideration not only of specialized services for alcohol dependence, but also of medical care and social welfare services that interact with and complement specialized alcohol services. During the past 30 years, significant progress has been made in the scientific study of alcohol dependence and its treatment. On the basis of evidence reviewed in this article, a number of conclusions appear warranted at this time:

1. People with alcohol-related problems are heterogeneous with respect to demographic features (e.g., age, gender, race/ethnicity), age of onset of heavy drinking, severity of alcohol dependence, comorbid psychopathology, genetic vulnerability, and other prognostic factors.
2. Any treatment for alcohol dependence is better than no treatment. The majority of those treated demonstrate improvement, but many improve with minimal treatment.
3. The intensity of treatment has not been shown to produce pronounced differences in outcome. Similarly, medical inpatient treatment, while more costly, is not demonstrably more effective than nonmedical residential or outpatient treatment. For patients with serious comorbid medical and psychiatric disorders, medical inpatient treatment may, nonetheless, be necessary. Continuing aftercare helps to maintain abstinence following short-term intensive rehabilitation in inpatient settings.
4. There is little evidence that any one treatment approach is superior. There is some support for certain kinds of behavior therapy, but the effectiveness of AA and disulfiram seem to depend on patient characteristics and compliance. Several new pharmacological interventions show promise as a basis for a new generation of ambulatory treatments, but they add little to the effect of nonpharmacological treatment.
5. Brief interventions for harmful drinkers are effective in reducing hazardous drinking and are feasible to implement in primary care settings.
6. A combination of early intervention, specialized treatment, and mutual help groups has the potential to reduce the rate of alcohol-related problems in a society.

Acknowledgments

The writing of this article was supported by grant P50 AA03510 from the U.S. National Institute on Alcohol Abuse and Alcoholism.

See also: Alcohol Consumption: Overview of International Trends; Alcohol: The Burden of Disease; Alcohol—Socio-Economic Impacts (Including Externalities).

Citations

Anton RF, O'Malley SO, Ciraulo DA, *et al.* (2006) Combined pharmacotherapies and behavioral interventions for alcohol dependence: The COMBINE Study: A Randomized Controlled Trial. *Journal of the American Medical Association* 295: 2003–2017.

Babor TF and Del Boca FK (eds.) (2003) *Treatment Matching in Alcoholism.* Cambridge, UK: Cambridge University Press.

Babor TF, Hofmann M, DelBoca FK, *et al.* (1992) Types of alcoholics: Evidence for an empirically-derived typology based on indicators of vulnerability and severity. *Archives of General Psychiatry* 8: 599–608.

Babor T, Caetano R, Casswell S, *et al.* (2003) *Alcohol: No Ordinary Commodity – Research and Public Policy.* Oxford, UK: Oxford University Press.

Carroll D, Nich C, Ball SA, *et al.* (2000) One-year follow-up of disulfiram and psychotherapy for cocaine-alcohol users: Sustained effects of treatment. *Addiction* 95: 1335–1349.

Cloninger CR (1987) Neurogenetic adaptive mechanisms in alcoholism. *Science* 236: 410–416.

Edwards G and Gross MM (1976) Alcohol dependence: Provisional description of a clinical syndrome. *British Medical Journal* 1: 1058–1061.

Edwards G, Marshall EJ, and Cook CCH (2003) *The Treatment of Drinking Problems: A Guide for the Helping Professions.* Cambridge, UK: Cambridge University Press.

Ewing JA (1984) Detecting alcoholism: The CAGE questionnaire. *Journal of the American Medical Association* 252: 1905–1907.

Finney JW, Hahn AC, and Moos RH (1996) The effectiveness of inpatient and outpatient treatment for alcohol abuse: The need to focus on mediators and moderators of setting effects. *Addiction* 91: 1773–1796.

Hesselbrock VM and Hesselbrock MN (2006) Are there empirically supported and clinically useful subtypes of alcohol dependence? *Addiction* 101(supplement 1): 97–103.

Kodl M, Fu SS, and Joseph AM (2006) Tobacco cessation treatment for alcohol-dependent smokers: When is the best time? *Alcohol Research and Health* 29: 203–207.

Kranzler HR (2000) Pharmacotherapy of alcoholism: Gaps in knowledge and opportunities for research. *Alcohol and Alcoholism* 35: 537–547.

Kranzler HR and Van Kirk J (2001) Naltrexone and acamprosate in the treatment of alcoholism: A meta-analysis. *Alcoholism, Clinical and Experimental Research* 25: 1335–1341.

McLellan AT, Grissom GR, Brill P, *et al.* (1993) Private substance abuse treatments: Are some programs more effective than others? *Journal of Substance Abuse Treatment* 10: 243–254.

Ouimette PC, Finney JW, Gima K, *et al.* (1999) A comparative evaluation of substance abuse treatment: Examining mechanisms underlying patient-treatment matching hypotheses for 12-step and cognitive–behavioral treatments for substance abuse. *Alcoholism, Clinical and Experimental Research* 23: 545–551.

Saunders JB, Aasland OG, Babor TF, *et al.* (1993) Development of the Alcohol Use Disorders Identification Test (AUDIT): WHO collaborative project on early detection of persons with harmful alcohol consumption – II. *Addiction* 88: 791–804.

Smart RG and Mann RE (2000) The impact of programs for high-risk drinkers on population levels of alcohol problems. *Addiction* 95: 37–52.

Timko C, Moos RH, Finney JW, *et al.* (2000) Long-term outcomes of alcohol use disorders: Comparing untreated individuals with those in Alcoholics Anonymous and formal treatment. *Journal of Studies on Alcohol* 61: 529–538.

Walsh DC, Hingson RW, Merrigan DM, *et al.* (1991) A randomized trial of treatment options for alcohol-abusing workers. *New England Journal of Medicine* 325: 775–782.

Whitlock EP, Polen MR, Green CA, *et al.* (2004) Behavioral counseling interventions in primary care to reduce risky/harmful alcohol use by adults: A summary of the evidence for the US Preventive Services Task Force. *Annals of Internal Medicine* 140: 557–568.

World Health Organization (1992) The ICD-10 Classification of Mental and Behavioural Disorders: Clinical Descriptions and Diagnostic Guidelines. Geneva, Switzerland: World Health Organization.

Further Reading

American Psychiatric Association (1994) *Diagnostic and Statistical Manual of Mental Disorders*. 4th edn. Washington, DC: American Psychiatric Association.

American Society of Addiction Medicine (2001) *Patient Placement Criteria for the Treatment of Substance-Related Disorders*. 2nd edn. Chevy Chase, MD: American Society of Addiction Medicine.

Babor TF and Higgins-Biddle JC (2001) *AUDIT The Alcohol Use Disorders Identification Test: Guidelines for Use in Primary Care*. 2nd edn. Geneva, Switzerland: World Health Organization.

Babor TF, Kranzler KR, Hernandez-Avlia CA, et al. (2003) Substance abuse: Alcohol use disorders. In: Tasman A, Kay J and Lieberman JA (eds.) *Psychiatry* In: Bloom FE and Kupfer DJ (eds.). *Psychopharmacology: The Fourth Generation of Progress*, pp. 1479–1484., Vol. 1, pp. 936–972. London: John Wiley & Sons.

Humphreys K (2004) *Circles of Recovery: Self-Help Organizations for Addictions*. Cambridge, UK: Cambridge University Press.

Institute of Medicine (1990) *Broadening the Base of Treatment for Alcohol Problems*. Washington, DC: National Academy Press.

McLellan AT, Kushner H, Metzger D, et al. (1992) The fifth edition of the Addiction Severity Index. *Journal of Substance Abuse Treatment* 9: 199–213.

Mendelson JH and Mello NK (eds) (1985) *Diagnosis and Treatment of Alcoholism*, 2nd edn. New York: McGraw-Hill.

Meyer RE (1986) How to understand the relationship between psychopathology and addictive disorders: Another example of the chicken and the egg. In: Meyer RE (ed.) *Psychopathology and Addictive Disorder*, pp. 3–16. New York: Guilford Press

Naranjo CA and Sellers EM (1986) Clinical assessment and pharmacotherapy of the alcohol withdrawal syndrome. In: Galanter M (ed.) *Recent Developments in Alcoholism* Vol. 4, pp. 265–281. New York: Plenum Press.

Peterson K (2004/2005) Biomarkers for alcohol use and abuse. *Alcohol Research & Health* 28: 30–37.

Vaillant GE (1983) *The Natural History of Alcoholism*. Cambridge, MA: Harvard University Press.

Relevant Websites

http://www.jointogether.org/ – Join Together.

http://ncadi.samhsa.gov/ – The U.S. government's National Clearinghouse on Alcohol and Drug Information.

http://www.who.int/substance_abuse/en/ – The World Health Organization, Management of Substance Abuse.

Blindness

S Resnikoff and R Pararajasegaram, World Health Organization, Geneva, Switzerland

Blindness is a health and social concern of significant public health dimensions that, until recently, has not received the attention it warrants on the global health agenda.

As will be seen, the majority of the world's blind live in developing regions and in the impoverished regions of rapidly economically developing countries. There has been, however, as seen in recent studies, a transition from infection- and nutrition-related causes of blinding eye diseases to those of a chronic nature that generally stem from noncommunicable disorders, referred to as the 'epidemiological transition.' This is in keeping with the demographic transition that is occurring at an enhanced pace in the developing regions of the world, consequent to their inevitable population momentum. These transitions have far-reaching consequences for population eye health, with all its implications in terms of underdevelopment, social costs, and poverty alleviation in general, and the quality of life of affected individuals and communities, in particular. The lowered life expectancy consequent to becoming blind is an illustrative example.

What Is Blindness?

There is no simple answer. The reason for this is that until recently there has been great variation in the definition of blindness from one country to another. This is despite the availability of a definition and classification dating back to 1972 that has found international acceptance and was included in the 10th revision of the WHO International Statistical Classification of Diseases Injuries and Causes of Death.

In this classification, blindness is defined as visual acuity of less than 3/60 (20/400 or 0.05) or corresponding field not greater than 10 degrees in the better eye, with best possible correction. Low vision is defined as visual acuity of less than 6/18 (20/70 or 0.30) but equal to or better than 3/60, or corresponding visual field not greater than 20 degrees in the better eye, with best possible correction.

Some of the definitions, such as 'best corrected' in the current classification, have been under review, because they do not reflect the true magnitude of uncorrected refractive error as a cause of visual impairment, including blindness. Such defective vision resulting from refractive error has remained masked as a result of the existing definition.

The use of the concept of 'presenting vision' instead of 'best corrected vision' will overcome this anomalous definition. The current definition is being amended. In addition, there is currently confusion over the use of the term 'low vision' to describe the various categories of visual impairment other than blindness. It has been recommended that the use of the term 'low vision' be avoided for use in this context.

Epidemiology

There are some limitations inherent in describing the epidemiology of visual impairment and blindness. These stem from the use of different definitions and visual cut-off points for the different categories of visual impairment in different studies. However, more recent epidemiological surveys have begun to use more standardized definitions and methodologies based on them. As such, the recent estimation would more closely reflect the real situation.

Magnitude and Causes of Visual Impairment

The estimate of the global magnitude of visual impairment in relation to the 2002 world population was updated using the most recent available data on blindness and low vision (Pascolini et al., 2004). The number of people globally who are visually impaired is an estimated 161 million, of whom 36.8 million are blind (Resnikoff et al., 2004). A more recent estimate based on presenting vision has revealed the true magnitude of visual impairment, now estimated at 314 million (Resnikoff et al., 2007), with an estimated 153 million cases due to uncorrected refractive error alone, of which 8.2 million are in the blind category.

Thus the most recent update indicates that globally there are 314 million persons who are visually impaired (when presenting vision is used in studies), of whom 45 million persons are blind.

Causes of Visual Impairment Including Blindness

According to WHO estimates (2002) (in, Resnikoff et al., 2004), the causes of blindness are as follows: cataract, 47.8%; glaucoma, 12%; age-related macular degeneration, 8.7%; trachoma, 3.6%; corneal opacity (various causes excluding trachoma), 5.1%; diabetic retinopathy, 4.8%; onchocerciasis, 1%; childhood blindness (various causes), 3.8%; and other causes, 12.9%.

The above conditions also predominate as causes of visual impairment not amounting to blindness. However, in light of the data that have been recently determined in relation to uncorrected refractive error, it is seen that this represents the major causes of visual impairment, if presenting vision rather than best corrected vision is used as the criterion, as has been recommended.

Figure 1 depicts the causes and their relative magnitude from a global perspective.

Inequity in Eye Health Status and Causes of Visual Impairment

There is wide variation in both the prevalence and underlying causes of visual impairment and blindness based on geographical location, demographic structure, gender, socioeconomic status, and health system development. An estimated 90% of the world's visually impaired persons live in developing parts of the world.

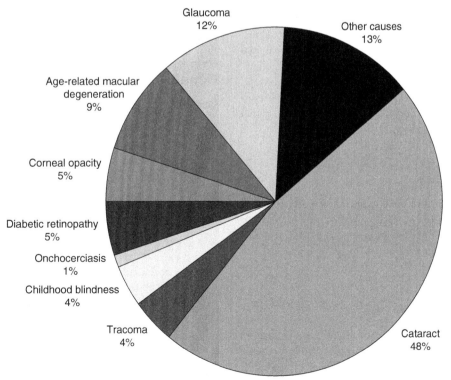

Figure 1   Global causes of blindness (best corrected visual acuity). with permission from Resnikoff S, et al. (2004) Global data on visual impairment in the year 2002. *Bulletin of the World Health Organization* 82: 844–851.

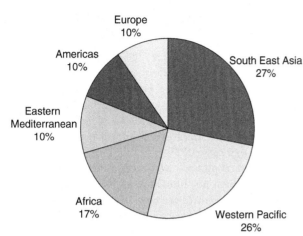

Figure 2   Regional distribution of visual impairment, by WHO regions.

Figure 2 illustrates the geographical distribution of global blindness.

Vision Impairment Across the Life Spectrum

Visual impairment is not equally prevalent across various age groups of the population. For instance, over 82% of all persons who are blind are 50 years and over. However, this cohort currently represents only 19% of the global population. Those persons 50 years and older therefore bear a disproportionate load of blindness.

At the other end of the life spectrum, blindness in childhood has a lower absolute prevalence, constituting only an estimated 1.4 million children, or 3.8% of global blindness. A child going blind in early childhood and surviving to, say, 50 years of age has many years of blindness ahead. Therefore in terms of 'years of blindness,' childhood blindness ranks second to blindness from cataract in adults, and merits to be addressed as a global priority in public health ophthalmology.

Gender Disparities

Gender variations have been reported in all age groups and in all regions of the world. Consistently, for reasons such as limited access and uptake of eye care services, females are at a higher risk than males of being visually impaired or blind.

Biological Determinants

Many of the causes that result in visual impairment and blindness have biological determinants such as genetic background, age, and gender. These are nonmodifiable, and prevention or treatment of these are related to biomedical interventions. These include treatment for cataract

and trichiasis (in trachoma) or a mix of interventions, as in glaucoma and diabetic retinopathy. Where underlying ecological determinants prevail such as in onchocerciasis and trachoma, medical treatment together with interventions such as vector control, personal hygiene, (e.g., face washing), and environmental improvement are employed.

Social Determinants

An understanding of the underlying social determinants of eye health is a necessary prerequisite not only for an understanding of the public health dimensions of the problem, despite the availability of appropriate knowledge, technology, and skills, but also for preventing and controlling the many determinants and diseases that lead to visual impairment.

However, when dealing with these conditions as causes of vision impairment and blindness in a population setting, the existence of social determinants is often overlooked. These include various barriers to uptake of services. Health illiteracy, poverty along with its related deprivations, physical and social distance from health facilities, and cultural beliefs and barriers predominate.

In general, these factors determine the availability, accessibility, and affordability of services even when they are provided. Compounding these determinants of visual impairment is the inequitable distribution of service in terms of geographic distribution, quality, cost, and accountability.

Prevention of Blindness: What Can Be Done?

Cataract

Cataract remains the leading cause of blindness, accounting for nearly half of all cases, as shown in **Figure 1**, except in the most developed countries.

This is certainly not due to the lack of an effective intervention.

Evidence-based, cost-effective interventions are being practiced to deal with the surgical management of cataract (Baltussen *et al.*, 2004). Removal of the affected lens of the eye and replacement with a synthetic posterior chamber intraocular lens (IOL) is standard practice the world over. Refinements in technology and approaches in IOL material and design ensure a near normal restoration of vision for the large majority of patients. In low- and middle-income countries, it has been estimated that the cost-effectiveness ratio of these surgical interventions are below US$200 per disability-adjusted life year (DALY) averted, and less than US$24 000 in high-income countries.

However, to be able to minimize the magnitude of cataract as a cause of blindness, interventions must go beyond technology to outcome-oriented interventions that vigorously address the various social determinants that predicate the high prevalence of cataract and other blinding conditions in developing countries. Even in these countries, studies have demonstrated the wide disparity in cataract surgical rates (defined as the number of cataract surgeries carried out per 1 million population annually), surgical outcome, and population coverage, not only between countries but also between regions in the same country.

The equitable provision of efficient and effective health systems delivering eye care should be an essential public health priority for all developing countries.

Trachoma

The SAFE strategy (Surgery, Antibiotics, Facial cleanliness, Environmental improvement) is an integrated approach based on the principles of primary health care recommended by WHO to help eliminate blinding trachoma in a sustainable manner. The four elements complement each other and comprise a mix of primary, secondary, and tertiary preventive interventions, with strong community involvement and educational activities.

Studies on the cost-effectiveness of these interventions are limited. However, the few reported studies point to a range of approximately US$4 to US$82 per DALY averted across trachoma-endemic areas, in the case of trichiasis surgery. In the case of antibiotic treatment, it has been estimated that across the endemic regions studied, the cost per DALY averted ranged between US$4000 to US$220 000, depending on whether the drug is part of a donation program or is calculated at the market price.

Diabetic Retinopathy

Diabetic retinopathy, already a leading cause of blindness in working-age populations in developed countries, is fast assuming epidemic proportions worldwide with the upsurge of diabetes mellitus even in developing countries. The causes of vision loss are multifactorial and are closely linked to the duration of diabetes. Other risk factors include uncontrolled blood sugar, high blood pressure, and increased blood lipids.

Besides controlling the disordered metabolic state, available interventions include periodic examination of the ocular fundus through dilated pupils, early identification of sight-threatening lesions, and treatment with laser photocoagulation. Health promotion and patient education are important supportive interventions. A multidisciplinary team approach to care of these patients is desirable. Extended follow-up with careful monitoring and tracking of

patients is important. In patients with some residual vision that is not amenable to further treatment, low-vision care should be offered.

Glaucoma

This comprises a group of conditions that lead to irreversible vision loss and blindness through damage to the optic nerve (optic neuropathy). WHO has estimated that 4.5 million persons are blind due to glaucoma (Resnikoff et al., 2004). Published projections indicate that by 2010, 4.5 million persons will be blind from open-angle glaucoma and 3.9 million from primary angle-closure glaucoma. Given the aging of the world population, these numbers are set to increase further by 2020 (Quigley and Broman, 2006).

Significant improvement in treatment interventions has been made in recent years, such as laser therapy, medication, and surgery to prevent vision loss from glaucoma. However, given the fact that the tools currently required for the identification, assessment, and management of early glaucoma are often lacking, particularly in poorer parts of the developing world, the management of glaucoma at a community level holds many challenges.

Childhood Blindness

Childhood blindness results from a number of causes that range from genetically determined and congenital conditions to micronutrient deficiency (vitamin A) and infective conditions (measles, ophthalmia neonatorum, rubella) to conditions requiring specialized surgical treatment such as childhood cataract, glaucoma, and retinopathy of prematurity. In developed and rapidly economically developing regions of the world, retinopathy of prematurity is more than an emerging problem. With increased survival of low birth weight and low gestational age infants, there is already an upsurge in vision loss from this cause.

Uncorrected refractive errors comprise a significant cause of vision impairment, particularly among certain ethnic groups. These have implications for child development and education, future employment prospects, and performance.

Considerable regional variations between and within countries exist with regard to the magnitude and causes of childhood blindness. Services for children are arranged through vision screening in schools and community centers with follow-up assessment and provision of spectacles.

A concerted primary eye care approach could control and minimize causes related to poverty and deprivation such as malnutrition, measles, and harmful traditional practices. Other causes such as cataract, glaucoma, and retinopathy of prematurity require specialized surgical care and management, including low vision care and inclusive education of affected children.

Uncorrected Refractive Errors

These include conditions such as myopia (nearsightedness), hypermetropia (farsightedness), and astigmatism. Age-related presbyopia also falls within this category. There are an estimated 153 million persons with visual impairment due to uncorrected refractive errors (not including presbyopia), in other words, presenting visual acuity less than 6/18 in the better eye. This comprises the commonest cause of visual impairment. The proportion of uncorrected refractive errors varies based on cultural norms, gender, and availability and affordability of services.

Services to correct disabling refractive errors should include identification of persons requiring correction, assessment and prescription of appropriate correction, and the provision of spectacles that are affordable and cosmetically acceptable.

Age-Related Macular Degeneration

This condition presents an emerging challenge given the rapidly escalating number of older populations globally. It is already the major cause of blindness in the developed countries. While there is greater knowledge regarding the cause and pathophysiology of the disease, efforts at prevention and treatment have not been promising until now. Ongoing research has suggested the potential value of newer treatment modalities, but the outcome of such treatment on a large scale has yet to be determined. In the interim, much can be gained through the provision of low-vision care to improve the functioning and quality of life of these patients.

Low Vision

The following definition was agreed upon to identify persons who could benefit from low-vision care:

> A person with low vision is someone who, after medical, surgical, and/or standard refractive intervention, has a corrected visual acuity in the better eye of less than 6/18 down to and including light perception or a central visual field of less than 20 degrees, but who uses or has the potential to use vision for the planning and/or execution of a task.

Currently there are no global estimates of the number of people with low vision who would benefit from low-vision services. Based on available data, this is estimated to be around 40–65 million. However, with the advancing age of the population and a concomitant increase in age-related chronic diseases such as glaucoma, diabetic retinopathy, and macular degeneration, the unmet need for low-vision services could rapidly escalate.

The coverage of low-vision services currently is extremely sparse, even in developed countries. Low-vision care needs to be developed in close collaboration with the correction of uncorrected refractive errors, and follow the same principles, such as affordability and acceptability.

Concepts of Primary Eye Care and the Domains of Prevention of Blindness

The basic principles of primary health care, as enshrined in the Alma Ata declaration (1978) and subsequent World Health Assembly resolutions, provide the basic framework for the development of health systems that could provide equitable, comprehensive, and sustainable eye care as an integral part of health care.

Primary health care, of which prevention of blindness needs to be an integral part, consists of:

> Essential health care based on practical, scientifically sound, and socially acceptable methods and technology made universally accessible to individuals and families in the community through their full participation and at a cost that the community and country can afford to maintain at every stage of their development in the spirit of self-reliance and self determination.

Primary eye care comprises a simple but comprehensive set of promotive, preventive, curative, and rehabilitative activities that can be carried out by suitably trained primary health-care workers, who in turn are supported by a referral system that ought to comprise secondary and tertiary level of services and in some regions provide mobile services.

Available Primary Eye Care Interventions to Eliminate Avoidable Blindness

Cataract, glaucoma, a corneal opacities (from various causes), diabetic retinopathy, trachoma, and onchocerciasis lend themselves to potential health promotion, prevention, treatment, and rehabilitative strategies.

Similar interventions are possible in the case of childhood blindness.

Another area in which primary-level services could provide effective support is in vision screening, early detection, and appropriate referral of persons of all age groups with uncorrected refractive error. This constitutes a large segment of the population across the life spectrum that could benefit from appropriate corrective services.

Economic Implications of Visual Impairment and Blindness

Studies on the economic losses to individuals and society from visual impairment and the economic gains from the application of cost-effective interventions to prevent blindness and restore sight provide supportive evidence for investment in blindness-prevention programs. The economic burden of avoidable visual impairment includes the direct costs in terms of resources spent in individual and community care, including the various components of the eye care system at all levels, and the indirect costs, which comprise a range of productivity losses, with their far-reaching implications, social and rehabilitative expenses, impaired quality of life, and premature death.

Studies have been published to highlight the economic aspects of some of the commoner individual blinding conditions such as cataract, trachoma, onchocerciasis, glaucoma, and diabetic retinopathy. Most of these have been carried out in developed countries.

For instance, an Australian study (Taylor *et al.*, 2004) assessed the overall economic impact of the five most prevalent visually impairing conditions (75% of all causes) in Australia (**Figure 3**). This included cataract, age-related macular degeneration, glaucoma, diabetic retinopathy, and errors of refraction. The economic analysis predicted an estimated direct cost of AU$1.824 billion (US$1.3 billion). Indirect costs were estimated to add a further AU$8 billion (US$5.6 billion) to the annual eye care budget for 2004. These estimates cannot be easily extrapolated to other parts of the world, however, due to different disease patterns, health-care costs, work force wage structures, and social security systems.

There has been an effort to calculate on a global basis the projected annual personal productivity loss of individuals over the period 2000–2020 (Frick and Foster, 2003). The conservative annual estimate amounts to US$42 billion for the year 2000. This figure was projected to rise to US$110 billion per year (in year 2000 dollars) by 2020, if then-current prevalence levels showed no decrease. If, however, the implementation of VISION 2020 showed successful outcomes (see 'VISION 2020: The right to sight'), it was estimated that the annual productivity loss would increase to only US$58 billion

(in year 2000 dollars). It was further estimated that the overall global saving that could accrue over 20 years would amount to US$223 billion.

Partnerships for Prevention of Blindness

Global and Regional Initiatives

Onchocerciasis Control Program (OCP)

This was established in West Africa in 1974. The objectives of this international collaboration were to eliminate onchocerciasis in the 11 countries covered by the program and consequently improve the socioeconomic condition of the people, who largely comprised an agrarian society.

African Program for Onchocerciasis Control

This was launched in December 1995 with the sole aim of eliminating onchocerciasis from the African countries where the disease continued to be endemic. The region covered extended to 11 countries beyond those included in OCP. While WHO serves as the executing agency, the fiscal agency is the World Bank.

The primary strategic objective was to create, by 2007, a system of community-directed distribution of ivermectin, as a microfilaricidal agent, donated at no cost by Merck. Much success has been achieved toward reaching this objective, and steps are underway to use community-directed distributors in the control of coexistent diseases such as lymphatic filariasis and trachoma that respond to periodic administration of appropriate medications.

Onchocerciasis Elimination Program for the Americas

This is a regional initiative for Brazil, Colombia, Ecuador, Guatemala, Mexico, and Venezuela, initiated in 1991. The goals are to eliminate morbidity and to interrupt transmission of river blindness. This is a partnership program, including the six countries, the Pan American Health Organization, the private sector, specialized institutions, and international nongovernmental developmental organizations. The program strategy is to provide sustained mass distribution of ivermectin every six months, with the aim of reaching at least 85% of the at-risk population.

WHO Global Alliance for the Global Elimination of (Blinding) Trachoma (GET 2020)

GET 2020 was constituted in 1997 to provide support and technical assistance to a number of international institutions and organizations, nongovernmental development organizations, and foundations in working toward elimination of trachoma as a public health problem, using the SAFE strategy. The Alliance meets on an annual basis and

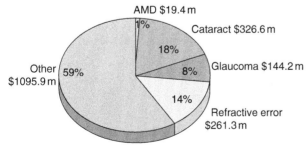

Total $1824.4m

AMD $19.4m — 1%
Cataract $326.6m — 18%
Glaucoma $144.2m — 8%
Refractive error $261.3m — 14%
Other $1095.9m — 59%

Figure 3 Cost of eye diseases, 2004, AU$, by condition. AMD, age-related macular degeneration. Source: Taylor H, *et al.* (2004) *Clear Insight: The Economic Impact and Cost of Vision Loss in Australia*. Melbourne: Center for Eye Research Australia.

involves concerned member state representatives. The agenda includes the sharing of information on the progress of national programs, research initiatives and results, future plans, and reports on available financial and in-kind resources.

VISION 2020: The Right to Sight

On January 18, 1999, WHO's then Director General, Dr. Gro Harlem Brundtland, launched the Global Initiative for the Elimination of Avoidable Blindness under the title 'VISION 2020: The Right to Sight.' The initiative was spurred by the dismal global data on blindness that became available in the mid-1990s. These data were compounded by the predicted near-doubling of the global magnitude of visual impairment and blindness by the year 2020, with many of the underlying causes being preventable or treatable. These predictions were based on demographic projections and a presumed relatively unchanged eye care delivery as part of national healthcare systems. Such a scenario was likely to be realistic in the developing countries, where the problem was greatest and the resources for eye care are severely limited. Moreover, these countries were beset with competing demands for resources from limited health budgets to control other priority diseases such as HIV/AIDS, malaria, tuberculosis, and childhood diseases.

The initiative was thus seen not only as a health challenge but also as a moral imperative that needed to be urgently addressed.

VISION 2020 is a collaborative effort conceived by the World Health Organization and the International Agency for the Prevention of Blindness and its constituent members. The objective was to support member countries by providing technical and financial support to realign and strengthen existing national programs or to initiate and develop new national programs aimed at the collective achievement of the common goal of eliminating avoidable blindness globally.

The initiative identified three strategic components as the Framework for Action:

● Cost-effective disease control;
● Human resource development;
● Infrastructure, including appropriate technology.

The overarching supportive elements included advocacy, public awareness campaigns, resource mobilization, and improved governance and management of health systems, including monitoring and evaluation for quality assurance.

Partnership development was a key factor.

The underlying guiding principle was delivering eye care as an integral part of primary health care.

Global political commitment to VISION 2020 was forthcoming in 2003 and 2006 through the unanimous adoption by the WHO member states of resolutions WHA 56.26, *Elimination of Avoidable Blindness*, and WHA 59.25, *Prevention of Avoidable Blindness and Visual Impairment*, respectively.

At the national level, a number of countries have signed national declarations of support, and outcome-oriented national action plans have been formulated and are being implemented.

Overall, there is greater global awareness of the dimension of the problem of visual impairment, including blindness, as a public health concern.

This has led to the all-important political commitment at all levels to eliminate avoidable blindness as a public health problem globally before 2020. It has also led to the development of partnerships among a variety of partners, such as WHO, member countries, international nongovernmental developmental organizations and institutions, academia, the corporate sector, and civil society.

The ultimate goal is to establish a sustainable, equitable, and comprehensive eye care system as an integral part of national health systems based on the principles of primary health care.

Citations

Baltussen R, Sylla M, and Mariotti SP (2004) Cost effectiveness analysis of cataract surgery: A global and regional analysis. *Bulletin of the World Health Organization* 82(5): 338–345.

Frick KD and Foster A (2003) The magnitude and cost of global blindness: An increasing problem that can be alleviated. *American Journal of Ophthalmology* 135(4): 471–476.

Pascolini D, Mariotti SPM, Pokharel GP, et al. (2004) 2002 global update of available data on visual impairment: a compilation of population-based prevalence studies. *Opthalmic Epidemiology* 11 (2): 67–115.

Resnikoff S, Pascolini D, Etyáale D, et al. (2004) Global data on visual impairment in the year 2002. *Bulletin of the World Health Organization* 82: 844–851.

Resnikoff S, Pascolini D, Mariotti SP, and Pokharel GP (2008) Global magnitude of visual impairment caused by uncorrected refractive errors in 2004. *Bulletin of the World Health Organization* 86: 63–70.

Taylor H, Keete J, and Mitchell P (2004) *Clear Insight: The Economic Impact and Cost of Vision Loss in Australia.* Melbourne, Australia: Center for Eye Research.

Further Reading

Johnson GJ, Minassian DC, Weale CA, and West SK (eds.) (2003) *The Epidemiology of Eye Diseases*, 2nd edn. London: Arnold.

Relevant Websites

http://www.cehjournal.org/ – *Community Eye Health Journal.*
http://www.icoph.org/ – International Council of Ophthalmology.
http://www.nei.nih.gov/ – National Eye Institute.
http://www.v2020.org/ – Vision 2020: The Right to Sight.
http://www.who.int/blindness/en/ – WHO, Prevention of Blindness and Visual Impairment.

Brain Tumours

R McKean-Cowdin, P Razavi, and S Preston-Martin, Keck School of Medicine of the University of Southern California, Los Angeles, CA, USA

Malignant brain and nervous system tumors account for 18 820 new cancer diagnoses each year in the United States, or 1.3% of all primary incident cancers, and 12 820 or 2.3% of annual cancer deaths (American Cancer Society, 2006). Each year more than 41 130 new benign or malignant primary brain tumors are diagnosed among residents of the United States (CBTRUS, 2005). Worldwide the incidence rate of primary malignant brain and nervous system tumors ranges from 5.8 per 100 000 person-years for males in developed countries (4.1 per 100 000 females) to 3.0 per 100 000 person-years for males in less developed countries (2.1 per 100 000 person-years females) (Ferlay et al., 2004). Brain tumors are the second leading cause of death from neurological disease, second only to stroke, and the eleventh most common cause of death from cancer in the United States. Five-year survival rates published by the American Cancer Society show that survival from 1974 to 2001 for all types of brain tumors combined significantly improved in the United States; however, the average survival rate from 1995 to 2001 was still only 33% (American Cancer Society, 2006). The average 5-year brain tumor survival rate for 22 European countries when including follow-up data through 1998 was 18% (Sant et al., 2003). However, differences in survival by country are likely to be heavily influenced by variation in histology types diagnosed in each country.

Benign tumors can result in similar symptoms and prognoses as malignant tumors. For this reason, many cancer registries have routinely included both benign and malignant intracranial tumors. The U.S. Surveillance, Epidemiology, and End Results (SEER) network of population-based cancer registries now reports both benign and malignant CNS tumors. Brain tumor patients may present with general symptoms, such as headaches and seizures, which result from an increase in intracranial pressure. One-third of patients present with headaches and one-fifth with seizures. Other symptoms may include specific motor, speech, or sensory deficits resulting from compression of the corresponding region of the brain; slow-growing tumors may present with change in character only.

The discussion in this article will include benign and malignant tumors of the brain, cranial nerves, and cranial meninges, which account for 95% of all CNS tumors and 93% of all nervous system tumors. For simplicity, this group of tumors will be called brain tumors or, when benign tumors are excluded, brain cancer. The term central nervous system tumors (or cancer) indicates that tumors of the spinal cord and spinal meninges are included along with brain tumors, and nervous system (NS) tumors indicates that tumors of the peripheral nerves are included as well. Three major histologic groups are used in the descriptive tables of this article, corresponding to International Classification of Diseases for Oncology (ICD-O-3) morphology codes 9530–9534 and 9537–9539 for gliomas, 9530–9534 and 9537–9539 for meningiomas, and 9540–9571 for nerve sheath tumors. The statistics reported on incidence will focus on data from Surveillance, Epidemiology, and End Results (SEER).

Classification

Anatomic Classification

Tumors of the central nervous system include tumors of the brain, cranial nerves, cerebral meninges, spinal cord, and spinal meninges. These subsites are represented by the International Classification of Diseases for Oncology (ICD-O) codes C70.0–C72.9. We will not include tumors of sites such as the eye and the pituitary gland, which appear to be etiologically distinct.

Histopathology

The WHO classification of tumors system has allowed for international standardization of CNS malignancies based on cell of origin and histopathologic features, including degree of anaplasia. Tumors are classified into one of four grades: grade 1 is benign, grade 2 is considered low grade, while grades 3 and 4 are considered high grade or malignant. The most common are tumors of neuroepithelial origin, including astrocytomas, oligodendrogliomas, mixed gliomas, ependymal tumors, choroid plexus tumors, glial tumors of uncertain origin, neuronal and mixed neuronal-glial tumors, neuroblastic tumors, pineal parenchymal tumors, and embryonal tumors. The majority of CNS primary tumors are of astroglial origin, called gliomas. In the United States, according to recent data from the Los Angeles County Cancer Surveillance Program, gliomas account for 55% and 40% of primary CNS tumors among men and women, respectively (**Table 1**). The astrocytic tumors account for 80% of gliomas and include astrocytomas (grade II), anaplastic astrocytomas (grade III),

Table 1 Average annual age-adjusted incidence by major histologic type of primary tumors of the brain, cranial nerves, or cranial meninges by gender and race, Los Angeles County, 1972–2002[a]

	Glioma			Meningioma			Nerve sheath tumor			All primary CNS tumors		
	Rate	CI	N	Rate	CI	N	Rate	CI	N	Rate	CI	N
Males												
Blacks	4.26	3.84,4.67	473	2.70	2.33,3.07	238	0.52	0.38,0.66	57	9.37	8.74,10.0	987
Latinos	4.56	4.23,4.89	1185	1.43	1.21,1.65	238	0.53	0.43,0.62	141	8.37	7.90,8.83	2016
Other Whites	7.59	7.36,7.81	4530	2.21	2.09,2.34	1266	1.40	1.30,1.49	855	13.64	13.34,13.94	8059
Chinese	3.07	2.37,3.77	80	1.17	0.72,1.62	28	0.72	0.39,1.05	19	6.16	5.15,7.17	157
Japanese	2.29	1.55,3.03	39	0.87	0.44,1.31	16	1.33	0.79,1.86	25	5.64	4.50,6.77	101
Filipino	2.44	1.80,3.09	58	2.03	1.38,2.68	39	1.15	0.69,1.61	25	7.11	5.95,8.27	152
Korean	2.68	1.77,3.58	40	1.15	0.47,1.83	13	0.71	0.25,1.18	10	5.72	4.32,7.12	78
Other races	2.17	1.59,2.75	92	1.38	0.86,1.91	40	0.82	0.53,1.12	34	5.21	4.23,6.19	191
All races	6.08	5.92,6.23	6497	2.03	1.94,2.13	1878	1.08	1.01,1.14	1166	11.29	11.08,11.50	11741
Females												
Blacks	2.89	2.59,3.18	387	4.20	3.82,4.57	506	0.50	0.38,0.62	67	9.08	8.55,9.62	1145
Latinos	3.58	3.32,3.83	997	3.13	2.88,3.39	660	0.68	0.57,0.78	181	8.79	8.38,9.20	2190
Other Whites	5.06	4.89,5.23	3478	3.97	3.82,4.12	2873	1.31	1.22,1.40	872	12.03	11.77,12.29	8454
Chinese	1.90	1.38,2.42	54	2.16	1.61,2.72	61	0.59	0.31,0.88	17	5.57	4.67,6.47	155
Japanese	1.52	0.96,2.07	30	2.28	1.63,2.93	48	0.81	0.44,1.17	19	5.59	4.56,6.62	117
Filipino	1.87	1.31,2.44	49	3.94	3.14,4.74	100	1.07	0.68,1.47	29	7.92	6.78,9.05	203
Korean	1.95	1.27,2.63	33	2.59	1.69,3.50	37	0.72	0.31,1.13	12	6.77	5.41,8.13	105
Other races	1.45	1.08,1.82	71	2.35	2.17,3.33	100	1.14	0.80,1.47	48	6.13	5.31,6.94	254
All races	4.10	3.99,4.22	5099	3.69	3.58,3.80	4385	1.03	0.97,1.09	1245	10.37	10.19,10.55	12623

[a]Data from University of Southern California/Los Angles County Cancer Surveillance Program (CSP), the population-based tumor registry for Los Angeles County. Age-adjusted rates are a weighted average of the age-specific rates, where the weights represent the age distribution of a standard population. Rates are adjusted by the direct method to the 2000 U.S. population and are calculated per 100 000 persons.

and glioblastoma multiforme (grade IV). These represent increasing grades of anaplasia and clinical virulence of tumors of astrocytic cells. Two clinical variants of glioblastoma multiforme (GBM), primary and secondary, have been described, with primary GBM representing the more common (75%) of the two forms. Primary GBM is believed to develop *de novo* and grows very aggressively without evidence of a malignant precursor lesion. Secondary GBM is believed to arise from a low-grade lesion that has undergone genetic alterations to transition to a high-grade tumor. Oligodendrogliomas are classified as tumors with a cellular morphology most closely resembling that of the normal oligodendrocyte. There are two grades of oligodendrogliomas in the WHO classification system, where grade II is the lowest grade of oligodendroglioma and grade III (anaplastic) is the highest.

Tumors in the cranium can also originate from structures surrounding the brain, including the meninges, cranial nerves exiting the brain, blood vessels, or primitive remnants left from early development. Tumors of the peripheral nerves represent a subheading of the WHO classification scheme that includes schwannomas, neurofibromas, and malignant peripheral nerve sheath tumors. Acoustic schwannomas, which originate from the eighth cranial nerve, account for 90% of CNS schwannomas and 8% of all CNS tumors. Using recent data from the Los Angeles Cancer Surveillance Program in the United States, tumors of the meninges account for approximately 16% and 35% of central nervous system tumors in men and women respectively (**Table 1**). These originate in the cells of the dura mater, which is the covering for the brain and spinal cord. Tumors of the last three subheadings include lymphomas and hemopoietic tumors, germ cell tumors, and tumors of the sellar region. Tumors of the sellar region include craniopharyngiomas, tumor-like processes growing from epithelial rests remaining from Rathke's pouch, the progenitor for the pituitary gland.

Molecular Genetic Characteristics

Advances in molecular genetics are of growing importance for the correct classification of brain tumors, as well as the prediction of patient prognosis (i.e., survival) and treatment response. Details have been described in recent reviews (Ohgaki, 2005). As with other human malignancies, the pathogenesis of brain tumors is known to be associated with inactivation of tumor suppressor genes (TSG) and/or the activation of oncogenes, which may occur through several mechanisms including gene mutation, chromosomal loss, chromosomal gain or amplification, and methylation. In the sections below, we focus on several of the more common molecular genetic characteristics of brain tumors.

Chromosomal loss

Molecular studies indicate that gliomas frequently have loss of several chromosomal regions, referred to as loss of heterozygosity (LOH), at chromosomal regions 1p, 9p, 10q, 17p, 19q, and 22q. Frequent LOH suggests that inactivation of tumor suppressor genes in these regions may contribute to the development of gliomas. LOH 10q is one of the most frequent genetic alterations in gliomas, occurring in 40–50% of astrocytomas (grades II–III) and 60–80% of glioblastomas. Loss of one specific tumor suppressor gene on chromosome 10, named phosphatase and tensin homolog (PTEN), is associated with high-grade tumors and has been observed in 15–40% of glioblastomas. Mutations in PTEN can cause disruptions in cellular growth, migration, apoptosis or cellular death, and interaction with the extracellular matrix. Chromosomal loss is also a common distinguishing feature of oligodendrogliomas. Loss of the short arm of chromosome 1 (1p) and the long arm of chromosome 19 (19q) is present in 50–90% of oligodendrogliomas and is considered a marker of better patient outcome. Oligodendrogliomas from patients without loss of 1p/19q may instead have loss of chromosomal regions 9p and 10q; these losses frequently occur in the presence of amplification (i.e., multiple copies) of the oncogene known as epidermal growth factor receptor (EGFR).

Loss of chromosomal region 17p or mutations in the tumor suppressor gene *p53* located in the 17p region is believed to play a major role in both the formation of low-grade glioma and in the transition of low-grade gliomas to malignant glioblastoma. This tumor suppressor gene is known to be involved in many types of cancer, potentially through a regulatory role in apoptosis and cell cycle control. TP53 mutations are the earliest detectable change in gliomas and have been observed in as many as 53% of low-grade and anaplastic astrocytomas (WHO grades II and III, respectively) and 65% of glioblastomas. TP53 mutations are more common among the secondary glioblastomas (65%) than primary glioblastomas (28%) (Ohgaki, 2005). Some studies suggest that there is no difference in survival between patients with or without a p53 mutation, while others suggest there may be a survival benefit.

Mutations or loss of part of the promoter of the tumor suppressor gene retinoblastoma (*RB1*) can decrease gene activity and therefore diminish its ability to regulate cell cycle control. Mutations in *RB1* have been detected primarily in high-grade gliomas, suggesting *RB1* mutations represent a late event in astrocytoma development. Cyclin-dependent kinase inhibitor-2A (*CDKN2A*, also known as *P16*) is a second tumor suppressor gene in the RB1 pathway that contributes to cell cycle regulation.

Loss of chromosomal regions of this tumor suppressor gene are found in high-grade gliomas and some types of oligodendrogliomas.

Chromosomal gain

The epidermal growth factor receptor gene (*EGFR*), located on chromosome arm 7p, is a pro-oncogene involved in cellular proliferation. Amplification or chromosomal gain through accumulation of multiple gene copies are rarely found in low-grade gliomas and anaplastic oligodendrogliomas (<10%) but frequently found (40%) in primary glioblastomas (Ohgaki, 2005). Overexpression of the protein coded by *EGFR* is less common (<10%) among secondary glioblastomas, but common in primary glioblastomas (>60%). The frequency of EGFR amplification in brain tumors in the United States is more common in white non-Hispanic cases than other racial/ethnic groups. The prognostic value of *EGFR* is controversial. Some studies suggest *EGFR* amplification or overexpression may contribute to radiotherapy resistance and to overall poor survival; however, these differences may be due to confounding by age, because EGFR is more common in older patients and survival significantly decreases with age. *EGFR* amplification was not associated with survival in a recent meta-analysis (Huncharek and Kupelnick, 2000); however, some studies suggest *EGFR* is predictive of poor prognosis when present in younger patients.

Demographic Patterns

Incidence and Mortality

From the 1970s through the mid-1990s, incidence rates of primary brain tumors steadily increased in the United States (**Figure 1**), leading to speculation that the number of people being diagnosed with brain tumors was rising due to changes in the environment or lifestyle exposures. Age-adjusted incidence rates of primary malignant brain tumors increased by 22% from 1973 to 2003, using data from nine U.S. SEER registries (SEER Program, 2006). However, two reports using SEER incidence data and the U.S. National Center for Health Statistics mortality data found that the changing patterns of incidence and mortality were best explained by increasing use of better diagnostic equipment, in particular computed tomography (CT) and magnetic resonance imaging (MRI) (Smith *et al.*, 1998; Legler *et al.*, 1999). Legler *et al.* found that from 1975 to 1995, incidence rates were significantly increasing only among children under 15 years of age and adults 65 years of age and older. During this same time period, mortality declined for the youngest age group and increased among the oldest age group. The difference in mortality by age may be explained in part by the fact that low-grade tumors that have better prognosis are more

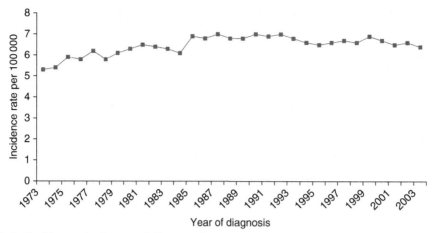

Figure 1   Age-adjusted incidence rates by year of primary malignant tumors for nine U.S. SEER registries combined, 1973–2003. Rates are per 100 000 and age-adjusted to the 2000 U.S. Standard Population (19 age groups – Census P25–1130).

common in children and high-grade tumors that have poorer prognosis are more common in adults. The authors also showed that use of CT and MRI procedures by doctors for their patients 65 years and older increased during the mid-1980s and early 1990s, suggesting greater use of available technology to diagnose patients.

Survival

Age-adjusted 5-year survival rates for all malignant primary brain tumors in the United States, as catalogued by the National Cancer Institute from 1989 to 1996 were 31% (Gurney and Kadan-Lottick, 2001). While this represents an improvement from rates observed in 1974–76 (23%), the survival rates remain extremely low. Five-year survival rates recently published by the American Cancer Society, show that the average survival rate from 1995 to 2001 is still only 33% (American Cancer Society, 2006). Similarly, the weighted 5-year brain cancer survival rate calculated for 22 European countries through 1998 was also low, reaching only 18%.

Survival rates are dependent on a number of patient and tumor characteristics, including age and histologic type of tumor. For example, the SEER 5-year survival rate for patients aged 0–19 years of age at diagnosis is 65%, while the rate for those aged 65–74 years or 75 years and older are 6.5% and 3.6%, respectively (Ries et al., 2000).

A study using SEER data that examined malignant brain tumor survival by histology (Davis et al., 1998) also found that survival declined with increasing age at diagnosis. For the most part, the survival rates between the sexes did not differ. The survival rate for patients with glioblastoma whose brain tumor was diagnosed between the years 1986 and 1991 was only 1% for all ages combined. The rate of survival was 34% for astrocytomas and 84% for pilocytic astrocytomas, which occur predominantly in children. Survival from medulloblastoma for

all age groups combined improved from 40% in the 1970s to 60%. The survival rates for oligodendroglioma also substantially improved to 65% between 1986 and 1991. Five-year survival rates remained similar over the 20 years for ependymomas (60%), mixed gliomas (51%), other gliomas (23%), and gliomas not otherwise specified (NOS) (17%).

It is thought that improved diagnostic abilities, treatment modalities, and earlier age at diagnosis may account for the improvements in survival of astrocytomas, medulloblastomas, and oligodendrogliomas over the last 20 years.

Incidence patterns of primary brain tumors by age, gender, and race are described using data from SEER.

Age

Incidence rates of primary brain tumors show a bimodal peak by age. Incidence rates of tumors vary by histologic type; however, for all tumor types combined, incidence rates peak in early childhood (generally by age 5 years), decline and increase again from approximately ages 25 through 75 years of age. The average annual age-specific incidence of brain tumors in nine SEER registries is shown in **Figure 2**.

Gender

Table 1 shows the age-adjusted annual incidence for the major histologic groups of primary brain tumors by sex and racial/ethnic group in Los Angeles County, CA for 1972–2002. For all histologic types and races combined, the rate is higher in men than in women. However, incidence rates vary considerably by histologic subtype. Glioma rates are higher in males than in females in each racial/ethnic group and meningiomas are higher in women.

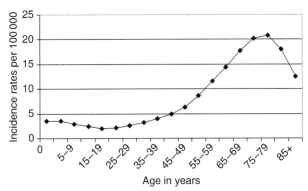

Figure 2 Average annual age-specific incidence rates for primary brain cancer for nine U.S. SEER registries combined, 1973–2003. Rates are per 100 000 and age-adjusted to the 2000 U.S. Standard Population (19 age groups – Census P25–1130).

Race and Ethnicity

The incidence of gliomas in the United States is highest in non-Spanish-surnamed Whites for males and females, while the incidence of meningiomas is highest in Blacks for males and females (see **Table 1**).

Environmental Factors

This section reviews recent findings from epidemiologic studies, which have investigated the association between human brain tumors and various potential risk factors.

N-nitroso Compounds (NOCs)

N-nitroso compounds (NOCs) and their precursors are experimental carcinogens (Lijinsky, 1992) that have been investigated as potential causes of brain tumors in humans. NOCs are divided into two major categories based on their chemical structure – nitrosamines and nitrosamides. Nitrosamines are carcinogenic in animal studies, but have never been shown to cause tumors in the brain or spinal cord. Nitrosamides are direct-acting agents that can cause DNA adducts and have been shown to be potent nervous system carcinogens in a variety of species. Ethylnitrosourea (ENU), a type of nitrosamide, has been shown to be a neurocarcinogen in rats, mice, rabbits, opossums, and monkeys through various routes of administration and when given in a single dose or through chronic low-dose exposure. Transplacental exposure is the most potent route of exposure, as only one-fiftieth (1/50) of the dose of ENU required to induce tumors in adult animals is necessary to cause 100% tumor induction in fetal animals (Ivankovic, 1979).

Population Exposure to NOCs

The major sources of population exposure to NOCs in the United States are tobacco smoke, cosmetics, automobile interiors, cured meats, and some types of pesticides (National Research Council Committee on Diet Nutrition and Cancer, 1982). Other sources of NOC exposure include soaps, shampoos, hand lotions, rubber baby bottle nipples, and pacifiers. Endogenous formation of NOCs in humans occurs in the stomach or bladder when both an amino compound and a nitrosating agent are present simultaneously. Food is a primary source of both highly concentrated nitrite solutions (e.g., from cured meats) and amino compounds (e.g., in fish and other foods, and in many drugs). Drinking water also contains nitrate (in the absence of vitamins), but this is a minor source unless levels are extraordinarily high.

Diet and Vitamin Supplementation

The majority of hypotheses regarding dietary factors and brain tumors have focused on cured meats (sources of N-nitroso compounds), antioxidants, and inhibitors of nitrosation, including vitamins C and E. Eight of ten epidemiologic studies that investigated the role of cured meats during pregnancy found a significant positive association between the frequency of maternal cured meat intake by the mother (individual or combined cured meats) and the risk of childhood brain tumors (CBT) (Baldwin and Preston-Martin, 2004). The individual foods most consistently found to be associated with increased risk for CBT were hot dogs and bacon. In a study of adults, serum levels of ascorbic acid (vitamin C) and alpha- and gamma-tocopherol (vitamin E) were both inversely related to glioblastoma risk (Schwartzbaum and Cornwell, 2000). Furthermore, high intake of fruits and vegetables has been associated with lower risk of childhood brain tumors in several studies of CBT (maternal intake of fruits and vegetables during pregnancy) and has also been reported in a number of studies of adult brain tumors.

The apparent reduction in risk of brain tumor development associated with fruits, vegetables, and vitamin intake may be interpreted as supportive of the N-nitroso hypothesis due to the inhibition of the endogenous formation of NOCs in the presence of vitamins C or E, or the apparent protective effect may be due to another mechanism such as the inhibition of free radical formation in the brain.

Radiation

High-dose exposure to ionizing radiation is the only established environmental cause of brain tumors. Several studies have shown an excess risk of brain tumors following exposure to high-dose therapeutic radiation (2500 cGy) for primary malignancies or benign conditions (Wrensch et al., 2002). Meningioma appears to be the most common brain tumor resulting from radiotherapy for other medical conditions; however, tumors of other histological types have occurred, including glioblastoma.

One of the strongest pieces of evidence supporting a role of therapeutic radiation and brain tumor risk comes from an Israeli cohort study of adults irradiated as children for tinea capitis (i.e. ringworm of the scalp); adults with a history of irradiation were at high risk of developing nerve sheath tumors of the head and neck (RR = 33.1 or exposed children were 33 times more likely to develop a nerve sheath tumor), intermediate risk of meningioma (RR = 9.5), and lowest risk of glioma (RR = 2.6). Recent updated results from this cohort show that risk remains elevated after 40 years of follow-up for both benign meningiomas and malignant brain gliomas (Sadetzki *et al.*, 2005).

The association between brain tumors and prior exposure to low-dose, diagnostic X-rays remains less certain. A Swedish case-control study found that X-rays of the head and neck were associated with increased risk of adult brain tumors (OR 1.64; 95% CI 1.04–2.58) and that this risk was strongest among individuals irradiated 5 or more years before tumor diagnosis (OR 2.10; 95% CI 1.25–3.53) (Hardell *et al.*, 2001). Epidemiologic studies have found that prior dental radiography, particularly in earlier decades when doses were high, was associated with subtentorial, intracranial meningiomas (Preston-Martin and White, 1990). Other studies, however, did not confirm these findings.

Electric and Magnetic Fields

In the 1990s, numerous studies of electric and magnetic fields were completed to investigate the potential association with child and adult brain tumor risk. Electric and magnetic fields induce weak electric currents in the body; however, they can neither break bonds nor heat tissue. Several studies that have explored the association between exposure to electromagnetic fields (EMFs) and brain tumor risk have been recently reviewed (Kheifets, 2001). Although early studies of childhood brain tumors and residential exposure (both from ambient fields and use of electrical appliances) were suggestive of an increased risk, findings from the most recent studies have produced inconsistent results. Methodologic limitations of studies have included small sample sizes, in particular small numbers of subjects with high levels of exposure; measurement errors; lack of a standardized reference interval for the evaluation of magnetic fields; and incomplete evaluation of potential confounding variables. Exposure to radiofrequency sources is difficult to quantify in the laboratory setting; their measurement in large epidemiologic populations is even more challenging.

Studies of residential exposure to EMF and adult brain tumors have provided little evidence that EMF is a risk factor for brain tumors. A meta-analysis of 29 studies of occupational sources of EMF and brain cancer found a small increase in risk among electrical workers (Kheifets *et al.*, 1995), but there was substantial heterogeneity in findings across studies due to differences in study design, occupations included, and exposure assessment methods.

Cellular Telephones and Other Radiofrequency Exposures

In recent years, public concern has focused on the potential risk of brain tumors due to cell phone usage. However, experimental data indicate that nonthermal radio frequency (RF) waves do not have enough energy to damage DNA, either directly or through epigenetic changes. Additionally, animal studies indicate RF exposure does not increase malignancies in rodents. Several early occupational studies did report associations between RF exposure and hematopoietic or brain cancers (Moulder *et al.*, 2005). Nevertheless, these studies did not provide adequate support for a causal relationship between RF and cancer, due to limitations in design and exposure assessment.

The majority of epidemiologic studies to date do not support an association between cell phone use and brain tumor risk. No excess risk was found in a number of large case-control studies. Two case-control studies did find an elevated risk of brain tumors on the side of the head where the phone was most often held (Muscat *et al.*, 2000; Hardell *et al.*, 2001); however, the conclusions for one of these studies was questioned due to the use of prevalent cases and other design issues. Data from the Interphone Study found no overall increase in risk for temporal glioma or meningioma among cellular phone users (Lonn *et al.*, 2005). Further, a Danish cohort found no increase in brain cancer or any other cancer incidence when including 450 085 mobile phone subscribers during the period of 1982–95 (Johansen *et al.*, 2001). However, a Finnish registry-based study found a significant association (OR 1.5; 95% CI 1.0–2.4) between gliomas and analog cellular phones (Auvinen *et al.*, 2002). No excess of brain cancer was found among employees of a cell phone manufacturing company or in a cohort study designed to examine cancer mortality in Korean War radar and radio technicians (Groves *et al.*, 2002).

Misclassification of exposure is a potential design limitation in all cell phone studies, because RF exposure levels have changed over time with changes in cell phone technology and RF exposure varies with a person's distance from cellular phone stations at the time they are using a cell phone. Current studies estimate risk for a maximum of 20 years of RF exposure; brain tumor risk for long-term cell phone usage of more than two decades is not known. Despite these limitations, these studies seemingly rule out large and immediate increases in brain cancer rates in cellular phone users.

Trauma

Several case reports and series provide anecdotal evidence that prior head trauma is associated with brain tumor development, but larger studies have not consistently confirmed this relationship. One report describes a case of malignant glioma occurring in the same spot where a man suffered a metal splinter injury 37 years earlier (Sabel *et al.*, 1999); most previous case reports of this sort have involved meningiomas. An international case-control study of head trauma and risk of gliomas and meningiomas found an increased risk of meningioma only among men who had a serious head injury 15–24 years prior to diagnosis (Preston-Martin *et al.*, 1998). Other investigators have found a weak relationship between trauma and meningiomas, suggesting that cellular proliferation due to repair of the dura may explain the increase in risk. However, recall bias is a concern when interpreting these studies because those who developed a brain tumor may be more likely to remember a previous head injury. Large studies from Sweden and Denmark have not confirmed a trauma–brain tumor risk relationship (Inskip *et al.*, 1998; Nygren *et al.*, 2001).

Infectious Agents

Several types of viruses cause brain tumors in experimental animals, including simian immunodeficiency as well as JC and BK viruses. In one of the earliest epidemiologic studies of brain tumors, astrocytomas were associated with positive antibody titers to *Toxoplasma gondii* (Schuman *et al.*, 1967); however, more recent studies have failed to confirm this association. It is believed that over 62% of the United States population have been exposed to Simian virus 40 (SV 40), a member of the *Polyomaviridae* family, through administration of polio vaccine contaminated with the virus between 1955 and 1963 (Shah and Nathanson, 1976). Early animal studies revealed the carcinogenic effect of the virus and recent studies detected specific SV40 complexes in brain cancer tissue, suggesting a possible SV 40 role in primary brain tumor pathogenesis (Eddy *et al.*, 1962). The tumorigenicity of other common polyomaviruses, including JC and BK viruses, have been well established through *in vitro* and animal experimental studies (Inskip *et al.*, 1995). While JC and BK viruses normally do not cause symptoms in healthy individuals, JC and BK viral DNA sequences have been isolated from a number of types of human brain tumors, including medulloblastoma, ependymoma, and gliomas.

Other studies have found associations between risk of maternal infections during pregnancy and childhood brain tumors. Bithell *et al.* found an increased risk of brain tumors among children of mothers who had chickenpox during the pregnancy (Bithell *et al.*, 1973). History of varicella-zoster infection was related to a reduced risk of adult gliomas if a history of chickenpox or shingles or serum levels of immunoglobulin G antibodies to the virus was used in the analysis (Wrensch *et al.*, 2002). In a recent case-control study, Wrensch *et al.* reported that glioma cases (particularly those with glioblastoma) had significantly lower levels of anti-varicella zoster

virus immunoglobulin G than controls and that cases were less likely than controls to report a history of chickenpox. However, no significant differences were noted between cases and controls for positivity to three other herpesviruses: Epstein-Barr virus, cytomegalovirus, and herpes simplex virus (Wrensch *et al.*, 2002).

Allergies, Epilepsy, and Other Medical Conditions

Several epidemiologic studies have reported a protective association between brain tumor risk and a history of asthma and other allergic conditions. This finding has been consistent across a number of large case-control studies conducted in various countries (Wrensch *et al.*, 2002). One study specifically reported an inverse association of autoimmune disease with both glioma and meningioma, with the greatest reduction in risk found among glioma patients with both asthma and diabetes (Brenner *et al.*, 2002). Three cohort studies using Swedish data provide limited support for this association (relative risk (RR) 0.45; 95% CI 0.19–1.07 and RR 0.45; 95% CI 0.11–1.92 among low-grade and high-grade gliomas, respectively) (Schwartzbaum *et al.*, 2003).

Recent studies of immunologic biomarkers and gliomas further support the association between allergic conditions and brain tumor risk. In a case-control study of adult glioma, Wiemels *et al.* found cases had significantly lower serum IgE levels than controls; this was particularly true among subjects reporting food allergies. However, it remains possible that differences in IgE levels were due to changes in IgE after the tumor was diagnosed (Wiemels *et al.*, 2004). Schwartzbaum *et al.* completed a population-based case-control study to investigate the association between GBM and common genetic changes in immune pathway genes. The study focused on genes coding for interleukins, which regulate and cause differentiation of cells of the immune system. Investigators found that people with a history of asthma, eczema, and fever were significantly less likely to be diagnosed with a GBM. Two genetic variants in the interleukin-4 receptor were associated with a greater chance of developing a GBM, while a single genetic variant in the interleukin-13 gene was associated with a lower risk of developing GBM (Schwartzbaum *et al.*, 2005). Additional molecular studies are needed to explore the biological basis of this association.

Occupational Exposures

Associations between employment in various occupations and industries and brain tumor risk have been investigated in numerous epidemiological studies, but few associations have been found consistently across studies. Further, results have been limited by difficulties in determining past workplace exposures and by small numbers of people who have been exposed to any specific agent.

Several epidemiological studies have investigated associations between employment in the petrochemical industry and brain tumor risk. One study found an excess of brain cancers among white men with 10 or more years of employment in a particular building complex of interest (Beall *et al.*, 2001). Another case-control study of workers at a petrochemical research facility found positive associations between gliomas and ionizing radiation, n-hexane, organometallics, and amines other than nitrosamines.

Epidemiological studies of brain tumor deaths have reported elevated risk of mortality due to brain tumors for a variety of occupations involving exposure to electromagnetic fields (EMFs). These include electrical or electronic engineers, electronics teachers, and electrical technicians and assemblers, electric utility workers, and workers in the communications industry. A recent review on this subject found that the quality of epidemiological studies of EMF exposure has improved and there is a large body of high-quality data on brain tumor risk and occupational EMF exposure (Ahlbom *et al.*, 2001). No excess brain tumor risk was seen in a cohort of British electrical utility workers (Sorahan *et al.*, 2001). A case-control study conducted in eight Canadian provinces, with emphasis placed on variations in EMF-related risk across different histological types found a pronounced risk for glioblastoma multiforme, but no association for astrocytoma or other brain tumors (Villeneuve *et al.*, 2002).

Smoking and Environmental Tobacco Smoke

Most studies of adult brain tumors have not established any relationship between smoking tobacco and brain cancer. However, a study of adult gliomas in the San Francisco Bay area found that male cases are more likely to report smoking unfiltered cigarettes than controls (Lee *et al.*, 1997). A second study reported that a history of active smoking was associated with a significant dose–response increase in risk of meningioma in men. In the same study, exposure to passive smoke from a spouse on the part of never smokers was associated with increased risk of brain tumors in both sexes (OR = 2.0) and risk increased with increasing duration of exposure (p for trend = 0.02) (Phillips *et al.*, 2005).

Overall, the epidemiologic data do not support an association between maternal smoking during pregnancy and risk of CBT (Boffetta *et al.*, 2000). However, the meta-analysis of ten studies found a small increase in risk for childhood brain tumors (OR 1.2; CI 1.1–1.4) in relation to father's smoking during pregnancy. An international collaborative population-based case-control study conducted in seven countries found a small association between paternal smoking before pregnancy and risk of childhood astroglial tumors (OR 1.4) (Cordier *et al.*, 2004). A recent prospective study of 1.4 million Swedish births found an association between maternal smoking during pregnancy and risk of CBT (RR 1.24; 95% CI 1.01–1.53) (Brooks *et al.*, 2004).

Alcohol

Findings relating to parental alcohol intake are mostly unremarkable. Most studies of adult brain tumors find no excess and possibly a reduced risk related to intake of wine and beer.

Use of Pesticides

Several epidemiologic studies have investigated home and occupational use of pesticides, insecticides, or herbicides as possible etiologic factors for brain tumors. Case-control studies have linked household pest exterminations to the development of childhood brain tumors, while others have found no association with parental pesticide use. A recent review indicated 14 of 17 studies of maternal and childhood pesticide exposure and CBT found positive associations (Zahm, 1999). One large case-control study found an excess risk of CBT related specifically to prenatal exposure to flea and tick products (Pogoda and Preston-Martin, 1997). A cohort study of licensed pesticide applicators (Blair *et al.*, 1983) found an excess risk of brain cancer. More studies are needed to confirm associations seen and to identify which compounds may relate to brain tumor development.

Summary of Environmental Risk Factors

The cause of most types of brain tumor remain unexplained. High-dose levels of ionizing radiation (IR) are the most clearly established cause of pediatric and adult brain tumors based on both experimental and epidemiologic data. However, few cases are likely to be explained by this factor because precautions are now taken to avoid exposing individuals to unnecessarily high doses of IR. A growing number of epidemiologic studies suggest a strong, protective association between brain tumor risk and a history of asthma and other allergic conditions. Other environmental factors have been less consistently associated with brain tumor risk. Occupational studies suggest that employment in the petrochemical industry or employment involving exposure to electromagnetic fields may increase risk. N-nitroso compounds and pesticide use in the home have been associated with risk of pediatric brain tumors in some studies, but challenges in recreating exposure years in the past limit the strength of conclusions that can be drawn from these data. Current evidence that cell phones, smoking history, or alcohol are risk factors for brain tumors is weak.

Host Factors

Familial Aggregation

The potential heritability and familial clustering of CNS tumors is well documented. The implication of such reports is that shared genes, environment, or gene–environment interaction could be responsible for some neoplasms, but reports estimate that familial gliomas account for 5% or fewer of total cases.

Neurogenetic Syndromes

Various hereditary syndromes have been associated with increased brain tumor risk, including neurofibromatosis-1 and -2, Von Hippel-Lindau disease, Li-Fraumeni syndrome, tuberous sclerosis, and Gorlin's syndrome. However, these hereditary syndromes are rare and are likely to account for few cases in a population-based series of CNS neoplasia.

Preventive Measures

Few causes of brain tumors in adults or children have been identified. Etiologic associations may be more likely to be detected if analyses are restricted to more homogeneous tumor sets with common morphologic and molecular genetic characteristics. For many subgroups, in order to obtain sufficient numbers of subjects it will become necessary to pool data from studies across geographic areas. We have the most to gain using this approach in studies of the etiology of gliomas, whose causes remain largely unknown. Gliomas appear far more morphologically and genetically diverse than do the other major categories of CNS tumors. Perhaps more is known about the etiology of meningiomas and nerve sheath tumors because each of these major groups represents a more homogeneous entity than do gliomas. Diet, genetics, and immunology will continue to be an important focus of the next generation of epidemiologic studies of brain tumors.

Citations

Ahlbom IC, Cardis E, Green A, Linet M, Savitz D, and Swerdlow A (2001) Review of the *epidemiologic literature on EMF and Health*. *Environmental Health Perspectives* 109 (supplement 6): 911–933.

American Cancer Society (2006) *Cancer Facts & Figures*. Atlanta, GA: Surveillance Research.

Auvinen A, Hietanen M, Luukkonen R, and Koskela RS (2002) Brain tumors and salivary gland cancers among cellular telephone users. *Epidemiology* 13: 356–359.

Baldwin RT and Preston-Martin S (2004) Epidemiology of brain tumors in childhood: A review. *Toxicology and Applied Pharmacology* 199: 118–131.

Beall C, Delzell E, Rodu B, Sathiakumar N, and Myers S (2001) Cancer and benign tumor incidence among employees in a polymers research complex. *Journal of Occupational and Environmental Medicine* 43: 914–924.

Bithell JF, Draper GJ, and Gorbach PD (1973) Association between malignant disease in children and maternal virus infections during pregnancy. *British Journal of Preventive Social Medicine* 27: 68.

Blair A, Grauman DJ, Lubin JH, and Fraumeni JF Jr (1983) Lung cancer and other causes of death among licensed pesticide applicators. *Journal of the National Cancer Institute* 71: 31–37.

Boffetta P, Tredaniel J, and Greco A (2000) Risk of childhood cancer and adult lung cancer after childhood exposure to passive smoke: A meta-analysis. *Environmental Health Perspectives* 108: 73–82.

Brenner AV, Linet MS, Fine HA, et al. (2002) History of allergies and autoimmune diseases and risk of brain tumors in adults. *International Journal of Cancer* 99: 252–259.

Brooks DR, Mucci LA, Hatch EE, and Cnattingius S (2004) Maternal smoking during pregnancy and risk of brain tumors in the offspring. A prospective study of 1.4 million Swedish births. *Cancer Causes and Control* 15: 997–1005.

CBTRUS (2005) *Statistical Report: Primary Brain Tumors in the United States, 1998–2002*. Hinsdale, IL: Central Brain Tumor Registry of the United States.

Cordier S, Monfort C, Filippini G, et al. (2004) Parental exposure to polycyclic aromatic hydrocarbons and the risk of childhood brain tumors: The SEARCH International Childhood Brain Tumor Study. *American Journal of Epidemiology* 159: 1109–1116.

Davis FG, Freels S, Grutsch J, Barlas S, and Brem S (1998) Survival rates in patients with primary malignant brain tumors stratified by patient age and tumor histological type: An analysis based on Surveillance Epidemiology, and End Results (SEER) data, 1973–1991. *Journal of Neurosurgery* 88: 1–10.

Eddy BE, Borman GS, Grubbs GE, and Young RD (1962) Identification of the oncogenic substance in rhesus monkey kidney cell culture as simian virus 40. *Virology* 17: 65–75.

Ferlay J, Bray F, Pisani P, and Parkin DM (2004) *Cancer Incidence Mortality, and Prevalence Worldwide, Verson 2.0. IARC CancerBase No. 5*. Lyon, France: IARC Press, 2004.

Groves FD, Page WF, Gridley G, et al. (2002) Cancer in Korean war navy technicians: Mortality survey after 40 years. *American Journal Epidemiology* 155: 810–818.

Gurney JG and Kadan-Lottick N (2001) Brain and other central nervous system tumors: Rates, trends, and epidemiology. *Current Opinions in Oncology* 13: 160–166.

Hardell L, Mild KH, Pahlson A, and Hallquist A (2001) Ionizing radiation, cellular telephones and the risk for brain tumours. *European Journal of Cancer Prevention* 10: 523–529.

Huncharek M and Kupelnick B (2000) Epidermal growth factor receptor gene amplification as a prognostic marker in glioblastoma multiforme: Results of a meta-analysis. *Oncology Research* 12: 107–112.

Inskip PD, Linet MS, and Heineman EF (1995) Etiology of brain tumors in adults. *Epidemiology Reviews* 17: 382–414.

Inskip PD, Mellemkjaer L, Gridley G, and Olsen JH (1998) Incidence of intracranial tumors following hospitalization for head injuries (Denmark). *Cancer Causes and Control* 9: 109–116.

Ivankovic S (1979) Teratogenic and carcinogenic effects of some chemicals during perinatal life in rats Syrian golden hamsters, and minipigs. *National Cancer Institute Monographs* 103–115.

Johansen C, Boice J Jr, McLaughlin J, and Olsen J (2001) Cellular telephones and cancer – A nationwide cohort study in Denmark. *Journal of the National Cancer Institute* 93: 203–207.

Kheifets LI (2001) Electric and magnetic field exposure and brain cancer: A review. *Bioelectromagnetics Supplement* 5: S120–131.

Kheifets LI, Afifi AA, Buffler PA, and Zhang ZW (1995) Occupational electric and magnetic field exposure and brain cancer: A meta-analysis. *Journal of Occupational and Environmental Medicine* 37: 1327–1341.

Lee M, Wrensch M, and Miike R (1997) Dietary and tobacco risk factors for adult onset glioma in the San Freidlin Bay Area (California USA). *Cancer Causes and Control* 8: 13–24.

Legler J, Ries L, Smith M, et al. (1999) Cancer surveillance series [corrected]: Brain and other central nervous system cancers: Recent trends in incidence and mortality. *Journal of the National Cancer Institute* 91: 1382–1390.

Lijinsky W (1992) *Chemistry and Biology of N-nitroso Compounds.* Cambridge, UK: Cambridge University Press.

Lonn S, Ahlbom A, Hall P, and Feychting M (2005) Long-term mobile phone use and brain tumor risk. *American Journal of Epidemiology* 161: 526–535.

Moulder JE, Foster KR, Erdreich LS, and McNamee JP (2005) Mobile phones, mobile phone base stations and cancer: A review. *International Journal of Radiation Biology* 81: 189–203.

Muscat JE, Malkin MG, Thompson S, et al. (2000) Handheld cellular telephone use and risk of brain cancer. *Journal of the American Medical Association* 284: 3001–3007.

National Research Council Committee on Diet Nutrition and Cancer (1982) *Diet, Nutrition and Cancer.* Washington, DC: National Academy Press.

Nygren C, Adami J, Ye W, et al. (2001) Primary brain tumors following traumatic brain injury – A population-based cohort study in Sweden. *Cancer Causes and Control* 12: 733–737.

Ohgaki H (2005) Genetic pathways to glioblastomas. *Neuropathology* 25: 1–7.

Phillips LE, Longstreth WT Jr, Koepsell T, Custer BS, Kukull WA, and van Belle G (2005) Active and passive cigarette smoking and risk of intracranial meningioma. *Neuroepidemiology* 24: 117–122.

Pogoda JM and Preston-Martin S (1997) Household pesticides and risk of pediatric brain tumors. *Environmental Health Perspectives* 105: 1214–1220.

Preston-Martin S and White SC (1990) Brain and salivary gland tumors related to prior dental radiography: Implications for current practice. *Journal of the American Dental Association* 120: 151–158.

Preston-Martin S, Pogoda JM, Mueller BA, et al. (1998) Prenatal vitamin supplementation and risk of childhood brain tumors. *International Journal of Cancer Supplement* 11: 17–22.

Ries LA, Eisner MP, and Kosary CL (2000) *SEER Cancer Statistics Review 1973–1977.* http://www-seer.ims.nci.nih.gov/Publications/ (accessed February 2008).

Sabel M, Felsberg J, Messing-Junger M, Neuen-Jacob E, and Piek J (1999) Glioblastoma multiforme at the site of metal splinter injury: A coincidence? Case report. *Journal of Neurosurgury* 91: 1041–1044.

Sadetzki S, Chetrit A, Freedman L, Stovall M, Modan B, and Novikov I (2005) Long-term follow-up for brain tumor development after childhood exposure to ionizing radiation for tinea capitis. *Radiation Research* 163: 424–432.

Sant M, Aareleid T, Berrino F, et al. (2003) EUROCARE-3: Survival of cancer patients diagnosed 1990–94: Results and commentary. *Annals of Oncology* 14(supplement 5): 61–118.

Schuman LM, Choi NW, and Gullen WH (1967) Relationship of central nervous system neoplasms to *Toxoplasma gondii* infection. *American Journal of Public Health and the Nation's Health* 57: 848–856.

Schwartzbaum J, Ahlbom A, Malmer B, et al. (2005) Polymorphisms associated with asthma are inversely related to glioblastoma multiforme. *Cancer Research* 65: 6459–6465.

Schwartzbaum JA and Cornwell DG (2000) Oxidant stress and glioblastoma multiforme risk: serum antioxidants, gamma-glutamyl transpeptidase, and ferritin. *Nutrition and Cancer* 38: 40–49.

Schwartzbaum J, Jonsson F, Ahlbom A, et al. (2003) Cohort studies of association between self-reported allergic conditions, immune-related diagnoses and glioma and meningioma risk. *International Journal of Cancer* 106: 423–428.

Shah K and Nathanson N (1976) Human exposure to SV40: Review and comment. *American Journal of Epidemiology* 103: 1–12.

Smith MA, Freidlin B, Ries LA, and Simon R (1998) Trends in reported incidence of primary malignant brain tumors in children in the United States. *Journal of the National Cancer Institute* 90: 1269–1277.

Sorahan T, Nichols L, van Tongeren M, and Harrington JM (2001) Occupational exposure to magnetic fields relative to mortality from brain tumours: Updated and revised findings from a study of United Kingdom electricity generation and transmission workers, 1973–97. *Occupational and Environmental Medicine* 58: 626–630.

Surveillance Epidemiology and End Results (SEER). *Program SEER*Stat Database: Incidence-SEER 9 Regs Public Use Nov 2005 Sub (1973–2003), Linked to County Attributes. Total US, 1969–2003 Counties.* http://www.seer.cancer.gov (accessed February 2008).

Villeneuve PJ, Agnew DA, Johnson KC, and Mao Y (2002) Brain cancer and occupational exposure to magnetic fields among men: Results from a Canadian population-based case-control study. *International Journal of Epidemiology* 31: 210–217.

Wiemels JL, Wiencke JK, Patoka J, et al. (2004) Reduced immunoglobulin E and allergy among adults with glioma compared with controls. *Cancer Research* 64: 8468–8473.

Wrensch M, Bondy ML, Wiencke J, and Yost M (1993) Environmental risk factors for primary malignant brain tumors: A review. *Journal of Neuro-oncology* 17: 47–64.

Wrensch M, Fisher JL, Schwartzbaum JA, Bondy M, Berger M, and Aldape KD (2005) The molecular epidemiology of gliomas in adults. *Neurosurgery Focus* 19: E5.

Wrensch M, Minn Y, Chew T, Bondy M, and Berger MS (2002) Epidemiology of primary brain tumors: Current concepts and review of the literature. *Neuro-oncology* 4: 278–299.

Zahm SH (1999) Childhood leukemia and pesticides. *Epidemiology* 10: 473–475.

Further Reading

Deitrich M, Block G, Pogoda JM, Buffler P, Hechts S, and Preston-Martin S (2005) A review: Dietary and endogenously formed N-nitroso compounds and risk of childhood brain tumors. *Cancer Causes and Control* 16(6): 619–635.

Ohgaki H and Kleihues P (2005) Epidemiology and etiology of gliomas. *Acta Neuropathologica (Berlin)* 109: 93–108.

Wrensch M, Bondy ML, Wiencke J, and Yost M (1993) Environmental risk factors for primary malignant brain tumors: A review. *Journal of Neuro-oncology* 17: 47–64.

Wrensch M, Fisher JL, Schwartzbaum JA, Bondy M, Berger M, and Aldape KD (2005) The molecular epidemiology of gliomas in adults. *Neurosurgery Focus* 19: E5.

Cerebrovascular Disease

V Feigin, The University of Auckland, Auckland, New Zealand
G Donnan, University of Melbourne, Melbourne, VIC, Australia

Introduction

Cerebrovascular disease is a heterogeneous disorder. It comprises of a number of distinct pathologies, including transient ischemic attack, stroke pathological types (ischemic stroke, intracerebral hemorrhage, subarachnoid hemorrhage) and etiological subtypes (e.g., cardioembolic, atherothrombotic, lacunar ischemic strokes, aneurysmal subarachnoid hemorrhage), and other intracranial vascular disorders (e.g., vascular malformations, unruptured aneurysms), each of which has different epidemiological and management features. Stroke is the most important and devastating clinical manifestation of all the cerebrovascular disorders.

Stroke is the second most common cause of death worldwide and the most frequent cause of disability in adults in many countries (Kaste *et al.*, 1997). It also has an enormous physical, psychological, and financial impact on patients, families, the health-care system, and society. The lifetime costs per stroke patient in various countries are estimated to range from US$59 800 to US$230 000. Moreover, stroke burden on families and societies is projected to rise from around 38 million disability-adjusted life years (DALYs) lost globally in 1990 to 61 million DALYs in 2020, largely due to aging of most populations. Although stroke mortality in Western populations has declined steadily over the last few decades, stroke incidence trends differ between the countries and the overall number of stroke survivors has tended to increase. The best management strategy to reduce burden of stroke is its prevention on both individual and population levels. Given that over half of survivors remain dependent on others for everyday activities, often with significant adverse effects on caregivers, reducing the impact of stroke, on caregivers as well as patients, is key to the maintenance of independence, quality of life, and burden on health services in populations.

Incidence and Prevalence

Stroke

In epidemiological research, stroke is commonly defined using the WHO definition of stroke, 'rapidly developing signs of focal (or global) disturbance of cerebral function, leading to death or lasting longer than 24 hours, with no apparent cause other than vascular'. Despite a continuous decrease in stroke mortality rates observed in many developed countries over the last few decades, globally stroke as a cause of death has moved from third to second place in the world and is now the leading cause of physical disability in adults aged 65 years and older. In recent years, there has been an unprecedented increase in stroke burden in developing countries (**Figure 1**). Although causes of the changing epidemiology of stroke are not

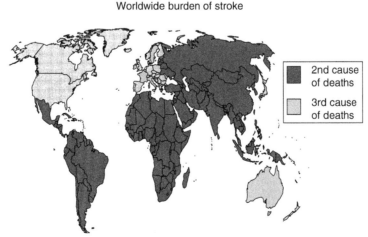

Worldwide burden of stroke

Figure 1 Worldwide stroke mortality.

fully understood, the importance of aging of the population has been postulated.

Why do we need stroke incidence studies? Good-quality stroke incidence studies are essential for evidence-based health-care planning and resource allocation in stroke, and they are also important for quantifying the burden of stroke. Monitoring trends in stroke incidence and outcomes allows projection of future stroke burden as well as an evaluation of effectiveness of various stroke prevention and management strategies. A physician who knows age- and sex-specific incidence rates of stroke in his or her area is able to tell their patients an exact probability (absolute risk) that an individual will have a stroke during a specified period of time (usually a year). For example, **Table 1** shows age- and sex-specific incidence rates of stroke types derived from a population-based study in Auckland, New Zealand in 2002–03 (Feigin *et al.*, 2006). As shown in the table, the absolute risk of having an ischemic stroke during 1 year for any man within the 65- to 74-year age band is approximately 0.6% (95% CI, 0.5–0.7%). In other words, one can say with 95% confidence that approximately 10–14 of 200 men of this age group would have an ischemic stroke during a year.

Of course, this absolute risk does not take into account other risk factors for stroke (for more information on absolute risk of stroke, see the section titled 'Risk factors'). This information can be used by doctors and patients for some decision-making (e.g., weighting benefits and risk of carotid endarterectomy against the background risk of stroke). Another useful utilization of good-quality stroke incidence data is for health-care planning. For example, if one knew the total stroke incidence rate in the population served, the number of hospital beds that are needed for acute stroke patients in the population could be calculated. For example, if stroke incidence rate in a given population is 1.5 per 1000 people per year (this is an average stroke incidence rate in developed countries), the total population is 200 000 residents, the expected or desirable percentage of hospitalization with acute stroke is between 80% and 95% with the average length of hospital stay in an acute stroke unit (ASU) of 6 days (bed turnover of 50 during a year), then one would need approximately five to six beds in the ASU to serve acute stroke patients in the population ($1.5 \times 200 \times 0.8{:}50 = 4.8$ beds; $1.5 \times 200 \times 0.95{:}50 = 5.7$ beds). Similar calculations can be used to compute an expected workload for CT/MRI head scanning of admitted stroke patients, number of staff members, medications, and diagnostic procedures that would be required for the hospitalized stroke patients per year. Knowing the total number of acute stroke patients in the population served and assuming that approximately 20% of acute stroke patients die within a month after stroke onset, 20% of survivors live in rest homes or private hospitals, 50% of survivors are discharged home, and only 30% of survivors remain independent in their activities of daily living (these figures are common in many developed countries), one can also approximate the number of out-patient services and stroke-associated costs needed in the community.

Stroke incidence data are commonly reported together with stroke mortality and/or stroke case-fatality data obtained in the same population-based study. While high mortality rates may be a reflection of high stroke incidence rates in the population (especially if incidence rates parallel mortality rates), high stroke case fatality is suggestive of either greater severity of stroke (e.g., a high proportion of hemorrhagic strokes or large cerebral infarcts) and/or poor management of stroke patients in the population. These data have clear practical implications. Finally, incidence rates by stroke subtypes may provide some information on the etiology of the stroke subtypes. For example, a high incidence of intracerebral hemorrhage is suggestive of high prevalence and/or poor control of hypertension in the population; high incidence of large anterior circulation infarctions (atherothrombotic strokes) is suggestive of high prevalence and/or poor

Table 1 Age- and sex-specific incidence rates of major pathological types of stroke per 100 000 population per year

Sex, age group (years)	Ischemic stroke	Intracerebral hemorrhage	Subarachnoid hemorrhage
	Rate (95% CI)	Rate (95% CI)	Rate (95% CI)
Men			
15–64	40 (34–47)	8 (6–12)	7.9 (6–11)
65–74	568 (486–663)	82 (54–123)	21 (10–47)
75–84	1013 (865–1186)	158 (106–235)	20 (6–61)
85+	1156 (854–1564)	55 (14–220)	55 (14–220)
Women			
15–64	28 (24–34)	6 (4–9)	8 (5–11)
65–74	333 (274–403)	70 (46–107)	13 (5–34)
75–84	832 (721–959)	150 (108–211)	35 (18–71)
85+	1307 (1090–1568)	180 (111–294)	34 (11–105)

Modified from Feigin V, Carter K, Hackett M, *et al.* (2006) Ethnic disparities in incidence of stroke subtypes: Auckland Regional Community Stroke Study, 2002–2003. *Lancet Neurology* 5(2): 130–139.

control of carotid artery stenosis in the population, etc. Data on incidence of various pathological types of stroke and its subtypes can also be used for more specific health-care planning and resource allocation (e.g., number of acute atherothrombotic strokes in the population can be used to calculate the expected number of emergency interventional procedures on carotid arteries; the number of patients with aneurysmal subarachnoid hemorrhage can be used to calculate the required number of neurosurgical services for these patients, etc.).

However, validity and generalizability of information about stroke incidence rates largely depend on the validity of the methods used to collect the data. Stroke mortality and hospitalization data commonly used in the past, while providing important information for trends and patterns of stroke mortality and hospitalization, cannot be generalized to the whole population, suffer from selection (hospital data) and classification (mortality data) biases, and therefore are of limited scientific value. Analyses limited to hospital cases, incomplete mortality data, or cases with varying criteria and definitions, may distort results due to nonstandardized measures and nonrepresentative study populations.

It is well recognized that population-based good-quality studies are the most reliable source of information on stroke incidence on a population level. However,

identifying all new stroke events in a population is particularly challenging, so such epidemiological studies are relatively rare compared with studies using mortality data, hospital-based stroke registers, or incidence studies in younger age groups only. Moreover, even among published population-based stroke incidence studies there are differences in the methodologies used to ensure completeness of case ascertainment and some studies claimed to be population- or community-based are not really population-based because they did not meet all the criteria for a population-based study. In 1987, Malmgren *et al.* published a list of 12 core criteria for ideal stroke incidence studies that were related to definitions, methods, and mode of data presentation, by which the quality of population-based studies of stroke could be judged. These criteria have been updated by Sudlow and Warlow (1996), and most recently by Feigin *et al.* (2003) (**Table 2**).

Although developed primarily for affluent developed countries, these criteria for an ideal stroke incidence study have been successfully utilized in recent stroke incidence studies in Chile and Georgia, suggesting that they can be of use in some less-affluent countries. However, these criteria may not be practical for stroke studies undertaken in other developing countries, where most strokes occur and resources are limited. To address the problem of

Table 2   Gold standards for an ideal stroke incidence study

Domains	Core criteria	Supplementary criteria
Standard definitions	• World Health Organization definition of stroke • At least 80% CT/MRI verification of the diagnosis of ischemic stroke, intracerebral hemorrhage, and subarachnoid hemorrhage[a] • First-ever-in-a-lifetime stroke	• Classification of ischemic stroke into subtypes (e.g., large artery disease, cardioembolic, small artery disease, other)[a] • Recurrent stroke[a]
Standard methods	• Complete, population-based case ascertainment, based on multiple overlapping sources of information (hospitals, outpatient clinics, general practitioners, death certificates)[b] • Prospective study design • Large, well-defined and stable population, allowing at least 100 000 person-years of observation • Follow-up of patients' vital status for at least 1 month[a] • Reliable method for estimating denominator (census data not more than 5 years old)[b]	• Ascertainment of patients with TIA, recurrent strokes and those referred for brain, carotid or cerebral vascular imaging[a] • 'Hot pursuit' of cases • Direct assessment of under-ascertainment[a] by regular checking of general practitioners' databases and hospital admissions for acute vascular problems and cerebrovascular imaging studies and/or interventions
Standard data presentation	• Complete calendar years of data; not more than 5 years of data averaged together[b] • Men and women presented separately • Mid-decade age bands (e.g., 55–64 years) used in publications, including ≥85 years old • 95% confidence interval around rates	• Unpublished 5-year age bands available for comparison with other studies

[a]New criteria.
[b]Updated and modified by Feigin and Carter (Feigin VL, Lawes CM, Bennett DA, and Anderson CS (2003) Stroke epidemiology: A review of population-based studies of incidence, prevalence, and case-fatality in the late 20th century. *Lancet Neurology* 2(1):43–53.) from Sudlow CLM and Warlow CP (1996) Comparing stroke incidence worldwide: what makes studies comparable? *Stroke* 27(3): 550–558, with permission.

accurate and comparable data in these countries, a step-wise approach to increasing detail in the data to be collected for stroke surveillance has recently been proposed by the WHO. This flexible and sustainable system includes three steps: standard (hospital-based case ascertainment for calculating hospital admission due to stroke), expanded population coverage (ascertainment of death certificates or verbal autopsy in the whole community to calculate mortality rates), and comprehensive population-based (additional ascertainment of nonfatal events to calculate incidence and case fatality in the community). These steps could provide vital basic epidemiological estimates of the burden of stroke in many countries around the world.

The first most reliable single-center population-based data on stroke incidence and outcomes came from Rochester, Minnesota, USA (Homer *et al.*, 1978). In this important study, stroke registration on the population level started in 1935 and continues until the present day, providing one of the most reliable sources of information on stroke incidence, outcomes, and risk factors, including trend data. The first international multicenter study on stroke incidence was carried out under the auspices of the WHO in 17 centers representing 12 countries in 1971–74. It is noteworthy that in this study registration of stroke cases was not restricted by age of stroke patients. This study demonstrated a relatively low stroke incidence in developing countries and rather moderate geographical differences in stroke incidence worldwide. Noticeable geographical variations in stroke incidence were also demonstrated in the WHO MONICA Project (1985–87), but this study registered stroke in people 25–74 years old only (in the majority of centers, only people aged 25–64 were registered). Interestingly, substantial geographical differences in the incidence of subarachnoid hemorrhage were also noted in this age group of the population at the study period.

In 1997, Sudlow and Warlow published a comprehensive overview of the 11 available (at that time) population-based stroke incidence studies from Europe (Oxfordshire, UK; Dijon, France; Umbria and Valle d'Aosta, Italy; Frederiksberg, Denmark; Söderhamn, Sweden; Warsaw, Poland); Russia (Novosibirsk), Australia (Perth), New Zealand (Auckland), and the United States (Rochester, Minnesota) (Sudlow and Warlow, 1997). Age- and sex-standardized annual incidence rates for subjects aged 45–84 years were similar (between approximately 300/100 000 and 500/100 000) in most places but were significantly lower in Dijon, France (238/100 000) and higher in Novosibirsk, Russia (627/100 000) (Sudlow and Warlow, 1997). The distribution of pathological types, when these were reliably distinguished, did not differ significantly between studies. Our recent overview of population-based stroke incidence studies (Feigin *et al.*, 2003) included 17 new studies (nine new stroke incidence studies published since

1990 and eight new studies on secular trends in stroke incidence) confirmed Sudlow and Warlow's findings (Sudlow and Warlow, 1997) of modest geographical variations in the incidence of total stroke and stroke pathological types. As shown in **Figures 2–6**, toward the end of the twentieth century and early in the twenty-first century, the incidence of all strokes combined, age-specific incidence, proportions of stroke subtypes, prevalence, and 1-month case fatality show, with a few exceptions, rather modest geographical variation between the studies included in the analyses, as compared to that observed in the MONICA Project.

Only population-based studies published after 1990 in which a CT/MRI or autopsy was done in more than 70% of cases were included in the analyses of stroke types. All stroke subtype analyses were based on cases classified by CT/MRI or autopsy findings for ischemic stroke (IS) and primary intracerebral hemorrhage (PICH), or cerebrospinal fluid examination and/or cerebral angiography for subarachnoid hemorrhage (SAH). The error bars are 95% confidence intervals. Box size is proportional to the number of events contributing to the analysis in each graph.

It has been suggested that the highest stroke incidence in Russia and Ukraine may be attributed to well-known social and economic changes that have occurred in these countries over the last decade, including changes in medical care, in access to vascular prevention strategies among those at high risk, and in the prevalence of risk factors. The reasons for the relatively high stroke incidence in Japan compared to other developed countries are not clear but may be related to genetic and environmental (e.g., diet, prevalence of cardiovascular risk factors, etc.) parameters. In this overview, the hospitalization rate of acute stroke patients ranged from 41% in Japan to 95% in Germany, averaging 81%, 1 month case fatality averaged 23%, and the prevalence of stroke per 1000 population in nine studies published after 1990 ranged from 5 to 11.

Over the last few years, data from new reviews and population-based stroke incidence studies have become available. Overall proportional frequency of pathological types of stroke and of ischemic stroke subtypes in white populations was reviewed by Warlow and colleagues (Warlow *et al.*, 2003). According to their review, atherothromboembolism accounts for half of all ischemic strokes, while intracranial small vessel disease and cardioembolism account for 25% and 20% ischemic strokes, respectively (**Figure 7**).

Rothwell and colleagues recently reported results of a population-based TIA/stroke incidence study that analyzed changes in TIA/stroke rates, outcomes, and risk factors in Oxfordshire, UK over the period 1981–2004. This was the first ideal population-based study that showed a significant reduction in stroke incidence

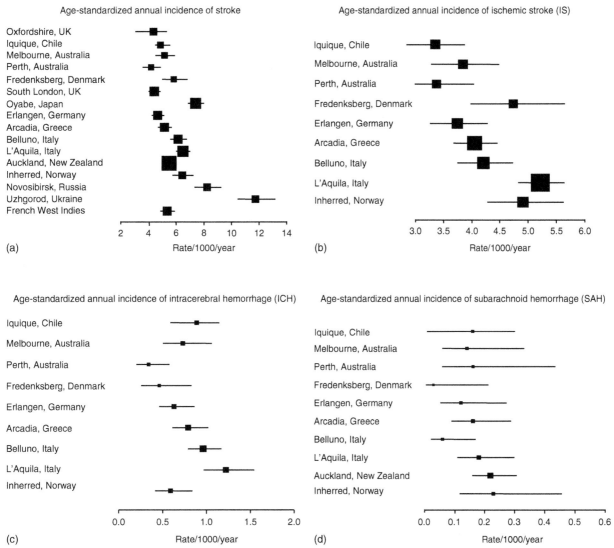

Figure 2 (a–d) Age-standardized annual incidence per 1000 population of all strokes combined and by pathological type in people aged 55 years and older. Reproduced from Feigin VL, Lawes CM, Bennett DA, and Anderson CS (2003) Stroke epidemiology: A review of population-based studies of incidence, prevalence, and case-fatality in the late 20th century. *Lancet Neurology* 2(1): 43–53, with permission.

(particularly for ischemic stroke and intracerebral hemorrhage) and mortality (but not case fatality) over the last 20 years, thus providing evidence that preventive strategies do actually reduce the incidence of stroke on the community level. It was also the first population-based study to document the predominance of acute cerebrovascular incidence (stroke and transient ischemic attack combined) over the incidence of acute coronary events (myocardial infarction and unstable angina combined) (relative incidence 1.2; 95% confidence interval, 1.1–1.3). Anderson and colleagues have recently completed the largest Auckland Regional Community Stroke (ARCOS) 2002–03 stroke incidence and outcomes study in Auckland, New Zealand and compared its results with two similar stroke population-based studies in Auckland

carried out in 1981–82 and 1991–92. This study showed modest declines in overall stroke incidence and attack rates in Auckland over the two decades. Two other recent publications based on the ARCOS 2002–03 study demonstrated substantial ethnic differences in trends and stroke subtype incidence rates in New Zealand (Carter *et al.*, 2003; Feigin *et al.*, 2006), with non-white populations (particularly Pacific and Maori people) experiencing a high and increased incidence rate and a greater risk of stroke (especially ischemic stroke and intracerebral hemorrhage) compared with New Zealand people of European descent. A decrease in stroke incidence rates was also recently observed in Tartu, Estonia (Vibo *et al.*, 2005). These and other ideal population-based studies (Feigi *et al.*, 2003) published after 1990 showed a decline in stroke incidence,

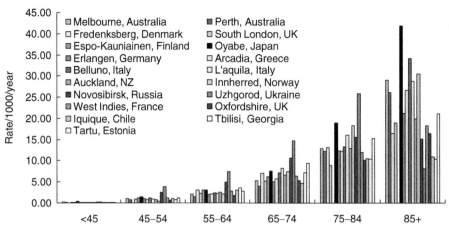

Figure 3 Age-specific annual incidence per 1000 population of all strokes combined in selected populations.

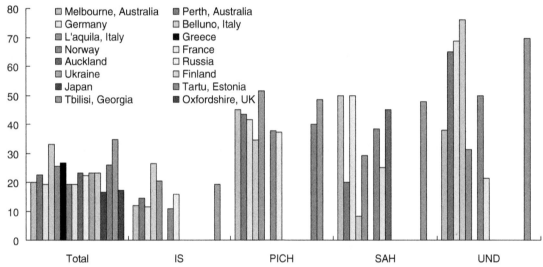

Figure 4 Case-fatality within 1 month of stroke onset by stroke type in selected populations. IS, ischemic stroke; PICH, primary intracerebral hemorrhage; SAH, subarachnoid hemorrhage; UND, undetermined. Reproduced from Feigin VL, Lawes CM, Bennett DA, Anderson CS (2003) Stroke epidemiology: A review of population-based studies of incidence, prevalence, and case-fatality in the late 20th century. *Lancet Neurology* 2(1): 43–53, with permission.

as summarized in **Table 3**. A stroke incidence and outcomes study by Lavados and colleagues in Iquique, Chile (the PISCIS Project) was the first population-based stroke incidence study in Latin America that met not only the standard (Sudlow and Warlow, 1997), but also the most rigorous criteria for an ideal stroke incidence study (Feigin and Carter, 2004). The key findings of this study were that stroke outcomes and incidence rates in a predominantly Hispanic-Mestizo population of the city of Iquique, Chile, are similar to those in other populations, but the proportion of intracerebral hemorrhage is somewhat higher. Another population-based stroke incidence study in less affluent countries was recently carried out in Tbilisi, Georgia (Tsiskaridze *et al.*, 2004). This study demonstrated

overall stroke incidence rates comparable to those reported in developed countries, but the proportion of hemorrhagic strokes and 1-month case fatality were greater than those in developed countries. **Table 4** summarizes key features of modern stroke incidence and prevalence.

Transient Ischemic Attack

Transient ischemic attack (TIA) is commonly diagnosed on the basis of presence of focal neurological symptoms relating to focal cerebral, brain stem, or retinal ischemia with abrupt onset and complete resolution within 24 h (usually within minutes). Although this definition of TIA

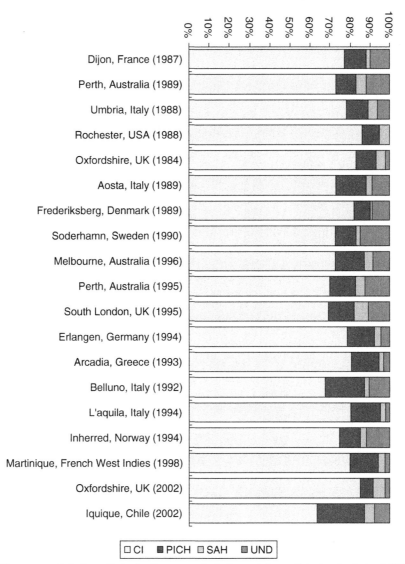

Figure 5 Proportional frequency of stroke pathological types in selected populations. IS, ischemic stroke; PICH, primary intracerebral hemorrhage; SAH, subarachnoid hemorrhage; UND, undetermined. Reproduced from Feigin VL, Lawes CM, Bennett DA, and Anderson CS (2003) Stroke epidemiology: A review of population-based studies of incidence, prevalence, and case-fatality in the late 20th century. *Lancet Neurology* 2(1): 43–53, with permission.

is commonly used in epidemiologic research, it should be noted that structural lesions in the brain relevant to TIA can be found in 30–67% of the patients (Winbeck *et al.*, 2004). TIA constitutes approximately 10–50% of stroke incidence but population-based data on TIA are scarce and inconsistent. The highest incidence rates of TIA (approximately 70 cases per 100 000 people per year) were reported in Rochester, Minnesota, USA (Brown *et al.*, 1998) and Northern Portugal (Correia *et al.*, 2006), the lowest (approximately 30 cases per 100 000 people per year) in Tartu, Estonia and Novosibirsk, Russia (Feigin *et al.*, 2000). Overall, 80% of all TIAs occur in the carotid artery and 20% in the vertebrobasilar distribution, with incidence rates increasing with age.

Risk Factors

A number of stroke risk factors have been identified and commonly described as well documented and less well documented, modifiable and nonmodifiable. The major established risk factors for stroke that can be addressed therapeutically are elevated blood pressure, cardiac disease, TIA, asymptomatic carotid stenosis, cigarette smoking, and diabetes mellitus. Less well-documented but also potentially controllable risk factors include low socioeconomic status, unhealthy diet/nutrition, alcohol abuse (especially binge drinking; the overall relationship between alcohol consumption and stroke is J-shaped), obesity, diabetes mellitus, physical inactivity, some blood disorders and lipid

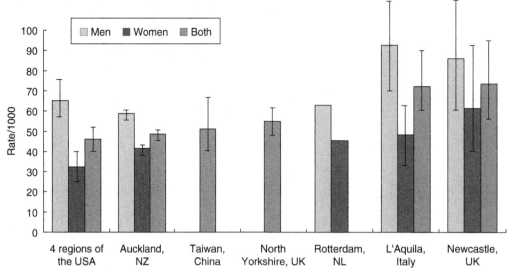

Figure 6   Age-standardized prevalence of stroke per 1000 people aged 65 years and older in selected populations. Reproduced from Feigin VL, Lawes CM, Bennett DA, and Anderson CS (2003) Stroke epidemiology: A review of population-based studies of incidence, prevalence, and case-fatality in the late 20th century. *Lancet Neurology* 2(1): 43–53, with permission.

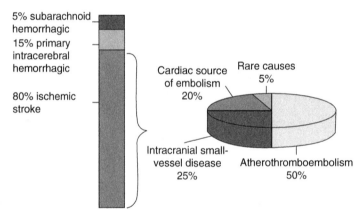

Figure 7   Overall proportional frequency of pathological types of stroke and of ischemic stroke subtypes in white populations. Reproduced from Warlow C, Sudlow C, Dennis M, and Sandercock P (2003) Stroke. *Lancet* 362: 1211–1224, with permission.

abnormalities, migraine with aura, hormone replacement therapy, oral contraceptives, drug abuse, inflammatory processes, and low personal and environmental temperature. Although some risk factors are similar for various stroke pathological types and subtypes (e.g., elevated blood pressure, cigarette smoking), some are more specific for particular types of stroke (e.g., unruptured intracranial aneurysms for SAH, atrial fibrillation for cardioembolic stroke). Non-modifiable but well-documented risk factors for stroke are increasing age (almost doubling for each successive decade), sex (men are at greater risk of stroke than women until the age of 65 years but women are at greater risk of stroke than men at older age). Some studies suggest that a parental history of stroke and genetic predisposition are also important risk factors for stroke. Current evidence

suggests that stroke and vascular risk factors have similar relative effects across the world, with modest interaction with ethnicity and nation (Feigin and Rodgers, 2004; Pearce *et al.*, 2004).

At least two-thirds of strokes are explained by identifiable risk factors and there is suggestive evidence that at least 80% of strokes can be prevented (Wald and Law, 2003). The modern approach to stroke prevention includes a combination of population-based (control of risk factors on the population level) and individual-based or high-risk strategies. The high-risk strategy includes identification and management of individuals with high risk of stroke or even preclinical individuals with high risk of developing some stroke risk factors (e.g., subjects with increased left atrial volume). Current American Heart

Table 3 Secular trends in stroke incidence rates in ideal population-based studies

Study region (city, country)	Period of study	Change in stroke incidence
Rochester, Minnesota, USA (Brown et al., 1996)	1955–89	30% decline
Fredericksburg, Denmark (Jorgensen et al., 1992)	1972–90	15% increase
Copenhagen, Denmark (Thorvaldsen et al., 1999)	1982–91	3% decline
Espoo-Kauniainen, Finland	1972–91	20% decline
Oyabe, Japan	1977–91	30% decline
Novosibirsk, Russia (Feigin et al., 1995)	1982–92	22% decline
Perth, Australia	1989–96	23% decline
Tartu, Estonia (Vibo et al., 2005)	1991–2003	18% decline
Auckland, NZ	1981–2003	11% decline
Oxfordshire, UK	1981–2004	29% decline

Table 4 Key features of modern stroke incidence and prevalence research

The overall age-standardized incidence of stroke in people aged 55 years and older ranges from 4.2 to 11.7 per 1000 person-years. The proportion of ischemic stroke ranges from 67 to 81%; intracerebral hemorrhage, 7 to 20%; and subarachnoid hemorrhage, 1 to 7%. The risk of ischemic stroke (including ischemic stroke subtypes) and intracerebral hemorrhage and the proportion of intracerebral hemorrhage in non-white populations is about two times greater than that in white populations

Two-thirds of stroke-related deaths occur in developing countries and there is some evidence that, at least in developed countries, acute cerebrovascular events (stroke and transient ischemic attack) are becoming more common events than acute coronary events (myocardial infarction and unstable angina)

Stroke incidence, prevalence, stroke-subtype structure, 1-month case fatality, and mortality rates show modest geographical variations, with the exception of Ukraine, Russia, and Japan, where incidence rates are highest, and Italy and the UK where prevalence rates are highest

The average age of patients affected by stroke is 70 years in men and 75 years in women, but it is substantially younger in non-white populations and developing countries. In developed countries, more than half of all strokes occur in people over 75 years of age. Approximately 25% of all strokes occur in people younger than 65 years, and 5% in people younger than 45 years

The age-standardized prevalence rate of stroke in people aged 65 years and older ranges from 5 to 7% and is tending to increase due to the aging of the population and improved survival; therefore, the overall burden of stroke is likely to continue to increase

In developed countries, overall case fatality within 1 month of stroke onset is approximately 23% and is higher for intracerebral hemorrhage (42%) and subarachnoid hemorrhage (32%) than for ischemic stroke (16%). Early stroke-related case fatality in developing countries is substantially greater than that in developed countries

Overall, there is a trend toward stabilizing or decreasing stroke incidence in some developed countries, but there is suggestive evidence that incidence of stroke is increasing in developing countries

Modified from Feigin VL, Lawes CM, Bennett DA, and Anderson CS (2003) Stroke epidemiology: A review of population-based studies of incidence, prevalence, and case-fatality in the late 20th century. *Lancet Neurology* 2(1): 43–53.

Association Guidelines for primary prevention of cardiovascular disease and stroke recommend risk factor screening in adults to begin at age 20 years, with blood pressure, body mass index, waist circumference, and pulse (to screen for atrial fibrillation) to be recorded at least every 2 years; and fasting serum lipoprotein profile (or total and high-density lipoprotein cholesterol if fasting is unavailable) and fasting blood glucose measured according to person's risk for hyperlipidemia and diabetes, respectively (at least every 5 years if no risk factors are present, and every 2 years if risk factors are present). For all adults 40 years of age and older or people with two or more risk factors (e.g. smoking, elevated blood pressure, total/LDL cholesterol, ECG documented left ventricular hypertrophy, or diabetes), the absolute risk of developing coronary heart disease and stroke can be calculated. Prediction charts have also been developed for selecting people with an increased risk of cardiovascular disease (stroke, TIA, coronary heart disease, congestive heart failure, or peripheral vascular disease) (**Figure 8**). Control of risk factors should be aimed to lower the absolute risk of developing coronary heart disease and stroke as much as possible. A stepwise implementation of evidence-based interventions with comprehensive and integrated action at the country level have recently been suggested by the WHO as the major means to the worldwide prevention and control of chronic diseases including stroke.

Stroke Outcomes

Clinical outcomes in stroke have often been classified into survival (death), impairment (signs and symptoms of the underlying pathology), disability (limitation in functional activities), handicap (disadvantage to the individual resulting from impairment and disability), and quality of life (patient's general well-being resulting from physical, psychological, and social aspects of life that may be affected by changes in health states). The recent International Classification of Functioning (ICF), Disability and Health (World Health Organization, 2001) describes outcomes in terms of body functioning, activities (related to tasks and actions by an individual) and participation (involvement in a life situation), and environment.

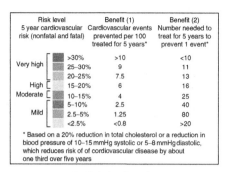

New Zealand cardiovascular
risk prediction charts

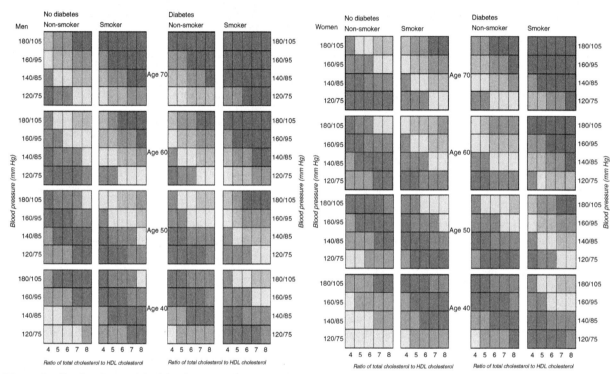

Figure 8   Absolute 5-year risk of developing cardiovascular disease and stroke. Adapted from Jackson R (2000) Updated New Zealand cardiovascular disease risk–benefit prediction guide. *British Medical Journal* 320(7236): 709–710, with permission.

According to the ICF (Salter *et al.*, 2005), functioning and disability are viewed as a complex interaction between the health condition of the individual and the contextual factors of the environment as well as personal factors. The picture produced by this combination of factors and dimensions is of 'the person in his or her world'. The classification treats these dimensions as interactive and dynamic rather than linear or static. It allows for an assessment of the degree of disability, although it is not a measurement instrument. It is applicable to all people, whatever their health condition. The language of the ICF is neutral as to etiology, placing the emphasis on function rather than condition or disease. It also is carefully designed to be relevant across cultures as well as age groups and genders, making it highly appropriate for heterogeneous populations. The ICF is currently considered as the standard measure of outcomes and has been shown to have reasonably good psychometric and administrative properties in the area of stroke rehabilitation and research. Accurate information on short-term and long-term stroke outcomes is important to the patients, their families, and health-care providers for setting up appropriate goals and expectations and developing appropriate management options (e.g., discharge plan, interventions).

Survival

On average, about one-quarter of stroke patients die within the 1st month after stroke onset, one-third within the first 6–12 months, and one-half within the first 2 years after stroke, with the average case fatality of 5% between years 1 and 10 and about 2% between years 10 and 21 after stroke, with older patients having the worse prognosis. Based on these and other similar population-based studies, cumulative case-fatalities have been estimated at 40 to 60% at 5 years, approximately 80% at 10 years, 90% at 15 years and 93% at 21 years. Stroke patients have nearly twice the mortality rates of the general population. The most important prognostic factors for death are increasing age, urinary incontinence, stroke severity, pre-stroke disability, and the presence of cardiovascular risk factors. While approximately two-thirds of deaths within the 1st month after the stroke onset are due to the direct effects of the brain lesion and another one-sixth due to recurrent stroke, among 1-month stroke survivors one-fifth of subsequent deaths between 30 days to 1 year, 1- to 5-year and 5- to 10-year periods are due to recurrent strokes and about one-third due to cardiovascular causes.

Functional Outcomes

Since stroke often results in activity limitations across multiple domains of functioning and some outcomes may have independent prognostic implications, it is important to exercise a multifocal approach to studying stroke outcomes and include patient-centered measures that evaluate different functions so that the impact of stroke on the patient as a whole can be understood and quantified. Although a relationship between impairment, disability, handicap, and quality of life has been documented, these relationships are not simple.

While the number of studies of outcomes (especially death, disability, and neurological impairments) in stroke survivors is substantial, there have only been three population-based studies evaluating medium- to long-term functional outcomes in stroke survivors. Two early population-based stroke incidence studies in Auckland (1981–82 and 1991–92) showed that approximately 55% of 3-year stroke survivors have incomplete recovery, and one third of them require assistance in at least one self-care activity (Bonita *et al.*, 1997). In the 1991–92 study (Hackett *et al.*, 2000), health-related quality of life (HRQoL measured by the SF-36 questionnaire) and basic activities of daily living were assessed in stroke survivors 6 years after stroke ($n = 639$) and compared to an age- and sex-matched general population ($n = 310$). The authors found that although the majority of stroke survivors (77%) were living at home, 42% of the patients were dependent in at least one aspect of basic care activities of daily living, and they had lower scores for the physical health, general health, vitality, and social function components of HRQoL compared with the general population. In the Perth Community Stroke Study (Australia, 1989–94) (Hankey *et al.*, 2002), 152 stroke patients (41% of acute stroke patients) survived to

5 years. Of survivors who were neither institutionalized nor disabled at the time of their initial stroke, 21 (14%) were institutionalized in a nursing home, and 47 (36%) were disabled at 5 years after stroke. In a larger and more recent population-based study in South London (UK 1995–2000) (Patel, 2001), of 639 registered stroke patients, 392 without previous disability survived and were assessed for disability at 3 months, of whom 34 (9%) were severely disabled and 60 (15%) moderately disabled. Of 225 survivors (35%) at 12 months after stroke, 11% had moderate or severe disability (Barthel Index <15).

As noted above, stroke is a heterogeneous disorder that consists of three major pathological types, each of which has differing short- to medium-term outcomes. However, data on the long-term functional outcomes and costs in survivors of different stroke subtypes are scarce, limited to 1-year follow-up, and are often inconsistent. There is good evidence that cost of stroke differs in different stroke subtypes, but there was only one population-based study that addressed this issue. In the population-based study in Australia, the total lifetime costs of all new strokes was estimated to be Aus $1.3 billion a year, of which ischemic stroke (IS) costs constituted 72% (Aus $937 million), intracerebral hemorrhage (ICH) 26% (Aus $334 million), and unclassified stroke 2% (Aus $30 million), with the average cost per case of Aus $44 428 (Dewey *et al.*, 2001, 2003). The lifetime cost per person of first strokes occurring in the USA was estimated to be $228 030 for SAH, $123 565 for ICH, $90 981 for IS, and $103 576 averaged across all stroke subtypes, and indirect costs accounted for 58% of lifetime costs (Taylor *et al.*, 1996).

To our knowledge, there are only three population-based studies that investigated health outcomes by stroke subtype (Patel, 2001; Sturm *et al.*, 2002). In the study in Perth (Australia) (Sturm *et al.*, 2002), handicap (measured by the London Handicap Scale) differed significantly with severity of disability (measured by the Barthel Index) in ischemic stroke subtypes (defined by the Oxfordshire stroke classification) at 12 months. In the Australasian study, incomplete recovery at 1 year after SAH was found in 46% of survivors, of which ongoing memory problems were recorded in 50%, mood abnormalities in 39%, and speech problems in 14%, while a substantial proportion of survivors had diminished level of HRQoL. No association between cognitive impairment and the Oxfordshire Community Stroke Project classification of stroke subtypes was found in the South London population-based study (Patel *et al.*, 2002).

Although prognostic factors of stroke outcomes have been the subject of much discussion in the literature, there have been only a few studies that addressed some aspects of this issue in the population-based setting (Hankey *et al.*, 2002; Patel *et al.*, 2002). In a population-based study in

Perth, Australia ($n = 152$), factors found to be associated with poor outcome (death or disability) at 5 years included increasing age, baseline disability, hemiparesis, and recurrent stroke (Hankey *et al.*, 2002). No predictors of complete recovery from SAH were determined in a population-based study of SAH in Australasia, but the follow-up period was restricted to 1 year and no other measures of disability and handicap were undertaken in this report. In a population-based study in the UK (Patel *et al.*, 2002), initial incontinence was found to be the best predictor of moderate or severe disability (Barthel Index <15) at 1 year after stroke; however, it remains unclear whether this association holds true in the long term. A useful model for predicting ipsilateral ischemic stroke after TIA has recently been developed by Rothwell and colleagues (**Figure 9**). These models allow clinicians to

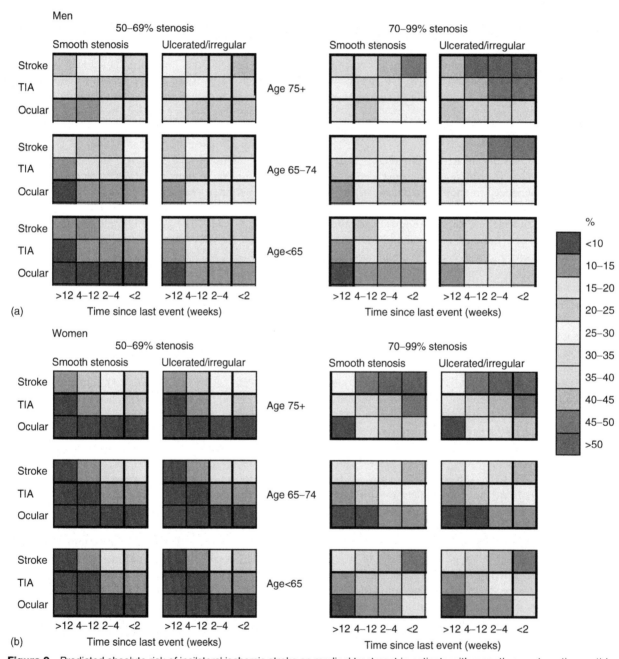

Figure 9 Predicted absolute risk of ipsilateral ischemic stroke on medical treatment in patients with recently symptomatic carotid stenosis by level and characteristics of stenosis. Reproduced from Rothwell PM, Mehta Z, Howard SC, Gutnikov SA, Warlow CP (2005) From subgroups to individuals: General principles and the example of carotid endarterectomy. *Lancet* 365(9455): 256–265, with permission.

take into account the many characteristics of an individual patient and their interactions, to consider the risks and benefits of interventions (e.g., carotid endarterectomy for stroke prevention) separately if needed, and to provide patients with personalized estimates of their likelihood of benefit. Although stroke incidence and mortality are known to be inversely related to socioeconomic status (SES) (Bennett, 1996; Engstrom *et al.*, 2001; Boden-Albala and Sacco, 2002; Avendano *et al.*, 2005), data on the relationship between SES and stroke functional outcomes are scarce. In a recent UK hospital-based study (Weir *et al.*, 2005), social deprivation was found to be strongly and inversely related to disability after stroke. Overall, about half of the patients who survive for 6 months after stroke are partially or totally dependent in their activities of daily living such as bathing, dressing, feeding, and mobility (10% need long-term nursing care). About one-third of patients surviving stroke for 1 year are unable to remain independent, and this proportion remains relatively unchanged in survivors followed for up to 5 years. However, functional recovery (lessening of disability or handicap) often continues long after specific neurologic deficits have ceased to change. Therefore patients and their families should never give up their fight for recovery and greater independence.

Management Strategies

Any acute stroke patient should be admitted to a hospital stroke unit as soon as possible (**Table 5**). There is robust evidence that stroke patients who receive organized inpatient care in a geographically defined acute stroke unit (ASU) are more likely to be alive, independent, and living at home 1 year after the stroke (Stroke Unit Trialists' Collaboration, 2001). All patients with acute stroke or TIA, irrespective of age or stroke severity or any other considerations, should be admitted to the ASU for initial evaluation and management. There are two major types of stroke units: (1) the ASU unit for acute care only (the average length of staying in such units is usually a few days) and (2) the comprehensive stroke unit that provides both acute care and rehabilitation (the average length of staying in such units is usually from several days to a few weeks). A mobile stroke team is usually not regarded as a stroke unit, although it is part of the organized stroke care. Current evidence shows superiority of the two types of acute stroke units over a mobile stroke team. The key elements of acute stroke units are the coordinated expert interdisciplinary team working in a geographically based setting with regular team meetings (at least weekly). The tasks of the team are to establish an accurate diagnosis, observe vital signs, maintain homeostasis, provide acute treatment, prevent complications, implement early

rehabilitation, initiate secondary prevention strategies, and develop the most appropriate discharge and rehabilitation plan. There is no evidence that extensive (and expensive!) laboratory monitoring of acute stroke patients is more effective than conventional management in the ASU. Current recommendations for management and rehabilitation of acute stroke patients are summarized in **Tables 5–8** (Feigin, 2005).

It is commonly accepted that all patients should have a follow-up plan at discharge from hospital. Follow-up may involve different community services. The patients should be reviewed at the stroke (neurovascular) clinic or have a home visit. At follow-up, the caregiver should be interviewed and an attempt made to minimize caregiver stress.

Although the duration of rehabilitation therapy is generally determined by the rate of functional recovery, the

Table 5 Acute stroke treatment

	Level of evidence[a]
All patients with suspected stroke/TIA should be referred to, and assessed by, the ASU team as soon as possible after the patient is considered for admission to hospital	A
All patients should have a CT head scan ASAP to confirm the diagnosis of stroke and stroke subtype	B
Unless there is absolute contraindication, or the patient has agreed to thrombolysis with Alteplase or an experimental hyperacute treatment, all patients with ischemic stroke should be given aspirin (150–300 mg) as soon as possible after onset	A
All patients with subarachnoid hemorrhage, potentially caused by intracranial aneurysm rupture, should be urgently evaluated by neurosurgeon for possible neurosurgical intervention	A
All patients should be closely monitored for hyperglycemia and hyperthermia ($\geq 37.5\,°C$); those with diabetes or raised blood-glucose concentration should receive insulin; in patients with hyperthermia, an antipyretic such as paracetamol or cooling devices such as cooling blankets or compresses may be considered to maintain body temperature in the normal range	B
All patients with deteriorating clinical state due to cerebellar hemorrhage should be considered for neurosurgical referral for possible intervention	B

[a]A, at least one randomized controlled trial as part of the body of literature of overall good quality and consistency addressing specific recommendation; B, availability of well-conducted clinical studies but no randomized clinical trials on the topic of recommendation; C, evidence obtained from expert committee reports or opinions and/or clinical experiences of respected authorities.

Table 6   Prevention and management of complications of acute stroke

	Level of evidence[a]
Each stroke patient should undergo swallowing assessment	B
Urinary catheters should be used with caution and alternative methods for the management of continence explored	C
All those involved in moving stroke patients should receive training in lifting, transferring, and moving and handling of the upper limb	C
In patients at high risk of deep vein thrombosis and/or pulmonary embolism, external compression stockings or intermittent pneumatic compression devices should be used where heparin/Clexane is contraindicated	B
Awareness of the possibility of depression and other related mood disorders should lead to prompt evaluation and treatment	B

[a]A, at least one randomized controlled trial as part of the body of literature of overall good quality and consistency addressing specific recommendation; B, availability of well-conducted clinical studies but no randomized clinical trials on the topic of recommendation; C, evidence obtained from expert committee reports or opinions and/or clinical experiences of respected authorities.

probability of improvement of movement in paralyzed limbs is maximal during the 1st month after stroke and decreases significantly after 6 months, whereas improvement of speech, domestic and working skills, and unsteadiness can continue for up to 2 years. Recovery of arm movement is usually less complete than that of leg movement, and complete lack of any movement at onset of stroke, or no measurable grip strength by 4 weeks, is associated with a poor prognosis for return of useful arm function (Katrak, 1990).

Conclusion

The epidemiology of stroke, like any other noncommunicable disorder, is changing over time. Reliable data on stroke incidence, prevalence, and risk factors are essential for evidence-based health care, therefore more good-quality stroke incidence, prevalence, outcomes, and risk factor studies in various regions and populations (especially in developing countries) are warranted. Despite a continuous decrease in stroke mortality rates observed in many developed countries over the last few decades, globally stroke as a cause of death has moved from third to second place in the world and is now the leading cause of physical disability in adults aged 65 years and older.

Table 7   Rehabilitation following acute stroke

	Level of evidence[a]
Rehabilitation should be started as soon as the patient's condition permits	B
Rehabilitation aims, with short- and long-term rehabilitation objectives, should be established and agreed by all parties including the patient and carers	C
Physiotherapy should aim to promote recovery of motor control, independence in functional tasks, optimize sensory stimulation, and prevent secondary complications such as soft tissue shortening and chest infections	C
The broad role of occupational therapy in the rehabilitation of stroke patients should be recognized. Early referral for assessment is appropriate	C
All patients with a communication problem resulting from stroke should be referred for speech and language therapy assessment and treatment	A
Intensive speech and language therapy should be initiated as soon as the patient's condition is stable and may be required to continue over the long term	B
Where intelligible speech is not a reasonable goal, the speech and language therapist should augment speech attempts and enable communication through means other than spoken language	B
Speech and language therapist should play a key role in swallowing assessment	C
Patients with diabetes, high blood cholesterol levels, and poor oral intake or who are significantly underweight should be referred to dietician	C
Active bowel and bladder management should be implemented. Catheters should be used only after full assessment. It is important to have regular bowel movements with at least one bowel emptying every 2–3 days. Continence services can be approached when required	C
Screening for depression and anxiety should be provided. Persistently (>6 weeks) depressed patients should be given antidepressant treatment	B

[a]A, at least one randomized controlled trial as part of the body of literature of overall good quality and consistency addressing specific recommendation; B, availability of well-conducted clinical studies but no randomized clinical trials on the topic of recommendation; C, evidence obtained from expert committee reports or opinions and/or clinical experiences of respected authorities.

Recent advances in stroke prevention and management offer an opportunity to reduce the burden of stroke. Urgent and practicable preventive measures, such as those recommended by the WHO, need to be implemented to limit the epidemic of stroke in developing countries.

Table 8 Secondary prevention of vascular events

	Level of evidence[a]
All patients with ischemic stroke or TIA should be given long-term aspirin (100–150 mg) for prevention of future vascular disease, unless contraindication to aspirin or warfarin is considered more appropriate. Other antiplatelet strategies which can be considered are aspirin plus dipyridamole or clopidogrel, particularly in situations of aspirin failure	A
All postacute patients with either ischemic stroke or primary intracerebral hemorrhage (when the patient is medically stable, which is usually within the first 5–10 days after stroke onset) should receive blood pressure-lowering therapy (preferably ACE inhibitor-diuretic combination) irrespective of initial blood pressure (hypertensive or nonhypertensive), age, and gender	A
Warfarin anticoagulation (INR 2–3) should be used where the stroke resulted from a cardiac source (e.g., atrial fibrillation), the patient has a good understanding of the treatment, and the patient is at low risk of hemorrhagic complications (e.g., low risk of falls, no alcohol abuse)	A
Carotid ultrasound should be organized in patients with severe ipsilateral disease who have no major comorbidities that reduce life expectancy and are prepared to accept the real early risk of surgery	A
Carotid endarterectomy for patients with high-grade carotid artery stenosis should be considered	A
Post-stroke or TIA patients who have a persistent elevation of cholesterol despite dietary modification and two fasting levels above 5 mmol/l should be considered for statin therapy to reduce the risk of further stroke	A
Secondary prevention of stroke should include adequate control of stroke risk factors, including lifestyle modifications (e.g., diet low in saturated fat, salt, and cholesterol; smoking abstinence; reasonable physical activity; etc.)	B

[a]A, at least one randomized controlled trial as part of the body of literature of overall good quality and consistency addressing specific recommendation; B, availability of well-conducted clinical studies but no randomized clinical trials on the topic of recommendation; C, evidence obtained from expert committee reports or opinions and/or clinical experiences of respected authorities.

Citations

Avendano M, Kunst AE, van LF, *et al.* (2005) Trends in socioeconomic disparities in stroke mortality in six European countries between 1981–1985 and 1991–1995. *American Journal of Epidemiology* 161(1): 52–61.

Bennett S (1996) Socioeconomic inequalities in coronary heart disease and stroke mortality among Australian men, 1979–1993. *International Journal of Epidemiology* 25(2): 266–275.

Boden-Albala B and Sacco RL (2002) Socioeconomic status and stroke mortality: Refining the relationship. *Stroke* 33(1): 274–275.

Bonita R, Solomon N, and Broad JB (1997) Prevalence of stroke and stroke-related disability. Estimates from the Auckland stroke studies. *Stroke* 28(10): 1898–1902.

Brown RD, Whisnant JP, Sicks JD, O'Fallon WM, and Wiebers DO (1996) Stroke incidence, prevalence, and survival: Secular trends in Rochester, Minnesota, through 1989. *Stroke* 27(3): 373–380.

Brown RD Jr, Petty GW, O'Fallon WM, Wiebers DO, and Whisnant JP (1998) Incidence of transient ischemic attack in Rochester, Minnesota, 1985–1989. *Stroke* 29: 2109–2113.

Carter KM, Anderson CP, Hacket MM, *et al.* (2003) Trends in ethnic disparities in stroke incidence in Auckland, New Zealand, during 1981 to 2003. *Stroke* 37(1): 56–62.

Correia MM, Silva MRM, Magalhaes RB, Guimaraes LP, and Silva MCP (2006) Transient ischemic attacks in rural and urban northern Portugal: Incidence and short-term prognosis. *Stroke* 37(1): 50–55.

Dewey HM, Thrift AG, Mihalopoulos C, *et al.* (2001) Cost of stroke in Australia from a societal perspective: results from the North East Melbourne Stroke Incidence Study (NEMESIS). *Stroke* 32(10): 2409–2416.

Dewey HM, Thrift AG, Mihalopoulos C, *et al.* (2003) Lifetime cost of stroke subtypes in Australia: findings from the North East Melbourne Stroke Incidence Study (NEMESIS). *Stroke* 34(10): 2502–2507.

Engstrom G, Jerntorp I, Pessah-Rasmussen H, Hedblad B, Berglund G, and Janzon L (2001) Geographic distribution of stroke incidence within an urban population: Relations to socioeconomic circumstances and prevalence of cardiovascular risk factors. *Stroke* 32(5): 1098–1103.

Feigin VL (2005) Managing stroke: key principles and updates. *New Zealand Family Physician* 32(4): 241–246.

Feigin V and Carter K (2004) Editorial: stroke incidence studies: One step closer to the elusive gold standard? *Stroke* 35: 2045–2047.

Feigin VL and Rodgers A (2004) Editorial comment – Ethnic disparities in risk factors for stroke: What are the implications? *Stroke* 35(7): 1568–1569.

Feigin VL, Wiebers DO, Whisnant JP, and O'Fallon WM (1995) Stroke incidence and 30-day case-fatality rates in Novosibirsk, Russia, 1982 through 1992. *Stroke* 26: 924–929.

Feigin VL, Shishkin SV, Tzirkin GM, *et al.* (2000) A population-based study of transient ischemic attack incidence in Novosibirsk, Russia, 1987–1988 and 1996–1997. *Stroke* 31(1): 9–13.

Feigin VL, Lawes CM, Bennett DA, and Anderson CS (2003) Stroke epidemiology: A review of population-based studies of incidence, prevalence, and case-fatality in the late 20th century. *Lancet Neurology* 2(1): 43–53.

Feigin V, Carter K, Hackett M, *et al.* (2006) Ethnic disparities in incidence of stroke subtypes: Auckland Regional Community Stroke Study, 2002–2003. *Lancet Neurology* 5(2): 130–139.

Hackett ML, Duncan JR, Anderson CS, Broad JB, and Bonita R (2000) Health-related quality of life among long-term survivors of stroke: Results from the Auckland Stroke Study, 1991–1992. *Stroke* 31(3): 440–447.

Hankey GJ, Jamrozik K, Broadhurst RJ, Forbes S, and Anderson CS (2002) Long-term disability after first-ever stroke and related prognostic factors in the Perth Community Stroke Study, 1989–1990. *Stroke* 33(4): 1034–1040.

Homer D, Whisnant JP, and Schoenberg BS (1987) Trends in the incidence rates of stroke in Rochester, Minnesota, since 1935. *Annals of Neurology* 22(2): 245–251.

Jackson R (2000) Updated New Zealand cardiovascular disease risk-benefit prediction guide. *British Medical Journal* 320(7236): 709–710.

Jorgensen HS, Plesner AM, Hubbe P, and Larsen K (1992) Marked increase of stroke incidence in men between 1972 and 1990 in Frederiksberg, Denmark. *Stroke* 23(12): 1701–1704.

Kaste M, Fogelholm R, and Rissanen A (1998) Economic burden of stroke and the evaluation of new therapies. *Public Health* 112: 103–112.

Katrak PH (1990) Shoulder shrug – a prognostic sign for recovery of hand movement after stroke. *Medical Journal of Australia* 152(6): 297–301.

Patel AT (2001) Disability evaluation following stroke. *Physical Medicine and Rehabilitation Clinics of North America* 12(3): 613–619.

Patel MD, Coshall C, Rudd AG, and Wolfe CD (2002) Cognitive impairment after stroke: Clinical determinants and its associations with long-term stroke outcomes. *Journal of the American Geriatrics Society* 50(4): 700–706.

Pearce N, Foliaki S, Sporle A, and Cunningham C (2004) Genetics, race, ethnicity, and health. *British Medical Journal* 328(7447): 1070–1072.

Stroke Unit Trialists' Collaboration (2001) Organised inpatient (stroke unit) care for stroke. *Cochrane Database of Systematic Reviews* 2001(2): CD000197.

Sturm JW, Dewey HM, Donnan GA, Macdonell RA, McNeil JJ, and Thrift AG (2002) Handicap after stroke: How does it relate to disability, perception of recovery, and stroke subtype? The North East Melbourne Stroke Incidence Study (NEMESIS). *Stroke* 33(3): 762–768.

Sudlow CLM and Warlow CP (1996) Comparing stroke incidence worldwide : what makes studies comparable? *Stroke* 27(3): 550–558.

Sudlow CL and Warlow CP (1997) Comparable studies of the incidence of stroke and its pathological types: Results from an international collaboration. International Stroke Incidence Collaboration. *Stroke* 28(3): 491–499.

Taylor TN, Davis PH, Torner JC, Holmes J, Meyer JW, and Jacobson MF (1996) Lifetime cost of stroke in the United States. *Stroke* 27(9): 1459–1466.

Thorvaldsen P, Davidsen M, Bronnum-Hansen H, and Schroll M (1999) Stable stroke occurrence despite incidence reduction in an aging population : Stroke trends in the Danish Monitoring Trends and Determinants in Cardiovascular Disease (MONICA) Population. *Stroke* 30(12): 2529–2934.

Tsiskaridze A, Djibuti M, van MG, et al. (2004) Stroke incidence and 30-day case-fatality in a suburb of Tbilisi: Results of the first prospective population-based study in Georgia. *Stroke* 35(11): 2523–2528.

Vibo RM, Korv JM, and Roose MM (2005) The Third Stroke Registry in Tartu, Estonia: Decline of stroke incidence and 28-day case-fatality rate since 1991. *Stroke* 36(12): 2544–2548.

Wald NJ and Law MR (2003) A strategy to reduce cardiovascular disease by more than 80%. *British Medical Journal* 326(7404): 1419.

Warlow C, Sudlow C, Dennis M, and Sandercock P (2003) Stroke. *Lancet* 362: 1211–1224.

Weir NU, Gunkel A, McDowall M, and Dennis MS (2005) Study of the relationship between social deprivation and outcome after stroke. *Stroke* 36(4): 815–819.

Winbeck KM, Bruckmaier K, Etgen TM, von Einsiedel HGM, Rottinger MM, and Sander DM (2004) Transient ischemic attack and stroke can be differentiated by analyzing early diffusion-weighted imaging signal intensity changes. *Stroke* 35(5): 1095–1999.

World Health Organization (2001) *International Classification of Functioning, Disability and Health*. Geneva, Switzerlanfd: World Health Organization.

Further Reading

Aho K, Harmsen P, Hatano S, Marquardsen J, Smirnov VE, and Strasser T (1980) Cerebrovascular disease in the community: Results of a WHO collaborative study. *Bulletin of the World Health Organization* 58(1): 113–130.

Anderson C, Carter KN, Hackett ML, et al. (2005) Trends in stroke incidence in Auckland, New Zealand, during 1981 to 2003. *Stroke* 36(10): 2087–2093.

Anonymous (1997) The World Health Report 1997 – Conquering suffering, enriching humanity. *World Health Forum* 18(3–4): 248–260.

Hackett ML and Anderson CS (2000) Health outcomes 1 year after subarachnoid hemorrhage: An international population-based study. The Australian Cooperative Research on Subarachnoid Hemorrhage Study Group. *Neurology* 55(5): 658–662.

Ionita CC, Xavier AR, Kirmani JF, Dash S, Divani AA, and Qureshi AI (2005) What proportion of stroke is not explained by classic risk factors? *Preventive Cardiology* 8(1): 41–46.

Jamrozik K, Broadhurst RJ, Lai N, Hankey GJ, Burvill PW, and Anderson CS (1999) Trends in the incidence, severity, and short-term outcome of stroke in Perth, Western Australia. *Stroke* 30(10): 2105–2111.

Lavados PM, Sacks C, Prina L, et al. (2005) Incidence, 30-day case-fatality rate, and prognosis of stroke in Iquique, Chile: A 2-year community-based prospective study (PISCIS project). *Lancet* 365 (9478): 2206–2215.

Morikawa Y, Nakagawa H, Naruse Y, et al. (2000) Trends in stroke incidence and acute case fatality in a Japanese rural area: The Oyabe Study. *Stroke* 31(7): 1583–1587.

Numminen H, Kotila M, Waltimo O, Aho K, and Kaste M (1996) Declining incidence and mortality rates of stroke in Finland from 1972 to 1991: Results of three population-based stroke registers. *Stroke* 27(9): 1487–1491.

Pearson TA, Blair SN, Daniels SR, et al. (2002) AHA guidelines for primary prevention of cardiovascular disease and stroke: 2002 Update: Consensus Panel guide to comprehensive risk reduction for adult patients without coronary or other atherosclerotic vascular diseases. American Heart Association Science Advisory and Coordinating Committee. *Circulation* 106(3): 388–391.

Rothwell PM, Coull AJ, Giles MF, et al. (2004) Change in stroke incidence, mortality, case-fatality, severity, and risk factors in Oxfordshire, UK from 1981 to 2004 (Oxford Vascular Study). *Lancet* 363(9425): 1925–1933.

Rothwell PM, Mehta Z, Howard SC, Gutnikov SA, and Warlow CP (2005) From subgroups to individuals: General principles and the example of carotid endarterectomy. *Lancet* 365(9455): 256–265.

Salter K, Jutai JW, Teasell R, Foley NC, and Bitensky J (2005a) Issues for selection of outcome measures in stroke rehabilitation: ICF body functions. *Disability and Rehabilitation* 27(4): 191–207.

Salter K, Jutai JW, Teasell R, Foley NC, Bitensky J, and Bayley M (2005b) Issues for selection of outcome measures in stroke rehabilitation: ICF participation. *Disability and Rehabilitation* 27(9): 507–528.

Taub NA, Wolfe CD, Richardson E, and Burney PG (1994) Predicting the disability of first-time stroke sufferers at 1 year. 12-month follow-up of a population-based cohort in southeast England. *Stroke* 25(2): 352–357.

Tempest S and McIntyre A (2006) Using the ICF to clarify team roles and demonstrate clinical reasoning in stroke rehabilitation. *Disability and Rehabilitation* 28(10): 663–667.

Cognitive Disorders of Aging

L D Ravdin, Weill Medical College of Cornell University, New York, NY, USA

As we age, changes in the physical aspects of our bodies have corresponding changes in function. Transformation in physical stature as a result of aging may be accompanied by reduced flexibility or decreased motor speed, and although it is not a welcome change, it is one with an observable correlate that is often understood or expected. In contrast, changes in cognition are not associated with any directly observable physical alteration, and as a result, they can be unexpected or a source of distress. However, there are in fact structural changes that occur in the brain as we age.

These changes over time result from loss of neurons that occurs throughout the life span, resulting in decreased brain weight and volume. This is influenced in part by genetics, but is also affected by the environment and lifestyle factors, such as nutritional status, alcohol consumption, tobacco usage, level of education, and history of trauma. These lifestyle factors may be associated with one's vulnerability to developing cognitive disorders with aging. For example, high levels of education have been associated with cognitive reserve, a concept that supposes that an individual's education and other life experiences create a supply of skills or a knowledge base that can be called upon in situations when cognitive functioning is challenged (i.e., following neuronal loss from injury or disease). In theory, individuals with greater cognitive reserve (e.g., better educated) may be able to sustain greater cerebral insult before cognition becomes noticeably compromised. On the contrary, factors such as cerebral insult sustained in one's lifetime (traumatic head injury) may increase risk for development of cognitive disorders in late life. Perhaps one of the most striking examples of this comes from the literature on professional boxers who, as a result of their occupation, sustain repeated blows to the head. Boxers with greater exposure to the sport have been found to be at increased risk for late life cognitive decline. More common everyday examples include increased vulnerability associated with the deleterious effects of a lifetime of chronic alcohol consumption, tobacco use, or prolonged nutritional deficiencies.

Patterns of Age-Related Cognitive Decline and Cognitive Disorders

It is difficult to gauge whether the changes one experiences in thinking abilities can be attributable to normal aging, or if there is an issue of greater concern. Normal age-related changes in cognition are not disabling, and generally present as more of a nuisance than a real problem. They do not interfere with an individual's ability to carry on conversations, manage finances, and coordinate other basic everyday activities. Differentiating normal age-related changes in cognition from disease-associated impairment can be a challenge, even for health-care practitioners. Not all aspects of thinking abilities decline with age. Studies show that over-learned verbal information, such as vocabulary, general fund of knowledge, and reasoning, tend to stay relatively intact until advanced old age. The degree to which these abilities do decline is relatively small and typically imperceptible by others. In comparison, performance-based skills, such as novel

Table 1 Common factors associated with changes in cognition

Lifestyle changes (retirement, residential move)
Death of spouse, relatives, friends
Diminution of social network
Sleep disturbance
Depression
Chronic pain
Sensory changes (i.e., reduced vision or hearing)
Medication side effects

problem solving or tests that involve speed of information processing, tend to show more significant age-related declines.

Perhaps the most frequent cognitive complaint of older adults is decreased memory, especially with advanced aging. Common complaints include entering a room and forgetting what you went in there for, forgetting names, and misplacing basic everyday objects such as glasses or keys. Many have referred to this in jest as 'senior moments,' given their increased frequency in older adults. These types of forgetting are similar to difficulties encountered in the early stage of a cognitive disorder, yet they differ in terms of frequency and severity. Although forgetting where you put your car key can be distressing, it is something that may be regarded as a normal memory failure or result of inattention. However, forgetting that you need the key to start the car, or confusion about how to use it, would be a better indicator of an issue that warrants medical attention.

Cognitive complaints can often signify other issues of clinical concern. **Table 1** shows common conditions that may initially present with complaints of cognitive difficulties. It has been said that if you think you have Alzheimer's disease (AD), you probably don't. The reasoning here is that those with disease-associated impairments in cognition are often not the ones who complain about it most; it is typically family members that are more concerned. Individuals with early dementia may be aware of a change in cognition but tend to minimize the impact on their everyday functioning. Lack of complaint should not be erroneously assumed to be indicative of a lack of impairment.

Loss of Mental Faculties Is Not a Normal Part of the Aging Process

Years ago, it was generally accepted that losing one's mental faculties was a normal part of the aging process referred to as senility. Many of those individuals previously identified as senile probably had what is now recognized as AD or some other form of dementia.

The term senility has fallen out of favor because its use implies an unknown etiology and, as a result, no specified treatment or progress. Instead, the term dementia is used as a way to describe impairment in cognition, usually in the domain of memory plus some other aspect of cognition, that interferes with an individual's ability to function independently. There have been major advances in the field of cognitive disorders in the past decade. Most notably, now there are treatment options for dementia, and although they were originally thought to simply delay disease progression, more recent evidence suggests that these agents may in fact be disease modifiers. In recent years, increasing efforts have focused on diagnosing dementia in its earliest stages, since treatment at the first indication of cognitive compromise may prove to be the most beneficial.

Mild Cognitive Impairment Is a Risk Factor for Dementia

The term mild cognitive impairment (MCI) has been used to describe cognitive decline greater than expected as compared to age-matched peers, yet not at a level consistent with a dementing disorder. In its original conception, the term implied mild memory changes (now referred to as amnestic MCI), but the concept has evolved to include difficulties in other cognitive domains (nonamnestic MCI) as well as mild changes in more than one cognitive domain (MCI-multidomain). MCI reflects cognitive difficulties in the context of otherwise normal functioning (no interruption in activities of daily living).

Individuals with MCI can be viewed as being in a transitional state between normal age-related decline and dementia, yet they may not necessarily progress to a dementing condition. Estimates vary, but numbers are as high as suggesting up to 40% of patients with MCI develop dementing conditions within three years of diagnosis. **Table 2** shows the annual rates of conversion from MCI to dementia over a 48-month period. The literature suggests that those with amnestic MCI are most likely to go on and develop AD at a rate of 15–25% per year. Those with MCI multidomain and nonamnestic MCI may progress to Alzheimer's or some other form of dementia (e.g., frontotemporal dementia, vascular dementia, Lewy body dementia) or other conditions associated with cognitive compromise.

AD Is the Most Common Form of Dementia

One hundred years ago, there was not as much concern about late life dementing disorders, mainly because people were not living long enough to get them. AD is an age-related disorder, and as a result the incidence has dramatically increased over the years as the population throughout the world is living longer. Numbers of affected individuals will differ across countries as a function of life expectancy. World-wide estimates suggest over 25 million people have dementia, and this estimate is expected to double every 20 years. These staggering projections are likely the result of numerous factors, including increased life expectancies, greater awareness, as well as the availability of treatments that are delaying the disease process and possibly extending the lives of affected individuals. AD is the most common form of dementia. The neuropathology of senile plaques and neurofibrillary tangles that are characteristic of the disease are also found to a much lesser degree in the brains of healthy older adults.

Aside from age, other hypothesized risk factors for development of AD include female gender, history of head trauma, and low levels of education. There are rare forms of AD that are associated with genetic risk factors, but the most common form of the disease is likely a result of a combination of genes and the environment. Genetic risk associated with the most common form of the disorder has been associated with the presence of a particular type of gene that makes a form of a protein present in all individuals. Presence of a specific form of this gene (Apolipoprotein-e4 allele; APOE-e4) has been associated with increased chance of developing late-onset sporadic AD. APOE is a susceptibility factor for development of AD; its presence does not determine who will get the disease. Given its low sensitivity and specificity as well as equivocal predictive value for an individual patient, testing for APOE (APOE genotyping) is not recommended for clinical purposes.

In AD, the primary symptoms of memory decline tend to come on slowly. It often takes a year or longer before

Table 2   Annual rates of conversion from mild cognition impairment (MCI) to dementia over 48 months

Time Elapse	MCI	Alzheimer Disease
Initial	100%	–
12 months	87%	13%
24 months	75%	25%
36 months	62%	38%
48 months	50%	50%

Adapted from Petersen RC, Smith GE, Waring SC, Ivnik RJ, Tangalos EG, and Kokmen E (1999) Mild cognitive impairment: Clinical characteristics and outcome. *Archives of Neurology* 56(3): 303–308. Copyright © (1999) American Medical Association. All rights reserved.

Table 3   Common forms of dementia

Alzheimer's disease
Vascular dementia (also referred to as multi-infarct dementia,
    Binswanger's disease)
Primary progressive aphasia
Dementia with Lewy bodies
Corticobasal degeneration
Posterior cortical atrophy
Infectious diseases (HIV dementia, syphilis, Creutzfeldt-Jakob
    disease)
Structural abnormalities (hydrocephalus, tumors)
Toxic substances (alcohol, exposure to heavy metals)

these symptoms come to medical attention. Symptoms of forgetfulness and confusion are often observed by family members, since the affected individual typically has diminished insight, and even if they admit to memory problems, they tend to minimize the impact on their everyday life. In its most common manifestation, AD is slowly progressive, and cognitive decline may occur over a period of 8 to 10 years or longer before death. AD is just one type of dementia. **Table 3** lists common forms of dementia. In the advanced stages, all progressive dementias present with very similar clinical manifestations, and it is difficult to distinguish among them.

Mixed Dementia (Primary Dementia Plus Vascular Disease) Is Likely Underdiagnosed

Perhaps the second most common form of dementia is that attributable to vascular disease. Aging of the cerebrovasculature (blood vessels in the brain) can result in cognitive difficulties ranging from mild deficits to a full-blown dementia (vascular dementia, also referred to as multi-infarct dementia or Binswanger's disease). These changes frequently occur in conjunction with Alzheimer's-like plaques and tangles, resulting in a mixed dementia (i.e., neuropathology of both AD and vascular dementia). Given the prevalence of age-related changes in the cerbrovasculature, and the fact that vascular disease risk factors have also been found to be associated with increased risk for AD, mixed dementias likely occur more frequently than they are recognized. In fact, some investigators have reasonably argued that mixed dementias may be the most common cause of late-life cognitive disorders. Although initially used to describe AD symptoms in the presence of cognitive impairment attributable to vascular disease, the term mixed dementia is also used to represent the combination of other primary dementing disorders and evidence of cerebrovascular compromise.

Cognitive Disorders Can Present Initially as Behavior or Personality Change

Not all cognitive disorders will present with complaints about memory or thinking as the primary symptom. Frontal systems dementias, such as Pick's disease or frontotemporal dementia, may initially present as changes in behavior or personality. In some cases, there may be an exacerbation of premorbid personality characteristics, or behavior may be uncharacteristic of the individual. Cognition may be affected, but deficits may be secondary to behavioral disturbances such as impulsivity, poor judgment, reduced initiative and planning, and impaired ability to organize. The individual is unable to engage and interact effectively with the environment, resulting in difficulties learning and conducting everyday activities independently. For example, someone with a frontal systems dementia may be able to conduct each element of food preparation in isolation, but because they are unable to plan, organize, and sequence the events appropriately, they cannot prepare a meal. Presence of these types of symptoms can help in determining the etiology of the cognitive disturbance. Visual hallucinations and misidentification syndromes (e.g., Capgras syndrome, the belief that loved ones have been replaced by imposters) in the early stages of a dementia may be of diagnostic significance. For example, these behaviors are more likely to be seen in the early stages of dementia with Lewy bodies (DLB) than some of the other forms of dementia. Patients with DLB also present with confusion and cognitive difficulties not unlike that observed in AD, although their symptoms may fluctuate throughout the day between periods of lucidness and confusion. In addition, patients with DLB can be differentiated from AD by the presence of motor symptoms similar to those observed in Parkinson's disease.

Dementia Can Occur in Conjunction with Movement Disorders

Cognitive disturbances associated with movement disorders can progress to a global dementia. In movement disorders such as Parkinson's disease, Huntington's disease, corticobasal degeneration, and progressive supranuclear palsy, cognitive difficulties can occur in conjunction with or following initial symptoms of a disturbance in motor systems. In keeping with slowing of motor functions (bradykinesia) often found in these disorders, the cognitive disturbance typically reflects slowing of thought processes referred to as bradyphrenia. Performance on timed tasks is often particularly affected, as are skills generally referred to as executive functions, which require organization and planning, rapid generation of responses, and task persistence. Cognitive deficits can be relatively mild but can advance to a full-blown dementia as the disease progresses, such that the cognitive disturbance may be indistinguishable from an Alzheimer's-type dementia in the advanced stages.

Not All Cognitive Disorders Are Progressive or Irreversible

The dementing disorders described thus far have generally referred to progressive and irreversible disturbances in cognition, the majority of which have a slow, insidious onset. Those characteristics do not appropriately describe all late-life cognitive disorders. Perhaps the best example of an acute alteration in mental status that is also reversible is delirium, which can closely follow medical illness and present as a sudden change in thinking abilities, reduced alertness, and confusion. This transient deficit has a fluctuating course throughout the day, but eventually resolves shortly after the disturbance that provoked it is alleviated. Delirium can be differentiated from dementia by several factors relating to the onset, course, and presentation (see **Table 4**). Delirium does not necessarily negate a subsequent diagnosis of dementia, and all else being equal, those with even mild symptoms of dementia are at greater risk for developing delirium relative to cognitively intact individuals.

There are several types of dementias generally referred to as reversible dementias (e.g., normal pressure hydrocephalus, depression, metabolic/endocrine disturbances), but it is important to note that cognitive decline associated

Table 4 Differential diagnosis of delirium versus dementia based on presenting features

Feature	Delirium	Dementia
Onset	Acute onset	Insidious onset
Arousal	Reduced consciousness (drowsy, semi-comatose)	Alert
Attention	Clouded attention	Intact attention
Symptom fluctuation	Fluctuating symptoms throughout the day	Insignificant daily fluctuations[a]
Behavioral changes	Agitation and aggression	Agitation and aggression usually not present until moderate to advanced stages

[a]Dementia with Lewy bodies can present with fluctuating cognitive symptoms.

with these conditions is not always completely reversible. For example, if unrecognized, untreated, or subject to significant delays in treatment, the cognitive disturbance in patients with normal pressure hydrocephalus can evolve into a dementing disorder indistinguishable from other dementias (e.g., AD). The dementia syndrome of depression is typically regarded as a reversible condition; however, late life depression may be a warning signaling the earliest stages of a dementing disorder. There is a substantial literature describing a relationship between depression and cerebrovascular disease, and depression has been regarded as a prodrome to dementia and a risk factor for development of cognitive disorders such as AD.

Differentiating Normal Cognitive Changes from Disease-Associated Impairment

The process of distinguishing between different cognitive disorders for the purpose of diagnosis includes consideration of demographic and clinical factors such as age, family history, onset and course of symptoms, and presence of other signs of dysfunction (e.g., presence and symmetry of motor abnormalities). Factors such as an acute onset versus a slowly evolving disturbance in cognition can signal particular etiologies. Neuroimaging can be helpful in identifying tumors or vascular lesions, and although there are no specific neuroimaging signs associated with primary dementing disorders, imaging may identify greater than expected atrophy (brain cell loss) for one's age. In some cases, it may be necessary to observe an individual over time to determine whether the disturbance is in fact progressive. The profile of cognitive functioning on neuropsychological measures (formal tests of cognitive abilities) can help inform diagnosis as well as treatment planning.

Neuropsychology: The Study of Brain Behavior Relationships

The field of neuropsychology involves investigation of how developmental changes across the life span, diseases, and injury to the brain affect cognitive functioning. Clinical neuropsychology consists of administration of various types of tests of thinking abilities, and the resulting information is compared to age- and education-matched normative data and interpreted in the context of an individual's demographic, medical, psychiatric, and social history. Many people are familiar with neuroimaging, structural assessment of the brain in the form of CT or MRI (magnetic resonance imaging), in which the structure of the brain is assessed at a given time point. Neuropsychology can be thought of as a functional assessment of the brain, putting the brain to work and measuring its functional abilities at a given point in time. In clinical practice, this information is used in conjunction with results of structural imaging, a physical exam, and a detailed medical history to explain cognitive and behavioral symptoms.

Cognitive Disorders Can Be Differentiated Based on Neuropsychological Profiles

Differences in the profile of cognitive functioning on neuropsychological tests give clues to the etiology of the cognitive deficit. For example, the memory changes in AD differ from those associated with vascular dementia. AD is characterized by rapid forgetting of new information. Basic attention is typically intact in the early stages, and as a result, the AD patient may be able to demonstrate learning (albeit at a rate compromised relative to premorbid expectation). Despite learning of material, recall of this information after a delay is markedly impaired. The AD patient may not even remember being given the information to begin with. In comparison, individuals with vascular cognitive impairment tend to have significantly greater difficulty learning at the point of acquiring the new information, particularly when there is no inherent structure in the information to be remembered (e.g., lists of words as compared to story recall). Nevertheless, when questioned about the material after a delay period, these individuals tend to recall the information they initially learned. Certain cognitive disturbances that may be present in a variety of disorders may be the predominant presenting symptom distinguishing a particular type of dementia, such as marked aphasia in the patient with primary progressive aphasia, visuospatial deficits in patients with posterior cortical atrophy, or marked behavioral disturbances and social inappropriateness in patients with Pick's disease.

Preservation of Cognitive Function with Aging

The phrase 'use it or lose it' implies that engaging in challenging cerebral activity will stimulate the brain and help to maintain mental fitness, and failure to do so will have undesirable consequences. Research supports this notion, with studies showing that seniors who stay active, mentally as well as physically, perform better on tests of cognitive functioning. Further, people who engage in mentally stimulating behaviors throughout their life are

believed to build cognitive reserve that may serve a protective role in preventing the development of late-life cognitive disorders. The literature suggests that other health and lifestyle factors may affect age-associated cognitive decline.

Studies have shown that higher fish consumption (at least once per week) in North Americans and Europeans was associated with reduced incidence of AD. Other studies have shown that eating fruits and vegetables high in antioxidants helps to fight off free radicals, which are detrimental to brain function. Alcohol consumption has been said to have an aging effect on the brain. While many sources cite benefits of modest consumption (particularly red wine) for cardiovascular health, excessive abuse has been associated with increased brain atrophy (wasting away of brain tissue) and cognitive dysfunction. Smoking is associated with changes in the cerebrovasculature, affecting blood flow to the brain and other vital organs.

Numerous clinical trials have been conducted to assess possible neuroprotective effects of prescription medications, herbal supplements, and hormones. Nonsteroidal anti-inflammatory drugs (NSAIDs) such as aspirin or ibuprofen have been investigated as potential agents to ward off cognitive decline based on the theory that brain inflammation plays a role in the development of late life cognitive disorders. It is unclear whether the preventative benefit observed in some studies with NSAIDs was due to other extrinsic factors, and their use is not recommended for preventing cognitive decline at this time. These agents should not be taken without a doctor's advice, since their use can cause severe bleeding and other complications. Early studies on estrogen were promising in terms of a protective effect on cognitive decline; however, later studies yielded contradictory findings. Given equivocal findings and the risks associated with use, more research needs to be done on hormones and cognition.

There is no one substance that will prevent dementia; other agents such as statins (used to control cholesterol) and herbal supplements (such as Ginkgo biloba) are regarded by some as neuroprotective, but the results of controlled experimental investigations in these types of agents have been regarded as equivocal due to methodological limitations (e.g., lack of statistical power) or inconsistent findings across studies. Ginkgo biloba is widely used throughout Europe for treatment of cognitive decline. Although a systematic review of Gingko biloba revealed a positive effect over placebo, specific recommendations for use in treating cognitive disorders are deferred awaiting further investigations. The GEM trial (Ginkgo Evaluation of Memory) is a large-scale (>3000 participants), double-blind, randomized controlled trial designed to investigate Ginkgo biloba in the prevention of dementia that completed recruitment in 2002 (DeKosky *et al.*, 2006). When the results of this well-designed 5-year trial are published, they may shed some light on the effectiveness of Ginkgo biloba in preventing late-life cognitive decline.

Sensory changes can mistakenly present as or exacerbate cognitive decline; failure to accurately hear what has been said or see clearly interferes with one's ability to process and retain information. Correcting hearing and vision as needed may improve one's ability to engage in the environment and acquire what is needed to process information efficiently. Systemic illness and medications used can also influence how well a person engages in the environment, having an indirect effect on cognitive abilities. Given the known effects of cerebrovascular disease on mental status as well as the association of vascular risk and changes with the development of late life cognitive disorders, Alzheimer's Disease International researchers advocate public health policies that address reducing modifiable risk factors for cerebrovascular disease (elevated cholesterol, tobacco use, diabetes). These risk factors not only are associated with diseases that threaten mental functioning, but have in and of themselves been associated with cognitive decline. Sleep and mood disturbances also influence how well an individual processes information and can present with changes in cognitive function that may be alleviated once the primary disturbance is treated. Perhaps the best plan for dementia prevention is consonant with recommendations to prevent other diseases: maintain your best health by paying attention to lifestyle factors that influence your physical and mental status (e.g., diet, exercise, alcohol/tobacco consumption, stress). In general, those that fare best tend to be those with a healthy attitude toward aging. Keeping active, both physically and mentally, may serve a protective role against cognitive decline associated with aging.

See also: Cerebrovascular Disease.

Citation

DeKosky ST, Fitzpatrick A, Ives DG, *et al.* (2006) The Ginkgo Evaluation of Memory (GEM) study: Design and baseline data of a randomized trial of Ginkgo biloba extract in prevention of dementia. *Contemporary Clinical Trials* 27(3): 238–253.

Further Reading

Attix DK and Welsh-Bohmer KA (2006) *Geriatric Neuropsychology: Assessment and Intervention.* New York: The Guilford Press.
Fillit HM, Butler RN, O'Connell AW, *et al.* (2002) Achieving and maintaining cognitive vitality with aging. *Mayo Clinic Proceedings* 77(7): 681–696.
Gauthier S, Reisberg B, Zaudig M, *et al.* (2006) International Psychogeriatric Association Expert Conference on Mild Cognitive Impairment. *Lancet* 367: 1262–1270.
Hayden KM, Zandi PP, Lyketsos CG, *et al.* (2006) Vascular risk factors for incident Alzheimer disease and vascular dementia: The Cache County study. *Alzheimer Disease and Associated Disorders* 20(2): 93–100.
McKeith IG, Dickson DW, and Lowe J (2005) Diagnosis and management of dementia with Lewy bodies: Third report of the DLB Consortium. *Neurology* 65(12): 1863–1872.
Petersen RC, Smith GE, Waring SC, Ivnik RJ, Tangalos EG, and Kokmen E (1999) Mild cognitive impairment: Clinical characteristics and outcome. *Archives of Neurology* 56(3): 303–308.
Petersen RC, Doody R, Kurz A, *et al.* (2001) Current concepts in mild cognitive impairment. *Archives of Neurology* 58: 1985–1992.
Rockwood K (2002) Vascular cognitive impairment and vascular dementia. *Journal of the Neurological Sciences* 203: 23–27.

Relevant Websites

http://www.alz.co.uk/ – Alzheimer's Disease International.
http://www.theaacn.org/links.html – American Academy of Clinical Neuropsychology.
http://www.the-ins.org/ – International Neuropsychological Society.
http://www.mayoclinic.com/ – Mayo Clinic (for Mild Cognitive Impairment).
http://www.ninds.nih.gov/ – National Institutes of Health/National Institute of Neurological Disorders and Stroke.
http://www.nia.nih.gov/ – National Institutes of Health/National Institute on Aging.
http://www.wpda.org/ – World Parkinson's Disease Association.

Head Trauma

J Knopman and R Härtl, New York-Presbyterian Hospital, New York, NY, USA

Introduction

Traumatic brain injury is graded as mild, moderate, or severe based on the Glasgow Coma Scale (GCS) score after resuscitation according to *Brain Trauma Guidelines* (Brain Trauma Foundation, 2000, 2004, 2006, 2007) (**Table 1**). Mild TBI is defined as a GCS score between 13 and 15. In most cases, it represents a concussion, and there is full neurological recovery, although some patients may reveal persistent short-term memory and concentration difficulties. Patients with moderate TBI are stuporous and lethargic with a GCS score between 9 and 13.

A comatose patient with a TBI unable to open his or her eyes or follow commands, with a GCS score of less than 9, by definition has a severe TBI. Over the past two decades, it has become increasingly clear that patients with TBI are very susceptible to posttraumatic arterial hypotension, hypoxia, and brain swelling. All major advances in the care of these patients have been achieved by reducing the severity of these secondary insults on the injured central nervous system. Rapid resuscitation of trauma patients in the field, direct transport to a major trauma center, and improved critical care management in the hospital with intracranial pressure/oxygenation (ICP) monitoring seem to have cut down the rate of mortality from up to 50% in the 1970s and 1980s to between 15% and 25% in most recent series (Palmer *et al.*, 2001; Fakhry *et al.*, 2004). The development of scientifically based management protocols for the treatment of patients with TBI holds considerable promise for further improvement in outcome. The goal of this article is to familiarize the reader with the basic principles of TBI management. In this article, we refer to recently published evidence-based documents containing guidelines for the prehospital and in-hospital surgical and medical management of patients with severe TBI. These *Guidelines* have been approved by the American Association of Neurological Surgeons (AANS) and the Congress of Neurological Surgeons (CNS) and can be accessed via the Internet at www.braintrauma.org.

Epidemiology

Approximately 1.6 million people sustain a TBI each year in the United States and 270 000 require hospitalization. With roughly 52 000 deaths per year, TBI is the most common cause of death and disability in young people and accounts for about one-third of all trauma deaths (Sosin *et al.*, 1995). The costs of TBI to society are immense; neurotrauma is a serious public health problem requiring continuing improvement in the care of injured patients. Motor vehicle accidents are the major cause of TBI, particularly in young people. Falls are the leading cause of death and disability from TBI in people older than 65 years.

Pathophysiology: Secondary Brain Damage

Neurological injury not only occurs during the impact (primary injury) but also evolves over the following hours and days (secondary brain injury). Within the first days and weeks after TBI, the brain is extremely vulnerable to decreases in blood pressure and oxygenation that are well tolerated by the noninjured central nervous system. These and other secondary insults to the brain can initiate a detrimental cascade of events. Posttraumatic brain swelling and edema leads to increased ICP and a reduction in cerebral perfusion pressure (CPP = MAP – ICP) and cerebral blood flow (CBF). If left untreated this can result in cerebral ischemia, which worsens the brain swelling and edema (**Figure 1**). The most important insults that may lead to secondary brain damage are listed in **Table 2**. Many of these insults are preventable. In the prehospital phase, hypoxia and arterial hypotension have been shown to be the most significant secondary insults. Arterial hypotension is defined as a single systolic blood pressure reading of less than 90 mmHg. A single hypotensive episode has been shown to be associated with increased morbidity and a doubling of the mortality rate

Table 1 Glasgow Coma Scale

	Eyes open	Best verbal response	Best motor response
6	–	–	Obeys commands
5	–	Oriented and converses	Localizes painful stimuli
4	Spontaneously	Disoriented and converses	Flexion withdrawal
3	To verbal command	Inappropriate words	Flexion abnormal
2	To painful stimuli	Incomprehensible sounds	Extension
1	No response	No response	No response

The GCS scoring system is routinely used as part of the neurological examination in severe TBI. Note that the GCS represents the best response elicited from the patient. The lowest score is 3 and the highest is 15. GCS scores < 9 indicate coma.

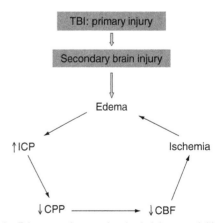

Figure 1 Primary and secondary brain injury can initiate a cascade of events that may lead to fatal outcome. Posttraumatic brain swelling and edema lead to increased intracranial pressure (ICP) and a reduction in cerebral perfusion pressure (CPP = MAP – ICP) and cerebral blood flow (CBF). If left untreated this can result in cerebral ischemia which worsens the brain swelling and edema. MAP, mean arterial pressure.

Table 2   Causes of secondary brain injury

Secondary insult	Critical values in TBI	Main cause
Arterial hypotension	Systolic blood pressure <90 mmHg	Blood loss, sepsis, cardiac failure, spinal cord injury, brain stem injury
Hypoxemia	Arterial O_2 saturation <90%, PaO_2 <60 mmHg, apnea, cyanosis	Hypoventilation, thoracic injury, aspiration
Hypocapnia	Sustained $PaCO_2$ <25 mmHg	Induced or spontaneous hyperventilation
Intracranial hypertension	ICP >20–25 mmHg	Mass lesion, cerebral swelling caused by vasodilation and/ or increased water content

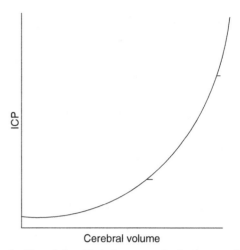

Figure 2   The relationship between cerebral volume and intracranial pressure after TBI.

(Chestnut *et al.*, 1993). This has been shown to be statistically independent of other predictive factors including age, GCS score, intracranial diagnosis, and pupillary status. Similarly, multiple episodes of hypotension may have a cumulative effect on morbidity and mortality. Manley *et al.* (2001) reported a fourfold increase in relative risk for mortality in patients who experience two or more episodes of intracranial hypotension. Therefore, the recommendation based on the CNS/AANS *Guidelines* is that the systolic pressure in patients with severe TBI be maintained above 90 mmHg to keep the cerebral perfusion pressure at approximately 60 mmHg. It is important to note that it may be necessary in certain situations to keep systolic pressure greater than 90 mmHg in order to maintain adequate CPP. It should also be noted that mean arterial pressure does not always correlate with systolic pressure. No studies have been conducted to examine these caveats, therefore, 90 mmHg systolic pressure should be considered a threshold, not an absolute goal.

Hypoxia runs in association with hypotensive episodes. Hypoxia was defined in studies as either apnea/ cyanosis in the field or a PaO_2 less than 60 mmHg. An analysis of a large prospectively collected data set from the Traumatic Coma Data Bank (TCDB) demonstrated that hypoxia occurred in 22.4% of severe TBI patients and was significantly associated with increased morbidity and mortality (Marmarou *et al.*, 1991; Chestnut *et al.*, 1993). Furthermore, a study conducted by Stocchetti *et al.* (1996) not adjusting for confounding factors determined that in patients with documented oxygen saturations less than 60%, the mortality rate was 50% and all survivors were severely disabled. This was in contrast to nonhypoxemic patients whose mortality was 14.3% with a 4.8% rate of disability. Jones *et al.* (1994) determined that duration of hypoxia was also found to be an independent predictor of mortality, but not morbidity.

The development of posttraumatic brain swelling may occur soon after the primary injury and plays a key role in the pathophysiological cascade that leads to irreversible brain damage. The brain is contained inside a rigid closed space, the skull. The skull is noncompliant, providing a fixed amount of space for the brain to occupy. As intracranial space is taken up by edema, blood, or any other mass-occupying lesion, the physiological pressure inside the skull can initially be maintained due to displacement of CSF and blood. After a certain point, this mechanism is exhausted and the ICP will increase. The challenge for the clinician treating patients with severe TBI and still controlled ICP is to determine on what point on the curve the patient is (**Figure 2**).

Brain swelling can be caused by vascular engorgement or an increase in brain water content, called brain edema. Depending on the underlying mechanism, it is possible to distinguish several types of brain swelling (Unterberg *et al.*, 2004):

● Swelling caused by hyperemia or venous congestion with increased cerebral blood volume;
● Vasogenic brain edema;
● Cytotoxic brain edema.

Disruption of the blood–brain barrier, within minutes after TBI, leads to accumulation of fluid in the extravascular compartment and vasogenic edema. Vasogenic edema can also develop later around areas of contused brain tissue and hemorrhage. Despite the effectiveness of steroids to treat vasogenic edema in patients with brain tumors, they have not proven to be of benefit in patients with TBI. The main type of brain swelling after TBI is caused by cytotoxic edema. This type of edema is characterized by a failure of sodium/potassium pumps to maintain intracellular homeostasis. This leads to influx of ions and water into cells and initiates a self-destructive cascade culminating in progressive ischemia and intracranial hypertension. Several pharmacologic agents that interfere with this cascade, such as calcium antagonists, free-radical scavengers, and N-methyl-D-aspartate antagonists have been tested, but none have been proven effective (Narayan *et al.*, 2002). The lack of pharmacologic agents that are available to treat patients with TBI reinforces the importance of optimal critical care management and monitoring and treatment of brain pressure, blood pressure, and oxygenation to maintain and improve cerebral perfusion.

Management of Patients with Severe Traumatic Brain Injury

Prehospital Management

The prehospital management of patients with severe TBI is outlined in **Table 3** and the principles are summarized in the *Guidelines* for the prehospital management of TBI (Brain Trauma Foundation, 2000). Rapid and physiologic resuscitation is the first priority in these patients. Following stabilization of airways, breathing, and circulation, the GCS score should be determined by direct verbal or physical interaction with the patient. Patients with a GCS score of less than 9 should be brought to a trauma center with the following TBI capabilities:

- 24-h CT scanning capability;
- 24-h available operating room and prompt neurosurgical care;
- The ability to monitor ICP and treat intracranial hypertension.

Comatose patients with a GCS score less than 9 should be intubated. All patients should have their oxygenation and blood pressure assessed at least every 5 min. Their oxygen saturation should be maintained above 90% and systolic blood pressure should be kept above 90 mmHg.

Initial Management in the Emergency Department

Maintaining brain perfusion is the guiding principle in managing comatose patients with severe TBI. The cornerstones of the resuscitation of the severely head-injured patient are:

- Resuscitation according to ACLS/ATLS protocol (airways, breathing, circulation);
- Primary survey with cervical spine control and brief neurologic assessment;
- Secondary survey with complete neurologic examination and determination of the GCS score.

Emergency room patients with mild or moderate TBI or suspected TBI need to be followed very closely for neurological deterioration, ideally with neuro-checks every 15 min in the acute period. A complete trauma workup following the ACLS/ATLS protocols should be initiated if there is any suspicion of associated injuries. Nausea or vomiting, progressive headaches, restlessness, pupillary asymmetry, seizures, and increasing lethargy should be interpreted as signs of neurological deterioration, and a head computed tomography (CT) scan should be obtained immediately. It is important to remember that with expanding intracranial mass lesions, pupillary changes can precede a significant change in mental status. Blood alcohol levels and urine toxicology screen should be considered in all patients presenting with TBI. Routine blood tests, including coagulation parameters, should be obtained in patients with moderate and severe TBI and in patients with associated injuries. Tetanus toxoid must be administered if there are any associated open wounds. Immobilization of the cervical spine using a hard collar is mandatory in all patients with TBI. All patients with severe TBI need radiographic evaluation of the craniocervical junction down to T1. Any complaint of neck pain in patients with mild or moderate TBI should also lead to a radiographic assessment of the cervical spine. A list of typical admission orders for a severe TBI patient is given in **Table 4**.

Table 3 Immediate assessment and treatment of patients with traumatic brain injury

Parameter	Critical findings	Immediate intervention
1. Resuscitation		
Oxygenation/ventilation	Apnea, cyanosis, oxygen saturation <90%	Intubation if hypoxemic despite supplemental O_2, not hyperventilation
Blood pressure	SBP <90 mmHg	Fluid resuscitation
2. Primary survey/postresuscitation		
Spinal stability	Pain, step-off, external signs of trauma to neck, mechanism	Immobilization, radiographs
Postresuscitation GCS score	<9	Intubation, normoventilation, head CT
Motor examination, pupillary diameter, light reflex, direct orbital trauma	Suspect cerebral herniation: flaccidity or motor posturing and asymmetrical or fixed and dilated pupils	Short-term hyperventilation ± mannitol, if herniation suspected
3. Placement of lines, urinary and gastric catheters, and cervical spine, chest, and pelvis radiographs		
Secondary survey/dedicated neurological examination		

GCS, Glasgow Coma Scale; CT, computed tomography; SBP, systolic blood pressure.

Table 4   Typical orders for patients with severe traumatic brain injury

Admit to neuro/trauma intensive care unit

Monitoring and notifications
- Check vital signs and neuro status q1h, call HO for change in neurological condition
- Check temperature q4h, call for T > 38.3 °C. If T > 38.3 °C, remove sheets, use cooling blankets, fan, and/or ice packings
- Monitor end tidal CO_2. Call for $PaCO_2$ < 30 mmHg
- Notify for SBP >180 or SBP < 90
- Specify ventriculostomy settings
- Monitor CPP, call for CPP < 60 mmHg
- Monitor CVP, call for CVP < 5 or CVP >10 mmHg
- If Swan Ganz catheter in place, measure cardiac parameters q4 h, call for wedge pressure <8 and >15 mmHg
- Strict I's and O's, call for UO >200 ml/h × 2 h

Activity
- Bedrest with HOB 30°
- Log roll, spine precautions
- Cervical collar

Nursing
- Foley catheter
- Knee-high stockings and/or pneumatic compression devices
- Daily weights
- 2–4 L O_2 per nasal cannula
- Orogastric tube, nasogastric tube if no basilar skull fracture

Diet
- Start tube feedings within 24–36 h after TBI

Maintenance IV fluids
- Normal saline @ 1–2 ml/kg/h, typically 80–120 ml/h

Medication
- Stool softener
- Docusate sodium (Colace) 200 mg PO bid

Antiemetic
- Reglan 10 mg IV q4 h prn nausea/vomiting

Analgesia
- Codeine 30–60 mg IM/PO q3 h prn
- Morphine 1–6 mg IV/IM q4–6 h prn or IV drip up to 5–10 mg/h
- Fentanyl (Sublimaze) 50–150 μg bolus, then 30–100 μg/h maintenance

Antipyretics
- Acetaminophen (Tylenol) 600–1000 mg PO/PR q6 h prn if T > 38.3 °C

Sedation
- Midazolam (Versed) drip 1–2 mg/h
- Lorazepam (Ativan) 1 mg IV/PO bid–tid
- Propofol (Diprivan) drip 5 μg/kg/min

GI prophylaxis
- Esomeprazole (Nexium) 40 mg IV/PO qd

Seizure prophylaxis
- Phenytoin (Dilantin) 100 mg IV/PO tid

Arterial hypertension
- Labetalol (Trandate) 10 mg IV q15 min for SBP >180 mmHg prn, hold for HR <60 beats/min
- Hydralazine (Apresoline) 10 mg IV q15 min for SBP >180 prn, hold for HR >90 beats/min; may increase ICP and CBF

Others
- Lidocaine protocol for suctioning

Labs
- CBC, Coags, T&C, SMA-10, Tox screen, ETOH level

Ventilator settings as indicated

General principles of the workup in patients with severe TBI are summarized below:

- Normocapnia should be maintained. Unless there are signs of cerebral herniation (pupillary asymmetry, dilated/fixed pupils, and/or extensor posturing or flaccidity to noxious stimuli) patients should not be hyperventilated and the arterial PCO_2 should be maintained around 35 mmHg.

- Isotonic fluids should be used for resuscitation to avoid free water overload.
- CT is the imaging study of choice to detect skull fractures and intracranial injury with hemorrhage and to assess the necessity of surgical evacuation of a mass lesion. A head CT scan can also demonstrate findings that are closely associated with intracranial hypertension such as obliterated basal cisterns, compressed cerebral ventricles, and midline shift.

- All comatose patients with an abnormal CT scan and a GCS score of 8 or less should undergo ICP monitoring.
- Once the patient has been stabilized, a careful physical examination should be conducted.

Computed tomography scan assessment

After resuscitation, all stable patients with severe TBI should receive a CT scan of the head as soon as possible to identify:

- A life-threatening mass lesion that requires surgical evacuation;
- Evidence of raised ICP;
- The degree of intracranial injury, to determine prognostic indicators of outcome.

Approximately 10% of initial head CT scans in patients with severe TBI will not show any abnormalities. The absence of abnormalities on CT scan at admission does not preclude increased ICP. Significant new lesions and increased ICP may develop in 40% of patients with initially normal head CT scan. In addition, in patients with normal CT findings, systolic blood pressure lower than 90 mmHg, age greater than 40 years, or motor posturing are at increased risk for intracranial hypertension according to The Brain Trauma Foundation.

Intensive Care Unit Management

Intracranial pressure and brain oxygen monitoring

Comatose TBI patients (GCS score 3–8) with abnormal CT scans should undergo ICP monitoring for the following reasons, as recommended by The Brain Trauma Foundation:

- Helps in the earlier detection of intracranial mass lesions;
- Can limit the indiscriminate use of therapies to control ICP, which themselves can be potentially harmful;
- Can reduce ICP by cerebrospinal fluid drainage and thus improve cerebral perfusion;
- Helps in determining prognosis;
- May improve outcome.

Elevated ICP is present in the majority of severely head-injured patients. Cerebral perfusion pressure (CPP) is defined as the mean arterial blood pressure minus ICP. This physiologic variable defines the pressure gradient driving cerebral blood flow and metabolite delivery and is therefore closely related to cerebral ischemia. A threshold for cerebral perfusion pressure of approximately 60 mmHg for adults is currently recommended, as noted in the *Guidelines* publications.

The CNS/AANS *Guidelines* recommend that ICP monitoring is appropriate in severe TBI patients (GCS score 3–8) with an abnormal CT scan, or a normal CT scan if two or more of the following are noted upon admission:

- Systolic blood pressure less than 90 mmHg;
- Age greater than 40 years;
- Unilateral or bilateral motor posturing.

ICP treatment should be initiated at an upper threshold of 20 or 25 mmHg. CPP should be maintained at approximately 60 mmHg. In the absence of cerebral ischemia, aggressive attempts to maintain CPP above 70 mmHg with fluids and pressors should be avoided because of the risk of adult respiratory distress syndrome (Robertson *et al.*, 1999). Increased ICP should be treated vigorously. A treatment algorithm for elevated ICP is outlined in **Table 5**.

Although ICP measurement is an important and predictive adjunct in the assessment of adequate cerebral perfusion, it gives no direct information on the cerebral blood flow and metabolism. Recent years have seen the development of additional monitoring systems to determine cerebral oxygenation and blood flow.

It has been demonstrated through studies by Bardt, Valadka, Van den Brink, and their respective groups that mortality is increased after TBI in patients who have increased duration of time of brain tissue oxygen tension ($P_{br}O_2$) below 15 mmHg. Clinical data have demonstrated preliminary evidence of the benefit of brain-tissue oxygen monitoring on patient outcome after TBI. A 2005 study by Stiefel *et al.* (2005) of 53 patients comparing those treated with both standard ICP/CPP parameters and the addition of oxygen-directed therapy goal at maintaining $P_{br}O_2$ over 25 mmHg found a significant decrease in mortality in those treated with oxygen therapy.

True guidelines for brain oxygen monitoring and treatment have yet to be established, as data are now emerging and questions still remain. One of the key topics of future investigation regards the correct placement of brain tissue oxygen monitoring probes with respect to the area of injury (most injured vs. least injured), and if meaningful clinical data can be garnered from measurement of brain oxygen levels outside a direct area of contusion.

Mannitol

Mannitol is effective for control of raised ICP after severe TBI. Limited data suggest that intermittent boluses may be more effective than continuous infusion. The mechanism of action of hyperosmolar agents such as mannitol are twofold: the immediate effect of plasma expansion results in decreased hematocrit and increased deformity of red blood cells, thereby decreasing viscosity and increasing cerebral blood flow/oxygenation. This rheological effect is followed by a more delayed and long-lasting osmotic effect, where a gradient is established to extract fluid from edematous cells. Randomized, non-placebo controlled trials by Cruz *et al.* (2001, 2002, 2004) have

Table 5   Management of elevated intracranial pressure (ICP) in the patient with severe traumatic brain injury

In all patients with GCS score <9	Add if ICP >20 mmHg	Add if ICP >25 mmHg	Add for persistent ICP >20 mmHg	Add for persistent ICP >20 mmHg and/or pupillary abnormalities
ICP monitoring Elevate head of bed 30°	Ventricular CSF drainage	Neuromuscular blockade: vecuronium (Norcuron), atracurium (Tracrium)	Moderate hypothermia, core temperature 34–36°C	High-dose propofol (Diprivan) infusion
Maintain euvolemia and hemodynamic stability, keep CVP 5–10 mmHg	Sedation: midazolam (Versed) or lorazepam (Ativan)	Mannitol 0.25–1.0 g/kg IV over 5–10 min q4–6 h prn. Serum osmolarity 300–320 mOsm/L; serum sodium 150–155 mEq/L	Hyperventilation to PaCO₂ 30–35 mmHg	Hyperventilation to PaCO₂ 25–30 mmHg
$PaCO_2$ >90 mmHg	Analgesia: fentanyl (Sublimaze) or morphine			Consider hypertonic saline bolus infusion Consider decompressive craniectomy
$PaCO_2$ 35–40 mmHg Systolic blood pressure >90 mmHg	CPP management: inotropic and pressor support to maintain CPP (dopamine (Intropin) 5–20 μg/kg/min, norepinephrine (Levophed) 0.05–0.5 μg/kg/min)			
CPP approximately 70 mmHg	Repeat head CT to exclude operable mass lesion			

CPP, cerebral perfusion pressure; CSF, cerebrospinal fluid; CT, computed tomography; CVP, central venous pressure; ICP, intracranial pressure; GCS, Glasgow Coma Scale.

demonstrated high dose mannitol (1.2–1.4 g/kg) to have beneficial effects on Glasgow Outcome Scores at 6 months when compared with conventional dose mannitol (0.6–0.7 g/kg) in three groups of severe TBI patients (temporal lobe hematomas, acute subdural hematomas, and impending brain death). Hypovolemia should be avoided by fluid replacement. Serum osmolarity should be kept below 320 mOsm to avoid renal failure. Euvolemia should be maintained by adequate fluid replacement. A Foley catheter has to be placed in these patients. ICP reduction reaches a maximum approximately 30–60 min after bolus infusion and persists between 90 min and 6 h. Mannitol together with furosemide (Lasix) may cause rapid diuresis and depletion of intravascular volume and electrolytes and is therefore not recommended.

Hypertonic saline

Hypertonic saline has found its place as a second-tier therapy in the treatment of intracranial hypertension resistant to conventional treatment maneuvers. Its use remained largely unexplored in humans until the last 20 years. Hypertonic saline has been used both as bolus infusion for treatment of acutely elevated ICP (up to concentrations of 23.4% NaCl) and as continuous infusion of 1.8–3% saline to increase serum osmolarity. Hypertonic saline decreases ICP through similar mechanisms as mannitol, but runs less of a risk for hypovolemia as it has plasma-expanding

capability without the subsequent effect of diuresis. Clinical data demonstrate that bolus infusion reliably decreases ICP in patients in whom mannitol has lost its efficacy. A hyperosmolar state with serum osmolarities well above 320 mOsm/L may develop but seems to be tolerated well as long as euvolemia and arterial normotension are maintained. Hypertonic saline infusion should only commence after preexisting hyponatremia has been ruled out in order to prevent central pontine myelinolysis (CPM). In normonatremic individuals, there have been no reported cases of CPM after hypertonic saline administration. More studies are needed to compare mannitol versus hypertonic saline in the treatment of ICP; however, one randomized trial by Battison et al. (2005) comparing equimolar concentrations demonstrated that hypertonic saline has a more profound effect on lowering ICP as well as longer duration of action.

Hyperventilation

Hyperventilation should not be used routinely in these patients because of the risk of further compromising cerebral perfusion. Hyperventilation can be used for brief periods when there is acute neurologic deterioration or if intracranial hypertension is refractory to other treatment interventions. Under these circumstances, intraparenchymal brain-tissue oxygen monitoring is utilized to titrate the degree of hyperventilation and to avoid cerebral ischemia (**Table 5**). The use of prophylactic hyperventilation ($PaCO_2 = 35$ mmHg) therapy during the first 24 h after severe TBI should be avoided because it can compromise cerebral perfusion during a time period when CBF is already decreased.

Prophylactic measures

Although some centers induce prophylactic hypothermia in patients with acute TBI, the literature has failed to demonstrate a consistently positive influence on morbidity or mortality. Hypothermia is not routinely employed as a first-line therapy for TBI, and its use is reserved for long-standing, refractory ICP elevation in posttraumatic patients.

In TBI patients, infection rates are increased in those on mechanical ventilation and with ICP monitoring devices. Prophylactic antibiotics are not recommended for ventilated patients so as not to select for resistant organisms. In addition, although ICP monitoring devices such as ventriculostomies should be inserted under sterile conditions, it is not recommended to continue a course of antibiotics for the duration of monitoring. It is routine to administer one to two doses of antibiotics during periprocedural insertion of these monitoring devices despite conflicting clinical studies.

Barbiturate coma

High-dose barbiturate therapy may be considered in hemodynamically stable, salvageable, severe TBI patients with intracranial hypertension refractory to maximal medical and surgical ICP-lowering therapy. Barbiturates appear to exert their cerebral protective and ICP-lowering effects through alterations in vascular tone, suppression of metabolism, and inhibition of free radical-mediated lipid peroxidation. The risk of arterial hypotension induced by peripheral vasodilation is high. Adequate barbiturate coma therapy results in the electroencephalographic pattern of burst suppression. Near-maximal reductions in cerebral metabolism and cerebral blood flow occur when burst suppression is induced.

High-dose propofol

Propofol (Diprivan) at low doses is commonly used for sedation in patients requiring mechanical ventilation. In recent years, high-dose propofol has gained popularity as an alternative to barbiturates in patients with intracranial hypertension refractory to maximal medical and surgical ICP-lowering therapy (Oertel *et al.*, 2002). The main advantage of propofol is that it is short-acting. Like other anesthetics, it can cause hypotension, and, even though ICP decreases, overall cerebral perfusion pressure may drop. High-dose use of propofol can result in propofol infusion syndrome, a multiorgan and metabolic crisis that was first identified in children, but can also occur in adults. The characteristics include hyperkalemia, hepatomegaly, metabolic acidosis, renal failure, myocardial failure, and rhabdomyolysis. Hepatic and pancreatic enzymes should be monitored while on propofol and this neurosedative should not be used in pediatric patients.

Glucocorticoids

Glucocorticoids have not been shown to improve outcome after severe TBI according to *Guidelines* publications. A recent large prospective randomized trial has shown that corticosteroids are associated with increased rates of severe disability and death when used in the treatment of patients with TBI (Edwards *et al.*, 2005).

Nutritional support

Studies have shown that the failure to achieve full nutritional support within the first week after severe TBI increases mortality. Tube feedings should ideally commence within the first 2 days after TBI.

Treatment of seizures

Posttraumatic seizures (PTS) can be divided into early (<7 days after trauma) and late seizures (>7 days after trauma). In recent TBI studies that followed high-risk patients up to 36 months, the incidence of early PTS varied between 4% and 25%, and the incidence of late PTS varied between 9% and 42% in untreated patients. Prophylactic use of phenytoin (Dilantin), carbamazepine (Tegretol), or phenobarbital is not recommended by *Guidelines* publications for preventing late PTS. Anticonvulsants may be used to prevent early PTS in patients at high risk for seizures following TBI. Phenytoin and carbamazepine have been demonstrated to be effective in this setting. However, the available evidence does not indicate that prevention of early PTS improves outcome following TBI. Routine seizure prophylaxis later than 1 week following TBI is therefore not recommended. If late PTS occurs, patients should be managed in accordance with standard approaches to patients with new-onset seizures. Routine seizure prophylaxis after TBI also raises concern for potential side effects such as drug fever and anaphylaxis. Fever may develop 1–8 weeks after exposure to phenytoin, phenobarbital, or carbamazepine.

Surgical Management of Acute Traumatic Brain Injury

The decision as to whether an intracranial lesion requires surgical evacuation can be difficult and is based on the patient's GCS score, pupillary examination findings, comorbidities, CT findings, age, and – in delayed decisions – ICP. Neurological deterioration over time is also an important factor influencing the decision to operate. Trauma patients presenting to the emergency department with altered mental status, pupillary asymmetry, and abnormal flexion or extension are at high risk for an intracranial mass lesion, and it is our practice to notify the operating room even before obtaining a CT scan that an emergency craniotomy will most likely be necessary.

Epidural Hematoma

The incidence of surgical and nonsurgical epidural hematoma (EDH) among TBI patients is approximately 3%. Among patients in coma, up to 9% harbored an EDH requiring craniotomy. The peak incidence of EDH is in the second decade and the mean age of patients with EDH is between 20 and 30 years of age. Traffic-related accidents, falls, and assaults account for the majority of all cases of EDH. EDH usually results from injury to the middle meningeal artery but can also be due to bleeding from the middle meningeal vein, the diploic veins, or the venous sinuses (**Figures 3** and **4**). In patients with EDH, one-third to one-half are comatose on admission or immediately before surgery. The classically described lucid interval, which describes a patient who is initially unconscious, then wakes up and secondarily deteriorates, is seen in approximately one-half of patients undergoing surgery for EDH. Clot thickness, hematoma volume, and midline shift (MLS) on the preoperative CT scan are related to outcome. Noncomatose patients without focal neurologic deficits and with an acute EDH with a thickness of less than 15 mm, an MLS less than 5 mm, and a hematoma volume less than 30 ml can be managed nonsurgically with serial CT scanning and close neurologic evaluation in a neurosurgical center (**Figure 5**). The first follow-up CT scan in stable nonsurgical patients should be obtained within 6–8 h after TBI. Temporal location of an EDH is associated with failure of nonsurgical management and should lower the threshold for surgery. Patients with a GCS score less than 9 and an EDH larger than 30 ml should undergo immediate surgical evacuation of the lesion. All patients, regardless of GCS score, should be considered for surgery if the volume of their EDH exceeds 30 ml. Patients with an EDH volume less than 30 ml should be considered for surgery but may be managed successfully without surgery in selected cases. Time from neurologic deterioration to surgery correlates with outcome. In these patients, surgical evacuation should be done as soon as possible, since every hour of delay in surgery is associated with progressively worse outcome.

Acute Subdural Hematoma

A subdural hematoma (SDH) is diagnosed on a CT scan as extracerebral, hyperdense, crescentic collections between the dura and the brain parenchyma (**Figures 3** and **4**). They can be divided into acute and chronic lesions. The incidence of acute SDH is between 12% and 29% in patients admitted with severe TBI. The mean age is between 31 and 47 years, with the vast majority of patients being male. Most SDHs are caused by motor vehicle-related accidents, falls, and assaults. Falls have been identified as the main cause of traumatic SDH in patients older than 75 years. Between 37% and 80% of patients with acute SDH present with initial GCS scores of 8 or lower. Clot thickness or volume and MLS on the preoperative CT scan correlate with outcome. *Guidelines* publications note that patients with SDH presenting with a clot thickness greater than 10 mm or MLS greater than 5 mm should undergo surgical evacuation, regardless of their GCS (**Figure 6**). Patients who present in a coma (GCS score < 9) but with a SDH with a thickness of less

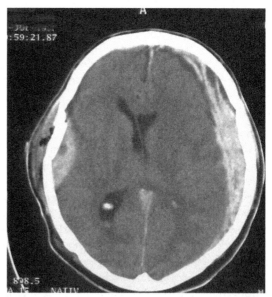

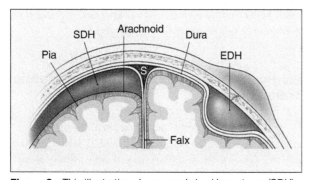

Figure 3 This illustration shows a subdural hematoma (SDH) below the dura mater on the left side. An epidural hematoma (EDH), between the dura mater and the skull, is shown on the right with a skull fracture and scalp hematoma overlying.

Figure 4 Head CT of a patient with a severe TBI. On the patient's right is an acute epidural hematoma with skull fracture and scalp hematoma overlying. On the patient's left side is an acute subdural hematoma. Note also the midline shift from left to right.

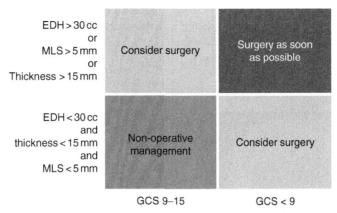

Figure 5 Graph showing considerations for nonoperative vs. operative management of epidural hematomas (EDH). These are based on Brain Trauma Foundation (2006) Guidelines for the surgical management of traumatic brain injury. *Neurosurgery* 58(supplement): S2–S10.

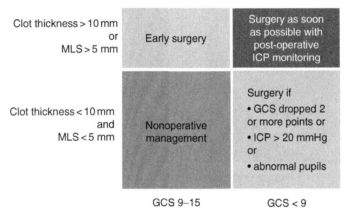

Figure 6 Graph showing considerations for nonoperative vs operative management of subdural hematomas (SDH). These are based on Brain Trauma Foundation (2006) Guidelines for the surgical management of traumatic brain injury. *Neurosurgery* 58(supplement): S2–S10.

than 10 mm and MLS less than 5 mm can be treated nonsurgically, providing that they undergo ICP monitoring, they are neurologically stable since injury, they have no pupillary abnormalities, and they have no intracranial hypertension (ICP >20 mmHg). In comatose patients or patients with progressive neurological deterioration surgical evacuation should be done as soon as possible.

Traumatic Parenchymal Lesions

Traumatic parenchymal mass lesions occur in up to 10% of all patients with TBI and 13–35% of patients with severe TBI. Most small parenchymal lesions do not require surgical evacuation. However, the development of mass effect from larger lesions may result in secondary brain injury, placing the patient at risk for further neurologic deterioration, herniation, and death. Parenchymal lesions tend to evolve over time and increase in size, which reflects the potentially devastating effect of secondary brain damage (**Figure 7(a), (b)**). Patients with

parenchymal mass lesions and signs of progressive neurologic deterioration referable to the lesion, medically refractory intracranial hypertension, or signs of mass effect on CT scan should be treated operatively. Comatose patients with frontal or temporal contusions greater than 20 ml in volume and with MLS of 5 mm or cisternal compression on CT scan, or both, and patients with any lesion greater than 50 ml in volume should be treated surgically (Mathiesen *et al.*, 1995). Patients with parenchymal mass lesions who do not show evidence of neurological compromise, have controlled ICP, and have no significant signs of mass effect on CT scan can be managed nonsurgically.

Depressed Skull Fractures

Depressed skull fractures complicate up to 6% of head injuries, and the presence of skull fracture is associated with a higher incidence of intracranial lesions, neurological deficit, and poorer outcome. Patients with open skull fractures depressed greater than the thickness of the skull should undergo surgical intervention to prevent infection. Patients with open depressed fractures should be covered with antibiotic prophylaxis according to *Guidelines* literature.

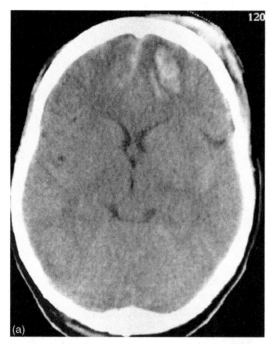

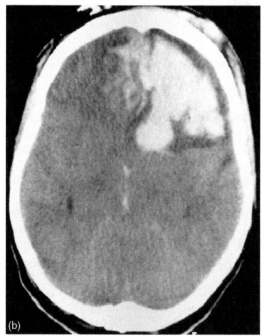

Figure 7 Traumatic parenchymal mass lesions occur in up to 10% of all patients with TBI and 13–35% of patients with severe TBI. Parenchymal lesions tend to evolve, which reflects the potentially devastating effect of secondary brain damage. This patient presented with a left-sided frontal contusion (a) that blossomed within 12 h and required surgical evacuation (b).

Decompressive Craniectomy for Control of Intracranial Hypertension

Decompressive procedures such as subtemporal decompression, temporal lobectomy, and hemispheric decompressive craniectomy are surgical procedures that have been used to treat patients with refractory intracranial hypertension and diffuse parenchymal injury. Decompressive craniectomy may be very effective if it is done early after TBI in young patients who are expected to develop postoperative brain swelling and intracranial hypertension.

Early Prognostic Indicators of Severe Traumatic Brain Injury

Outcome from TBI is frequently described using the Glasgow Outcome Scale at 6 months following TBI (**Table 6**). This is a widely accepted and standardized scale that is of value for the clinical description of patients and also for medicolegal documentation and research purposes.

The most important early presenting factors influencing outcome from severe TBI are:

- Age;
- GCS score;
- Pupillary examination findings;
- Arterial hypotension;
- CT scan findings.

Studies show that the probability of poor outcome increases with decreasing admission GCS score in a continuous manner below a GCS score of 9.

Patients with very low GCS scores have a mortality rate between 70% and 90%, but up to 10% may survive with Glasgow Outcome Scale scores of 4 or 5. Increasing age is a strong independent factor in prognosis from severe TBI, with a significant increase in poor outcome in patients older than 60 years of age. This is not explained by the increased frequency of systemic complications in older

Table 6   Glasgow Outcome Scale

Score	Rating	Definition
5	Good recovery	Resumption of normal life despite minor deficits
4	Moderate disability	Disabled but independent. Can work in sheltered setting
3	Severe disability	Conscious but disabled. Dependent for daily support
2	Persistent vegetative	Minimal responsiveness
1	Death	Nonsurvival

patients. The pupillary diameter and the pupilloconstrictor light reflex can prognosticate outcome from severe TBI. Bilaterally unreactive pupils following resuscitation on admission are associated with a greater than 90% chance of poor outcome. A systolic blood pressure less than 90 mmHg measured after severe TBI on the way to the hospital or in hospital has been associated with an almost 70% likelihood of poor outcome. Combined with hypoxia, this likelihood increases to 79%. A single recording of arterial hypotension doubles the rate of mortality from severe TBI. Among these early prognostic indicators of outcome, arterial hypotension is the only factor that can be significantly affected by therapeutic intervention.

The CT scan findings associated with poor outcome from severe TBI are:

- Compressed or absent basal cisterns;
- Traumatic subarachnoid hemorrhage;
- MLS greater than 5 mm.

Following admission, ICP greater than 20 mmHg is a poor prognostic indicator. The rate of mortality from epidural hematoma requiring surgery is around 10%. The rate of mortality from acute SDH is between 40% and 60%. The mortality rate among patients with acute SDH presenting to the hospital in coma with subsequent surgical evacuation is between 57% and 68%.

Conclusion

The mortality rate from severe TBI has been reduced from up to 50% in the 1970s and 1980s to between 15% and 25% in most recent series. This improvement should be attributed to more effective resuscitation in the field, rapid transport of TBI patients to trauma hospitals, more widely accepted ICP monitoring, and improvements in critical care management. In a recent study by Palmer *et al.* (2001) of 93 patients with severe TBI, the 6-month mortality rate was reduced 50% by the introduction of evidence-based protocol for the management of severe TBI. The treatment protocol supported ICP monitoring, adequate volume resuscitation, aggressive treatment of low blood pressure and oxygenation, avoidance of extreme hyperventilation, and early nutritional intervention. New paradigms such as direct measurement of brain tissue oxygenation hold early promise for more specific and effective management of cerebral metabolism after TBI. Multidisciplinary clinical pathways based on evidence-supported treatment guidelines for TBI streamline patient care, standardize critical care management, and hold the potential for significantly improving patient outcome and reducing hospital costs. Medical personnel in the prehospital and in-hospital setting should be aware of and trained in these principles of TBI care.

Citations

Battison C, Andrews PJ, Graham C, *et al.* (2005) Randomized, controlled trial on the effect of a 20% mannitol solution and a 7.5% saline/6% dextran solution on increased intracranial pressure after brain injury. *Critical Care Medicine* 33: 196–202 discussion 257–198.

Brain Trauma Foundation (2000) Guidelines for the management of severe traumatic brain injury. *Journal of Neurotrauma* 17: 449–554.

Brain Trauma Foundation (2000) Hyperventilation. *Journal of Neurotrauma* 17: 513–520.

Brain Trauma Foundation (2004) Update notice: guidelines for the management of severe traumatic brain injury: Cerebral perfusion pressure. *Neurotrauma and Critical Care News* 3: 3.

Brain Trauma Foundation (2006) Guidelines for the surgical management of traumatic brain injury. *Neurosurgery* 58 (supplement): S2–S10.

Bullock MR and Povlishock JT (eds.), Brain Trauma Foundation (2007) Guidelines for the Management of Severe Traumatic Brain Injury. 3rd edn. *Journal of Neurotrauma* 24 (supplement 1): 1–106.

Chesnut R, Marshall L, Klauber M, *et al.* (1993) The role of secondary brain injury in determining outcome from severe head injury. *Journal of Trauma* 34: 216–222.

Cruz J, Minoja G, and Okuchi K (2001) Improving clinical outcomes from acute subdural hematomas with the emergency preoperative administration of high doses of mannitol: a randomized trial. *Neurosurgery* 49: 864–871.

Cruz J, Minoja G, and Okuchi K (2002) Major clinical and physiological benefits of early high doses of mannitol for intraparenchymal temporal lobe hemorrhages with abnormal papillary widening: A randomized trial. *Neurosurgery* 51: 628–637.

Cruz J, Minoja G, Okuchi K, *et al.* (2004) Successful use of new high-dose mannitol treatment in patients with Glasgow Coma Scale scores of 3 and bilateral abnormal pupillary widening: a randomized trial. *Journal of Neurosurgery* 100: 376–383.

Edwards P, Arango M, Balica L, *et al.* (2005) Final results of MRC CRASH, a randomised placebo-controlled trial of intravenous corticosteroid in adults with head injury-outcomes at 6 months. *Lancet* 365: 1957–1959.

Fakhry SM, Trask AL, Waller MA, *et al.* (2004) Management of brain-injured patients by an evidence-based medicine protocol improves outcomes and decreases hospital charges. *Journal of Trauma* 56: 492–499; discussion 499–500.

Jones PA, Andrews PJD, Midgely S, *et al.* (1994) Measuring the burden of secondary insults in head injured patients during intensive care. *Journal of Neurosurgery and Anesthesiology* 6: 4–14.

Manley G, Knudson M, Morabito D, *et al.* (2001) Hypotension, hypoxia, and head injury: Frequency, duration, and consequences. *Archives of Surgery* 136: 1118–1123.

Marmarou A, Anderson RL, Ward JD, *et al.* (1991) Impact of ICP instability and hypotension on outcome in patients with severe head trauma. *Journal of Neurosurgery* 75: 159–166.

Mathiesen T, Kakarieka A, and Edner G (1995) Traumatic intracerebral lesions without extracerebral haematoma in 218 patients. *Acta Neurochirica (Wien)* 137: 155–163 discussion 163.

Narayan RK, Michel ME, Ansell B, *et al.* (2002) Clinical trials in head injury. *Journal of Neurotrauma* 19: 503–557.

Oertel M, Kelly DF, Lee JH, *et al.* (2002) Efficacy of hyperventilation, blood pressure elevation, and metabolic suppression therapy in controlling intracranial pressure after head injury. *Journal of Neurosurgery* 97: 1045–1053.

Palmer S, Bader M, Qureshi A, *et al.* (2001) The impact on outcomes in a community hospital setting of using the AANS traumatic brain injury guidelines. Americans Associations for Neurologic Surgeons. *Journal of Trauma* 50: 657–664.

Robertson CS, Valadka AB, Hannay HJ, *et al.* (1999) Prevention of secondary ischemic insults after severe head injury. *Critical Care Medicine* 27: 2086–2095.

Sosin D, Sniezek J, and Waxweiler R (1995) Trends in death associated with traumatic brain injury. *Journal of the American Medical Association* 273: 1778–1780.

Stiefel MF, Spiotta A, Gracias VH, et al. (2005) Reduced mortality rate in patients with severe traumatic brain injury treated with brain tissue oxygen monitoring. *Journal of Neurosurgery* 103: 805–811.

Stocchetti N, Furlan A, and Volta F (1996) Hypoxemia and arterial hypotension at the accident scene in head injury. *Journal of Trauma* 40: 764–767.

Unterberg AW, Stover J, Kress B, et al. (2004) Edema and brain trauma. *Neuroscience* 129: 1021–1029.

Further Reading

Anonymous (2000) Early indicators of prognosis in severe traumatic brain injury. *Journal of Neurotrauma* 17: 535–627.

Bardt TF, Unterberg AW, Hartl R, et al. (1998) Monitoring of brain tissue PO$_2$ in traumatic brain injury: effect of cerebral hypoxia on outcome. *Acta Neurochirurgica Supplement* 71: 153–156.

Cohen J, Montero A, and Israel Z (1996) Prognosis and clinical relevance of anisocoria-craniotomy latency for epidural hematoma in comatose patients. *Journal of Trauma* 41: 120–122.

Hartl R, Ghajar J, Hochleuthner H, et al. (1997) Hypertonic/hyperoncotic saline reliably reduces ICP in severely head-injured patients with intracranial hypertension. *Acta Neurochirurgica Supplement (Wien)* 70: 126–129.

Haselsberger K, Pucher R, and Auer L (1988) Prognosis after acute subdural or epidural haemorrhage. *Acta Neurochirurgica Supplement (Wien)* 90: 111–116.

Horn P, Munch E, Vajkoczy P, et al. (1999) Hypertonic saline solution for control of elevated intracranial pressure in patients with exhausted response to mannitol and barbiturates. *Neurological Research* 21: 758–764.

Lee E, Hung Y, Wang L, et al. (1998) Factors influencing the functional outcome of patients with acute epidural hematomas: Analysis of 200 patients undergoing surgery. *Journal of Trauma* 45: 946–952.

Munar F, Ferrer AM, de Nadal M, et al. (2000) Cerebral hemodynamic effects of 7.2% hypertonic saline in patients with head injury and raised intracranial pressure. *Journal of Neurotrauma* 17: 41–51.

Qureshi AI, Suarez JI, Bhardwaj A, et al. (1998) Use of hypertonic (3%) saline/acetate infusion in the treatment of cerebral edema: Effect on intracranial pressure and lateral displacement of the brain. *Critical Care Medicine* 26: 440–446.

Qureshi AI, Suarez JI, Castro A, et al. (1999) Use of hypertonic saline/acetate infusion in treatment of cerebral edema in patients with head trauma: Experience at a single center. *Journal of Trauma* 47: 659–665.

Sakas D, Bullock M, and Teasdale G (1995) One-year outcome following craniotomy for traumatic hematoma in patients with fixed dilated pupils. *Journal of Neurosurgery* 82: 961–965.

Schatzmann C, Heissler HE, Konig K, et al. (1998) Treatment of elevated intracranial pressure by infusions of 10% saline in severely head injured patients. *Acta Neurochirurgica Supplement (Wien)* 71: 31–33.

Shackford SR, Bourguignon PR, Wald SL, et al. (1998) Hypertonic saline resuscitation of patients with head injury: A prospective, randomized clinical trial. *Journal of Trauma* 44: 50–58.

Valadka AB, Gopinath SP, Contant CF, et al. (1998) Relationship of brain tissue PO$_2$ to outcome after severe head injury. *Critical Care Medicine* 26: 1576–1581.

Van den Brink WA, van Santbrink H, Steyerberg EW, et al. (2000) Brain oxygen tension in severe head injury. *Neurosurgery* 46: 868–876; discussion 876–878.

Vialet R, Albanese J, Thomachot L, et al. (2003) Isovolume hypertonic solutes (sodium chloride or mannitol) in the treatment of refractory posttraumatic intracranial hypertension: 2 mL/kg 7.5% saline is more effective than 2 mL/kg 20% mannitol. *Critical Care Medicine* 31: 1683–1687.

Wilberger JJ, Harris M, and Diamond D (1990) Acute subdural hematoma: Morbidity and mortality related to timing of operative intervention. *Journal of Trauma* 30: 733–736.

Hearing Disorders

R Burkard, University at Buffalo, Buffalo, NY, USA

Introduction

Humans need their auditory system for communication. In those born without adequate hearing, speech and language will not fully develop unless the hearing loss is identified early and proper intervention is initiated in a timely manner. In adults, the development of a hearing loss can cause significant communication difficulty, which appears to be especially problematic in a noisy environment. In this article, we discuss hearing and hearing loss. Topics range from physics (acoustics) through biology (anatomy and physiology) and pathophysiology (hearing loss) to (re)habilitation (treatment).

Hearing Health-Care Professionals

Audiologists

Audiologists are nonmedical clinicians who evaluate hearing, fit hearing aids and other devices, and perform aural (re)habilitation. The entry-level clinical degree for this specialization in the United States is presently a doctorate, in many instances a specialized degree called an audiology doctorate (AuD), but often other doctoral degrees, including the PhD, the ScD, or the EdD. Specific requirements for the practice of clinical audiology differ in different countries.

Otolaryngologists

Otolaryngologists are medical/surgical specialists who treat medical conditions affecting the ear. In the United States, board certification in Otolaryngology requires a medical degree (MD or doctor of osteopathy, DO) and a residency in otolaryngology. Some otolaryngologists do a fellowship in otology to specialize in the ear, and others specialize in ear/brain disorders, completing a neuro-otology fellowship. While specific details of certification no doubt differ across countries, in all cases clinical practice requires a medical degree and specialty training in otolaryngology.

Anatomy and Physiology of Hearing

The ear is a remarkably complex structure. Entire textbooks are devoted to this topic (e.g., Pickles, 1988), and herein we can provide only the most superficial of descriptions.

The Outer Ear

The outer ear is the portion of the ear that can be seen by casual inspection. It consists of the pinna (what we generally call the 'ear'), which is attached to a bowl-shaped structure called the concha. The concha ends at the ear canal, most correctly called the external auditory meatus. The ear canal ends at the eardrum (the tympanic membrane), which serves as the boundary between the outer and middle ears. The outer ear amplifies the level of some sounds due to its physical properties. Having two ears (one at each side of the head) means that sounds arriving at the ears may differ in level or timing – cues used by the brain to determine where the sound is coming from.

The Middle Ear

The middle ear includes the tympanic membrane, three small bones (called ossicles), and several small muscles (and tendons). The three ossicles (from lateral to medial) are the malleus, the incus, and the stapes. The malleus is connected to the eardrum laterally, and it articulates medially with the incus. The incus connects with the stapes, and the small stapes footplate inserts into the inner ear at the oval window. The eustachian tube connects the middle-ear space to the back of the throat, and when working correctly, it allows for pressure equalization across the eardrum. The main purpose of the middle ear is to maximize the flow of sound energy between the air medium in the outer ear and the fluid medium of the inner ear, and it converts the acoustical energy in the outer ear into mechanical energy. The maximization of energy flow into the inner ear is achieved by several mechanisms, including the area ratio of the eardrum versus the stapes footplate, which amplifies the pressure at the stapes footplate, as well as a lever ratio due to the length of the malleus versus that of the incus. These factors offset the loss of energy that occurs when sound crosses from air to fluid, which would reflect most of the sound energy if the middle ear were not present. The two muscles in the middle ear are the tensor tympani and the stapedius – the latter contracts in humans in response to loud sounds, producing the acoustic (or stapedial) reflex, which helps protect the ear from noise damage, and this reflex can be used to identify various disorders of hearing.

The Inner Ear

The inner ear is a complex and delicate organ housed in the temporal bone of the skull. The inner ear is a lot like a Tootsie Pop – crunchy on the outside, chewy on the inside. Its crunchy outer shell is called the bony labyrinth and contains both the end organ of hearing (the cochlea) and the five end organs of vestibular function (the three semicircular canals, the saccule, and the utricle). This article discusses only the chewy inside, the cochlea. The cochlea is composed of three fluid-filled chambers: The scala vestibuli, the scala media, and the scala tympani. The scala tympani and vestibuli are connected at the helicotrema and contain a fluid called perilymph, which is like extracellular fluid – an ultrafiltrate of blood, being high in sodium content and low in potassium content. In contrast, the scala media contains endolymph, which has the ionic content of intracellular fluid and is high in potassium and low in sodium. This unique ionic content of the scala media is due to the ionic pump of the stria vascularis, a highly vascularized organ at the lateral wall of the scala media. Two membranes form the upper and lower boundaries of the scala media, Reissner's membrane and the basilar membrane. Sitting on the basilar membrane is the organ of Corti. Specialized cells, called inner and outer hair cells, sit on top of support cells that rest on the basilar membrane. The stereocilia (hairlike structures on the apical end, or the top, of inner and outer hair cells) that protrude from the top of the hair cells are covered by the tectorial membrane. When the basilar membrane vibrates in response to sound, the vibration creates a shearing action at the top of the hair cells, leading to a bending of the stereocilia. This bending, in turn, opens up ion channels that cause excitation (depolarization) of the hair cell, which results in a release of neurotransmitter at the base of the hair cells, which leads to excitation of the auditory nerve fibers that innervate the base of the hair cells. Thus, the hair cells of the inner ear convert (i.e., transduce) mechanical energy into electrical energy. The cochlea also performs a frequency analysis of incoming sound. The portion of the cochlea close to the stapes footplate, called the base, is sensitive to high-frequency (high-pitch) sounds, whereas the portion of the cochlea far away from the stapes (called the apex) is sensitive to low-frequency (low-pitch) sounds. The pattern of hearing loss can often tell us where damage has occurred in the inner ear.

The Central Auditory Nervous System

Ultimately, the organ of hearing is the brain, not the ear, as we cannot actually perceive sound if we don't have a brain. The central auditory nervous system begins with the auditory nerve fibers that innervate the hair cells. These fibers converge inside the cochlea as a portion of the eighth cranial nerve (vestibular fibers form the rest of the eighth cranial nerve). The eighth cranial nerve projects to the lateral aspect of the pontomedullary junction (the region in the part of the brain called the brainstem, where the medulla oblongata and the pons adjoin), projecting to the first nucleus of the brain that responds to sound: the cochlear nucleus. From here, fibers from the cochlear nuclei on both sides of the brain project to the superior olivary complex, then to the inferior colliculus via the lateral lemniscus. Fibers from the inferior colliculus project to the primary thalamic nucleus of hearing, the medial geniculate body, and from there to primary auditory cortex in the temporal lobe. The auditory nerve and central portions of the auditory system contribute to the generation of auditory evoked potentials (AEPs), which are electrical responses to sound that can be recorded with noninvasive (e.g., surface) electrodes. Several AEPs are useful for site-of-lesion testing and intraoperative monitoring (i.e., monitoring sensory and/or motor function during surgical procedures that put a sensory or motor or brain system at risk, with the goal of reducing the incidence and severity of systemic damage; see the section titled 'Special and Advanced Tests'), which specifically includes electrocochleography (EcochG; recording of AEPs detected by an electrode near the inner ear to monitor specific electrical responses that arise from the inner ear and the auditory nerve) and auditory brainstem response (ABR). AEPs (including EcochG and ABR) can be used to measure hearing threshold. The acoustic reflex is also useful for site-of-lesion testing. This reflex is mediated by a pathway that includes the cochlea, auditory portion of the eighth cranial, cochlear nucleus, superior olivary complex, motor nucleus of the seventh cranial (facial) nerve, motor division of the seventh nerve, and stapedius muscle.

Measurement of Hearing

Why Measure Hearing?

Trauma, noise, various drugs, and numerous genetic and disease entities can cause hearing loss. When a patient with a hearing loss comes into a clinic, a hearing evaluation is performed to determine where in the auditory system the loss is occurring (i.e., the site of lesion). Batteries of tests are often needed to successfully determine the site of lesion. Some of these tests are not specifically tests of hearing and include a detailed case history, perhaps some blood tests, and in some instances imaging evaluations.

Medical or surgical interventions for hearing loss are often a double-edged sword – they can (and it is hoped they most often do) improve hearing, but in some cases they can and do impair hearing further. As practitioners in the helping professions may periodically be sued, documentation of baseline hearing function is necessary to document improvement, as well as for medicolegal purposes. It should also be noted that hearing loss can result from treatment of problems unrelated to hearing,

such as aminoglycoside usage for bacterial infections and radiation and use of platinum-based chemotherapy agents for the treatment of various types of cancer.

Finally, much of human communication occurs along the oral–aural route (speech and hearing), and hearing loss may not only have health implications but may also lead to communication problems. If an infant is born with a substantial hearing loss (or if hearing loss develops shortly after birth), it may produce a substantial delay in, or even a complete failure to develop, oral–aural communication. For this reason most states in the United States have implemented universal newborn hearing screening programs. It is clear that identification of hearing loss early in life, followed by appropriate intervention, can greatly reduce the communication deficits resulting from hearing loss.

Acoustics 101

As a sensory system, hearing is typically tested by presentation of a sound and evaluation of the response of the auditory system. This response could be a mechanical response (in the case of some acoustic impedance testing), an electrical response (in the case of AEPs), a voluntary motor response (as in the case of behavioral audiometry, in which patients push a button or raise their hand when they hear the sound), or a reflexive motor response (such as the acoustic reflex). In all these cases, the response has meaning only if the health professional has a rather detailed knowledge of the stimulus, that is, the physics of sound.

There are really three aspects of sound: (1) its frequency content, (2) its amplitude, and (3) its temporal pattern. The simplest sound, and the basis for the audiogram, is the sinusoid, also called a sine wave or a pure tone. The sine wave has energy at only one frequency. Frequency is defined in terms of how many times it vibrates in 1 s. The unit of vibration is the Hertz (Hz), and a vibrator that oscillates back and forth 1000 times in 1 s vibrates at 1000 Hz. Sometimes the unit is the kilohertz (kHz), which is 1000 vibrations per second. Thus, 1000 Hz is 1 kHz. In general, as a sine wave's frequency increases, its pitch increases. The amplitude of a sound can be reported in a number of different units, such as sound power, sound intensity, or sound pressure. For clinical purposes, sound pressure is used most often. Pressure is force per unit area: In the metric system, the unit of pressure is the pascal (Pa); 1 Pa is defined at 1 newton (force) per square meter (area). The range of sound pressures from the lowest sound level that humans can barely hear, to the sound level that causes pain, can exceed six or seven orders of magnitude (1 000 000–10 000 000 times). To make the units more user friendly (and because human sensory systems are typically ratio-based), sound pressure is typically expressed as a ratio (the numerator is the pressure of interest, and the denominator is a value historically chosen to be close to human threshold: 0.000 02 Pa). This ratio is then converted to a decibel (dB) value by taking 20 times its base 10 logarithm. These units are called decibels of sound pressure level (dB SPL). In this way, a pressure range of 10 000 000 is converted to 140 dB. Lower dB values reflect lower sound pressures.

The time pattern of a stimulus is another way that sound can be manipulated. For example, instead of a tone's being turned on continuously, it can be turned on and off, with, for example, a 1-s on time and a 1-s off time.

Pure-Tone Audiogram

A pure-tone audiogram plots the threshold of hearing over frequency (see **Figure 1**). The audiogram is usually obtained using a device called an audiometer. A pure-tone audiometer allows the practitioner to change the frequency of the sinusoid, change stimulus level (usually in 5-dB steps), route the sound to different transducers (earphone, maybe a bone vibrator, discussed later, or speakers), and to turn the signal on and off. Thresholds are usually obtained in octave intervals (with a few near-half-octave frequencies) between 125 Hz and 8000 Hz. As an octave is a doubling, the tested frequencies at octave intervals include 125, 250, 500, 1000, 2000, 4000, and 8000 Hz. In many audiometers, frequencies are also available that are close to half-octave intervals and often include: 750, 1500, 3000, and 6000 Hz. Threshold is usually determined as the lowest level at which the patient can hear some criterion proportion (e.g., half or more) of presentations. The sound-level axis (y-axis) is plotted in dB hearing level (dB HL), rather than dB SPL. A measure of 0 dB HL represents the average threshold of a group of

normal-hearing listeners for that frequency and for a specific earphone and measurement system. To calibrate an audiometer and an earphone in order to determine dB HL, a coupler (an artificial ear), a microphone, and a sound level meter may be used to measure the dB SPL for each frequency at a given dB setting. The dB SPL that corresponds to the average hearing threshold of a group of normal-hearing listeners at each frequency represents the 0 dB HL value. Fortunately, the American National Standards Institute and international groups such as the International Electrotechnical Commission and the International Standards Organization publish and periodically update standard corresponding values of dB SPL and dB HL.

Figure 1 also shows that there are different symbols for different transducers. Practitioners almost always test each ear individually with an earphone and use the symbols O and X for the unmasked right and left ears, respectively. Sometimes sound called a masking noise is presented to the opposite ear to prevent sound from crossing over from the test ear to the nontest ear, and different symbols are used when masking noise is presented to the opposite ear (Δ and □ , for right and left ear, respectively). To bypass the outer and middle ear, in cases when a conductive hearing loss is suspected, a bone vibrator is placed on the mastoid (the bone behind the ear) or the forehead. This mode of testing is called bone conduction. Masking, or introducing an acoustical signal (such as a noise) in the nontest ear to prevent the patient's hearing (and thus responding to) the test stimulus in the nontest ear, can be particularly important when bone conduction is used. For right and left mastoid bone conduction without masking, the symbols used

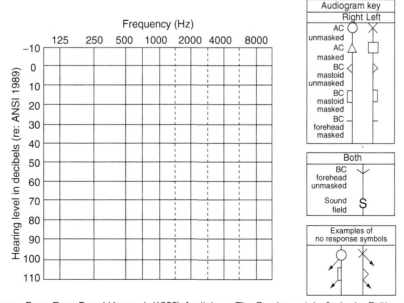

Figure 1 The audiogram. From Bess F and Humes L (1995) *Audiology: The Fundamentals*, 2nd edn. Baltimore, MD: Williams and Wilkins.

are < and >, respectively; with masking, the symbols are [and], respectively. The pattern of audiometric threshold, for both ears, across frequency, and for air versus bone conduction, not only portrays the magnitude of hearing loss but also provides valuable site-of-lesion information. Thresholds up to 25 dB HL are considered normal. Thresholds ranging from 25 to 40 dB HL are considered mild hearing loss, and thresholds ranging from 40 to 55 dB HL are labeled moderate hearing loss. 'Moderate-severe hearing loss' is the label for thresholds ranging from 55 to 70 dB HL, and a severe hearing loss encompasses the range of 70–90 dB HL. Finally, thresholds greater than 90 dB HL are labeled a profound hearing loss, and people with thresholds exceeding 90 dB HL across frequency are considered legally deaf.

Speech Tests

Two types of speech test are used in everyday clinical evaluation of hearing loss. The first is the speech recognition threshold, which evaluates the lowest level of a speech signal at which an individual can accurately repeat roughly half of the speech stimuli. In many clinics, these tests use two-syllable words with equal stress on each syllable (called spondees). The speech recognition threshold should numerically agree with either the average threshold of 500, 1000, and 2000 Hz, or the best threshold of these three, should the hearing loss vary substantially across this frequency range.

The other common test is called speech discrimination, which (most typically) presents single-syllable stimuli at a comfortable listening level. Speech discrimination is reported as a percentage correct. Normal-hearing listeners show a very high percentage correct (in the mid-90s or above). With progressively greater magnitudes of hearing loss, the expected speech discrimination score decreases. Unusually low speech discrimination scores for a given hearing loss might indicate a retrocochlear problem (see the section titled 'Neural or Retrocochlear Hearing Loss'), whereas a very good speech discrimination score in the presence of a substantial hearing loss might indicate that the patient's reported hearing loss is exaggerated.

Acoustic Impedance

One type of hearing loss, a conductive loss (see the section titled 'Conductive hearing loss'), is produced by a reduction in sound energy reaching the inner ear. This reduction in sound energy can occur in either the outer or the middle ear, or both. While some causes of conductive loss can be seen by casual inspection of the outer ear (e.g., atresia of the external auditory meatus, or ear canal, in which blockage of the ear canal results from incomplete development of the outer ear) or by looking into the ear canal with an otoscope (a small, hand-held device with a speculum and light source for illuminating and viewing the ear canal and ear drum and which can reveal a hole in the tympanic membrane), it is often not possible to identify conductive losses, especially those originating in the middle ear, by such inspection. Measures of acoustic impedance, a complex mathematical construct that refers to the opposition to the flow of acoustic energy, can identify a number of causes of conductive hearing loss. A tympanogram is a measure of the transfer of sound energy through the middle ear as one varies the resting pressure in the ear canal. In this procedure, a probe encased in a compliant, disposable probe tip is placed snugly into the ear canal. Once an airtight seal is achieved, a (typically) low-frequency tone is presented through an earphone in the probe tip, and the sound pressure in the ear canal is monitored via a microphone also located in the probe tip. Some fairly simple mathematical calculations yield the acoustic impedance (the opposition to the flow of energy), acoustic admittance (the inverse of acoustic impedance), or real and imaginary components of impedance or admittance. A manometer is used to change the air pressure in the ear canal, and the acoustic impedance or admittance is plotted across air pressure of the ear canal. Some typical tympanograms are shown in **Figure 2**. Whether there is a peak in the tympanogram, where that peak is, and how high or shallow the peak is all provide information about the nature of the conductive hearing loss. A normal response is shown in **Figure 2(a)**; note that this tympanogram has a peak at or near ambient air pressure. This contrasts with **Figure 2(b)**, which has a peak at a negative pressure (in this case, −200 daPa). A flat tympanogram is shown in **Figure 2(c)**. This can be caused by fluid in the middle ear (called otitis media). **Figures 2(d)** and **2(e)** have peaks near ambient pressure, but the peaks are either abnormally shallow (**Figure 2(d)**) or too deep (**Figure 2(e)**). A shallow tympanogram can be caused by a disorder called otosclerosis, in which a bony growth on the ossicles leads to a stiffening of the middle-ear system. A deep tympanogram can be produced either by a healed perforation of the eardrum or by a break in the ossicles (called an ossicular disruption), which is often caused by head trauma. Additional information can be gleaned by varying the frequency of the probe tone. Multifrequency tympanometry is well beyond the scope of this article, and the interested reader is referred to Fowler and Shanks (2002).

Another common use of acoustic impedance measures is to obtain the acoustic reflex. In response to a suitably intense sound, the stapedius muscle (which is attached to the stapes) contracts, stiffening up the middle-ear and increasing the acoustic impedance (decreasing the acoustic admittance) at the tympanic membrane. The acoustic reflex is a bilateral reflex (the reflex occurs in both ears with single-ear stimulation) and can be measured by recording the change in acoustic impedance or

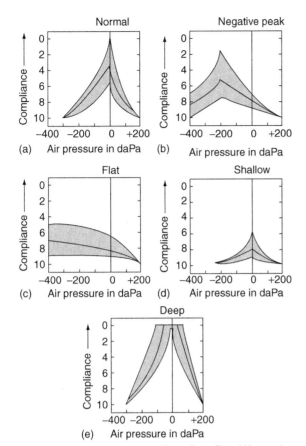

Figure 2 Tympanogram types. From Bess F and Humes L (1995) *Audiology: The Fundamentals*, 2nd edn. Baltimore, MD: Williams and Wilkins.

admittance in response to stimuli (tones or noise) to the same or the opposite ear (called the uncrossed and crossed reflex, respectively). Acoustic reflex threshold across frequency, the pattern of crossed and uncrossed responses, and numerous other variables provide important information for site-of-lesion testing, not only for problems with hearing, but also for facial nerve disorders (because the stapedius muscle is innervated by the seventh cranial, or facial, nerve).

Special and Advanced Tests

There are many special tests of hearing, and only a few of the more commonly used ones can be described in this article.

A number of years ago, it was determined that some of the cells in the inner ear, called outer hair cells, contract in response to sound (Brownell *et al.*, 1985). In one test, sounds are generated that cause the outer hair cell contractions, which can be recorded in the ear canal by a sensitive microphone. These inner-ear-produced sounds are called otoacoustic emissions (OAEs). OAEs are currently in use for newborn hearing screening and

are also useful for site-of-lesion testing (Prieve and Fitzgerald, 2002).

A number of AEPs can be recorded from near the ear or from the scalp. EcochG and ABR have the most clinical utility. EcochG is done with electrodes near the cochlea and includes several subcomponents: the summating potential (SP), the cochlear microphonic (CM), and the compound action potential (CAP). The SP and the CM represent hair cell responses, and the CAP represents the output of the auditory nerve. The CAP can be used for threshold evaluation but in the United States has largely been replaced for threshold estimation by the ABR. EcochG is very useful for intraoperative monitoring during surgery involving the eighth cranial nerve, for example, to determine whether any damage is occurring to the cochlea or auditory nerve. The ABR can be recorded with noninvasive scalp electrodes (see Burkard and Secor, 2002). It can be used to screen hearing (including newborns), to determine hearing threshold, for site-of-lesion testing, and for intraoperative monitoring of cochlear, auditory nerve, and auditory brainstem function (Don and Kwong, 2002; Martin and Mishler, 2002; Sininger and Cone-Wesson, 2002).

Disorders of Hearing

Hearing loss can be classified in a variety of ways: by whether it is unilateral (one ear) or bilateral (both ears), by its severity (mild, moderate, severe, or profound), by its configuration (whether it is equal across frequency or greater in the high or the low frequencies), and by site of lesion. The following paragraphs describe the categorizations of hearing loss that identify where in the auditory system the hearing loss has occurred.

Conductive Hearing Loss

Should a hearing loss be caused by an abnormality in the outer and/or middle ear, it is classified as a conductive loss. Audiometrically, a purely conductive hearing loss is usually at most a moderate hearing loss. For a pure conductive hearing loss, hearing by bone conduction is normal, whereas thresholds are elevated (worse) via air conduction, leading to what is commonly called an air–bone gap. Individuals with a conductive loss have very good speech discrimination abilities once the speech signal is presented at a sufficiently intense sound level. Many types of conductive hearing loss can be treated medically or surgically.

Otitis media is a very common type of conductive hearing loss in children. It can start with negative pressure in the middle ear, indicated by a tympanogram with a negative peak pressure (see **Figure 2(b)**). Fluid often fills the middle-ear space, leading to a flat tympanogram (see **Figure 2(c)**). Most children have one or more bouts of otitis media, and an 'ear infection' is a very common reason children see their physician.

Otosclerosis tends to occur in young to middle-aged adults. It involves the creation and resorption of bone in the middle ear and leads to a hearing loss when it affects the motion of the ossicles (such as fixing the stapes footplate where it inserts into the cochlea).

Sensory Hearing Loss

In the past, a sensory hearing loss was often referred to as a sensorineural hearing loss, but due to advances in site-of-lesion testing, practitioners now differentiate those losses affecting the sensory end organ (the cochlea, hence a sensory loss) from those affecting the acoustic portion of the eighth nerve (a neural loss).

Sensory loss, as indicated above, is a hearing loss that is localized to the inner ear. In those relatively common instances in which the hair cells of the inner ear are damaged, there is not only a loss of hearing sensitivity (i.e., threshold is elevated) but also a degradation in the ability to understand speech signals (i.e., a decrement in speech discrimination ability), which is often exacerbated by a noisy background. In the case of a sensory hearing loss, there is an equivalent elevation of bone-conduction threshold and air-conduction threshold and hence no air–bone gap. It is uncommon for sensory hearing loss to be reversible by medical or surgical treatment, and in most cases treatment involves counseling, amplification (a hearing aid or cochlear implant), and therapy, referred to as aural rehabilitation. In cases of noise-induced hearing loss, where the noise exposure can be reduced, it is certainly true that an ounce of prevention is worth a pound of cure.

Meniere's disease refers to a tetrad of symptoms that include a (typically) low-frequency hearing loss, episodic vertigo (a sense of spinning – see the section titled 'Dizziness and Vertigo'), roaring tinnitus (ringing in the ears, see the section titled 'Tinnitus'), and a feeling of fullness in the ear. It should be emphasized that these symptoms fluctuate over time. One well-supported theory suggests that Meniere's disease is caused by a buildup of the endolymphatic fluid in the scala media, and the condition is sometimes called endolymphatic hydrops.

Mixed Hearing Loss

A mixed hearing loss has a conductive and a sensory component. Some auditory pathologies can have a conductive and a sensory component. Similarly, there is nothing preventing a given individual from having two causes of hearing loss: one leading to a conductive hearing loss (such as otitis media) and another leading to a sensory loss (such as noise exposure). In a mixed hearing loss, there is a hearing loss via bone conduction, but there is a greater hearing loss via air conduction (and yes, in a mixed loss, there is an air–bone gap).

Neural or Retrocochlear Hearing Loss

For a neural (sometimes called a retrocochlear, for 'beyond the cochlea') hearing loss, the loss is localized beyond the cochlea, at the level of the eighth nerve or in the auditory nervous system. In many cases, a neural loss means involvement of the auditory nerve. In such cases, the most common lesion is a tumor in the eighth nerve, often incorrectly called an acoustic neuroma, and correctly called a vestibular schwannoma. Due to pressure and vascular compromise, the response of the auditory nerve is affected, leading to an audiogram that looks remarkably like a sensory loss. Hearing loss due to vestibular schwannoma can be quite mild in severity. It is in most instances unilateral, and the patient's speech discrimination ability is poorer than would be expected if the loss were sensory. Special tests (such as ABR testing, specialized acoustic reflex tests, tests of vestibular function, and imaging) are needed to identify a vestibular schwannoma. Surgery can successfully remove such a tumor, and while the vestibular nerve must be sacrificed, in some cases the auditory nerve can be saved and some level of hearing maintained in the ear.

Other types of hearing loss are thought to represent neural disorders. Auditory neuropathy or dys-synchrony (AN/AD) is thought to occur in the auditory nerve (although some argue it occurs in the inner hair cells). There is no unique audiometric configuration for patients with AN/AD; they present with grossly abnormal or missing acoustic reflexes and ABR, normal OAEs, and poor speech perception abilities, especially in noise. Central auditory processing disorder is another type of hearing loss that is thought to affect the central auditory system, although a site of lesion has not been clearly demonstrated. Those with this disorder can register perfectly normal hearing abilities on conventional audiometric tests but show complicated patterns of abnormalities in response to filtered speech and speech tests in which one speech stimulus is presented to one ear and another speech signal is presented to the opposite ear (called dichotic listening tests), as well as degraded performance on tests of temporal patterns.

Associated Disorders

Depending on the particular cause of a hearing loss, there may be accompanying problems. One common symptom associated with hearing loss is ringing in the ear, or tinnitus. Due to the close proximity of the cochlea to the vestibular end organs, some causes of hearing loss are associated with a form of dizziness known as vertigo.

Tinnitus

Tinnitus is a remarkably common problem in those with hearing loss. In a few instances, it does appear that individuals can have tinnitus without a clinically significant hearing loss. Most patients have subjective tinnitus, that is, tinnitus can be perceived only by the individual who has it. However, there are a number of causes of tinnitus in which the astute clinician can hear the tinnitus. While in many patients the tinnitus is well tolerated, a substantial portion of those suffering this malady are tormented by the phantom sound, have difficulty concentrating and sleeping, and may be depressed. Treatments such as the use of maskers to hide the tinnitus, or various behavioral therapy regimens, help some, but not all, tinnitus sufferers.

Dizziness and Vertigo

A fairly common clinical symptom of those with a vestibular end-organ disorder is dizziness. For this dizziness to be specifically related to the vestibular end organ, it must involve the sensation of the room or the patient spinning, and it is then called vertigo. Light-headedness or a sense of imbalance can be caused by disorders of the vestibular system but might also be caused by disorders of the brain and/or the vascular system.

Treatment of Some Common Hearing Disorders

Otitis media is often treated by antibiotics although it is not always the result of a bacterial infection. Another common treatment of otitis media is to surgically place polyethylene tubes into the tympanic membrane. This relieves the pressure and often the pain by allowing the fluid to drain from the middle ear.

As described above, otosclerosis is abnormal bone growth and resorption in the middle ear, which leads to a conductive hearing loss, most often by fixation of the stapes footplate into the oval window of the cochlea. Very good results are often achieved by performing a stapedectomy (removal of the stapes) and replacing the structure with a prosthesis. Trauma can lead to a disarticulation of the ossicles (an ossicular disruption), which can likewise be treated by the use of an appropriate prosthesis.

In most cases of sensory hearing loss, loss of the hair cells means the hearing loss is permanent. If a noise-induced hearing loss is identified at a fairly early stage, patients should be counseled to protect their remaining hearing. The appropriate use of hearing protection while at work or during loud recreational or home activities (e.g., hunting; riding snow mobiles; using chain saws, lawn mowers, or snow blowers) may prevent further decrements in hearing. In many cases of sensory hearing loss, the use of a hearing aid, or an assistive listening device, can help reduce the communication problems associated with a hearing loss. Counseling is an important part of fitting a patient with amplification, as the amplification makes sounds louder, not necessarily clearer, and the hearing aid (or other amplification device) is not as clever as mother nature and often cannot separate the signal of interest from background noise. When a hearing loss becomes severe enough, a hearing aid may not provide adequate help, and a cochlear implant might be needed. This is literally an electronic ear, in which sound is processed and routed to an array of electrodes placed inside the cochlea, and the electrodes directly stimulate auditory nerve fibers. Cochlear implants can be implanted in patients at virtually any age (from infants through geriatrics), and many individuals have great success with them.

Meniere's disease, as described already, is a hearing disorder that includes fluctuating (often low-frequency) hearing loss, roaring tinnitus, a feeling of fullness in the ear, and episodic vertigo. This disorder (in particular, the episodic vertigo) can be very traumatizing to the patient, and myriad treatments have been used: a low-salt diet, endolymphatic shunt surgery (whereby endolymph is routed out of the scala media by a shunt), destruction of the inner ear (by aminoglycoside administration or surgical intervention), and section of the vestibular nerve. Each of these approaches (and others) has (or has had) its proponents.

The vestibular schwannoma is a benign tumor and in most cases grows quite slowly. The problem is that as it grows, it compresses the nerve and/or the blood supply. As it in most if not all cases arises from either the inferior or the superior vestibular nerve inside the internal auditory meatus, the symptoms experienced by the patients might reflect dysfunction of the vestibular system (e.g., dizziness or a sense of imbalance), the auditory system (hearing loss, tinnitus), or the facial nerve (unilateral facial muscle weakness or abnormal taste sensation). As the tumor enlarges, it can distend the lateral brainstem, and myriad other neurologic symptoms may be manifested. In many cases, removal of the tumor is the treatment of choice. During surgery, the vestibular nerve is sacrificed, but because the vestibular system on the opposite side is intact, a full recovery of balance function is likely. The auditory nerve is often sacrificed but can sometimes be saved if the tumor is small enough. A complete unilateral section of the auditory nerve leads to unilateral deafness. A hearing aid or cochlear implant is useless for such a nerve section, but brainstem implants are under development that may offer hope. While unilateral deafness might cause some difficulties in localizing sounds or understanding speech in noise, in most cases there is good functional hearing ability via the remaining ear. However, in neurofibromatosis type II, bilateral eighth nerve tumors can develop, and if tumors must be removed bilaterally, postsurgically the patient is not only bilaterally deaf (and in serious need of the brainstem implants under development) but also has absent vestibular function bilaterally.

Incidence of Hearing Loss

Davis (1998) reported that for births occurring between 1985 and 1990 in England, the prevalence of significant permanent hearing loss ($\geq$40 dB HL) was 133 per 100 000 live births (~0.13%), while 24 per 100 000 live births (0.024%) are deaf ($\geq$95 dB HL).

In early life, a very common cause of (conductive) hearing loss is otitis media. This is a middle ear infection in which fluid (which might be sterile fluid or might have a high bacterial count) builds up in the middle ear. The child may or may not have a fever but will often be irritable, as the condition can be quite painful. It has been estimated that up to 90% of all infants have at least one bout of otitis media during the first 6 years of life (Meyerhoff *et al.*, 1997).

As humans age, the incidence of hearing loss increases. Age-related hearing loss is typically sensory, and age-related sensory hearing loss is called presbycusis. The prevalence of presbycusis increases with advancing age; it is estimated that 30–35% of those age 65–75 years have age-related hearing loss, and this increases to 40% of those older than 75 years (McFadden, 2001).

Summary

Audiologists and otolaryngologists are two professionals who are involved in both the diagnosis and treatment of hearing loss. To understand hearing and hearing loss, one must have a firm grasp of the anatomy and physiology of the auditory system, as well as the physical aspects of sound (acoustics). Hearing is measured in many ways: by the lowest level at which tones of varying frequency can be heard (a pure-tone audiogram), by measures of threshold and understanding of speech presented above threshold (speech recognition and speech discrimination tests), by measures of the amount of sound that is reflected off the eardrum (tympanometry and acoustic reflex testing), and a multitude of more-specialized tests. Hearing loss is quantified by not only its severity (e.g., mild, moderate, severe), but by configuration (e.g., equal across frequency, greater in the higher frequencies), whether it involves one or both ears, and site of lesion (conductive, sensory, mixed, retrocochlear). There are many causes of hearing loss. In some instances (such as conductive hearing loss), the hearing loss is medically treatable, while in other instances, assistive devices (hearing aids, cochlear implants), combined with various counseling or (re)habilitation approaches, are required.

Citations

Brownell W, Bader C, Betrand D, and de Ribaupierre Y (1985) Evoked mechanical responses of isolated cochlear outer hair cells. *Science* 227: 194–196.

Burkard R and Secor C (2002) Overview of auditory evoked potentials. In: Katz J (ed.) *Handbook of Clinical Audiology*, 5th edn., pp. 233–248. Baltimore, MD: Lippincott, Williams and Wilkins.

Davis A (1998) Epidemiology of hearing impairment. In: Ludman H and Wright T (eds.) *Diseases of the Ear*, 6th edn., pp. 129–137. London: Arnold.

Don M and Kwong B (2002) Auditory brainstem response: Differential diagnosis. In: Katz J (ed.) *Handbook of Clinical Audiology*, 5th edn., pp. 274–297. Baltimore, MD: Lippincott, Williams and Wilkins.

Fowler C and Shanks J (2002) Tympanometry. In: Katz J (ed.) *Handbook of Clinical Audiology*, 5th edn., pp. 175–204. Baltimore, MD: Lippincott, Williams and Wilkins.

Martin W and Mishler T (2002) Intraoperative monitoring of auditory evoked potentials and facial nerve electromyography. In: Katz J (ed.) *Handbook of Clinical Audiology*, 5th edn., pp. 323–348. Baltimore, Lippincott: Williams and Wilkins.

McFadden S (2001) Genetics and age-related hearing loss. In: Hof P and Mobbs C (eds.) *Functional Neurobiology of Aging*, pp. 597–603. New York: Academic.

Meyerhoff W, Marple B, and Roland P (1997) Tympanic membrane, middle ear, and mastoid. In: Ludman H and Wright T (eds.) *Diseases of the Ear*, 6th edn., pp. 155–194. London: Arnold.

Pickles J (1988) *An Introduction to the Physiology of Hearing*, 2nd edn. London: Academic.

Prieve B and Fitzgerald T (2002) Otoacoustic emissions. In: Katz J (ed.) *Handbook of Clinical Audiology*, 5th edn., pp. 440–466. Baltimore, MD: Lippincott, Williams and Wilkins.

Sininger Y and Cone-Wesson B (2002) Threshold prediction using auditory brainstem response and steady-state evoked potentials with infants and young children. In: Katz J (ed.) *Handbook of Clinical Audiology*, 5th edn., pp. 298–322. Baltimore, MD: Lippincott, Williams and Wilkins.

Further Reading

Berlin C (1998) *Otoacoustic Emissions: Basic Science and Clinical Applications*. San Diego, CA: Singular.

Desmond A (2004) *Vestibular Function: Evaluation and Treatment*. New York: Thieme.

Hood L (1998) *Clinical Applications of the Auditory Brainstem Response*. San Diego, CA: Singular.

Katz J (2002) *The Handbook of Clinical Audiology*, 5th edn. Baltimore, MD: Lippincott, Williams and Wilkins.

Ludman H and Wright T (1998) *Diseases of the Ear*, 6th edn. London: Arnold.

Sininger Y and Starr A (2001) *Auditory Neuropathy: A New Perspective on Hearing Disorders*. San Diego, CA: Singular.

Snow J (2004) *Tinnitus: Theory and Management*. Hamilton, Ontario: Decker.

Speaks C (1996) *Introduction to Sound: Acoustics for the Hearing and Speech Sciences*, 2nd edn. San Diego, CA: Singular.

Yost W (2000) *Fundamentals of Hearing: An Introduction*, 4th edn. New York: Academic.

Relevant Websites

http://www.asha.org/default.htm – American Speech-Language-Hearing Association.

http://www.ata.org/ – American Tinnitus Association (ATA).

http://www.shhh.org/ – Hearing Loss Association of America (formerly called Self Help for the Hard of Hearing).

http://www.nidcd.nih.gov/ – National Institute of Deafness and Communicative Disorders.

http://www.nia.nih.gov/ – National Institute on Aging.

http://www.vestibular.org/ – Vestibular Disorders Association.

HIV/AIDS of the Central Nervous System

S S Spudich, University of California at San Francisco, San Francisco, CA, USA

Introduction

Neurological disorders have been a leading cause of morbidity associated with HIV and the immunosuppression characterizing AIDS since early in the disease epidemic. HIV-associated neurological disorders may affect any portion of the neuroaxis, manifesting as disorders of the brain, spinal cord, peripheral nerve, and muscle. The etiologies of neurological disease in this setting include opportunistic and other comorbid infections, malignancies, vascular disorders, nutritional diseases, and direct infection with HIV-1 itself. Neurological diseases affecting either the central or peripheral nervous system occur in the majority of infected individuals and are the initial presenting illnesses of AIDS in 7–20% of patients. Neurological disorders in the context of HIV infection are associated with increased expenses related to medical care and increased mortality compared to patients without nervous system complications, and lead to impairment ranging from painful extremities or mild cognitive difficulties to frank dementia or coma and death. Thus, the public health burden of HIV-related neurological diseases is extremely high, though the importance of these relative to other complications of HIV/AIDS varies depending on geographic and medical setting.

Although the frequency of severe neurological disorders has declined dramatically in settings where highly active antiretroviral therapy (HAART) and prophylactic anti-infective agents are in common widespread use, the spectrum of neurological disorders afflicting patients who progress to severe immunodeficiency has remained constant through the course of the epidemic, with diversity depending on geographic and demographic factors. In the setting of HAART use, new clinical syndromes have developed, related specifically to the robust but abnormally regulated inflammatory reaction seen in the context of reconstitution of the immune response. Consequently, though clinicians are used to a certain spectrum of neurological conditions – many of which are treatable – in the context of HIV/AIDS, diagnosis in any particular case may be challenging and complex. Diagnosis and appropriate treatment of these disorders depends on understanding the main predisposing factors to each condition and the presentation of disease in each segment of the nervous system. A discussion of the most common disorders affecting the central nervous system (CNS) in HIV-infected patients is presented below.

Stages of Neurological Complications of HIV

As outlined in **Figure 1**, distinct neurological diseases occur at different stages of infection with HIV. During the earliest phases of infection, approximately 2 weeks after exposure to virus, the majority of patients experience systemic signs and symptoms of fever, rash, headache, and lymphadenopathy. In a subgroup of these patients, such systemic symptoms may be followed within 2–4 weeks by disorders involving the nervous system, including meningitis, encephalitis, focal cranial nerve palsy, or sensory or motor symptoms of acute peripheral neuropathy. These syndromes are usually self-limited and resolve without specific therapy. The first 7–10 years after infection are usually a period of relative clinical latency in terms of overt disease. The predominant neurological conditions that may present during this period include peripheral neuropathy, inflammatory demyelinating neuropathies, mononeuritis multiplex, myopathies, and episodes of aseptic meningitis. These conditions and those that occur during the period of acute infection are thought to be autoimmune-mediated in the setting of an aberrant systemic immune response. During the late stages of HIV infection in the setting of declining systemic immunity, patients develop more debilitating and morbid complications relating either to HIV infection itself or to opportunistic infections, which are conditions related to suppressed immunity. Both focal brain lesions that present difficulty with specific neurological functions and diffuse brain involvement leading to cognitive and motor difficulties present during this time. The specific diagnosis of each of these conditions depends on typical signs and symptoms as well as clinical and demographic parameters. Many serious central nervous system complications of HIV and AIDS may be reversed or treated with appropriate therapy, either pathogen-specific therapy or with the immune reconstitution that can occur with institution of antiretroviral therapy.

Focal Brain Diseases

Patients harboring a focus of tumor, infection, or demyelination present with focal brain dysfunction referable to the cerebral location of the lesion, such as difficulty moving one side of the body (hemiparesis), inability to see a part of the visual world (hemi- or quadrantanopsia), poor comprehension or production of language (aphasia), or incoordination of an extremity (ataxia). Often, more than one focal lesion affecting distinct brain structures may confound attempts at localization or appear as a more diffuse brain disorder (see 'Diffuse Brain Diseases' section). Among the focal brain disorders afflicting individuals in the developed world with AIDS, cerebral toxoplasmosis, primary central nervous system lymphoma (PCNSL), and progressive multifocal leukoencephalopathy (PML) are most common. Where *Mycobacterium tuberculosis* is endemic (Asia, Africa, Central and South America), cerebral complications of tuberculosis are another major etiology of focal lesions. Less common focal brain lesions in patients with advanced immunosuppression include infectious abscesses due to *Staphylococcus* and *Streptococcus* species, nocardia, cytomegalovirus, *Aspergillus*, mucor, *Candida*, or amoeba. Noninfectious focal lesions include glioma, ischemic stroke, and hemorrhagic stroke. The more uncommon brain lesions are usually diagnosed either in the setting of extraneural infection (e.g., pulmonary cavitary fungal lesions or septicemia) or through the use of brain biopsy, a procedure with low morbidity when appropriately performed.

The majority of common focal brain lesions in patients with AIDS cause an expansion of tissue with surrounding swelling. These most commonly include cerebral toxoplasmosis and PCNSL in developed countries, and tuberculosis in many areas of the resource-limited world. Focal brain lesions that cause no expansion of tissue are most commonly attributable to progressive multifocal leukoencephalopathy (PML) in the setting of JC virus infection in the central nervous system. **Table 1** summarizes the typical clinical features of focal neurological disorders seen in HIV.

Cerebral Toxoplasmosis

Focal encephalitis/abscesses occurring in the context of reactivation of infection with the parasite *Toxoplasma gondii* have historically been the most common cause of focal central nervous system lesions in patients with AIDS in the developed world. Approximately 33% of patients with advanced immunosuppression (CD4 counts <200 cells/μl) who are not on antitoxoplasma prophylaxis will develop toxoplasma encephalitis at

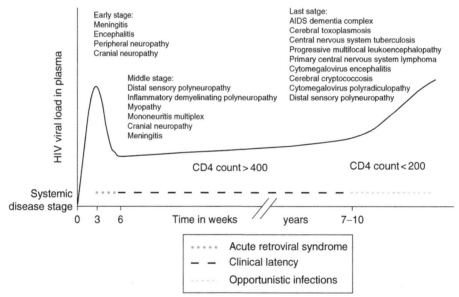

Figure 1   Diseases of the central and peripheral nervous system associated with different stages of HIV infection. CD4 count refers to CD4+ T lymphocytes in cells/mm³.

Table 1   Clinical features of focal brain lesions in AIDS

	Temporal progression	Level of alertness	Fever	Typical symptoms
Cerebral toxoplasmosis	Days	Reduced	Possible	Severe headache, any focal deficit
Primary CNS lymphoma	Days/weeks	Variable	Absent	Moderate headache, any focal deficit
Progressive multifocal leukoencephalopathy	Week	Preserved	Absent	Painless deficit, spasticity, cortical blindness
Central nervous system tuberculosis	Weeks	Reduced	Possible	Headache, cranial nerve palsies, myelopathy
Stroke	Acute	Variable	Possible	Any focal deficit, possibly history of zoster rash

some time during their disease course, though incidence depends somewhat on the relative prevalence of seropositivity for *T. gondii*, which varies widely with geographic region (less than 10% in areas of Britain to greater than 70% in Nigeria). Though domesticated and undomesticated cats are the definitive hosts for the responsible parasite, humans usually become infected through ingestion of undercooked infected tissue of pigs or sheep, the intermediate zoonotic hosts.

Clinically, cerebral toxoplasmosis is characterized by the rapid development over days of neurological signs or symptoms in the setting of headache and low-grade fever. Since the condition is related to reactivation of latent chronic infection, IgG antibodies indicating previous exposure are present in the blood in at least 95% of patients with cerebral toxoplasmosis, although in some rare cases serology may be negative. Typically, either CT or MRI imaging shows contrast-enhancing lesions (single or multiple) involving the cortex or basal ganglia and thalamus, surrounded by extensive areas of edema, which may extend through white matter tracts, mimicking other conditions (see **Figure 2**). The contrast enhancement is typically ring enhancing around the border of the primary lesions, though there may be enhancement in the center (a target sign). Diagnosis is usually made based on the typical clinical course, presence of positive serology, and typical neuroimaging features on CT

or MRI imaging. Reliable information about adherence to potential prophylaxis against toxoplasma reactivation (trimethoprim-sulfamethoxazole is effective in preventing both *Pneumocystis carinii* pneumonia and toxoplasmosis) also helps guide diagnosis in this setting. If all of these features are consistent with potential toxoplasmosis, patients are treated with prompt initiation of induction therapy with sulfadiazine (clindamycin may be used in sulfa-intolerant patients), pyrimethamine, and folinic acid to prevent myelosuppression, then closely observed. Clinical improvement should be evident within a few days, usually first marked by the patient as improvement in headache. Radiological improvement is typically apparent within weeks. Without improvement after 2 weeks (or with continued deterioration during early therapy), alternate diagnoses should be considered.

Toxoplasmosis is perhaps the most amenable to treatment of all neurological manifestations of HIV, with the potential for lesions to macroscopically entirely resolve with little or no sequelae if there are no mechanical complications relating to transient mass effect or the rare vasculitic or hemorrhagic involvement. Patients should be treated with induction-dose therapy for 4–6 weeks after diagnosis, then continually treated with the same anti-infective medications at reduced doses for life or until the CD4 count has been over 200 cells/µl for more than 6 months in the context of complete resolution of

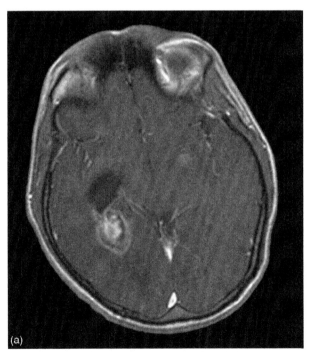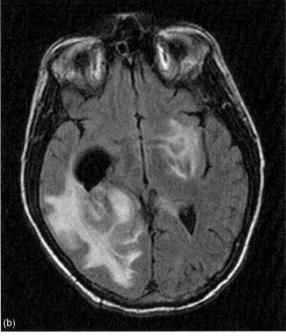

Figure 2   MRI images of a patient with cerebral toxoplasmosis. T1-weighted image with gadolinium (a) shows typical outline of the lesion with contrast on left side of image, appearing as a slightly serpiginous border around the lesion core, and a target-appearing central area of additional enhancement (enlarged dark area next to lesion represents an expanded lateral ventricle due to the lesion's blockade of cerebrospinal fluid drainage); an additional lesion enhances more diffusely in the basal ganglia on the opposite side. Fluid-attenuated inversion recovery (FLAIR) image (b) demonstrates extensive bright signal surrounding both lesions, which reflects dramatic cerebral edema extending through the white matter, typical of toxoplasmosis.

symptoms referable to cerebral toxoplasmosis. Without secondary prophylaxis, cerebral toxoplasmosis recurs in 30–50% of patients; even in the setting of chronic suppressive therapy, treatment failure occurs in up to 10%, likely in part due to inconsistent adherence.

Central Nervous System Tuberculosis

In regions of the resource-limited world where infection with *Mycobacterium tuberculosis* is endemic or epidemic, extrapulmonary – including CNS – involvement is a significant cause of morbidity and death in patients with AIDS. Though meningitis with headache, neck stiffness, and decline in the level of consciousness is the most common manifestation of CNS infection with tuberculosis (TB), focal lesions may develop in the setting of tuberculomas, intraparenchymal tubercular abscesses, and sites of vascular infection or inflammation leading to cerebral infarction. Such extrameningeal manifestations of CNS TB are common in HIV infection, and TB is the most common cause of HIV-associated focal brain lesions in parts of India and Africa.

CNS TB typically presents over weeks, with development of cranial nerve palsies, small-vessel strokes, and increased intracranial pressure, indicating a predilection for inflammatory collections in the basilar meninges and along cranial nerve sheaths. Increased intracranial pressure leads to visual compromise and optic disc swelling in many patients, and involvement of the spinal cord may result from transverse myelitis, vasculitis, or spinal tubercular abscesses. Importantly, severely immunocompromised patients may have less overt symptomatology of meningeal irritation than immunocompetent hosts. CSF may demonstrate elevations in opening pressure, white blood cell count (predominantly lymphocytes or neutrophils), and protein (usually >100 mg/dl), along with low glucose levels, but fails to manifest one or more of these findings in at least 10% of patients with AIDS. CSF acid-fast stains are only positive in 25% of specimens, and mycobacterial cultures are more sensitive but require several weeks for incubation. PCR for TB is at present the most effective diagnostic method for CNS TB available from the CSF. Neuroimaging may be nonspecific; the most common CT finding is enlargement of the cerebral ventricles (hydrocephalus), which is present in up to 80% of patients. A more distinctive thickening of the meninges, especially those adjacent to the base of the brain, marked by robust enhancement after the administration of contrast, is seen in 60% of those with CNS TB. Other findings, including focal areas of infarction, or either smoothly or ring-enhancing lesions, may also be seen in HIV-infected patients with concomitant CNS TB infection.

CNS tuberculosis often, but not always, occurs in the company of pulmonary or disseminated multiorgan infection. The approach to treatment is similar in CNS disease as for extraneural involvement, including multidrug therapy tailored to the possibility of drug-resistant organisms in relevant geographic settings. Of drugs commonly used, isoniazid and pyrazinamide typically penetrate well into the CNS, while rifampin and ethambutol do not. However, in the setting of meningeal inflammation and disruption of the blood–brain barrier, drugs may effectively enter the CNS, and the combination of these four drugs may be successful in cases where organisms are susceptible. In some cases, including TB-related overt cerebral edema in children, addition of corticosteroids may have some therapeutic benefit.

Primary Central Nervous System Lymphoma

Primary CNS lymphoma (PCNSL), the most common CNS malignancy in AIDS patients, refers to lymphoma that arises in the nervous system in the absence of systemic lymphoma. AIDS-related PCNSL is usually B cell in origin, arising in association with the oncogenic infection Epstein-Barr virus, and accounts for 15% of non-Hodgkin's lymphoma in patients with AIDS. PCNSL is one of the most common neurological AIDS-defining illnesses and will develop in 3% of patients with AIDS at some point during the course of infection. Although in the pre-HAART era, PCNSL was almost exclusively described in patients with extremely advanced immunosuppression (CD4 counts <50 cells/μl), we and others have recently seen patients with pathologically confirmed PCNSL presenting with CD4 counts in higher ranges (200–350 cells/μl), possibly reflecting more restricted immune responses in the setting of prior low CD4 nadirs.

The clinical syndrome of PCNSL may differ slightly from toxoplasma encephalitis, in that the course is slightly more indolent, usually causing recognizable signs and symptoms over the course of weeks rather than days. Systemic signs of fever, weight loss, and malaise may be present, though headache is usually less prominent than in cerebral toxoplasmosis. However, there is enough overlap between the presentation of PCNSL and that of other causes of cerebral mass lesions that these may be clinically indistinguishable. Usually, radiological appearance is helpful in identifying whether a lesion is consistent with PCNSL, but not in differentiating between this and other causes of focal lesions with mass effect. The lesions may be single or multiple, may enhance solidly or along the rim of lesions with contrast, and are accompanied by surrounding edema (see **Figure 3**). Typical locations of PCNSL lesions include the cerebral white matter, the surfaces of the cerebral ventricles, and the corpus callosum. CT or MRI appearance may be indistinguishable from that of toxoplasma encephalitis.

A recommended diagnostic and therapeutic approach to cerebral mass lesions that are of undetermined etiology has been to initially treat for the most common infectious

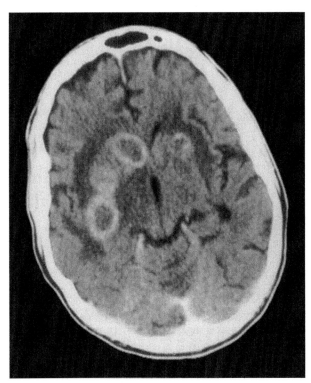

Figure 3 CT with contrast of patient with primary central nervous system lymphoma. Note thick ring enhancement surrounding multiple lesions in basal ganglia and on right side of image, abutting the ependymal surface. These images are indistinguishable from those seen in toxoplasmosis. Image provided courtesy of Dr. Steven Feske.

cause (toxoplasmosis in the developed world or tuberculosis in areas of the resource-limited world), and watch carefully for clinical improvement in the first few days after initiation of therapy, with a high suspicion of alternate diagnoses if the patient is toxoplasma serology-negative (where tuberculosis is less common) or does not respond within days with clinical improvement or indeed continues to decline on therapy. In patients with one of these factors, rapid employment of brain biopsy is usually required for diagnosis, although where available, further diagnostic testing may be helpful. If positron emission tomography (PET) or single-photon emission computed tomography (SPECT) is performed, the lesions of PCNSL are hypermetabolic or thallium-avid, versus lesions from foci of infections, which are bland on radionuclide imaging. Furthermore, the presence of Epstein-Barr virus (EBV) DNA detected in spinal fluid by PCR is both sensitive (80–98%) and specific (88–100%) for PCNSL in HIV-infected patients, likely relating to the reactivation of latent EBV infection associated with this condition. Although often brain biopsy is necessary in the diagnostic evaluation of PCNL, combining suggestive results of radionuclide imaging with PCR detection of EBV in the CSF is considered adequate evidence of PCNSL to warrant definitive treatment in some cases.

PCNSL can be a devastating condition, which was associated with a mean survival of only a few months after diagnosis in the pre-HAART era, even in those treated with aggressive whole-brain radiation for symptom palliation. In the context of immune restoration on antiretroviral therapy, survival has improved and regression of lesions has been reported with chemotherapy, including high-dose intravenous methotrexate. The optimal regimens for therapy and the definitive long-term prognosis of PCNSL in patients with HIV are an area of active investigation.

Progressive Multifocal Leukoencephalopathy

Although progressive multifocal leukoencephalopathy (PML) is caused by brain infection with a viral organism (JC virus), the painless, slowly progressive loss of function associated with this disorder is distinct from the clinical presentation of most other forms of cerebral infection. This classic clinical presentation can be obscured, however, by the presence of multiple active conditions in patients with severe immunosuppression, making access to neuroimaging and CSF sampling crucial for diagnostic certainty. Latent kidney infection with JC virus is ubiquitous and seemingly benign in the immunocompetent host. In the setting of impaired cell-mediated immunity, including hematological malignancies, organ transplantation, and HIV infection, JC virus seems to be activated to enter and infect cells of the host CNS. Up to 5% of patients who meet criteria for AIDS will develop PML during their lifetime, and although it typically affects patients with advanced immunosuppression, at least 10% of patients develop PML with CD4 counts over 200 cells/μl.

The absence of headache and fever in typical PML reflects the lack of an inflammatory response to JC virus infection of oligodendrocytes, cells within the central nervous system that are responsible for maintenance of myelinated axons primarily traversing the white matter of the brain. Oligodendrocyte infection and dysfunction leads to single or multiple expanding areas of demyelination, most marked in the large white matter tracts. Clinically, PML is characterized by the smoothly progressive development of neurological dysfunction over weeks, typically manifesting as hemi-body weakness or sensory loss due to involvement of the frontal or parietal white matter, hemifield visual loss due to a lesion in the occipital subcortical white matter, gait disorders due to involvement of the cerebellar peduncles, or abnormalities of bulbar functions such as swallowing or articulation due to brainstem disease.

In typical PML, neuroimaging demonstrates characteristic lesions, mostly confined to white matter, which appear dark on CT scans and T1-weighted MRI images, and bright on T2-weighted MRI sequences (see **Figure 4**). These may be subcortical or involve the white matter

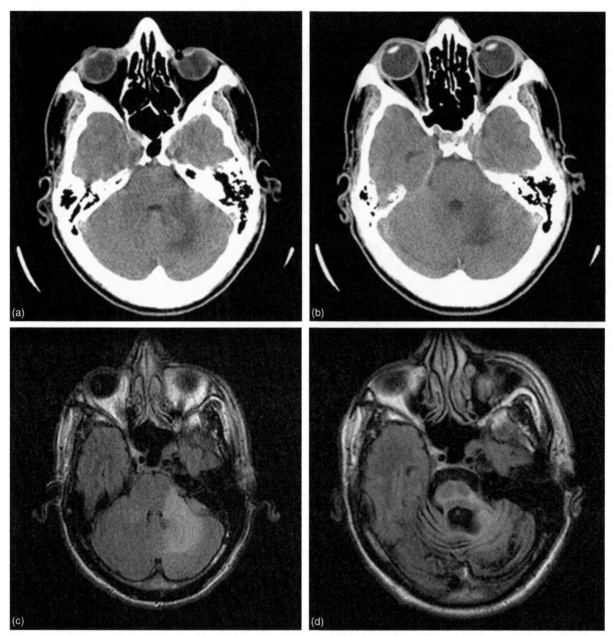

Figure 4 Brain images of a patient with progressive multifocal leukoencephalopathy (PML). CT scans without contrast (a) and after the administration of contrast (b) indicate a hypodense lesion (dark) in the cerebellum on the right side of the image which does not measurably enhance with contrast. FLAIR MRI obtained at presentation (c) shows a large area of increased (bright) signal in the affected area of the cerebellum, suggestive of demyelination due to a predilection for white matter and lack of mass effect. MRI obtained 18 months later (b) demonstrates striking atrophy in the brainstem and cerebellum as sequelae of PML, despite this patient's survival and clinical stabilization in response to combination antiretroviral therapy.

tracts of the deeper white matter and posterior fossa. They are not surrounded by edema or characterized by the displacement of structures, which indicates mass effect, and they only rarely enhance (less than 10%) when contrast is administered. CSF should be examined for the presence of JC virus and for other potential etiologies, but is typically relatively normal or may have a mild pleocytosis (fewer than ten cells) or slightly elevated protein, a nonspecific finding in chronic asymptomatic

HIV infection. Demonstration of JC virus in the CSF by PCR is close to 100% specific for PML, but only partially sensitive in the current era, ranging from 58 to 92%. Thus, a negative CSF JC virus PCR warrants re-evaluation with additional lumbar punctures and occasionally brain biopsy for confirmation of diagnosis if neuroimaging and clinical presentation are typical.

Although a number of therapies, including cidofovir, cytarabine, and topotecan, have failed to show efficacy in treatment of PML, treatment with HAART has a beneficial impact on the outcome of this condition in most cases. Before the availability of HAART, PML was associated with survival of approximately 3–6 months after diagnosis, with only 10% of patients surviving at 1 year. With the advent of HAART, 50% of patients are alive at 1 year after diagnosis. Approximately 50% of patients with PML started on effective HAART experience a halt in the progression of neurological deficits from PML, and in some cases improvement in function. Ironically, however, immune reconstitution in response to HAART has also been associated with novel phenotypes of CNS disease associated with JC virus infection, including inflammatory lesions that may appear in conjunction with immune recovery as reflected in a rising CD4 count. Clinically, patients may develop fulminant progression of previously indolent disease, associated with marked clinical signs of cerebral inflammation, including headache, seizures, and fever. On neuroimaging, lesions associated with PML in the context of this immune reconstitution inflammatory syndrome (IRIS) may appear to be centered in the white matter but are surrounded by edema and typically dramatically enhance with the administration of contrast, as shown in **Figure 5**. Pathologic evaluations in cases of PML IRIS have demonstrated an atypical inflammatory cell infiltrate in demyelinating lesions, which simultaneously harbor JC virus. Due to the inflammation detected in these lesions, corticosteroid therapy has been employed as adjunctive therapy to HAART, without consistent benefit. Those patients who survive the acute period of decline during

PML IRIS have a similar prognosis to patients with PML who have an uneventful course of immune recovery with the initiation of HAART.

Stroke

Stroke due to cerebrovascular ischemia or hemorrhage is characterized by the development of a focal neurological deficit of acute onset. The incidence of stroke is increased in HIV-infected individuals, though the reason for this predilection remains unclear. Possible contributory factors include abnormalities in lipid levels associated with antiretroviral therapy, autoimmune or inflammatory factors affecting coagulation and thrombosis, and the role of specific infections that lead to cerebral vasculopathy or cerebral embolism. Varicella-zoster virus (VZV) infection may lead to vascular inflammation or bland infection with resultant vessel occlusion and cerebral infarction. This usually presents with hemi-body deficits contralateral to a trigeminal distribution herpes zoster rash. Although it is usually associated with dermatologic evidence of VZV, the neurological deficit may be remote from the zoster rash by up to 1 year. CSF may demonstrate mild elevations in protein and white blood cell count and be positive for VZV DNA by PCR. Treatment is for typical stroke in conjunction with antiviral therapy with acyclovir or foscarnet, with or without the addition of corticosteroids. Neurosyphilis and TB meningitis are also associated with vasculitis and stroke, with a predilection for small penetrating vessels, and *Aspergillus fumigatus*

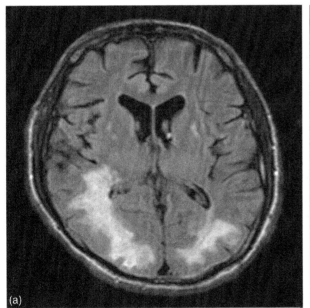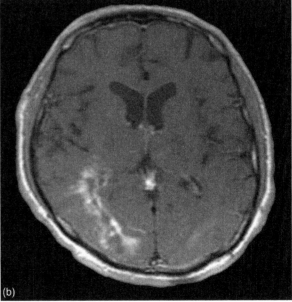

Figure 5   MRI scans of a patient with immune reconstitution inflammatory syndrome (IRIS) associated with PML. (a) FLAIR image shows extensive white matter abnormality extending throughout bilateral hemispheres, atypical for isolated demyelination due to appearance of mass effect (effacement of sulci and asymmetry of ventricles). (b) T1 image with gadolinium shows area of feathery enhancement within lesion on left side of image, a finding rare in typical PML but which is commonly seen in IRIS-associated PML.

causes cerebral vasculitis, often complicated by arterial rupture and hemorrhage. Bacterial endocarditis with typical and atypical organisms is more common than in the HIV-uninfected population, due both to immunosuppression and risk factors such as intravenous drug abuse, if present.

Diffuse Brain Diseases

Patients with pathology involving diffuse areas of the cerebral hemispheres or the meninges and intrathecal compartment present clinically with alterations in cognition. Behavioral and memory abnormalities in the setting of preserved consciousness may be the presenting manifestation of profound CNS dysfunction in patients with AIDS. Alternately, abnormal thinking and memory may be accompanied by signs of symmetric tendon reflex and motor system abnormalities, decline in the level of consciousness, or headache and symptoms of meningeal irritation. The main distinction between the clinical presentation of diffuse lesions and those of the focal disorders described above is the lack of discrete deficits referable to one or more areas of the brain. While there may be lesions apparent on neuroimaging or even pathological studies in the diffuse disorders, the clinical manifestations of these lesions are less distinct and instead part of a larger syndrome where cognitive changes are the predominant feature.

AIDS Dementia Complex

AIDS dementia complex (ADC), also termed HIV-associated cognitive-motor complex, AIDS dementia, or HIV dementia is a syndrome of cognitive and motor dysfunction that is caused by HIV-1 itself, rather than by an opportunistic organism. A significant portion of the 40 million HIV-infected individuals worldwide are therefore at risk for what might be considered premature dementia, since long-term chronic exposure of the nervous system to HIV leads to overt ADC in up to 30% of untreated patients or those failing to recover immune function on antiretroviral therapy. Although ADC has declined in incidence since the advent of HAART in the developed world, the prevalence of this disease has not dropped as significantly, perhaps related to prolonged survival. Furthermore, though previous dogma had suggested that ADC was less prevalent in resource-limited settings than in the developed world, recent well-executed studies indicate that similar proportions of HIV-infected patients in Africa meet diagnostic criteria for ADC, as do untreated patients in the United States and Europe.

Although a small number of patients present with ADC as the first AIDS-defining illness, more commonly ADC develops in the setting of late-stage disease when overt immunosuppression, opportunistic diseases, and generalized wasting may already be evident. Dementia is usually subacute, developing over months, in contrast to most other forms of diffuse brain dysfunction affecting patients with advanced AIDS. Usually the disease presents at low CD4 counts (<200 cells/µl), though a disorder termed mild cognitive motor dysfunction (MCMD) has been recently detected in a large proportion of HAART-treated patients at higher or even normal CD4 counts. Though milder in phenotype than ADC, MCMD can still lead to impairment of quality of life and productive function at work or in society.

The cognitive manifestations of AIDS dementia complexes reflect its injury to the subcortical regions, including deep gray matter structures and white matter of the brain. Patients develop psychomotor slowing, leading them to complain that it takes longer than usual to complete a simple household or work-related task. The interviewer may note overt clinical psychomotor slowing in terms of delay in answering questions and performing tasks associated with the examination. Patients also complain of difficulty simultaneously juggling multiple tasks or concepts at work, related to impairment of higher executive function. Memory difficulties, beginning with needing to keep lists and appointment books and eventually leading to confusion such as getting lost in previously familiar surroundings are frequent complaints.

These cognitive symptoms are typically associated with the development of slow clumsy or still limb and extremity movement, affecting both coordination of the upper limbs as well as mobility and balance. Examination reveals slowed fine movements of the fingers, impaired ability to repetitively direct limb movement to a target, increased muscular tone, unsteadiness of gait, and brisk tendon reflexes. In association with these cognitive and motor signs, patients often demonstrate alterations and behavior, usually characterized by apparent apathy, a diminished display of emotion, and lack of interest in their surroundings. Abulia, or a reduction in the production of spontaneous speech, is a characteristic sign.

The spectrum of ADC ranges from mild symptoms or signs of cognitive or motor dysfunction to extreme incapacity characterized by mutants and complete inability to walk or spontaneously move the legs. A staging system that factors not only signs and symptoms in the ADC spectrum, but also functional capacity is useful for the classification and monitoring of patients with this disease. In the staging system, stage 0.5 indicates equivocal or subclinical disease, whereas stage 4 disease indicates a nearly vegetative condition (see **Table 2**). In addition, differential diagnosis may be different in different stages of disease. In early-stage disease, in particular, depression is high on the differential diagnosis with ADC. The clinical overlap between the main cognitive and behavioral features of AIDS dementia complex and those of

Table 2   AIDS dementia complex staging

ADC stage	Characteristics
Stage 0 (normal)	Normal mental and motor function
Stage 0.5 (equivocal/ subclinical)	Minimal or equivocal symptoms or mild signs of cognitive or motor dysfunction characteristic of AIDS dementia complex, without impairment of work or capacity to perform activities of daily living (ADL); normal gait and strength
Stage 1 (mild)	Unequivocal symptoms, signs, neuropsychological test performance indicating intellectual or motor impairment characteristic of ADC but able to perform all but the more demanding aspects of work or ADL; walks without assistance
Stage 2 (moderate)	Cannot work or maintain demanding aspects of daily life but able to perform basic activities of self-care; ambulatory but may require a single prop
Stage 3 (severe)	Major intellectual incapacity (cannot sustain complex conversation, considerable slowing of all output) or motor disability (cannot walk unassisted)
Stage 4 (end stage)	Nearly vegetative; intellectual and social comprehension are at a rudimentary level; nearly or absolutely mute; paraparetic or paraplegic with double incontinence

Adapted from Price R and Brew B (1988) The AIDS dementia complex. *Journal of Infectious Diseases* 158: 1079–1083; Sidtis JJ and Price RW (1990) Early HIV-1 infection and the AIDS dementia complex. *Neurology* 40: 323–326.

depression lead to diagnostic confusion, or missed ADC diagnosis, in many cases. Thorough examination for the presence of the motor disturbance typical of ADC may be helpful, and the differential diagnosis should be expanded to include or confirm the diagnosis of ADC. In later stages of disease, usually stage 2 or higher, multifocal lesions (such as in the setting of advanced PML) or other diffuse conditions, may mimic the clinical findings of ADC.

Diagnosis

After history and neurological exam raises the possibility of ADC, helpful diagnostic information may result from neuropsychological evaluation, laboratory testing, and neuroimaging. Often, detailed neuropsychological testing reveals subtle deficits that are consistent with the patient's or acquaintances' complaints, but are not detected on general office examination. Neuropsychological testing is useful chiefly for definition of the domains of cognition that may be affected in any given individual, allowing identification of patterns suggesting a subcortical dementia (which would be consistent with ADC) versus a chiefly cortical dementia (more suggestive of Alzheimer's disease), a deficit suggestive of focal disease or difficulties more likely referable to a mood disorder. Of course, patterns may overlap, and detection of suggestive abnormalities on evaluation does not necessarily indicate whether the process is active or static. Thus, in some cases, serial neuropsychological testing has utility in demonstrating a progression in deficits. Typically, patients with even early ADC have particular difficulty with tests requiring trailmaking, copying and substitution of digit symbols, placing shaped pegs into a pegboard, tapping fingers rapidly, and walking briskly, reflecting difficulty with executive function, psychomotor speed, and motor coordination and control.

In conjunction with neuropsychological testing, laboratory evaluation is important in approaching the patient with ADC. This mainly involves analysis of the likelihood of ADC based on the patient's current CD4 count and plasma HIV RNA burden, and exclusion of other causes of dementia or delirium. In most patients with ADC, the CD4 count is low (<200 cells/µl) and the viral load is elevated (more than 1000 copies/µl), reflecting the later stages of immunosuppression and loss of viral suppression that characterizes overt AIDS. However, there are rare exceptions to this standard, with reported cases of patients with ADC-like cognitive impairment without any other obvious etiologies at CD4 counts above 350 cells/µl, or with apparently suppressed plasma HIV RNA levels. In at least one case, a patient with ADC in the context of an undetectable HIV RNA in the plasma was found to have an extremely elevated CSF HIV RNA level. Such findings indicate the utility of considering other markers as risk factors or coincident diagnostic laboratory findings for ADC, including CSF-specific markers that may more specifically indicate or reflect nervous system disease.

Due to the presence of anatomic and physiologic blood–brain and blood–CSF barriers, the nervous system is compartmentalized from the systemic circulation in terms of molecular, drug, and viral exchange. As a result, CNS HIV infection is often compartmentalized from systemic infection, reflected in distinct viral loads in the two compartments in most patients (approximately one log higher in the blood than the CSF in untreated patients), differing dynamics of viral decay in response to therapy, and often diverging genotypic and phenotypic characteristics of HIV species. Thus, examination of CSF can reveal a more direct reflection of CNS HIV infection than sampling of blood alone. In patients with advanced immunosuppression, ADC severity and HIV encephalitis correlate with HIV RNA levels in the CSF. However, many patients with a high CSF viral burden are asymptomatic and neurologically normal on examination, especially in the earlier stages of HIV infection. Furthermore, the presence of any neuroinflammatory response (such as that due to concurrent neurosyphilis or the presence of a CNS opportunistic infection) can raise the CSF HIV RNA level even in the absence of ADC. Thus elevated CSF HIV RNA is not specific for the presence of neurological disease. CSF HIV-1 measurement may be useful in helping to clarify the possible activity of HIV in the CNS in patients who have ongoing neurological disease in the context of suppressed systemic viral loads or in monitoring the response to therapy in patients with known neurological disease, but is not a current part of routine clinical practice.

In evaluation of a patient with possible ADC, CSF analysis is crucial in order to exclude disease due to conditions besides HIV itself. As a result, patients with neurological disease in the setting of HIV and immunosuppression should almost always receive a routine lumbar puncture (though the presence of focal cerebral lesion with mass effect or bleeding diathesis or clotting dysfunction are contraindications to lumbar puncture due to the risk of brain herniation or intrathecal or epidural bleeding). CSF protein and white blood cell count are often mildly elevated in ADC, but may also be elevated in asymptomatic untreated HIV infection as well as other CNS conditions such as neurosyphilis. CSF markers of inflammation, macrophage activation, and neuronal injury including neopterin, beta-2-microglobulin, quinolinic acid, monocyte chemoattractant protein-1, and neurofilament light chain are elevated in ADC but are also nonspecific for this disease. Disease-specific CSF studies that should be considered are cryptococcal antigen detection, CSF venereal disease research laboratory (VDRL) for syphilis, Gram stain and routine culture, and examination for particular organisms by culture (mycobacteria, fungal), stain (India ink, acid fast bacilli), or PCR analysis (CMV, VZV, EBV) depending on risk factors, demographics, and clinical presentation.

Although neuroimaging may be unremarkable in ADC, several findings on CT or MRI support the diagnosis. Atrophy of the brain, as reflected in large ventricles and sulci is evident in the majority of patients with ADC, but also in many patients with asymptomatic HIV infection. Bilateral periventricular white matter abnormalities, characterized by nonenhancing hypodense lesions on CT or areas of increased signal on T2-weighted MRI sequences that appear normal on T1 and do not enhance with contrast or more specifically suggestive of ADC. **Figure 6** demonstrates the typical MRI findings in a patient with ADC. More biochemically based imaging such as MR spectroscopy may be more sensitive and specific than anatomic imaging done for the diagnosis of ADC.

Treatment

Although the detailed steps in pathogenesis from initial HIV infection to the characteristic findings of neuronal loss, white matter pallor, and HIV encephalitis in ADC are not entirely understood, the clinical and pathologic abnormalities are known to improve in response to combination antiretroviral therapy employed in treatment of systemic infection. HAART's effects on HIV may be caused by direct reduction of CNS HIV viral burden, indirect suppression of neurotoxic cytokines related to inflammatory and immune responses, or both mechanisms. Clearly, however, ADC incidence is much reduced in the era of antiretroviral therapy in the developed world, and patients may experience a halt in the progression of ADC or reversal of deficits in the context of successful HAART and immune reconstitution. In most situations, any HAART regimen effective in suppressing plasma virus and maintaining or elevating CD4 counts seems to be effective in treating the CNS. Given the potential compartmentalization of CNS HIV, in certain situations drug with favorable CNS penetration may be preferred if a patient has known ADC. Of currently available drugs, these include zidovudine, abacavir, stavudine, nevirapine, and some protease inhibitors (with the important exceptions of indinavir and lopinavir) in combination with ritonavir. In addition, in cases of patients who may harbor resistant virus, assessment of resistance mutations present in CSF HIV viral species may be important for effective treatment of the CNS.

Other Diffuse Brain Diseases

Besides ADC, a number of conditions may develop in patients with advanced AIDS that manifest predominantly as altered cognition. These often, if not always, present with additional signs and symptoms that leave the clinician to suspect specific conditions distinct from ADC.

Cytomegalovirus Encephalitis

In patients with extremely advanced AIDS (CD4 count <50), a syndrome of acute or subacute onset of confusion may develop in the setting of CNS infection with cytomegalovirus (CMV). Often, the clinical presentation includes striking impairments of short-term memory, accompanied by nystagmus, cranial neuropathies, and ataxia, reflecting the predilection of this infection to provoke ventriculoencephalitis involving ependymal surfaces of the ventricles and thus midline structures of the brain and brain stem. In addition, patients often have fluctuations in their level of arousal, seizures, and constitutional symptoms of fever, headache, and malaise that are distinct from the typical presentation of ADC. CMV disease of the nervous system usually develops in the setting of active CMV infection at other sites, including the esophagus, lung, and most commonly, the eye.

Related to the fact that overt clinical CMV CNS infection is characterized by ventriculoencephalitis, CSF may

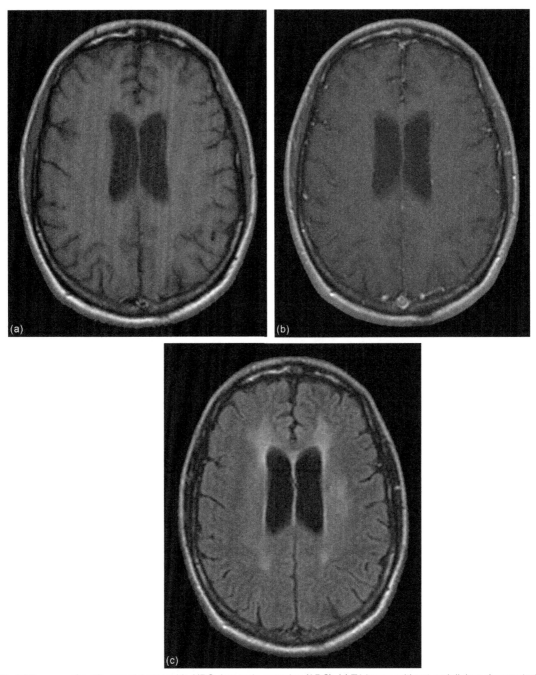

Figure 6 MRI scans of a 40-year-old man with AIDS dementia complex (ADC). (a) T1 image without gadolinium demonstrates enlarged ventricles for age and diffuse cerebral atrophy which are hallmarks of ADC. (b) T1 image with gadolinium shows no areas of enhancement with contrast. (c) FLAIR image shows symmetric areas of periventricular T2 hyperintensity in periventricular white matter which are not apparent in (a); these are typical in character and location for lesions seen in ADC.

be markedly inflammatory in nature. Abnormalities include elevations in white blood cell count, protein level, and occasionally low glucose. In contrast to other forms of viral encephalitis, a polymorphonuclear predominance may be found in the CSF, although this is not always present. Extremely helpful in specific diagnosis of CNS disease due to CMV is the detection of CMV DNA by PCR in the CSF, though a distinct syndrome of CMV polyradiculomyelitis that leads to groin and leg pain, incontinence, and lower extremity weakness is also accompanied by this finding. MRI may be normal or may show evidence of ventriculitis, with contrast enhancement along the linings of the cerebral ventricles and T2 hyperintense signal in midline structures and the brainstem (**Figure 7**).

Pathologic studies have in fact demonstrated histological evidence of CMV infection in a quarter of brains of

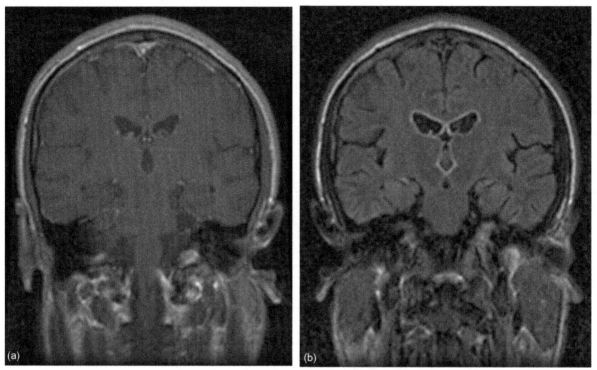

Figure 7 Coronal MRI images of a patient with CMV encephalitis. Note the thin rim of contrast enhancement lining cerebral ventricles in T1 image with gadolinium (a), with more extensive bright signal visible in cerebral tissues adjacent to ventricles on FLAIR image, indicating inflammation of ependymal surfaces (b).

AIDS patients at autopsy, the majority of whom had no evidence of the distinct ventriculoencephalitis syndrome. Thus, the spectrum of effects in CMV infection in the brain may range from asymptomatic to severe disease. In its severe form, CMV encephalitis should be treated with IV ganciclovir, foscarnet, or a combination of these therapies. Even with aggressive therapy, many patients sustain permanent memory loss, seizure disorders, and cognitive impairment.

Central Nervous System Cryptococcal Infection

Cryptococcus neoformans is the most common fungal organism leading to neurological disease. Though in some developed areas, the incidence of CNS cryptococcal infection is low (2–5%), it may be the most common CNS opportunistic infection worldwide since its prevalence in patients with AIDS reaches 38% in areas of the resource-limited world with the highest HIV prevalence. CNS infection is related to exposure to the ubiquitous encapsulated yeast that is found in the soil. Cryptococci are spread through inhalation from the environment and can cause disease ranging from lung abscesses to skin infections, though cerebral cryptococcosis is the most common and usually severe form of the infection.

Cryptococcal infections of the CNS may occur in non-AIDS immunocompromised or immunocompetent hosts; in this setting, disease commonly manifests as stiff neck, confusion, fever, and headache. However, cryptococcosis in AIDS patients presents with a much wider spectrum of disease, ranging from headache alone to confusion, headache, and drowsiness, which may rapidly progress to coma. Hallmarks of cryptococcal infection are loss of hearing or vision, often reported by patients prior to diagnosis, due in part to infiltration of cryptococcal organisms directly into the IInd (optic) or VIIIth (auditory) cranial nerves. Not uncommonly, cognitive and/or cranial nerve abnormalities present in the absence of any headache and/or meningeal signs (60–75% of patients have no signs of meningeal irritation). The minimal meningeal signs and symptoms on history and examination reflect the typically limited inflammatory reaction related to CNS infection with cryptococcus in AIDS, leading to the designation as cerebral cryptococcosis rather than cryptococcal meningitis. Reflecting this lack of inflammation in typical disease, CSF may have few or no white blood cells and normal protein levels, especially in advanced immunosuppression. India ink stains for rapid identification of the fungal capsule often reveal an enormous burden of organisms even when there is little or no inflammatory reaction. Cryptococcal antigen titers are positive in the CSF in at least 72% of cases. CT scans of the brain are usually normal or reveal only enlarged ventricles and sulci, suggesting communicating hydrocephalus. MRI more commonly shows abnormalities, revealing better characterization of hydrocephalus and often

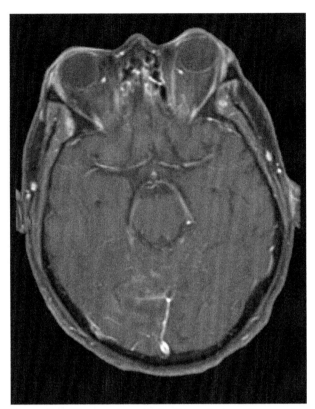

Figure 8 MRI scan of a patient with cerebral cryptococcosis. Although patients with cerebral cryptococcosis may have normal-appearing neuroimaging or scans that solely indicate communicating hydrocephalus, in some cases patients develop focal lesions in the cerebellum and occipital lobes that enhance with gadolinium and may represent focal cerebritis adjacent to collections of infected cerebrospinal fluid, as is evident in this case.

meningeal enhancement. In some cases, focal lesions are evident, including small globular lesions within the basal ganglia, or areas of inflammation in the posterior areas of the brain and cerebellum that enhance with contrast and likely represent focal cerebritis (see **Figure 8**).

A predominant portion of the symptoms of headache, confusion, and visual disturbance noted in cryptococcal meningitis are due directly to increased intracranial pressure caused presumably by failure of proper CSF drainage in the setting of a large burden of cryptococcal organisms. Communicating hydrocephalus is a significant cause of irreversible neurological deficits and death in this condition; an opening pressure of greater than 350 mm H_2O on initial diagnostic examination is one of the most salient predictors of increased disease-related mortality. Serum cryptococcal antigen is invariably positive in the setting of CNS disease in patients with AIDS. However, even when a diagnosis is clear from clinical presentation and cryptococcal antigenemia, spinal tap for opening pressure is necessary for evaluation and therapeutic management of this condition. Serial cryptococcal antigen titers are not useful to monitor response to therapy in

either CSF or blood, though serial examination of the opening pressure is helpful.

An important development in the spectrum of illness that may present with CNS cryptococcal disease has been a new phenotype of disease associated with the recovery of the immune system in response to treatment with effective HAART. As with PML, the characteristics of cerebral cryptococcosis in the setting of immune reconstitution may include a dramatic syndrome of meningitis with fulminant symptoms of meningismus, headache, nausea, vomiting, and fever. Lumbar puncture may reveal a predominantly inflammatory CSF characterized by a pleocytosis of more than 50 cells/mm^3 (predominantly lymphocytes). These presentations usually occur at least 6 weeks after the initiation of therapy in the context of a marked rise in CD4 cell count and are most common in patients who are extremely immunosuppressed (<50 cells/μl) at the time of initiation of HAART. In some reported cases, presentations are of a change in the otherwise typical low-grade course of known cryptococcal infection, whereas in some cases this fulminant meningitis presents in the context of a previously unidentified latent infection. Though such presentations and those of other forms of IRIS have added complexity to the questions of when to start HAART in patients with known opportunistic infections, most clinicians initiate HAART early in such cases as long as patients can be monitored carefully for unusual inflammatory complications.

Neurosyphilis

Though syphilis had been decreasing in prevalence through the latter part of the twentieth century, in parallel with the rising worldwide prevalence of HIV/AIDS it reemerged as an important coinfection affecting up to one-quarter of those infected with HIV. Symptomatic nervous system infection with *Treponema pallidum* presents in less than 3% of HIV-uninfected persons, predominantly in the context of late-stage systemic syphilis. However, neurosyphilis is more common and develops much earlier in the course of infection in patients with concomitant HIV infection. Though *T. pallidum* notoriously causes protean manifestations throughout the neuroaxis, in HIV-infected patients neurosyphilis tends to be either asymptomatic, or to present with meningitis, VIIth and VIIIth cranial nerve palsies, meningovascular involvement, or ocular disease. Thus, neurosyphilis may be associated with delirium or confusion in the context of overt meningeal symptoms or a syndrome of cerebral vasculitis, although syphilitic gummas may occur, causing more focal deficits, and myelopathy may occur.

In the setting of the most typical form of neurosyphilis in HIV, the serum rapid plasma reagin (RPR) and confirmatory *T. pallidum* hemagglutination assay (TPHA) test are positive, indicating current or past active infection.

CSF usually reveals a lymphocytic pleocytosis of up to several hundred cells/mm^3 and moderately elevated protein. As these are common findings in even asymptomatic HIV infection, more direct evidence of treponemal infection should be sought. The CSF Venereal Disease Research Laboratory (VDRL), a non-treponemal test, is diagnostic of current or past neurosyphilis if positive, but is negative in 30–70% of cases. The treponemal test FTA-ABS is highly sensitive, so a negative result can exclude the diagnosis of syphilis. However, for many labs this test is not readily available. Since laboratory confirmation of neurosyphilis is not always possible, most clinicians recommend definitive therapy in the context of known systemic syphilis infection and suspicion of CNS involvement based on typical clinical symptoms and findings. Therapy options for neurosyphilis include a 10- to 14-day course of any of the following: penicillin IV every 3–4 h, procaine penicillin IM with probenecid orally, or ceftriaxone IV daily. CSF should be reexamined every 6 months after treatment to monitor for a decline in CSF WBC and until CSF VDRL becomes nonreactive, if initially positive.

Spinal Cord Disorders

In the context of HIV infection, diseases affecting the spinal cord lead to difficulty with gait due to lower-extremity weakness, increased muscle tone in the legs, or a combination of these. Accompanying these motor symptoms may be sensory abnormalities such as loss of joint position sense in the limbs, a discrete sensory level below which sensation is abnormal, painful paresthesias in the legs or the groin, and a variable degree of urinary or anal sphincter dysfunction. The typical patterns and associated symptoms of disease help to distinguish the etiologies of myelopathy in the clinical setting of HIV/AIDS.

Vacuolar Myelopathy

Vacuolar myelopathy is the term used to describe the most common spinal disorder in AIDS. The condition appears to be attributable to HIV infection itself, rather than dysfunction caused by an opportunistic disease. However, the pathology reveals vacuolization of the white matter of the spinal cord, in the absence of direct cord infection with HIV. As a result, the pathogenesis of vacuolar myelopathy, like that of ADC in the brain, seems related to immune-mediated or metabolic neuronal injury in the setting of active HIV infection.

Clinically, there is a spectrum of overlap between patients developing spinal cord disease and dementia in the setting of AIDS, leading the symptoms and signs of myelopathy to be included in the diagnostic criterion for ADC. The myelopathy in this case is diffuse rather than dysfunctional at a focal spinal level. These symptoms are of a gradually progressive (over months to years) spasticity and weakness of the lower extremities, leading to impaired gait, accompanied by urinary retention or incontinence. Sensory changes, if present, may be mild and related to posterior column (enervating joint position and vibratory sensation) dysfunction or often to concomitant underlying peripheral neuropathy. Brisk deep tendon reflexes are found in the limbs, though ankle jerks may be relatively diminished in the presence of neuropathy. Though dementia often develops in parallel, in some patients stiff and weak lower extremities are the predominant finding.

Since obtaining tissue from the spinal cord directly is almost impossible in life, diagnosis of vacuolar myelopathy rests on the presence of the correct clinical scenario in the absence of alternate conditions. Patients tend to develop vacuolar myelopathy when they are not on HAART, when plasma HIV RNA levels are uncontrolled, and when CD4 counts are lower than 200 cells/μl. CSF should be sampled for evidence of HTLV-1/2 infection and syphilis, and blood levels of vitamin B_{12} should be examined. Spinal cord imaging should be performed to rule out compressive lesions. In HIV-associated vacuolar myelopathy, imaging is generally normal or shows cord atrophy.

The best current available treatment for vacuolar myelopathy is HAART and viral suppression. While in some cases, myelopathy due to HIV does not improve with HAART to the extent that cognitive abnormalities regress in ADC, our clinical experience and that of others indicates that some patients have substantial recovery of motor function and diminution in spasticity. Adjunctive therapies such as corticosteroids or intravenous immune globulin are not helpful.

Focal Myelopathies

Several spinal cord disorders in HIV/AIDS cause distinct impairments at the level of the spinal cord, leading to characteristic dysfunction of motor, sensory, and sphincter function at that level and below. Varicella zoster virus (VZV) is known to cause acute myelitis in approximately 1% of patients within approximately 3 weeks following an outbreak of herpes zoster. Typically, the spinal level affected is adjacent to the nerve root associated with the dermatomal rash, with infection directly infiltrating the cord at the site of entry of the nerve. The clinical presentation is a very rapidly developing (over days) focal myelopathy after a reported zoster rash. CSF typically reveals a lymphocytic pleocytosis and may yield a positive PCR test for VZV DNA. MRI of the cord shows a T2 hyperintense lesion in the cord at the affected level. IV acyclovir is the first-line therapy for all CNS VZV infections, though foscarnet is needed in cases of acyclovir resistance.

Corticosteroids are often used as additional therapy, although their effectiveness is unclear. CMV and herpes simplex virus can also cause myelitis in rare cases. Diagnosis is usually facilitated by detection of the responsible virus through PCR studies.

Additionally, compressive lesions may affect the spinal cord in patients with HIV and AIDS. Their frequency is usually related to the degree of immunosuppression, and their clinical presentation is that of severe back pain in the setting of bilateral limb weakness and incontinence. Metastatic lymphoma causes compressive lesions in the setting of systemic disease. TB may lead to intraspinal tuberculomas as well as cord compression due to Pott's disease (tubercular infection of the vertebral bodies). Finally, acute bacterial abscesses occur in patients due to increased susceptibility from immunosuppression in the setting of IV drug abuse or indwelling catheters.

Conclusions

Central nervous system disease in HIV is a source of considerable morbidity for patients, especially once they reach the levels of immunosuppression associated with AIDS. These disorders also may present particular challenges for practitioners who may be experienced in infectious conditions or disorders of the nervous system, but not both. Although some aspects of these disorders may be changing over time and in response to the increasing availability of HAART, the bulk of neurological manifestations of AIDS fall within a limited spectrum. Careful evaluation of the clinical context, the patient's history, and clinical examination, combined with crucial examination of CSF and neuroimaging, where possible, will yield a diagnosis in most patients. If antiretroviral therapy is available, such treatment in conjunction with targeted anti-infectious therapy against the offending pathogen leads to improvement in survival and reversal of deficits in many cases.

See also: Mental Health and Physical Health (Including HIV/AIDS); Specific Mental Health Disorders: Mental Disorders Associated With Aging.

Further Reading

Ammassari A, Cingolani A, Pezzotti P, *et al.* (2000) AIDS-related focal brain lesions in the era of highly active antiretroviral therapy. *Neurology* 55: 1194–1200.

Berger JR and Levy RM (1997) *AIDS and the Nervous System,* 2nd edn. Philadelphia, PA: Lippincott-Raven.

d'Arminio Monforte A, Cinque P, Vago L, *et al.* (1997) A comparison of brain biopsy and CSF-PCR in the diagnosis of CNS lesions in AIDS patients. *Neurology* 244: 35–39.

d'Arminio Monforte A, Duca PG, Vago L, *et al.* (2000) Decreasing incidence of CNS AIDS-defining events associated with antiretroviral therapy. *Neurology* 54: 1856–1859.

d'Arminio Monforte A, Cinque P, Mocroft A, *et al.* (2004) Changing incidence of central nervous system diseases in the EuroSIDA cohort. *Annals of Neurology* 55: 320–328.

Di Rocco A (1999) Diseases of the spinal cord in human immunodeficiency virus infection. *Seminars in Neurology* 19: 151–155.

Gendelman HE, Grant I, Everall I, *et al.* (2005) *The Neurology of AIDS,* 2nd edn. Oxford, UK: Oxford University Press.

Gonzalez-Scarano F and Martin-Garcia J (2005) The neuropathogenesis of AIDS. *Nature Reviews in Immunology* 5: 69–81.

Harrison MJG and McArthur JC (1995) *AIDS and Neurology.* New York: Churchill Livingstone.

McArthur JC, Brew BJ, and Nath A (2005) Neurological complications of HIV infection. *Lancet Neurology* 4: 543–555.

Navia B and Price RW (2005) An overview of the clinical and biological features of the AIDS dementia complex. In: Gendelman HE, Grant I, Everall I, *et al.* (eds.) *The Neurology of AIDS,* 2nd edn., pp. 339–356Oxford, UK: Oxford University Press.

Navia BA, Jordan BD, and Price RW (1986a) The AIDS dementia complex: I. Clinical features. *Annals of Neurology* 19: 517–524.

Navia BA, Cho ES, Petito CK, and Price RW (1986b) The AIDS dementia complex: II. Neuropathology. *Annals of Neurology* 19: 525–535.

Price RW (1996) Neurological complications of HIV infection. *Lancet* 348: 445–452.

Sacktor N, Lyles RH, Skolasky R, *et al.* (2001) HIV-associated neurologic disease incidence changes: Multicenter AIDS Cohort Study, 1990–1998. *Neurology* 56: 257–260.

Bacterial Meningitis

D van de Beek and J de Gans, University of Amsterdam, Amsterdam, The Netherlands

Introduction

Meningitis is an infection of the fluid that surrounds the brain and spinal cord (cerebrospinal fluid, CSF). Most patients with bacterial meningitis also have inflammation of the brain (meningoencephalitis) because of the close anatomic relation between CSF and the brain. Bacterial meningitis is a potentially lethal disease and is therefore a medical emergency. A diagnosis of bacterial meningitis is often considered, but the disease can be difficult to recognize. Controversies remain for emergency medicine and primary care providers who need to accurately diagnose patients with bacterial meningitis and administer antibiotics and adjunctive therapies rapidly for this life-threatening disease. Treatment recommendations for antimicrobial therapy are changing as a result of emergence of antimicrobial resistance, and the management of the critically ill neurologic patient with bacterial meningitis may pose important dilemmas. In this article we provide an overview of bacterial meningitis dealing with such important aspects as the changing epidemiology and diagnostic and therapeutic decisions in the emergency evaluation and treatment of patients with bacterial meningitis.

Epidemiology

The estimated incidence of bacterial meningitis is 0.6 to 4 per 100 000 per year in developed countries, and may be up to ten times higher in other parts of the world (van de Beek *et al.*, 2006). The epidemiology of bacterial meningitis has substantially changed over the last two decades. Meningitis due to *Haemophilus influenzae* type b has nearly been eliminated since routine childhood vaccination was initiated in many developed countries (**Figure 1**), and the introduction of conjugate vaccines against seven serotypes of *Streptococcus pneumoniae* has reduced the burden of childhood pneumococcal meningitis substantially (Peltola, 2000; Whitney *et al.*, 2003). In some regions of the world, invasive infections due to *Neisseria meningitidis* serogroup C have increased over the last 10 years,

prompting the introduction of routine immunization with meningococcal serogroup C protein-polysaccharide conjugate vaccines (Snape and Pollard, 2005). The main consequence of these kinds of routine vaccination programs in developed countries is that the age-specific incidence of bacterial meningitis has decreased in children, thus increasing the fraction of patients that are adults. The most common etiologic agents now are *S. pneumoniae* and *N. meningitidis*, which cause 80 to 85% of all cases (Saez-Llorens and McCracken, 2003; van de Beek *et al.*, 2004).

S. pneumoniae primarily causes respiratory infections, including otitis media, sinusitis, and pneumonia. Groups at increased risk of pneumococcal infection include children, elderly, immunocompromised patients (including those with human immunodeficiency virus type 1 infection), smokers, and certain other demographic groups. In contrast, *N. meningitidis* most commonly causes meningitis in young adults. Nasopharyngeal carriage of meningococci is an important factor that leads to the development of invasive disease. The estimated prevalence of meningococcal carriage is 5–10% under nonepidemic conditions (Snape and Pollard, 2005).

Another epidemiological trend is emergence of antibiotic-resistant strains of *S. pneumoniae* (Whitney *et al.*, 2003). Pneumococcal resistance to penicillin, due to changes in its penicillin-binding proteins, was first reported in 1965. The prevalence of such resistance was limited until an epidemic of highly resistant pneumococci occurred in South Africa in 1977. Since then, resistance has developed

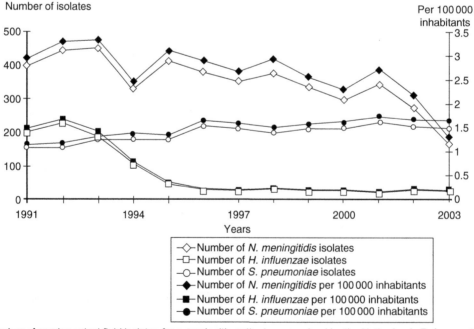

Figure 1   Number of cerebrospinal fluid isolates from meningitis patients as received by the Netherlands Reference Laboratory for Bacterial Meningitis from 1991 through 2003. In the Netherlands, routine vaccination with the conjugate *Haemophilus influenzae* type b vaccine started in 1993. From van de Beek D and de Gans J (2006) Dexamethasone in adults with bacterial meningitis. *Drugs* 66: 415–427.

worldwide, and in some regions it occurs in a frequency up to 70%. Reports of reduced susceptibility of pneumococci to several antibiotics, including broad-spectrum cephalosporins, have also been published. In response to this epidemiological trend, recommendations for suspected and confirmed bacterial meningitis have necessarily evolved.

Clinical Presentation

When a patient presents to a physician for an emergent evaluation, the patient's history and signs and symptoms can help to estimate the probability of meningitis. A wide variety of patient complaints may be elicited from patients with meningitis, and symptoms such as headache, nausea, and vomiting demonstrated poor sensitivity and specificity for the diagnosis of meningitis (van de Beek *et al.*, 2004). The 'classic triad' of fever, neck stiffness, and change in mental status was found to be present in 44% of patients with bacterial meningitis; 95% of patients with bacterial meningitis presented with at least two signs or symptoms of headache, fever, neck stiffness, and alterations in mental status. At least one of these four elements was present in 99% of patients, so aspects of history and physical exam can be used to heighten suspicion for meningitis even if they cannot alone rule out the diagnosis.

Meningeal signs such as Kernig's sign or Brudzinski's sign are physical exam findings often documented when evaluating a patient for possible meningitis (Thomas *et al.*, 2002). Kernig's test involves flexing the hip and extending the knee, and a positive result is recorded when pain is elicited in the back and legs. Brudzinski's neck test is

typically performed in the supine position where the head is passively flexed and is interpreted as positive when flexion at the hips to lift the legs is elicited in response. A prospective study found that none of these signs accurately identified patients with meningitis, although this study included only adults. There was no correlation with moderate meningeal inflammation or with microbial evidence of infection, and Kernig's sign and Brudzinski's sign were found to have poor sensitivity (5%) with high specificity (95%). Thus, also these classic signs lack the adequate sensitivity to perform as screening tests to rule out meningitis, but when present they are concerning for an underlying meningitis and should be followed up with appropriate additional testing.

Diagnostic Lumbar Puncture

Once an initial patient evaluation with history and physical findings has been completed, lumbar puncture (LP) is the diagnostic procedure of choice if the diagnosis of bacterial meningitis cannot be ruled out (van de Beek *et al.*, 2006). Characteristic findings in the CSF are typically used to make the diagnosis of meningitis (Fitch and van de Beek, 2007). With the urgent nature of this testing to make the diagnosis of meningitis, one of the issues facing physicians is whether neuroimaging, in most cases computed tomography (CT), is required before LP. CT before lumbar puncture will detect brain shift and is therefore recommended as a precaution in selected patients before lumbar puncture to avoid the likelihood of further brain shift (**Figure 2**). Therefore, cranial imaging should precede lumbar puncture in patients with new

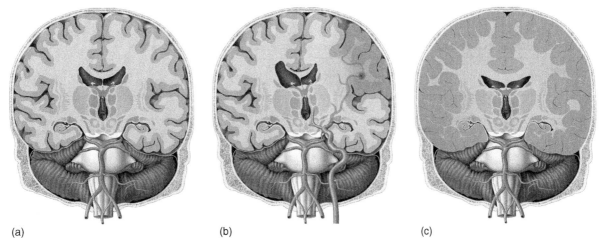

(a)   (b)   (c)

Figure 2 Cranial imaging to evaluate potential contraindications for lumbar puncture should be focused on identifying signs of a focal space-occupying lesion, evidence of brain shift, and/or signs of severe diffuse brain swelling. (a) Normal brain, (b) meningitis-associated cerebral infarct causing significant brain shift, and (c) diffuse brain swelling associated with severe infection. Initial lumbar puncture should not be performed when computed tomography findings of significant brain shift are found, and empiric therapy for meningitis should be continued. From Fitch MT and van de Beek D (2007) Emergency diagnosis and treatment of adult meningitis. *Lancet Infectious Diseases* 7: 191–200.

onset seizures, with immunocompromised state, with signs suspicious for space-occupying lesions, or with moderate or severe impairment of consciousness (van de Beek *et al.*, 2006). When these criteria are followed, the indications for cranial imaging before lumbar puncture are often present (45% of patients with bacterial meningitis). Initial lumbar puncture may also be harmful in patients with coagulopathy, because of hazard of needle-induced subarachnoid hemorrhage or the development of spinal subdural and epidural hematomas. Importantly, if imaging is performed before lumbar puncture, therapy should precede it (see later discussion).

When lumbar puncture is completed and findings demonstrate increased white cell count in the CSF, thus confirming a diagnosis of meningitis, clinicians would like to determine which patients are at risk for the truly life-threatening bacterial meningitis versus those with a typically less concerning viral meningitis (Nigrovic *et al.*, 2007). CSF findings are present in nearly all patients, although normal CSF parameters do occur. Individual predictors for the presence of bacterial meningitis are a glucose level $<1.9 \, \text{mmol} \, \text{l}^{-1}$, a ratio of CSF glucose to blood glucose <0.23, a protein level $>2.20 \, \text{g} \, \text{l}^{-1}$, a white cell count $>2000/\text{mm}^3$, or a CSF neutrophil count $>1180/\text{mm}^3$ (Spanos *et al.*, 1989).

Gram staining and culture of CSF can identify the causative pathogen in approximately 80–85% of the patients (van de Beek *et al.*, 2006). The sensitivity of bacterial antigen tests is limited; however, these tests may be helpful in patients with suspected bacterial meningitis and negative Gram staining and culture of CSF. A promising diagnostic tool in cases of suspected bacterial meningitis and negative CSF cultures is the amplification of bacterial DNA by polymerase chain reaction (PCR). Although high diagnostic sensitivity and specificity have been reported, further refinements and particularly a reduction of the false-positive rates are needed before PCR can be routinely recommended in the diagnosis of bacterial meningitis.

Antimicrobial Therapy

A delay in antimicrobial therapy (e.g., due to imaging, transfer to another hospital, or stabilization of vital signs) has been associated with an increased risk for adverse clinical outcome in adults with bacterial meningitis. Therefore, if imaging precedes lumbar puncture, blood cultures should be drawn and antimicrobial therapy with adjunctive dexamethasone initiated before imaging is performed (van de Beek *et al.*, 2006).

The choice of initial antimicrobial therapy is based on the most common bacteria causing the disease based on age and/or clinical setting and on antimicrobial susceptibility patterns (**Table 1**). Also important are pharmacokinetics and pharmacodynamics of the antimicrobial agents, particularly the penetration into the CSF.

Once culture results and susceptibility testing are available, antimicrobial therapy can be modified for optimum treatment. With worldwide increases in prevalence of penicillin-resistant pneumococci, combination therapy of vancomycin plus a third-generation cephalosporin (either ceftriaxone or cefotaxime) has become the standard approach to empiric antimicrobial therapy.

Respiratory isolation for 24 h is indicated for patients with suspected meningococcal infection. Isolation is not required for patients with signs of pneumococcal infection (otitis, pneumonia) or with bacteria other than *N. meningitidis* identified by Gram staining. Close contacts of the patient must receive chemoprophylaxis to eradicate meningococcal carriage.

Table 1   Recommendations for initial antibiotic therapy in patients with suspected or proved community-acquired bacterial meningitis. Empirical antibiotic therapy in adults with suspected community-acquired bacterial meningitis

Predisposing factor	Common bacterial pathogens	Initial management
Age		
<1 month	*Streptococcus agalactiae, Escherichia coli, Listeria monocytogenes, Klebsiella* species	Ampicillin plus cefotaxime or ampicillin plus an aminoglycoside
2–60 years	*Neisseria meningitidis, Streptococcus pneumoniae*	Vancomycin plus cefotaxime/ceftriaxone[a]
>60 years	*N. meningitidis, S. pneumoniae, L. monocytogenes*, aerobic Gram-negative bacilli	Vancomycin plus cefotaxime/ceftriaxone plus ampicillin[b]
With risk factor present[c]	*S. pneumoniae, L. monocytogenes, Haemophilus influenzae*	Vancomycin plus cefotaxime/ceftriaxone plus ampicillin[b]

[a]In regions with very low rates of penicillin resistance (<1%), monotherapy with penicillin may be considered, although many experts recommend combination therapy for all patients until the results of in vitro susceptibility testing are available.
[b]In areas with very low penicillin-resistance and cephalosporin-resistance rates, combination therapy of amoxicillin and third-generation cephalosporin may be considered.
[c]Alcoholism, altered immune status.
Reproduced from van de Beek D, de Gans J, Tunkel AR and Wijdicks EFM (2006) Community-acquired bacterial meningitis in adults. *New England Journal of Medicine* 354: 46–55.

Adjunctive Corticosteroid Therapy

Inflammation from any source in the central nervous system is poorly tolerated, and such inflammatory responses within the enclosed spaces of the brain and spinal cord have been demonstrated to lead to destructive secondary effects in basic science models. The CSF is effectively sterilized a few hours after beginning appropriate antimicrobial therapy, and Gram stain and culture are often negative within hours of antibiotic administration. The intense inflammatory response to bacterial infection within the enclosed spaces of the brain and spinal cord is thought to lead to significant morbidity and mortality despite effective antibiotic therapy. Therefore, pharmacologic attempts to modulate this inflammatory response may be an essential component of a successful strategy to treat this life-threatening disease, and dexamethasone is the only currently accepted adjunctive therapy for the treatment of patients with bacterial meningitis that has proven clinical efficacy.

In 2007, an updated Cochrane analysis on the efficacy and safety of adjunctive corticosteroid therapy included 20 randomized clinical trials (RCTs), involving 2750 patients (van de Beek *et al.*, 2007). In this analysis, adjuvant corticosteroids were associated with lower case fatality rates and lower rates of severe hearing loss and long-term neurological sequelae. The use of corticosteroids was not associated with an increase of adverse events. The effect of corticosteroids was evident in adults with bacterial meningitis. In children the beneficial effect was less convincing, although there was a trend toward a beneficial effect on hearing loss in non-*H. influenzae* meningitis.

The Cochrane analysis found a clear difference in efficacy of corticosteroids between high- and low-income countries (Molyneux *et al.*, 2002). Therefore, the use of adjunctive corticosteroids is recommended for children in high-income countries. For children in low-income countries, the use of corticosteroids was associated neither with benefit nor with harmful effects.

The available studies also do not address two other important issues concerning the corticosteroid regimen: the minimum duration of corticosteroid therapy and the maximum length of time after parenteral antibiotic therapy for commencement of corticosteroid therapy. In a post hoc analysis of an RCT of corticosteroids involving 301 adults with bacterial meningitis, the beneficial effect of dexamethasone on mortality in patients with pneumococcal meningitis was attributable to a reduction in systemic complications (de Gans and van de Beek, 2002). This could imply that the effect of dexamethasone is not restricted to the first hours after administration, although there are no clinical data to support this. In experimental pneumococcal meningitis, CSF bacterial concentrations at the start of therapy appeared to be more important than the timing of dexamethasone therapy in influencing the antimicrobial-induced inflammatory response.

Concerns have been raised over the interference by corticosteroids on CSF eradication of meningeal pathogens by reducing the blood–brain barrier permeability and thereby the penetration of antibiotics in the subarachnoid space. In both children and adults with acute bacterial meningitis, treatment of dexamethasone did not reduce vancomycin levels in the CSF; however, therapeutic failures have been described in adults treated with standard doses of vancomycin and adjunctive dexamethasone. Therefore, patients with pneumococcal meningitis who are treated with vancomycin and dexamethasone should be carefully observed throughout therapy.

Complications

Complications develop in the majority of patients with bacterial meningitis and may be difficult to predict. Therefore, monitoring in a neurological-neurosurgical intensive care unit is recommended in order to recognize changes in consciousness or the development of new neurologic signs, to monitor for subtle seizures, and to more effectively treat severe agitation (van de Beek *et al.*, 2006). Bacterial meningitis is often associated with septic shock, which is an important predictor for outcome.

A common cause of a decline of consciousness in the patient with bacterial meningitis is clinical evidence of meningoencephalitis. The release of proinflammatory mediators in the subarachnoid space leads to an inflammatory response in the central nervous system, which contributes to increased blood–brain barrier permeability, cerebral edema, and increased intracranial pressure. For patients with decline of consciousness, or for those who fail to improve after initiation of appropriate antimicrobial therapy, brain imaging is indicated. The indication for repeated imaging is often arbitrarily based on the clinical status of the patient, the time frame between decline of consciousness and initiation of adequate therapy, and results of previous imaging. On neuroimaging, early signs of brain edema are disappearance of sylvian fissures and narrowing of ventricular size. In patients with an advanced stage of brain edema and raised intracranial pressure, basal cisterns and sulci may become obliterated. Several supportive therapies have been described in such patients, although no therapy has proven clinical efficacy. Osmotic diuretics to control intracranial pressure may be an option, although there are no definitive data on the efficacy of this approach.

Seizures and acute hydrocephalus are other frequent causes of a deteriorating level of consciousness. Patients with seizures or clinical suspicion of prior seizure should receive anticonvulsant therapy, but the low incidence of this complication does not justify prophylactic treatment. In patients with acute and non-obstructive (communicating) hydrocephalus, a lumbar puncture can allow measurement of CSF pressure.

Focal neurological abnormalities (i.e., hemiparesis, monoparesis, or aphasia) are most commonly caused by stroke, seizures, or a combination of both. Cranial nerve abnormalities are caused by the meningeal inflammatory process or by an increase of CSF pressure. The most frequent cranial nerve abnormality is involvement of the eighth cranial nerve, reflected by hearing loss. A cochlear implant may be needed in some severely affected patients.

Outcome

Community-acquired bacterial meningitis is a severe disease with high fatality and morbidity rates (Saez-Llorens and McCracken, 2003; van de Beek *et al.*, 2006). Meningitis caused by *S. pneumoniae* has the highest case fatality rates, reported from 19 to 37%. Of those who survive, up to 50% develop long-term neurologic sequelae, including cognitive impairment and developmental delays (van de Beek *et al.*, 2002). For meningococcal meningitis, mortality and morbidity rates are lower, with rates up to 5 and 7%, respectively. The strongest risk factors for an unfavorable outcome in patients with bacterial meningitis are those indicative of systemic compromise, impaired consciousness, low CSF white cell count, and infection with *S. pneumoniae*.

Citations

de Gans J and van de Beek D (2002) Dexamethasone in adults with bacterial meningitis. *New England Journal of Medicine* 347: 1549–1556.

Fitch MT and van de Beek D (2007) Emergency diagnosis and treatment of adult meningitis. *Lancet Infectious Diseases* 7: 191–200.

Molyneux EM, Walsh AL, Forsyth H, *et al.* (2002) Dexamethasone treatment in childhood bacterial meningitis in Malawi: A randomised controlled trial. *Lancet* 360: 211–218.

Nigrovic LE, Kuppermann N, Macias CG, *et al.* (2007) Clinical prediction rule for identifying children with cerebrospinal fluid pleocytosis at very low risk of bacterial meningitis. *Journal of the American Medical Association* 297: 52–60.

Peltola H (2000) Worldwide *Haemophilus influenzae* type b disease at the beginning of the 21st century: Global analysis of the disease burden 25 years after the use of the polysaccharide vaccine and a decade after the advent of conjugates. *Clinical Microbiology Reviews* 13: 302–317.

Saez-Llorens X and McCracken GH Jr. (2003) Bacterial meningitis in children. *Lancet* 361: 2139–2148.

Snape MD and Pollard AJ (2005) Meningococcal polysaccharide-protein conjugate vaccines. *Lancet Infectious Diseases* 5: 21–30.

Spanos A, Harrell FE Jr., and Durack DT (1989) Differential diagnosis of acute meningitis: An analysis of the predictive value of initial observations. *Journal of the American Medical Association* 262: 2700–2707.

Thomas KE, Hasbun R, Jekel J, and Quagliarello VJ (2002) The diagnostic accuracy of Kernig's sign, Brudzinski's sign, and nuchal rigidity in adults with suspected meningitis. *Clinical Infectious Diseases* 35: 46–52.

van de Beek D, Schmand B, de Gans J, *et al.* (2002) Cognitive impairment in adults with good recovery after bacterial meningitis. *Journal of Infectious Diseases* 186: 1047–1052.

van de Beek D, de Gans J, Spanjaard L, Weisfelt M, Reitsma JB, and Vermeulen M (2004) Clinical features and prognostic factors in adults with bacterial meningitis. *New England Journal of Medicine* 351: 1849–1859.

van de Beek D and de Gans J (2006) Dexamethasone in adults with bacterial meningitis. *Drugs* 66: 415–427.

van de Beek D, de Gans J, Tunkel AR, and Wijdicks EFM (2006) Community-acquired bacterial meningitis. *New England Journal of Medicine* 354: 46–55.

van de Beek D, de Gans J, McIntyre P, and Prasad K (2007) Corticosteroids in acute bacterial meningitis. *Cochrane Database of Systematic Reviews* 1: CD004405.

Whitney CG, Farley MM, Hadler J, *et al.* (2000) Increasing prevalence of multidrug-resistant *Streptococcus pneumoniae* in the United States. *New England Journal of Medicine* 343: 1917–1924.

Whitney CG, Farley MM, Hadler J, *et al.* (2003) Decline in invasive pneumococcal disease after the introduction of protein-polysaccharide conjugate vaccine. *New England Journal of Medicine* 348: 1737–1746.

Relevant Websites

http://www.ninds.nih.gov/ – American National Institutes of Health, National Institute of Neurological Disorders and Stroke.

http://www.meningvax.org – Information concerning the meningitis vaccination project of the World Health Organization.

http://www.meningitis.ca – Meningitis Research Foundation, Canada.

http://www.meningitis.org – Meningitis Research Foundation, UK.

Metabolic Myopathies

M Tarnopolsky, McMaster University, Hamilton, ON, Canada

Background

The metabolic myopathies represent a group of muscle disorders characterized by impairments in intermediary metabolism. The three main categories of disease include the mitochondrial myopathies, fatty acid oxidation defects (FAODs), and glycogen storage diseases (GSDs). Myoadenylate deaminase deficiency (AMPD1) has been considered by some to be a metabolic myopathy; however, its prevalence of almost 2% in the general population, and the documentation of completely asymptomatic individuals, renders its pathogenicity in question. Although there are a number of medications that can impair muscle metabolism (e.g., statins), these are generally grouped within the category of toxic myopathies and will not be considered further in this article. The focus of the article will be on the three major categories of inborn errors of metabolism as described above. It is important to recognize these conditions, because interventional strategies may be effective in preventing rhabdomyolysis and the severe consequence of potential renal failure. Furthermore, in conditions such as mitochondrial myopathies there may be multisystem involvement with very severe consequences, and genetic counseling may be appropriate. Finally, multisystem disorders such as the mitochondrial myopathies may be mislabeled as multiple sclerosis (MS), nonspecific encephalopathy, or vasculitis, and accurate diagnosis can avoid inappropriate therapeutic interventions such as β-interferon for MS or cyclophosphamide for vasculitis. A list of the more common metabolic myopathies is found in **Table 1**.

Although some consider the metabolic myopathies to be rare entities, it has been estimated that mitochondrial cytopathies affect about 1 in 8000 in the population. Although the FAODs and GSDs are comparatively less common (McArdle's disease = ~1/100 000; carnitine palmitoyl transferase (CPT) deficiency ~1/300 000, respectively), they do represent one of the more common causes of exercise-induced rhabdomyolysis, and prompt recognition by the treating physician is important.

The purpose of this article is to present a brief overview of the more common metabolic myopathies to provide the clinician with the tools to recognize symptoms, organize appropriate diagnostic testing, and be familiar with the available treatment options. Given space constraints, the reader will be referred to comprehensive and contemporary reviews. Other reviews of metabolic myopathies in general can be found in the references by Tarnopolsky (2006) and Tein (1996).

General Features of the Disorders and Inheritance

Mitochondrial Disorders

Mitochondrial disorders represent a diverse group of conditions with a primary defect in electron transport chain function. Although other conditions, such as amino acid and fatty acid oxidation defects, also occur in the mitochondria, they are not traditionally considered part of the mitochondrial disorders. Many of the mitochondrial myopathies were originally characterized by acronyms based upon the phenotypic presentation. For example, MELAS refers to Mitochondrial Encephalomyopathy, Lactic Acidosis, and Stroke-like episodes. The era of mitochondrial medicine expanded rapidly after the identification of a point mutation responsible for Leber's hereditary optic neuropathy (LHON, G11778A), chronic progressive external ophthalmoplegia (CPEO, mitochondrial DNA deletions) and MELAS (A3243G). Since that time there has been a massive proliferation of the number of point mutations in the mitochondrial genome ascribed to phenotypic characteristics.

In addition to the vast array of mutations found within the maternally inherited mitochondrial DNA (mtDNA), there is an increasing recognition of the mitochondrial disorders arising from mutations within the nuclear genome and following Mendelian genetic inheritance patterns. For example, the mutations responsible for a number of autosomal recessive conditions have been found, including myo-neuro-gastrointestinal encephalomyopathy (MNGIE, thymidine phosphorylase), complex I (NDUF) and IV (SURF-1) Leigh's disease, mtDNA depletion (dGuOK, TK) and some forms of mtDNA deletion syndromes (polymerase gamma, twinkle, ANT). Autosomal dominant inheritance patterns have also been seen in rare cases of mtDNA deletion syndromes.

Irrespective of the mutation, many of the cellular consequences of mitochondrial dysfunction can be linked to a decrease in aerobic energy production and/or an increased production of free radicals. Given that the mitochondrion is the final common pathway for the oxidative decarboxylation of fats, proteins, and carbohydrates, it is understandable that mitochondrial dysfunction can impair cellular energy metabolism, which can be particularly apparent during periods of superimposed metabolic stress (exercise, infection, prolonged fasting). Given the ubiquitous presence of mitochondria in all tissues except red blood cells, there is often widespread tissue involvement (mitochondrial

Table 1 Metabolic myopathies in skeletal muscle

Major category	Examples
Mitochondrial myopathy	MELAS, MERRF, mtDNA deletion, Kearn-Sayre syndrome, complex I deficiency, cytochrome b mutations, cytochrome c oxidase mutations
Fatty acid oxidation defect	CPT I, CPT II, TFP, MCAD, VLCAD, glutaric aciduria II
Glycogen storage disease	McArdle's (GSD V), Tarui's (GSD VII), Pompe's (GSD II), phosphorylase b kinase, lactate dehydrogenase, phosphoglycerate mutase, phosphoglycerate kinase (deficiency)
Myoadenylate deaminase deficiency	AMPD1 mutations

MELAS, mitochondria encephalomyopathy lactic acidosis and stroke-like episode; MERRF, myoclonus epilepsy and ragged red fibers; mtDNA, mitochondrial DNA; CPT, carnitine palmitoyl transferase; TFP, trifunctional protein; MCAD, medium chain acyl-COA dehydrogenase deficiency; VLCAD, very long acyl-COA dehydrogenase deficiency; GSD, glycogen storage disease.

cytopathies); however, most patients will have varying degrees of muscle symptoms (decreased endurance or weakness), and these forms can be termed 'mitochondrial myopathies.' Recent reviews of the mitochondrial cytopathies can be found in Tarnopolsky and Raha (2005) and Dimauro *et al.* (2006).

Fatty Acid Oxidation Defects

FAODs ultimately impair β-oxidation of lipid within the mitochondrial matrix. The main defects that have been identified include transport of long-chain fat across the mitochondrial membrane (i.e., CPT deficiency); transport of carnitine into the cell (i.e., carnitine transporter deficiency); and the majority of defects attributed to mutations in β-oxidation directly (i.e., long-chain acyl-CoA dehydrogenase (LCAD), medium-chain acyl-CoA dehydrogenase (MCAD), and trifunctional protein (TFP) deficiencies). These disorders are inherited with an autosomal recessive inheritance pattern. The more severe variants present in infancy or childhood with a primary liver or encephalopathic picture, while the adult-onset forms are predominantly myopathic. The main FAODs presenting in adulthood include CPT II, TFP, and very-long-chain acyl-CoA dehydrogenase deficiencies. Further reading in this area can be found in the reviews by Tein (1996) and Vockley *et al.* (2002).

Glycogen Storage Disease

GSD refers to a group of disorders characterized by genetic mutations in glycogen synthesis, glycogenolysis, or glycolysis. The pathology results from an inability to break down glycogen to maintain plasma glucose concentration (e.g., hepatic forms such as hepatic phosphorylase deficiency or glucose-6-phosphatase deficiency), abnormal tissue storage and cirrhosis (e.g., branching enzyme deficiency), or the myopathic forms that inhibit muscle glycogenolysis or glycolysis (e.g., McArdle's disease, Tarui's disease, etc.). The hepatic forms usually result in hypoglycemia as the main clinical manifestation, with type IV also leading to cirrhosis due to the accumulation of abnormal nonbranched glycogen molecules. The myopathic forms usually result in muscle cramping and premature fatigue particularly during high-intensity exercise when there is the obligatory use of anaerobic pathways. Some of the myopathic forms of GSD result in fixed muscle weakness such as Pompe's disease (GSD II), whereas others such as McArdle's disease (GSD V) may develop a more indolent proximal myopathy later in life. With the exception of phosphorylase b kinase deficiency and phosphoglycerate kinase deficiency, which are X-linked recessive conditions, the remainder of the GSDs are autosomal recessive in their inheritance pattern.

The more common myopathic forms of GSD, in approximate order of frequency, include phosphorylase deficiency (McArdle's disease, GSD V), acid maltase deficiency (Pompe's disease, GSD II), phosphorylase b kinase deficiency (GSD VIII), and phosphofructokinase (PFK) deficiency (Tarui's disease, GSD VII). Less common myopathic forms include debranching enzyme (GSD III), phosphoglycerate kinase (GSD IX), phosphoglycerate mutase (GSD X), and lactate dehydrogenase (GSD XI) deficiencies.

Clinical Presentation

It is important to note that many of the metabolic myopathies present with symptoms during exercise. During higher intensity exercise such as sprinting, or at the onset of aerobic exercise, there is predominantly an anaerobic component, with the adenylate kinase/myoadenylate deaminase pathway being quantitatively the least important, followed by the CK-mediated pathway of phosphocreatine hydrolysis, and anaerobic glycolysis and glycogenolysis (**Figure 1**).

With endurance-type activity, the proportion of oxidized fuels changes as a function of exercise intensity, training status, and gender; however, at moderate-intensity exercise (less than 50% of maximal aerobic capacity (VO_{2max})), the main sources of fuels are plasma free fatty acids and blood-borne glucose. As the intensity of exercise increases there is proportionately greater utilization of intramuscular glycogen and intramyocellular lipids, with almost exclusive utilization of intramuscular glycogen at intensities closer to a 10-km or marathon race

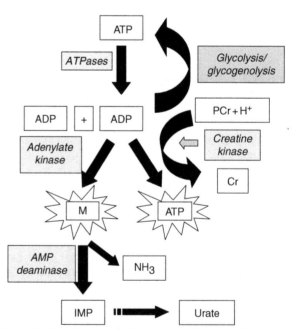

Figure 1 The three anaerobic energy pathways in skeletal muscle.

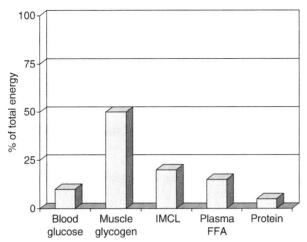

Figure 2 The major fuel sources in skeletal muscle during submaximal endurance exercise. Each value is a proportion of the total energy expenditure. FFA , free fatty acids; IMCL, intramyocellular lipids.

pace. The mitochondria are obligatory for the oxidative metabolism of carbohydrate fat and protein, thus representing the final common pathway of aerobic energy transduction. The main fuel sources during endurance activity at approximately 65% of the VO_{2max} are presented in **Figure 2**.

Under normal circumstances, the ATP content of skeletal muscle is tightly regulated and does not decrease; however, with the metabolic myopathies it is possible to reach a state of metabolic crisis and induce rhabdomyolysis, which can lead to myoglobinuria and subsequent renal failure. A list of some of the causes of myoglobinuria is found in **Table 2**. A list of the common symtoms of the metabolic myopathies is presented in **Table 3**.

Mitochondrial Disorders

There is extreme phenotypic and genotypic heterogeneity in the mitochondrial cytopathies. For example, patients with the MELAS A3243G gene mutation can present with later adult-onset deafness and diabetes, or in infancy with fatal encephalomyopathy with seizures and stroke-like episodes. Conversely, patients with a wide array of specific point mutations, mtDNA deletions, and nuclear defects can present with encephalopathy, muscle fatigue or ptosis and hearing loss. Due to the impairment in aerobic energy transduction, most patients have very low maximal oxygen uptake (VO_{2max}), which renders daily activities much more stressful and taxing and patients often present with exercise intolerance. Although the exercise intolerance is often overshadowed by more significant neurological symptoms, most adult patients will have quite severe exercise intolerance, often dating back to childhood. These individuals were often labeled as being 'the worst athlete in the school' and

Table 2 Neuromuscular diseases causing myoglobinuria

More common	Less common
CPT II	mtDNA deletion
McArdle's disease (GSD V)	Mitochondrial cytochrome
Toxic myopathies (alcohol, statins)	oxidase defect
Some muscular dystrophies (with unaccustomed exercise)	Familial recurrent myoglobinuria
	Other GSDs
Extreme overexertion in dehydrated state (e.g., hot/humid environment)	Other FAODs (VLCAD, TFP)
Viral myositis (e.g., Coxsackie, influenza A and B)	Inflammatory myopathies

CPT, carnitine palmitoyl transferase; GSD, glycogen storage disease; FAOD, fatty acid oxidation defect; VLCAD, very long acyl-COA dehydrogenase deficiency; TFP, trifunctional protein.

Table 3 Clinical symptoms and history suggesting metabolic myopathies

History	Possible disorder
Pigmenturia	GSDs, FAODs
Myalgias/cramps with endurance sports	FAODs, mtDNA defects, ? AMPD1 deficiency
Myalgias/cramps with power/sprint sports	GSDs, ? AMPD1 deficiency
Symptoms triggered by fasting or superimposed illness	FAODs, mtDNA defect
Gouty arthritis	GSDs
Nausea/vomiting with exercise	GSD VII, mtDNA defect
Multiple system involvement	mtDNA defect
Family history:	
X-linked	Phosphorylase b kinase
Maternal	mtDNA
Sporadic	mtDNA deletions
Autosomal recessive/consanguinous	CPT II, most GSDs, AMPD deficiency

GSD, glycogen storage disease; FAOD, fatty acid oxidation defect; AMPD1, myoadenylate deaminase deficiency; mtDNA, mitochondrial DNA; CPT II, carnitine palmitoyl tranferase-2 deficiency.

frequently avoided physical activity. Unlike the FAODs and GSDs, it is rare for patients to have rhabdomyolysis with resultant myoglobinuria; however, this can be seen in cytochrome b, cytochrome c oxidase (COX), and MELAS A3260G mutations.

In addition to exercise intolerance, patients with mitochondrial myopathies frequently have headache, nausea, and vomiting induced by exercise and can become frankly encephalopathic. We have seen one pedigree with the MELAS A3260G gene mutation where exercise-induced deafness was a characteristic feature. The symptoms of exercise intolerance are much worse when individuals have a superimposed infection or are in the fasted state, which are conditions where a greater reliance on mitochondrial energy function is required.

In addition to exercise intolerance and the extensive list of other clinical features that can accompany these disorders (ptosis, ophthalmoplegia, hearing loss, stroke-like episodes, migraine, headaches, cardiomyopathy,-ataxia, encephalopathy, etc.), another muscle-related symptom can be fixed weakness. We have had several pedigrees with the MELAS A3243G gene mutation where fixed proximal weakness to the point of respiratory failure was a presenting feature. In most patients, however, strength is reasonably well preserved, and the factors predisposing some patients to severe weakness are currently unclear.

Fatty Acid Oxidation Defects

Many patients with myopathic FAODs are asymptomatic without the superimposition of a metabolic stress. In children, the two main metabolic stressors are superimposed illnesses, such as viral illness, or prolonged fasting, nausea, and vomiting with decreased fluid and caloric intake, where significant weakness, lethargy, and even encephalopathy can occur. The adult myopathic forms of FAOD usually present during endurance type activity, particularly if it is prolonged, performed in the fasted state, or with a superimposed viral illness. These individuals can often perform high-intensity activity for short periods of time without difficulty; however, when the utilization of lipid becomes more important, such as during longer-term endurance activity, they often experience cramps, muscle discomfort, and inability to continue the activity. There is often pigmenturia later in the day or the next day following such an activity, and the muscles remain very sore for several days. In some cases severe myalgias with rhabdomyolysis and renal failure can be the presenting symptom of FAOD.

Glycogen Storage Disease

As mentioned previously, the infantile and childhood forms of GSD often present with hypoglycemia and an encephalopathic picture. McArdle's disease (GSD V) is exclusively a myopathic condition with muscle cramps and pigmenturia induced by higher-intensity exercise, such as climbing stairs or sprinting for a bus. Other disorders, such as Tarui's disease and phosphorylase b kinase deficiency (GSD VIII), are usually predominantly myopathic; whereas all of the other myopathic forms can have more severe pediatric onset, with hepatomegaly and more severe progressive proximal myopathy in addition to exercise intolerance. Patients with Pompe's disease (GSD II) have predominantly fixed proximal weakness and respiratory insufficiency rather than exercise-induced discomfort. Patients with McArdle's disease and Tarui's disease have a compensatory increase in flux through the adenylate kinase/myoadenylate deaminase pathway, with a subsequent increase in uric acid, and can present with myogenic hyperuricemia and gout.

Diagnostic Testing

The main diagnostic tests for the metabolic myopathies include blood tests (serum CK activity, lactate, acyl-carnitine), urine testing (organic acids, myoglobin), muscle biopsy (light and electron microscopy, enzymology), exercise testing, genetic testing, and magnetic resonance spectroscopy. These should be conducted at a center with experience in these disorders and the ability to collect and process samples appropriately. For example, delays in freezing the muscle biopsy, delays in serum lactate determination, and timing of sample acquisition are only a few examples of situations in which false-positive or -negative tests can occur. A summary of the common diagnostic tests can be found in **Table 4**.

Table 4 Common tests for metabolic myopathies

Disease	*Testing*
Mitochondrial disease	Elevated lactate Abnormal urine organic acids (3-methyl glutaconic, fumarate) Low exercise capacity (decreased VO_2) Impaired muscle deoxygenation (near infra-red spectroscopy) MRI findings (strokes, white matter changes) MR spectroscopy (elevated lactate, decreased phosphocreatine) Muscle biopsy (ragged red fibers, COX negative fibers) Muscle enzymology Specific gene mutations (mtDNA deletion (PCR), Southern blot, A3243G (PCR-RFLP))
Fatty acid oxidation defect	Elevated creatine kinase during event (normal between) +/− carnitine concentration Acyl-carnitine profile (GS-MS-MS) Urine organic acids (dicarboxylic acids) Decreased glucose and ketone during event Muscle biopsy (increased lipids) Enzyme analysis (muscle +/− fibroblasts) specific mutation (ser113leu (PCR-RFLP))
Glycogen storage disease	Elevated creatine kinase (even at rest (McArdle's)) +/− elevated uric acid 'Second wind' with exercise test No increase in lactate with exaggerated ammonia response to forearm exercise testing Muscle biopsy = increased glycogen Muscle enzyme activity Specific mutation analysis (R49X)

Mitochondrial Disorders

The serum lactate determination is one of the more important blood tests. This indicator is elevated in approximately 70% of patients. It is important that the blood be collected on ice and promptly analyzed. An elevated lactate has high specificity (>0.9) but lower sensitivity (~ 0.7) for mitochondrial cytopathies. False-positive tests can occur in diabetics and in patients who ate a high-carbohydrate meal within $2\,h$ of collection. Patients with MELAS may have elevated plasma glucose level or impaired glucose tolerance given their propensity towards insulin resistance in type 2 diabetes. Serum CK activity may be elevated but is rarely more than five times the upper limit of normal. Urine testing includes organic acid assessment with elevations noted in ethylmalonic acid, 3-methyl glutaconic acid, and fumarate.

The muscle biopsy can show ragged red fibers (sub-sarcolemmal accumulation of mitochondria on modified Gomori trichrome staining), COX-negative fibers, and accumulation of neutral lipids. At the electron microscopic level, pleomorphic mitochondria often containing para-crystalline inclusions are a feature of mitochondrial dysfunction. Although some of the mitochondrial myopathies will show defects in specific enzyme activity in fibroblasts and platelets, the vast majority are detectable only with biochemical assays of electron transport chain enzyme activity in skeletal muscle homogenates or isolated mitochondria. A selected defect in complex IV activity would prompt a search for mutations associated with complex IV assembly (SCO2) or mutations in the mitochondrial (COI, II, III) or nuclear-encoded (COIV, COVb) sub-units. Conversely, multiple enzymatic defects would prompt a search for transfer RNA or mtDNA mutations.

Specific mutation analysis can be completed if a given gene mutation is strongly suspected from the history or if a mutation is known in a family. Mutation analysis can be performed using polymerase chain reaction–restriction fragment length polymorphism (PCR-RFLP), allele specific oligonucleotide, and a host of other tests to identify the point mutation. Often, a test panel is completed as a function of the clinical phenotype. For example, a patient with stroke-like episodes, seizures, and muscle fatigability would probably start with a screen for MELAS A3243G, T3271C. A patient with CPEO would prompt a search for mtDNA deletions by Southern blot or long-range PCR. If a mutation is not identified, mtDNA sequencing can be completed in approximately one day of the entire genome (16 569 base pairs).

Exercise testing in mitochondrial myopathies usually demonstrates a markedly reduced VO_{2max} or an abnormally high respiratory exchange ratio (indicative of early lactate production) with cycle ergometry testing (for a review, see Tarnopolsky, 2004). A variety of testing modalities have been employed with forearm exercise testing, including near infrared spectroscopy or direct venous blood gas measurements, to demonstrate the lack of deoxygenation due to decreased oxygen consumption by defective mitochondria. Phosphorus (^{31}P) magnetic resonance spectroscopy has also been used to demonstrate an increased reliance on phosphocreatine hydrolysis or a delay in the postexercise phosphocreatine recovery. A review of the diagnostic criteria for the mitochondrial cytopathies can be found in Naviaux (2004).

Fatty Acid Oxidation Defects

Blood tests including CK, lactate, and glucose can be completely normal in asymptomatic individuals with FAODs. During an acute metabolic crisis, there is often hypoketotic hypoglycemia and an increase in serum CK activity. Other findings such as hyperkalemia can be associated with an acute episode of rhabdomyolysis. If the rhabdomyolysis induces renal failure, a delayed increase in urea and creatinine and other markers such as metabolic acidosis and hyperkalemia can accompany the acute renal failure.

More definite blood testing can be completed using liquid chromatography–tandem mass spectroscopy (LC/MS/MS) characterizing the acyl-carnitine profile. Occasionally, in the non-stressed situation, but more often during an acute event, the acyl-carnitine signature can yield the definitive diagnosis. A reduction in serum total and free carnitine can also be documented in many cases.

Urine testing during an acute myopathic event may show myoglobin, in which case admission and standard rhabdomyolysis protocols must be employed. During this time, dicarboxylic acids can be identified in the urine using gas chromatography/mass spectroscopy (GC/MS). Enzymatic testing in fibroblasts is usually much more informative than with the mitochondrial cytopathies and specific enzyme pathways (CPT II) or functional assays with medium- or long-chain substrates can be used to help identify a biochemical defect. The molecular defects can be screened using standard procedures once either an acyl-carnitine profile or biochemical tests suggest a specific mutation. In some cases, such as a classic presentation of CPT II deficiency, it may be appropriate to screen by checking for the most common mutation (ser113leu) through a variety of genetic methods as mentioned previously.

Exercise testing is often normal, although the VO_{2max} can be somewhat diminished; however, this is neither sensitive nor specific. Occasionally, a high respiratory exchange ratio during low-intensity exercise may indicate the increased reliance upon carbohydrates, although this finding cannot rule in or rule out a FAOD. A muscle biopsy may show an increase in neutral lipids but may also be completely normal, with no other structural alterations. Reviews of the FAODs can be found in Tein (1996).

Glycogen Storage Disease

The serum CK activity is invariably elevated in patients with McArdle's disease at all times and may be variably elevated in the other GSDs. During an acute metabolic crisis the CK activity is invariably elevated to values that can exceed 100 000 U/L. The elevation of CK activity and the resultant risk for renal abnormalities are no different from those seen for FAODs, and these patterns alone cannot be used to determine the etiology of the rhabdomyolysis during an acute event. Serum uric acid may be elevated due to myogenic hyperuricemia, and this can trigger gouty arthritis. A unique feature of PFK deficiency is the presence of hemolytic anemia. Urine testing is totally normal except during acute rhabdomyolysis, where the expected myoglobin is often present.

The muscle biopsy often shows an increase in glycogen concentration as determined by periodic acid-Schiff staining. Histological enzyme assays are routinely available for phosphorylase and PFK activity and can confirm a diagnosis in the appropriate clinical context. Electron microscopy usually shows increased glycogen concentration, and in the case of Pompe's disease, it is membrane bound within lysosomes.

Forearm ischemic, semi-ischemic, and aerobic exercise testing have been described and debated; however, all of these methods demonstrate a failure of lactate to increase with an exaggerated ammonia response (Tarnopolsky et al., 2003). Aerobic exercise testing shows rapid increase in heart rate, rating of perceived exertion, and early fatigue and cramping. If an individual with McArdle's disease slows down and continues to exercise, there is often a 'second wind' that occurs when blood-borne substrates become available and the heart rate falls, and it becomes easier to continue to exercise. The VO_{2max} is often significantly reduced in patients with myopathic GSD.

Magnetic resonance spectroscopy using ^{31}P spectra can demonstrate a lack of acidosis in most cases with distal defects in glycolysis (PFK, phosphoglycerate kinase, phosphoglycerate mutase deficiencies) showing a characteristic increase in phosphomonoesters.

If a specific genetic mutation is known in the family or strongly suspected based on the aforementioned testing, mutation analysis is available for most of the disorders. For example, for a North American Caucasian patient with classic symptoms of muscle cramps with high-intensity exercise and rhabdomyolysis, an initial genetic screen for the most common mutation (R49X) may be prudent.

Treatment

Mitochondrial Disorders

The mitochondrial myopathies result in a decrease in aerobic energy transduction through the electron transport chain, an increase in free radical production, and an increased reliance on alternative energy stores. Consequently, therapeutic strategies have traditionally focused on these areas. Strategies that have been used to either bypass specific defects or enhance the flux through the electron transport chain have included; succinate and riboflavin to bypass complex I; coenzyme Q10 as an antioxidant and electron acceptor from complex I and II; antioxidants such as vitamin E, vitamin C, α-lipoic acid and coenzyme Q10. In an attempt to provide an alternative energy supply, some have tried oral creatine monohydrate supplementation with variable success. Studies using dichloroacetate to reduce lactate levels have not been rewarding, and a major side effect of peripheral neuropathy has been seen. Consequently, its use is only advocated during acute severe events with very high lactate concentration. Reviews of nutritional therapies and pharmacological therapies can be found in the following references (Mahoney et al., 2002; DiMauro et al., 2006).

Studies have demonstrated improvement in function in patients following an endurance exercise training program and there is theoretical evidence that higher intensity weight training can activate satellite cells and lessen the mutational burden particularly in sporadic mitochondrial cytopathies (Taivassalo and Haller, 2005). There are a variety of genetic strategies that have been attempted *in vitro*; however, to date these are not applicable to the clinical scenario (Dimauro et al., 2006).

Fatty Acid Oxidation Defects

The mainstay of therapy is to avoid exercise during the fasting state or during periods of superimposed infection. If an individual has a flu-like illness with vomiting and diarrhea and can not consume carbohydrates, careful monitoring is required, sometimes with emergency admission and intravenous treatment with glucose-containing fluids. Most patients can avoid problems with more frequent, higher-carbohydrate feedings, and in some more severe cases cornstarch at night may be required. The consumption of a high-carbohydrate diet including carbohydrate loading and carbohydrates before and during exercise is a mainstay of therapy. Although riboflavin and medium-chain triglyceride oil have been advocated, their efficacy has not yet been demonstrated conclusively in a randomized double-blind trial.

Glycogen Storage Disease

Lifestyle adjustment is probably the best treatment for GSDs, including avoiding brief bursts of high-intensity activity. Interestingly, progressive aerobic conditioning improves functional capacity in such cases, likely by improving fitness and 'raising the bar' for the exercise metabolic

Table 5 Treatments for metabolic myopathies

Disease	Treatment
Mitochondrial disease	Progressive exercise training
	Avoid fasting and no exercise during illness
	Antioxidants (vitamin C, vitamin E, alpha lipoic acid)
	Cofactors (coenzyme Q_{10})
	Alternative substrates (creatine monohydrate)
Fatty acid oxidation defect	Progressive exercise training
	Avoid fasting and no exercise during illness
	Carnitine (only if low or transporter defect)
	High-carbohydrate diet
	? Medium chain triglyceride oil
	Carbohydrate before and during exercise
	Riboflavin
Glycogen storage disease	Progressive exercise training
	Pyridoxine
	Creatine monohydrate
	High-protein diet (>20% of energy)
	Pre-exercise carbohydrates

crisis threshold (Haller *et al.*, 2006). The consumption of sucrose or glucose 15 to 20 min prior to exercise can provide an exogenous source of glucose and improve exercise capacity in patients with glycogenolytic defects (Vissing and Haller, 2003). In contrast, patients with defects in glycolysis do worse with glucose ingestion, because it inhibits lipolysis and they can't take advantage of the exogenous glucose (due to the block in glycolysis). Pyridoxine (vitamin B6) supplementation has been advocated in the specific entity of McArdle's disease due to the fact that it is stored in conjunction with the enzyme phosphorylase (which is missing in this entity); however, it has not been evaluated by a rigorous clinical trial. High-protein diets have also been advocated to up-regulate alternative fuel utilization; again, randomized double-blind trials have not been completed. One randomized double-blind trial did demonstrate benefits from the use of creatine monohydrate in low to moderate doses with an impairment of exercise capacity in higher doses (see two papers by Vorgerd and colleagues).

A summary of the treatment strategies for metabolic myopathies can be found in **Table 5**.

See also: Multiple Sclerosis; Muscular Dystrophies.

Citations

DiMauro S, Hirano M, and Schon EA (2006) Approaches to the treatment of mitochondrial diseases. *Muscle and Nerve* 34(3): 265–283.

Haller RG, Wyrick P, Taivassalo T, and Vissing J (2006) Aerobic conditioning: An effective therapy in McArdle's disease. *Annals of Neurology* 59(6): 922–928.

Mahoney DJ, Parise G, and Tarnopolsky MA (2002) Nutritional and exercise-based therapies in the treatment of mitochondrial disease. *Current Opinion in Clinical Nutrition and Metabolic Care* 5(6): 619–629.

Naviaux RK (2004) Developing a systematic approach to the diagnosis and classification of mitochondrial disease. *Mitochondrion* 4: 351–361.

Taivassalo T and Haller RG (2005) Exercise and training in mitochondrial myopathies. *Medicine and Science in Sports and Exercise* 37(12): 2094–2101.

Tarnopolsky MA (2004) Exercise testing as a diagnostic entity in mitochondrial myopathies. *Mitochondrion* 4(5–6): 529–542.

Tarnopolsky MA (2006) What can metabolic myopathies teach us about exercise physiology? *Applied Physiology, Nutrition, and Metabolism* 31(1): 21–30.

Tarnopolsky MA and Raha S (2005) Mitochondrial myopathies: Diagnosis, exercise intolerance, and treatment options. *Medicine and Science in Sports and Exercise* 37(12): 2086–2093.

Tarnopolsky M, Stevens L, MacDonald JR, et al. (2003) Diagnostic utility of a modified forearm ischemic exercise test and technical issues relevant to exercise testing. *Muscle and Nerve* 27(3): 359–366.

Tein I (1996) Metabolic myopathies. *Seminars in Pediatric Neurology* 3(2): 59–98.

Vissing J and Haller RG (2003) The effect of oral sucrose on exercise tolerance in patients with McArdle's disease. *New England Journal of Medicine* 349(26): 2503–2509.

Vockley J, Singh RH, and Whiteman DA (2002) Diagnosis and management of defects of mitochondrial beta-oxidation. *Current Opinion in Clinical Nutrition and Metabolic Care* 5(6): 601–609.

Vorgerd M, Grehl T, Jager M, et al. (2000) Creatine therapy in myophosphorylase deficiency (McArdle disease): a placebo-controlled crossover trial. *Archives of Neurology* 57(7): 956–963.

Vorgerd M, Zange J, Kley R, et al. (2002) Effect of high-dose creatine therapy on symptoms of exercise intolerance in McArdle disease; double-blind, placebo-controlled crossover study. *Archives of Neurology* 59(1): 97–101.

Further Reading

Quinlivan R and Beynon RJ (2004) Pharmacological and nutritional treatment for McArdle's disease (glycogen storage disease type V). *Cochrane Database of Systematic Reviews* 3: CD003458.

World Muscle Society (2004) NMD gene tables. *Neuromuscular Disorders* 14(1). http://www1.elsevier.com/homepage/sah/nmd/doc/genetables.html (accessed August 2007).

Relevant Websites

http://www.spiralnotebook.org/ – The Spiral Notebook: Short Takes on Carnitine Palmitoyl Transferase Deficiency.

http://www.mdausa.org/ – U.S. Muscular Dystrophy Association (MDA).

http://www.neuro.wustl.edu/neuromuscular/ – Washington University at St. Louis Neuromuscular Disease Center.

Migraine

A May, University of Hamburg, Hamburg, Germany

The Clinical Picture

Migraine is an idiopathic headache disorder characterized by moderate to severe, often unilateral and pulsating headache attacks, which are typically aggravated by physical activity. The individual attacks are accompanied by a loss of appetite (almost always), nausea (80%), vomiting (40–50%), light sensitivity (photophobia, 60%), noise sensitivity (phonophobia, 50%) and odor hypersensitivity (10%). If the headaches are unilateral, they can change sides within an attack or from attack to attack. The diagnostic criteria for migraine attacks and the migraine aura are presented in **Table 1**. The duration of attacks is typically 4 to 72 h; at least five attacks must have occurred before the diagnosis can be established. The frequency and duration of migraine attacks varies widely between individuals, though the median frequency is around one attack per month and median duration is roughly 24 h. In up to 15% of cases, the migraine headache is preceded by a recurrent disorder manifesting itself in attacks of reversible focal neurological symptoms, usually developing gradually over a period of 5 to 20 min and lasting for less than 60 min. This neurological sign known as an aura consists mostly of visual phenomena, typically jagged zig-zag lines that move slowly across the visual field, often followed by visual loss (scotoma). Cortical spreading depression (CSD) has been suggested to underlie migraine visual aura, based on the slow spread of clinical and electrophysiological events in animal experiments.

Most patients suffer from migraine attacks without aura. However, there are several migraine syndromes with particular aura features and migraine syndromes with uncommon histories or complications. These syndromes have their own diagnostic criteria; the subclassification of these syndromes is outlined in **Table 2**. These diagnostic criteria for migraine syndromes are also available on the homepage of the IHS (International Headache Society) (www.i-h-s.org).

In children, migraine attacks can be shorter (e.g., for only 1 or 2 h) and the accompanying symptoms can be more prominent, including syndromes such as abdominal migraine or periodic syndromes in childhood.

Epidemiology and Genetics

Migraine is one of the most frequent headache disorders. About 6 to 8% of males and 12 to 14% of females suffer from migraine attacks. The lifetime prevalence in females may be up to 25%. Before puberty, the prevalence of migraine is about 5% both in boys and girls. The highest incidence of migraine attacks occurs between the ages 35 and 45, potentially the most productive period of life, with a female preponderance of three to one. The median duration of untreated migraine attacks is 18 h; the median attack frequency is one per month.

Table 1 Diagnostic criteria of migraine according to the IHS classification (2004)

A. At least five attacks fulfilling criteria B–D
B. Headache lasting 4–72 h (untreated or unsuccessfully treated)
C. Headache has at least two of the following characteristics:
   1. unilateral location
   2. pulsating quality
   3. moderate or severe pain intensity
   4. aggravation by or causing avoidance of routine physical activity (e.g., walking or climbing stairs)
D. During headache at least one of the following occurs:
   1. nausea and/or vomiting
   2. photophobia and phonophobia
E. Not attributed to another disorder

Table 2 Subclassification of migraine according to the IHS classification (2004)

1.1 Migraine without aura
1.2 Migraine with aura
   1.2.1 Typical aura with migraine headache
   1.2.2 Typical aura with non-migraine headache
   1.2.3 Typical aura without headache
   1.2.4 Familial hemiplegic migraine
   1.2.5 Sporadic hemiplegic migraine
   1.2.6 Basilar-type migraine
1.3 Childhood periodic syndromes that are commonly precursors of migraine
   1.3.1 Cyclical vomiting
   1.3.2 Abdominal migraine
   1.3.3 Benign paroxysmal vertigo of childhood
1.4 Retinal migraine
1.5 Complications of migraine
   1.5.1 Chronic migraine
   1.5.2 Status migrainosus
   1.5.3 Persistent aura without infarction
   1.5.4 Migrainous infarction
   1.5.5 Migraine-triggered seizure
1.6 Probable migraine
   1.6.1 Probable migraine without aura
   1.6.2 Probable migraine with aura
   1.6.3 Probable chronic migraine

Epidemiological and twin studies indicate that migraine and in particular migraine with aura is an inherited disease. However, multiple genes must be involved. Familial hemiplegic migraine (FHM) is a dominantly inherited disease in which the affected family members have severe and long-lasting migraine auras sometimes leading to hemiplegia or even loss of consciousness. Several years ago a French group and a Dutch group independently identified a gene locus on chromosome 19 as the responsible culprit. Several genetic loci have been identified by now, encoding P/Q calcium channels, Na^{2+}/K^+ pump, and a neuronal voltage-gated sodium channel. Consequently, FHM is considered a 'channelopathy,' but whether these genetic variants play a role in non-hemiplegic migraine with aura and in migraine without aura is not known.

The Burden of Migraine

Migraine attacks can have a profound effect on the quality of life of the sufferer. In the long term, migraine may cause emotional changes and result in coping strategies that interfere with work, social, and family life. Consequently, the results of health-related quality-of-life studies demonstrate that migraine has a considerable impact on functional capacity, resulting in disrupted work and social activities. The impact of migraine on many quality of life parameters is similar to that of other chronic conditions, such as osteoarthritis, diabetes, and depression.

The direct costs of migraine (due to medical care) are small compared with the indirect costs caused by absence from work and reduced productivity. Many migraineurs, however, do not seek medical attention, have not been accurately diagnosed by a physician, or do not use prescription medication. Epidemiological studies reveal that migraine is often underdiagnosed and undertreated. Identifying and treating appropriate patients will reduce the impact of migraine on the individual level and the burden of migraine on the society.

Diagnosis

The diagnosis of migraine is based on the typical patient's history (see above: clinical picture) and a normal neurological examination. Further investigations, in particular brain imaging, are necessary if secondary headache is suspected (e.g., if the headache characteristics are atypical), when the course of headache attacks changes, or if persistent neurological or psychopathological abnormalities are present. In particular, a diagnostic investigation including imaging of the brain in migraine is recommended when

- the neurological examination is not normal
- typical migraine attacks occur for the first time after the age of 40
- frequency or intensity of migraine attacks continuously increases
- the accompanying symptoms of migraine attacks change
- new psychiatric symptoms occur in relation to the attacks.

Comorbid neuropathologies in migraine may involve mood disorders, such as depression and anxiety, as well as epilepsy and essential tremor. Epidemiological data suggest that migraine may be associated with subclinical vascular brain lesions and that migraine may be a risk factor for cerebral ischemia. However, prospective data evaluating the association between specific headache forms and stroke are sparse. In a recent prospective study including nearly 40 000 women, an increased risk of total and ischemic stroke was found for migraineurs with aura. However, the absolute risk increase was low, with 3.8 additional cases per year per 10 000 women.

Treatment

The medical treatment of migraine includes both acute therapy aimed at aborting the attacks and prophylactic therapy aimed at reducing attacks in the long term.

Acute Therapy

Several large randomized, placebo-controlled studies have been undertaken to establish the best drug treatment regimen for the acute management of migraine. In most of these trials, successful treatment of migraine attacks was defined as one or a combination of the following criteria:

- pain free after 2 h
- improvement of headache from moderate or severe to mild or none after 2 h
- consistent efficacy in two out of three attacks
- no headache recurrence and no further drug intake within 24 h after successful treatment (so-called sustained pain relief or pain free).

Analgesics and antiemetics

Analgesics are the preferred drugs of choice for mild or moderate migraine attacks. Evidence of efficacy in migraine treatment in at least one placebo-controlled study has been obtained for acetylsalicylic acid (ASA) up to 1000 mg, for ibuprofen from 200 mg to 800 mg, for diclofenac from 50 mg to 100 mg, 1000 mg for metamizol, and 1000 mg for paracetamol. In addition, the fixed combination of ASA, paracetamol, and caffeine is effective in acute migraine treatment and is also more effective than either of the single substances alone. In order to prevent drug overuse headache, the intake of simple analgesics should be restricted to 15 days per month and the intake of combined analgesics to 10 days per month. Coxibs are not recommended for acute migraine treatment because of cerebrovascular adverse side effects. Opioids are of only minor efficacy; no modern controlled trials are available for these substances. **Table 3** presents an overview of analgesics with efficacy in acute migraine treatment.

The use of antiemetics in acute migraine attacks is recommended for the treatment of vegetative symptoms and because it is assumed that these drugs improve the resorption of analgesics. However, prospective, placebo-controlled randomized trials to prove this assumption are lacking. There is no evidence that the fixed combination of an antiemetic with an analgesic or with a triptan is more effective than the analgesic or triptan alone. Regarding ergot alkaloids, the only compound with sufficient evidence of efficacy is ergotamine tartrate 2 mg (oral or suppositories). Ergot alkaloids can induce drug overuse headache very fast and at very low doses. Therefore, their use must be limited to 10 days per month. Major side effects include nausea, vomiting, paresthesia, and ergotism. Contraindications are cardiovascular and cerebrovascular diseases, Raynaud's disease, arterial hypertension, renal failure, and pregnancy and breastfeeding.

Triptans (5-HT$_{1B/1D}$-agonists)

The 5-HT$_{1B/1D}$ agonists sumatriptan, zolmitriptan, naratriptan, rizatriptan, almotriptan, eletriptan, and frovatriptan (ordered by year marketed), so-called triptans, are specific migraine medications and should not be used for other headache disorders, except for cluster headache. The efficacy of all triptans has been proven in large placebo-controlled trials of which several meta-analyses have been published. It should be noted that in about 60% of nonresponders to NSAIDs, triptans are effective. Triptans can be effective at any time during a migraine attack.

Table 3 Migraine therapy according to the task force of the EFNS (2006)

Acute therapy
1. Acetylsalicylic acid
2. Ibuprofen
3. Naproxen
4. Acetaminophen
5. Dihydroergotamin
6. Triptans
Preventive therapy
1. Beta blockers (Metoprolol or Propranolol)
2. Flunarizine
3. Valproic acid
4. Topiramate

However, there is evidence that the earlier triptans are taken, the better the efficacy. However, a strategy of strictly early intake may lead to frequent drug treatment in certain patients. The use of triptans is restricted to a maximum of 10 days per month. Otherwise, there is a danger of developing a drug overuse headache.

Preventive Therapy

Prophylactic drug treatment of migraine is possible with several drugs. Substances with good efficacy and tolerability are beta blockers, calcium channel blockers, antiepileptic drugs, NSAIDs, and antidepressants. The use of all these drugs, however, is based on empirical data rather than on proven pathophysiological concepts. The decision to introduce a prophylactic treatment has to be carefully discussed with the patient. A prophylactic drug treatment of migraine should be considered and discussed with the patient when

- the quality of life, business duties, or school attendance are severely impaired
- frequency of attacks per month is two or higher
- migraine attacks do not respond to acute drug treatment
- frequent, very long, or uncomfortable auras occur.

A migraine prophylaxis is regarded as successful if the frequency of migraine attacks per month is decreased by at least 50% within 3 months. For therapy evaluation, a headache diary is mandatory. The drugs of choice, according to the consensus of the task force, are outlined in **Table 3**.

Specific Situations

Menstrual migraine

Headaches may occur as a result of natural ovarian cycles, or in response to the withdrawal of exogenously administered estrogen. For some women, these headaches are more severe, are of longer duration, and lead to greater disability than those occurring at other times in the menstrual cycle. Consequently, one prophylactic treatment regimen of menstrual migraine involves estrogen replacement therapy. Supplemental estrogen may be administered in the late luteal phase of the natural menstrual cycle or during the pill-free week of traditional combination oral contraceptives. In menopause, hormonally associated migraine is most likely due to estrogen-replacement regimens. However, evidence regarding the safety and efficacy of hormonal replacement/modulating regimens is limited, and evidence particularly is lacking regarding its long-term dangers or side effects. Consequently, hormonal treatment of migraine is not a preferred treatment strategy for most women with migraine. Alternatively, Naproxen sodium (550 mg twice daily) has been shown to reduce pain including headache in the premenstrual syndrome.

Migraine in pregnancy

Migraine does not increase the risk of complications of pregnancy either for the mother or for the fetus. Several retrospective studies have shown a tendency for migraine to improve with pregnancy. Between 60 and 70% of women either go into remission or improve significantly, mainly during the second and third trimesters. It seems as if women with migraine onset at menarche and those with perimenstrual migraine are more likely to go into remission during pregnancy. It is in the first trimester that the fetus is at the greatest risk from drugs. Fortunately, most of the pregnant migraineurs experience fewer or even no migraine attacks. However, migraine often recurs post partum. There are no specific clinical trials evaluating drug treatment of migraine during pregnancy; most of the migraine drugs are contraindicated. If migraine occurs during pregnancy, only paracetamol is recommended. Triptans and ergot alkaloids are contraindicated. The use of prophylactic agents during pregnancy should be the exception, not the rule, and preferably only during the second and third trimesters; only magnesium and metoprolol are recommended.

Migraine in children and adolescents

Pediatric headache is a common health problem in children, with a significant headache reported in more than 75% by the age of 15 years. Pediatric migraine occurs in up to 10% of children and in up to 28% of adolescents between the ages of 15 and 19 years. Nevertheless, migraine diagnosis and treatment in these age groups present unique challenges. The attacks are shorter in children than in adolescents, the headache is less specific (may be holocranial, may lack photo- or phonophobia, abdominal pain is frequently associated). Children with migraine miss more school days in a school year than their matched controls. Non-drug treatments (relaxation training, self-hypnosis, and biofeedback) have been shown to have good efficacy as prophylactic measures. The only analgesics with evidence of efficacy for acute migraine treatment in children and adolescents are ibuprofen 10 mg per kg body weight and paracetamol 15 mg per kg body weight. The only antiemetic for use in children up to 12 years is domperidon. For migraine prophylaxis, flunarizine and propranolol in low doses showed positive effects in controlled trials. Other drugs have not been studied or did not show efficacy in appropriately designed studies.

The Pathophysiological Puzzle

Migraine has long been considered a vascular headache, based on the idea that changes in vessel diameter or gross changes in cerebral blood flow would trigger pain and

could, in part, explain the mechanism of action of vasoconstrictor drugs, such as ergotamine. Modern theories explaining the peripheral pain mechanisms suggest, based on experimental and clinical data, an activation of the trigeminal innervation of the cranial circulation with involvement of vasoactive neuropeptides, such as calcitonin gene-related peptide. To account for the periodicity and other clinical features in migraine, a primary dysfunction of central brain structures seems more likely.

Early studies have emphasized a dysfunction of the cerebrovascular regulation in headache, while little attention has been given to the central processing of headache. Recent data incorporating genetic, electrophysiological, and neuroimaging techniques have revolutionized our understanding of the pathophysiology of migraine and provided unique insights into this syndrome. Modern imaging studies point, together with the clinical picture, toward a central triggering cause, possibly based on genetic variations. The early functional imaging work has recently been reworked and implies involvement of highly specific activation of the brainstem in migraine, though it is still unclear whether in a permissive or triggering manner. Additionally, most studies show that information processing is abnormal in migraineurs. The best documented abnormality is an interictal lack of habituation in migraineurs, with normalization during the headache state. Together with a diminished energy reserve found in MR-spectroscopy studies, a possible role of increased energy consumption in attack generation has been suggested. Following this line of thought, migraine is understood as a paroxysmal central nervous system dysfunction.

Regarding the development of head pain, both vascular and neuronal mechanisms have been proposed. A much discussed scenario begins with CSD, which in turn activates the trigeminovascular system and causes headaches. As most of the migraine patients never experience an aura, silent CSD attacks have been proposed to explain why these patients suffer from recurrent attacks. In summary, modern concepts suggest that migraine is, in essence, a neurovascular headache, and that the susceptibility to CSD and to migraine is probably genetically determined.

See also: Cerebrovascular Disease; Seizure Disorders; Specific Mental Health Disorders: Child and Adolescent Mental Disorders.

Further Reading

Bolay H, Reuter U, Dunn AK, *et al.* (2002) Intrinsic brain activity triggers trigeminal meningeal afferents in a migraine model. *Nature Medicine* 8(2): 136–142.

Diener HC, Steiner TJ, and Tepper SJ (2006) Migraine—the forgotten epidemic: Development of the EHF/WHA Rome Declaration on Migraine. *Journal of Headache and Pain* 7(6): 433–437.

Evers S, Afra J, Frese A, *et al.* (2006) EFNS guideline on the drug treatment of migraine–report of an EFNS task force. *European Journal of Neurology* 13(6): 560–572.

Ferrari MD, Roon KI, Lipton RB, *et al.* (2001) Oral triptans (serotonin 5–HT(1B/1D) agonists) in acute migraine treatment: A meta-analysis of 53 trials. *Lancet* 358(9294): 1668–1675.

Goadsby PJ (2005) Advances in the understanding of headache. *British Medical Bulletin* 73–74(1): 83–92.

Goadsby PJ (2005) Migraine pathophysiology. *Headache* 45 (supplement 1): S14–S24.

Goadsby PJ (2006) Recent advances in the diagnosis and management of migraine. *British Medical Journal* 332(7532): 25–29.

Headache Classification Committee of the International Headache Society (2004) The International Classification of Headache Disorders, 2nd edn. *Cephalalgia* 24(supplement 1): 1–160.

Kelman L (2004) The aura: A tertiary care study of 952 migraine patients. *Cephalalgia* 24(9): 728–734.

Kurth T, Slomke MA, Kase CS, *et al.* (2005) Migraine, headache, and the risk of stroke in women: A prospective study. *Neurology* 64(6): 1020–1026.

Lance JW and Goadsby PJ (2005) *Mechanism and Management of Headache.* Oxford, UK: Butterworth-Heinemann Ltd.

Lipton RB, Stewart WF, and Von Korff M (1994) The burden of migraine: A review of cost to society. *Pharmacoeconomics* 6(3): 215–221.

Lipton RB, Stewart WF, Diamond S, *et al.* (2001) Prevalence and burden of migraine in the United States: Data from the American Migraine Study II. *Headache* 41(7): 646–657.

Lipton RB and Bigal ME (2006) Migraine and cardiovascular disease. *Journal of the American Medical Association* 296(3): 332–333.

Olesen J, Tfelt–Hansen P, and Welch K (2006) *The Headaches.* Philadelphia, PA: Lippincott Williams & Wilkins.

Relevant Websites

http://www.aacfp.org – The American Academy of Craniofacial Pain.

http://www.americanheadachesociety.org – The American Headache Society.

http://www.i-h-s.org – The International Headache Society.

http://www.headaches.org – The National Headache Foundation.

http://www.who.int/mediacentre/factsheets/fs277/en/ – The World Health Organization: Headache Disorders.

Multiple Sclerosis

C M Poser, Harvard Medical School, Boston, MA, USA

Introduction

Multiple sclerosis (MS) is an inflammatory-degenerative disease of the central nervous system (CNS). Its primary target is the myelin sheath via a mechanism that has yet to be explained. The degenerative phase causes destruction of axons and neurons. Except for secondary involvement of the facial nerve in its course within the brainstem, and the nucleus of the trigeminal nerve, it does not affect the peripheral nervous system. It was described well over a hundred years ago, but many of its aspects are still not known. Its pathogenesis is poorly understood and its long-term treatment is ineffectual. Much of its curious epidemiology is unexplained and its genetic transmission unknown. MS is the most common disease of the CNS of the young adult. The first symptoms usually appear at ages 20 to 40. The number of MS patients in the United States has been estimated at about 300 000, a prevalence of 100/100 000. This is probably inaccurate for two reasons: it includes as many as 20–25% of people who have been misdiagnosed as having MS based on the misinterpretation of the magnetic resonance imaging (MRI), and it obviously also does not count the substantial number of persons who have the asymptomatic form of the disease.

The course of the disease is extremely unpredictable and its clinical presentation is variable, but its predilection for certain parts of the CNS, which include the optic nerves, the brainstem, cerebellum, and cervical spinal cord, eventually provide a characteristic constellation of signs and symptoms.

The Classification of the Inflammatory Demyelinating Diseases

Some neurologists have recently suggested that MS is a part of a spectrum of idiopathic inflammatory demyelinating diseases that differ only in chronicity and severity. For example, acute disseminated encephalomyelitis (DEM) and Marburg's disease are grouped under the rubric of 'fulminant,' whereas Devic's and Balo's diseases are included with relapsing myelitis in the group of 'restricted distribution.' Such a scheme ignores the pathology of these conditions and seems to have no logical basis. A revised updated classification of the inflammatory demyelinating diseases is presented in **Table 1**. Marburg's disease is nothing more than acute MS, as is Balo's concentric sclerosis, the latter characterized by alternating bands of demyelination. The extremely rare Schilder's diffuse sclerosis 1912 type has very large lesions. All three of these diseases are often erroneously diagnosed (and treated) as MS because of misread MRIs. Devic's disease (neuromyelitis optica) is believed to be a variant of DEM (Poser and Brinar, 2004). All the lesions in

Table 1   The inflammatory demyelinating diseases

Multiple sclerosis	Disseminated
Marburg's disease (acute	encephalomyelitis
MS)	Acute, recurrent and
Chronic MS: Acute	multiphasic
hemorrhagic	Relapsing-remitting type
leukoencephalitis	Acute and recurrent optic
Secondary progressive type	neuritis
Primary progressive type	Acute and recurrent
Balo's concentric sclerosis	neuromyelitis optica
	Recurrent neuromyelitis optica
	with Schilder's 1912 diffuse
	sclerosis endocrinopathies
	Acute and recurrent transverse
	myelitis

every condition listed under 'MS' in **Table 1** exhibit the pathognomonic sharply demarcated edge between normal tissue and demyelination. The various types of DEM differ from MS not only in the absence of the typical plaques but also on the basis of clinical and pathological indices.

Epidemiology

Latitude and Prevalence

One of the most enduring myths of the epidemiology of MS is that of the direct relationship between latitude and its prevalence. **Table 2** makes it clear that prevalence of the disease varies greatly between areas of similar latitude. However, MS prevalence is higher in northern than in southern Europe, as it is in the Americas. This is most likely due to differences in the ethnicity of the populations: MS is much more frequent in persons of both direct (Swedes, Danes, Norwegians, Icelanders) and indirect Scandinavian descent (English, Irish, Russian, Norman, etc.), including Americans in the northern tier of states, many of whom are of Scandinavian origin. The latitude gradient seen in African Americans in the United States, which parallels that of Caucasians but at somewhat lower level, has been explained by the increasing mixture of Caucasian genetic material with progression to the north (**Figure 1**) (Poser, 1994). There are also many exceptions to the prevalence/latitude rule that militate against it, as is well exemplified by the data in **Table 2** for Croatia, Israel, Kuwait, and South Africa. There is a great difference in MS prevalence between three small villages in the Korski Gotar region of Croatia despite an identical environment (**Figure 2**). The disease is extremely rare in Hindus living in Mumbai, but not uncommon in Parsis living in the same city. No convincingly documented cases of MS have ever been reported in North or South American Indians, in Samis (Lapps), Eskimos, Australian Aborigines, Maoris, Melanesians, Micronesians, or

Table 2   Latitude and prevalence of MS

Location	Latitude	Prevalence[a]
Iceland	65°N	99
Shetland Islands	61°N	129
Winnipeg, Canada	50°N	35
Seattle, USA	47°N	69
Croatia	45°N	
Cabar		194
Vrbovsko		27
Parma, Italy	44°N	12
Olmsted County, MN, USA	44°N	122
Copparo, Sardinia	44°N	31
Asahikawa, Japan	44°N	2.5
Hobart, Tasmania	43°S	68
Hautes Pyrénées, France	43°N	40
Boston, USA	42°N	41
Sassari, Sardinia, Italy	41°N	69
Alcoy, Spain	39°N	17
Seoul, Korea	38°N	2
Malta	36°N	4
Cape Town, South Africa	36°S	
Afrikaner		11
Colored/Oriental		3
Charleston, SC, USA	33°N	14
Newcastle, Australia	33°S	32.5
Israel (immigrants)	32°N	
Sephardi		9.5
Ashkenazi		36
New Orleans, LA, USA	30°N	6
Kuwait (Arabs)	30°N	
Kuwaiti		9.5
Palestinian		24
Okinawa, Japan	26°N	2
Hong Kong	23°N	1
Bombay (Parsi)	19°N	26

[a]Per 100 000 inhabitants.
Modified from Poser C (1994) The epidemiology of multiple sclerosis. A general review. *Annals of Neurology* 36 (S2): S180–193.

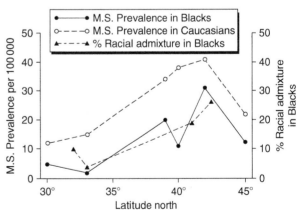

Figure 1   Prevalence of MS in African-Americans. The percentage of racial admixture based on blood group studies parallels the increase in latitude. Reprinted with permission from Poser C, *An Atlas of Multiple Sclerosis*. London: Parthenon Publishing Group, 1998. Fig. 11, p. 52.

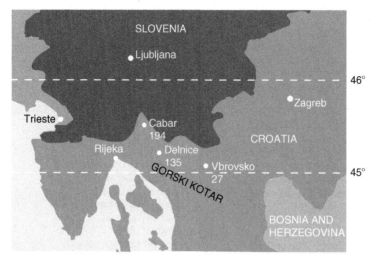

Figure 2   Map of the Gorski-Kotar region of Croatia. The peoples of Cabar and Delnice are descendants of north Germans; those of Vbrovsko from southern Slavs. Courtesy of Dr. E. Materljan and Prof. J. Sepcic, University of Rijeka, Croatia.

Polynesians. The disease occurs much less frequently in Orientals and is extremely rare in black Africans. There is one well-publicized example of a latitude gradient that has defied explanation: the prevalence of MS in Tasmania is twice that of southern Australia, and has remained that way for 30 years despite a lack of discernible ethnic difference between the populations.

Several reports claim that MS is increasing in frequency. It is hard to know whether this is a true increase or whether it is due to a combination of factors, such as greater awareness of the disease in physicians and the general population, and greater use (and misuse) of imaging. Longer life expectancy and earlier diagnosis may have added to the number of cases, but it is also possible that the disease has in fact become more common.

Genetics

The striking differences in prevalence in similar environments strongly suggest an important role for genetic factors. There is a familial occurrence rate of about 15%. The age-adjusted risk is higher in siblings (3%), parents (2%), and children (2%) than in second- and third-degree relatives. There is only a 35% concordance in monozygotic twins, but it is the same as in siblings for dizygotic pairs. Children of conjugal pairs with MS have a much higher prevalence rate (20%), but adopted offspring or other nonbiological relatives have no increased risk (Sadovnick, 1994).

Because of these indications, numerous studies of genetic markers have been carried out, but to date few secure candidates or regions have been identified. Many studies of the class II major histocompatibility complex (MHC) alleles of the human leukocyte antigen (HLA) system and their genotypes have been carried out, but at the family level have been disappointing. Some of these have suggested an association between the MHC alleles

DR15 and DQ6 (DRB1* 1501 and DBQ2 *0602) and the gene for tissue necrosis factor encoded within the same linkage group. A specifically different association (with DR4 and its DRB 1*O405-DQA1 *0301-DQB1*0302 genotype) is seen in Mediterranean populations, primarily Sardinians. There is strong evidence indicating that MS is a polygenic disease.

The Vikings and the Genetic Origin of MS

The highest prevalence rates for MS are found in Iceland, Scandinavia, the British Isles, and the countries settled by their descendants. This suggests that the Vikings may have been instrumental in disseminating the genetic susceptibility to the disease (Poser, 1994a). The Norwegian and Danish Vikings raided in most European countries and settled in large numbers in Normandy ('the land of the Northmen'), Sicily, and southern Italy. They also founded Dublin in Ireland and York in England. They traveled west and settled in Iceland and the Faroe Islands. The Swedish Vikings originating in Götland went to the southeast, along the river routes to the Caucasus and the Black and Caspian Seas, and penetrated into Persia, India, and as far as China. They founded Kiev and Novgorod and established Ukraine and the Russian state. Called 'Varangians,' they were active in all the military activities of the Byzantine Empire. As early as the tenth century, the Vikings engaged in trade with the Arabs; Arab coins dating from that period have been found in tombs in Iceland and Norway. Vikings from Scandinavia and Iceland, as well as their descendants from England and France, were Crusaders. In fact, the Palestinians born and raised in Kuwait, who have an unexpectedly high prevalence of MS, originated in what had been part of the Latin Kingdom established after the First Crusade. Russians from the Ukraine, and thus of Viking origin, settled in a separate community near what is now Beijing, China, and formed an elite regiment of the Mongol army that participated in the conquests of western Asia and much of southeastern Europe, reaching the gates of Vienna in the thirteenth century. Although the Vikings had a fearful reputation as raiders and plunderers, most of them settled in the areas they had conquered and eventually were integrated into the local population. The practice of capturing and keeping local women as wives or concubines, or selling them as well as other Vikings as slaves, mostly to Arabs, were important factors in this genetic dissemination throughout the world.

Environmental Factors

Genetics alone cannot account for the differences in MS observed in various situations; therefore, it is likely that some environmental factors also influence the acquisition of the disease. Many studies of an enormous variety of possible agents and factors that could influence the acquisition or development of the disease have been carried out in various countries, with almost no results. Most of the agents and factors are meaningless, since they are completely lacking in biological plausibility (**Table 3**) (Lauer, 1994). Usually these factors are related to the clinical onset rather than the acquisition of MS.

Table 3   Environmental factors for MS

Variable	Rs[a]
Latitude	0.865[b]
Precipitation	0.566[c]
Low temperature	0.868[b]
Rainy climate	0.695[b]
Forestation (all types)	0.249
Coniferous forests	0.638[b]
Pig farming	0.575[c]
Lack of sheep	0.537[c]
Indo-European ancestry	0.686[b]
Christian culture	0.686[b]
Pork consumption	0.639[b]
Beef consumption	0.582[c]
Consumption of cow's milk	0.758[b]
Low consumption of fish	−0.382[d]
Consumption of smoked food	0.819[b]
Industrialization	0.663[b]
Life expectancy	0.353[d]
Low infant mortality	0.617[b]
Small population <20 years	0.525[c]

[a]Rs = Risk correlation coefficient.
[b]$p < 0.001$.
[c]$p < 0.01$.
[d]$p < 0.05$.
Modified from Lauer K (1994) Multiple sclerosis in the old world: The new old map. In: Firnhaber W and Lauer K (eds.) *Multiple Sclerosis in Europe. An Epidemiological Update*. p. 19. Alsbach/Bergstrasse: Leuchtturm Verlag.

Ultraviolet Rays: A Protective Factor?

In recent years, some investigators have focused attention on the intensity of sunshine and ultraviolet rays as possible protection against the acquisition of MS, pointing to the very low prevalence or total absence of the disease in African Blacks, Australian Aborigines, and other highly melanotic ethnic groups. This overlooks the fact that the disease is also completely unknown in non- or lightly pigmented groups such as Samis, Inuits, and Eskimos, and that their heavy clothing would effectively screen out the supposedly protective ultraviolet rays. There is no question that MS is extremely rare in African Blacks, but there have been at least four autopsy-proven cases in Senegal. In South Africa, most neurologists are still unwilling to accept the diagnosis in their black patients, thus making the disease seem even rarer.

Migrations

The influence of environmental factors is most apparent in considering the effects of migration on prevalence and incidence rates. Frenchmen living in Africa have a considerably lower prevalence rate than those living in France. The children of West Indian and Asian immigrants to the United Kingdom have the same incidence and prevalence rates as native-born Englishmen, and the Israel-born children of both Ashkenazi and Sephardic Jews also have the same prevalence rates, although their parents' rates are quite different. Most Martinican Blacks who developed MS had spent significant periods of time in metropolitan France before acquiring the disease. The situation in Hawaii illustrates what appears to be a unique, contradictory situation in which the presumably same environment exerts opposite effects on different ethnic groups (Alter *et al.*, 1971). For persons of Japanese extraction living in Hawaii or in California there is an increased risk of MS compared with those living in Japan (6.5 vs. 2.1); for Caucasians raised in Hawaii it appears to offer some protection against MS (10.5 vs. 34.4). It is difficult to conceive of environmental factors having such a disparate effect unless the genetic make-up of the individual also plays a role in the equation. The existence of a premorbid genetic marker such as the MS 'trait' could provide an explanation. Epidemiological studies have demonstrated the primary importance of genetic factors modified by an as yet unrecognized environmental one.

The MS 'Trait': A Premorbid Marker of Genetic Susceptibility

The remarkably low rate of concordance of MS in monozygotic twins has never been fully explained, but it indicates the possibility of a systemic condition called the MS 'trait' (MST) (Poser, 2006), which is quite different from asymptomatic MS and may never develop into the disease. It results from the action of an antigenic challenge to the immune system of a genetically vulnerable person that does not cause damage to the nervous parenchyma. A subsequent environmental viral-antigenic event in some MST-carriers can change the trait into the disease. This event could be an infection, which need not be symptomatic, or a vaccination. The MS may become symptomatic, remain asymptomatic, or be manifested only by lesions visible by MRI. It is likely that the development of the MST, called 'activation,' occurs early in life, whereas the transition from MST to MS, called 'acquisition,' takes place at puberty in most patients, when the immune system is made more vulnerable by the outpouring of female sex hormones. Differences in prevalence between prepuberal migrants, the locally born children of migrants, and their population of origin may also be explained by the MST. Thus, the Hawaii-born Japanese who carries the MST develops MS when he is exposed to an antigenic challenge that is not present in Japan; but the MST-bearing Caucasian does not encounter the appropriate viral antigen, which does not occur in Hawaii, and never develops MS.

Etiology

MS has been described as a disease of unknown etiology, implying the existence of a single cause. A number of infectious agents have been reported as potential etiological agents. They include the corona, measles, Epstein-Barr, herpes simplex type 6, and canine distemper viruses; the human T-cell lymphotrophic virus (HTLV)-l, an 'MS-associated agent'; and, most recently, chlamydia. None of these has been confirmed, but the idea lingers on, despite exhaustive searches by competent investigators using sophisticated techniques. Nevertheless, so-called 'epidemics' in Iceland and in the Faroe Islands continue to be cited as evidence of the infectious nature of the disease, its introduction to the islands ascribed to the arrival of asymptomatic British troops in 1941. The data show a peak of clinical disease onset starting in 1941 and purport to find a direct relationship between the occurrence of MS in natives and British soldiers billeted in their homes. These studies unfortunately are based on the meaningless date of clinical onset; recalculation of the data using the putative date of acquisition at puberty (age 14) clearly show a peak before 1941.

It is important to differentiate between age of clinical onset and age of acquisition of the disease for all etiological and epidemiological investigations. Clinical onset simply means the appearance of symptoms of an already existing disease. The putative date of acquisition of MS has been generally accepted as being at puberty in most if not all patients. This was deduced from the study of MS in English immigrants to South Africa, noting that the disease rarely developed in those who had immigrated before age 15, compared to the number that would have developed it in England (Dean and Kurtzke, 1971). Similar studies confirmed this observation. In support of this concept, and because MS is almost twice as common in women, is that the secretion of female sex hormones, which play an important role in enhancing immune responses, significantly increases in both girls and boys at puberty. Furthermore, many new environmental factors that may influence disease acquisition may be encountered at the same time, including new school, sport, and social activities.

From all of the information that is currently available, it is much more likely that MS is the result in a genetically susceptible subject of the activation of the immune system by different viral agents, which initiates a pathogenetic cascade that is not fully understood and which eventually leads to the destruction of the myelin sheath and the axon.

Pathogenesis

Much of what is known about the pathogenesis of MS comes from studies of experimental allergic encephalomyelitis (EAE), an imperfect model of MS but the equivalent of human DEM. In common with EAE, a major alteration of the blood–brain barrier (BBB) is, if not the first, certainly an early and obligatory step in the development of the MS lesion, but EAE does not lead to the formation of the characteristic plaques of MS. In fact, the BBB appears to be injured quite early in the course of illness. Inflammation of capillary and venule walls can be seen in the normal-appearing white matter (NAWM), but it is insufficient to lead to leakage of water and immunoactive substances into the brain parenchyma.

In its early phase MS has several of the features of an autoimmune disease. Although the immune system of MS patients has many abnormalities, the exact pathogenesis remains obscure, and the various schemes that have been proposed are a mixture of fact and speculation. It is unclear whether the immunological alterations are part of the pathogenetic cascade or its results. Ebers (1998) put it succinctly: "It is sobering to realize that despite decades of cellular immunology research of the survey type, no specific abnormality that characterizes or defines MS has been identified."

The stimulus for this immunological response is probably an antigenic challenge from an infection, or possibly a vaccination, involving the phenomenon of molecular mimicry. (This is a phenomenon in which some component peptides of the active antigenic molecule are immunologically indistinguishable from a myelin antigen, and hence an appropriate response to infection produces an inappropriate action against some component of the myelin sheath.) A key role has been suggested for tumor necrosis factor, immune complexes, and adhesion molecules, the last named in particular, in the loss of impermeability of the BBB. As a result of the alteration in the BBB, immunoactive T-lymphocytes penetrate into the brain parenchyma. Other immunoactive substances in serum, including complement and interferon-gamma, as well as B-lymphocytes and macrophages, also cross the now permeable BBB and by a still unknown mechanism attack the oligodendroglial–myelin complex. Various cytokines secreted by T-cells have been proposed as the agents of myelinoclasia. The role of the oligodendrocyte in the pathogenetic cascade also remains in dispute, and many consider this rather than the myelin sheath to be the primary target of the process.

The primary effects of MS are inflammation and edema. Myelin destruction does not necessarily follow. Spontaneous resolution of the inflammation and edema without destruction frequently occurs, and provides a logical explanation for the very short duration of some symptoms. Remyelination occurs even in the earliest lesions, but is generally relatively inefficient and much too slow to account for clinical improvement within only a few hours or days. Another explanation may be the activation of alternative or supplementary physiological pathways.

After myelin is destroyed, it is replaced by a glial scar. It is such scars that have given MS its name. In addition to the probable role of the T-cell in causing the inflammatory reaction, antibodies against myelin components also play a crucial role in pathogenesis. The destruction of myelin releases a number of its structural components, including cholesterol, fatty acids, myelin basic protein, myelin-associated glycoprotein, myelin-oligo-dendrocyte glycoprotein, proteolipid protein, phospholipids, cerebrosides, sphingomyelin, and gangliosides. These substances may enter the bloodstream via the permeable BBB and, in turn, provoke an immune response from systemic lymphocytes, thereby causing a vicious cycle that results in a self-perpetuating condition. This may explain the intermittent progression of the disease. In MS, periods of immune activity, probably stimulated by nonspecific viral infections, are believed to alternate with periods of immunoquiescence. The current status of our understanding, or lack thereof, of the role of the immune system in MS has been summarized by Cedric Raine (1994) as follows:

> "In sum, while no single immune system molecule can he assigned as unusual to the CSF of MS, and, while there appears to he nothing unique about the manner in which the CNS responds to inflammation, the true uniqueness of the situation in MS is probably related to the many normally sequestered, specific antigens within the myelin sheath and the biology of the myelinating cell, the oligo-dendrocyte."

A generalized pathogenetic scheme is depicted in **Figure 3**.

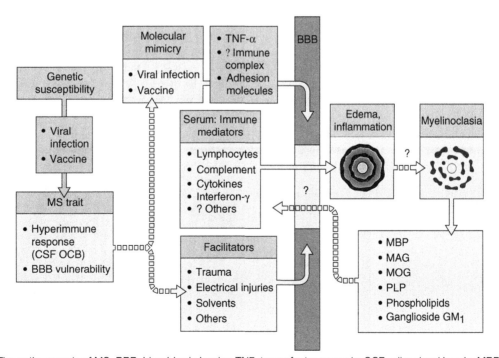

Figure 3 The pathogenesis of MS. BBB, blood-brain barrier; TNF, tumor factor necrosis; OCB, oligoclonal bands; MBP, myelin basic protein; MAG, myelin-associated glycoprotein; MOG, myelin-oligodendroglia protein; PLP, proteolipid protein. Reprinted with permission from Poser C, *An Atlas of Multiple Sclerosis*. London: Parthenon Publishing Group, 1998. fig.14, p. 53.

Pathology

The pattern of destruction of myelin is unique to MS and is seen in none of the other demyelinating (e.g., DEM) or dysmyelinating (e.g., metachromatic or adrenoleukodystrophy) diseases: it consists of plaques that are sharply demarcated from the normal white matter surrounding them (**Figure 4**). They have been aptly described as "cut out with a cookie cutter." In contrast, the inflammatory lesions in DEM are almost invariably perivascular and often become confluent. Unless the pathognomonic sharp edge of the MS lesion is captured by the biopsy, it may be impossible to differentiate it from DEM.

Plaques are most commonly seen in the optic nerves and chiasm, the periventricular centrum semiovale, the brainstem, the cerebellar hemispheres, and the cervical spinal cord. Although most plaques are seen in the white matter, they may involve the subcortical U-fibers and extend into gray matter. The cortex, thalamus, the basal ganglia, and the dentate nuclei may all be affected. Lesions of the sensory nucleus of the trigeminal nerve, the intraparenchymal portion of the facial, and some of the connections of the acoustic nerve are frequently involved, but peripheral nerves are spared. Asymmetry of the lesions is the rule.

Inflammatory cellular infiltrates and edema are almost invariably seen in the walls of small blood vessels and the surrounding parenchyma at the edges of the plaques. Similar changes in the walls of capillaries and venules can also be seen in the NAWM. One of the earliest changes is separation of the myelin lamellae by vesicular edema, fragmentation of the sheath, invasion by macrophages that engulf the myelin debris, and eventual denudation of the axon. Most of the plaques show periaxile demyelination, the axon appearing intact, but older lesions clearly show axonal and neuronal degeneration. Clumps of large abnormal gemistocytic astrocytes

may be seen near the lesions; these are occasionally mistaken for astrocytomas.

The MS variants, Marburg's acute MS, Balo's concentric sclerosis, and Schilder's 1912 type diffuse sclerosis, all exhibit the same pathological features (Poser and Brinar, 2004).

Physiology

Normal motor and sensory function depend upon the rapid propagation of the nerve impulse along myelinated nerve fibers, measured in milliseconds. The myelin sheath is interrupted at regular intervals by the nodes of Ranvier, where the axon is denuded. Because the axon has a high resistance to the electrical impulse, which makes the speed of conduction too slow, an alternative mechanism takes over. It is called 'saltatory conduction,' in which the electrical impulse jumps from one node of Ranvier to the next while achieving the required conduction velocity. However, if the distance between the available nodes is too great because of destruction of some myelin segments, the impulse cannot bridge the gap, and saltatory conduction is no longer possible. The electrical impulse must then travel via the slow axonal route (**Figure 5**). Once the axon itself is destroyed, conduction is obviously no longer possible and the deficit, if any, becomes permanent.

In some MS patients signs or symptoms appear because nerve conduction slows when body temperature is elevated as a result of either ambient heat or fever. The latter is a common cause of pseudoexacerbations. A body temperature increase of as little as 1 °C may be sufficient to cause such signs and symptoms, which disappear upon cooling. Until recently, this was used diagnostically by means of the hot bath test.

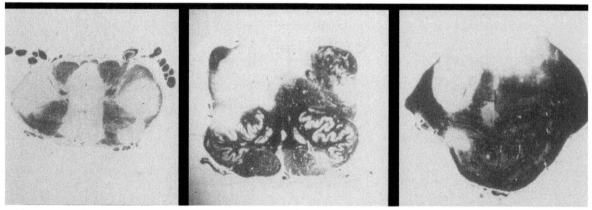

Figure 4   MS: sections of spinal cord and brainstem (celloidin, Weigert). Note the sharp edges of the areas of demyelination. Reprinted with permission from Poser C, *An Atlas of Multiple Sclerosis*. London: Parthenon Publishing Group, 1998. fig. 44, p. 70.

Clinical Aspects

The Clinical Course

Several clinical types have been recognized: relapsing-remitting, primary, and secondary progressive. However, the pathological end result, that is, the sharply bordered plaques of demyelination, is noted in all of them. Some investigators believe that these clinical types represent different diseases or genetic variants of MS, but it is much more likely that the differences in evolution indicate the aggressivity of the disease process, the patient's susceptibility, and the accumulation of lesions in eloquent areas of the CNS. Many MS lesions remain silent, and a number of routine autopsy series have shown that asymptomatic MS may be as common as the diagnosed condition, with a prevalence of 100/100 000.

Signs and Symptoms

Table 4 summarizes the symptoms of MS at onset in six series, in three of which the diagnosis was confirmed at autopsy. The disease is almost twice as common in women as in men, and the clinical onset is most frequent in the third and fourth decades. Certain neurological complaints in a person under the age of 40 are tantamount to making the diagnosis of MS: a Lhermitte symptom (tingling going down the back when flexing the neck), trigeminal neuralgia, hemifacial spasms, unilateral intention tremor, or binocular diplopia which disappears when closing either eye. Similarly, certain abnormalities of the neurological examination of a young person are also common enough in MS to be of diagnostic value: temporal pallor of the optic disk, unilateral hyperreflexia and a Babinski sign, a significant decrease in position and/or vibratory sensation at the ankles, or some dysmetria on finger-to-nose testing. Dating the clinical onset of MS is often important in epidemiological studies and clinical trials; many patients – and physicians – ascribe symptoms to MS that are unrelated. Table 5 lists the only signs and symptoms that should be considered for that purpose. MS patients may well suffer from headaches, positional vertigo, seizures, back and neck pain, for example, but such signs and symptoms are not part of the MS syndrome. In addition to signs and symptoms indicating involvement of different parts of the CNS, or dissemination in space, and dissemination in time (symptoms appearing at different times) are characteristic of about 2/3 of patients. True exacerbations or bouts appear spontaneously or may follow some kind of viral infection but must be differentiated from pseudo-exacerbations that result from fever, elevated ambient temperature, or some metabolic derangement.

The correlation between the number, site, and size of MS lesions, as revealed by neuroimaging and at autopsy, and clinical manifestations is poor. Many plaques involve so-called 'silent' areas of the brain. Furthermore, the disease process must impair conduction in a critical

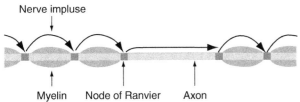

Figure 5 Saltatory conduction in MS. Reprinted with permission from Poser C, *An Atlas of Multiple Sclerosis.* London: Parthenon Publishing Group, 1998. fig. 51, p. 76.

Table 4 Frequency of symptoms of MS in various countries

Clinical feature	United States[a] (n = 25)	Canada (n = 54)	Denmark (n = 60)	Norway[a] (n = 31)	England[a] (n = 55)	Germany (n = 120)
Remission	68.0	76.5	81.7	74.2	72.7	80.0
Pyramidal tract	100.0	83.3	100.0	100.0	98.2	90.0
Ocular	92.0	85.2	75.0	80.6	83.6	76.7
Urinary	52.0	53.7	71.7	87.1	92.7	55.8
Nonequilibratory	76.0	68.5	81.7	80.6	80.0	69.2
Vibration/position	64.0	64.8	51.7	64.5	78.2	76.7
Nystagmus	68.0	37.0	56.7	67.7	72.7	39.2
Paresthesiae	68.0	87.0	83.3	54.8	70.9	61.7
Dysarthria	52.0	33.3	40.0	61.3	52.7	28.3
Gait ataxia	60.0	46.3	60.0	67.7	45.5	45.0
Mental/cognitive	44.0	15.7	48.3	51.6	41.8	52.5
Duration of illness						
Mean (years)	14.0	6.8	8.3	16.5	12.4	13.1
Median (years)	11.0	4.0	6.0	15.0	12.0	12.0
Range (months–years)	2–32	1–43	2–48	3–37	2–36	12–45

[a]Autopsied cases.

Table 5   Symptoms to be used to determine clinical onset

A. Definite (all symptoms must last at least 24 h)

Optic/retrobulbar neuritis	Tranverse myelitis
Monoparesis	Trigeminal neuralgia (< age 40)
Binocular diplopia	Scanning speech
Unilateral intention tremor	Acute, painless urinary retention
Urinary urgency/	Non-positional vertigo
incontinence (men)	Paresthesiae of one limb
Useless hand syndrome	Hemifacial spasms
Gait ataxia	Oscillopsia
Unilateral dysmetria	Monocular color blindness
Fecal incontinence	

B. Possible (a definite symptom or abnormal sign must appear within 2 years)

Blurred vision	Extreme fatigue
Positional vertigo	Lhermitte symptom
Facial palsy	Dysarthria
Painless urinary frequency (men)	Organic sexual impotence (men)

number of fibers in order to produce neurological dysfunction. The available fibers in the affected tract above this number constitute the safety factor. If the signs and symptoms are due to inflammation and edema only, which is almost always the case at the onset of a bout, they will be reversible; it is only when the safety factor is breached, that is, when the number of demyelinated or destroyed fibers exceeds the required minimum, that signs and symptoms become permanent. **Figure 6** depicts the mechanism that explains the relapsing-remitting course that develops into secondary progression.

Clinically Isolated Syndromes Suggestive of MS

Many clinicians now contend that the first manifestation of MS often is optic neuritis, transverse myelitis, or a cerebellar syndrome. Rather than waiting for the confirmatory second episode and fulfilling the classic criteria of dissemination in time and in space, specific, expensive, lifelong treatment is initiated on such flimsy evidence.

Diagnosis

Diagnostic Criteria

Because MS is such a variable disease, many diagnostic schemes incorporating a variety of confirmatory tests and procedures have been proposed, but none are accurate and specific enough to eliminate the main differential diagnostic considerations. This applies to the McDonald *et al.* scheme which is widely used (2001). Although it relies heavily on magnetic resonance imaging (MRI), it still endorses the traditional principles

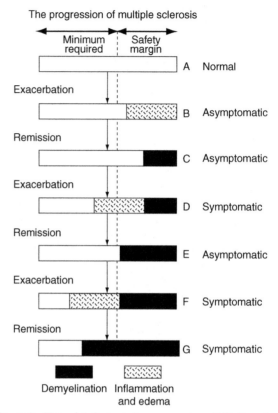

The progression of multiple sclerosis

Figure 6   The safety factor in the progression of MS. Symptoms occur only when the safety factor is decreased: temporarily by edema and inflammation, permanently by demyelination and/or axonal destruction. Reprinted with permission from Poser C, *An Atlas of Multiple Sclerosis*. London: Parthenon Publishing Group, 1998. fig. 52, p. 76.

of dissemination in both time and space as the basic diagnostic characteristics.

Among its improvements over previous schemes are the following: the first criteria for primary progressive MS, the recommendation that brainstem auditory and sensorimotor evoked potential studies no longer be considered of diagnostic value, retaining only the visual ones; and most important, the notation that spinal cord lesions should be at least 3 mm but not exceed the length of two vertebrae. The McDonald *et al.* scheme also warns against forming the diagnosis on the results of a brain biopsy. Unfortunately, however, this scheme is heavily dependent on MRI, for which a series of quantitative measures are offered, in the complete absence of descriptive, qualitative images. These MRI criteria were not derived from a series of clinically well-established cases of MS, but rather on the retrospective review of the MR images of patients who had a clinically isolated syndrome (CIS) and subsequently suffered from a second episode, thus presumably establishing the diagnosis of MS.

The diagnosis of MS remains a clinical one, and usually a careful history coupled with the neurological examination by an experienced neurologist will be sufficient and not require confirmatory procedures. It is regrettable that in the last few years the diagnosis of MS has been based almost exclusively on the interpretation of the MRI by the radiologist. Not only is the latter not necessarily specially trained or experienced but often has been given only a minimum of clinical information.

Examination of the Cerebrospinal Fluid

Examination of the cerebrospinal fluid (CSF) as an adjunct for the diagnosis of MS has become increasingly rare but remains an essential procedure when other conditions such as Lyme disease, sarcoidosis, HTLV-I-associated paraparesis, AIDS, and neurosyphilis must be ruled out. Thus it remains a useful confirmatory test for MS. The CSF is usually acellular, and the total protein level normal. A protein level above 75 mg% and a white cell count above 15 should raise serious doubts about the diagnosis of MS. Measurement of the level of IgG is important. The simplest and most reliable measurement is the percentage of total CSF protein: less than 15% is considered normal. However, an elevated CSF IgG is nonspecific. It is often observed in many other conditions affecting the nervous system. A more useful examination is the search for oligoclonal bands in the gammaglobulin fraction of protein. To be significant, there must be at least two bands, and none in a coincidental immunoelectrophoresis of the patient's serum. These bands are present in over 90% of cases and do not vary with disease activity or lack thereof, but are not MS-specific and may be noted in other conditions, including disseminated encephalomyelitis. In the latter, however, they may disappear in time, which never happens in MS.

Visual Evoked Potential Studies

Pattern-reversal visual evoked responses are particularly useful in identifying optic nerve and chiasmatic lesions in patients who have had no symptoms or signs of involvement of the visual system, because they may be delayed in 75% of such patients, including those with normal visual acuity. The critical measurement is that of the peak, designated as P100. The amplitude of the response is of little portent. Interocular differences in P100 delay are usually meaningless. Because the response is modified by changes in visual acuity, it is imperative that the patient wear prescribed corrective lenses during the test. Delay in P100 is far from specific for MS lesions of the optic system; in addition to poor fixation and changes in visual acuity, many other conditions may give false-positive results. Among these are glaucoma, alcohol ingestion, cerebrovascular disease, spinocerebellar degeneration, all types of optic atrophy, and the use of many commonly prescribed drugs.

Neuroimaging

Computed tomography

Despite the general availability of MRI in most countries, computed tomography (CT) scanning will undoubtedly remain for many years to come the only neuroimaging procedure available in the poorer areas of the world. Doubling or tripling the dose of intravenous iodinated contrast medium and delaying imaging for one or two hours have greatly enhanced the ability of CT to reveal MS lesions (**Figure 7**).

Magnetic resonance imaging

The introduction of magnetic resonance imaging (MRI) has revolutionized the diagnostic process of MS, but it has proved to be a mixed blessing. Only too often today, the clinician will ignore the history and neurological abnormalities in favor of the radiologist's report. Approximately 5–15% of clinically definite MS patients have normal MRIs on repeated examination. The correlation between the number, site, and size of MRI white-matter areas of increased signal intensity (AISI) and the clinical signs and symptoms of MS is unreliable. The often-used term 'burden of disease,' based on the number and size of lesions, is misleading, as many AISIs may be seen that have persisted for years in clinically normal subjects.

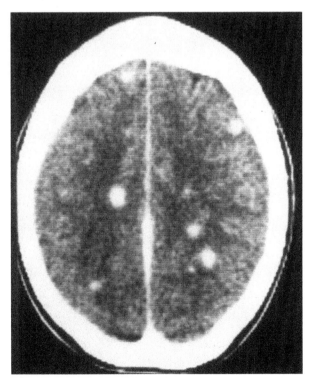

Figure 7   Double dose iodine contrast delayed CT scan in MS. Reprinted with permission from Poser C, *An Atlas of Multiple Sclerosis*. London: Parthenon Publishing Group, 1998. fig. 68, p. 87.

Attempts to establish reliable MRI diagnostic criteria have largely been unsuccessful, because the pattern and characteristics of images associated with MS are nonspecific and are also seen in many other diseases. No pattern of lesions, including the ovoid and perpendicular periventricular lesion, is specific enough to be diagnostic of MS (**Figure 8**).

The MRI guidelines that are available are all quantitative; they consist of numbers of lesions without any indications of the details, location, distribution, or size of the images. As new treatments become available, accuracy of diagnosis assumes even greater importance, and correctly distinguishing between MS and other demyelinating conditions producing AISIs on T2-weighted MRIs becomes crucial. By far the most common problem in differential diagnosis is posed by DEM, which may be of the recurrent or polyphasic type and indistinguishable from MS in fulfilling the classical criteria of dissemination in time and in space. None of the published clinical and radiological diagnostic criteria make it possible to differentiate between MS and DEM. Characteristic illustrative MR images of DEM are available: the eight patterns in **Figure 9** represent essentially all those that have been published (Poser, 1994). MR images of DEM have often been

erroneously misinterpreted as Marburg's or Balo's disease, or as brain tumors that have been subjected to the risks of a biopsy. Another helpful differential point is that in DEM ring-like gadolinium enhancement will be seen for almost all the lesions, whereas in MS very few of the AISIs will enhance (**Figure 10**).

Treatment

Symptomatic

Effective drugs have been available for a long time for the treatment for some of the typical problems such as spasticity, the control of urinary urgency and frequency, erectile dysfunction, the pain of trigeminal neuralgia, and the characteristic and disabling severe fatigue. Both oral and intravenous corticosteroids have successfully shortened relapses in many patients (Poser and Brinar, 2002).

Specific

A new era of specific therapy was introduced about ten years ago with the use of the immunomodifying

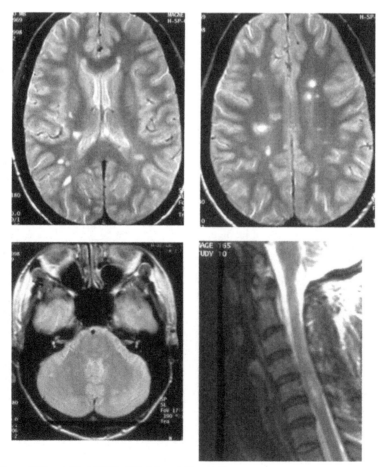

Figure 8   Common pattern of T2-weighted MRI in MS. It is not diagnostic.

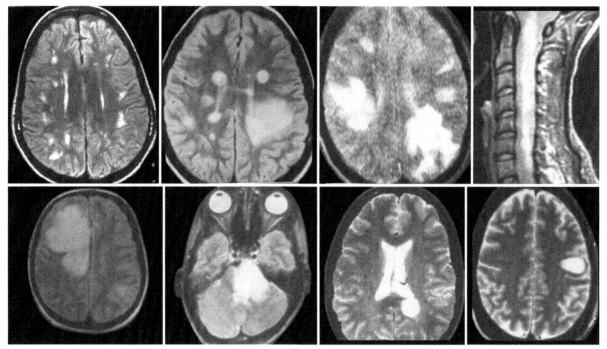

Figure 9 Eight examples of patterns of T-2 weighted MRIs in disseminated encephalomyelitis. They represent all those that have been published and can be used to rule out MS. Reprinted with permission from Poser C, *An Atlas of Multiple Sclerosis*. London: Parthenon Publishing Group, 1998. fig. 100, p. 109–110.

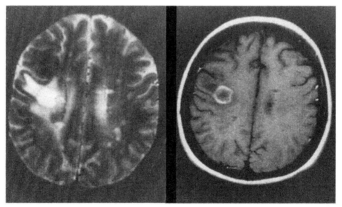

Figure 10 T-2 weighted MRI of disseminated encephalomyelitis (left) and T-1 gadolinium ring-like enhancement of the newest part of the lesion (right). Courtesy of Prof. V. Brinar, University of Zagreb, Croatia.

parenteral drugs β-interferon and glatiramer acetate and, to a limited extent, the immunosuppressant mito-xanthrone. These drugs have several possible modes of action on the immune system, but the exact mechanisms of action in MS have not been identified. Despite their side effects, their high cost, and the tendency of some of them to produce antibodies, these lifelong treatments have been used with unbridled enthusiasm and, unfortunately, in some patients whose MS diagnosis was based entirely but erroneously on the MRI interpretation. Although there is convincing evidence that the immunomodula-tory and immunosuppressant drugs produce statistically

significant decreases in both the number of relapses and of new lesions on MRI, they do not modify the long-term course of the disease (Confavreux *et al.*, 2000).

Another result of the availability of these medications is the practice of initiating treatment after a CIS, such as a single episode of optic neuritis, myelitis, or an isolated cerebellar dysfunction. Rather than wait for a confirma-tory second clinical bout, MRI criteria of dubious validity are used to sustain the diagnosis of MS, with the justifica-tion that treatment should be started as soon as possible to prevent damage. The fact that the disease has almost always been present for 10 or 15 years is ignored. A great many clinical trials of potential therapeutic agents are in progress. Much attention has been devoted to monoclonal antibodies and to oral tolerization as potential therapeutic agents, but so far results have been disappointing.

Support Systems

Many MS sufferers pursue productive and enjoyable lives despite their disease. Patients should be encouraged to continue working as long as possible or to seek accommodations to their limitations. Participation in sports, even if confined to a wheelchair, is possible; horseback riding is popular with MS patients. Also available are wheelchair basketball teams and 'sitdown' skiing. People with MS must be able to depend upon their immediate families for moral support. In many places however, there are specialized MS clinics that offer comprehensive care, including medications, psychiatric and social service counseling, and physical and occupational rehabilitation. Some patients belong to peer groups whereas others avoid them; in some cities, there are day centers run by the local MS society. Other services that may be available are transportation and the loan of wheelchairs and walkers. Wheelchair-bound patients require access to restaurants, museums, theaters, and other public facilities via ramps and elevators, but many cities have yet to recognize this need.

Citations

Alter M, Okihiro M, Rowley W, et al. (1971) MS among Orientals and Caucasians in Hawaii. Neurology 21: 122–130.

Confavreux C, Vukusic S, Moreau T, et al. (2000) Relapses and progression of disability in multiple sclerosis. New England Journal of Medicine 343: 1430–1438.

Dean G and Kurtzke J (1971) On the risk of multiple sclerosis according to the age of immigration to South Africa. British Medical Journal 3: 725–729.

Ebers G (1998) Immunology. In: Paty D and Ebers G (eds.) Multiple Sclerosis, p. 410. Philadelphia, PA: Davis.

Lauer K (1994) Multiple sclerosis in the old world: The new old map. In: Firnhaber W and Lauer K (eds.) Multiple Sclerosis in Europe. An Epidemiological Update, p. 19. Alsbach/Bergstrasse, Germany: Leuchtturm Verlag.

McDonald W, Compston A, Edan G, et al. (2001) Recommended diagnostic criteria for multiple sclerosis: Guidelines from the international panel on the diagnosis of multiple sclerosis. Annals of Neurology 50: 121–127.

Poser C (1994) The epidemiology of multiple sclerosis. A general review. Annals of Neurology 36(S2): S180–193.

Poser C (1994a) The dissemination of multiple sclerosis: A Viking saga? A historical essay. Annals of Neurology 36(S2): S321–343.

Poser C (2006) The multiple sclerosis trait and the development of multiple sclerosis: Genetic vulnerability and environmental effect. Clinical Neurology and Neurosurgery 108: 227–233.

Poser C and Brinar V (2002) The symptomatic treatment of multiple sclerosis. Clinical Neurology and Neurosurgery 104: 231–235.

Poser C and Brinar V (2004) The nature of multiple sclerosis. Clinical Neurology and Neurosurgery 106: 139–171.

Raine C (1994) The immunology of multiple sclerosis. Annals of Neurology 36(S1): S61–72.

Sadovnick A (1994) Genetic epidemiology of multiple sclerosis: A survey. Annals of Neurology 36(S2): S194–203.

Muscular Dystrophies

M Astejada, M C Malicdan, and I Nishino, National Center of Neurology and Psychiatry, Tokyo, Japan

Introduction

Muscular dystrophy (MD), as described by Walton and Nattrass in 1954, is a heterogeneous group of inherited primary diseases of the muscle, clinically characterized by progressive muscle weakness and wasting. Histologically, it is unified by the presence of necrotic and regenerating processes, often associated with an increased amount of connective and adipose tissues (Emery, 2001). Following this definition, the discussion will be focused on dystrophinopathies, Emery-Dreifuss muscular dystrophies, congenital muscular dystrophies, limb-girdle muscular dystrophies, and fascioscapulohumeral muscular dystrophy. The heterogeneity of these different disorders included is often delineated by a combination of clinical, genetic, molecular, and pathological aspects, which will be thoroughly discussed in this article.

Dystrophinopathies

Dystrophinopathies are X-linked progressive hereditary degenerative diseases of skeletal muscles caused by an absence or deficiency of dystrophin, a sarcolemmal protein. Dystrophin and the associated proteins form a complex integral framework connecting the intracellular actin cytoskeleton to the extracellular matrix, stabilizing the sarcolemma from mechanical stresses during muscle contraction (**Figure 1**). The responsible gene is located on the short arm of the X chromosome at locus *Xp21*. It is an extremely large gene, comprising more than 2.5 million base pairs and 79 exons. Out-of-frame mutation of dystrophin can result in Duchenne muscular dystrophy (DMD), while in-frame mutation causes its milder allelic form, Becker muscular dystrophy (BMD). In both DMD and BMD, the most common mechanism of mutation is large-scale deletion.

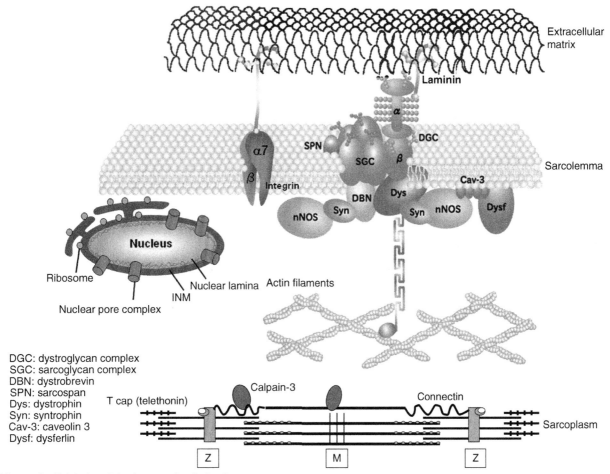

DGC: dystroglycan complex
SGC: sarcoglycan complex
DBN: dystrobrevin
SPN: sarcospan
Dys: dystrophin
Syn: syntrophin
Cav-3: caveolin 3
Dysf: dysferlin

Figure 1 Related proteins in muscular dystrophy.

Duchenne Muscular Dystrophy

Named after a French physician in 1861, DMD is one of the most common muscular dystrophies occurring in approximately 1 in 5000 male births. Symptoms are usually recognized by 2 years of age when an apparent delayed motor development is noted. In over 50% of cases, walking is delayed until 18 months and affected boys never learn to run normally. Muscle involvement is often bilateral and symmetrical. As knee and hip extensor weakness progresses, the child employs the Gowers' maneuver, whereby he climbs up his thighs with both hands to extend his hips and trunk in assuming a standing position. In most cases, calf muscle hypertrophy (**Figure 2**) is observed. Cardiac and central nervous system involvement is clearly evident, with cardiomyopathy and low IQ associated in some cases. Creatine kinase (CK) is usually elevated, with levels greater than ten times the upper normal limits during the early stages; it never reaches a normal level, even during the terminal stage. Pathologically, fiber size variation associated with clusters of necrotic and regenerating processes (**Figure 3a**) is often observed, with complete absence of dystrophin on

immunostaining (**Figure 3c**). This disease is slowly progressive and most patients are wheelchair-bound by 15 years of age. Previously, death occurred at around 20 years of age due to respiratory failure; however, improvement in respiratory care has prolonged life expectancy. Most patients now live to around 30 years of age and die from cardiac complications. Female DMD has also been reported due to X chromosome translocation involving the dystrophin gene locus. In other instances, Turner syndrome (this syndrome encompasses several conditions, most commonly monosomes X. In females, normally there are XX sex chromosomes, but in this syndrome, there is only one X chromosome which is fully functional. As a result, the karyotype is labeled |45, X|| instead of 46, XX|) is associated with DMD due to complete or partial absence of an X chromosome or nonrandom X chromosome inactivation.

Becker Muscular Dystrophy

Becker muscular dystrophy, named after a well-known German geneticist, occurs in approximately one out of 30 000 male births. Although the same dystrophin gene is mutated, the clinical features of BMD vary greatly from DMD-like phenotype to no subjective weakness. The onset of disease is much later. Muscle cramp and calf hypertrophy are frequently noted. Cardiac abnormalities may also be seen, but mental retardation is rare. Creatine

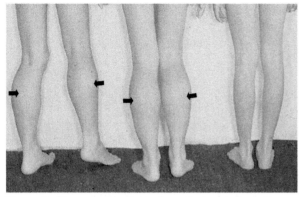

Figure 2 Two muscular dystrophy patients showing calf hypertrophy (arrows). Normal sibling is shown on the rightmost figure.

kinase is elevated. Muscle biopsy findings include an active necrotic and regenerative process with endomysial fibrosis. In milder cases, type 2 fiber can be hypertrophic, while type 1 fibers are atrophic. Patchy dystrophin immunostaining is diagnostic (**Figure 3d**). The presence of some measure of functioning dystrophin in BMD patients allows a more benign course and most affected individuals lose ambulation only after 20–30 years of illness.

Female carriers of both DMD/BMD can also be symptomatic with elevated serum creatine kinase and muscle weakness with mosaic pattern of dystrophin immunostaining. Some carriers develop cardiomyopathy later in life.

For initial diagnosis of dystrophinopathies, multiplex polymerase chain reaction (PCR) should be performed. This method can detect deletion in 60% in all DMD and 85% in all BMD patients, while Southern blots and quantitative PCR can be used to detect duplication. The algorithm in diagnosis of dystrophinopathies is shown in **Figure 4**. Prenatal diagnosis could be performed by DNA studies on chorionic villus sampling at 8–10 weeks gestation and cultured amniotic fluid cells at 12–16 weeks gestation.

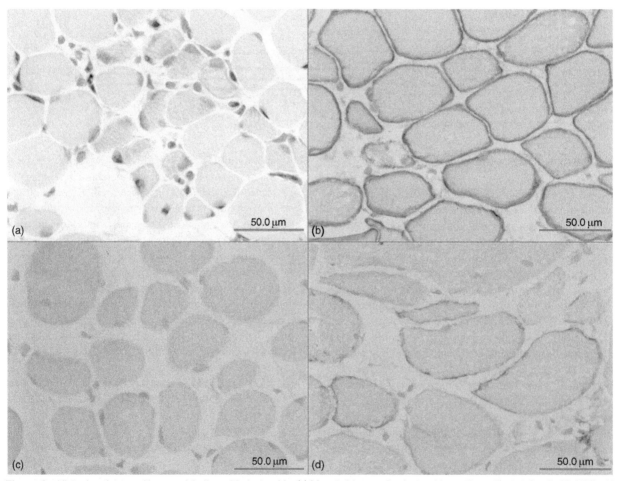

Figure 3 Histochemistry and immunolabeling with dystrophin. (a) Muscle biopsy of a dystrophinopathy patient stained with H&E×40 showing clusters of regenerating fibers with fiber size variation. (b) Normal: dystrophin is located at the sarcolemma on all fibers. (c) DMD: no dystrophin staining appreciated. (d) BMD: patchy sarcolemmal dystrophin staining.

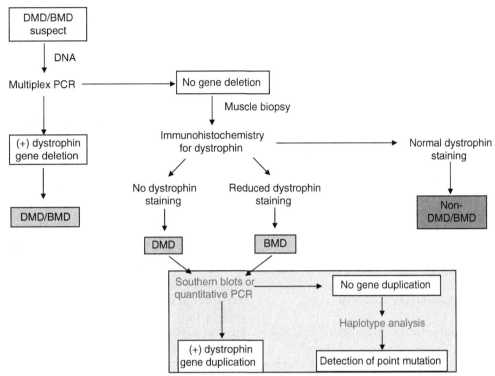

Figure 4 Algorithm in the diagnosis of dystrophinopathies. Southern blots and haplotype analysis are optional.

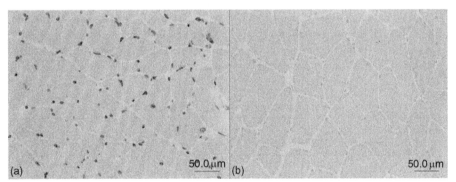

Figure 5 Immunostaining with emerin. (a) Normal: emerin is located at the nucleus. (b) X-EDMD: nuclear staining with emerin is not observed. Magnification ×20; indirect immunoperoxidase labeling with emerin monoclonal antibody.

Emery-Dreifuss Muscular Dystrophy

Emery-Dreifuss muscular dystrophy (EDMD) was coined by Rowland in 1979 after the two physicians who detailed, described, and differentiated the disease from DMD/BMD. It is characterized by a triad of early joint contractures, progressive humeroperoneal muscle wasting, and cardiomyopathy with conduction block. There are three modes of inheritance: X-linked recessive (X-EDMD), autosomal dominant (AD-EDMD), and autosomal recessive (AR-EDMD). X-EDMD is often caused by a nonsense mutation in the *EMD* gene, which is located on the X chromosome at locus *Xq28*, resulting in the absence of an inner nuclear

protein emerin (**Figure 5**). The clinical onset of disease is usually in the first or second decade of life with joint contractures involving the elbows, Achilles tendon, and posterior neck appearing before any significant muscle weakness. The nature of the early onset contracture is still not understood at present. Muscle weakness initially involves the humeroperoneal areas and later involving the scapular and pelvic muscles. In most cases of X-EDMD, cardiac abnormalities appear later than muscle involvement, generally after 20–30 years of age. In contrast, both AD-EDMD and AR-EDMD are included in a group of diseases collectively known as laminopathies, which stem from missense mutation of the Lamin A/C (*LMNA*) gene located on chromosome *1q21.2-q21.3*, resulting in a nonfunctional nuclear lamina protein. As reported by Bonne *et al.* in 2000, the clinical presentation of the autosomal form, including the age of onset and severity of disease, is much more heterogeneous than X-EDMD. Joint contractures occur after muscle weakness. Cardiac conduction defects in EDMD can manifest as sinus bradycardia, first-degree atrioventricular block, Wenckebach phenomenon, third-degree atrioventricular block, and bundle-branch block. Atrial and ventricular arrhythmias are frequent. In AD-EDMD, the risk of ventricular tachyarrhythmia and dilated cardiomyopathy manifested by left ventricular dilation and dysfunction is higher than in XL-EDMD. Serum CK is moderately elevated. Muscle biopsy often reveals nonspecific features such as fiber size variation with necrotic and regenerating process.

Congenital Muscular Dystrophy

First described by Batten in 1903, congenital muscular dystrophy (CMD) is a group of clinically heterogeneous autosomal recessive inherited muscle diseases characterized by hypotonia at birth, generalized muscle weakness, frequently multiple contractures, and necrotic and regenerating process on muscle biopsy. The clinical spectrum ranges from a very severe form, often resulting in early infant death, to relatively mild conditions, where the patient survives into adulthood. The recent advances of molecular genetics have led to a more comprehensive classification of CMD based on the clinical presentation,

genetic abnormality, and the primary biochemical protein defects (**Table 1**). Presently, nine genes responsible for the different type of CMD have been identified. Importantly, the frequency of each subtype varies widely among different ethnic groups.

Laminin 2 (Merosin) Deficiency

Laminin $\alpha2$ deficiency comprises 40–50% of all CMD in European countries. However, in Japan, it accounts for only a few percent. Laminin $\alpha2$, encoded by the *LAMA* gene, is a glycoprotein in the basement membrane, which binds to a number of macromolecules including agrin, nidogen, and collagen IV in the extracellular matrix and serves as ligand to two transmembrane proteins, alpha dystroglycan and integrin (**Figure 1**). Laminin $\alpha2$ is expressed in muscle, cerebral blood vessels, developing white matter tracts, and Schwann cells. Affected children present with hypotonia, weakness, and respiratory and feeding problems at birth or in the first few months of life. Contractures can occur but severe arthrogryposis is rare. Sitting without support is the maximal motor ability attained. Calf hypertrophy and facial muscle weakness can be observed in the neonatal period. Brain magnetic resonance imaging (MRI) invariably shows white matter changes in patients after 6 months, despite normal mentation. However, structural brain anomalies are also observed in some cases, causing mental retardation and epilepsies (Muntoni and Voit, 2004). Demyelination of the motor nerve is also observed in some patients with

Table 1   Classification of congenital muscular dystrophy with recognizable gene loci

Disorder	Abbreviation	Gene locus	Gene	Protein	CNS involvement
Merosin deficient CMD	MDC1A	6q2	Laminin alpha 2 (LAMA2)	Laminin $\alpha2$	+
Congenital muscular dystrophy 1B	MDC1B	1q42	?	?	?
Congenital muscular dystrophy 1C	MDC1C	19q13	Fukutin-related protein (FKRP)	Putative glycosyltransferase	−/+
Congenital muscular dystrophy 1D	MDC1D	22q	LARGE	Putative glycosyltransferase	+
Fukuyama CMD	FCMD	9q3	FUKUTIN (FKTN)	Fukutin	+
Muscle eye–brain disease	MEB	1p32–34	POMGnT1	O-linked mannose beta 1,2-N-acetyl-glucosaminyltransferase	+
Walker Warburg syndrome	WWS	9q34	POMT1	O-mannosyltransferase	+
Ullrich disease	UCMD	21q22 and 2q37	Collagen VI (COL 6A1, COL6A2/ COL6A3)	Collagen 6 $\alpha1$, collagen 6 $\alpha2$, collagen 6 $\alpha3$	−
Integrin $\alpha7$ deficiency	ITGA7	12q13	INTEGRIN $\alpha7$	Integrin $\alpha7$	−
Rigid spine syndrome	RSM1	1p35–36	Selenoprotein N1 (SEPN1)	Selenoprotein N	−
Marinesco-Sjögren syndrome	MSS	5q31	SIL1	BIP-associated protein or BAP	+

reduced motor nerve conduction velocity. Serum CK is invariably elevated, usually more than ten times the normal values in the early stages. Failure to thrive occurs in 80% of the cases, from weakness of the muscles involved in swallowing often resulting in aspiration pneumonia. Coupled with frequent infection, respiratory muscle weakness eventually leads to respiratory failure, necessitating ventilatory support. Mild to moderate cardiac hypokinesia is seen in a small portion of MCD1A patients. Immunostaining techniques can readily demonstrate the absent or partial reduction of merosin. However, in the latter cases, further test is warranted for careful interpretation.

Fukuyama Congenital Muscular Dystrophy

Currently, five genes (*FKTN*, *POMGnT1*, *POMT1*, *FKRP*, and *LARGE*) are identified encoding proteins and glycosyltransferases involved in the glycosylation of α-dystroglycan. Collectively, disorders resulting from mutation in these genes are called α-dystroglycanopathies. The common pathologic mechanism governing these diseases is aberrant glycosylation of α-dystroglycan, which might explain the existing phenotypic overlap between the different forms. Immunolabeling reveals complete absence or reduced α-dystroglycan. Among them, Fukuyama congenital muscular dystrophy (FCMD) is caused by mutation in *FKTN* gene. This disease, originally described by Fukuyama and his collaborators in 1960, is the most frequent CMD in Japan, accounting for 60% of cases. Virtually all FCMD patients are Japanese. This is because only the Japanese share the common 3 kb retrotransposal insertion in the 3′ UTR of the *FKTN* gene. Seventy-five percent of FCMD cases in Japan are attributable to homozygous 3 kb retrotransposal insertion into the 3′ UTR of the fukutin gene and 25% have compound heterozygous mutations of the 3 kb insertion at the 3′ UTR and a mutation in the coding sequence. The classical features include hypotonia, generalized weakness, facies, mental retardation, and ocular anomalies. Motor improvement is often observed in a brief period between ages 2 and 8 years. Typically, the patient sits independently but never walks. This is followed by progressive weakness with subsequent respiratory failure. Brain changes are often due to abnormal neuronal migration, resulting in profound mental retardation and epilepsy. Dilated cardiomyopathy typically develops in the second decade of life. Life expectancy averages approximately 20 years but with the advent of more sophisticated respiratory equipment, survival into the third decade is increasingly possible. Recently, a patient with a homozygous 1bp insertion was reported from Turkey. This patient had severe brain and eye abnormalities and died 15 days after birth.

Muscle Eye Brain Disease

Muscle eye brain disease (MEB) due to mutation in the *POMGnT1* gene was first described in Finland in 1977, but presently, worldwide distribution including Japan and Korea is known. The clinical spectrum of brain and muscle involvement is similar to that described in FCMD patients but typically with more severe eye dysfunction manifested as poor visual alertness during the neonatal period. Despite the loss of glycosylated α-dystroglycan and laminin α-2 binding capacity, the expression of core α-dystroglycan is preserved in MEB.

Walker-Warburg Syndrome

Walker-Warburg syndrome, first described in 1942, is the most severe form of the α-dystroglycanopathy associated with life expectancy of less than 3 years. Although mutation in *FKTN* and *FKRP* account for a small fraction of WWS, mutation in POMT1 has also been recently identified in a well-characterized cohort of WWS patients, suggesting genetic heterogeneity. The characteristic feature of marked weakness is compounded by the severe brain and eye anomalies.

Congenital Muscular Dystrophy 1C

Fukutin-related protein (FKRP) is ubiquitously expressed throughout the human body with the highest levels in the skeletal and cardiac muscles. Recently, *FKRP* gene mutation has been considered to be associated with the widest phenotypic spectrum of muscular dystrophy ranging from *in utero* onset and early fetal lethality in WWS or MEB to late adult onset, slowly progressive limb-girdle muscular dystrophy (LGMD2I). Mutation in this gene, which is associated with reduced immunolabeling of α-dystroglycan, is likewise responsible for congenital muscular dystrophy 1C (MDC1C). The hallmark is severe muscle weakness and early onset of respiratory insufficiency. Serum CK levels are always elevated (20–75 times). Intelligence and brain MRI are normal. Heart involvement is less prominent, in contrast to LGMD2I. A considerable number of MDC1C/LGMD2I patients have been identified in European and Middle Eastern countries, but only a few patients have been found in Japan.

Congenital Muscular Dystrophy 1D

Loss of function mutation in the *LARGE* gene, as depicted in the myodystrophy (*Large*^myd^) mouse, displays a severe, progressive muscular dystrophy and mild cardiomyopathy, in addition to retinal and peripheral and central nervous system involvement. Recently, recessive mutation in the human homolog *LARGE* gene has been identified to be responsible for congenital muscular dystrophy 1D (MDC1D), which is congenital muscular dystrophy associated with profound mental retardation brought about by white matter changes and subtle structural abnormalities on brain MRI. Pathologically, there is reduced immunolabeling of α-dystroglycan and reduced molecular weight of α-dystroglycan on immunoblot with preserved laminin binding ability.

Ullrich Congenital Muscular Dystrophy

Collagen VI, a ubiquitously expressed extracellular matrix protein, forms microfibrils in close association with the basal lamina around the muscle fibers. This protein interacts with several other matrix constituents. It is composed of three chains, α1, α2, and α3, encoded by the genes *COL6A1* and *COL6A2* on chromosome *21q22.3* and *COL6A3* on chromosome *2q37*. Recessive mutation in any of the three genes causes Ullrich congenital muscular dystrophy (UCMD). Originally reported by Ullrich in 1930 as congenital atonic-sclerotic muscular dystrophy, the typical phenotype is represented by a combination of early-onset severe muscle weakness with proximal joint contractures and distal joint hyperextensibility. Normal intelligence is also an integral feature of the disease. Characteristic round facies, lid lag, and prominent ears are also often observed. Progressive functional deterioration is mostly due to increased contractures, which subsequently involves even the distal joint in later stages. Respiratory insufficiency invariably develops in the first or second decade. Serum CK is normal or mildly elevated. Pathological features in the muscle biopsy range from mildly myopathic with occasional necrotic and regenerating fibers to overtly dystrophic with profound endomysial and perimysial fibrosis. Collagen VI immunolabeling reportedly shows three different patterns of abnormalities: Complete deficiency, partial deficiency, and sarcolemma-specific collagen VI deficiency (SSCD). Complete deficiency is associated with recessive mutation, while SSCD is associated with dominant mutations. An increasing number of patients has recently been recognized. Most likely, this is one of the major CMDs, accounting for 10–20% of CMD cases.

Rigid Spine Syndrome

The clinical phenotype of rigid spine syndrome was initially described by Victor Dubowitz. Following linkage study, Moghadaszadeh *et al.* identified selenoprotein N gene (*SEPN1*) as the causative gene for this disease. It encodes an endoplasmic reticulum glycoprotein with the highest expression in the fetal tissues, suggesting its functional role in the developing muscular system. Severely affected patients present as floppy infants with weak suckling, poor neck flexion, and they never achieve ambulation. However, in more mildly affected children, symptoms may present in infancy or childhood with delayed motor development or frequent falls. In such cases, ambulation is usually maintained into adulthood. The hallmark of this syndrome is spinal rigidity and scoliosis due to contractures of the spine extensor muscles, which may develop between the ages of 3 and 12 years. Serum CK is normal or mildly elevated and muscle imaging reveals selective involvement of medial thigh muscles with relative sparing of rectus femoris and gracilis. Vital capacity decreases over time due to the stiffness of the rib cage with compounding diaphragmatic weakness. Pathologically, fiber size variation with mild necrotic and regenerating process, type 1 fiber predominance, and atrophy may be observed. Many specimens would show unevenness of intermyofibrillar network in oxidative staining, sometimes with overt core-like features.

Integrin 7 Deficiency

Integrins are a major laminin α2 receptor in the muscle fibers. The accurate expression and localization of integrin α7β1 is laminin α-2-dependent. Primary deficiency of integrin α7 is rare, and so far causative mutation in *ITGA7* has only been identified in three patients. These patients manifested as mild congenital myopathy with delayed motor milestones. Muscle biopsies revealed only mild variation in fiber size. Direct diagnosis through immunolabeling of integrin α7 seems to be hindered by the developmental regulation and interindividual variation observed in the first 2 years of life wherein expression of the protein employing the available antibodies is frequently low.

Marinesco Sjögren Syndrome

Marinesco-Sjögren syndrome is a rare disorder that is inherited as an autosomal recessive genetic condition. The major features of this disorder are cerebellar atrophy causing ataxias, congenital cataracts, and psychomotor retardation. Other cardinal features include myopathies, short stature, and hypergonadotrophic hypogonadism. Muscle pathology is characterized by fiber size variation, necrotic fibers, rimmed vacuoles with marked connective tissue, and fat replacement. The underlying causative gene *SIL1* encodes for a co-chaperone for HSPA5 (also called BiP), which is a chaperone for the heat-shock protein

70 (HSP70) (Antonen *et al.*, 2006). Recently, researchers have suggested that disturbed SIL1–HSPA5 interaction and protein folding is most likely the primary pathogenesis in Marinesco Sjögren syndrome.

Limb-Girdle Muscular Dystrophies

The limb-girdle muscular dystrophies (LGMDs) are a group of genotypically and phenotypically heterogeneous muscular dystrophies (Bushby, 1999). They are characterized by weakness of the proximal muscles in the upper and lower extremities. Involvement is usually first evident in either the pelvic or, less frequently, the shoulder girdle, often with asymmetry of wasting when the upper limbs are first involved. Pathologically, findings include variation in fiber size, dystrophic process, internal nucleation, and endomysial fibrosis.

The identification of the DAP complex and the characterization of the complex's role in the pathogenesis of many LGMDs has provided a new basis for the distinction and classification of these muscular dystrophies (**Table 2**). Presently, there are 16 different loci identified, seven autosomal dominant causing type 1 LGMD and 14 autosomal recessive causing type 2 LGMD. Further genetic heterogeneity exists for both autosomal dominant and autosomal recessive LGMD, as established by further linkage studies.

LGMD2 cases are more common, having a cumulative prevalence of 1:15 000 with a number of geographical differences. Moreover, these are more severe, with some

resembling DMD phenotype. Four of the recessive forms have been associated with defects in genes coding for the sarcoglycan complex, which along with dystrophin helps anchor muscles to the extracellular matrix. More devastating mutations in these same genes can cause severe childhood autosomal muscular dystrophy (SCARMD). In contrast, only a relatively small proportion of LGMD, around 10%, is autosomal dominant in inheritance.

Calpainopathy

Calpainopathy (LGMD2A) involves mutations in the *CAPN3* gene, which encodes the muscle-specific protein calpain-3. It is characterized mainly by a symmetric, very selective atrophic involvement of limb-girdle and trunk muscles, with the gluteus maximus and thigh adductors being most affected. Clinically, calf hypertrophy is rarely observed, but Achilles tendon contractures are common. Scapular winging is usually present from the early stages, though it may be asymptomatic. Onset of symptoms occurs between the ages of 8 and 15 years, but adult onset is not uncommon. Progression of calpainopathy is variable. Most patients may have normal mobility in childhood with a very slowly progressive course of disease. Confinement to a wheelchair occurs at the earliest typically 11–28 years after onset. Anterior distal leg and distal arm muscles are relatively spared. While the first location of detectable muscle weakness was in the pelvifemoral muscles, muscle CT scanning in some patients showed early involvement of the gastrocnemius muscle, which was usually asymptomatic, though early inability to walk on

Table 2 Present classification of limb girdle muscular dystrophy (LGMD)

Disease name	Abbreviation	Gene locus	Gene name	Gene product
Autosomal dominant limb-girdle muscular dystrophy	LGMD1A	*5q31*	TTID	Myotilin
	LGMD1B	*1q21.2*	LMNA	Lamin A/C
	LGMD1C	*3p25*	CAV3	Caveolin 3 (CAV3)
	LGMD1D	*7q*		?
Familial dilated cardiomyopathy with conduction defect and muscular dystrophy	LGMD1E	*6q23*		?
	LGMD1F	*7q32.1–32.2*		
	LGMD1G	*4p21*		?
Autosomal recessive limb-girdle muscular dystrophy				
Calpain-deficient LGMD	LGMD2A	*15q15.1–21.2*	CAPN3	Calpain 3 (CAPN3)
Dysferlin-deficient LGMD	LGMD2B	*2p13.3-p13.1*	DYSF	Dysferlin (DYSF)
	LGMD2G	*17q11–12*	TCAP	Telethonin
Manitoba Hutterite dystrophy	LGMD2H	*9q31–33*	TRIM32	Tripartite motif-containing protein-32
	LGMD2I	*19q13.3*	FKRP	Fukutin-related protein
	LGMD2J	*2q31*	TTN	Titin
LGMD with mental retardation and reduced α-dystroglycan	LGMD2K	*9q34.1*	POMT1	Protein O-mannosyltransferase 1
α-Sarcoglycanopathy	LGMD2D	*17q21*	SGCA	α-Sarcoglycan
β-Sarcoglycanopathy	LGMD2E	*4q12*	SGCB	β-Sarcoglycan
γ-Sarcoglycanopathy	LGMD2C	*13q12*	SGCG	γ-Sarcoglycan
δ-Sarcoglycanopathy	LGMD2F	*5q33–34*	SGCD	δ-Sarcoglycan

tiptoe is an important clinical clue. Respiratory, but not cardiac, complications have been reported.

The majority of patients with *CAPN3* mutations had a variable degree of calpain-3 protein deficiency determined by immunoblot analysis. The probability of having LGMD2A is high when patients have a complete calpain-3 deficiency and progressively decreases with increasing amounts of protein detected. Patients with severe, early-onset disease usually have no calpain-3 protein, but absent or markedly reduced protein levels are also detected in patients with adult onset. However, almost all patients with normal calpain-3 levels have late or adult onset of the disorder. Given the heterogeneity of the mutations seen in this very large gene, muscle biopsy will probably still prove a more straightforward starting point for diagnosis than mutation detection, though this will remain necessary for carrier detection and prenatal diagnosis where this is required.

Dysferlinopathy (LGMD2B)

Dysferlinopathy (LGMD2B) is secondary to mutations in the dysferlin gene. In this disease, CK levels are often 20–150 times above the normal range at presentation. Disease onset usually is in the late teens, and progression of illness is slow. Commonly, patients have inability to stand on tiptoes because of the predominant distal lower limb involvement. Dysferlin localizes to the muscle fiber membrane and is expressed from very early in human development. This gene is involved in two forms of muscular dystrophy: LGMD2B and the predominantly distal muscular dystrophy, Miyoshi myopathy. The underlying means by which mutations in this gene are responsible for these different phenotypes is not known. Interestingly, both forms (LGMD2B and Miyoshi) can co-exist in the same family.

Sarcoglycanopathies

There are five known sarcoglycans (α, β, γ, δ, and possibly ε) (**Figure 1**) at the muscle fiber membrane that forms part of the DAPC, and genetic defects affecting four (α-, β-, γ-, and δ-sarcoglycan) of these proteins cause specific type 2 LGMDs, also known as sarcoglycanopathies (LGMD2C, 2D, 2E, and 2F). The most characteristic clinical features of this group include calf hypertrophy, involvement of scapular and deltoid muscles at onset of disease, and cardiomyopathy. Symptoms mostly occur during childhood, although the onset can occur in adulthood. Progression of the disease ranges from very mild to very severe.

α-Sarcoglycanopathy (LGMD2D) patients commonly present with difficulty running and climbing stairs; like in dystrophinopathy, however, they can present with

muscle cramps or exercise intolerance. Toe-walking is an early feature in fewer than half of the patients. Other patients have delayed walking, implying an earlier onset, but adult-onset cases have also been reported. Calf hypertrophy is seen in almost all patients at some stage. Facial, ocular, and velopharyngeal muscles are spared. Progression of the disease is usually faster with earlier presentation, but some intrafamilial variability has been observed.

γ-Sarcoglycanopathy (LGMD2C) patients have similar presentation as those having LGMD2D. They have proximal lower limb weakness, frequent calf hypertrophy, variability in severity, which may be intrafamilial, predominantly with childhood onset, no cardiac involvement, and normal intelligence (Noguchi *et al.*, 1995).

β-Sarcoglycanopathy (LGMD2E) patients with this myopathy have a broad range of clinical severity, even within the same family. The mean age at onset usually is at 7–8 years. Patients with an adult onset usually have a milder phenotype; ambulation is still possible in some patients in the sixth decade. More severe forms have earlier onset during childhood and faster progression.

Patients with δ-sarcoglycanopathy (LGMD2F) tend to show a very severe clinical course. Age at onset ranges from 4 to 10 years, with confinement to a wheelchair between 9 and 16 years and death between 9 and 19 years.

Limb-Girdle Muscular Dystrophy 2G

Limb-girdle muscular dystrophy 2G (LGMD2G) has been shown to be secondary to mutations in the gene encoding telethonin. Patients typically present early in the second decade with difficulty climbing stairs and running, although foot-drop is also an early feature. Proximal and distal lower-limb weakness is therefore present from the onset, while in the upper limbs the proximal musculature is more severely affected. Confinement to a wheelchair occurs approximately 18 years after onset. Creatine kinase may be mildly or moderately elevated. Muscle biopsies show a considerable number of rimmed vacuoles.

Limb-Girdle Muscular Dystrophy 2H

Limb-girdle muscular dystrophy 2H (LGMD2H), linked to chromosome *9q31–33*, has been shown to be caused by mutations in the gene encoding a tripartite motif-containing protein-32 (TRIM32) among Hutterites. The initial report was from Jerusalem *et al.* in 1973, where two brothers from an inbred Hutterite colony with nonprogressive weakness from infancy were diagnosed as having sarcotubular myopathy. Affected individuals presented with proximal lower limb weakness between 8 and

27 years of age, with elevated serum creatine kinase concentration (2–30 times normal). Facial and proximal upper limb muscles, predominantly the trapezius and deltoid were affected as disease progressed. Mild distal limb muscle (brachioradialis and anterior peroneal muscle) involvement was also seen. Most patients have remained ambulant late into adult life.

Limb-Girdle Muscular Dystrophy 2I

Limb-girdle muscular dystrophy 2I (LGMD2I) is caused by mutation in the gene encoding fukutin-related protein (FKRP). Age at onset ranges from 6 months to 40 years. The disorder can be phenotypically variable. Patients can present with hypotonia, waddling gait, or difficulty in climbing stairs, weakness in the hip and shoulder girdle muscles, calf hypertrophy, tight Achilles tendon, and elevated serum creatine kinase. Young boys can resemble DMD or BMD phenotype. Some patients show signs of cardiomyopathy on electrocardiogram. In the consanguineous Tunisian family originally reported by Driss *et al.* (2000), however, the patients had symmetric proximal muscle weakness and wasting in all four limbs but no heart involvement.

Limb-Girdle Muscular Dystrophy 2J

Limb-girdle muscular dystrophy 2J (LGMD2J) is caused by homozygous mutation in the titin gene (*TTN*). Heterozygous mutation in the titin gene causes tardive tibial muscular dystrophy (TMD). Mutation in the titin gene also causes dilated cardiomyopathy type 1G (CMD1G). As reported by Udd *et al.* in a consanguineous Finnish pedigree, 8 out of 20 members had a severe limb-girdle muscular dystrophy inherited in an autosomal recessive pattern, with an onset in the first to third decades involving all proximal muscles, although some patients developed distal muscle involvement. Severe disability with loss of ambulation occurs on the third to sixth decades. There was no facial muscle involvement or cardiomyopathy. The findings were compatible with the hypothesis that the severe LGMD phenotype was the homozygous manifestation of a dominant gene that in the heterozygous state caused the milder distal myopathy. In patients with homozygous mutations, complete loss of calpain-3 is seen, which may be a secondary downstream effect of deficiency of the TMD gene protein and results in phenotypic overlap with LGMD2A.

Limb-Girdle Muscular Dystrophy 2K

Limb-girdle muscular dystrophy 2K (LGMD2K), caused by mutation in the gene encoding protein O-mannosyltransferase-1 (POMT1), is an early-onset myopathy, which is allelic to Walker-Warburg syndrome, and is mostly found in Turkish families. All patients acquire early motor milestones, excluding congenital muscular dystrophy. Age at onset ranges from 1 to 6 years, with difficulty in walking and climbing stairs. Other features include slow progression, proximal muscle weakness, mild muscle hypertrophy, increased serum creatine kinase, microcephaly, and mental retardation.

Limb-Girdle Muscular Dystrophy 1A

Limb-girdle muscular dystrophy 1A (LGMD1A), secondary to mutations in the myotilin-encoding gene, is an autosomal dominant disorder characterized by adult onset of proximal muscle weakness, beginning in the hip girdle and later progressing to the shoulder girdle region. Distal muscle weakness may occur later. Progression of the disease is very slow, and very few patients progress to wheelchair confinement.

Limb-Girdle Muscular Dystrophy 1B

Limb-girdle muscular dystrophy 1B (LGMD1B) is caused by *LMNA* mutations. In affected individuals, symmetric weakness starts in the proximal lower-limb muscles before the age of 20 years. In the third or fourth decade, upper-limb muscles gradually become affected as well. Early contractures of the spine are absent, and contractures of elbows and Achilles tendons are either minimal or late, distinguishing this disorder from Emery-Dreifuss muscular dystrophy. Like EDMD, however, cardiac involvement is also prominent, mostly in the form of atrioventricular conduction blocks. A minority of patients also have dilated cardiomyopathy (van der Kooi *et al.*, 1997). While cardiac problems very rarely precede muscle symptoms, in some patients their muscle symptoms are recognized only in retrospect.

Limb-Girdle Muscular Dystrophy 1C

Limb-girdle muscular dystrophy 1C (LGMD1C) is an autosomal dominant muscular dystrophy, associated with a severe deficiency of caveolin-3 in muscle fibers (up to 95% reduction). The clinical features are usually mild, comprising calf hypertrophy and muscle pain on exertion. Age of onset is around 5 years and disease progression is variable, as patients can remain ambulant up to adulthood. Episodes of exertional muscle cramps are noted in some patients. Serum creatine kinase levels are elevated four- to 25-fold.

The remaining LGMDs are only defined by a chromosomal localization since the genes associated with these dystrophies have not yet been cloned. LGMD1D has been mapped to chromosome *7q*. Onset is between the second and sixth decades, with hip girdle preceding shoulder girdle involvement. Creatine kinase is elevated and muscle biopsy shows fiber splitting and fibrosis. LGMD1E, mapped to *6q23*, characteristically is associated with cardiomyopathy, conduction defects, with or without muscle weakness. It is also referred to as dilated cardiomyopathy 1F (CMD1F). It has been identified in a large family of French-Canadian descent. LGMD1F, linked to chromosome *7q32.1–32.2*, has been described in one Spanish family. Proximal muscle weakness is seen during the onset of the disease, involving distal muscles in the later stage. Muscle biopsy revealed myopathic changes and sometimes rimmed vacuoles. LGMD1G, mapped to chromosome *4p21*, was described in a Brazilian Caucasian family. Clinical presentation is rather homogenous: patients present with cramps early in the course, gradually developing proximal myopathy. Contractures produce limited flexion of fingers and toes.

Despite the recent advances in the molecular characterization of LGMDs, a clear method of classification is not yet available. In the future, when all the causative genes and their respective protein products are identified, a new method of classification may be feasible.

Facioscapulohumeral Muscular Dystrophy

Facioscapulohumeral (FSH) muscular dystrophy is an autosomal dominant form that affects muscles of the face (facio), scapula (scapulo), and upper arms (humeral). Although extraocular muscles are not affected, weakness in muscles around the eye (i.e., orbicularis oculi) may be evident when patients sleep with their eyes slightly open, a symptom that may manifest itself before other symptoms develop. There is also difficulty in whistling or blowing. Distal extremity muscles also can be affected, and the weakness is often asymmetric. There is a wide range of clinical severity, with symptoms that can include cardiac, cognitive, visual, and auditory impairments. Symptoms may develop in early childhood and are usually noticeable in teenage years. Life expectancy is normal, but some affected individuals become severely disabled. Nearly all cases are associated with a distal *4q35* deletion.

Clinical diagnosis of FSHD is based initially on the pattern of muscle involvement, but genetic tests, which can detect FSHD with a 98% success rate, are now preferred. Because there are no known genes in this region, a novel position effect has been postulated to explain the disease phenotype. Although the specific gene responsible for FSHD has not been identified, FSHD is associated with a deletion of 3.3-kb repeats

(called D4Z4) mapped to the telomeric end of the long arm of chromosome 4. This region, termed *4q35*, normally has 11–150 D4Z4 repeats, but in patients with FSHD, the number of repeats is fewer than 11. Although it was thought until recently that the severity of clinical presentation increased as the number of D4Z4 repeats under 11 decreased, this has recently been challenged. The telomeric D4Z4 repeats have most recently been thought to affect anchoring of chromosome 4 to the inner nuclear membrane. If true, FSHD would resemble other MDs, such as Emery-Dreifuss muscular dystrophy, that are nuclear in origin.

See also: Metabolic Myopathies; Multiple Sclerosis.

Citations

Antonen A, Mahjneh I, Hämäläinen R, *et al.* (2006) The gene disrupted in Marinesco Sjögren syndrome encodes SIL1, an HSPA5 cochaperone. *Nature Genetics* 37: 1309–1311.

Bonne G, Mercuri E, Muchir A, *et al.* (2000) Clinical and molecular genetic spectrum of autosomal dominant muscular dystrophy due to mutations of the lamin A/C gene. *Annals of Neurology* 48: 170–180.

Bushby KM (1999) The limb-girdle muscular dystrophies-multiple genes, multiple mechanisms. *Human Molecular Genetics* 8(10): 1875–1882.

Driss A, Amouri C, Hamida CB, *et al.* (2000) A new locus for autosomal recessive limb girdle muscular dystrophy in a large consanguineous Tunisian family maps to chromosome *19q13.3*. *Neuromuscular Disorders* 10: 240–246.

Emery A (2001) *The Muscular Dystrophies.* New York: Oxford University Press.

Muntoni F and Voit T (2004) The congenital muscular dystrophies in 2004: a century of exciting progress. *Neuromuscular Disorders* 14: 635–649.

Noguchi S, McNally EM, Ben Othmane K, *et al.* (1995) Mutations in the dystrophin-associated protein gamma-sarcoglycan in chromosome 13 muscular dystrophy. *Science* 270: 819–821.

van der Kooi AJ, van Meegen M, Ledderhof TM, *et al.* (1997) Genetic localization of a newly recognized autosomal dominant limb-girdle muscular dystrophy with cardiac involvement (LGMD1B) to chromosome *1q11–21*. *American Journal of Human Genetics* 60: 891–895.

Further Reading

Bonnenmann CG and Bushby KM (2004) The limb girdle muscular dystrophies. In: Engel AG and Franzini-Armstrong C (eds.) 3rd edn. 1077–1121*Myology*, 3rd edn., pp. 1077–1121. New York: McGraw-Hill.

Hayashi YK (2005) X-linked form of Emery-Dreifuss Muscular dystrophy. *Acta Myologica* 24: 98–103.

Nishino I and Ozawa E (2002) Muscular dystrophies. *Current Opinion in Neurology* 15: 539–544.

Voit T and Tome F (2004) The congenital muscular dystrophies. In: Engel AG and Franzini-Armstrong C (eds.) 3rd edn. 1203–1238*Myology*, 3rd edn., pp. 1203–1238. New York: McGraw-Hill.

Neurodevelopmental Disorders

E Klimkeit, N Rinehart, and J Bradshaw, Monash University, Clayton, VIC, Australia

Introduction

The brain's frontal regions are slow to mature, and they are vulnerable to neurodevelopmental disorders such as autism as well as neurodegenerative disorders of aging such as Parkinson's and Huntington's disease. The frontostriatal system involved in neurodevelopmental disorders comprises the dorsolateral prefrontal cortex, the lateral orbitofrontal cortex, the anterior cingulate, the supplementary motor area, and the basal ganglia. These areas are involved in a number of functions, such as executive functions (that is, functions such as self-monitoring, planning, organization, flexibility of thinking, and inhibition), motivation, control of complex behaviors, and sequencing movements. Below we outline the particular frontostriatal areas involved in six different development disorders, how they are characterized clinically, neuropsychologically, and genetically, and how they are best treated. The six disorders are attention-deficit/hyperactivity disorder (ADHD), autism spectrum disorders (ASDs), depression, schizophrenia, Tourette's syndrome (TS), and obsessive–compulsive disorder (OCD).

Attention-Deficit/Hyperactivity Disorder

ADHD is an early-onset behavioral disorder comprising problems with inattention, impulsivity, distractibility, and excessive motor activity. It is classified in the *Diagnostic and Statistical Manual of Mental Disorders* as three major subtypes: predominantly inattentive (20–30%), predominantly hyperactive (less than 15%), and combined (50–75%). ADHD occurs in approximately 1–10% of school-aged children. Boys are more frequently diagnosed than girls, with ratios ranging from 2:1 to 9:1.

Clinical Features

Diagnosis of ADHD is based on the presence of a sufficient number of symptoms present before the age of 7, and the report that these symptoms impair the child's functioning in at least two settings (home, school). Other than high levels of distractibility and inattention, children with ADHD tend to be disorganized, struggling to follow routines and to complete tasks. They tend to interrupt others, struggle to follow rules, and are often impulsive. Hyperactive children have difficulty remaining seated and are constantly restless and fidgety. These behaviors wax and wane and are influenced by the environment. Symptoms are typically worse in situations requiring sustained attention or mental effort, or those that are not appealing or novel.

Between 50 and 80% of children with ADHD also meet diagnostic criteria for other disorders, and generally the presence of such a comorbid disorder indicates a more serious problem and worse prognosis. The most common comorbid disorders are other externalizing disorders, such as oppositional defiant disorder and conduct disorder, followed by internalizing disorders, such as mood disorders, anxiety disorders, and specific learning disorders. Language and speech disorders and OCD are also common. While almost half of individuals with TS also have ADHD, the reverse is not the case.

ADHD symptoms usually reduce with maturation but persist to adulthood in 30–50% of cases. ADHD is a major risk factor for later personality and psychiatric disorders, delinquency, substance abuse, driving accidents and speeding violations, and difficulties in adult social relationships, marriage, and employment. Most of these developmental risks are exacerbated by the presence of comorbid aggression/conduct problems.

Treatment

Stimulant medications like methylphenidate and dextroamphetamine are the most commonly used treatment. They have a positive effect for approximately three-quarters of children with ADHD at least in the short term. Stimulant medications are primarily dopaminergic (although they also affect noradrenergic and serotonergic systems), and treatment is associated with a reduced risk of later substance abuse. Contrary to popular belief that the effects of stimulant medication are paradoxical because ADHD children appear 'slowed down,' normally developing children respond to stimulants in the same way, with improved cognitive function and reduced motor activity.

Antidepressants (tricyclics like imipramine, desipramine; a norepinephrine [noradrenaline] reuptake inhibitor antidepressant, atomoxetine) are alternative treatments if children have intolerable side effects or are unresponsive to stimulants. These particular antidepressants primarily act on norepinephrine transmission.

Education of parents about the disorder, training in managing problem behaviors, learning how to manage stress, and social supports are useful for parents of ADHD children and result in reported improvements in the child's behavior. Treatment involving medication is better than behavioral treatment alone. Behavior therapy may be a useful adjunct to medication by improving other associated difficulties such as social problems.

Neuropsychology

Executive functioning problems are indicated, with an emphasis on inhibitory deficits and problems with sustaining attention. These individuals typically show slow, variable, and inaccurate responding. They are impaired on tasks requiring inhibition of a response and of distracting stimuli, as well as in thinking flexibly, specifically being able to change response strategies when task demands change (change of set). Planning, word generation, withholding premature responses, working memory, and sustained attention are also deficient. Poor performance on many of these tasks is normalized through stimulant medication. While in the past the inattentive subtype was thought to be characterized more by problems with processing speed and selective attention, it now appears that the underlying neuropsychological deficits are more similar to than different from those with the combined subtype.

Neuroimaging

ADHD is associated with smaller whole-brain volumes, smaller right prefrontal cortex, and structural anomalies in the basal ganglia, cerebellum, and corpus callosum. Functional imaging studies indicate low striatal and frontal activity, particularly on the right, that is partially reversible with stimulant medication. These regions are involved in higher, executive function, such as working memory, rule-based learning, and planning. The right prefrontal cortex is important in editing one's behavior, spatially focusing attention, resisting distraction, and developing an awareness of self and time. Lesions in the prefrontal cortex cause poor attention regulation, hyperactivity, and impulsivity. The basal ganglia act in switching off automatic responses, in coordination, and in selecting deliberate actions.

Genetics

While environmental factors such as birth complications, maternal alcohol, and tobacco use have been indicated, ADHD has a strong genetic component, with heritability estimates ranging from 61 to 98%. The mode of inheritance, however, is not clear. Like most psychiatric conditions, ADHD is a complex disorder with several genes, each of minor or moderate effect.

Disruption in dopaminergic pathways has been proposed for ADHD, and several dopaminergic genes have been implicated (DRD4, DRD5, DAT1). The dopaminergic system influences motor control, reward, and cognition, and is indicated by the primarily dopaminergic effects of stimulant medication. Dopamine receptors are present in the striatum and dorsolateral prefrontal cortex, areas shown in imaging studies to function abnormally. Problems in the dopaminergic system may also help explain the slow responding, poor timing, and clumsiness in ADHD.

The noradrenergic and serotonergic systems are also implicated, and clearly, multiple neurotransmitters may be involved. The study of the role of neurotransmitters is complicated by the interrelationship between neurotransmitter systems: a change in one results in a change in another. Noradrenergic projections are dense in the frontal cortex and cingulate gyrus, regions that subserve alertness and attentional control. Norepinephrine is implicated in working memory, behavioral inhibition, and attention. Low concentrations of norepinephrine in certain regions of the prefrontal cortex are associated with poor concentration, poor self-control, and greater motor activity. Serotonergic deficiency is associated with impulsivity and aggression, and serotonin is important in mood control, sleep, appetite, memory and learning, and control of attention and locomotion.

Depression

Depression, the 'common cold' of psychiatry, has a lifetime risk of between 10 and 20%, with females at twice the risk of males. The mean age of onset of a depressive disorder is between adolescence and the mid-twenties. It is more debilitating than the sadness that everyone sometimes experiences, and different even from grief of bereavement. It may have morbid consequences, with depression being the most common diagnosis in individuals who suicide.

Clinical Features

Major depressive disorder (MDD) is characterized by depressed mood of at least two weeks' duration (depressed or irritable mood in children/adolescents) or loss of interest or pleasure in all activities. In addition, a number of other symptoms must be present: individuals with MDD often become preoccupied with suicide, plagued by guilt and a sense of worthlessness. They often have difficulty thinking clearly, concentrating, remembering, or making decisions. They may have difficulties with sleeping: they may feel sapped of energy and have trouble sleeping, or instead may want to eat and sleep excessively. They may also have symptoms of psychomotor agitation or retardation (psychomotor symptoms are rare in children/adolescents). MDD can present with psychotic features, usually consistent with depressive themes. It can also, rarely, present with catatonic features (immobility), melancholic features (lack of reactivity to pleasurable stimuli with worsening of symptoms in the morning, psychomotor retardation, and early morning awakening; this is rare in children/adolescents), and atypical features (reactive mood, increased appetite, excessive sleep, leaden paralysis).

Approximately 3–6% may develop a less acute but more chronic dysthymic disorder where symptoms of depressed mood and at least two other symptoms (poor appetite or overeating, insomnia or hypersomnia, low energy or fatigue, low self-esteem, poor concentration, or difficulty making decisions and feelings of hopelessness) are present most of the day, more days than not for a period of at least 2 years (1 year in children/adolescents). Bipolar disorder, characterized by episodes of mania (marked by a decreased need for sleep, rapid speech, delusions of grandeur, and engaging in self-destructive activities such as spending sprees and promiscuous sex), typically commences following one or more depressive episodes. It is rarer than unipolar depression, estimated at 1–1.5%.

Depression is comorbid in approximately 60% of cases, with anxiety disorders being the most common comorbidities. Substance abuse, eating disorders, conduct disorders, and ADHD are also often comorbid. Comorbid disorders such as anxiety (but not substance abuse) often precede depression.

Only two-thirds respond to treatment; 15% fail to recover (with the episode lasting for 2 or more years). Among those who respond to treatment one-third will relapse during remission. Of those that recover, 75% will have a recurrent episode. Only 11% ever have a single episode. Those with depression can expect four to six episodes during a lifetime.

Treatment

Cognitive behavior therapy (CBT) and interpersonal therapy (IPT) are the two empirically validated psychotherapies for adolescent and adult depression. CBT focuses on developing a less distorted/negative thinking style and more adaptive coping behaviors, while IPT focuses on improving effective communication. However, severe depression usually requires antidepressant medication. There are added benefits with combined psychotherapy and medication treatment. In very severe treatment-resistant depression, or with severe illness/suicidality, electroconvulsive therapy (ECT) is used, involving induction of brief seizures. It is an efficacious rapid treatment, but benefits need to be maintained with maintenance treatment (e.g., maintenance ECT or antidepressant medication). Transcranial magnetic stimulation, the use of a powerful magnetic field to stimulate brain areas such as the prefrontal cortex, also temporarily ameliorates symptoms.

Antidepressant medications act primarily on serotonin (the serotonergic system plays a role in control of appetite, sleep, memory and learning, control of attention and locomotion, muscle contraction, and endocrine regulation) and norepinephrine. Older tricyclic antidepressants are primarily noradrenergic and especially indicated where psychomotor retardation is prominent, as in the melancholic type. Tricyclics are no more effective than placebo in adolescents, where psychomotor symptoms and melancholic depression are rarely seen. In this group, the newer SSRIs (selective serotonin reuptake inhibitors) are more effective than tricyclics, suggesting that serotonin may be more important in childhood depression. There is recent controversy over the use of SSRIs in children and adolescents, in terms of safety and efficacy. Only fluoxetine (i.e., Prozac/Lovan) was considered to have an acceptable risk–benefit ratio by the Food and Drug Administration, and warning labels have been issued for antidepressants. Lithium remains the standard treatment for bipolar disorder. Some antiepilepsy drugs are also used as mood stabilizers in bipolar disorder.

Neuropsychology

Depressed individuals are slower in cognitive processing and responding. Cognitive deficits have also been observed, such as concentration difficulties and learning and memory problems (especially verbal memory); and reduced executive functioning with an emphasis on flexibility of thinking or shifting attentional set. Individuals with depression are also often impaired in planning, word generation, working memory, and inhibition of irrelevant information. While some difficulties disappear in remission (e.g., verbal fluency), others continue to manifest (e.g., inhibition of irrelevant information). Fewer difficulties are apparent in younger individuals. The neuropsychological difficulties in bipolar disorder are similar, but more severe than in unipolar depression.

Neuroimaging

Structural imaging reveals ventricular enlargement (correlating with cognitive and psychomotor retardation) similar to Alzheimer's disease, Huntington's disease, and schizophrenia, together with periventricular white matter lesions, decreased striatal volume, temporal lobe anomalies, and smaller frontal lobe volume. Smaller hippocampus (involved in learning and memory) and enlarged amygdala (involved in emotional functioning) are also reported. Functional imaging studies show lower activity in the anterior cingulate, left dorsolateral prefrontal cortex, amygdala, and striatum. Increased orbitofrontal activity reflects inhibitory processes and rumination.

These brain areas mediate the affective aspects (e.g., orbitofrontal cortex, amygdala, hippocampus), psychomotor aspects (e.g., dorsolateral prefrontal cortex), and cognitive/executive function aspects (anterior cingulate and dorsolateral prefrontal cortex).

Genetics

Individuals with major depression are more likely to have relatives suffering from anxiety, depression, and alcohol abuse. There may be overlapping genetic association between mood disorders and alcohol abuse. While relatives of individuals with bipolar disorder are at increased risk of depression, the reverse is not true. Depression has heritability estimates around 40–70%. Environmental risk factors for depression include stressful life events and childhood neglect/abuse, absence of social support, and low maternal support in childhood.

Various genes have been investigated in depression, including those affecting neurotransmitters such as serotonin and norepinephrine and those that control activities of certain hormones, with unclear findings. Some studies find that stress interacts with serotonin transporter genes in predicting depression, while others do not. Neurotoxic effects, possibly from cortisol released during stress, may damage hippocampal cells (part of the limbic system involved in memory and emotion), resulting in depressive symptoms. After a few weeks of antidepressant treatment the hippocampus may regain mass (neurogenesis). Possibly neuroprotective proteins are also implicated. Depression probably involves an interaction of several genes with environmental events.

Tourette's Syndrome

TS is a severe form of tic disorder, marked by multiple motor tics and one or more vocal tics that are present for at least 1 year. Tics are sudden rapid, recurrent, purposeless movements or vocalizations/utterances. TS is more commonly found in boys than girls (3:1 ratio) and affects less than 1% of the population. Motor tics usually develop before vocal tics, and these symptoms typically progress over time, becoming more severe and complex. Onset is usually during childhood or early adolescence, and is by definition before age 18. Tics typically develop prior to age eight, peak by puberty, and decline substantially thereafter. In some cases symptoms disappear entirely by adulthood.

Clinical Features

Simple motor tics include eye blinking, neck jerking, grimacing, and coughing, whereas simple vocal tics include throat clearing, sniffling, grunting, and barking.

Complex tics include licking, head shaking, throwing, biting, jumping, compulsive touching, compulsive copying of another's actions (echopraxia) or speech (echolalia), obscene gestures (copropraxia), and socially unacceptable utterances (coprolalia). However, coprolalia occurs in less than 15% of cases. Tics are experienced as irresistible but can be suppressed for periods of time, though with an increasing build up of tension. Most individuals are aware of an urge similar to the urge to sneeze or scratch an itch. Tics constantly change in number, frequency, and severity, and are typically exacerbated by stress or boredom and reduced during concentration.

Tics can cause embarrassment and interfere with social interactions, and can sometimes be quite uncomfortable and painful. Self-injurious behavior such as biting, scratching, cutting, or hitting are also seen in TS. Some individuals with TS have speech dysfluencies that resemble stuttering. The majority of individuals with TS have symptoms of ADHD, OCD, or both, at some time during the course of their condition. There is considerable overlap between TS and OCD, in that in both conditions the repetitive behaviors are considered to be involuntary (although for both there is some degree of voluntary control), tension is experienced if the behavior is inhibited, and relief is reported as the behavior is carried out. TS is also comorbid with problems of poor impulse control and an inability to control anger, learning disorders, and anxiety and depression.

Treatment

Management involves medication, behavior or cognitive therapy, and for a minority of severe cases, surgery (involving for example, making multiple lesions in the cingulum and beneath the head of the caudate nucleus). The main aim of treatment is to achieve a degree of control of tics allowing the individual to function as normally as possible and to relieve tic-related embarrassment or discomfort. Most cases of tic disorders such as TS are mild and are considered not to require medication. Behavioral therapy such as biofeedback, habit reversal (e.g., practicing muscular movements opposite to the tic) and relaxation training (to help relieve stress that aggravates tics) has been suggested to help. Cognitive therapy and supportive psychotherapy are also helpful in avoiding depression and social isolation and improving family support. Habit reversal is superior to supportive psychotherapy in reducing tic severity, but both improve life satisfaction and psychosocial functioning. Most psychotherapeutic interventions (with the exception of habit reversal) have, however, not been systematically evaluated. Often it is the comorbid conditions like ADHD that cause greater impact, and these comorbid disorders are often the reason for seeking help. Medications useful in treating tics target dopaminergic systems by blocking dopamine receptors. Thus antipsychotics (e.g., 'typicals' like haloperidol and newer 'atypicals' like risperidone) are considered the most effective anti-tic agents, but are often associated with unwanted side effects. Variable efficacy has also been shown for antihypertensives such as clonidine.

Neuropsychology

Increased rates of eye blinking and poor handwriting (similarly found in ADHD) suggest mild impairment in motor control. There is some evidence for difficulties with respect to visuomotor integration (e.g., copying complex designs) and in motor coordination, as well as deficits in eye movement control. Early studies suggested executive function deficits. However, these deficits may be related to the comorbid symptomatology of OCD and ADHD. Studies comparing neuropsychological performance of individuals with TS with and without comorbid ADHD or OCD symptomatology, suggest more extensive impairments in those with comorbid disorders and only mild cognitive deficits in the 'pure' form. There is debate that rather than widespread executive deficits, deficits in TS may be more inhibitory in nature, though whether this is so, and precisely which inhibitory processes are involved, requires further investigation.

Neuroimaging

The main brain areas implicated are the basal ganglia (especially the caudate nucleus) and the inferior prefrontal cortex. Caudal volume correlates inversely with tic severity and obsessive–compulsive symptoms. Neuroimaging studies show anomalies of the basal ganglia and activation changes in the ventral striatum, orbitofrontal cortex, and anterior cingulate. The basal ganglia normally gate release of behaviors, with TS probably reflecting excess facilitation of unintended (and inhibition of intended) actions. Tics involve activity of not just motor areas, but also oculomotor, language, limbic, and cognitive/executive areas. During periods of tic suppression, decreased activity is observed in the ventral globus pallidus, putamen, and thalamus, and increased activation in areas involved in the inhibition of unwanted impulses: the prefrontal, parietal, temporal, and cingulate cortical areas. Prior to tic occurrence paralimbic areas are activated (anterior cingulate, insular cortex, supplementary motor area – receiving input from basal ganglia – and parietal cortex) and as the tic commences, sensorimotor activation occurs in the superior parietal cortex and cerebellum. Interestingly, paralimbic and associated areas are implicated not only in tic generation, but also with movements triggered internally by unpleasant sensations such as pain or itching.

Genetics

While environmental factors such as infection, maternal stress, and nausea during the first trimester of pregnancy may influence expression of TS, it also has a strong genetic component. Monozygotic twins have concordance rates of 50–70% (that is, if one identical twin has TS there is a 50–70% probability that the other will also have TS) and dizygotic twins around 10–20%. The disorder's familial characteristics have been interpreted in terms of autosomal dominant transmission with high but incomplete penetrance and variable expression; thus, not everyone who inherits the genetic vulnerability will show the same severity of symptoms, or even any symptoms at all. Males are more likely than females to show genetic vulnerability to tic expression. However, the exact mode of inheritance is not yet known, and some researchers propose an additive model of gene inheritance where many genes are likely to contribute to the expression of TS. Many chromosomal locations have been proposed – for example, on chromosomes 4, 5, 8, 11, and 17 – likely influencing dopamine receptor subtypes and/or controlling neuronal development. Some forms of OCD may be genetically linked to TS, and a genetic relationship of ADHD to TS has also been proposed.

Obsessive–Compulsive Disorder

OCD is characterized by uncontrolled, recurrent, intrusive thoughts, impulses, and images (obsessions), accompanied by feelings of urgency or catastrophe, leading to repetitive, time-consuming and ritualistic behavior (compulsions), which are an antianxiety attempt to avert fear or distress. The obsessions and compulsions cause marked distress, are time consuming, or interfere with the individual's normal routine, job, or social activities. There is often variable insight into the reasonableness of the obsessions and compulsions. The disorder is equally common in males and females, and age of onset is typically around or before puberty in males and in the 20s in females. Lifetime prevalence is estimated to be around 2.5%.

Clinical Features

OCD is considered an anxiety disorder that is typically chronic rather than acute. Unlike obsessive–compulsive personality disorder, with its characteristic perfectionism and scrupulosity, where individuals derive pleasure from their obsessions and compulsions, those with OCD feel distress and anxiety. The frequency of common obsessions has been calculated as: fear of contamination (e.g., becoming contaminated by handling money), 45%; pathological doubt (e.g., wondering whether one has left the oven on), 42%; somatic concerns, 36%; need for exactness, symmetry, or evenness, 31%; fear of committing acts of aggression, which unlike in psychopathy are not carried through, 28%; sexual or religious obsessions (e.g., a recurrent pornographic image), 26%. Individuals with obsessions usually attempt to suppress such thoughts or to neutralize them through another thought or action, i.e., compulsions. For *compulsions*, the figures are: checking (63%), washing or cleaning (50%), counting (36%), need to ask or confess (31%), symmetry and precision until position or number of repetitions are 'just right' (28%), and hoarding (18%). Factor analysis suggests the following groupings: aggressive and somatic obsessions with checking compulsions; preoccupations with symmetry and exactness involving counting, ordering, and arranging rituals; fears of contamination or illness with washing or cleaning rituals; sexual and religious obsessions. The last, unlike the others which may change over time, tend to be particularly stable.

Because obsessions are distracting, they may result in inefficient performance in tasks that require concentration. In addition, many individuals may avoid objects or situations related to the content of the obsessions, and for some, performing compulsions may become a major activity leading to severe disruption to occupational functioning and relationships. Disorders commonly comorbid with OCD include depression (67% lifetime rate), simple phobia (22%), social phobia (18%), eating disorder (17%), problems with alcohol (14%), panic disorder (12%) and TS (7%).

Treatment

The tricyclic antidepressant clomipramine, which has serotonergic and noradrenergic action, and the selective serotonin reuptake inhibitors (fluoxetine, sertraline, paroxetine, citalopram, and fluvoxamine) are effective treatments. There is controversy over whether clomipramine is more effective than the SSRIs. Behavioral treatments such as exposure and response prevention (this involves gradually learning to tolerate the anxiety associated with not performing the ritual behavior) are effective, compared to control relaxation treatments. Cognitive therapy challenges irrational beliefs and is as effective as exposure treatments. Cognitive behavior treatments are associated with greater long-term gains (despite not entirely eliminating symptoms) than medication treatments, where relapse is highly probable upon stopping medication. Randomized controlled trials are required to clarify whether or not there is any additional benefit of medication and psychological treatment. For patients with severe OCD who do not respond to medication or psychological treatments, psychosurgery (anterior capsulotomy, anterior cingulotomy, subcaudate tractotomy, or limbic leucotomy) is a last resort.

Neuropsychology

Individuals with OCD respond more slowly, and their performance on set shifting, response inhibition, and motor suppression tasks (measures of executive function) correlates negatively with the frequency and intensity of their compulsive behaviors. There is some evidence of selective deficits in pattern recognition and spatial memory, set shifting, and reversal of response set, with largely intact planning and decision processes.

Neuroimaging

Specific brain regions are implicated; the basal ganglia (particularly the caudate and striatum), orbitofrontal cortex, and anterior cingulate, plus perhaps temporal lobe and amygdala, which may provide the emotional features. Caudate volume is reduced and overactivity of the orbitofrontal cortex, anterior cingulate, and right striatum is observed. However, there are many inconsistencies in the literature. These brain areas play an important role in the inhibition of inappropriate responses, for executive functioning, for overriding predominant response patterns, and for error monitoring and detection.

Genetics

OCD has heritability estimates around 27–65%. While the mode of inheritance remains unclear, it is likely to be polygenic with a number of vulnerability genes, including at least chromosomes 4, 5, and 7. Very recent studies indicate significant associations between OCD transmission and a locus on chromosome 9 that may be crucial for controlling the excitatory neurotransmitter glutamate. Genes of the serotonin and dopamine systems (5HTTLPR, 5HT1Dβ, DRD4) are also implicated in OCD. The relationship between OCD and TS may imply a common genetic background, although the TS genes may not be the only mode of acquisition of OCD. Environmental factors such as pre- and perinatal events and infection also play a role in its expression.

Autism Spectrum Disorders

ASDs such as autism and Asperger's disorder onset within the first 3 years of life. The prevalence of autism and Asperger's disorder are around 10–12 per 10 000, with Asperger's disorder possibly more prevalent than autism. Both autism and Asperger's disorder are more common in boys than girls (4:1), with perhaps a greater preponderance of affected males to females for Asperger's disorder.

Clinical Features

Autism is defined by impairments in social and communication function, and repetitive and stereotyped behavioral patterns. Areas of social disturbance include poor eye contact, reduced ability to interpret emotional states, failure to develop peer relations, and deficiencies in social-emotional reciprocity (e.g., not participating in social play, impaired awareness of the needs of others). For a diagnosis of autism, a child must, before 3 years of age, exhibit abnormal or delayed functioning in at least one of the following areas of social interaction: social use of language, symbolic play, or imaginative play. Core communication deficiencies include either a delay or total lack of expressive language, as well as a marked impairment in nonverbal behavior. Where individuals develop language, they often have problems in initiating or sustaining conversations. Developmentally inappropriate echolalia (copying another's speech) and pronoun reversal, reduced prosody and intonation, and impairments in the use of figurative language are also associated with autism. Restricted, repetitive, and stereotyped behaviors manifest as an intense preoccupation with a single subject or activity, adherence to nonfunctional routines or rituals, stereotypies, and motor mannerisms, e.g., hand or finger flapping, and body rocking. Disturbances in sensory modulation may also be observed; for example, under- and overreactivity to sensory stimuli.

Treatment

ASDs are lifelong conditions and therefore treatments need to be tailored to the individuals' particular developmental needs. In general, treatments meet criteria for best practice if they include a combination of educational, behavioral, communication, and social skills training approaches, together with medication if indicated. For example, a comprehensive treatment plan might include: teaching new skills using positive reinforcement; the provision of an individually designed school-based educational program; social skills training tailored to the child's intellectual and language abilities; and skills training for the parents of children with autism to provide them with appropriate skills to promote their development. Medication may be prescribed to target specific symptoms, e.g., neuroleptic medication or SSRIs to treat anxiety, while lithium and other mood stabilizers may reduce episodes of disruptive, aggressive, and self-injurious behavior.

Neuropsychology

There are three main cognitive theories of autism and Asperger's disorder: theory-of-mind, the executive dysfunction theory, and the theory of weak central coherence. Deficiencies in theory-of-mind – that is, the ability to understand that other people have unique perspectives and thoughts that are sometimes contextually independent – may be linked to the social-communicative deficits. Weak central coherence, a deficit in the ability to integrate details into a coherent global perception, may be linked to the tendency to be preoccupied with parts of objects and to miss the 'bigger picture.' Executive functioning refers to the role of the frontostriatal circuits in coordinating cognitive-motor output so that behavior is

well timed, planned, adaptable, appropriate, and relevant. The repetitive, stereotyped, and restricted behaviors may be due, in part, to deficient executive functioning. Movement abnormalities in ASDs, in particular gait (walking) abnormalities, may be underpinned by disruption to neural circuitry involving the basal ganglia and cerebellum.

Neuroimaging

No consistent neuroimaging marker has been identified for ASDs. Structural changes in the brains of individuals with autism include: a slightly increased average brain volume; decreased gray matter volumes in the limbic system (important for social cognition); reduced neuron numbers in the vermis of the cerebellum; and gross structural changes in the cerebellum and the parietal lobes (important for efficient attention). Consistent with the executive functioning and neuromotor impairments associated with ASDs, functional imaging has revealed decreased activation in the highly interconnected cortical and subcortical frontal structures, including lateral and medial premotor cortex, frontal eye fields, caudate, dorsolateral prefrontal cortex, and anterior cingulate, suggesting disruption to multiple frontostriatal circuits.

Genetics

The concordance for autism in monozygotic twins is 60% for autistic disorder and 92% for ASDs. For dizygotic twins the concordance for either diagnosis is up to 10%. If an older sibling has autism, the risk that a subsequent full sibling will have autism is about 5%. Studies of individuals with autism suggest that chromosome 15q11-q13 is a candidate region for genetic risk factors. There is also an increased frequency of the chromosome 4B null allele, and of variant serotonin transporter gene alleles on chromosome 17q11-q12. Autism is associated with defined environmental causes, such as rubella and cytomegalovirus, fetal infections, perinatal brain injury, toxins, and specific genetic abnormalities such as tuberous sclerosis and fragile X syndrome, in less than 10% of cases.

Schizophrenia

Schizophrenia is characterized by psychosis (disturbances in thinking and perception), apathy, withdrawal, and cognitive impairment. Schizophrenia affects emotional reactivity, interpersonal relations, perceptual processes, attention, information processing, and thought. Its psychosocial impact is devastating at an individual, family, and societal level. The prevalence of schizophrenia is between 0.5–1.5%. Recent studies suggest a small, but significantly higher, incidence of schizophrenia among men compared with women when stringent classification criteria are applied. Onset is typically in young adulthood, later in females.

Clinical Features

Individuals experience a combination of 'positive' and 'negative' symptoms, which interfere with interpersonal relations, work or education, or self-care over (at least) a six-month period. Key 'positive symptoms' include: delusions (distortions of thought content), hallucinations (perceptual anomalies), and disorganized thinking, language, and behavior. An example of a delusion might be the belief that someone has inserted a thought into one's head or broadcast a thought from one's own mind to others'. Hallucinations are commonly auditory – for example, 'hearing voices' that are so intense that they are interpreted as being of external origin. Disorganized thinking, measured clinically by the patients' verbal output, is often referred to clinically as the single most important feature of schizophrenia. 'Negative' symptoms essentially refer to restrictions in the range and intensity of one's ability to express emotion (affective flattening), a reduced ability to produce fluent thoughts and ideas (alogia), and a reduced ability to form and achieve particular life goals. The negative symptoms of schizophrenia account for the increased suicide rate, estimated at 10% of all those diagnosed with the disorder. The main determinants of quality of life are depression and negative symptoms (not active psychosis).

Depending on the constellation and type of positive and negative symptoms, the disorder may be subtyped as paranoid, disorganized, or catatonic. Individuals may shift between positive and negative symptom types during the progression of the disease – for example, commencing with an exacerbating phase of largely positive symptoms, followed by a plateau phase, where the severity and frequency of positive symptoms stabilize, followed by a remission of hallucinations, delusions, and disorganized behavior with evolution of worsening negative symptoms. Individuals may experience a single psychotic episode followed by more or less total recovery, or suffer repeated psychotic episodes with subtotal recovery, or, more commonly, experience a course progressing to chronic disability.

Treatment

The first line of treatment is pharmacotherapy. While in the past pharmacotherapy was concentrated on controlling positive symptoms using neuroleptic medications that block dopamine D2 receptors, atypical antipsychotic medications (e.g., clozapine) are now more commonly prescribed and are more effective than conventional antipsychotics, as well as yielding a more acceptable side-effect profile. Antidepressants and mood stabilizers (e.g., lithium) are commonly used in treatment. Compliant medication use sets the scene for effective psychosocial interventions, including family psychoeducation, social skills training, cognitive-behavior therapy, and substance abuse treatments.

Neuropsychology

Schizophrenia is associated with multiple cognitive deficits, including executive dysfunction (most notably working memory), problems with attention, concentration, psychomotor speed, learning, and memory. Working memory problems and attentional difficulties may underlie the positive and negative symptoms. For example, distortions in perception and thinking may emerge from a difficulty in being able to hold and manipulate cognitive information long enough to reference an actual experience, as compared to emergent associated memory. Similarly, negative symptoms such as a reduced ability to set and execute daily goals may be underpinned by a difficulty in maintaining an initial plan of action. Many of the cognitive deficits associated with schizophrenia manifest during remission, and are therefore considered as core features as opposed to state deficits apparent only during psychotic phases. As for autism, research using retrospective video footage has identified subtle neuromotor features that are apparent prior to clinical onset. Additionally, upper-body bimanual coordination deficits have been systematically documented.

Neuroimaging

Structural and functional brain imaging studies reveal three consistent neuropathological findings: (1) hypofrontality (i.e., decreased neural activity in the frontal regions); (2) enlargement of the lateral ventricles and decreased brain tissue (for example, gray and white matter deficits have consistently been found in the left superior temporal gyrus and the left medial temporal lobe); and (3) reduced hippocampal volume. Impairments in the dorsolateral prefrontal cortex are responsible for core cognitive deficits, most notably working memory. The hypometabolism of the dorsolateral prefrontal cortex and anterior cingulate are linked to negative symptom severity, while hypermetabolism of the temporolimbic cortex has been linked to positive symptomatology. Abnormalities have also been reported in neuron density, number, and size in the nucleus accumbens, substantia nigra, thalamus, locus coeruleus, pedunculopontine nucleus, basal ganglia, thalamus, and corpus callosum. The highly salient clinical feature of disorganized thinking is thought to be underpinned by a neuronal disconnectivity between the multiple neural sites identified in schizophrenia.

Genetics

Schizophrenia is highly heritable. The monozygotic co-twin of an affected individual has an estimated risk of 60–84%, whereas that of a dizygotic co-twin is around 14%. There is an 8% risk if a sibling has the disorder, and 12% if one parent and 40% if both parents are sufferers. There are likely to be multiple susceptibility genes, each with small effects, or several such genes, each with moderate effects. Linkage analysis has identified 5q, 6p, 8p, 13q, 15q14, and 22q as promising genetic susceptibility regions. Chromosomes 3, 9, and 20 have also been implicated. The location of a schizophrenia susceptibility locus at chromosome 22q11 has been suggested by recent genome-wide linkage studies. Approximately 20–30% of individuals with 22q11 microdeletions develop schizophrenia or a related psychiatric condition (e.g., schizoaffective disorder).

Conclusion

There are many similarities across the neurodevelopmental disorders, in terms of high rates of comorbidity and the fact that the mode of inheritance is typically unclear, usually with a number of genes implicated. The neuropsychology deficits and implicated brain areas overlap, and how each disorder manifests may depend on how the frontostriatal system is compromised as a result of both genetic predisposition and environmental factors.

Acknowledgments

This article is based on Bradshaw, *Developmental Disorders of the Frontostriatal System*, with extensive updates from new material, the most important of which appears in the further reading section.

See also: Historical Views of Mental Illness; Specific Mental Health Disorders: Child and Adolescent Mental Disorders; Specific Mental Health Disorders: Eating Disorders; Specific Mental Health Disorders: Personality Disorders; Specific Mental Health Disorders: Psychotic Disorders; Specific Mental Health Disorders: Trauma and Mental Disorders.

Further Reading

Abramowitz JS (1997) Effectiveness of psychological and pharmacological treatments for obsessive-compulsive disorder: A quantitative review. *Journal of Consulting and Clinical Psychology* 65(1): 44–52.

Aouizerate B, Guehl D, Cuny E, et al. (2004) Pathophysiology of obsessive-compulsive disorder: A necessary link between phenomenology, neuropsychology, imagery and physiology. *Progress in Neurobiology* 72: 195–221.

Bradshaw JL (2001) *Developmental Disorders of the Frontostriatal System: Neuropsychological, Neuropsychiatric and Evolutionary Perspectives.* Hove, UK: Psychology Press.

Cohen DJ and Volkmar FR (1997) *Handbook of Autism and Pervasive Developmental Disorders,* 2nd edn. New York: Wiley & Sons.

Fitzgerald M, Bellgrove M, and Gill M (2007) *Handbook of Attention Deficit Hyperactivity Disorder.* London: John Wiley and Sons.

Fombonne P (2003) Epidemiological surveys of autism and other pervasive developmental disorders. *Journal of Autism and Developmental Disorders* 33: 365–382.

Fonagy P, Target M, Cottrell D, Phillips J, and Kurtz Z (2002) *What Works for Whom? A Critical Review of Treatments for Children and Adolescents.* New York: The Guilford Press.

Jankovic J (2001) Medical progress: Tourette's syndrome. *The New England Journal of Medicine* 345(16): 1184–1192.

Levinson DF (2006) The genetics of depression: A review. *Biological Psychiatry:* 60: 84–92.

Mueser KT and McGurk SR (2004) Schizophrenia. *Lancet* 363(9426): 2063–2072.

Riccio CA, Homack S, Jarrat KP, and Wolfe ME (2001) Differences in academic and executive function domains among children with ADHD predominantly inattentive and combined types. *Archives of Clinical Neuropsychology* 21: 657–667.

Sheppard DM, Bradshaw JL, Purcell R, and Pantelis C (1999) Tourette's and comorbid syndromes: Obsessive compulsive and attention deficit hyperactivity disorder. A common etiology? *Clinical Psychology Review* 19(5): 531–552.

Singer HS (2005) Tourette's syndrome: From behavior to biology. *Lancet Neurology* 4: 149–159.

Stein DJ (2002) Obsessive-compulsive disorder. *Lancet* 360: 397–405.

Parkinson's Disease

A D Korczyn, Tel-Aviv University, Ramat-Aviv, Israel

Introduction

Parkinson's disease (PD) is one of the more common chronic neurological diseases of old age. It is a prototypical disease in the sense that the understanding of its pathophysiology and treatment development have advanced hand-in-hand at a very impressive rate during the past 50 years, following a long dormant period since its first description by James Parkinson in 1817 (Parkinson, 1817; Korczyn, 1995). However, the new developments have not solved the main problems of the causation of the disease and how the disease process can be slowed.

Clinical Features

PD is considered to be primarily a disease of the 'extra-pyramidal' motor system. It has an insidious onset, slowly progressing to eventual severe disability. The cardinal motor symptoms include tremor at rest, poverty or slowness of movement, rigidity, and loss of postural reflexes. None of these four primary manifestations is specific to PD, and therefore the clinical diagnosis can only be tentative. The slow evolution and the lack of other features (e.g., pyramidal, sensory, or marked autonomic disturbances) support the diagnosis, although some vegetative symptoms and particularly constipation are common even early during disease development (Korczyn, 1989, 1990). The clinical diagnosis is also supported by a positive response to levodopa.

Several other brain diseases mimic PD. The assumption that vascular brain disease can result in similar manifestations was favored several years ago, leading to the clinical designation of 'arteriosclerotic parkinsonism.' This nosologic entity has been disfavored but has recently re-emerged. Historically, the encephalitis pandemic of the 1920s resulted in a multitude of cases with postencephalitic parkinsonism. Nine decades after the disappearance of new cases of lethargic encephalitis, parkinsonism is rarely a consequence of encephalitis (Nisipeanu and Korczyn, 2002).

Other disorders with extrapyramidal features resembling PD include progressive supranuclear palsy, multiple system atrophy (previously known as olivopontocerebellar atrophy and Shy-Drager syndrome) and corticobasal ganglionic degeneration, all of which can frequently be suspected by the existence of specific clinical features. However, several reports indicate that the accuracy of the clinical diagnosis is limited and that as many as one-quarter or one-third of patients who were clinically diagnosed as having PD will be found at autopsy to have alternative diagnoses (Koller, 1992).

Even after exclusion of all these other nosologic entities, the question remains as to whether PD is a single disease (Korczyn, 1999). One of the main streams of recent advances during the past decade has been the identification of genetic mutations that are clinically indistinguishable from PD. In some cases, mutation carriers have no known affected family members, and these are designated as sporadic PD unless genetic tests have been performed. For most sporadic cases, environmental causes are sought but account for only a minority of cases. Thus PD is heterogeneous also in its pathogenesis (genetic vs. nongenetic), and therefore it is not really a single disease.

In addition to the motor abnormalities, patients with PD frequently have affective and cognitive disturbances. Depression is common in PD and in many patients predates the extrapyramidal features (Cummings, 1992; Treves *et al.*, 1995). The nature of the association of the motor and affective features is still unclear, but for reasons discussed below it is quite likely that depression should be regarded as one of the features of PD rather than just one of its complications.

Dementia also commonly occurs in PD patients; prevalence data suggest that at least 50% of PD cases will eventually develop significant cognitive impairment (Aarsland *et al.*, 1996; Korczyn, 2001). This too seems to be an integral part of the spectrum of clinical manifestations of PD, as discussed below.

Neuropathology and Neurochemistry

The pathological hallmark of PD was considered to consist of intracellular eosinophilic inclusions called Lewy bodies. These occur inside neurons in the substantia nigra, presumably in dopamine (DA)-containing cells. Lewy bodies probably accumulate in neurons undergoing degeneration. The number of DA neurons in the substantia nigra progressively diminishes in PD. It is important to note that only DA neurons in the substantia nigra whose axons are destined to go to the putamen (less so to the caudate) in the nigrostriatal tract are affected, while other dopaminergic tracts are spared, with progressive loss of DA in the striatum. Clinical symptoms first appear when DA content in the striatum is reduced by about 70%. This may imply that a long preclinical stage, of 20 years or more, predates the appearance of motor symptoms.

Other neurotransmitter systems are also affected in PD. These include norepinephrine (NE) loss in the cell bodies of the locus coeruleus, serotonin (5-hydroxytryptamine, 5-HT) loss in the raphe nuclei, and cholinergic cell loss in the nucleus basalis of Meynert. These deficiencies probably contribute to the affective and cognitive changes in PD but may also contribute to motor dysfunction. However, it is clear that most motor disturbances are primarily related to DA deficits, because replacement of endogenous DA can dramatically alleviate the motor disability.

Until recently, it was impossible to demonstrate the DA deficiencies during life. However, this was changed by the use of positron emission tomography (PET) and single photon emission tomography (SPECT). Using radioactive tracer techniques, it can be demonstrated that DA marker accumulation is reduced in the corpus striatum in PD, presumably because of the loss of DA terminals that normally take up these markers. PET and SPECT correlate with the side of the clinical abnormalities in unilateral parkinsonism, and may be sensitive enough to detect the progression of the disease (Bhatt *et al.*, 1991).

While the complete chemical composition of Lewy bodies is not yet known, they definitely contain parkin, ubiquitin, and synuclein. Antibodies against these substances, particularly anti-synuclein antibodies, will stain all Lewy bodies in the substantia nigra and frequently additional ones in the brain stem, olfactory bulb, and in the cortex. Anti-synuclein staining in the substantia nigra relates to motor dysfunction. Braak *et al.* (2004) have suggested a sequential progression of the pathology in PD, starting in the dorsal motor nucleus of the vagus and the olfactory bulb, than appearing in other brainstem nuclei and the substantia nigra, and only at a late stage in the cerebral cortex. Interestingly, staining in neurites is also seen. These Lewy neurites (Braak *et al.*, 1996) may suggest axonal dysfunction as an important part of the pathophysiology of PD.

Pathophysiology

The pathophysiology of PD is still rather clouded. The dopaminergic denervation of the basal ganglia (and particularly the striatum) is obviously central in the movement abnormalities. 'Motor loops' involving the basal ganglia, subthalamic nucleus, thalamus, and cortex have been described (Bergman *et al.*, 1990). However, their function is poorly understood. How the loss of dopamine causes tremor at rest, enhanced tone both at rest and during action, and bradykinesia or hypokinesia still needs to be fully explained. The pathophysiology of the fourth cardinal feature of PD, loss of postural reflexes, is even less clear. Some gains were made through the use of kinematic studies, such as of arm trajectories. These quantify the defects and demonstrate some unexpected findings (e.g., regarding the importance of visual feedback), explaining how the 'motor loops' incorporate sensory information (Flash *et al.*, 1991).

The nigrostriatal pathway activates, in the corpus striatum, dopaminergic receptors. Five subtypes have been identified and, while the most important seem to be of the D2 type, the role of D1 receptors in normal brain activity is unclear, and therefore the functional correlate of activation of these receptors is not established. In particular, it is not clear whether activation of D1 receptors is important for the elicitation of dyskinesias or other motor complications occurring commonly in advanced stages of the disease in patients who are treated by levodopa.

Pathogenesis of PD

There is no consensus on the pathogenesis of the disease. The fact that only a selected population of neurons die off may suggest the involvement of a toxin affecting these cells. Drugs are known that can selectively damage catecholaminergic neurons – for example, 6-hydroxydopamine (6-OHDA). This substance is uptaken by the DA transporters, and it is concentrated in DA cells and causes their degeneration. Because 6-OHDA does not cross the blood–brain barrier (BBB), it cannot account for human PD. (However, it is an important experimental tool in the study of PD and drug development.) But another chemical, MPTP, has been identified as causing in humans a disorder quite similar to PD in many characteristics. The mechanisms of MPTP toxicity have been explored in depth and, although there is no doubt that this chemical only accounts for very few cases of PD, the possible existence of MPTP-like chemicals has been explored.

Epidemiological and toxicological studies have inconsistently suggested an environmental toxin (Stevenson *et al.*, 1989). The possibility of endogenous production of a substance similar to MPTP in its mechanism of action is still debated (Tanner and Langston, 1990).

The substantia nigra and globus pallidum are rich in iron; the iron concentration increases with age and particularly in PD. This may suggest involvement of this metal in neurotoxicity, perhaps through a process of lipid peroxidation.

Genetics

About 10% of patients with PD report first-degree relatives with the same disorder. Although they constitute only a small portion, these cases are important in many ways. During the past two decades, several genes have been identified that account for monogenic forms. In addition to being able to help in genetic counseling, these genes have been very important in understanding the mechanism underlying the neurodegenerative processes in PD. For example, the first gene to be described, α-synuclein, could have either point mutation or overexpression (duplication or triplication). The protein synuclein was found to be a major component of the Lewy bodies. It is likely that this protein, once mutated or overexpressed, will be more likely to be misfolded, thus evading the usual mechanisms of intracellular protein metabolism. In attempt to be removed from the cell, it is directed into the Lewy bodies. Another gene that was found to be associated with PD is parkin, coding for an enzyme responsible for intracellular degradation of proteins (such as α-synuclein). Another gene, PINK1, codes for a mitochondrial enzyme (mitochondrial dysfunction has long been thought to be a cause of PD). The most common genetic abnormality underlying PD is the LRRK2 gene, which may account for 1–2% of PD cases and in some ethnic groups much more frequently. The genetic heterogeneity associated with PD is helpful in discovering mechanisms of neurodegeneration. But even more surprising is the finding of pathologic heterogeneity: Patients carrying the parkin mutations usually do not have Lewy bodies, while in families with LRRK2 mutations, some members may contain Lewy bodies in nigral neurons while others do not. These observations shatter the view

Table 1   Genetic mutations causing parkinsonism

Gene	Inheritance	Onset	Map position	Gene
PARK1	Dominant	40–50	4q21	α-synuclein
PARK2	Recessive	20–40	6q25	Parkin
PARK3	Dominant	60–70	2p13	?
PARK4	Dominant	30–40	4q21	α-synuclein triplication and duplications
PARK5	Dominant	40–60	4p14	Ubiquitin C-terminal Hydrolase L1
PARK6	Recessive	30–40	1p35–37	PINK1
PARK7	Recessive	30–40	1p38	DJ-1
PARK8	Dominant	50–70	12cen	LRRK2
PARK9	Recessive	30–40	1q36	ATP13A2
PARK10	Dominant (?)	50–60	1p32	?
PARK11	Dominant (?)	60–70	2q34	?

that PD is a Lewy body disease, as if patients without Lewy bodies must have a 'different disease' to explain their parkinsonism. Several other mutations have been described (**Table 1**) (Polymeropoulos et al., 1997; Gasser et al., 1998; Kitada et al., 1998; Kruger et al., 1998; Leroy et al., 1998; Bonifati et al., 2002; Hicks et al., 2002; Singleton et al., 2003; Pankratz et al., 2003; Paisan-Ruiz et al., 2004; Valente et al., 2004; Zimprich et al., 2004; Ramirez et al., 2006).

Treatment of PD

The basic treatment of PD is by replacement of the deficient DA using levodopa. Levodopa is absorbed from the gastrointestinal tract and transported through the blood–brain barrier by active amino acid transport mechanisms. In the brain, as well as in the periphery, levodopa is metabolized to DA by an enzyme, 1-amino acid decarboxylase. This enzyme can be blocked by the substances benserazide and carbidopa. Employing either of these inhibitors can prevent the peripheral conversion of levodopa to DA, thus diverting larger amounts of levodopa to the brain, where it is taken up by dopaminergic terminals to be used in dopamine synthesis. Most patients today are treated by a combination of levodopa and one of those enzyme inhibitors. By preventing the peripheral conversion to DA, undesirable side effects such as orthostatic hypotension and nausea are minimized.

A second enzyme involved in levodopa metabolism is catechol O-methyltransferase (COMT). The inactivation of DA after its release into the synaptic cleft involves both reuptake by DA terminals and metabolism. COMT inhibitors, tolcapone and entacapone, are used clinically together with levodopa because they prevent peripheral metabolism of levodopa. By prolonging the half-life of levodopa, they minimize fluctuation of serum concentration which may cause subsequent adverse events. The reuptake is performed by specialized DA transporter molecules in the membrane. Inhibitors of this transporter, as well as those of COMT, may prolong the action of DA.

Levodopa replacement is extremely effective in controlling much of the disability in PD. It is most efficacious against rigidity and hypokinesia, but tremor also responds. However, postural instability does not respond well to dopaminergic therapy.

Because the progressive loss of DA neurons continues despite levodopa treatment, patients become less and less mobile as time elapses since the last dose was ingested, manifesting as end-of-dose hypokinesia. Therefore patients gradually require higher doses of the drug. These increments may cause significant problems, particularly peak-dose dyskinesias. Basically, these reactions are to be expected because when brain DA concentrations are very high, the patient is in a state opposite to the baseline DA deficiency.

Treating patients who reach this stage can be done by dividing the daily dose into several smaller administrations. While initially three daily doses of levodopa are sufficient to control symptoms, as the disease advances six or more doses may be required. In normal subjects, levodopa will never produce dyskinesias. Presumably this is because terminals of the nigrostriatal pathways in the corpus striatum take up any excessive DA and either store or degrade it to inactive metabolites. This buffering mechanism will necessarily fail in PD because of the progressive loss of DA neurons and terminals (Karstaedt and Pincus, 1992). The loss of this buffering capacity may be responsible also for the eventual and most problematic complication of therapy, the so-called 'on-off' phenomenon. Patients fluctuate from being normal in their function, or even dyskinetic as a manifestation of excessive DA stimulation ('on'), to severe parkinsonian hypokinesia and rigidity ('off'). As the disease advances, these fluctuations come on unexpectedly ('random on-off'). Once buffering capacity is lost, pharmacokinetic factors (e.g., levodopa serum concentration) determine the clinical response state (Korczyn, 1973). Motor fluctuations could be due to erratic absorption of levodopa from the gastrointestinal tract (possibly related partly to competition by amino acids derived from dietary proteins), distribution factors, or transportation across the blood–brain barrier. Attempts to reduce such fluctuations, which are of some benefit, include a low-protein diet (Karstaedt and Pincus, 1992), gastric administration of levodopa at a constant rate or by duodenal infusion (Antonini et al., 2007; Samanta and Hauser, 2007), controlled-release levodopa preparations, and administration of direct-acting dopamine agonists (DAA) (Rascol et al., 2000), either orally or, in advanced stages, as water-soluble DAA (e.g., rotigotine, lisuride, and apomorphine) (Parkinson Study Group, 2003; Pahwa et al., 2006; Korczyn, 2007; Poewe et al., 2007).

The revolutionary introduction of levodopa into the therapeutics of PD was so dramatic that its impact is unlikely to be superseded by another drug any time soon. However, as is discussed above, this treatment does not solve all the problems. One critical question relates to the time at which levodopa therapy should be initiated. The basic aim of levodopa therapy is to replace endogenous DA. It is thus a symptomatic therapy that, however, also masks to some extent the relentless progression of neuronal cell loss. However, it is still unclear whether levodopa treatment itself accelerates or retards this loss. There are suggestions that levodopa reduces the oxidative stress that results from excessive burden on the remaining neurons. Alternatively, it is possible that the pharmacological concentrations of extrinsic levodopa will contribute to the formation of toxic free radicals inside neurons. Therefore, diverging views exist on whether levodopa should be started immediately upon diagnosing PD, or delayed as much as possible, with the aid of other types of therapy (Rascol et al., 2002).

Monoamine oxidase (MAO), the enzyme that metabolizes several catecholamines and indolamines, exists in two forms. MAO-A metabolizes not only dopamine but also NE and 5-HT, whereas MAO-B does not metabolize either NE or 5-HT. Selective inhibitors of MAO-B, and particularly selegiline (deprenyl) and rasagiline, are effective against MPTP toxicity. In PD patients, selegiline and rasagiline provide symptomatic benefit (Olanow and Calne, 1992). This may be related to an ampfetamine-like action in releasing DA from terminals or, more likely, by preventing DA reuptake. Interestingly, it has been shown that newly diagnosed PD patients can be maintained on MAO-B inhibitors alone for a long period (Landau, 1990; Olanow and Calne, 1992), although the significance of this observation is still unclear (Bonucelli and Del Dotto, 2006).

Monotherapy with selegiline or rasagiline is not efficacious in more advanced cases. At present, many patients are being treated with selegiline or rasagiline in addition to levodopa. The usefulness of this combination in retarding the progression of the disease has not been convincingly demonstrated, although rasagiline is useful in moderating the motor fluctuations in advanced stages of PD (Bonucelli and Del Dotto, 2006).

Direct-acting dopamine agonists (DAA) are important in the treatment of PD. These include apomorphine, bromocriptine, pergolide, cabergoline, and lisuride, as well as newer agents such as rotigotine, ropinirole, and pramipexole. Theoretically, the use of such agents could be advantageous. In initial stages, they relieve the excessive burden on remaining DA neurons without being subject to metabolism into toxic free radicals inside DA neurons, as has been hypothesized for levodopa. In later stages, it is easier to maintain constant levels at receptor sites because these drugs do not depend on active transport in the gut and through the BBB. Particularly cabergoline, which has a very long biological half-life, may be advantageous in PD patients who develop motor fluctuations or off symptoms at night (Inzelberg et al., 1995). Similar benefit may occur if percutaneous administration of DA agonists is applied, such as rotigotine and lisuride.

However, DAA have significant drawbacks and side effects. Their potency is lower than that of levodopa. Therefore they can be used as monotherapy in the initial stages of the disease but will have to be supplanted by levodopa in subsequent years. Ergoline derivatives are not very specific and interact with several subtypes of DA receptors as well as with 5-HT and other receptors. D1 stimulation may contribute to the occurrence of dyskinesias, while 5-HT and D4 stimulation may be conductive to hallucinations and other psychiatric manifestations. Ropinirole and pramipexole, two synthetic nonergoline compounds, are specific to DA (particularly D2 type) receptors and were therefore expected to be advantageous. Unfortunately, this does not seem to be the case, and the frequency of these psychiatric adverse events is identical. In addition, DA agonists act also at the periphery, and this may contribute to significant side effects such as orthostatic hypotension and nausea and leg edema (Rascol et al., 2007). A behavioral syndrome consisting of gambling, uncontrolled shopping or eating, and hypersexuality has been reported and may be rather severe (Weintraub et al., 2006). These behavioral effects were termed dopamine dysregulation syndrome and are probably related to the effect of dopamine agonists on D3 and D4 receptors, since in animals quetiapine, a dopamine agonist that activates these receptors selectively, has been shown to induce stereotypic 'compulsive' behavior. Also, recently cardiotoxic effects were described for two agents, cabergoline and pergolide, leading to the withdrawal of pergolide from the market (Roth, 2007).

Surgical interventions of PD are also available. These include ablative and transplanting approaches. Targets for functional stereotactic neurosurgical lesions that reduce tremor are the ventrolateral thalamus and the posteroventral pallidum. Within the last decade, accumulating evidence has proved that subthalamic stimulation is very effective in the treatment of PD, reducing both the parkinsonian symptoms and dyskinesias, and allowing reduction of drug dosage (Sailer *et al.*, 2007). Whether subthalamic stimulation should be initiated at an early stage of the disease is still an open question. There has been extensive interest in transplanting DA tissue into the caudate or putamen in PD. Originally, autologous tissue was used, but the benefits, if any, were offset by the significant complications (Windner and Rechcronal, 1993). This approach was discarded. In newer experiments, dopaminergic transplants were used in which the tissue was removed from aborted fetal midbrains. The use of stem cells is presently being explored (Sontag *et al.*, 2005). It is difficult to assess the success of this approach, because frequently the patients who have been recruited had a poor prognosis to start with and also because this intervention is associated with a high placebo factor (Korczyn, 1993). However, the main question may not necessarily be whether neurons are generated, survive, and produce and release dopamine, but whether the release of dopamine can be properly regulated, since otherwise on-off dyskinesias will result.

Cognitive Changes in PD

The prevalence of frank dementia in PD is far greater than that in the general population. PD dementia may be preceded by mild memory loss, transient confusional episodes, vivid dreams, or hallucinosis. Clinically, the dementia of PD differs from that of Alzheimer disease (AD). PD patients rarely develop dysfunctions of the isocortical association areas, such as dysphasia or agnosia, and may resemble a 'frontal' type of dementia, with dysexecutive symptoms. But while the differentiation between cortical and subcortical dementia is of some theoretical interest, individual PD patients may develop a clinical AD-like picture.

Cell loss in PD is not limited to DA neurons. The degeneration of cholinergic neurons in the nucleus basalis of Meynert, as well as 5-HT, NE, and somatostatin deficiencies are well-documented, and glutamatergic deficiency may also exist. These deficiencies are similar to those observed in AD and therefore suggest similarities in pathogenesis and treatment, as well as a clinical overlap.

During the past decade, it has become obvious that Lewy bodies are not limited to the substantia nigra in PD, but may occur in a widespread distribution, extending to the cortex. Diffuse Lewy body disease is a pathological entity whose clinical correlates have been tentatively defined (McKeith *et al.*, 2005). Patients commonly have cognitive decline and parkinsonian features, and either one may dominate the picture. Therefore, it seems that Lewy body disease can first manifest itself as parkinsonism (if the lesions primarily affect the substantia nigra) or cognitive decline (if predominantly the cortex is affected). There seems to be a continuum in this respect, and the question is whether factors can be identified that are responsible for which region is more affected.

The main risk factors for dementia in PD include older age and severity of motor symptoms (Giladi *et al.*, 2000).

Treatment of the cognitive changes of PD is unsatisfactory. The cholinergic defect suggests that drugs with antimuscarinic action may be detrimental, and these include not only specific antiparkinsonian agents such as benzhexol or trihexyphenidyl but also antidepressants such as amitriptyline. Contrariwise, cholinomimetic agents such as rivastigmine, widely used in AD, may be of significant value in dementia associated with PD (Giladi *et al.*, 2003; Emre *et al.*, 2004). Treatment of hallucinations and delusions similarly poses difficult problems because the use of D2 blockers may well result in motor exacerbation. Clozapine, a specific D4 blocker, has been suggested as an efficacious treatment of this condition (Rabey *et al.*, 1995).

Depression in PD

Exactly how frequently depression occurs in PD is a question that is difficult to answer. There is quite a spectrum of figures in the literature, which diverge depending on (1) the criteria used to diagnose depression, (2) possible inclusion or exclusion of demented patients or those with parkinsonism due to causes other than PD (e.g., vascular etiology and progressive supranuclear palsy), and (3) the severity of the neurological impairment. In addition, referral bias to specialized centers probably results in excessive numbers of depressed patients in these centers. However, and regardless of these factors, it is safe to conclude that depression is rather common in PD. Because depression is potentially treatable, this conclusion is of significant importance.

Several tests are available for diagnosing depression. These include neuropsychological evaluations, self-reports, projection tests, and others. However, while all these tests have important roles in research, none is superior to the clinical assessment by a competent clinician. Nor is such a test likely to ever be developed, because the manifestations of PD are so varied. The clinical evaluation of the affective state of PD patients may be difficult because the motionless face, the slowness of movement, and the bradyphrenia that may create an erroneous impression of depression even if this is absent. The distinction from depressive motor retardation is also important (Treves *et al.*, 1995).

Decision about the therapeutic approaches should be based not solely, perhaps not even primarily, on an objective measure but rather on the context and repercussions of the affective state of the patient.

Based on the above, every patient with PD must be assessed for possible depressive symptomatology, and adequate consideration should be given to the therapeutic implications. The therapeutic consideration regarding depression in PD may differ from those for major depression. In the latter situation, massive treatment with 5-HT reuptake inhibitors or tricyclic antidepressants is recommended, with the expected benefits occurring only several weeks later. However, in the parkinsonian patient who is depressed, less aggressive therapy is usually sufficient, and high doses may in fact cause intolerable side effects.

The present knowledge of therapeutic options for parkinsonian depression is limited because of the scarcity of drug evaluations in this condition, let alone of comparative studies of different agents. Tricyclic antidepressants (TCAs) have marked antimuscarinic effects. These are potentially advantageous for the PD patient because they reduce the motor symptoms, particularly the tremor. Another feature of TCAs is their anxiolytic action, and of course this is helpful in those patients manifesting anxiety symptomatology. A third relevant feature is the soporific effect of TCAs, which is of significant value in those patients suffering from insomnia (although some patients respond to TCAs with increased alertness and restlessness).

The antimuscarinic action of TCAs, already alluded to, may unfortunately lead to disorientation and confusion. This is particularly true when patients with more limited cognitive reserves are being treated (i.e., those with incipient or actual dementia), when relatively high doses are prescribed, or when employed together with antiparkinsonian drugs with antimuscarinic actions.

Selective 5-HT reuptake blockers include clomipramine, fluvoxamine, fluoxetine, and citalopram. Fluoxetine and fluvoxamine lack antimuscarinic actions and thus may be particularly useful in those patients for whom the use of anticholinergic drugs is contraindicated. Although these newer drugs do have specific actions, it remains to be demonstrated that this is of practical significance.

The use of nonselective monoamine oxidase inhibitors (MAOIs) is of course well-established for the treatment of depression; although they have a bad reputation regarding safety, they continue to be used. Ever since it was realized that DA deficiency is responsible for PD, attempts were made to treat it by MAOIs, but the response is limited. It is probably true that MAOIs can successfully be used in PD patients who are depressed, with expected mild benefits also in the motor function.

The use of electroconvulsive therapy is reserved to patients with severe depression. Previous reluctance to use this treatment in the elderly seems to have been excessive, but there is only anecdotal information on its use in PD. Some case reports suggested improvement in both affective and motor symptomatology.

Meager data exist suggesting an independent antidepressant action of levodopa. Bromocriptine is also reputed to have some antidepressant activity, although, again, this largely depends on nonsystematic observations. However, newer dopamine agonists drugs used in the treatment of PD have mood-elevating actions.

Citations

Aarsland D, Tandberg E, Larsen JP, and Cummings JL (1996) Frequency of dementia in Parkinson's disease. *Archives of Neurology* 53: 538–542.

Antonini A, Isaias IU, Canesi M, *et al.* (2007) Duodenal levodopa infusion for advanced Parkinson's disease: 12-month treatment outcome. *Movement Disorders* 22: 1145–1149.

Bergman H, Wichmann T, and Delong MR (1990) Reversal of experimental parkinsonism by lesions of the subthalamic nucleus. *Science* 249: 1436–1438.

Bhatt MH, Snow BJ, Martin WRW, Pate BD, and Calne DB (1991) Positron emission tomography suggests that the rate of progression of idiopathic parkinsonism is slow. *Annals of Neurology* 29: 673–677.

Bonifati V, Rizzu P, Van Baren MJ, *et al.* (2002) Mutations in the DJ-1 gene associatd with autosomal recessive early-onset parkinsonism. *Science* 299: 256–259.

Bonucelli U and Del Dotto P (2006) New pharmacologic horizons in the treatment of Parkinson disease. *Neurology* 67: 530–538.

Braak H, Braak E, Yilmazer D, de Vos RA, Jansen EN, and Bohl J (1996) New aspects of pathology in Parkinson's disease with concomitant incipient Alzheimer's disease. *Journal of Neural Transmission* 48: 1–6.

Braak H, Ghebremedhin E, Rueb U, Bratzke H, and Del Tredici K (2004) Stages in the development of Parkinson's disease-related pathology. *Cell and Tissue Research* 318: 121–134.

Cummings JL (1992) Depression and Parkinson's disease: Review. *American Journal of Psychiatry* 149: 443–454.

Emre M, Aarsland D, Albanese A, *et al.* (2004) Rivastigmine for dementia associated with Parkinson's disease. *New England Journal of Medicine* 351: 2509–2518.

Flash T, Inzelberg R, Schechtman E, and Korczyn AD (1991) Kinematic analysis of upper limb trajectories in Parkinson's disease. *Acta Neuropathol* 81: 691–694.

Gasser T, Muller-Myhsok B, Wszolek ZK, *et al.* (1998) A susceptibility locus for Parkinson's disease maps to chromosome 2p13. *Nature Genetics* 18: 262–265.

Giladi N, Treves TA, Paleacu D, *et al.* (2000) Risk factors for dementia, depression and psychosis in long-standing Parkinson's disease. *Journal of Neural Transmission* 107: 59–71.

Giladi N, Shabtai H, Gurevich T, Benbunan B, Anca M, and Korczyn AD (2003) Rivastigmine (Exelon) for dementia in patients with Parkinson's disease. *Acta Neurologica Scandinavica* 108: 368–373.

Hicks AA, Petursson H, Jonsson T, *et al.* (2002) A susceptibility gene for lae-onset idioipathic Parkinson's disease. *Annals of Neurology* 52(5): 549–555.

Inzelberg R, Nisipeanu P, Rabey JM, and Korczyn AD (1995) Long-term tolerability and efficacy of cabergoline, a new long-acting dopamine agonist in Parkinson's disease. *Movement Disorders* 10: 604–607.

Karstaedt PJ and Pincus JH (1992) Protein redistribution diet remains effective in patients with fluctuatin parkinsonism. *Archives of Neurology* 49: 149–151.

Kitada T, Asakawa S, Hattori N, *et al.* (1998) Mutations in the parkin gene cause autosomal recessive juvenile parkinsonism. *Nature* 392: 605–608.

Koller WC (1992) How accurately can Parkinson's disease be diagnosed? *Neurology* 42(Suppl): 6–16.

Korczyn AD (1973) Pathophysiology on drug-induced dyskinesias. *Neuropharmacology* 11: 601–607.

Korczyn AD (1989) Autonomic nervous system dysfunction in Parkinson's disease. In: Calne DB (ed.) *Parkinsonism and Aging*, pp. 211–219. New York: Raven Press

Korczyn AD (1990) Autonomic nervous system disturbances in Parkinson's disease. In: Streifler MB, Korczyn AD, Melamed E, and Youdim MBH (eds.) *Advances in Neurology: Parkinson's Disease: Anatomy, Pathology, Therapy*, pp. 463–468. New York: Raven Press

Korczyn AD (1993) Placebos and other biases in clinical trials in dementia. Guidelines for Drug Trials in Memory Disorders. *Aging* 39: 135–141.

Korczyn AD (1995) Parkinson's disease. In: Bloom FE and Kupfer DJ (eds.). *Psychopharmacology: The Fourth Generation of Progress*, pp. 1479–1484. New York: Raven Press.

Korczyn AD (1999) Parkinson's disease: one disease entity or many? In: Muller Hpa (ed.) *Diagnosis and Treatment of Parkinson's Disease – State of the Art*, pp. 107–111. New York: Springer, Wien

Korczyn AD (2001) Neuropsychiatric manifestations in Parkinson's disease. In: Calne DCS (ed.) *Parkinson's Disease: Advances in Neurology*, pp. 395–404. Philadelphia, PA: Lippincott Williams & Wilkins

Korczyn AD (2007) Transdermal therapy in Parkinson's disease. *Lancet Neurology* 6: 475–476.

Kruger R, Kuhn W, Muller T, *et al.* (1998) Ala39Pro mutation in the gene encoding a-synuclein in Parkinson's disease. *Nature Genetics* 18: 106–108.

Landau WM (1990) Pyramid sale in the bucket shop; datatop bottoms out. *Neurology* 40: 1337–1339.

Leroy E, Boyer R, Auburger G, *et al.* (1998) The ubiquitin pathway in Parkinson's disease. [letter]. *Nature* 395(670): 451–452.

McKeith IG, Dickson DW, Lowe J, *et al.* (2005) Diagnosis and management of dementia with Lewy bodies: third report of the DLB Consortium. *Neurology* 65(12): 1863–1872.

Nisipeanu P and Korczyn AD (2002) Parkinson's disease diagnosis, clinical management. In: Factor SA and Weiner WJ (eds.) *Dopamine Agonists*, pp. 379–397. New York: Demos.

Olanow CW and Calne DB (1992) Does selegiline monotherapy in Parkinson's disease act by symptomatic on protective mechanisms? *Neurology* 42(Suppl. 4): 13–26.

Pahwa R, Factor SA, and Lyons KE; Quality Standards Subcomitee of the American Academy of Neurology (2006) Practice Parameter: treatment of Parkinson disease with motor fluctuations and dyskinesias (an evidence-based review): report of the Quality Standards Subcommittee of the American Academy of Neurology. *Neurology* 66: 983–995.

Paisan-Ruiz C, Jain S, Evans EW, *et al.* (2004) Cloning of the gene containing mutation that cause PARK8-linked Parkinson's disease. *Neuron* 44(4): 595–600.

Pankratz N, Nichols WC, Uniacke SK, *et al.* (2003) Significant linkage of Parkinson disease to chromosome 2q36–37. *American Journal of Human Genetics* 72(4): 1053–1057.

Parkinson J (1817) An Essay on the Shaking Palsy. In: Rowland W (ed.) London.

Poewe WH, Rascol O, and Quinn N; SP 515 Investigators (2007) Efficacy of pramipexole and transdermal rotigotine in advanced Parkinson's disease: a double-blind, double-dummy, randomized controlled trial. *Lancet Neurology* 6: 513–520.

Polymeropoulos MH, Lavedan C, and Leroy E (1997) Mutation in the a-synuclein gene identified in families with Parkinson's disease. *Science* 276: 2045–2047.

Rabey JM, Treves TA, Neufeld MY, Orlov E, and Korczyn AD (1995) Low-dose clozapine in the treatment of levodopa induced mental disturbances in Parkinson's disease. *Neurology* 45: 432–434.

Ramirez A, Heimbach A, Grundemann J, *et al.* (2006) Hereditary parkinsonism with dementia is caused by mutations in ATP13A2, encoding a lysosomal type 5 P-type ATPase. *Nature Genetics* 38(10): 1184–1191.

Rascol O, Brooks DJ, Korczyn AD, *et al.*; Group FtS (2000) A five-year study of the incidence of dyskinesias in pathients with early Parkinson's disease who were treated with ropinirole or levodopa. *New England Journal of Medicine* 342: 1484–1491.

Rascol O, Goetz C, Koller W, Poewe W, and Sampaio C (2002) Treatment interventions for Parkinson's disease: an evidence based assessment. *Lancet* 359: 1589–1598.

Roth BL (2007) Drugs and valvular heart disease. *New England Journal of Medicine* 356: 6–9.

Sailer A, Cunic DI, Paradiso GO, *et al.* (2007) Subthalamic nucleus stimulation modulates afferent inhibition in Parkinson disease. *Neurology* 68: 356–363.

Samanta J and Hauser RA (2007) Duodenal levodopa infusion for the treatment of Parkinson's disease. *Expert Opinion on Pharmacotheraphy* 8: 657–664.

Singleton AB, Farrer M, Johnson J, *et al.* (2003) [alpha]-Synuclein locus triplication causes Parkinson's disease. *Science* 302(5646): 841.

Stevenson GB, Heafield MTE, Waring RH, and Williams AC (1989) Xenobiotic metabolism in Parkinson's disease. *Neurology* 39: 883–887.

Tanner CM and Langston JW (1990) Do environmental toxins cause Parkinson's disease? A critical review. *Neurology* 40(Suppl 3): 17–30.

The Parkinson Study Group (2003) A controlled trial of rotigotine monotherapy in early Parkinson's disease. *Archives of Neurology* 60: 1721–1728.

Treves TA, Paleacu D, and Korczyn AD (1995) Treatment of depression in Parkinson's disease. In: Koller WC (ed.) *Therapy of Parkinson's Disease*. New York, Basel, Hong Kong: Marcel Dekker.

Treves TA, Paleacu D, Rabey JM, Korczyn AD. Depression inventories in Parkinson's disease. In: Przuntek H PHK, Kloty P, Korcyzn AD (eds.) *Instrumental Methods and Scoring in Extrapyramidal Disorders*, pp 31–43. Springer.

Valente EM, Abou-Sleiman PM, Caputo V, *et al.* (2004) Hereditary early-onset Parkinson's disease caused by mutations in PINKI. *Science* 304 (5674): 1158–1160.

Weintraub D, Siderowf AD, Potenza MN, *et al.* (2006) Association of dopamine agonist use with impulse control disorders in Parkinson disease. *Archives of Neurology* 63: 969–973.

Windner H and Rechcronal S (1993) Transplantation and surgical tratment of Parkinsonian syndromes. *Current Opinion in Neurology and Neurosurgery* 6: 344–349.

Zimprich A, Biskup S, Leitner P, *et al.* (2004) Mutations in LRRK2 cause autosomal-dominant parkinsonism with pleomorphic pathology. *Neuron* 44(4): 601–607.

Poliomyelitis

T J John, Christian Medical College, Vellore, India

What Is Polio? Definitions, Description of the Disease, and Surveillance

Polio is the abbreviation for the disease poliomyelitis, caused by poliovirus. It typically causes a mild enteric or febrile infection, but it can spread systemically and affect the nervous system. The early twentieth-century technical term was acute anterior poliomyelitis or paralytic poliomyelitis, and its diagnosis was clinical without laboratory support. The site of pathology in typical paralytic poliomyelitis is the anterior horn motor neurons in the gray (*polios*) matter of the spinal cord (*myelos*). When motor neuron death and local inflammation reaches a threshold, limb paralysis occurs. In 20–30% of subjects, recovery from paralysis occurs, but in the majority, paralysis is permanent, leading to muscle atrophy and joint deformities. Other infections (such as other enteroviruses or West Nile virus) may cause limb muscle paralysis known as acute flaccid paralysis (AFP) syndrome, but only that caused by polioviruses (antigenic types 1, 2, or 3, one species of the genus *Enterovirus*, family Picornaviridae) is poliomyelitis; hence laboratory confirmation test has become essential to the diagnosis of polio. Indeed, when paralysis of a facial nerve occurs due to poliovirus infection, it is still called poliomyelitis, even though the site of pathology is not in the spinal cord. Thus, the term poliomyelitis is now based on etiology rather than symptoms.

Most poliovirus infections are asymptomatic (subclinical). Infection with minor symptoms is termed nonparalytic polio. Only one in 160–200 persons infected with poliovirus type 1, and one in about 1000 infected with type 2 or 3, develop paralysis. One infection is sufficient for lifelong immunity, but immunity is type-specific.

Poliovirus attaches to cell surfaces via the poliovirus receptor (PVR), a membrane protein (CD155) of the immunoglobulin superfamily. Only polioviruses bind to PVR, which is expressed mainly on the nasopharyngeal mucosa, Peyer's patch M cells of small intestines, and the anterior horn motor neurons of the spinal cord and medulla oblongata. These are the main anatomic sites where polioviruses multiply inside the host. Almost all cultured human and primate cells express PVR, support growth of polioviruses and develop cytopathology (CPE), and have become the standard cells for virus isolation, detection, and cultivation for clinical and research purposes. The human PVR gene has been introduced into transgenic mice, and a fibroblastic cell line from them (L20B cells) has become very useful in primary isolation of polioviruses from clinical specimens.

Infection with poliovirus was essentially universal until the advent of vaccination. Polio was first clinically recognized in 1840 and an 1887 Swedish polio epidemic was described in 1891. No country was able to control or interrupt polio transmission solely by sanitation, clean water supply, personal hygiene, or very high living standards. Although dogma is that transmission was primarily through contaminated water and food (fecal–oral) there is compelling evidence to show that direct person-to-person transmission during ordinary social contact is a critical factor during outbreaks. Polio is highly contagious and can be transmitted via the respiratory route by inhalation of droplets or aerosols containing virus expelled through saliva or nasal secretions. Polio has now been eliminated from most of the world through vaccination, and this article will focus on the development of the polio vaccine and eradication efforts.

In developing countries, acute flaccid paralysis (AFP) in children under 15 years of age is monitored. From children with AFP, stool samples collected within 2 weeks of onset are sent to a poliovirus diagnostic laboratory for virological investigation. Globally laboratories are networked in three tiers: Global reference centers, national or regional reference laboratories, and local diagnostic laboratories. Poliovirus isolates are typed locally and submitted to the next higher level for differentiation as wild or vaccine-derived.

The World Health Organization (WHO) has established performance standards for surveillance sensitivity, stool collection, and virus isolation. Every country has its own polio elimination certification committee and when 3 consecutive years pass without any wild virus isolation, that country is certified to have achieved success. Countries are aggregated by WHO into six regions, and some regions (the Americas, Western Pacific, and Europe) have achieved regional elimination. The surveillance, stool collection, and laboratory standards are satisfactory in the four currently polio-endemic countries.

The Rise and Fall of Polio in the Twentieth Century: The Need for a Vaccine

Until the 1930s, polio was predominantly in infants and young children and called infantile paralysis. In countries with high birth rates and crowded living, about half of paralytic cases occurred in infancy and the remaining mostly before the age of 5. Infants were often infected during the first few months of life when maternal antibody protected them from disease (passive immunity), while the infection itself induced long-lasting active immunity. The total incidence of clinical disease was low and in younger children.

As nations became richer with improved living standards and housing, many children escaped infection in early childhood and remained nonimmune. Poliovirus spread rapidly during summer and fall, particularly when older, susceptible children aggregated for school or social activities such as summer camps. During the 1930s–1950s, the age range in Europe and North America shifted to older children, while the incidence of clinical polio increased. In older children and young adults, poliovirus increasingly affects the brain stem, resulting in more lethal respiratory paralysis or bulbar polio in contrast to the limb paralysis of spinal polio seen in infants. These annual outbreaks, suddenly paralyzing or killing healthy children and adolescents, caused much anxiety. This shift was originally attributed to improving sanitation, but in retrospect better housing with less crowding and fluctuating birth rates may have been more important. As improved sanitation, hygiene, and water supplies did not reduce the risk of polio, scientists and opinion leaders realized that polio could only be prevented by vaccination. The development of polio vaccines has indeed led to a tremendous decrement in the incidence of polio, while providing important lessons about bioethics, the nature of scientific discourse, and the selection of appropriate vaccines for different populations.

Early Poliovirus Research, the Development of the Inactivated Polio Virus Vaccine, and the Debate About the Vaccine

Early Research

Spinal cord extracts were inoculated into monkeys and the disease was replicated by Landsteiner and Popper in 1908. Through primate experiments the three known antigenic types (or serotypes) were identified. The infectious agent of polio was found in the feces of infected children, identifying the gastrointestinal tract as one major site of infection, and indeed monkeys were infected by oral feeding and the infectious agent (not as yet identified as a virus) recovered from feces. Thus the paradigm of poliovirus fecal–oral transmission in humans arose, which had important repercussions on future vaccine development and use. Subsequent early poliovirus vaccine attempts (1930s–1950s) were sometimes crude, sometimes sophisticated, sometimes ethically dubious, and largely unregulated. In the 1930s, Brodie and Park as well as Kolmer used monkey spinal cord preparations to inoculate children without knowing of the three antigenic types, nor that the cord myelin would induce allergic encephalomyelitis, and without reliable markers for complete virus inactivation or attenuation. The results were disastrous, as no protection was demonstrated and some children developed polio after inoculation. Poliovirus vaccine development identified the need for state regulations for quality, safety, and disease surveillance (monitoring and measuring vaccine efficacy and adverse reactions) as general principles for the current era.

In 1947–48, Isabel Morgan inoculated monkeys with formalin-inactivated virus from infected monkey neuronal tissues, which protected them from serotype-specific disease, providing proof-of-principle evidence for a killed virus vaccine. In the early 1950s, Hammon and colleagues showed that injected human serum gamma globulin protected against polio paralysis, demonstrating that serum antibodies protect against disease, and vaccination research was resurrected.

Cell Culture Adaptation of Polioviruses

Enders, Robbins and Weller discovered in 1949 that polioviruses could be grown in human and animal cell culture, for which they received the 1954 Nobel Prize. This led to several unsuccessful attempts to create either killed (inactivated) virus vaccine or live (attenuated) virus vaccine, using cell culture-grown virus stock. The prototype vaccines had residual neurovirulence and were unsuitable for

human use. All these early studies lacked stringent laboratory standards or ethical clearance for human use. Rectifying such obvious errors, Jonas Salk and Albert Sabin succeeded in developing satisfactory inactivated and live vaccines, respectively, during the late 1950s. These vaccines were developed with private agency funding in North America.

In 1921 Franklin Delano Roosevelt, who became President of the United States in 1932, developed paralytic polio of both legs at the age of 39. Roosevelt's law partner Basil O'Connor formed a National Foundation for Infantile Paralysis (NFIP) in 1938, with Roosevelt as its patron. Innumerable local chapters were organized, and gave all sectors of society the opportunity to participate in a national fight against polio, which was seen as the nation's most important challenge in children's health. Millions of small contributions were donated to NFIP with the catchy name of the March of Dimes (a dime being a tenth of a dollar coin). NFIP thus became the largest private philanthropic institution in the United States and indeed the world. Funds were liberally distributed nationally for the treatment and rehabilitation of affected persons, building treatment facilities in hospitals, purchasing necessary equipment, particularly the expensive iron lungs (Drinker apparatus, for noninvasive ventilation-assistance by alternate application of positive and negative air pressure), training of health-care personnel, and for research. O'Connor believed in the idea of a polio vaccine developed through science that would be the final answer to the crippling disease. It turned out he was right and his detractors, mostly renowned virologists who were experts in their own field but not necessarily in the ways of the world, were wrong.

Despite Roosevelt's death in 1945, contributions to the NFIP increased as cases of polio also increased. The NFIP had a Research Committee that guided research, but its work on a vaccine was slow, and O'Connor established an Immunization Committee that focused on vaccine development. Jonas Salk and Albert Sabin, among others, were recipients of NFIP funds for research. However, only Salk took the direct route of research toward a vaccine.

Salk's Success in Creating the Inactivated Polio Vaccine

Salk, unlike most polio experts, believed that an inactivated virus preparation would be both safe and immunogenic. Salk and Thomas Francis had already developed and proved that killed influenza virus vaccine was safe and effective. Others discounted this approach as earlier viral vaccines used live attenuated viruses (smallpox, rabies, yellow fever). In 1952, Salk showed that formaldehyde-inactivated polioviruses were highly immunogenic both in animals and in children. Despite opposition, O'Connor and NFIP research director Harry Weaver established a new Vaccine Advisory Committee, which funded Thomas Francis to conduct a field trial of an inactivated vaccine. Bulk concentrated vaccine was made in Canada by Connaught Laboratories and supplied to U.S. vaccine manufacturers who prepared vials of both vaccine and a placebo. Children were given three doses 1 month apart. The results showed inactivated polio vaccine (IPV) to be completely safe and highly effective. Vaccine efficacy correlated well with vaccine potency, and vaccine batches that induced high frequencies of antibody response showed 80–90% protection. In April 1955, the result was publicized and immediately the U.S. Government licensed IPV for wide usage.

IPV owes its birth to Basil O'Connor, Harry Weaver, and Thomas Francis in addition to Jonas Salk. They demonstrated vision, conviction, maneuvering ability, and an astute understanding of immunology. IPV was truly a people's vaccine, developed by people's money and Salk was a public hero, who was (partly consequently) shunned by the scientific establishment.

Once IPV was licensed, new problems arose. The NFIP bought up all the vaccine made by various manufacturers and gave it free of charge first to the placebo recipients in the trial, and then to children in the first and second grades of school, who were the most vulnerable age group. This upset the medical profession, the U.S. government, and to a certain extent, the pharmaceutical industry, as it was akin to socialized medicine, contrary to the principles of private, free-market enterprise. In contrast, the Canadian government manufactured, distributed, and regulated a plentiful, low-cost IPV of high quality. In the United States, the drug companies prevailed and six of them began marketing their product directly to doctors. Gradually, the selling price also rose. Obviously, IPV safety demanded full inactivation of the virus, which was not the case with a few batches made in the United States by private manufacturers. Due to faulty quality and manufacturing controls, a number of U.S. children developed polio after taking IPV, leading the U.S. Government to establish vaccine safety testing and polio surveillance standards, the principles of which are still used today. While no further mishaps occurred, these events fueled the schism between IPV supporters and live vaccine protagonists.

From 1955 to 1961, IPV was used exclusively in the United States and Canada. The effect on polio incidence was immediate and remarkable. In the United States, a 90% reduction occurred within 4 years and 99% within the next 4 years. However, vaccination coverage had not reached 90% and the greater decline than accounted for by vaccination was interpreted as the result of indirect effect on virus circulation, or the herd effect of vaccination (Stickle, 1964). Studies in Houston, Texas, showed vaccine efficacy remaining at 96% through 2 consecutive

years, likely due to the direct protective effect and added herd effect (Melnick *et al.*, 1961).

In 1962, the live vaccine, developed by Sabin and other live-vaccine proponents, was licensed in the United States and it gradually replaced IPV, which was no longer manufactured in the United States from 1965. For children with immune system defects, IPV was imported from Canada where IPV continued to be used in some provinces while others switched to live vaccine. Today the situation is the reverse, as will be described in the section titled 'Use of IPV in countries outside North America: Demonstration of herd effect.'

Use of IPV in Countries Outside North America: Demonstration of the Herd Effect

The original IPV trial included parts of Canada and Finland. Upon release of the trial results, Finland embarked on a nationwide vaccination program using IPV made by the Dutch public sector vaccine manufacturer and when IPV coverage reached approximately 60% in 1961, disease incidence became zero and poliovirus could no longer be detected in sewage, confirming the absence of excretion by infected individuals and to the high degree of a herd protective effect. Many other European countries introduced IPV during the late 1950s and brought down the incidence of polio rapidly.

Safety and Efficacy of IPV

While Salk had originally formulated IPV with a mineral oil adjuvant, which led to high antibody levels after a single dose, the NFIP found the local inflammatory response to the adjuvant unacceptable, and it persuaded Salk to make adjuvant-free vaccine to be given in three doses. Without adjuvant, IPV was rendered totally safe from any serious adverse reaction; anaphylaxis, although theoretically possible, has not been reported, and the minor local reactions of many injected vaccines are usually absent.

The efficacy of IPV, as measured by the proportion of the vaccinated being protected when exposed to infection, was moderate to high in the original trial, and with subsequent manufacturing refinements is over 99%. Poliovirus neutralizing antibody is a reliable surrogate for protection from disease. After receiving three doses of IPV at intervals of 4 weeks or more, nearly 100% of children become antibody-positive and protected. The vast majority of vaccinated children develop antibody titers in greater than 1:256, whereas with the live vaccine the antibody response is quite variable and usually below 1:128.

Basic Properties of the Original IPV

The key to the success of the IPV was the presence of the capsid protein (D antigen) that acts as the viral ligand that binds PVR on the host cell. IPV contained approximately 20, 2, and 4 D antigen units of poliovirus types 1, 2, and 3, respectively, in a liquid form without adjuvant. Residual traces of formaldehyde acted as a preservative, and in multidose vials an added alcoholic preservative (2-phenoxyethanol) provided protection against the multiplication of accidentally introduced organisms. Residual traces of antimicrobials used in the cell culture were also present. Aluminum salts and Thiomersal, both of which have been used for inactivated bacterial and toxoid vaccines, are absent from IPV.

In some countries, IPV was given as stand-alone vaccine, while in others it was presented as a combination vaccine containing DTP and IPV.

IPV Technology Improvements

Although the United States replaced IPV with oral polio vaccine (OPV), Dutch scientists continued to improve the vaccine. After demonstrating that IPV immunogenicity was due to the D antigen, they established standards for antibody responses in animal models. In order to improve vaccine yield, innovative techniques such as growing host cells on polystyrene beads in fermentation tanks were developed, so as to increase the total surface area of host cells and thus virus yield from cell culture. While the original Salk vaccine possessed about 20, 2, and 4 D antigen units of poliovirus types 1, 2, and 3, respectively, they established that the optimum vaccine antigen potency was 40, 8, and 32 D antigen units, respectively. This formulation was called enhanced potency IPV (e-IPV or IPV-E) to distinguish it from the original product, and since 1991 all manufacturers have adopted this formulation. Other advances have included the adoption of human diploid cells or Vero cells (of vervet monkey kidney origin) for virus production, so as to avoid the risk of contaminating viruses in primary monkey kidney cells that have theoretical potential for inducing tumors.

Safety and Efficacy of New Formulation IPV

Nearly all high-income nations and a few middle-income nations use IPV, and their experience confirms the efficacy and safety of the product. Only the low-income countries cannot afford IPV, as it has higher production costs than OPV and the limited global supply is currently all purchased by richer nations. Only five companies in the world make IPV (four in Europe and one in North America). OPV, on the other hand, is made by many companies in Asia, Europe, and Latin America.

IPV is one of the safest vaccines in current use. Apart from injection site discomfort, no serious adverse events have been reported to be due to IPV. Although anaphylaxis is listed as a potential adverse reaction,

it has not been reported (to the author's knowledge) anywhere.

IPV induces immune response according to the prime-boost principle. Therefore, a minimum of two and an optimum of three doses should be offered for primary vaccination, followed by one or more booster doses after long intervals. The presence of even moderate titers of maternal antibody in the young infant tends to dampen the antibody response to IPV, reducing the frequency of responders and the antibody titer. Therefore, wherever possible, the first dose of IPV should be given at or after 8 weeks (2 months) of age. The recommended age for commencing vaccination with DTP and OPV in developing countries (under the Expanded Program on Immunization, EPI, designed by WHO) is 6 weeks. IPV may be given at 6 weeks, provided two more doses are given to complete the primary series and a booster dose is given during the 2nd year of life.

The interval between the first and second doses also affects the immune response, as a 4-week interval is inferior to 8 weeks. The EPI schedule is to give the second dose of DTP and OPV 4 weeks after the first, namely at 10 weeks of age. IPV may be given in this schedule, but for predictable immune response three doses must be given and followed by at least one booster during the 2nd year of life.

The WHO has consistently stated that developing countries must use OPV. Thus, data on IPV efficacy and in developing countries is mostly limited to short-term research studies. All but one such study have shown that IPV efficacy in developing countries is as good as in developed countries. This is in contrast to OPV, which has very large degree of variation in vaccine efficacy, illustrated by the frequent occurrence of polio in children in some countries even after taking the recommended three doses (and more). In contrast, there has not been even a single report of a child developing polio after receiving three e-IPV doses.

Countries Using IPV in National Vaccination Programs

Only a few countries continued to use IPV when OPV became the vaccine of choice according to WHO. However, a number of countries have now switched to IPV because of the rare but continued occurrence of OPV-associated polio. As of 2006, Andorra, Australia, Austria, Belgium, Canada, Denmark, Finland, France, Germany, Greece, Hungary, Iceland, Ireland, Israel, Italy, Luxemburg, Monaco, Portugal, Netherlands, Norway, New Zealand, Slovakia, Slovenia, South Korea, Spain, Sweden, Switzerland, UK, and the United States exclusively use IPV.

In addition, in many countries in Latin America and Asia, IPV is registered as an alternative to OPV, but used mainly in the private sector health-care system. In many countries listed above, IPV is given to children as one component of a combination vaccine – using DTP as the base platform, but may contain hepatitis B vaccine, and/or *Haemophilus influenzae* type b vaccine. All such combinations use the acellular pertussis (aP) vaccine, whereas many developing countries continue to use whole cell killed pertussis (wP) bacterial vaccine. Currently no combination vaccine containing DTwP vaccine is available on the market, although such a combination vaccine was available before DTaP vaccine became the accepted one in most high-income countries.

The Live, Attenuated Oral Polio Vaccine

The Early History of the OPV

During the early vaccine development period of the 1930s through 1950s, two schools of thought existed, one favoring inactivated virus and the other live, attenuated virus for vaccine. Both approaches were funded by the NFIP, including Sabin and Salk. Concerns about insufficient attenuation of live vaccine were fueled not only by the early monkey experiments, but also by the experience of Koprowski, who conducted studies on a live vaccine in relative secrecy for the Lederle company. He administered prototype vaccines to children (without proper ethical review) in both the United States and in Ireland, but residual neurovirulence showed that the attenuation was incomplete.

After IPV licensure in 1955, the NFIP ended funding for an attenuated live vaccine. Through other funding, Sabin completed the attenuation of all three poliovirus strains in a series of elegant investigations that included testing for neurovirulence via direct inoculation of candidate strains of poliovirus into monkey spinal cord. Of note, the live attenuated vaccine that was shed in feces (and possibly respiratory secretions) after vaccination had the capacity to immunize other people, but also to revert to a more virulent neurotropic virus.

By the time Sabin had completed his work in 1959–60, IPV had been adopted in the United States, Canada, and Europe, removing the opportunity for a large-scale OPV trial in these regions. Sabin donated his strains to the Soviet Union where OPV was adopted, with a dramatic decline in polio incidence there and in Eastern Europe. The WHO experts who reviewed OPV were also supporters of the live virus vaccine strategy and concluded that the OPV was effective and safe. Based on this information, the U.S. Government approved the live vaccine (first in monovalent forms, and then a trivalent form) in 1962, and the WHO endorsed it for use globally. In retrospect, many have criticized this decision because the shed virus can establish transmission and circulation, resulting in virulent virus derived from the vaccine strain.

Monovalent and Trivalent OPVs: Balancing the Infection Rates

In July 1961, the American Medical Association (AMA), perhaps influenced by the strong live vaccine lobby, passed a resolution that IPV should be replaced in the United States with the oral live vaccine OPV upon its licensure. In September, type 1 vaccine (monovalent, mOPV-1) was licensed, and by 1962, so were types 2 and 3 vaccines (mOPV-2 and mOPV-3).

When 10^5 virus doses (median cell culture infectious dose, or $CCID_{50}$) of any of the monovalent vaccines was given to children, 80–100% responded with antibody production, proving effective intestinal infection and protection against the wild-type infection by the same serotype. However, when all three were included in a trivalent preparation (tOPV), the response was reduced, particularly for types 1 and 3, as type 2 infection was dominant over the others; type 1 is the least infectious and type 3 is intermediate. Robertson and colleagues in Canada made a balanced tOPV in which the highest (10^6) content of type 1, the lowest (10^5) of type 2, and intermediate ($10^{5.5}$) content of type 3 were mixed in one dose, with optimum results, but not near-100% responses. Type 2 is dominant in terms of infection frequency and antibody response; type 1 is the least infectious, and type 3 falls between the two. Thus, the tOPV content is balanced for 10:1:3 ratios of types 1, 2, and 3. When three doses were given, virtually all children tested in developed countries responded to all three virus types. The U.S. government licensed the tOPV in 1963, although the safety and effects of tOPV had not yet been established with the same rigor as IPV. Indeed, many pediatricians practiced a sequential schedule of one dose of Salk IPV vaccine followed by one or more doses of the OPV so as to prevent any untoward problem from OPV. By 1963, polio had already declined by some 99% in the United States, a fact that did not seem to attract much attention.

Efficacy of Trivalent OPV: Geographic Variations

The immune responses induced by vaccines are, in general, relatively uniform across various human populations, with rare exceptions. Hence, it was anticipated that children in all populations and countries would respond to OPV also in a satisfactory manner. That was not the case. As OPV was introduced in Africa and Asia in the early 1960s, response rates were lower than expected and several problems emerged. Potential reasons for this include low antibody response rates, loss of vaccine viability due to inadequate refrigeration, and possible interference by concurrent infection with other enteroviruses.

Inadequate refrigeration affects many vaccines and not just OPV, and this problem did not explain low antibody response rates when vaccine was properly shipped and stored. In addition, research has not shown that concurrent infection with other viruses is operant; indeed, no enterovirus other than poliovirus binds to PVRs, hence enterovirus interference has no biological plausibility. Investigations in the author's laboratory in the late 1960s and 1970s confirmed very low vaccine efficacy of OPV in India, particularly against types 1 and 3 polioviruses. Concurrent or antecedent infection with echo- or cox-sackie viruses did not affect the frequency of response. The problem was identified as low frequency of fecal virus shedding – the tell-tale sign of intestinal infection – of vaccine virus take. When a dose of tOPV was fed to Indian children, approximately 60–65% developed type 2 virus infection with an antibody response; roughly 25–30% responded to type 3, and 20–25% responded to type 1. The mean frequency of response to any poliovirus was 37–40% in South India, as against approximately 80% in the United States, South Africa, or Russia. Each additional dose improved the response rate according to an arithmetic proportional increment; thus in the Unites States, 16 of the remaining 20% would respond to the second dose and 3 of the remaining 4% would respond to a third dose, adding up to 99% with three doses of OPV. In India, a second OPV dose would seroconvert roughly 24% after the second dose and 14% after the third dose, for a total of 78% after three doses, lower than the 80% seroconversion with one dose in the United States. With five doses, the response would be 92%, lower than that of two doses in the United States. To achieve 99% response, it would take (theoretically) nine doses of OPV. This anomaly was first reported in South India in 1972 and since then vaccine-failure polio has been found to be widespread in many developing countries, especially in the tropical and subtropical zones. This striking variation in immune response to a vaccine was unprecedented and of uncertain reason. It was clear that the variation was geographical – with varying response frequencies in different locales – the worst in heavily populated communities with very poor sanitation and hygiene.

Perhaps the world's lowest OPV efficacy is in the adjacent northern Indian states of Uttar Pradesh and Bihar. A team of WHO officials determined the per-dose efficacy of tOPV against type 1 poliovirus as just 9%, with the protective efficacy after three doses only 24% (Grassly et al., 2006). Thus, children fully vaccinated with the WHO-recommended three OPV doses were inadequately immunized. Consequently, the majority of children with polio in recent decades were by definition fully immunized yet still susceptible, and consequently innumerable children had suffered paralytic polio that could have been prevented with additional OPV doses or the use of IPV. As an oral vaccine without the need of injection, it would have been very easy to give five to seven doses of OPV during infancy, thus protecting at least the majority of vaccinated children. When seroconversion rates to three doses of fully potent tOPV are measured, the problem becomes clear, in that 20–30% of vaccinated children remain without antibody responses against types 1 and 3 polioviruses, yet more than 90% seroconvert to type 2. Thus the problem is the biological response to the type 1 and 3 components of the vaccine, not the vaccine's potency. Unlike IPV where the immune response is of the prime-boost type, with OPV the vaccine viruses have to infect the child before an immune response can occur. Should infection fail to occur, then no protective antibody will develop and the child remains susceptible to polio. Each additional dose of OPV infects some more children, reducing their immunity gap.

In contrast to the experience in India and other developing countries, nearly all children seroconvert to all three serotypes of poliovirus in North America, Europe, Japan, and Australia with three doses of the balanced tOPV. Thus, the reputation of tOPV in all rich nations (with low birth rates and good sanitation and hygiene) is that it is highly efficacious with three doses. There have not been any cases of polio in children in rich countries if they have received three doses of OPV.

When poliovirus transmission was interrupted in Brazil in 1990, the mean number of OPV doses consumed by under-5 children was nine. In India, only when the mean number of doses reached or exceeded nine did the transmission of type 2 wild virus cease, later followed by cessation of type 1 and type 3 transmission in most states. Recently, it has been shown that there are locations in India where the per-dose vaccine efficacy is approximately 10% where wild-type 1 transmission continued, even after the mean number of OPV doses in under-5 children reached 15. The very low vaccine efficacy of OPV has been identified as the major reason for the inability to interrupt poliovirus transmission even in 2007, which is 7 years after the target year for global eradication.

The reason for this geographic variation in vaccine efficacy does not appear to be genetic or ethnic, but is apparently related to gastrointestinal factors associated with poor environmental sanitation and personal hygiene, as other theories relating to the cold chain and concurrent infections have been eliminated.

Attempts to Improve the Vaccine Efficacy of OPV

Four methods have been tried to improve vaccine efficacy (VE) of OPV in developing countries. The first was to increase the virus content of each OPV dose tenfold, which increases seroconversion rates, but at least three doses are still required to achieve very high response frequencies, and the cost of production also rises. By doubling the type 3 virus content in tOPV, marginally better response rates were obtained; however, this new-formulation OPV was unsuccessful in eliminating type 3 poliovirus transmission in parts of India where it continues to circulate in 2007. Moreover, the safety of enhanced potency OPV has not been established.

The second method was to simply increase the number of doses given to each child. Since each dose acts as an infectious inoculum, those who did not get infected previously get another chance each time the vaccine is given. In developing countries, at least five doses must be given as primary series, requiring at least five contacts between a health worker and the infant, which fortunately fits within the schedule for the global EPI. Countries such as Oman and Taiwan, and the Tamil Nadu state in India, which adopted this schedule rapidly, controlled polio and even interrupted wild virus transmission.

The third method has been to give the three doses of OPV over an 8-week period (4 weeks between doses) in annual drives, or pulses. Rather than improving vaccine efficacy, this method improves the inhibitory herd effect of OPV on the wild poliovirus transmission in the community. After the pulse, the speed of wild virus circulation slows down and for a period of time all children enjoy low incidence; by the time this effect wears down, the next annual pulse is due. The principle here is that pulse vaccination reduces the size of the susceptible pool of children by a sharp short vaccination effort. Unfortunately, this method has not been widely accepted by any country. A hidden advantage of pulse vaccination is that the remaining 10 months are available for the health staff to improve the performance of EPI in the community.

The fourth approach, currently widely practiced in Asia and Africa, is to give monovalent OPV, which avoids the intertype interference seen with tOPV. Since type 2 wild virus has been eliminated from circulation globally, mOPV-1 or mOPV-3 can be used where type 1 or 3 wild virus is still circulating. The infection rate for a specific type of mOPV is higher than what would occur for that specific type when given in tOPV. In its rebirth, mOPV type 1 is made with 10^6 $CCID_{50}$ per dose (the same as in tOPV), whereas the original had only 10^5 $CCID_{50}$, potency. Thus two improvements are combined in this approach: One, monovalent vaccine to avoid competition by other types, and two, enhanced potency to improve infection frequency.

Intertype Interference Between OPV Vaccine Viruses

As the infection rate of each poliovirus type is lower when given as tOPV than as mOPV, this phenomenon indicates that some form of intertype interference occurs. The reason for this is not understood. The site of infection of orally fed OPV polioviruses appears to be at the Peyer's

patches of ileum, as PVRs are found on the M cells of Peyer's patches but not elsewhere in the small intestinal mucosa. Although over 10^5 virus particles of each type are fed in a dose of OPV, and there are innumerable M cells in the ileum, actual take does not occur every time vaccine is fed, and for unknown reasons type 2 infection is more common than type 1 or 3. However, when mOPV type 1 or 2 is given, the take rate improves to the level of type 2 in tOPV, suggesting some degree of PVR competition by the three types, with type 2 most successful. The idea of a balanced tOPV preparation arose out of this observation: The formula of 10:1:3 was originally set for the proportions of the three types in tOPV, but later it was changed to 10:1:6 to improve the type 3 take rate.

In tropical settings where the take rates are low, there is yet another curious phenomenon. When children seroconvert to one type, they are more likely to seroconvert to another type, than those who did not. This has been interpreted to suggest that the intertype interference is weaker than the inhibitory factor(s) already present in the intestines of tropical children. In other words, if one type is able to reach the site with PVR, overcoming the barrier of the inhibitory factor(s), then another type is more likely to reach that site.

Safety of OPV: Vaccine-Associated Paralytic Polio

When IPV was introduced in the United States in 1955, there was concern about incomplete inactivation of virus particles, which in fact plagued the very early commercial batches of IPV when it was first licensed. When OPV was licensed (with the strong recommendation of the American Medical Association), the general belief was that it was completely safe as intra-spinal-cord injection did not cause paralysis in monkeys. However, soon after OPV licensure, suspicion arose among public health officials that children were developing paralytic polio within one polio incubation period, or vaccine-associated paralytic polio (VAPP). An expert committee examined all evidence on cases that had occurred within 24 months of the introduction of OPV and concluded that VAPP cases were temporally associated with OPV administration, but there was no laboratory test then available to prove such association to be causal. Today there is ample laboratory evidence proving that such cases are indeed caused by one or another of the three OPV viruses.

This problem was further examined by another WHO expert committee, which came to the conclusions that OPV does induce polio in a rare child given OPV; the frequency is geographically nonuniform; VAPP occurs not only in OPV-vaccinated children but also in children who directly or indirectly acquired vaccine virus infection from vaccinated children. Such VAPP in unvaccinated children is called contact VAPP to distinguish it from VAPP in vaccinated children. WHO estimates that developing countries using OPV may have an annual total of 250–500 cases of VAPP.

As OPV contains live infectious viruses, it is no surprise that they may, albeit rarely, spread to susceptible children near the vaccinated child. If transmission occurs beyond that second generation into a state of widespread circulation, the viruses would have regained two characteristics reduced drastically but not completely during attenuation, namely neurovirulence and transmissibility. Since OPV is fed by mouth and infection is in the intestines, the term enterovirulence is sometimes applied to the infection efficiency. Vaccine-derived virus that has regained enterovirulence may cause sporadic or epidemic polio. Such outbreak-associated viruses are named circulating vaccine-derived polioviruses (cVDPV). Episodes of cVDPV-caused polio outbreaks have occurred in Egypt, Dominican Republic and Haiti, Madagascar (thrice), Philippines, China, Indonesia, the United States, Nigeria, and Myanmar. All of them except the one in Egypt have been detected since 2000, suggesting that such episodes may be anticipated at the frequency of at least one per year as long as OPV is in use anywhere. Declined or declining coverage with OPV (leaving more susceptible children) seems to set the stage for its emergence/evolution. Continued use of OPV at very high coverage is the necessary deterrent against cVDPV.

Individuals with B cell defects and consequent immunodeficiency are prone to two adverse events with OPV. They have significantly more risk of VAPP, and some of them develop chronic infection and may continue fecal shedding of vaccine-derived poliovirus with increased neurovirulence over months or years. Such viruses are called immunodeficiency-associated VDPV (iVDPV). There has been one instance in which an iVDPV strain spread to several children, thus acting like cVDPV, showing that any VDPV is a potential source for transmission, circulation, and consequent polio outbreak.

Genetics of Wild and Vaccine Viruses

When Sabin developed attenuated strains of polioviruses by laboratory cultivation under selected conditions, only phenotypic differences were known between wild and vaccine viruses. Vaccine polioviruses did not grow well above 39 °C, whereas wild polioviruses grew efficiently at 40 °C. Plaque sizes were larger for wild than vaccine strains. Wild viruses caused severe inflammation, neuronal death, and paralysis in monkeys inoculated by intraspinal cord vaccination, whereas vaccine viruses did not cause any of them.

Subsequent knowledge regarding viral genetics has explained some of these phenotypic differences, sometimes even identifying the exact genetic changes associated with the attenuation. A single nucleotide G → A substitution at position 480 (in the 5′ untranslated or noncoding) region (UTR) is sufficient to render the Sabin type 1 strain neurovirulent in the monkey and in the transgenic mouse model. Similarly, A → G substitution at position 481, and U → C substitution at position 472 in 5′ UTR are critical for regaining neurovirulence for Sabin types 2 and 3, respectively. In addition, there are 56 other nucleotide substitutions distinguishing the wild parent and attenuated Sabin type 1, but only a few of them appear to contribute to the attenuation phenotype. Among the three types of Sabin strains, type 1 is the least likely to revert to neurovirulence. For types 2 and 3 just one additional mutation is also contributory to attenuation; hence these types tend to show genetic reversion more often than type 1. Type 3 revertants are commonest in vaccinated VAPP cases, whereas type 2 revertants are more common among contact VAPP cases.

The Global Eradication of Poliomyelitis

The Concept and Definition of Polio Eradication

Human mastery over infectious diseases takes several forms, such as specific etiologic diagnosis, specific therapy against the pathogen, and prevention (all at individual level) as well as control (community level, large or small), elimination (country or regional level), eradication or extinction (global level). Eradication is achieving and maintaining zero infection incidence worldwide by targeted intervention against the pathogen, such that there should be no risk of infection even in the absence of any intervention, particularly vaccination. The biologic criteria for eradicable infectious diseases include lack of a nonhuman reservoir, availability of intervention tactic or tool to reduce its reproductive rate (mean number of infections generated from one infected individual) to below 1 over time and also the availability of diagnostic tool(s) to monitor progress and certify eradication. To date, the only precedent for eradication is smallpox using smallpox vaccination and case-monitoring as intervention tools; there is no precedent for extinction (as smallpox virus, *variola* is held in viable form in frozen state in at least two countries). Currently, another disease is under eradication efforts – the parasitic disease Guinea worm ulcer (dracunculiasis) – here its transmission between the definitive and intermediate hosts is targeted for interruption such that eradication will also mean extinction as the life cycle is interrupted.

Eradication requires wide political support, cooperation of all affected countries, and a willingness to pay for the costs of eradication efforts by affording agencies. Rightly or otherwise, these prerequisites were fulfilled for polio, setting the stage for the goal of the global polio eradication initiative created during the second half of the 1980s.

History of the Eradication Effort and Its Progress

A global effort to eradicate poliomyelitis is currently under way. After the introduction of IPV and OPV, and the establishment of national vaccination programs during the late 1950s and early 1960s, all polio disappeared in countries using IPV, and polio due to wild (natural) polioviruses disappeared in some countries using OPV. Vaccine-induced polio (VAPP) continued to occur at very low incidence level. By the mid-1980s, some 68 countries were wild-polio-free, while 125 countries remained endemic (with periodic outbreaks). In the western hemisphere, wild-type polio outbreaks had been eliminated or drastically reduced in incidence, due to good national vaccination programs. In Asia and Africa, polio remained mostly uncontrolled despite the availability of the vaccines and attempts to adhere to the WHO-designed Expanded Program of Immunisation (EPI) which was established between 1974 and 1978. The failure to control polio was a stark reminder of the lack of success of EPI, but instead of fixing that problem, polio was singled out for a global onslaught in the 125 polio-endemic countries. That decision was not made by any special global public health think tank, but it was arrived at through serendipity.

In 1984, Rotary International (RI) resolved to provide financial assistance to all developing countries to purchase and give five doses of OPV to all under-5 children. This commitment started in 1985, so as to enable the world to achieve an undefined polio-free world by 2005, the centenary of RI's establishment. Polio was a highly visible and evocative problem of children of special concern to the Rotary movement, as many members of RI were involved in rehabilitation of the disabled in Asian and African countries.

Assured of financial assistance by RI, the Pan-American Health Organization (PAHO, the regional WHO body for the Americas) resolved to eliminate polio in the Americas by 1990, and established vaccination and monitoring systems to achieve the same. Where polio occurred despite high routine vaccination rates in South and Central America, two annual OPV campaigns for all under-5 children were conducted, irrespective of prior vaccination. Clinical and virological surveillance was also established to monitor progress and finally to certify elimination in the Americas. While PAHO was on the road to success, the WHO had to address the reality of uncontrolled polio in Africa and Asia. WHO designed a global polio eradication goal and plan of action in 1988, with a target date of 2000. A global polio eradication initiative (GPEI) was established by the WHO, with participation by the UN, WHO, UNICEF, the U.S. Centers for Disease Control and Prevention, and RI and a total direct budget of US$2 billion.

The WHO and CDC provided technical guidance and also design of interventions including vaccination and monitoring of progress; WHO, UNICEF, and RI participated in implementation of action in developing countries that needed assistance; all partners raised funds from rich-country governments, bilateral aid agencies, and philanthropic organizations. In many developing countries, the costs of vaccine delivery and other logistical support (utilizing health system institutions and personnel) were met by the governments themselves, assisted by the partners in GPEI.

The Overall Global Polio Eradication Strategy

The following four-item overall strategy was adapted from PAHO:

1. To reach and maintain consistent high routine vaccination coverage in infancy and early childhood;
2. To offer supplementary vaccination by large-scale campaigns;
3. To establish adequate clinical and virologic surveillance to effectively monitor progress and the ultimate success;
4. To provide local-level, small-scale mop-up vaccination when stray instances of persistent virus occurred.

While transplanting the PAHO experience to Asia and Africa, attention was not paid to certain details. GPEI ignored the strengthening of EPI and the poor vaccine efficacy of tOPV, and went ahead with the remaining three elements of the eradication strategy. This approach was successful in most countries or regions with reasonably high routine immunization coverage, but failed where routine coverage was extremely low, such as in Nigeria and Uttar Pradesh and Bihar states in India, where, even in 2007, the task of eradication remains unfinished. In retrospect, had routine coverage (where low) been improved through strengthening EPI, these eradication failures might have been avoided.

The world's last wild poliovirus type 2 was isolated in Uttar Pradesh, India, in October 1999, and can now be considered globally eradicated. As mentioned above, the vaccine efficacy of tOPV is very high against type 2 wild virus, which accounts for the success against that type. This picture shows that adequate vaccine coverage with tOPV could have interrupted all transmission, if only the vaccine had satisfactory vaccine efficacy. The delay in interrupting transmission of types 1 and 3 wild viruses in India is also in part due to very low vaccine efficacy of tOPV against these two virus types.

By 2000, the Western-Pacific–East-Asia and European regions were also declared polio eliminated (in addition to the Americas), leaving only Southeast Asia, Eastern Mediterranean, and African regions with some endemic polio (types 1 and 3). In total, 119 of the original 125 polio-endemic countries had achieved elimination status, with just six remaining endemic for polio, namely, India, Pakistan, and Afghanistan in Asia and Egypt, Nigeria, and Niger in Africa. By 2005, Egypt and Niger eliminated polio, leaving just four countries with some loci or the other with wild virus transmission. As of 2007, types 1 and 3 continue to be endemic in these four countries.

The Risk of Importation of Polioviruses from Endemic to Polio Free Countries

Although only Nigeria, India, Pakistan, and Afghanistan continue to be endemic for polio types 1 and 3, the wild poliovirus type 1 has traveled to territories that had earlier eliminated them. Such importation has occurred in neighboring countries (e.g., from India to Nepal, Bangladesh and Myanmar; from Nigeria to Niger, Chad, Sudan, Ethiopia, and Somalia) and also to distant continents (e.g., from India to Angola, Namibia, and Central African Republic of Congo; from Nigeria to Yemen and Saudi Arabia, and from the latter to Indonesia; from Pakistan to Australia). Some countries had only sporadic cases after importation, while others had widespread outbreaks. Thanks to the high-quality surveillance system, these importations were quickly identified and quelled with supplementary OPV (tOPV or mOPV-1). Where the outbreaks were large (e.g., in Yemen, Indonesia, and Bangladesh), OPV campaigns in under-5 children, covering the entire country, had to be conducted on average seven times in order to dislodge the virus. The current target of the GPEI is to interrupt transmission of wild viruses in these four countries in 2008. Since 2005, Saudi Arabia insists on proof of recent polio vaccination for *Hajj* pilgrims, especially from currently or recently polio-affected countries. From 2007–08, wild poliovirus will be counted a globally notifiable infection, in order to minimize the probability of intercountry transmission.

The Posteradication Global Scenario: How It Will Be Defined and the Potential Role of IPV

As mentioned earlier, the working definition of eradication is zero incidence of infection pertaining only to the wild polioviruses. As long as live virus vaccine (OPV) is used, VAPP, cVDPV, and iVDPV may continue to occur; hence, true eradication has been redefined as zero incidence of infection with wild and vaccine polioviruses. This requires discontinuing the use of OPV, but stopping is also not without risk. Most cVDPV outbreaks have occurred where the coverage of OPV, especially in multiple doses per child, had declined. Abrupt stoppage will result in a period of time when vaccine-shedding children and unvaccinated children (new birth cohorts) would

overlap and if vaccine virus gets into the latter group, potentially cVDPVs will develop.

The current plan of the GPEI is to stockpile large amounts of mOPVs, so that any cVDPV outbreak could be immediately doused. On the other hand, many experts believe that reintroduction of OPV into the community after it had been withdrawn is too risky and perhaps even unethical for that reason. They have proposed a transition into using IPV in the EPI system, to achieve high (over 80%) coverage in infants, and then and then only to withdraw OPV.

The prospects of introducing IPV on a large, even global, level may be improving, as there is renewed interest in IPV in many countries. Earlier in this article, the countries using exclusively IPV were listed. With increasing demand, newer vaccine manufacturers are gearing up for increasing production and supply. After resisting registering (licensing) of IPV in India for five decades (for reasons elaborated earlier), the national regulatory authority in India has licensed it as of June 2006, signaling a change in perception regarding the two vaccines. Virtually all of Europe has begun using IPV and has stopped the entry of OPV in their territories. The IPV has been licensed in several Asian and a few Latin American countries and is gaining popularity in the private sector health-care system. IPV seems to be the vaccine of the future.

Discontinuation of Polio Immunization After Eradication

By definition, eradication is qualified by the absence of any further need of intervention, as the pathogen does not exist in human communities or the environment. Thus the world discontinued smallpox vaccination once it was eradicated and thus certified in 1978. Indeed, the economic benefit of not vaccinating against the disease is one major incentive for the investment of the cost of eradication. For polio, the savings have been calculated at $1 billion per annum if the world stopped all polio immunization. Since the GPEI journey began, the world has changed in some ways due to terrorism. There are some issues that worry world experts in this regard.

Obviously, immunization (using IPV) has to be continued until all risk from cVDPV is gone, a few to several years after discontinuing OPV. Most likely, IPV will be used as a combination vaccine with DPT, Hib, and HBV. Within the overall cost of a national immunization program, the additional cost of IPV in such combination form will be so small that it will not be as attractive a saving for a country. In view of the lurking fear of the use of wild poliovirus as a weapon of bioterrorism, the self-perceived vulnerable countries are unlikely to stop IPV. Even if all stocks of wild and vaccine strains of polioviruses are destroyed (extinction, an unlikely event), polioviruses can be synthesized in the laboratory because its genome is small and its sequence is known. Therefore the threat of deliberate introduction will remain real in the current world scenario of confrontational politics between various incompatible ideologies and military approaches to resolve them. If one is forced to predict, the likelihood is that all rich nations will continue to opt for IPV while some low-income countries may discontinue it.

By describing the history and science behind the historic events surrounding the development of polio vaccines, we hope that these lessons can be applied to the challenges of the future.

Citations

Grassly NC, Fraser C, Wenjer J, et al. (2006) New strategies for the elimination of polio from India. *Science* 314: 1150–1153.

Melnick JL, Benyesh-MelnickPena R, and Yow M (1961) Effectiveness of Salk vaccine: Analysis of virologically confirmed cases of paralytic and nonparalytic poliomyelitis. *Journal of the American Medical Association* 175: 1159–1162.

Stickle G (1964) Observed and expected poliomyelitis in the United States, 1958–1961. *American Journal of Public Health* 54: 222–229.

Further Reading

Heymann D (2006) Global polio eradication initiative. *Bulletin of the World Health Organization* 84: 595.

John TJ (2004) The golden jubilee of vaccination against poliomyelitis. *Indian Journal of Medical Research* 119: 1–17.

Jublet B and Agre JC (2000) Characteristics and management of postpolio syndrome. *Journal of the American Medical Association* 284: 412–414.

Kew O, Sutter R, de Gourville E, and Pallansch M (2005) Vaccine-derived polioviruses and the endgame strategy for global polio eradication. *Annual Review in Microbiology* 59: 587–635.

Relevant Websites

http://www.polioeradication.org – About global polio eradication.

http://www.cdc.gov/doc.do/id/0900f3ec802286ba – About polio and vaccination.

Rabies

H Wilde, S Wacharapluesadee, T Hemachudha, and V Tepsumethanon, King Chulalongkorn Memorial Hospital, Bangkok, Thailand

Introduction

Rabies is usually transmitted to humans by dog or bat bites, and is uniformly fatal. The virus, a single-stranded RNA Lyssavirus, invades nerves en route to the brain. The bite site and severity and the inoculum size are determinants of the infection risk and incubation period. Immediate wound cleansing and the prompt use of anti-rabies immunoglobulin and rabies vaccine are life-saving. Older vaccines are being replaced by safe, effective, and less costly tissue culture products. New reduced-dose intradermal administration schedules have made them more affordable (Wilde *et al.*, 1999). Elimination of canine rabies in uncontrolled dog populations represents a major public health challenge.

Epidemiology

Extent of the Disease and Routes of Transmission

Rabies is generally transmitted through the bite of an infected mammal to another mammal. Rabies is believed to be capable of infecting all mammals. Both historically and currently, rabies was and is transmitted to humans primarily by canines, as well as by agriculturally important species such as cattle, horses, and sheep. Unless prevented by the measures described below, death inevitably results when the infection reaches and destroys its target, the central nervous system.

Rabies, and closely related Lyssaviruses, can be found throughout the world except in Greenland, Antarctica, and some isolated islands. Australia, previously considered rabies-free, harbors a Lyssavirus in fruit- and insect-eating bats, which causes a fatal rabies-like illness in humans (Warrilow, 2005) (**Figure 1**). Regions with large unsupervised dog populations present the greatest risk, since canines are the principal route of infection to humans. Vampire bat rabies in Central and South America is a hazard to humans and cattle. Worldwide rabies reporting is incomplete. The number of annual human deaths is unknown but is thought to be well over 50 000. Nearly 50% of these deaths are in children. They are less able to defend themselves against biting animals than adults, and are more likely to be bitten on high-risk body parts such as the face, head, and hands (WHO, 2005).

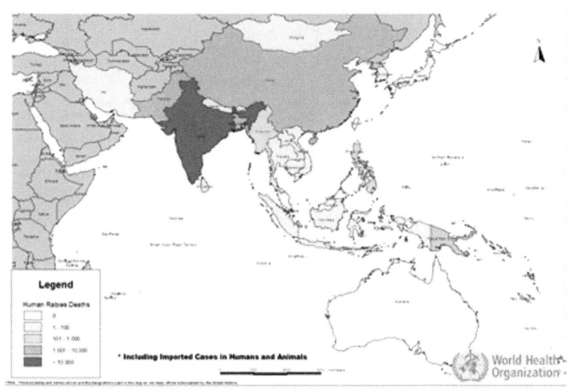

Figure 1   Human rabies deaths (2004). Source: World Health Organization (2004), with permission from Dr Fx Meslin.

Rabies is responsible for more deaths than polio, yellow fever, Japanese encephalitis, SARS, or meningococcal meningitis. India alone had an estimated 30 000 annual rabies deaths during past decades. Pakistan estimates over 5000 (Wilde *et al.*, 2005). Rabies is emerging again in China, which was virtually rabies-free during the reign of Mao Zedong. Japan, Taiwan, Malaysia, Singapore, and South Korea eliminated canine rabies decades ago. No other Asian countries have succeeded in doing so. Rabies can also be transmitted through the inhalation of bat secretions (e.g., in people exploring caves that house bats) and, rarely, through the transplantation of infected tissues. Rabies has also occurred in people who have bats in their homes without a history of bites.

New Lyssaviruses are Being Discovered

There may still be undetected bat Lyssaviruses related to classical rabies virus in many parts of the world. Bats do not often interact with people, but transmission to humans and pets has been documented in The Americas, Europe, and Australia. Indigenous bat Lyssaviruses have now been identified in the Philippines, Thailand, Siberia, Central Asia, and Cambodia, as well as in Australia. The United Kingdom, previously considered rabies-free, recently experienced a human death from a European bat Lyssavirus.

Importance of Animal Vector Control

Dogs, cats, and other mammalian rabies vectors are occasionally transported from rabies-endemic regions to rabies-free ones. The recent introduction of rabies by Indonesian fisherman to previously rabies-free Flores Island resulted in an ongoing rabies outbreak with over 100 human deaths (**Figure 2**). Recreational hunters in the 1990s in the eastern United States unknowingly transported rabid raccoons from Florida to a hunting reserve, which led to a widely reported epidemic of rabies, with many animal and some human deaths that traveled up the East Coast of the United States. Thus, in order to eliminate rabies expansion through animal transport, animal control measures within countries and at national boundaries must be maintained.

Canines remain the most important animal vector for transmission of rabies to humans. We know virtually all that is needed to eliminate canine rabies, but cultural, political, and economic barriers have prevented implementation. Sustained vaccination of over 70% of the canine population can control rabies. In order to regularly vaccinate a large canine population, given their short life spans and rapid reproduction rates, canine numbers must be made manageable. This can only be done when societies and governments are motivated to enforce vaccination regulations and to reduce stray dog populations (**Figure 3**). It requires funding, legislation, and energetic enforcement. The World Health Organization (WHO) publishes detailed guidelines for human and veterinary professionals (WHO, 2005). Hindu and Buddhist countries have religious barriers to some control measures. These will have to be overcome by developing humane means of canine population control and education toward responsible pet ownership. Some efforts in this direction are now underway by the WHO, enlightened animal rights organizations, and governments.

Oral vaccination of foxes with bait containing vaccine has virtually abolished fox rabies in Europe. Efforts are being made in North America to apply this to foxes, skunks, and raccoons. There is as yet no strategy for controlling rabies in bats and most wildlife.

Clinical Diagnosis of Rabies

Rabies generally presents in one of two forms, 'furious' (**Figures 4** and **5**) or 'paralytic' (**Figure 6**). Diagnosis of canine and feline rabies is not difficult when it is of the furious form. Irritability, aggression, increased salivation, indiscriminate biting, and damaged and inflamed oral structures are obvious signs of the disease. The paralytic form of rabies (approximately 30% in dogs) presents diagnostic problems. The clinical picture is similar to other infections such as canine distemper. Euthanasia and histological examination of the animal's brain is not always possible or available, and it is best to start post-exposure prophylaxis (PEP) immediately in a possibly exposed human if rabies is suspected. A free interactive computer program can aid in the clinical diagnosis of canine rabies (www.soonak.com).

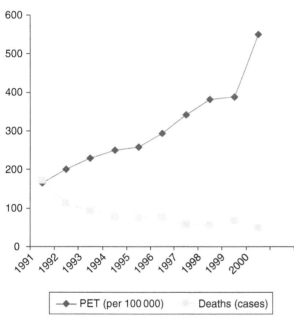

Figure 2 Human rabies deaths and PET per 100 000 population in Thailand.

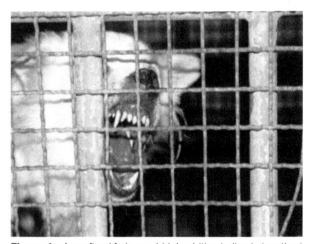

Figure 4 A confined furious rabid dog biting indiscriminantly at the cage.

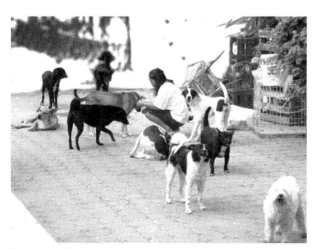

Figure 3 Street scene in Bangkok showing citizen feeding stray dogs, the main reservoir of rabies in southeast Asia.

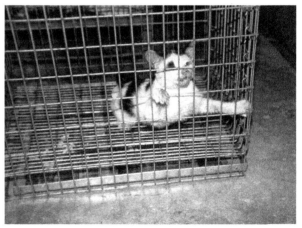

Figure 5 A cat with furous rabies. Such an animal can inflict incredibly severe wounds to several people when found at a market. All will become full-blown cellulites within hours.

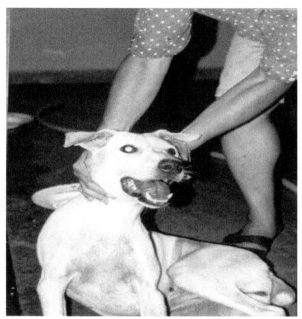

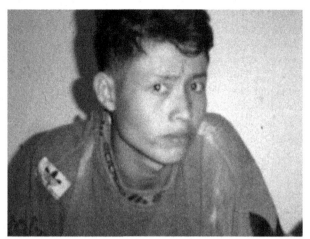

Figure 7 This anxious looking young man is seen in the OPD where he presented with fever, headache, some phobic spasms and aerophobia. He was bitten by a street dog 18 days earlier and had no treatment. He died within 3 days of encephalitic rabies.

Figure 6 A dog with paralytic rabies. It looks pitiful and several persons can become exposed to saliva in attempts to hand-feed such an animal.

The 'furious' human form is characterized by a prodrome manifesting as a feeling of impending doom, pain, or abnormal sensation in or near the bite site (Hemachudha *et al.*, 2002) (**Figure 7**). It is seen in 70% of cases. Other symptoms may be vague, such as anxiety, fever, headache, muscle aches, or even diarrhea. This is followed by the neurological phase, consisting of alternating intervals of agitation, aggression, and coherent calmness. Within a few days, coma ensues with respiratory failure, leading to rapid demise unless life is prolonged by intensive cardiopulmonary support. Several cases of humans surviving this stage have been reported, but they are the very rare exception, and there are only two long-term survivors known. Hydrophobic and aerophobic spasms of the neck and diaphragm may occur intermittently and may not appear together (**Figures 8** and **9**). Autonomic dysfunction may start early but usually becomes prominent in the neurological phase with excessive salivation, fluctuating blood pressure, cardiac arrythmia, pupillary dysfunction, and neurogenic pulmonary edema. Hallucinations and seizures are not usual in dog-related cases but are frequently seen in bat rabies (Hemachudha *et al.*, 2002).

One-third of human cases present as the paralytic form resembling Guillain-Barré syndrome (GBS), due to a different host response to the infection (not to differences in the infecting virus). It is difficult to diagnose without experience and sophisticated laboratory help. Nerve electrophysiological studies are identical to those seen with GBS, and thus efforts to identify the virus or its RNA in sputum, urine, tissues, or cerebrospinal fluid

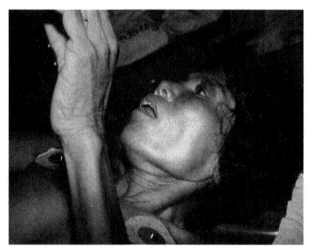

Figure 8 Patient with furious rabies. Note contracted muscles in neck due to phobic spasms. She lived for 2 weeks in the ICU with cardio-pulmonary support but died of multisystem failure. PCR of saliva was positive but she never showed antibodies in her CSF.

may be required to confirm the diagnosis. Phobic spasms can be seen in only half of paralytic cases. Survival time is shorter in the furious form than in the paralytic form (mean of 5 versus 11 days). Rabies can also present in atypical ways, particularly when associated with bat exposure. Rabies must be considered in any patient presenting with unclear encephalopathy. Use of illicit or 'recreational' drugs, medications, or alcohol may mislead clinicians. Rapid deterioration to coma suggests rabies. Constant rigidity of muscles is the hallmark of tetanus. Acute hepatic porphyria can be excluded by appropriate tests. A history of recent animal encounters (which may be absent in cryptic bat cases), fever, muscular paralysis with

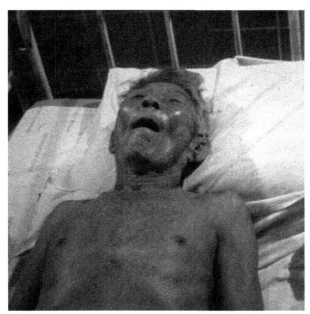

Figure 9 A near-terminal patient with furious rabies. He was fanned and shows facial and neck-muscle spasms.

preserved consciousness and intact sensory function, urinary incontinence, percussion myoedema, inspiratory spasms, and respiratory failure suggest paralytic rabies (Hemachudha *et al.*, 2002, 2005; Jackson, 2006).

Rabies awareness is inadequate in non-endemic countries. This became evident from recent transplantation-related cases in Germany and the United States. One case was diagnosed as drug abuse-related psychosis and the other as drug intoxication and a possible subarachnoid hemorrhage. The history that the former person had just returned from India having experienced a dog bite and that the latter had been bitten by a bat were not elicited or were disregarded. They were used as tissue donors for 10 recipients, of which 7 died of rabies. Interestingly, one of the survivors was a liver transplant recipient who had been previously vaccinated against rabies and had an anamnestic rabies-neutralizing antibody response.

Laboratory Diagnosis

The most secure method of diagnosis is by examination of brain tissue. Antemortem laboratory diagnosis of rabies in animals is not recommended since distribution of virus in organs may be variable, and shedding in saliva, urine, and spinal fluid is intermittent. Postmortem brain examination needs to demonstrate rabies antigen by direct fluorescent antibody (DFA) test, immunohistochemistry, or molecular methods. The DFA test is the gold standard; indeed, there were no false-negative results in a prospective study of 8987 brain impression smears (Tepsumethanon *et al.*, 1997). Brain tissue, dried on filter paper, can be kept at

room temperature for many days for rabies virus RNA detection. These techniques are available in many tertiary care centers and referral laboratories. To be of clinical value, results must be rapidly available, sensitive, and specific, since they will contribute to evidence-based postexposure prophylaxis decisions for exposed patients. In contrast to the above-mentioned methods, detection of classical Negri bodies in histopathological specimens is neither sensitive nor specific. Knowledge of the genetic sequences of rabies virus is useful for epidemiological surveillance and the study of transmission dynamics, as there are strains of rabies that circulate predominantly in foxes, bats, and other species.

Rapid antemortem laboratory diagnosis in humans is important for formulating ethical and rational management decisions (Hemachudha and Rupprecht, 2004). Reverse transcription polymerase chain reaction (RT-PCR) and other diagnostic molecular techniques can be performed, with results known within a day. Saliva, cerebrospinal fluid, urine, hair follicles, and tears should be used simultaneously owing to the intermittency of virus secretion. Negative results require repeat testing when there is a clinical suspicion of rabies. Brain imaging studies such as computerized tomography (CT) or magnetic resonance imaging (MRI) are most useful in excluding other diseases. MRI findings are usually localized to the brainstem, hippocampus, and hypothalamic regions, but are not sufficiently unique to make a specific diagnosis of rabies, they may be normal early after onset of clinical symptoms.

Brain necropsy can be done via the superior orbital fissure using a kidney or liver biopsy needle. It is invaluable when a complete necropsy is impossible.

Postexposure Prophylaxis (PEP)

The principles of postexposure prophylaxis (PEP) are (1) to cleanse the bite wound and (2) to provide the bite victim with antibodies to the rabies virus. Antirabies antibody prevents the virus from infecting cells and prevents death if virus is present before nerve cell invasion occurs.

PEP requires immediate cleansing of bite wounds with flowing water and soap and later with antiseptic agents. Washing with water may decrease the size of the virus (inoculum), while soap and antiseptic agents may denature the virus, thus preventing infection. This is followed by risk evaluation and the administration of a course of tissue culture vaccine (see **Table 1**). It takes 7–10 days for a significant level of vaccine-induced natural antibody to form. Unfortunately, this may leave sufficient time for the virus to invade peripheral nerve cells. Once inside nerve cells, it cannot be reached by antirabies antibody and can travel through the nerve cell centrally to the

Table 1   Guide for rabies postexposure prophylaxis

Category: Type of contact with a suspected or confirmed rabid domestic or wild animal, or animal not available for observation	Recommended treatment
I Touching or feeding animal, licks over intact skin	No treatment if reliable history[a]
II Nibbling over uncovered skin, minor scratches or abrasions without bleeding, licks on broken skin	Administer vaccine immediately;[b] stop treatment if animal healthy 10 days later or if animal examined and found rabies-free by laboratory tests
III Single or multiple transdermal bites or scratches, contamination of mucous membranes by saliva (licks)	Administer rabies immunoglobulin and vaccine immediately;[c] stop treatment if animal remains healthy for 10 days or if animal is euthanized and found negative for rabies by appropriate laboratory tests

[a]A history obtained from a small child may be unreliable.
[b]If an apparently healthy dog or cat is from a low rabies risk area and is placed under close observation, it may be justified to delay specific treatment. This observation period applies only to dogs and cats. Except in the case of threatened or endangered species, other domestic or wild animals should be euthanized and their tissues examined using appropriate laboratory techniques. Exposure to rodents, rabbits, and hares seldom, if ever, requires specific antirabies treatment.
[c]Immunoglobulin is administered into and around the bite sites.
Modified from WHO (2005) *WHO Expert Consultation on Rabies, First Report*. Technical Report 931. Geneva: WHO.

brain. Passive immunity must therefore be provided as soon as possible after the bite by aggressively injecting antirabies immunoglobulin (RIG) into and around the bite wounds to neutralize virus (WHO, 2005). Immunoglobulin, if injected intramuscularly at a distant site from the wound, is nearly useless. This was first reported in 1963 and was recently confirmed in our laboratory. A vaccine series is then started to induce active immunity with host antibody production. Consultation with an expert is mandatory when unusual problems are encountered. Various RIG preparations are available, as discussed below. PEP is costly and often substandard in many endemic regions of the world, and thus prevention through vector control is both more cost-effective (WHO, 2005) and efficacious.

Delay in starting PEP must be avoided at all cost. Rabies incubation periods may be as short as a few days or as long as many years, depending on the site of the bite, host factors, and size of the inoculum (Hemachudha and Rupprecht, 2004). **Table 1** summarizes the approach to rabies-exposed patients. It is best to initiate PEP unless immediate laboratory studies of the responsible animal exclude rabies. If the animal is observed and later found free of the virus, the vaccine series can be discontinued. There are no contraindications to rabies PEP (WHO, 2005). An infected wound can be injected safely with RIG as long as antibiotics are also used to treat bacterial infection. A vaccine history in the responsible dog is not an absolute justification for not providing PEP to a bite victim, unless the vaccination has been thoroughly documented and more than one annual dose had been administered.

Table 2 lists current WHO-recognized vaccines, which are tissue and avian culture products, as well as some older preparations derived from animal neuronal tissues, which had the potential to induce autoimmune neurological syndromes. Additional modern vaccines are now appearing from India, China, and South America.

Table 2   Rabies vaccines

- HDCV France, Germany, Canada, India
- PVRV France, India, Columbia, China
- PCEC Germany, India, Japan
- PDEV Switzerland, India
- PHKC China, Russia, central Asian republics
- SMB *South America, Vietnam, Cambodia*
Boldfaced entries are WHO-recognized products.
Black entries are recognized locally only.
Italic entries are WHO-condemned products.

HDCV, human diploid cell vaccine; PVRV, purified vero cell rabies vaccine; PCEC, purified chick embryo cell vaccine; PDEV, purified duck embryo vaccine; SMB, suckling mouse brain vaccine; Semple, semple sheep brain-derived vaccine.

WHO has approved four postexposure vaccine schedules using tissue culture vaccines (WHO, 2005). These are:

1. The 'gold standard' Essen Regimen, which consists of one intramuscular full-dose injection on days 0, 3, 7, 14, and 28 after the exposure;
2. The Zagreb regimen, which consists of two full-dose intramuscular injections on day 0 and one dose each on days 7 and 21;
3. The Thai Red Cross Intradermal Regimen, which consists of two injections of 0.1 mL of any WHO-recognized tissue culture vaccine at two different lymphatic drainage sites on days 0, 3, 7, and 28; and
4. The Oxford Intradermal Regimen, which consists of one injection of 0.1 mL of any WHO-recognized tissue culture vaccine at eight different body sites on day 0, at four sites on day 7, and at one site on days 28 and 90.

Intramuscular injections of vaccine must be administered in the deltoid or lateral thigh regions, avoiding fat. Intradermal vaccines are injected into arms or legs and, in the case of the Oxford Regimen, into the abdominal and intrascapular regions. The appearance of a split-skin 'bubble' at the injection site demonstrates successful intradermal and not subdermal administration (as in tuberculin testing). Reduced-dose intradermal PEP (schedules 3 and 4) significantly decrease the cost of vaccination and are used at rabies control clinics of several developing countries. Many studies have shown equivalent immunogenicity and efficacy (WHO, 2005). WHO-recognized tissue culture vaccines have excellent safety records. Adverse reactions with tissue culture vaccines are minor and equivalent to those seen with Expanded Program for Immunization (EPI) vaccines such as those against polio, mumps, and measles. Transient erythema, discomfort, and itching at injection sites as well as mild regional lymphadenopathy are reported with injections. Mild transient fever, headache, and malaise are also seen. Human diploid cell rabies vaccine (HDCV) and, very rarely, other tissue culture vaccines may cause mild serum-sickness-like reactions in individuals who have had a prior rabies series and are later given frequent boosters. These are not due to the viral components of the vaccine (Fischbein *et al.*, 1993).

Vaccines alone will protect the vast majority of exposed patients, but it is not possible to predict which victim will die if not given passive immunization with RIG. The provision of passive immunity to protect severely exposed patients during the first critical days can be life-saving. Patients with facial, head, and hand bites are at the highest risk of death, and they represent a high-priority group if RIG immunoglobulin is in short supply (**Figure 10**). The original unpurified equine or sheep serum-derived antisera had a deservedly bad reputation for serum sickness and anaphylaxis. Second-generation, highly purified equine antirabies immunoglobulins (ERIG) contain whole IgG molecules. They have an acceptable safety margin, causing only 1–7% serum sickness reactions, depending on the product and batch.

An effort was then made to reduce the serum sickness rate by further purification and splitting the antibody using pepsin digestion. This reduced the serum sickness rate only slightly. We have, however, become aware of several cases of treatment failure where split equine or human IgG products were used. Human rabies immunoglobulin (HRIG) appears to be as effective as the whole IgG ERIG and has virtually no adverse reactions. It is, however, in extremely short supply and is very expensive, and therefore is not available where it is needed the most, as in poorer rabies-endemic countries. A new equine product has been chromatography-purified, pepsin-digested and heat-inactivated. It is safe, but its efficacy is controversial. Several new manufacturers of ERIG have emerged in Thailand, India, South America, and China. Some products are undergoing WHO preapproval studies and may appear on the international market in the near future. In our view, it is unfortunate that most of these are pepsin-digested split IgG products. Monoclonal rabies antibody technology has emerged and monoclonal antibodies have been found to be safe and highly effective in animal experiments, and are now undergoing human studies. It will take time for such products to become commercially available. HRIG and ERIG must remain on the WHO essential drug list until we have a safe, effective and affordable monoclonal product commercially available (Goudsmit *et al.*, 2006).

Pre-Exposure Vaccination (PREP)

Human and equine rabies immunoglobulins are not available in many rabies-endemic regions, and PEP is often not carried out to WHO standards. Pre-exposure prophylaxis (PREP) is therefore recommended for travelers, workers in certain occupations who are likely to come in contact with infected animals, and laboratory workers exposed to Lyssaviruses. One study from Thailand showed that 9% of tourists had unanticipated or unwanted canine contact, suggesting that vaccination of tourists to endemic regions should be more widely considered. Recent studies have demonstrated that immunity following WHO-recommended tissue culture vaccine injections is very long-lasting. One study showed that neutralizing antibodies can be detected as long as two decades after completing a PREP or PEP series. Booster injections then result in an accelerated antibody response. WHO recommends one intramuscular or intradermal booster injection on days 0 and 3 in an individual who has experienced a possible rabies exposure after having had a reliable history of PREP or PEP with a WHO-recognized tissue culture rabies vaccine (WHO, 2005). An alternate method is to administer intradermal injections of 0.1 mL vaccine at four sites (deltoid and

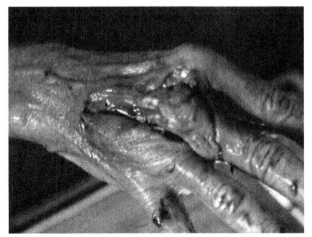

Figure 10 The hand of an elderly housewife bitten by a street dog she tried to feed and which escaped. She required two tendon repairs after wound-care and injection of all wounds with diluted immunoglobulin.

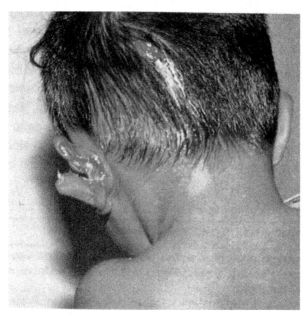

Figure 11 Dog bite in a child. They are often bitten on the head, face, and hands and represent almost half of the worldwide human rabies deaths.

lateral thigh) at one sitting. This saves clinic costs and travel time but has not yet been WHO-approved. Laboratory scientists at high risk of rabies, such as those working with potentially rabid animals or live virus, are still advised to have either periodic antibody titer determinations or a booster every 5 years. Some diplomatic missions, nongovernmental organizations, military, and UN teams recommend PREP for their staff when transferred to rabies-endemic countries.

Many countries are failing to control canine rabies. Since children represent half of rabies deaths (WHO, 2005), this has led to suggestions to include rabies vaccine as part of the childhood EPI in high-risk regions. Cost–benefit considerations and priority of funds for other vaccinations have, however, prevented implementation (**Figure 11**).

Management of Human Rabies

Treatment of human rabies was the subject of a Canadian and U.S. CDC-sponsored conference in Toronto in 2002. The expert consensus was that only comfort care should be provided, given the uniformly fatal prognosis (Jackson *et al.*, 2003). Intensive curative efforts should be reserved for a time when promising new technologies become available. We have as yet no known proven antiviral agents against Lyssaviruses. However, the survival of a 15-year-old girl, bitten by a bat who had not received PEP, has created hope. Treatment consisted of intensive care and induced deep coma with ketamine and benzodiazepine to

lessen excitotoxicity as well as ribavarine. This patient was unusual in that she had neutralizing antibodies on admission in both serum and spinal fluid but no demonstrable viable virus or viral RNA. Her case was similar to the other survivor, a 6-year-old (reported in 1972), who had a bat bite and early antibodies in serum and spinal fluid. He was treated with supportive care only and made a full recovery. His virus could not be isolated, either. These bat-derived agents could have been of less virulence, or both subjects may have managed to mount an unusually rapid and aggressive immune response that controlled their disease. By way of example, we recently treated a rabies patient who received the coma induction regimen with ketamine and ribavarine, never developed neutralizing antibodies, and died of multisystem failure on the eighth hospital day. Ample virus was identified throughout his hospital course. Approximately 25% of our dog-related human patients developed serum-neutralizing antibodies regardless of the form of rabies. However, none had neutralizing antibodies in CSF. Similar coma-induction regimens have been applied to 11 other patients in the United States, Europe, Asia, and Canada without success.

Acknowledgments

This work was supported in part by a grant from The National Center for Genetic Engineering and Biotechnology of Thailand. The authors have no conflicts of interest to declare.

Citations

Fischbein DB, Yenner KM, Dreesen DW, *et al.* (1993) Risk factors for systemic hypersensitivity reactions after booster vaccinations with human diploid cell rabies vaccines, a nationwide prospective study. *Vaccine* 14: 1390–1394.

Goudsmit J, Marissen WE, Weldon WC, *et al.* (2006) Comparison of an anti-rabies human monoclonal antibody combination with human polyclonal anti-rabies immune globulin. *Journal of Infectious Diseases* 15(193): 796–801.

Hemachudha T and Rupprecht C (2004) Rabies. In: Roos K (ed.) *Principles of Neurological Infectious Diseases*, pp. 151–174. New York: McGraw Hill

Hemachudha T, Wacharapluesadee S, Lumlertdaecha B, *et al.* (2002) Human rabies: A disease of complex neuropathogenetic mechanisms and diagnostic challenges. *Lancet Neurology* 1(2): 101–109.

Hemachudha T, Wacharapluesadee S, Mitrabhakdi E, Wilde H, Morimoto K, and Lewis RA (2005) Pathophysiology of human paralytic rabies. *Journal of NeuroVirology* 11: 93–100.

Jackson AC (2006) Rabies: New insights into pathogenesis and treatment. *Current Opinion in Neurology* 19(3): 267–270.

Jackson AC, Warrell MJ, and Rupprecht CE (2003) Management of rabies in humans. *Clinical Infectious Diseases* 36(1): 60–63.

Tepsumethanon V, Lumlertdacha B, Mitmoonpitak C, *et al.* (1997) Fluorescent antibody test for rabies: Prospective study of 8987 brains. *Clinical Infectious Diseases* 25: 1459–1461.

Warrilow D (2005) Australian bat lyssavirus: A recently discovered new rhabdovirus. *Current Topics in Microbiology and Immunology* 292: 25–44.

WHO (2005) *WHO Expert Consultation on Rabies, First Report*. Technical Report 931. Geneva, Switzerland: WHO.

Wilde H, Khawplod P, Khamoltham T, *et al.* (2005) Rabies control in South and Southeast Asia. *Vaccine* 23: 2284–2289.

Wilde H, Tipkong P, and Khawplod P (1999) Economic issues in post-exposure rabies treatment. *Journal of Travel Medicine* 4: 238–242.

Relevant Websites

http://www.rabiescontrol.org – Alliance for Rabies Control.

http://www.soonak.com/AIRE.htm – Artificial Intelligence Rabies Expert (software to assist with the diagnosis of rabies).

http://www.cdc.gov/rabies – Centers for Diseases Control, Rabies.

http://www.who.int/globalatlas/default.asp – WHO, Global Health Atlas.

http://www.who.int/rabies – WHO, Human and Animal Rabies.

http://www.who.int/rabnet – WHO, Rabnet, Human and Animal Rabies, An Interactive and Information Mapping System.

http://www.who.int/zoonoses – WHO, Zoonoses and Veterinary Public Health.

Seizure Disorders

S C Schachter, Harvard Medical School, Boston, MA, USA

Introduction

Epilepsy is a common and often debilitating neurological disorder among persons of all ages and socioeconomic backgrounds. Epilepsy is unique inasmuch as its full impact on the affected individual extends beyond seizures, the primary symptom of epilepsy, to include associated cognitive, behavioral, affect, interpersonal, cultural, and societal aspects. While current medical therapies successfully eliminate seizures in up to two-thirds of patients, a substantial proportion of persons with epilepsy have inadequate seizure control and a disproportionate psychosocial burden. This article provides an overview of the epidemiology of epilepsy, how it is diagnosed and treated, the psychosocial aspects associated with epilepsy, and challenges for improving the health and well-being of persons with epilepsy in developing countries.

Epidemiology of Epilepsy

Epilepsy is one of the most common neurological disorders and has been recognized since antiquity. An estimated 2 to 4 million people in the United States have epilepsy, including 1 of 50 children, 1 of 100 adults, and 1 million women of childbearing age (Hauser and Hesdorffer, 1990; Devinsky and Yerby, 1994). In addition, 200 000 new cases are diagnosed every year. In 2000, the annual cost of epilepsy in the United States was reported as $12.5 billion (Begley *et al.*, 2000). Worldwide, approximately 50 million persons have epilepsy, the majority of whom cannot afford or do not have access to appropriate medical therapy.

Epilepsy can develop at any age, though a disproportionate number of cases begin in the young and elderly. Because the prevalence of epilepsy among the elderly is steadily increasing in many countries as their population ages, it has been predicted that within a few decades more than half of the patients in developed countries who develop epilepsy will be over the age of 65. Contributing factors to the onset of epilepsy in this age group are Alzheimer's disease and other degenerative conditions of the central nervous system, cerebrovascular disease, brain tumors, head injuries, and alcohol or drug abuse.

Epilepsy is not benign and is associated with an increased risk of mortality. Causes of death among persons with epilepsy include accidental deaths (for example, drowning), sudden and unexplained death in epilepsy, status epilepticus (a condition of repeated seizures without recovery), underlying brain disease (such as brain tumors), and suicide. People with uncontrolled seizures are also at increased risk for injuries, such as bone fractures and burns.

Diagnosis and Medical Management

A seizure is a sudden change in behavior that may or may not be apparent to others. Not all sudden changes in behavior are seizures, and not all seizures are epileptic seizures. Whereas epileptic seizures result when the electrical activities of neuronal networks in the brain suddenly become hypersynchronized, non-epileptic seizures resemble epileptic seizures but actually reflect the response of an otherwise normal brain to a systemic physiological change, the behavioral manifestations of a psychiatric disorder, or other neurological conditions besides epilepsy. Consequently, while all patients with epilepsy have seizures, the converse may not be true. The most common causes of non-epileptic seizures are syncope (fainting); transient global amnesia (a condition characterized by prolonged loss of recent memory); metabolic disorders, including hyponatremia, hypoglycemia, and hypocalcemia; movement disorders, generally referred to as paroxysmal dyskinesias; sleep disorders; panic attacks; and psychogenic seizures, which are usually attributed to stressful psychological conflicts or major emotional trauma, such as sexual or physical abuse in childhood, a death, or divorce (**Table 1**). Of these conditions, non-epileptic seizures resulting from syncope and psychogenic causes are perhaps the most difficult to differentiate from epileptic seizures.

The purpose of the initial medical evaluation of a patient who has had his or her first seizure is to exclude other conditions that cause non-epileptic seizures and to determine if there is an underlying brain lesion, as assessed by computed tomography (CT) or magnetic resonance imaging (MRI). Initial laboratory studies include glucose, calcium, and magnesium levels, hematology, renal function tests, and toxicology screens. Electroencephalograms (EEGs) are helpful to support a diagnosis of epilepsy and to help classify a patient's epileptic seizure type as generalized or partial, as discussed below. However, initial EEGs may be normal in over half of patients with epilepsy.

Epilepsy is operationally defined as the tendency for a person to have recurrent epileptic seizures. The causes of epilepsy vary according to the age at onset of epilepsy, and include congenital brain malformations, inborn errors of metabolism, brain trauma, brain tumors, stroke, intracranial infection, vascular malformations, and cerebral degeneration. However, up to half of patients with epilepsy do not have an identifiable underlying cause when evaluated with currently available diagnostic tests.

Epilepsy is usually diagnosed after a patient has had two or more epileptic seizures. The goals of therapy are to treat the underlying cause, if known and if remediable to treatment, and to completely suppress further seizures from occurring without causing troublesome side effects from the therapy. Antiepileptic drugs (AEDs) are the

Table 1   Commonly occurring nonepileptic seizures

Breath-holding attacks (infants and children)
Cerebrovascular disease
Migraine and head pains
Movement disorders
Nonepileptic myoclonus
Psychiatric disorders
Sleep disorders
Syncope (fainting)
Toxic-metabolic or infectious states

Adapted from Brodie MJ, Schachter SC, and Kwan P (2005) *Fast Facts–Epilepsy*, 3rd edn. Oxford, UK: Health Press.

primary form of seizure-suppression therapy, and must be taken on a daily basis. Initial treatment achieves seizure freedom in up to 70% of patients, but prognosis for seizure control in the other 30% of patients is less favorable. These patients usually require numerous trials of AEDs, either as monotherapy or combination therapy, often require higher AED dosages, and typically must endure daily side effects. Such patients are said to have medically intractable epilepsy and may be candidates for adjunctive nonpharmacological treatments, including vagus nerve stimulation, brain surgery, special diets, stress reduction techniques, or investigational drugs or brain stimulation devices. Patients with medically intractable seizures require frequent visits to health-care professionals and periodic reassessment with EEGs and MRI scans, particularly if there is progressive worsening of the patient's neurological examination or cognitive function, or an increase in seizure frequency or severity. For all these reasons, the human and financial costs associated with medically intractable epilepsy are much greater than when epilepsy readily comes under control with initial therapy or goes into remission.

Physicians usually select an AED according to the patient's seizure type, which in turn is based on the description of the seizure as obtained from the patient and/or eyewitnesses. Other considerations for selecting an AED are the pharmacokinetic profile of the drug, the patient's age and comorbid medical and psychiatric conditions, whether the patient is a woman of childbearing potential, the potential for adverse effects and drug–drug interactions, and cost. With the exception of medical emergencies, therapy is usually initiated with a low dose and increased slowly until seizures are completely controlled, or until bothersome side effects occur that persist, at which time the dose is lowered to minimize side effects.

The two main seizure types are generalized and partial seizures, as shown in **Table 2**. Generalized seizures affect both sides of the brain simultaneously when the seizure begins and are usually not associated with identifiable brain pathology. Absence seizures, myoclonic seizures, and generalized tonic-clonic seizures are among the subtypes of generalized seizures.

- Absence seizures cause the sudden onset of staring with impaired consciousness. They typically begin in childhood, last between 5 to 10 s, and may occur dozens if not hundreds of times a day, particularly in association with boredom and hyperventilation. Up to 90% of patients undergo a spontaneous remission of their epilepsy before reaching adulthood.
- Myoclonic seizures consist of sudden, brief, shock-like contractions affecting the arms, legs, face, or trunk, often occurring in the early morning.
- Generalized tonic-clonic seizures (also called grand mal seizures or convulsions) may begin with a loud

Table 2 Classification of seizure types

I. Partial seizures
    A. Simple partial seizures
    B. Complex partial seizures
        1. Simple partial seizures at onset, followed by impairment of consciousness
        2. With impairment of consciousness at onset
    C. Partial seizures evolving to secondarily generalized seizures
II. Generalized seizures
    A. Absence seizures
    B. Myoclonic seizures
    C. Clonic seizures
    D. Tonic seizures
    E. Tonic-clonic seizures
    F. Atonic seizures

Adapted from Commission on classification and terminology of the International League Against Epilepsy (1981) Proposal for revised clinical classification of epileptic seizures. *Epilepsia* 22: 489–501.

noise or scream. The arms and legs then stiffen (tonic phase), the patient falls to the ground, and the patient's lips and skin appears dusky (cyanotic). After 60 to 90 s, the arms and legs start to jerk (convulse), eventually in unison, for an additional 1 to 2 min (clonic phase). Bloody, frothy sputum may be seen coming from the mouth. After the clonic phase ends, the patient appears to be in a deep sleep, and then wakes up gradually over minutes to hours, often sleepy, confused and complaining of a severe, throbbing headache.

At their onset, partial seizures affect a restricted area of cortex (the outer layer of the brain) and usually suggest the presence of an underlying brain lesion, whether or not apparent on CT or MRI scans. Symptoms that patients with partial seizures experience when the seizure begins may not be apparent to others and are called simple partial seizures – 'simple' meaning that consciousness is not impaired. Patients may refer to these symptoms as auras or warnings, and they may include nausea, fear, jerking of one side of the body, or a metallic taste. Many other symptoms may occur with simple partial seizures as well. Other patients do not have a conscious warning at the start of their partial seizures and abruptly lose consciousness. This type of partial seizure is called a complex partial seizure – 'complex' meaning that consciousness is impaired. Complex partial seizures (known in the past as temporal lobe seizures and psychomotor seizures) are the most common type of seizure experienced by adults with epilepsy. During complex partial seizures, patients typically appear awake but do not meaningfully interact with people or objects around them and do not respond normally to instructions or questions. They appear to stare and either remain still or demonstrate repetitive nonpurposeful behaviors (called automatisms), such as chewing, lip smacking, repeating words or phrases, aimless walking

or running, or undressing. If patients are forcibly restrained or redirected during complex partial seizures, they may become aggressive. Complex partial seizures typically last less than 3 min and may be immediately preceded by a simple partial seizure or followed by a tonic-clonic seizure. After complex partial seizures, patients may appear confused or somnolent, and may complain of a headache. Because their consciousness is impaired, patients have no memory of what happened during complex partial seizures.

Besides identifying the type(s) of seizure a patient has, clinicians determine whether a patient has an identifiable epilepsy syndrome, which is defined by specific seizure types, age of epilepsy onset, family history, response to particular AEDs, and prognosis.

The number and availability of pharmacological (AED) and nonpharmacological treatment options for patients with epilepsy have steadily increased over the past 10 to 20 years, as briefly described below. Successful use of AEDs requires detailed knowledge of their pharmacodynamic and pharmacokinetic properties, an understanding of the pertinent published safety and efficacy studies, and individualized therapy to a particular patient. Recently published guidelines from the American Academy of Neurology and the American Epilepsy Society for the use of the newer AEDs in the treatment of new-onset and medically refractory seizures are based on published studies of efficacy, tolerability, and safety in adults and children (French *et al.*, 2004a, 2004b). However, there are numerous clinical situations requiring an AED treatment decision for which there are few if any relevant clinical studies. In such circumstances, expert opinion can provide some direction to the clinician. The most recent compilation of expert opinion was based on data obtained in 2004 from 48 American epilepsy specialists covering all of the newer AEDs except for pregabalin (Karceski *et al.*, 2005).

To be effective, AEDs must enter the brain; consequently, AEDs often cause dose-related side effects that are due to brain dysfunction, such as sleepiness, trouble with balance, or double vision. Side effects are a major cause of medication intolerance and noncompliance, particularly within the first 6 months of therapy.

If a trial of the first AED is unsuccessful either because seizures are not controlled or side effects are bothersome, then a second AED, also appropriate for the patient's seizure type(s), is prescribed. The second AED is usually titrated to a tolerable and effective dosage before the first AED is tapered and stopped, unless the first AED caused a side effect requiring immediate discontinuation. While it is preferable to maintain a patient on a single AED rather than AED combinations because of enhanced compliance, lower medications costs, and generally fewer complications, some patients have better seizure control on combinations of AEDs than on individual drugs.

The selection of AEDs for women of childbearing potential is particularly important because all AEDs can potentially cause birth defects, especially when taken in combination. The overall risk of birth defects in the offspring of women with epilepsy who take an AED is approximately twice the expected rate, and risks are higher with combination therapy. The most frequently occurring birth defects are neural tube defects, cleft lip and palate, heart defects, and reduced brain size. Physicians often recommend that women on AEDs take between 0.4 and 4 mg/day of folic acid for a prolonged period before conceiving to reduce the risk of birth defects, but the health benefits of this practice to the fetus have not been proven in this population.

Currently available AEDs suppress the occurrence of seizures, but there is no evidence that they cure epilepsy or prevent the onset of seizures in patients at high risk, such as those who suffer a serious brain injury. Therefore, patient adherence to the AED dosing schedule on a daily basis is crucial for maintaining seizure control. Failure to take medications as prescribed can lead to an increase in seizures and/or medication side effects. Causes of noncompliance include memory lapses, complicated AED regimens, denial of illness, and fixed incomes. Patients must be educated about the importance of regularly taking seizure medication.

Primary care physicians or emergency room physicians often make the initial diagnosis of epilepsy and begin therapy. Patients are often referred to neurologists for further diagnostic evaluation and additional therapeutic trials if seizures do not respond to initial therapy, or to assess the feasibility of withdrawing AEDs if they have been seizure-free for 2 or more years. Epileptologists are neurologists who specialize in epilepsy, and are usually located at centers that have access to investigational treatments and sophisticated surgical procedures for the evaluation and treatment of medically intractable epilepsy. The psychosocial consequences of epilepsy, described later, may require the involvement of other specialists, such as psychiatrists, psychologists, neuropsychologists, social workers, and vocational counselors.

Antiepileptic Drugs

Antiepileptic drugs vary based on their mechanisms of action on brain neurons, the seizure type(s) they effectively control, pharmacokinetic properties, side effect profile, teratogenicity, and propensity for drug–drug interactions.

Carbamazepine (CBZ) blocks voltage-dependent sodium channels on neuronal membranes, thereby preventing neurons from firing as rapidly as needed to sustain a seizure. CBZ is used for partial seizures and generalized tonic-clonic seizures, and should be initiated at 100 to 200 mg daily and increased by 100 to 200 mg every 3 to 14 days as needed for seizure control, typically over a period of 1 to 2 months. Common side effects are double vision, headache, dizziness, and nausea and vomiting, which can be lessened by use of a controlled-release formulation. Other possible side effects include mild or serious rashes and reversible decreases in white blood cells. Potentially fatal effects on bone marrow or liver are fortunately very rare. CBZ can cause birth defects, including spina bifida. One of the difficulties in administering CBZ arises from its effects on increasing the metabolism of other drugs; hence, drug–drug interactions are common.

Ethosuximide (ESM) works by reducing calcium currents in neurons of the thalamus, a deep nuclear structure in the brain. ESM is a first-line treatment for patients with absence seizures. The usual starting dose is 250 to 500 mg daily, with 250-mg dose increments over 2 to 3 weeks as needed for seizure control. Side effects are infrequent and include hiccups, nausea and vomiting, abdominal pain, lack of appetite, headache, dizziness, drowsiness, and unsteadiness. Allergic rashes occur infrequently.

Felbamate (FBM) has several mechanisms of action and is effective against partial seizures as well as generalized seizures that occur with a particularly severe epilepsy syndrome in children called the Lennox-Gastaut syndrome. As with other AEDs, dosing is advanced slowly to minimize side effects, which include insomnia, headache, nausea and vomiting, loss of appetite, sleepiness, weight loss, and dizziness. FBM is associated with an elevated risk of potentially fatal bone marrow suppression and hepatitis. While routine monitoring of liver and blood counts is recommended, the results do not predict potentially fatal toxicity. Consequently, FBM is now primarily used in patients with Lennox-Gastaut syndrome, and only when the benefits of treatment are judged to outweigh the risks. FBM can affect other drugs by increasing their metabolism in the liver.

Gabapentin (GBP) binds to voltage-gated calcium channels on neurons, inhibiting the flow of calcium ions, and is effective against partial seizures. The usual starting dose is 300 mg daily, which is increased by 300 mg every 3 days as needed for seizure control to the maximum tolerated dose. Typical side effects are drowsiness, dizziness, weight gain, fluid retention, and trouble with balance. GBP has no known effects on other drugs. Because GBP is excreted by the kidneys, dosage requirements for patients with kidney dysfunction are less.

Lamotrigine (LTG), like CBZ, blocks voltage-dependent sodium channels on neuronal membranes and is effective against partial seizures and generalized tonic-clonic seizures. Dosing is initiated at 25 to 50 mg daily, and increased slowly to reduce the likelihood of rash, especially in patients who also are taking valproate. Common side effects are rash, headache, nausea and vomiting, insomnia, dizziness, double vision, trouble with balance, and tremor. Severe, potentially life-threatening, skin reactions occur in up to 1 in 1000 adults and 1 in 100 children. Recent data from a pregnancy registry suggest an increased risk to babies of isolated cleft lip or palate when LTG is taken during the first trimester of pregnancy.

Levetiracetam (LEV) affects the currents of two inhibitory neurotransmitters in the brain – GABA and glycine – although whether these actions account for the mechanism of action of LEV is unclear. It is effective against partial and generalized seizures, including myoclonic and absence seizures. The starting dosage is 500 to 1000 mg daily, which is increased by 1000 mg every 2 weeks as tolerated and needed for seizure control. Patients with kidney dysfunction require lower dosages. Side effects include somnolence, headache, lack of appetite, nervousness, and, less frequently, agitation, aggression, anxiety, or depression. LEV has no effects on other drugs.

Oxcarbazepine (OXC) works similarly to CBZ and LTG on neuronal membranes. It is quickly metabolized in the body to an active metabolite. OXC is used to treat partial seizures and generalized tonic-clonic seizures. Dosage is started at 150 to 600 mg daily in adults and increased every 1 to 2 weeks as tolerated and as needed to control seizures. Side effects include drowsiness, dizziness, headache, double vision, nausea and vomiting, trouble with balance, and rash.

Phenobarbital (PB) amplifies the inhibitory effect of GABA on brain neurons and is used for partial seizures, generalized tonic-clonic seizures, and myoclonic seizures. PB is the least expensive AED, but is generally viewed as a second-line drug because many patients experience side effects, such as sleepiness, depression, and agitation. An intravenous form of PB is useful for seizure emergencies. Adult dosages range from 60 to 240 mg/day. PB has been associated with birth defects and drug–drug interactions.

Phenytoin (PHT) blocks voltage-dependent neuronal sodium channels and is used for partial seizures and generalized tonic-clonic seizures. An intravenous formulation is useful for seizure emergencies. Typical dose-related side effects are rash, trouble with balance, slurred speech, and sleepiness. Long-term use may cause swelling of the gums (gingival hyperplasia), hair growth, acne, thinning of the bones, and peripheral nerve dysfunction. Very serious side effects, such as hepatitis, bone marrow suppression, swelling of the lymph nodes, and a potentially fatal rash, are very rare. On the other hand, drug–drug interactions are common. Phenytoin has been associated with birth defects.

Pregabalin (PGB) works in a similar manner as GBP, and is effective for the treatment of partial seizures. The starting dose is 150 mg/day, with subsequent titration every week to an effective and tolerable maintenance dose. Common side effects are dizziness, sleepiness, headache, trouble with balance, weight gain, and peripheral fluid retention. PGB has no known effects on other drugs. Because PGB is excreted by the kidneys, target dosages for patients with kidney dysfunction are lower than in patients with normal kidney function.

Primidone (PRM) is converted by the liver to PB and another active compound. PRM is used for partial seizures and generalized tonic-clonic seizures, but it is considered a second-line treatment because of sedating side effects and reduced sex drive. The initial dose is usually 125 mg at bedtime, with 125 mg increments every 3 to 5 days as needed for seizure control and as tolerated. PRM causes drug–drug interactions.

Sodium valproate (VPA) has several mechanisms of action, and is effective for all seizure types. The initial dosage is 500 to 1000 mg/day, with subsequent titration as needed and tolerated. Tremor is a dose-related side effect; weight gain and hair thinning may also occur. Rarely, serious effects on platelet counts, the pancreas, and the liver may be seen. VPA has been associated with birth defects, especially neural tube defects. VPA inhibits the metabolism of a number of drugs, including PHT, PB, the primary metabolite of CBZ, and LTG; therefore, drug–drug interactions are common.

Tiagabine (TGB) augments the effects of the inhibitory neurotransmitter GABA and is used to treat partial seizures. Treatment commences with 4 to 8 mg daily, and the dosage is increased weekly or more slowly by 4 to 8 mg as needed for control of seizures and as tolerated. Side effects are related to daily dose and rate of titration, and include dizziness, fatigue, muscle weakness, nervousness, tremor, impaired concentration, lethargy, and depression. Drug–drug interactions may occur, and required doses are reduced in patients with significant liver dysfunction.

Topiramate (TPM) has several mechanisms of action and is used for partial seizures, generalized tonic-clonic seizures, and myoclonic seizures. Treatment is initiated at 25 to 50 mg/day and increased by 25 to 50 mg every 1 to 2 weeks as needed for seizure control and as tolerated. Side effects include a language disorder characterized by word-finding difficulty, slowing of cognition, trouble with balance, dizziness, fatigue, numbness and tingling, reduced appetite, and weight loss. Rare side effects include kidney stones, decreased sweating, and acute angle closure glaucoma. Drug interactions may occur, especially with hormonal contraceptives, PHT, and CBZ.

Zonisamide (ZNS) has several mechanisms of action and is used for partial seizures and generalized seizures. The starting dose is 100 mg daily for adult patients, which is usually increased every 2 weeks as needed and tolerated. Typical side effects are lack of appetite, dizziness, trouble with balance, fatigue, sleepiness, and confusion. Rare side effects include kidney stones and decreased sweating. Drug interactions may occur.

Nonpharmacological Therapies

Several nonpharmacological therapies are available for selected patients whose seizures do not satisfactorily respond to AEDs. These include brain surgery, vagus nerve stimulation, dietary approaches, such as the ketogenic diet and the modified Atkins diet, and a variety of stress-reduction techniques. Ongoing treatment with AEDs is generally maintained. Among the nonpharmacological therapies, brain surgery offers the greatest potential for complete seizure control, especially when seizure onset can be localized with sophisticated EEG testing to the inner part of the temporal lobe and when the underlying pathology is determined by brain imaging studies to be a condition known as mesial temporal sclerosis. With the exception of stress-reduction techniques, nonpharmacological therapies generally require extensive and expensive evaluations and are primarily offered at comprehensive epilepsy centers.

Psychosocial Aspects of Epilepsy

Patients with epilepsy often experience an unsatisfactory quality of life because of a variety of epilepsy-related psychosocial factors, such as stigma and psychiatric comorbidity.

Stigma adversely affects patients with epilepsy, especially those with difficult-to-control seizures, and particularly in developing, resource-poor countries. Perceived and enacted stigma impact on nearly all everyday activities of persons with epilepsy, such as attending school, driving, working, enjoying recreational activities, establishing social relationships, and obtaining insurance. Even patients who are seizure-free and well informed about their disorder may experience unemployment and underemployment, driving restrictions, difficulty obtaining life and health insurance, and social stigmatization.

Psychiatric comorbidity is common in patients with epilepsy. The most frequent associated psychiatric condition is depression, occurring in 10–20% of patients with controlled seizures and up to 60% of patients with medically intractable epilepsy. Depression is underdiagnosed and undertreated in patients with epilepsy, in part because of the largely unjustified concern that all antidepressant drugs could exacerbate seizures. Undertreatment is a major problem, because suicide is a frequent cause of death in patients with epilepsy, occurring up to 10 times more frequently than in the general population.

Up to 25% of patients with epilepsy have anxiety, most commonly in the form of a generalized anxiety disorder. The severity of anxiety may not correlate with seizure frequency. Ironically, severe anxiety may develop after a patient with epilepsy becomes seizure-free. Apart from having an anxiety disorder, living with fear is common among people with epilepsy and is often reported as 'the worst thing about having epilepsy' (Fisher *et al.*, 2000a, 2000b). Specific fears include dying from a seizure, public embarrassment, losing employment, and being involved in an automobile accident.

Reducing the Global Burden of Epilepsy

The recognition that epilepsy is a multifaceted disorder consisting of seizures, underlying brain dysfunction, and numerous psychosocial complications has prompted major efforts around the world to identify and overcome the barriers to optimum quality of life for persons with epilepsy.

Public health initiatives have sought to improve education about epilepsy among health-care practitioners, ministers, teachers, rescue personnel, and the general public. For example, epilepsy-related initiatives of the United States Centers for Disease Control and Prevention have focused on improving care; enhancing communication and combating stigma; self-management, disease surveillance and prevention research; increasing public awareness and knowledge; and strengthening partnerships with other organizations such as the Epilepsy Foundation (Schachter, 2001). Reducing stigma is the primary objective of Out of the Shadows, a global campaign of the International League Against Epilepsy, the World Health Organization, and the International Bureau for Epilepsy, but this effort can be particularly challenging among cultures that continue to view epilepsy as the result of supernatural forces, as was more pervasive centuries ago.

In addition to education, public health agencies are attempting to improve access to appropriate medical care for the millions of patients with epilepsy worldwide who currently have no access to treatment or cannot afford appropriate medications.

See also: Specific Mental Health Disorders: Depressive and Anxiety Disorders.

Citations

Begley CE, Famulari M, Annegers JF, *et al.* (2000) The cost of epilepsy in the United States: As estimate from population-based clinical and survey data. *Epilepsia* 41: 342–351.

Brodie MJ, Schachter SC, and Kwan P (2005) *Fast Facts–Epilepsy,* 3rd edn. Oxford, UK: Health Press.

Devinsky O and Yerby MS (1994) Women with epilepsy: Reproduction and effects of pregnancy on epilepsy. *Neurologic Clinics of North America* 12: 479–495.

Fisher RS, Vickrey BG, Gibson P, *et al.* (2000a) The impact of epilepsy from the patient's perspective I: Descriptions and subjective perceptions. *Epilepsy Research* 41: 39–51.

Fisher RS, Vickrey BG, Gibson P, *et al.* (2000b) The impact of epilepsy from the patient's perspective II: Views about therapy and health care. *Epilepsy Research* 41: 53–61.

French JA, Kanner AM, Bautista J, *et al.* (2004a) Efficacy and tolerability of the new antiepileptic drugs I: Treatment of new onset epilepsy: Report of the Therapeutics and Technology Assessment Subcommittee and Quality Standards Subcommittee of the American Academy of Neurology and the American Epilepsy Society. *Neurology* 62: 1252–1260.

French JA, Kanner AM, Bautista J, *et al.* (2004b) Efficacy and tolerability of the new antiepileptic drugs II: Treatment of refractory epilepsy: Report of the Therapeutics and Technology Assessment Subcommittee and Quality Standards Subcommittee of the American Academy of Neurology and the American Epilepsy Society. *Neurology* 62: 1261–1273.

Hauser WA and Hesdorffer DC (1990) *Epilepsy: Frequency, Causes, and Consequences.* New York: Demos.

Karceski S, Morrell MJ, and Carpenter D (2005) Treatment of epilepsy in adults: Expert opinion, 2005. *Epilepsy & Behavior* 7(Supplement 1): S1–S64.

Schachter SC (2001) Ongoing epilepsy program activities at the Centers for Disease Control and Prevention. *Epilepsy & Behavior* 2: 381–383.

Brodie MJ, Schachter SC, and Kwan P (2005) *Fast Facts–Epilepsy*, 3rd edn. Oxford, UK: Health Press.

Jacoby A, Snape D, and Baker GA (2005) Epilepsy and social identity: The stigma of a chronic neurological disorder. *Lancet Neurology* 4: 171–178.

Kanner AM and Barry JJ (2003) The impact of mood disorders in neurological diseases: Should neurologists be concerned? *Epilepsy & Behavior* 4(Supplement 3): 3–13.

Kwan P and Brodie MJ (2000) Early identification of refractory epilepsy. *New England Journal of Medicine* 342: 314–319.

Levy RH, Mattson RH, Meldrum BS and Perucca E (eds.) (2002) *Antiepileptic Drugs,* 5th edn. Philadelphia, PA: Lippincott Williams and Wilkins.

Loring DW, Meador KJ, and Lee GP (2004) Determinants of quality of life in epilepsy. *Epilepsy & Behavior* 5: 976–980.

Meinardi H, Scott RA, Reis R, and Sander JW (2001) The treatment gap in epilepsy: The current situation and ways forward. *Epilepsia* 42: 136–149.

Schachter SC (2006) Quality of life for patients with epilepsy is determined by more than seizure control: The role of psychosocial factors. *Expert Review of Neurotherapeutics* 6: 111–118.

Schachter SC and Andermann L (eds.) (2003) *The Brainstorms Village: Epilepsy in our World.* Philadelphia, PA: Lippincott Williams and Wilkins.

Wyllie E, Gupta A and Lachhwani DK (eds.) (2006) *The Treatment of Epilepsy.* Philadelphia, PA: Lippincott Williams and Wilkins.

Further Reading

Artama M, Auvinen A, Raudaskoski T, Isojarvi I, and Isojarvi J (2005) Antiepileptic drug: use of women with epilepsy and congenital malformations in offspring. *Neurology* 64: 1874–1878.

Asconape JJ (2002) Some common issues in the use of antiepileptic drugs. *Seminars in Neurology* 22: 27–39.

Barry JJ and Jones JE (2005) What is effective treatment of depression in people with epilepsy? *Epilepsy & Behavior* 6: 520–528.

Beyenburg S, Mitchell AJ, Schmidt D, Elger CE, and Reuber M (2005) Anxiety in patients with epilepsy: Systematic review and suggestions for clinical management. *Epilepsy & Behavior* 7: 161–171.

Boro A and Haut S (2003) Medical comorbidities in the treatment of epilepsy. *Epilepsy & Behavior* 4(supplement 2): 2–12.

Relevant Websites

http://www.epilepsy.com – Epilepsy.com.
http://www.epilepsyfoundation.org – Epilepsy Foundation.
http://www.who.int/mental_health/management/globalepilepsycampaigner – Global Campaign Against Epilepsy: Out of the Shadows.
http://www.ilae.org/ – International League Against Epilepsy.

Sleep Disorders

A Culebras, Upstate Medical University, Syracuse, NY, USA

Introduction

Sleep is a function of the brain. As such, sleep develops, matures, and declines in consonance with other functions of the brain. Sleep is a universal phenomenon exhibited by most vertebrates. The ultimate physiological function of sleep remains enigmatic and unknown despite extensive research of this ubiquitous brain activity. Sleep intervenes in functions of growth, regeneration, and memory. In the new classification of sleep disorders, more than 80 clinical sleep disorders are codified.

Experiments have shown that sleep deprivation causes an increasing constellation of brain alterations leading to death in lower mammals if prolonged sufficiently.

Severely sleep-deprived individuals have a strong tendency to fall asleep and appear slow when performing mental or motor tasks. Their motor responses are delayed, with increasing apathy, reduced motivation, decreased concentration, and poor memory as unavoidable microsleeps break the continuity of consciousness. Most individuals require between 6 and 8 h of sleep at night. In Mediterranean countries, the daytime siesta allows subtraction of an equivalent amount of time from nocturnal asleep.

Sleep is a preprogrammed function of the brain modulated by the circadian rhythm. In the adult individual, nocturnal sleep progresses in stages and cycles. In the first half of the night the four stages of nonREM sleep predominate, whereas in the second half, REM (rapid eye movement) sleep or dream sleep is more prevalent. The fetus spends much of its time in REM sleep and the infant shows a great abundance of REM sleep. By 2 years of age, sleep has become consolidated to the nocturnal period with approximately 25% of the total time asleep in REM sleep. In old age, total sleep requirements continue to be 6–8 h every 24 hours, but deep stages of non-REM sleep decline while REM sleep remains at 20–25% of total sleep.

The nocturnal evolution of sleep stages can be recorded with polysomnography, a technique central to the sleep laboratory that combines recording of brain waves, eye movements, electrocardiography, electromyography, respiratory motions, and saturation of oxygen. Videotaping of the individual asleep is an integral part of polysomnography.

Sleep is important in medicine because it influences quality of life, while its disorders provoke family pathology, disturb work routines, alter social activities, reduce quality of life, and affect the health of the individual. Sleep disorders are prevalent and pervasive. Excessive daytime somnolence may lead to motor vehicle accidents, poor academic performance, reduced work productivity, and social decline. Sleep disorders medicine counts with diagnostic tools centered in the sleep laboratory to diagnose sleep disorders, and sleep specialists can procure comprehensive management of most sleep afflictions.

Sleep research focuses in brain mechanisms and the consequences of sleep-related alterations. Over the years, landmarks in sleep research have included the discovery of changes in brain waves during sleep, the discovery of the sleep cycles and of REM sleep, the localization of REM mechanisms to the brainstem, and the discovery of hypocretin (also called orexin), a neurotransmitter necessary for alertness produced by the hypothalamus.

History

Sleep was often assumed to be a passive response to reduced cerebral stimulation during mental and cerebral inactivity. Berger's demonstration of changes in the electroencephalogram (EEG) during sleep provided the first definite evidence that the brain is not passive during sleep. In the twentieth century, studies of encephalitis lethargica, hypothalamic and thalamic stimulation, and the reticular activating system of the brain provided major advances in the understanding of the neuroanatomical substrate of sleep and wakefulness. The discoveries of rapid eye movement (REM) sleep, the association of dreaming with REM sleep, and the periodic cycles of REM and non-REM sleep throughout the night led to a new view of sleep as an active process with distinctive neurophysiological substrates underlying the two major sleep states, non-REM and REM sleep.

Physicians have known for centuries that sleep disturbance is often a sign of disease, but the recognition that primary sleep disorders are common, serious, and often treatable occurred mainly in the second half of the twentieth century. The first sleep clinics devoted specifically to diagnosis and treatment of a broad range of sleep disorders appeared in the 1970s. Also, in the United States, the Association of Sleep Disorders Centers, organized in 1975, provided a focus for development of the field of sleep disorders medicine. Subsequent major events included the publication of specialized journals. As the breadth of the field expanded, it became apparent that a nosology devoted to sleep disorders was required. The Association of Sleep Disorders Centers published the first classification of sleep disorders in 1979. A more comprehensive classification published by the American Sleep Disorders Association in 1990 as the International Classification of Sleep Disorders was revised in 2000, and updated in 2005 by the American Academy of Sleep Medicine (**Table 1**). By the end of 2006, 3445 professionals were diplomates of the American Board of Sleep Medicine (**Figure 1**). The first board exam on sleep given by the American Board of Medical Specialties took place in November 2007.

The Sleep Center

Patients with sleep disorders are evaluated by sleep specialists in sleep centers and tested in the sleep laboratory with polysomnography, a technique that records sleep parameters such as brain waves, eye movements, muscle tone, and breathing patterns. Sleep laboratory testing with nocturnal and daytime polysomnography is an indispensable procedure for the evaluation of patients with sleep-disordered breathing, pathological excessive daytime sleepiness, and complex motor disorders. Titration of positive airway pressure apparatuses can only be done in conjunction with polysomnography. Polysomnography involves at a minimum a full night stay in the sleep laboratory attended by properly trained technicians.

Laboratories accredited by the American Academy of Sleep Medicine use digital equipment and computer-assisted scoring techniques. Some night tests will be

Table 1   International Classification of Sleep Disorders

1. Insomnia
2. Sleep-related breathing disorders
3. Hypersomnias of central origin not due to a circadian rhythm sleep disorder, sleep-related breathing disorder, or other cause of disturbed nocturnal sleep
4. Circadian rhythm sleep disorders
5. Parasomnias
6. Sleep-related movement disorders
7. Isolated symptoms, apparently normal variants, and unresolved issues
8. Other sleep disorders

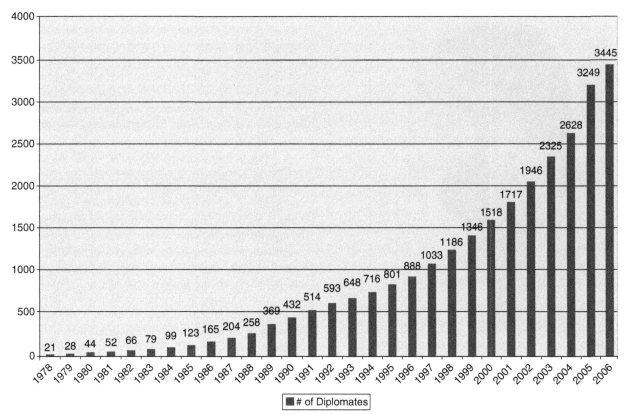

Figure 1 The number of diplomates of the American Board of Sleep Medicine has grown steadily over the years. Courtesy of American Academy of Sleep Medicine (2005) *International Classification of Sleep Disorders, 2nd edn. Diagnostic and Coding Manual*. Westchester, IL: American Academy of Sleep Medicine.

followed by daytime nap tests, also known as multiple sleep latency test (MSLT), or maintenance of wakefulness test (MWT). Patients report to the laboratory at 8.00 or 9.00 p.m. and are discharged the following morning at 8.00 a.m. or at 3.00–5.00 p.m. if a daytime test has been recorded. Scoring is usually done by a trained technician and the interpretation is carried out by the physician.

Actigraphy is a technique used to record body motion. Periods of quiescence during the 24-h period are associated with sleep, whereas periods of motion are associated with wakefulness.

Major Sleep Disorders

Sleep Apnea

Sleep apnea, also known as sleep-disordered breathing, is a very common disorder and the major sleep-related risk factor for cerebrovascular disease. Sleep apnea syndrome affects 2% of women and 4% of men (Young *et al.*, 1993). It appears more frequently past the age of 45 years and is more common in obese individuals. Loud disruptive snoring is a marker of sleep apnea and in itself a source of disease (Partinen *et al.*, 1985). Frequent symptoms are lapses in respiration, restless sleep, excessive daytime

somnolence, and depression. In addition, sleep apnea can increase the risk of stroke and myocardial infarction (Yaggi *et al.*, 2005). Epidemiological studies have shown a dose–response relationship between the severity of sleep apnea and the odds ratio for development of systemic hypertension (Nieto *et al.*, 2000). Sleep apnea is diagnosed with polysomnography in the sleep laboratory. Treatment with noninvasive positive airway ventilation is generally successful (**Figure 2**). For mild forms of sleep apnea, the application of mandibular advancement devices can be beneficial. Surgery removing excessive tissues in the oropharynx may be considered for individuals who cannot tolerate noninvasive equipment or who have obvious obstruction to airflow in the oropharynx by redundant tissue growth. There is proof that successful correction of sleep apnea with noninvasive positive airway pressure ventilation lowers mean blood pressure (Becker *et al.*, 2003). Excessive daytime somnolence generally improves with successful treatment of sleep apnea.

Narcolepsy

Narcolepsy is characterized by excessive sleepiness. Associated manifestations are cataplexy, sleep paralysis, and hallucinatory dreams at sleep onset (hypnagogic

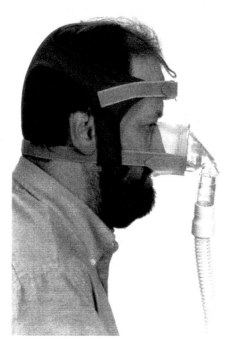

Figure 2 Continuous positive airway pressure (CPAP) application at night reverses in most cases the symptoms of sleep apnea. An air compressor delivers air at a specified pressure through a flexible hose to the mask. Oxygen and a humidifier may be added. Reproduced from Culebras A (1996) *Clinical Handbook of Sleep Disorders*. Boston: Butterworth-Heinemann, with permission from Butterworth-Heinemann.

hallucinations). Men and women are equally affected. Onset is typically in the second or third decade of life, although childhood onset may occur and some patients are not diagnosed until middle age. Changes in sleep schedule, psychological stress, head trauma, or infections sometimes appear to precipitate symptoms.

Excessive sleepiness in narcolepsy is associated with repeated naps or lapses into sleep. Sleep tends to occur in boring or monotonous situations and may be temporarily forestalled by physical activity and mental stimulation. Patients often report episodes of amnesia with automatic behavior during which they may carry out complex nonsensical activities such as mixing inappropriate foods, writing incomprehensible sentences, or driving to the wrong destination. Accidents due to sleepiness and automatic behavior may occur while driving or operating dangerous equipment.

Cataplexy, a unique feature of narcolepsy, is characterized by sudden loss of muscle tone usually provoked by strong emotion, particularly laughter lasting a few minutes. Consciousness is preserved and memory is intact. Respiratory and oculomotor muscles are not affected. In some patients, episodes of cataplexy may occur almost continuously, a condition referred to as status cataplecticus. Cataplexy rarely precedes the onset of excessive sleepiness but may develop simultaneously with sleepiness or with a delay of 1–30 years.

Hypnagogic hallucinations are vivid perceptual experiences that occur at sleep onset, often associated with fear or dread. Sleep paralysis is a transient, generalized inability to move or to speak during the transition between sleep and wakefulness. The experiences are often frightening. Disrupted nocturnal sleep with frequent awakenings is common in patients with narcolepsy. Many patients report that narcolepsy seriously affects interpersonal, marital, work, and social relationships.

A large segment of patients with otherwise typical features of narcolepsy do not have cataplexy, a condition referred to as monosymptomatic narcolepsy. In rare cases, narcolepsy is the consequence of brain tumors, stroke, multiple sclerosis, and other neurological disorders that damage the hypothalamus.

Patients with narcolepsy have excessive REM sleep both during the night and day, along with vivid dreaming. Discovery of the involvement of the hypothalamic hypocretin-releasing system in narcolepsy has improved the understanding of the ultimate etiology of the disorder. Hypocretin is a brain neurotransmitter that enhances alertness (Baumann *et al.*, 2005). Various injuries to the hypothalamic hypocretin-secreting cell group, from surgical injury to head trauma to immunologic aggression would explain narcolepsy and its gradations of severity (Mignot *et al.*, 2002). The diagnosis of narcolepsy is made clinically and confirmed with sleep laboratory tests that show excessive presence of REM sleep in daytime recordings. Treatment is symptomatic with a variety of agents that enhance daytime alertness, reduce REM sleep, or improve the continuity of sleep at night.

Insomnia

Insomnia is characterized by repeated difficulty with sleep initiation, duration, consolidation or quality despite adequate time and opportunity to sleep. Insomnia should incorporate daytime impairment as a result of faulty sleep. Primary insomnia includes psychophysiological insomnia, idiopathic insomnia, and paradoxical insomnia or sleep state misperception. Psychophysiological insomnia is one of the most common forms of insomnia. It develops as a result of chronic, somatized tension anxiety and negative conditioning to sleep. The individual with psychophysiological insomnia has focused attention on the inability to sleep, which is perceived to be the only source of distress. Other emotional or mental concerns are minimized. The search for contributing factors such as stress, caffeine ingestion, and poor sleep hygiene is generally fruitful. Not uncommonly there is a triggering factor such as divorce or the death of a relative followed by perpetuating factors at the core of which is the negative conditioning to sleep.

Patients respond initially to hypnotic medications but long-term results are more favorable with cognitive behavioral modification and similar techniques imparted by psychologists. These methods include sleep restriction consolidation, sleep hygiene education, relaxation therapy, stimulus control therapy, and correction of distorted perception of sleep. Sleep laboratory tests are only exceptionally of value in the diagnosis of insomnia.

Restless Legs

The diagnosis of restless legs syndrome (RLS) is based on the clinical history. Essential criteria are an urge to move the legs usually accompanied or caused by uncomfortable or unpleasant sensations in the legs, onset or exacerbation with rest, relief with movement, and evening or night presentation. Supportive clinical features of the diagnosis of RLS are family history, favorable response to dopaminergic therapy, and periodic limb movements (PLMs). These are repetitive limb movements that occur mostly in sleep in up to 80% of the patients. PLMs can appear in other disorders, particularly in the normal elderly population. The diagnosis of RLS can be supported by the sleep laboratory evaluation when periodic limb movements appear, as it does in most nocturnal tracings of patients with RLS. The diagnosis is confirmed with the favorable response to dopaminergic drugs.

Parasomnias

Parasomnias are undesirable physical events or experiences occurring at sleep onset, within sleep or during arousal from sleep. Common parasomnias are somnambulism or sleepwalking (SW) and sleep terrors. Patients exhibiting these disorders tend to have more than one parasomnia because of a shared pathogenic substrate, a strong familial predisposition and precipitating factors in common that include sleep deprivation, insufficient sleep syndrome, and sleep apnea. Parasomnias generally appear in the developmental age, although some start also later in life, posing problems of differential diagnosis with organic neurological or psychiatric disorders.

Sleep walking consists of a series of complex behaviors initiated during an arousal from slow-wave sleep that may culminate in walking behavior, coupled with an altered state of consciousness and impaired judgment. Episodes tend to occur during the first third of the night and may occur several times per night. Additional infrequent behaviors are eating, performing sexual intercourse, urinating, or most dramatically climbing out a window and injuring oneself or others (homicidal behavior). Sleep walking is frequent in childhood (17%), peaking by age 12 with no gender difference. Adult sleep walkers (4% prevalence) are most often men. Co-occurrence of enuresis and sleep terrors is high in relatives of patients with sleep walking.

Sleep terrors consist of abrupt arousals from deep sleep accompanied by a cry or scream with autonomic nervous system activation and behavioral manifestations of intense fear. Characteristics are confusion, retrograde amnesia, occurrence during the first part of the night, and precipitation by spontaneous or other disorder-related sleep deprivation.

Nightmares or anxiety dreams are frightening events with dream content that awaken the individual from REM sleep. Following awakening, the subject is oriented to the environment with clear sensorium. Dream content usually involves an experience of immediate and credible threat to survival, security, or self-esteem. Dream anxiety attacks occur in REM sleep. There is good recall for the disturbing dream and no displacement from the bed; injuries are quite rare.

REM sleep behavior disorder is a REM sleep parasomnia characterized by violent behaviors driven by a dream (Scheck et al., 1987). Patients are most often men who punch, kick, thrash about, get out of bed, move furniture, and perform other complex movements while in REM sleep. Not uncommonly, injuries are inflicted to the bed mate or patient. REM sleep behavior disorder has been associated with Parkinson disease (Comella et al., 1998) and other neurodegenerative disorders. Treatment with medications is generally satisfactory.

Circadian Dysrhythmias

Sleep is optimal in both quality and quantity only when it occurs during a proper time-frame in a 24-h day cycle governed by the circadian rhythm. Similarly, wakefulness is optimal at certain hours during the 24-h period. The timing of sleep and wake is a complex function of both circadian and homeostatic processes. Attempts at falling asleep or staying awake at physiologically inappropriate times will result in sleep–wake disturbance. This is the consequence of misalignment of the intrinsic sleep–wake propensity of a person and the 24-h physical and social environment. The intrinsic rhythm may be abnormally shifted relative to the environmental time-cues (delayed or advanced sleep phase disorder), become disrupted (irregular sleep–wake disorder), or have different periodicity (free-running type). The physical environment may change faster than the adaptation ability of the intrinsic sleep–wake rhythm (jet lag), or an individual may choose to disregard the intrinsic rhythm and voluntarily choose to stay awake at an inappropriate time (shift-work disorder). All these disturbances fall within the category of the circadian dysrhythmias, a group of intrinsic or acquired disorders of sleep and wakefulness.

Social Implications

Sleep–wake disorders decrease the quality of life and disrupt social activities. In addition there is a risk of

Table 2   Principles of sleep hygiene

DO

  Go to bed at the same time every day

  Get up at the same time every day

  Sleep sufficiently to be satisfied with sleep

  Use the bed only for sleep or sex

  Exercise regularly but not before going to bed or late in the evening

  Adhere to a regular meal schedule

  Read or listen to soft music before turning the lights out

  Use a twin bed if your bedmate is a restless sleeper

  Eliminate or attenuate physical disturbances (i.e., noise, light, heat, cold). Use ear plugs and eye shades if necessary

DON'T

  Eat, drink or smoke in bed

  Watch television in the bedroom

  Drink caffeine-containing beverages past 12 noon

  Use alcohol as a hypnotic. Excessive alcohol may cause rebound insomnia when the hypnotic effects dissipate while asleep

  Nap irregularly or frequently during the day

  Nap in the evenings

medicolegal troubles (Mahowald *et al.*, 2005). Academic decline is a distinct risk in sleepy subjects. Many individuals have no respect for sleep compliance or ignore the basic rules of sleepy hygiene. Sleep deprivation results when sleep hygiene is violated. The basic principles of sleep hygiene are listed in **Table 2**.

Individuals with excessive daytime somnolence and a tendency to fall asleep driving should not drive until the problem has been solved or brought under control. Situations that increase drowsiness and risk of accidents are driving at night, driving alone, or along monotonous stretches of road. If sleepy, the driver should stop the car and take a brief nap. All other measures are of no useful relief.

Past the age of 45 years, individuals tolerate poorly circadian rhythm violations and work shift schedules. Consideration should be given to eliminate shift work past this age. Jet lag is best alleviated by adopting immediately the sleep–wake schedule of the destination with the aid of a short-duration hypnotic, if necessary.

Citations

Baumann CR and Bassetti CL (2005) Hypocretins (orexins) and sleep-wake disorders. *Lancet Neurology* 4: 673–682.

Becker H, Jerrentrup A, Ploch T, *et al.* (2003) Effect of nasal continuous positive airway pressure treatment on blood pressure in patients with obstructive sleep apnea. *Circulation* 107: 68–73.

Comella CL, Nardine TM, Diederich NJ, and Stebbins GT (1998) Sleep-related violence, injury, and REM sleep behavior disorder in Parkinson's disease. *Neurology* 51(2): 526–529.

Mahowald MW and Schenck CH (2005) Violent parasomnias: Forensic medicine issues. In: Kryger MH, Roth T and Dement WC (eds.) *Principles and Practice of Sleep Medicine*, 4th edn., pp. 960–968. Philadelphia, PA: Elsevier/Saunders

Mignot E, Lammers GJ, Ripley B, *et al.* (2002) The role of cerebrospinal fluid hypocretin measurement in the diagnosis of narcolepsy and other hypersomnias. *Archives of Neurology* 59: 1553–1562.

Nieto FJ, Young TB, Lind BK, *et al.* (2000) Association of sleep-disordered breathing, sleep apnea, and hypertension in a large community-based study. *Journal of the American Medical Association* 283: 1829–1836.

Partinen M and Palomaki H (1985) Snoring and cerebral infarction. *Lancet* 2: 1325–1326.

Schenck CH, Bundlie SR, Patterson AL, and Mahowald MW (1987) REM sleep behavior disorder: a treatable parasomnia affecting older adults. *Journal of the American Medical Association* 257: 1786–1789.

Yaggi HK, Concato J, Kernan WN, Lichtman JH, Brass LM, and Mohsenin V (2005) Obstructive sleep apnea as a risk factor for stroke and death. *New England Journal of Medicine* 353: 2034–2041.

Young T, Palta M, Dempsey J, *et al.* (1993) The occurrence of sleep-disordered breathing among middle-aged adults. *New England Journal of Medicine* 328: 1230–1235.

Further Reading

American Academy of Sleep Medicine (2005) *International Classification of Sleep Disorders*, 2nd edn. *Diagnostic and Coding Manual*. Westchester, IL: American Academy of Sleep Medicine.

Culebras A (2006) *Sleep Disorders and Neurological Disease*, 2nd edn. New York: Informa Healthcare.

Jouvet M and Delorme F (1965) Locus coeruleus et sommeil paradoxal. *Comptes Rendues des Séances et Mémoires de la Société de Biologie* 159: 895–899.

Kryger MH, Roth T and Dement WC (eds.) (2005) *Principles and Practice of Sleep Medicine*, 4th edn. Philadelphia, PA: Elsevier/Saunders.

Relevant Websites

http://www.dentalsleepmed.org – Academy of Dental Sleep Medicine (ADSM).

http://www.aan.com – American Academy of Neurology, Sleep Medicine Section.

http://www.aasmnet.org – American Academy of Sleep Medicine (AASM).

http://www.absm.org – American Board of Sleep Medicine (ABSM).

http://www.aptweb.org – Association of Polysomnographic Technologists (APT).

http://www.apss.org – Associated Professional Sleep Societies Annual Meeting (APSS).

http://www.brpt.org – Board of Registered Polysomnographic Technologists (BRPT).

http://www.sleepresearchsociety.org – Sleep Research Society (SRS).

http://www.wasm.org – World Association of Sleep Medicine (WASM).

http://www.wfneurology.org – World Federation of Neurology, Sleep Research Group.

Specific Mental Health Disorders: Child and Adolescent Mental Disorders

A J Flisher, S Hatherill, and Y Dhansay, University of Cape Town, Cape Town, South Africa

Introduction

Reviews of the prevalence of child and adolescent psychiatric disorders indicate that about one in five children and adolescents suffer from such disorders (**Table 1**) some examples of which are provided in **Table 2** (World Health Organization, 2005b; Patel *et al.*, 2008). This estimate appears to be applicable to both genders, a range of ages within childhood and adolescence, all social classes, and both high-, low-, and middle-income countries. In this article, we have confined ourselves to psychiatric disorders in the narrow sense of the term. We have not addressed intellectual or learning disabilities.

Etiology

Whether a mental disorder develops in an individual and arises depends on the interplay between risk and protective factors. Risk factors are factors that increase the probability of developing a mental disorder, while protective factors moderate the effects of exposure to risk in the presence of one or more risk factors. For example, a person may have a strong family history of depression and thus be genetically predisposed to suffer from depression. Loss of a parent in adolescence may serve as another risk factor, which may then precipitate a major depressive episode. However, if such a person has strong connections with other family members, school, and community, such a depressive episode may be averted. In this case, the adolescent may experience a normal grieving process, which does not significantly adversely affect academic progress, relationships with peers, and physiological concomitants such as appetite disturbance and fatigue. This exemplifies the complex interaction of risk and protective factors at different ecological levels (**Table 3**) (World Health Organization, 2005b).

Public Health Significance

It is important to recognize that these disorders do not represent minor and transient responses to the normal challenges faced by children and adolescents. If this were the case, child and adolescent mental disorders would have limited public health significance. On the contrary, they are associated with a great degree of impairment and burden, longitudinal course into adulthood, long-term economic implications, associations with risk behavior, and stigma, each of which will be addressed below.

Impairment and Burden

The term impairment refers to interference with psychological or physical functions in one or more of the following domains: Interpersonal relationships, academic/work performance, social and leisure activities, and the ability to enjoy and obtain satisfaction from life. By definition, impairment always accompanies the presence of a psychiatric disorder, as impairment is a necessary condition for existence of a psychiatric disorder according to the diagnostic systems in common use. Indeed, if impairment is not included in the diagnostic criteria, the prevalence of child and adolescent psychiatric disorders in the general population would be two or three times the generally accepted prevalence. However, the extent of impairment varies according to diagnosis, with phobias being the least likely to be associated with impairment, followed by anxiety disorders and finally major depressive disorder and externalizing disorders such as conduct disorder and attention deficit hyperactivity disorder. Furthermore, the extent of impairment is correlated with factors, independent of the nature of the psychiatric disorder. These include the extent of comorbidity, either a long or short duration of psychopathology, psychosocial adversity (in generalized anxiety disorder), and mothers' ratings of the extent of conduct features (in children with conduct disorder).

Angold *et al.* (1998) reported that there is a positive association between impairment and parental perceived burden of care, although the direction of the causality has yet to be elucidated. The perceived burden of care was predicted by the child or adolescent's total symptom score, the child or adolescent's level of impairment, the presence of externalizing disorders (as opposed to internalizing disorders), and the existence of preexisting mental health problems on the part of the parent.

A further aspect of burden is the burden imposed by the disability suffered by the child or adolescent with a psychiatric disorder. This can be quantified by the disability-adjusted life years (DALYs) that are lost, which includes loss due to both mortality and disability, for each disorder. We do not have estimates of the DALYs

Table 1   Selected studies of the prevalence of child and adolescent psychiatric disorders in children and adolescents

Setting	Age range (years)	Prevalence (%)
Australia	18–24	27.0
Brazil	7–14	12.7
Canada, Ontario	4–16	18.1
Ethiopia	1–15	17.7
Germany	12–15	20.7
India	1–16	12.8
Hawaii	13–19	26.0
Japan	1–16	15.0
Netherlands	13–18	8.4
Spain	8, 11, 15	21.7
Switzerland	1–15	22.5
United Kingdom	13–15	29.4
United States		
• High-risk Native Americans, Northern Plain reservation	14–16	29.4
• North Carolina	13	12.7
	14	9.7
	15	14.2
	16	12.7
• Service users in five sectors of care, San Diego, CA	12–15	57.4

Data from Patel V, Flisher AJ, Nikapota A, and Malhotra S (2008) Promoting child and adolescent mental health in low and middle income countries. *Journal of Child Psychology and Psychiatry*; World Health Organization (2005b) *Child and Adolescent Mental Health Policies and Plans: Mental Health Policy and Service Guidance Package.* Geneva: World Health Organization and citations therein.

lost due to child and adolescent psychiatric disorders in childhood and adolescence specifically. However, among 15–44-year-olds, we know that five of the ten leading causes of DALYs lost are psychiatric disorders (unipolar depressive disorders, alcohol use disorders, self-inflicted injuries, schizophrenia, and bipolar mood disorder) (Murray and Lopez, 1996). Furthermore, there is an important mental health or behavioral contribution to the etiology of a further three of the ten leading causes DALYs lost (HIV/AIDS, road-traffic accidents, and violence). It is probable that similar findings are applicable to childhood and adolescence. Such data have contributed to an increased appreciation of the public health importance of psychiatric disorders.

Longitudinal Course of Mental Disorders in Childhood and Adolescence

There are two types of studies that address the longitudinal course of child and adolescent psychiatric disorders. First, there are studies that look back, by documenting the proportions of people with disorders in adulthood that had an age of onset in childhood or adolescence. The most

sophisticated of these studies was conducted by Kessler *et al.* (2005). They reported that 75% of all adults with psychiatric disorder had an age of onset of 24 years or less, 50% had an age of onset of 14 years or less, and 25% had an age of onset of 7 years or less. For anxiety disorders, the corresponding ages were 21, 11, and 6 years or less.

Second, there are studies that look forward. There is good evidence of continuity of disorders that manifest themselves in childhood or adolescence into adulthood. In major depressive disorder, for example, depressed adolescents are at two to seven times increased odds of being depressed as adults. Furthermore, about one-third of children or adolescents with a major depressive disorder will later develop bipolar disorder, and this is more likely if there is a family history of bipolar disorder, psychotic symptoms, or a manic response to antidepressants. Attention deficit hyperactivity disorder has three possible outcomes in adulthood, each of which occurs in about one-third of children with the disorder: (1) Developmental delay, in which over the course of time the individual no longer manifests impairing symptoms; (2) continual display, in which impairment related to ADHD persists into adulthood, although there are insufficient signs and symptoms for the diagnosis to be conferred; and (3) developmental decay, in which the diagnosis remains applicable in adulthood, often accompanied by other psychopathology such as substance abuse and personality disorder. Autistic disorder almost always is associated with lifelong impairment. However, there is considerable variation in outcome, with about 15% achieving independence in adulthood and a further 15–20% being able to function independently with periodic support.

In conclusion, there is evidence from retrospective and prospective studies of considerable continuity of psychiatric disorders from childhood to adulthood. This clearly provides support for increased resources to be allocated to child and adolescent psychiatric services, although evidence is currently sparse that early intervention will result in improved long-term prospects.

Long-Term Economic Implications of Child and Adolescent Mental Disorders

Given the continuity of psychiatric disorders from childhood or adolescence into adulthood, one would expect that there would also be economic implications of child and adolescent psychiatric disorders that would persist into adulthood. Such economic costs can be direct or indirect. The former are generally easier to evaluate and reflect pharmaceutical costs, primary health-care costs, emergency department visits, and outpatient and inpatient care. The latter are generally more difficult to evaluate and reflect the caregiver costs, unemployment, decreased productivity, and increased demand on the education, social services, and criminal justice systems. Existing data on the

Table 2 Examples of some common and/or important child and adolescent mental disorders

Attention deficit hyperactivity disorder (ADHD)	A persistent pattern of inattention and/or hyperactivity-impulsivity that is more frequent and severe than typically observed in children at a comparable level of development
Autistic disorder	The essential features are onset before the age of three; qualitative impairment in social interaction; qualitative impairment of verbal and nonverbal communication; and disturbed motor behavior or activities as manifest, for example, by stereotyped body movements
Conduct disorder	Repetitive and persistent pattern of behavior, lasting at least 12 months, in which the basic rights of others and major age-appropriate societal norms or rules are violated
Delirium	Transient and usually reversible mental disturbance that has fluctuating symptoms that usually develop over hours or days. Clinical features include the following: fluctuating awareness and attention; disturbed sleep–wake cycle; restlessness, irritability, anxiety, emotional lability OR decreased psychomotor activity; disorientation; disorganized thinking; memory impairment; and hallucinations and other perceptual disturbances
Generalized anxiety disorder	The essential feature of this disorder is excessive or unrealistic anxiety or worry, for example about achieving and about future events such as wars or world catastrophes
Major depressive disorder	A major depressive disorder is present if there is an onset of either depressed or irritable mood or loss of interest in former pleasurable activities lasting for a period of at least 2 weeks, accompanied by several of the following: increased or decreased appetite; insomnia or hypersomnia; increased or decreased motor activity; difficulty concentrating with fall-off in school work; feelings of worthlessness or guilt; fatigue or loss of energy; and suicidal thoughts or behavior
Obsessive-compulsive disorder	In this disorder, there is the presence of obsessions or compulsions or both, which are recognized as excessive or unreasonable
Panic disorder	There are recurrent panic attacks in which intense fear is accompanied by acute somatic symptoms of anxiety
Posttraumatic stress disorder (PTSD)	This disorder is present if there are recurrent, distressing, and intrusive images or flashbacks of the traumatic experience; marked avoidance of particular people, places, or other reminders of the experience; and symptoms of anxiety or increased sympathetic arousal as manifest, for example, by difficulty sleeping, poor concentration, exaggerated startle response, and restlessness. Depression, anxiety, and conduct disorder may accompany PTSD, or be an alternative outcome to traumatic experiences
Schizophrenia	In schizophrenia one finds delusions, hallucinations, disorganized speech, catatonic behavior, and negative symptoms
Separation anxiety disorder	There is excessive and persistent anxiety (lasting for at least 4 weeks) about separation from those to whom the child is attached

long-term economic implications of child and adolescent psychiatric disorders are scanty and confined to the direct costs of a subset of disorders in the US and the UK (Romeo et al., 2005). However, the existing data confirm that the long-term costs associated with child and adolescent psychiatric disorders are large. For example, the treatment costs for youth with ADHD are approximately double those for youth without ADHD; the cumulative costs of public services utilized through to adulthood by individuals with antisocial behavior in childhood were ten times higher than for those with no antisocial behaviors by the age of 28 years, and the annualized cost in adulthood for those who suffered from both depression and conduct disorder was more than double that of the group with major depression alone (Romeo et al., 2005).

It can be seen that the potential economic impact of successfully implementing proven prevention and early intervention strategies for children with disruptive behavior disorders is enormous (World Health Organization, 2005b). The characteristically recurring nature of the mood disorders and the strong evidence for their continuity into adult life would seem to suggest an equally compelling argument for early intervention and even

prevention in an effort to divert children from a possible trajectory of lifelong difficulties associated with substantial individual and societal costs.

Associations with Risk Behavior

There is robust international evidence that there is covariation between risk behaviors such as violent behavior, sexual behavior, suicidal behavior, dangerous road-related behavior, and use of tobacco, alcohol, and other drugs (Flisher et al., 2000). Furthermore, this cluster of risk behaviors appears to share common correlates, for example psychiatric disorder (Flisher et al., 2000). This has been established both for the cluster as a whole and individual components of the cluster. What is not clear is the direction of the causal relationship. Thus, the psychiatric disorder could cause the risk behavior or the risk behavior could cause the psychiatric disorder or they could both be caused by other factors. It is probable that the nature of the relationship varies according to the particular risk behaviors and psychiatric disorders in question. However, whatever the nature of the relationship, there are clear implications for public health. Specifically, preventive, promotive, or

Table 3   Selected risk and protective factors for mental health of children and adolescents

Domain	Risk factors	Protective factors
Biological	Exposure to toxins (e.g., tobacco and alcohol) in pregnancy Genetic predisposition Head trauma Hypoxia at birth and other birth complications HIV infection Malnutrition Other illnesses	Age-appropriate physical development Good physical health Good intellectual functioning
Psychological	Learning disorders Maladaptive personality traits Sexual, physical, and emotional abuse and neglect Difficult temperament	Ability to learn from experiences Good self-esteem High level of problem-solving ability Social skills
Social a) Family	Inconsistent care giving Family conflict Poor family discipline Poor family management Death of a family member	Family attachment Opportunities for positive involvement in family Rewards for involvement in family
b) School	Academic failure Failure of schools to provide an appropriate environment to support attendance and learning Inadequate/inappropriate provision of education	Opportunities for involvement in school life Positive reinforcement from academic achievement Identity with a school or need for educational attainment
c) Community	Lack of community efficacy Community disorganization Discrimination and marginalization Exposure to violence Lack of a sense of place Transitions (e.g., urbanization)	Connectedness to community Opportunities for constructive use of leisure Positive cultural experiences Positive role models Rewards for community involvement Connection with community organizations including religious organizations

From World Health Organization (2005b) *Child and Adolescent Mental Health Policies and Plans: Mental Health Policy and Service Guidance Package.* Geneva: World Health Organization.

treatment interventions that address either risk behavior or psychiatric disorders would benefit from addressing the other aspect.

Stigma

The term stigma is derived from a Greek word and refers to a mark that denotes a shameful quality in the individual thus marked. It is a complex phenomenon that is modified by the culture and contexts in which it occurs. There are five interrelated processes that combine to create stigma: (1) people identify and label human characteristics, and differences that are regarded as relevant and consequential are determined; (2) stereotyping takes place in that the labeled person is associated with undesirable characteristics; (3) there is separation of the stigmatized group (them) from those who are stigmatizing (us); (4) the stigmatized group experiences discrimination and loss of status; and (5) the stigmatizing group exercises power. The association of mental illness with irrational, dangerous, and unpredictable behavior and the misconception that mental illness is not a true illness has resulted in those with psychiatric disorders being subject to stigmatization. Psychiatric patients and their families are doubly

challenged: They are faced with the struggle caused by their impairment and they are confronted with chronic stress caused by the stigma that is associated with psychiatric disorders. As a result of these challenges, they are deprived of the opportunities such as good schooling and wide social networks, which in turn adversely affect self-esteem, and hence academic performance and economic well-being. Children and adolescents are particularly vulnerable to stigma for four main reasons (World Health Organization, 2005b):

- They are less likely to be able to advocate on their own behalf;
- Immature cognitive development results in children and adolescents being more likely to think dichotomously about opposites such as good and bad, and thus more likely to temper negative with other, less negative or positive, responses, and hence accept negative labels;
- The stigma suffered by children and adolescents may also affect the parents, which in turn could affect the quality of parenting that they are able to offer;
- There is limited understanding of child and adolescent psychiatric disorders, which implies that symptoms that are attributable to a psychiatric disorder may be

attributed to other causes, such as passive aggression in the case of depression or overt oppositionality in the case of attention deficit hyperactivity disorder; and their psychiatric disorders may persist into adulthood, which implies that any effects of stigma may persist for equally long.

Interventions for Child and Adolescent Mental Disorders

Mental Health Promotion

The aim of mental health promotion is to enhance positive mental health, which can be defined as the:

> ... capacity to achieve and maintain optimal psychological functioning and well-being. It is directly related to the level reached and competence reached and competence achieved in psychological and social functioning ... Child and adolescent mental health includes a sense of identity and self-worth; sound family and peer relationships; an ability to be productive and to learn; and a capacity to use developmental challenges and cultural resources to maximize development (Department of Health, Republic of South Africa, 2003: 4).

The focus is on enhancing protective factors through goals such as strengthening individuals, strengthening communities, and removing barriers to good mental health (**Table 4**) (Funk *et al.*, 2005). What is the relevance of mental health promotion for child and adolescent mental disorders? The relevance is that mental health promotion interventions arguably also contribute to reducing the prevalence of child and adolescent mental disorders. However, the empirical justification for this statement is currently somewhat flimsy, partly because of the methodological challenges of demonstrating outcomes of upstream interventions (such as those mentioned above) on downstream outcomes such as specific disorders in specific individuals (Patel *et al.*, 2008).

Mental Disorder Prevention

In contrast to mental heath promotion, mental disorder prevention aims to reduce the prevalence of specific disorders, by focusing on risk factors. There are a number of interventions for specific disorders that have been shown to be effective, at least for populations in high-income countries. Examples of disorders and interventions that have been shown to be effective include (Durlak and Wells, 1997; World Health Organization, 2004):

- Alcohol misuse: School-based individual-level education and skills training combined with a mass media campaign, parent education and organization program, training community leaders and local policy changes;

Table 4 Examples of child and adolescent mental health promotion interventions

Domain	Interventions
Strengthening individuals	Develop self-efficacy (the perception that one can achieve desired goals through one's own action)
	Encourage self-determination
	Enhance life skills of adolescents
	Foster belief in the future
	Improve the quality of parent–infant relationship
	Nurture a clear and positive identity
	Promote competencies in the social, emotional, cognitive, behavioral, and moral domains
	Recognize positive behavior
Strengthening communities	Develop facilities and structures to enable constructive and healthy use of leisure time of children and adolescents
	Establish prosocial norms
	Improve social connectedness of schools and neighborhoods
	Promote bonding (emotional attachment and commitment) with family, peer group, school, community, and culture
	Provide opportunities for prosocial involvement with family, peers, and adults
Removing barriers to good mental health	Develop and implement economic policies that reduce poverty
	Develop and implement legislation that protects the human rights of children and adolescents, for example around trafficking and sexual and physical abuse
	Improve access to good-quality education and health services

Funk M, Gale E, Grigg M, Minoletti A, and Yasamay MT (2005) Mental health promotion: An important component of a national mental health policy. In: Herman H, Saxena S, and Moodie R (eds.) *Promotion Mental Health: Concepts, Emerging Evidence, Practice*, pp. 216–225. Geneva, Switzerland: World Health Organization.

- Anxiety: Teaching skills to manage anxiety symptoms more effectively;
- Conduct disorder: Child or adolescent behavior management, social skills for child or adolescent, multimodal school programs, and prenatal or early childhood programs;
- Depression: Improving cognitive and problem-solving skills, group interventions that focus on cognitive style and problem solving;
- Pathological eating behavior: Increasing self-esteem and improving general eating habits and behavior;
- Schizophrenia: Low-dose neuroleptic medication and cognitive behavior therapy;
- Suicide: School-based intervention with school suicide policy, teacher consultation and training, education to parents, stress management and life skills curriculum, and a crisis team.

Treatment

It is important to develop a comprehensive treatment plan for each child or adolescent and the family, which requires psychiatric services. This plan should:

- address each problem or disorder that was identified in the assessment;
- aim to modify all modifiable etiological factors in the biological, psychological, and social domains;
- involve both the family and the child or adolescent in treatment;
- include all contributory settings, especially the school;
- make use of the unique contributions of all appropriate members of the clinical team.

There is a rapidly expanding evidence base on the efficacy and effectiveness of interventions for child and adolescent mental disorders. Specifically, there is good evidence of the effectiveness of certain antidepressant and antipsychotic agents and of psychotherapy (especially behavioral and cognitive behavioral treatments for anxiety and mood disorders) (Evans *et al.*, 2005).

The Current Response

We have argued above that the public health significance of child and adolescent mental disorders is enormous, and that there is evidence that preventive and treatment interventions (at least) can be effective. In light of these considerations, the response on the part of the health and other systems has been insufficient to meaningfully address the gap between the need for interventions and the available services. Only 7% of countries worldwide had a clearly articulated, stand-alone child and adolescent mental health policy (World Health Organization, 2005a). However, a larger proportion of countries have child and adolescent mental health content integrated into other policies, and/or have child and adolescent mental health programs. The proportions of counties with any child and adolescent mental health policy or programs are lowest in the Africa region, where 33% have the former (generally integrated into policy documents from other sectors such as child protection, social welfare, education, or human rights), while 6% have the latter (World Health Organization, 2005a). The corresponding figures for Europe are 96% and 67%. It is ironic that those countries with the largest proportion of children and adolescents are least likely to have a child and adolescent mental health policy. Other selected key aspects of the current situation include:

- There are no countries that have a data information system for child and adolescent mental health service outcomes at the national level.
- In the vast majority of countries outside of North America and Europe, systems for the care of children and

adolescents with mental disorders do not exist, and when they do exist they are based in hospitals or custodial settings with minimal or no community-based services.

- Even when services are present, there are considerable barriers to accessing it, such as stigma, lack of transportation, inability to pay for services, inability of the service providers to communicate effectively in the service users' home language, and lack of public knowledge about mental disorders in children and adolescents.
- In countries in all economic categories, these services are generally paid for by temporary and vulnerable sources of funding such as the service user (or their family), nongovernmental organizations and international grants, as opposed to more stable government funding.

The Way Forward

The first step in responding to the scenario is to develop a child and adolescent mental health policy with an associated plan. The WHO has published a guideline on how to develop a child and adolescent mental health policy and plan (World Health Organization, 2005b), which provides a step-by-step approach that can be used by policy makers

Table 5   Key standards for child and adolescent mental health service planning and provision

Core features of child and adolescent mental health services
- Include child and adolescent mental health in primary health care practices
- Provide a continuum of services
- Balance promotion, prevention, treatment, and rehabilitation
- Prioritize children and adolescent most at risk

Evidence and service planning
- Assess levels of service provision and need regularly
- Use this information to plan and commission appropriate services
- Involve parents/families and communities in service planning

Range of services, staffing, and facilities
- Offer early intervention and mental health promotion in all facilities
- Coordinate and integrate services across health, education, social care, youth justice, and voluntary sector agencies
- Use a multidisciplinary team approach
- Train, supervise, and support all staff to provide a full range of interventions
- Ensure that care is developmentally appropriate
- Keep children's mental health-care facilities separate from adults
- Offer services as near to home as possible and in child-centered settings, such as schools, youth clubs, the media, and the family

Adapted from Dawes A, Lund C, Kafaar Z, Brandt R, and Flisher AJ (2004) Norms for South African Child and Adolescent Mental Health Services (CAMHS) *Report for the Directorate: Mental Health and Substance Abuse National Department of Health* (Tender number DOH 48/2003–2004) Cape Town: Human Sciences Research Council and University of Cape Town.

and planners. The steps for developing a policy are as follows: gather information and data for policy development; gather evidence for effective strategies; undertake consultation and negotiation; exchange with other countries; set out the vision, values, principles and objectives of the policy; determine the areas for action; and identify the roles and responsibilities of the various stakeholders. The steps for developing a plan are as follows: determine the strategies and time frames; set indicators and targets; determine the manor activities; and determine the costs, available resources and the budget. The plan should be backed up by sufficient resources and political will to ensure widespread implementation.

It is not appropriate to specify in detail the outcomes of the process of developing policies and plans for a country, province, region, or district. Indeed, as is obvious from the steps that have just been listed, this would contradict the letter and spirit of the guidelines. However, a broad consensus has emerged in recent years as to the key standards that should characterize a child and adolescent mental health service, whether in a high-, middle-, or low-income country, which are summarized in **Table 5**.

Conclusion

Far from being minor or transient variations in response to childhood adversity, or a medicalization of society's intolerance of challenging childhood behaviors or inadequate parenting, it has become increasingly apparent that mental disorders presenting for the first time in childhood and adolescence represent serious conditions associated with markedly impaired functioning and significantly lower quality of life, for both the child or adolescent and their families. Even child or adolescent disorders traditionally viewed as mild, such as the anxiety disorders, are increasingly being construed as possible precursors of more serious and enduring mental health problems. In a substantial proportion of cases, psychiatric diagnosis in childhood or adolescence foreshadows psychiatric diagnosis in adulthood. An alternative view would suggest that child and adolescent psychiatric disorders provide us with a tantalizing window of opportunity for changing this gloomy trajectory. The exciting challenge for child mental health services is the prevention and early detection of these disorders; the implementation of evidence-based interventions with both short- and long-term clinical and cost effectiveness; and the development of mental health systems that ensure equitable access to such interventions. We are in the earliest stages of meeting this challenge and exploiting this opportunity.

See also: Child Abuse/Treatment; Mental Health and Substance abuse; Mental Health Policy; Historical Views of Mental Illness; Specific Mental Health Disorders: Eating Disorders; Specific Mental Health Disorders: Mental Disorders Associated With Aging; Specific Mental Health Disorders: Trauma and Mental Disorders.

Citations

Angold A, Messer S, Stangl D, *et al.* (1998) Perceived parental burden and service use for child and adolescent psychiatric disorders. *American Journal of Public Health* 88: 75–80.

Department of Health, Republic of South Africa (2003) *National Policy Guidelines for Child and Adolescent Mental Health.* Pretoria, South Africa: Department of Health Republic of South Africa.

Dawes A, Lund C, Kafaar Z, Brandt R, and Flisher AJ (2004) *Norms for South African Child and Adolescent Mental Health Services (CAMHS) Report for the Directorate: Mental Health and Substance Abuse National Department of Health* (Tender number DOH 48/ 2003–2004) Cape Town, South Africa: Human Sciences Research Council and University of Cape Town.

Durlak JA and Wells AM (1997) Primary preventive mental health programs for children and adolescents: A meta-analytic review. *American Journal of Community Psychology* 17: 5–18.

Evans DL, Foa EB Gur RE, *et al.* (eds.) (2005) *Treating and Preventing Adolescent Mental Health Disorders: What We Know and What We Don't Know. A Research Agenda for Improving the Mental Health of Our Youth.* Oxford, UK: Oxford University Press.

Flisher AJ, Kramer RA, Hoven CW, *et al.* (2000) Risk behavior in a community sample of children and adolescents. *Journal of the American Academy of Child and Adolescent Psychiatry* 39: 881–887.

Funk M, Gale E, Grigg M, Minoletti A, and Yasamy MT (2005) Mental health promotion: An important component of a national mental health policy. In: Herrman H, Saxena S, and Moodie R (eds.) *Promoting Mental Heath: Concepts, Emerging Evidence, Practice,* pp. 216–225. Geneva, Switzerland: World Health Organization.

Kessler R, Bergland R, Demler O, Jin R, and Walters EE (2005) Lifetime prevalence and age-of-onset distribution of DSM-IV disorders in the National Comorbidity Survey Replication. *Archives of General Psychiatry* 62: 593–602.

Murray C and Lopez A (1996) *The Global Burden of Disease.* Boston, MA: Harvard School of Public Health WHO and World Bank.

Patel V, Flisher AJ, Hetrick S, and McGorry P (2007) The mental health of young people: A global public health challenge. *Lancet* 369: 1302–1313.

Patel V, Flisher AJ, Nikapota A, and Malhotra S (2008) Promoting child and adolescent mental health in low and middle income countries. *Journal of Child Psychology and Psychiatry* 49: 313–334.

Romeo R, Byford S, and Knapp M (2005) Economic evaluations of child and adolescent mental health interventions: A systematic review. *Journal of Child Psychology and Psychiatry* 46: 919–930.

World Health Organization (2004) *Prevention of Mental Disorders: Effective Interventions and Policy Options: Summary Report.* Geneva, Switzerland: World Health Organization.

World Health Organization (2005a) *Atlas: Child and Adolescent Mental Health Resources: Global Concerns. Issues for the Future.* Geneva, Switzerland: World Health Organization.

World Health Organization (2005b) *Child and Adolescent Mental Health Policies and Plans: Mental Health Policy and Service Guidance Package.* Geneva, Switzerland: World Health Organization.

Further Reading

Breinbauer C and Maddelino M (2005) *Youth: Choices and Change: Promoting Healthy Behaviors in Adolescence.* Washington, DC: PAHO.

Kazdin A and Weisz J (2003) *Evidence-Based Psychotherapies for Children and Adolescents.* New York: Guildford Press.

World Health Organization (2001) *The World Health Report 2001: New Understanding, New Hope.* Geneva, Switzerland: World Health Organization.

Relevant Websites

http://www.aacap.org – American Academy of Child and Adolescent Psychiatry.

http://www.hcp.med.harvard.edu/icpe/ – International Consortium in Psychiatric Epidemiology.

http://www.mentalhealth.samhsa.gov/cmhs/surgeongeneral/ – Mental Health: Report of the Surgeon General (USA).

http://www.who.int/topics/mental_health/en/ – World Health Organization mental health page.

http://tinyurl.com/bs8zl – World Development Report 2007: Development and the Next Generation.

Specific Mental Health Disorders: Depressive and Anxiety Disorders

I B Hickie, The University of Sydney, Sydney, NSW, Australia

Introduction

Following the development of standardized diagnostic systems in the early 1980s (e.g., Research Diagnostic Criteria of Spitzer and colleagues and the DSM-III of the American Psychiatric Association) and their incorporation into large-scale epidemiological studies, there has been widespread acceptance of the dimensional nature of the common anxiety and depressive disorders. Such dimensional concepts can be readily incorporated into large-scale population-health and health service development plans. Importantly, they place an emphasis on detection and active management of the very common mild and moderately severe cases. In this environment, the center of clinical management is shifted from specialist care settings (for more severe, prolonged, treatment-resistant, comorbid and medically complicated) to primary care.

These broad concepts of depression and anxiety have predictive value for key outcomes such as response to available treatments, disability, and premature death. They incorporate the key symptom domains (e.g., affective, cognitive, sleep–wake cycle, somatic, behavioral, and self-harm) and they can also be readily incorporated into public and professional education campaigns as well as everyday clinical practice. For example, simple checklists can be widely circulated through e-health, media, print, and health-care distribution systems (see **Figure 1** for an example from the SPHERE-program in Australia).

Clinical debate as to the best ways to describe the relationship between different anxious and depressive phenotypes (e.g., mixed anxiety and depression, generalized anxiety and its relationship to dysthymia (symptoms of depression), and major depression), and between different depressive dimensions (e.g., major versus minor depression and unipolar versus bipolar spectrum disorders) will continue until more discrete pathophysiological pathways are identified. The development of future international diagnostic systems (e.g., DSM-V) has signaled this necessary move from over reliance on imprecise cross-sectional phenotypes to diagnostic categories based on putative causal paths.

A great deal of academic effort has been expended in epidemiological and clinical studies that seek to differentiate anxiety from depressive disorders or subtype the multiple and complex presentations of these conditions. These efforts have reflected traditional but simplistic belief systems about causality (e.g., psychosocial vs. biological) or the relevance of subtyping to the selection of specific medical or psychological therapies (e.g., only certain subtypes of depression benefit from one or other antidepressant medication; only psychological therapies should be provided to persons with anxiety disorders). In the absence of discrete biological or psychosocial markers of illness risk, illness onset, diagnostic subtypes, predictors of response to specific treatments, or illness course, we continue to work with broad syndromal concepts rather than valid or discrete diagnostic categories. Consequently, anxiety and depressive syndromes typically co-occur when studied either cross-sectionally or longitudinally, and generic terms such as common mental disorders are used.

Another important development in the clinical theorizing about common mental disorders has been the development of clinical staging models. Within this paradigm there is clear recognition that those at risk (Stage 0: as a result of exposure to relevant biological or psychosocial risks) or those with earlier and less severe manifestations of illness (Stage I: subthreshold symptoms with disability; and II: first clear episode with disability) are very common and likely to respond well to a range of information, e-health, and brief clinical interventions. These all have the potential advantages of being able to be delivered to large numbers of persons at relatively low cost either directly or with the assistance of a wide range of community agencies. They are particularly relevant to application in primary health care, education, and workplace settings. Specialized health-care workforces are more likely to be engaged preferentially in the provision of care to persons with more severe illnesses, those who have failed to respond to simpler clinical interventions, or those with major physical health, substance misuse, or other social complications of their conditions.

Burden of Depressive and Anxiety Disorders

Anxiety and depressive disorders are among the most common health conditions. At least one in ten persons will report symptoms and associated reduction in work or social function in any 12-month period. When combined with co-occurring harmful use of alcohol or other substances (which is particularly important for men), the estimates increase to one in five adults in any 12-month period, as shown in **Table 1**. As depression is common right across the lifespan, lifetime risk for depression may be as high as 30% for men and 40% for women.

There is no doubt that one of the most important drivers to public, professional, and health policy attention to the importance of depression and anxiety has been the improved measures of health-related disability used in association with the global burden of disease studies. For the first time, the real impact of these common conditions could be directly compared with that of other health problems. To the surprise of many, the overwhelming

How do you know if someone has depression?

Are you depressed?

For more than TWO WEEKS have you: Yes   No

1. Felt sad, down or miserable most of the time?
2. Lost interest or pleasure in most of your usual activities?

If you answered 'Yes' to either of these questions, complete the symptom checklist below.

Behaviors	Thoughts
Stopped going out	"I'm a failure."
Not getting things done at work	"It's all my fault."
Withdrawn from close family and friends	"Nothing good ever happens to me."
Relying on alcohol and sedatives	"I'm worthless."
Stopped doing things you enjoy	"Life is not worth living."
Unable to concentrate	

Feelings		Physical
Overwhelmed	Guilty	Tired all the time
Unhappy, depressed	Indecisive	Sick and run down
	Disappointed	Headaches and muscle pains
Irritable	Miserable	Churning gut
Frustrated	Sad	Can't sleep
No confidence		Poor appetite/weight loss

If you answered 'Yes' to question 1 and/or 2 and ticked 3 or more of the above symptoms, you probably have a depressive illness.

Figure 1   Continued

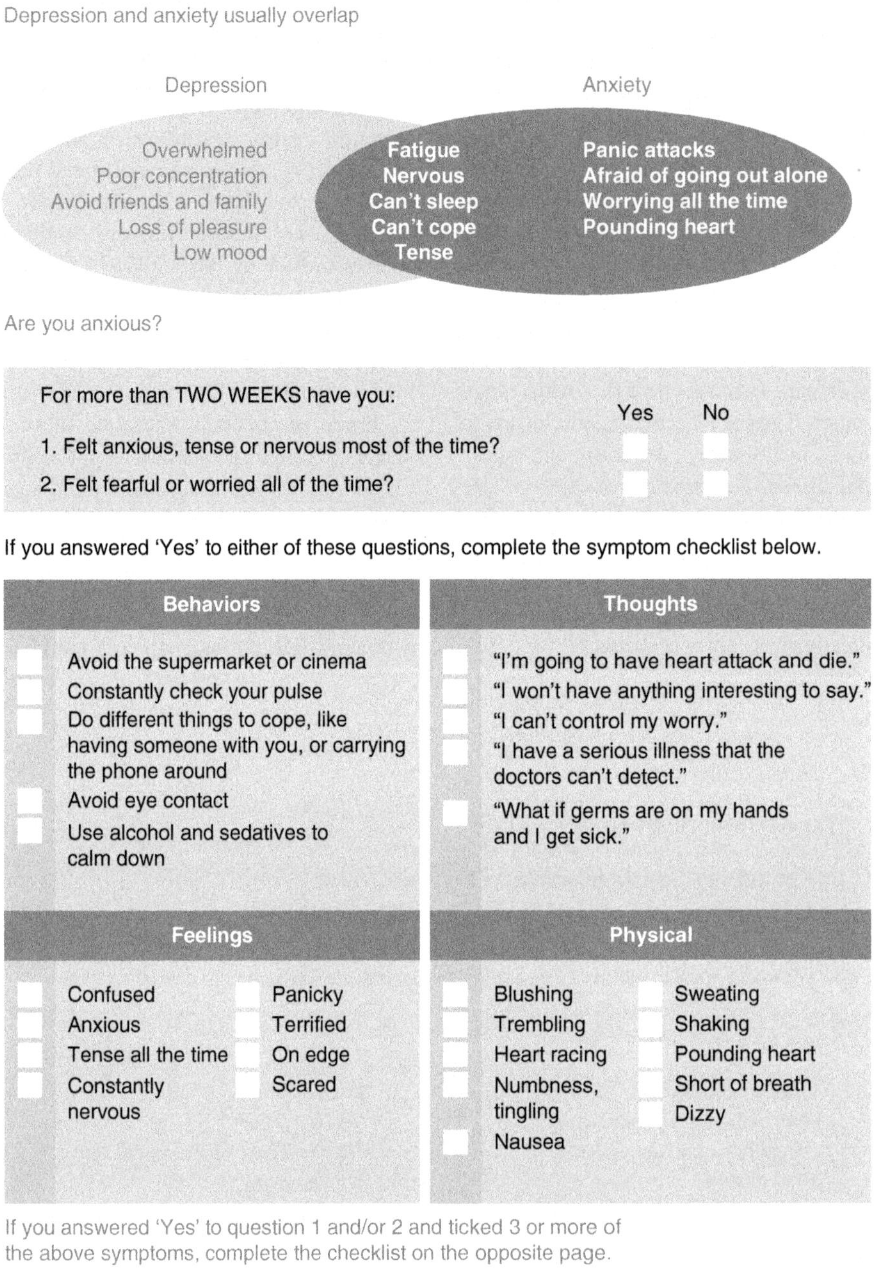

Depression and anxiety usually overlap

Depression		Anxiety
Overwhelmed	Fatigue	Panic attacks
Poor concentration	Nervous	Afraid of going out alone
Avoid friends and family	Can't sleep	Worrying all the time
Loss of pleasure	Can't cope	Pounding heart
Low mood	Tense	

Are you anxious?

For more than TWO WEEKS have you:	Yes	No
1. Felt anxious, tense or nervous most of the time?	☐	☐
2. Felt fearful or worried all of the time?	☐	☐

If you answered 'Yes' to either of these questions, complete the symptom checklist below.

Behaviors	Thoughts
☐ Avoid the supermarket or cinema	☐ "I'm going to have heart attack and die."
☐ Constantly check your pulse	☐ "I won't have anything interesting to say."
☐ Do different things to cope, like having someone with you, or carrying the phone around	☐ "I can't control my worry."
☐ Avoid eye contact	☐ "I have a serious illness that the doctors can't detect."
☐ Use alcohol and sedatives to calm down	☐ "What if germs are on my hands and I get sick."

Feelings		Physical	
☐ Confused	☐ Panicky	☐ Blushing	☐ Sweating
☐ Anxious	☐ Terrified	☐ Trembling	☐ Shaking
☐ Tense all the time	☐ On edge	☐ Heart racing	☐ Pounding heart
☐ Constantly nervous	☐ Scared	☐ Numbness, tingling	☐ Short of breath
		☐ Nausea	☐ Dizzy

If you answered 'Yes' to question 1 and/or 2 and ticked 3 or more of the above symptoms, complete the checklist on the opposite page.

Figure 1 Sphere checklist. Reproduced from Hickie I and Scott L (2007) *Understanding Depression*. Sydney: Educational Health Solutions, with permission.

contribution of unipolar major depression demanded attention.

In 2000, depression was the leading cause of disability as measured by years lived with disability (YLDs) and the fourth leading contributor to the global burden of disease (DALYs – disability-adjusted life years, which is the sum of years of potential life lost due to premature mortality and the years of productive life lost due to disability). By the year 2020, depression is projected to become the second highest cause of DALYs calculated for all ages and both sexes. Today, depression is already the second

cause of DALYs in the age category 15–44 years for both sexes combined.

Not only is depression the major cause of health-related disability internationally, but its contribution is only likely to increase in both developing and developed nations (see Mathers and Loncar, 2006; The Lancet Series on Global Mental Health, 2008). Given the lack of population-based campaigns to reduce this impact and the increasing recognition of the contribution of early-onset anxiety and depressive disorders to other health conditions (e.g., vascular disease) and other key risk factors

Table 1   Twelve-month prevalence and severity of DSM-IV and WMH-CIDI disorders in 9282 respondents*

	Total	Severity		
		Serious	Moderate	Mild
Anxiety disorders				
Panic disorder	2.7(0.2)	44.8(3.2)	29.5(2.7)	25.7(2.5)
Agoraphobia without panic	0.8(0.1)	40.6(7.2)	30.7(6.4)	28.7(8.4)
Specific phobia	8.7(0.4)	21.9(2.0)	30.0(2.0)	48.1(2.1)
Social phobia	6.8(0.3)	29.9(2.0)	38.8(2.5)	31.3(2.4)
Generalized anxiety disorder	3.1(0.2)	32.3(2.9)	44.6(4.0)	23.1(2.9)
Posttraumatic stress disorder[a]	3.5(0.3)	36.6(3.5)	33.1(2.2)	30.2(3.4)
Obsessive-compulsive disorder[b]	1.0(0.3)	50.6(12.4)	34.8(14.1)	14.6(5.7)
Separation anxiety disorder[c]	0.9(0.2)	43.3(9.2)	24.8(7.5)	31.9(12.2)
Any anxiety disorder[d]	18.1(0.7)	22.8(1.5)	33.7(1.4)	43.5(2.1)
Mood disorders				
Major depressive disorder	6.7(0.3)	30.4(1.7)	50.1(2.1)	19.5(2.1)
Dysthymia	1.5(0.1)	49.7(3.9)	32.1(4.0)	18.2(3.4)
Bipolar I and II disorders	2.6(0.2)	82.9(3.2)	17.1(3.2)	0(0)
Any mood disorder	9.5(0.4)	45.0(1.9)	40.0(1.7)	15.0(1.6)
Impulse control disorders				
Oppositional defiant disorder[c]	1.0(0.2)	49.6(8.0)	40.3(8.7)	10.1(4.8)
Conduct disorder[c]	1.0(0.2)	40.5(11.1)	31.6(7.5)	28.0(9.1)
Attention-deficit/hyperactivity disorder[c]	4.1(0.3)	41.3(4.3)	35.2(3.5)	23.5(4.5)
Intermittent explosive disorder	2.6(0.2)	23.8(3.3)	74.4(3.5)	1.7(0.9)
Any impulse control disorder[c,e]	8.9(0.5)	32.9(2.9)	52.4(3.0)	14.7(2.3)
Substance disorders				
Alcohol abuse[a]	3.1(0.3)	28.9(2.6)	39.7(3.7)	31.5(3.3)
Alcohol dependence[a]	1.3(0.2)	34.3(4.5)	65.7(4.5)	0(0)
Drug abuse[a]	1.4(0.1)	36.6(5.0)	30.4(5.8)	33.0(6.8)
Drug dependence[a]	0.4(0.1)	56.5(8.2)	43.5(8.2)	0(0)
Any substance disorder[a]	3.8(0.3)	29.6(2.8)	37.1(3.5)	33.4(3.2)
Any disorder				
Any[d]	26.2(0.8)	22.3(1.3)	37.3(1.3)	40.4(1.6)
1 disorder[d]	14.4(0.6)	9.6(1.3)	31.2(1.9)	59.2(2.3)
2 disorders[d]	5.8(0.3)	25.5(2.1)	46.4(2.6)	28.2(2.0)
≥3 disorders[d]	6.0(0.3)	49.9(2.3)	43.1(2.1)	7.0(1.3)

Source: http//www.oie.int/eng/info/en_esomonde.htm

*Values are expressed as percentage (standard error). Percentages in the three severity columns are repeated as proportions of all cases and sum to 100% across each row.

[a]Assessed in the part 2 sample ($n = 5692$).

[b]Assessed in a random one third of the part 2 sample ($n = 1808$).

[c]Assessed in the part 2 sample among respondents in the age range 18 to 44 years ($n = 3199$).

[d]Estimated in the part 2 sample. No adjustment is made for the fact that 1 or more disorders in the category were not assessed for all part 2 respondents.

[e]The estimated prevalence of any impulse control disorder is larger than the sum of the individual disorders because the prevalence of intermittent explosive disorder, the only impulse control disorder that was assessed in the total sample, is reported herein for the total sample rather than for the subsample of respondents among whom the other impulse control disorders were assessed (part 2 respondents in the age range 18–44 years). The estimated prevalence of any impulse control disorder, in comparison, is estimated in the latter subsample. Intermittent explosive disorder had a considerably higher estimated prevalence in this subsample than in the total sample.

(e.g., tobacco, alcohol, substance misuse, overweight), international and national health bodies have increasingly moved to develop more appropriate responses (Lancet series on Global Mental Health, 2007).

A more critical discourse has developed with regards to the accuracy of these health burden predictions. Typically, the attention of the international health community has been focused on those more traditional physical health areas (e.g., infectious diseases, cardiovascular diseases, and cancer) that make large contributions to premature death rather than ongoing disability. The largely hidden disability associated with common forms of anxiety and depression is often more evident to those with a wider community focus on education, training, employment, welfare, housing, and legal services than those who work within general health or specialist mental health-care settings. The specific ways in which mental health leads to poor physical health outcomes has been significantly underestimated (Lancet Series on Global Mental Health, 2007) (**Tables 2** and **3**).

A basic risk relationship exists between increasing severity and duration of anxious and depressive symptoms and a range of adverse outcomes, including impairment of daily functions, premature death, increased rates of misuse of alcohol, tobacco, and other drugs, and poor physical health (notably increased rates of cardiovascular disease). The significance of these common conditions has been a surprise to many national and international health policy

bodies. However, this is the predictable impact from disorders that commence in adolescence or early adult life, are associated with significant decrements in daily function (particularly reductions in education, training, and employment), persist or frequently recur, go largely untreated, lead to secondary medical morbidity and harmful use of alcohol and other substances, and do not result typically in major decrements in life expectancy. That is, a pattern of chronic ill health and disability is established just at that point in the life cycle where communities expect to receive the greatest returns on previous investments in childhood health and education. **Figure 2** demonstrates that the per capita incident non-fatal burden attributable to mental health (primarily

Table 2   Ten leading causes of DALYs, by income group, 2030 (baseline scenario)

Income group	Rank	Disease or injury	Percent total DALYs
World	1	HIV/AIDS	12.1
	2	Unipolar depressive disorders	5.7
	3	Ischemic heart disease	4.7
	4	Road traffic accidents	4.2
	5	Perinatal conditions	4.0
	6	Cerebrovascular disease	3.9
	7	COPD	3.1
	8	Lower respiratory infections	3.0
	9	Hearing loss, adult onset	2.5
	10	Cataracts	2.5
High-income countries	1	Unipolar depressive disorders	9.8
	2	Ischemic heart disease	5.9
	3	Alzheimer and other dementias	5.8
	4	Alcohol use disorders	4.7
	5	Diabetes mellitus	4.5
	6	Cerebrovascular disease	4.5
	7	Hearing loss, adult onset	4.1
	8	Trachea, bronchus, lung cancers	3.0
	9	Osteoarthritis	2.9
	10	COPD	2.5
Middle-income countries	1	HIV/AIDS	9.8
	2	Unipolar depressive disorders	6.7
	3	Cerebrovascular disease	6.0
	4	Ischemic heart disease	4.7
	5	COPD	4.7
	6	Road traffic accidents	4.0
	7	Violence	2.9
	8	Vision disorders, age-related	2.9
	9	Hearing loss, adult onset	2.9
	10	Diabetes mellitus	2.6
Low-income countries	1	HIV/AIDS	14.6
	2	Perinatal conditions	5.8
	3	Unipolar depressive disorders	4.7
	4	Road traffic accidents	4.6
	5	Ischemic heart disease	4.5
	6	Lower respiratory infections	4.4
	7	Diarrheal diseases	2.8
	8	Cerebrovascular disease	2.8
	9	Cataracts	2.8
	10	Malaria	2.5

Reproduced from Mathers CD and Loncar D (2006) Projections of global mortality and burden of disease from 2002 to 2030. *PLoS Medicine* 3: 2011–2030, with permission.

Table 3 The leading causes of disability worldwide, 1990

(As measured by years of life lived with a disability, YLD)	Total YLDs (millions)	Percent of total
All causes	472.7	
1. Unipolar major depression	50.8	10.7
2. Iron-deficiency anemia	22.0	4.7
3. Falls	22.0	4.6
4. Alcohol use	15.8	3.3
5. Chronic obstructive pulmonary disease	14.7	3.1
6. Bipolar disorder	14.1	3.0
7. Congenital anomalies	13.5	2.9
8. Osteoarthritis	13.3	2.8
9. Schizophrenia	12.1	2.6
10. Obsessive-compulsive disorders	10.2	2.2

Reproduced from Lopez AD and Murray CJL (1998) The global burden of disease, 1990–2020. *Nature Medicine* 4: 1241–1243, with permission.

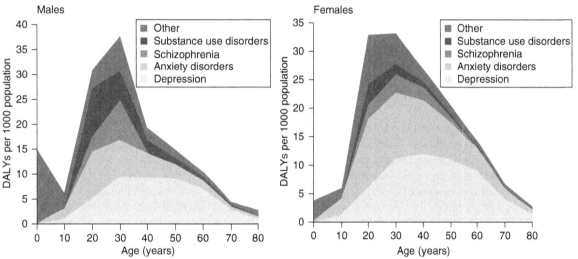

Figure 2 Incident YLD rates per 1000 population by mental disorder, age and sex, Victoria, 2001. Reproduced from Victorian Government (2001) Current report – Mortality & Morbidity report & DALY worksheets 2001 – http://www.health.vic.gov.au/healthstatus/bodvic/bod_current.htm with permission.

depression and anxiety) is far greater in early adulthood than at any other age. Depressive disorders also commonly accompany other medical conditions, particularly in aging populations. When depression does co-occur with other common medical conditions, the degree of resultant disability is higher than for any other combination of health conditions. This is illustrated in **Figure 3**, those with depression and another chronic condition had much lower mean health scores when compared with people who had only a chronic condition. These patterns were consistent even after adjusting for other sociodemographic variables.

Risk Factors

Each of the major risk factor domains (genes, family environment, and individual-specific environment)

influence depressive and anxiety disorders in a distinct manner. There is also a complex interaction between these risk factors that is still to be unraveled. What is absolutely clear is that social determinants affect mental health throughout life. People who are at the lower end of the socioeconomic ladder experience twice the risk of serious illness and premature death as those near the top. This effect is not limited to lower-income countries but rather is consistent across the spectrum of society. Specifically, the most disadvantaged groups in any community experience greater incidence of depression, drug use, anxiety, hostility, and feelings of hopelessness, which all rebound on physical health.

Our understanding of the specific nature of both the biological and social risk factors to anxiety and depression have advanced significantly in recent years. At this time, we have moved well beyond the simplistic nature vs nurture debates of previous decades. On the basis of

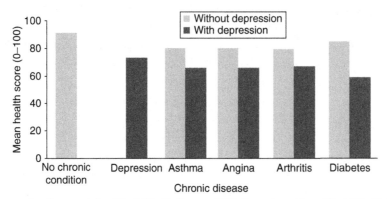

Figure 3   Mean health score by disease status, World Health Survey 2003. Reproduced from World Health Organization (2007) Statistical Information System. Ten statistical highlights in global public health. http://www.who.int/whosis/whostat2007_10highlights. pdf (accessed January 2008).

extensive twin and other genetically informative population and family studies, it is clear that at least 30% of the population-based risk to depressive disorders in adults can be attributed to additive genetic factors. Of the 70% of risk that is not readily attributed to genetic factors, most (up to 60%) is due to current (or unique) environmental factors rather than childhood (about 10%) experiences.

For those anxiety and depressive disorders that are present in early adult life, it appears that many of the genetic influences are shared in common and that overt differences in clinical presentation may be attributed to differential exposure to other environmental risk factors (e.g., personal trauma, dysfunctional parenting styles, or other interpersonal factors). Importantly, it is now clear that the pattern of genetic and environmental risk factors varies across the life span, with new genetic and environmental factors (particularly related to vascular disease and neurodegenerative disorders) beginning to emerge in later life.

Perhaps the most significant development in our understanding emerged with the publication of longitudinal studies demonstrating the additional risks that occur when an individual has both specific polymorphisms of genes of biological relevance to anxiety and depression (e.g., selective serotonin transporter) and exposure to specific childhood (e.g., maltreatment) or adult (e.g., recent interpersonal stressors) environmental factors (Caspi and Moffitt, 2006). These specific gene–environment interactions have long been postulated but not previously documented. They allow us to move beyond simplistic genetic or environmental models of adult mental health problems to focus on the actual pathways that may be relevant. Inherent in these emerging models is the complex dance between genetic substrates and the timing and extent of relevant environmental exposures, as shown in **Figure 4** (see discussion in Caspi and Moffit, 2006). This more detailed knowledge may assist us in designing more targeted preventative and early intervention strategies. Certainly it has already led to a much more active reconsideration of the roles

of specific environmental risk factors and the ways in which such risks may help us (in combination with other new neuroscience technologies such as structural and functional brain imaging) to better understand the biological mechanisms underpinning common anxiety and depressive disorders.

Age of Onset of Anxiety and Depression

For the common forms of anxiety and depression, the typical age of onset is the teenage or early adult years. Seventy-five percent of the common conditions commence before the age of 25 years. While various forms of anxiety are common in childhood, many are closely associated with perturbations in family and kin environments and do not necessarily persist into adulthood. Temperamental characteristics, such as social inhibition or social anxiety, which are the precursors of adult disorders, are often evident in early childhood and the preadolescent period. These temperamental characteristics appear to have their own genetic (e.g., polymorphism of the serotonin transporter gene) and/or other neurobiological determinants (e.g., heightened amygdala response to fearful stimuli).

The phenotypes associated with the onset of the more classical mood disorders begin to emerge in the adolescent era. There has been some debate about the variation in symptom patterns in younger persons with an emphasis on features such as increased somatic features of anxiety, irritability, inattention, brief and unstable mood variations, disturbed sleep–wake cycle, and persistent fatigue states. The disorders are also least likely to be identified or treated by health professionals during this period. Consequently, the age for first active treatment is often at least a decade after onset of the clinical manifestations of the disorder. By that time, the condition is likely to have become chronic or recurrent and to be associated with significant alcohol or other substance misuse, tobacco use, or other markers of social disability (reduced

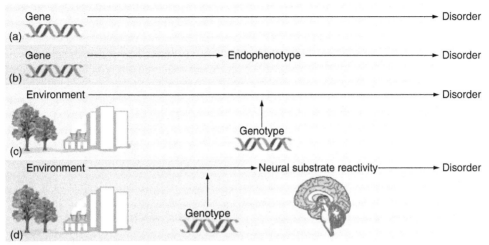

Figure 4 Approaches to psychiatric genetics research. (a) The gene to disorder approach assumes direct linear relations between genes and disorder. (b) The endophenotype approach replaces the disorder outcomes with intermediate phenotypes. (c) The gene–environment interaction approach assumes that genes moderate the effect of environmental pathogens on disorder. (d) Neuroscience complements the latter research by specifying the proximal role of nervous system reactivity in the gene–environment interaction. Reproduced from Caspi A and Moffitt TE (2006) Gene-environment interactions in psychiatry: Joining forces with neuroscience. *Nature Reviews Neuroscience* 7: 583–590, with permission.

educational achievement, reduced employment, and dysfunctional interpersonal relationships).

While many subtyping models of depressive disorders have been developed by clinicians, largely on the basis of cross-sectional phenotypic studies and short-term treatment trials, a system that simply differentiates early-onset (typically before 25 years of age) from late-onset cases (typically after 60 years) appears to have closer links with basic patterns of pathophysiology. It is also likely to be of greater utility in terms of increasing public awareness of relevant risk factors and the value of pursuing different preventive strategies or treatment regimens at different ages.

For early-onset depressive disorders, the emphasis will inevitably continue to be on development of universal prevention programs in childhood and the early adolescent period. When combined with early identification and treatment of major anxiety disorders in childhood and the early school years as well as identification and active management of significant anxiety and depressive disorders during the secondary school period, there is an opportunity for major reductions in lifetime burden estimates. Given the emerging evidence of the adverse effects of untreated depression on critical brain regions such as the hippocampus and the positive effects of some treatments on brain growth factors (e.g., antidepressant and second-generation antipsychotics that increase levels of brain-derived neurotrophic factor), we will increasingly see an emphasis on not just 'symptom reduction' and social recovery but also brain protection for those with early-onset disorders. **Figure 5** shows the level of hippocampal reduction in association with early- and late-onset depression.

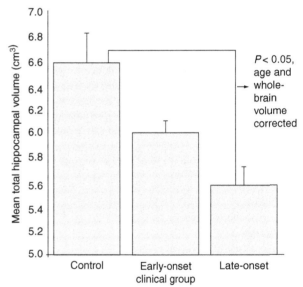

Figure 5 Hippocampal reduction in association with early- and late-onset depression demonstrating that hippocampal reduction is more severe in late-onset depression. Reproduced from Hickie I, Naismith S, Ward PB, *et al.* (2005) Reduced hippocampal volumes and memory loss in patients with early- and late-onset depression. *British Journal of Psychiatry* 186: 197–202, with permission.

For those with late-onset depressive disorders, it is now evident that different genetic, vascular, and other medical and environmental risk factors play major roles. Typically, the onset rate of new anxiety and depressive disorders declines with increasing age. Onsets in this age range are typically due less to changing psychosocial circumstances than the onset of physical illness, brain changes, and/or social isolation or decreased participation due to ill health. Neuroimaging and neurocognitive research indicate that the patterns of brain change demand not only traditional antidepressant therapies but an increased emphasis on improved vascular and general medical health. Importantly, new opportunities for prevention arise in this age range. The clearest relates to improved vascular health, but this may well be complemented by a variety of other behavioral (increased exercise), dietary, and supplement (increased folate, B group vitamins, antioxidants and omega-3 fatty acids), employment, and socialization strategies.

Recent Neurobiological Models of Depression

For the last 50 years, our neurobiological theories of depressive disorders have rested largely on circumstantial evidence of altered serotonin, norepinephrine, or dopamine neurotransmission. These functional monoamine models assume structural integrity within relevant frontal, subcortical, and temporal lobe nuclei and their connecting white matter tracts. However, there has always been an uneasy fit between this pharmacological model and the delay in clinical response, lack of difference in clinical outcomes associated with different neuropharmacological entities, benefits of medications that do not act principally on the monoamine systems, and evidence of progressive structural brain changes in persons with both unipolar and bipolar depressive disorders.

In the last 25 years, structural and functional brain imaging techniques have clearly demonstrated that substantive regional brain alterations occur in both early- and late-onset major depressive disorders, as well as bipolar disorder. These regional brain changes are likely to reflect various alterations to the neural microcircuitry, including neuronal, glial cell, and synaptic components. In addition to regional changes affecting cortical and subcortical nuclei, disruption of white matter tracts and reduction in size of the frontal lobes, subcortical nuclei, and the hippocampus have all been detected and linked with key phenotypic features such as psychomotor change, cognitive impairment, and poorer illness outcomes.

Given the epidemiological linkages of mid-life depression with late-life cognitive impairment and dementia, there is now a need to reconsider the underlying nature of this association. Previously, it was assumed that such associations were unlikely to be causal but more likely to reflect shared risk factors, such as small vessel cerebrovascular disease or other late-life neurodegenerative processes. However, the clear demonstration of reduced hippocampal size and the likely association between such reductions and duration of untreated illness suggests that structural brain changes in depression may create a unique neurobiological vulnerability to later-life dementia syndromes.

Consistent with these findings in human studies, relevant neurobiological correlates of depression have emerged in animal models. Some of the most interesting include impaired hippocampal neurogenesis, impaired synaptogenesis, and altered glial cell structure and function. The therapeutic effect of antidepressant medicines in rat models appears to be dependent on restoration of normal patterns of neurogenesis in the hippocampus. Additionally, small changes in absolute cell numbers are associated with major changes in critical neurocircuit functioning.

Evidenced-Based Interventions

Community and health development programs for underresourced communities with poor physical health status often ignore the importance of common mental health conditions, despite the direct and large contributions of poor mental health to lack of sustainable change in health and economic indicators. In contrast, these communities often place high worth on programs that promote such concepts as emotional and social well-being, reduction in premature death due to suicide, injury, and accidents, as well as increased achievements in education, employment, and social participation as a result of promotion of better mental health alongside active identification and management of common mental health problems.

Delivery of Evidence-Based Treatments through Collaborative Care Models

As a consequence of the prevalence of anxiety and depression, the lack of investment in mental health care historically, negative community attitudes, and the patterns of organization of health systems established in the nineteenth and early twentieth centuries, even in the best-resourced health systems, only a minority of those affected receive any care, let alone evidence-based treatments (see The Lancet Series on Global Mental Health, 2008). Future health service planning needs urgently to look at new methods of service delivery (e.g., e-health informational and clinical services – web examples of beyondblue, blue pages, moodgym, reachout central; reliance on educational and primary care-based workforces and promotion of collaborative care models) if we are ever to make substantial progress.

Two of the most important considerations here relate to the maintenance of choice in access to preferred treatments as well as the promotion of continuous improvement in the quality of services provided. Community surveys continue to highlight strong consumer preferences for increased access to nonpharmacological treatments, self-care strategies, detailed information about treatment options and self-monitoring tools. The emphasis on preference for psychological treatments is not limited to developed countries. The planning for delivery of adequate nonpharmacological strategies in developing countries has not been sufficiently addressed. Another major consideration is the continued emphasis in many primary care treatment settings on the short-term use of inexpensive sedatives and hypnotics rather than engagement in active antidepressant therapy. Negative community attitudes toward the use of antidepressant medicines persist and are reinforced by media and some professional stereotypes that overemphasize side effects, capacity for dependence, and links with self-harm or violence to others.

Of perhaps greater importance than the long-standing debate on the relative merits of pharmacological as compared with other modes of treatment has been the neglect of the issues of ensuring adequate adherence to any evidence-based therapy to achieve full remission and prevent recurrence. While such issues have been highlighted within clinical trial environments, they require significant restructuring of health-care systems (with greater use of information technologies, recall systems, and active monitoring tools) and greater emphasis on engaging consumers and carers in long-term rather than short-term treatment plans.

There is now no doubt that collaborative (or stepped) care models of clinical service, as shown in **Table 4**, deliver on the twin objectives of active engagement and continuous quality improvement. Sadly, even in well-resourced countries many professional groups and third-party insurance systems continue to promote more limited fee-for-service or other disjointed service models. In some national and private insurance systems, health care for mental disorders may be actively excluded or care severely restricted. The next major challenge for improved care for mental disorders such as anxiety and depression will be active recognition by health-care systems that when poorly managed these conditions are chronic, disabling, and costly to treat. In contrast, when actively managed with the appropriate and ongoing mix of psychological and medical care, costs are minimized and good health and economic outcomes are achieved.

Impact of Increased Treatments on Suicide Rates

One of the most important arguments for increasing access to treatments for those with anxiety and depressive disorders is to reduce premature death due to suicide, accident, and other injuries and other medical complications such as coronary heart disease. The most impressive evidence for the benefit to be derived by increased treatment of mild and moderately severe depressive disorders

in recent years has been the associated decline in suicide rates in proportion to the increase in access to care, as demonstrated in **Figure 6**. While this interpretation has been debated, sufficient evidence has accumulated across a large number of countries and treatment settings to support this interpretation (policy references). Of concern have been the recent reports that decreased provision of treatments to young persons in the United States and Europe (after regulatory bodies issued specific warnings about the potential dangers associated with antidepressant therapy) has now been associated with an upward spike in deaths due to suicide. International suicide prevention research has typically focused on other large community, demographic, and social factors (including reducing access to lethal means), while placing less emphasis on those clinical care factors that have a strong evidence base. These more recent studies suggest that particularly in well-resourced and socially stable countries, greater emphasis should now be placed on improved access to evidence-based care.

Matching Pathophysiological Models to Clinical Practice

The most recent large clinical effectiveness trials – Sequenced Treatment Alternatives to Relieve Depression (STAR*D) – provide even more reason to challenge the existing pharmacological dogma. What is most impressive in these studies is the marked effect of prolonged duration of pharmacological treatment. Independent of the specific characteristics of the treatment provided, fewer than 30% responded in the first 12 weeks of SSRI treatment, while another 20–30% responded in the next 14 weeks, and a further 12–20% responded in the last phase, as shown in **Figure 7**. This prolonged time course of additional clinical benefits is consistent with the view that full recovery depends on fundamental changes in underlying cellular or circuit elements.

To date, we do not have evidence from clinical studies that clinical recovery is linked directly to increases in hippocampal or other regional brain volumes or specific markers of neurogenesis or synaptogenesis. In the interim, the clear indication is that acute treatments may need to be prolonged to achieve maximal neurobiological benefits. Additional considerations include more active consideration of proposed neuroprotective compounds. These include not only the traditional psychopharmacological agents such as lithium carbonate, but also the second-generation antipsychotics that have been shown both to increase brain-derived neurotrophic factor (BDNF) as well as reduce brain changes during the early phases of psychotic disorders. Other potential augmentation or treatment strategies include folic acid, antioxidants, statins, and omega-3 fatty acids.

Table 4 Clinical staging model framework for psychotic and severe mood disorders

Stage	Definition	Target populations and referral sources	Potential interventions
0	Increased risk of psychotic or severe mood disorder No symptoms currently	• First-degree teenage relatives of probands (subjects/patients under study/concern)	• Improved mental health literacy • Family education, drug education • Brief cognitive skills training
1a	Mild or non-specific symptoms (including neurocognitive deficits) of psychosis or severe mood disorder. Mild functional change or decline	• Screening of teenage populations • *Referral by*: primary care physicians; school counsellors	• Formal mental health literacy • Family psychoeducation, formal CBT • Active substance misuse reduction
1b	Ultra high risk: moderate but subthreshold symptoms, with moderate neurocognitive changes and functional decline to caseness (GAF, <70)	• *Referral by*: educational agencies; primary care physicians; emergency departments; welfare agencies	• Family psychoeducation, formal CBT • Active substance misuse reduction • Omega-3 fatty acids • Atypical antipsychotic agents • Antidepressant agents or mood stabilizers
2	First episode of psychotic or severe mood disorder Full threshold disorder with moderate to severe symptoms, neurocognitive deficits and functional decline (GAF, 30–50)	• *Referral by*: primary care physicians; emergency departments; welfare agencies; specialist care agencies; drug and alcohol services	• Family psychoeducation, formal CBT • Active substance misuse reduction • Atypical antipsychotic agents • Antidepressant agents or mood stabilizers • Vocational rehabilitation
3a	Incomplete remission from first episode of care. Patient's management could be linked or fast-tracked to Stage 4	• Primary and specialist care services	• As for Stage 2, but with additional emphasis on medical and psychosocial strategies to achieve full remission
3b	Recurrence or relapse of psychotic or mood disorder, which stabilizes with treatment at a GAF level, or with residual symptoms or neurocognition below the best level achieved after remission from the first episode	• Primary and specialist care services	• As for Stage 3a, but with additional emphasis on relapse prevention and strategies to detect early warning signs
3c	Multiple relapses, provided worsening in clinical extent and impact of illness is objectively present	• Specialist care services	• As for Stage 3b, but with emphasis on long-term stabilization
4	Severe, persistent *or* unremitting illness, as judged by symptoms, neurocognition, and disability criteria Patient's management could be fast-tracked to this stage at first presentation, based on specific clinical and functional criteria (from Stage 2), or because of failure to respond to treatment (from Stage 3a)	• Specialized care services	• As for Stage 3c, but with emphasis on clozapine, other tertiary treatments, and social participation despite ongoing disability

Reproduced from McGorry PD, Hickie IB, Yung AR, *et al.* (2006) Clinical staging of psychiatric disorders: A heuristic framework for choosing earlier, safer and more effective interventions. *Australian and New Zealand Journal of Psychiatry* 40: 616–622, with permission.

Primary and Indicated Preventative Interventions

Some of the key social risk factors (e.g., dysfunctional parenting; physical, sexual, or emotional abuse) to adult anxiety or depression are clearly operative in early life and, hence, it is a key period for consideration of relevant primary preventative health programs. Of greatest interest from a broad population health perspective are those broad social, community, and family-based approaches that promote both good physical and mental health in pregnancy and throughout the early years. Prenatal identification of cases of anxiety and depression, which can lead not only to immediate treatment of the mother, but also to active engagement of the partner and extended family with consequent increased practical and emotional support following the birth, has obvious appeal (see beyondblue, the National Depression Initiative and beyondblue postnatal

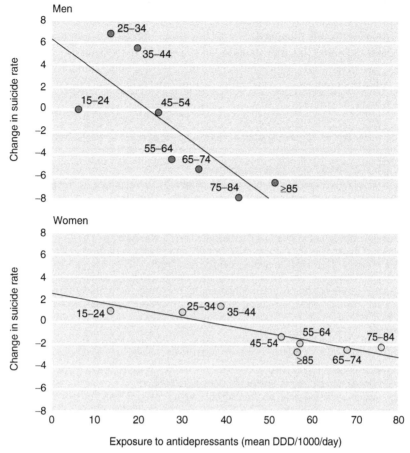

Figure 6 Change in suicide rate in men and women by age and exposure to antidepressants. Reproduced from Hall WD, Mant A, Mitchell PB, *et al.* (2003) Association between antidepressant prescribing and suicide in Australia, 1992–2000: Trend analysis. *British Medical Journal* 326: 1008–1011, with permission.

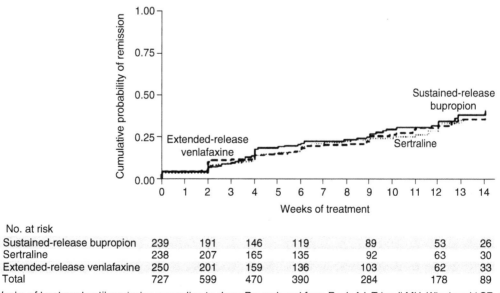

No. at risk						
Sustained-release bupropion	239	191	146	119	89	53	26
Sertraline	238	207	165	135	92	63	30
Extended-release venlafaxine	250	201	159	136	103	62	33
Total	727	599	470	390	284	178	89

Figure 7 Weeks of treatment until remission according to drug. Reproduced from Rush AJ, Trivedi MH, Wisniewski SR, *et al.* (2006) Bupropion-SR, Setraline, or Venlafaxine-XR after failure of SSRIs for depression. *The New England Journal of Medicine* 354: 1231–1242, with permission.

depression, Beyondblue Schools Research Initiative, 2007). For similar reasons, increased detection and treatment of postnatal depression has been extensively promoted.

Most population health planning (including most health service systems) has made little provision for early intervention and indicated prevention particularly for these adolescent and early adulthood cases of depression and anxiety. The challenge of youth mental health is now recognized internationally. Traditional health systems tend to focus on child health needs (infectious diseases, nutrition, immunization, management of developmental difficulties) and then the needs of adults in mid

Table 5   A consumer and carer agenda for people whose lives have been affected by depression and related disorders

A. Within health-care services
• Development of more responsive primary and specialist care sectors
• Education of health-care professionals to ensure that they do not contribute to the stigmatization of people with depression or anxiety
• Development of improved information resources for people provided with treatments
• Provision of more information about services and treatments available
• Advocacy for improved access to non-pharmacological forms of care at low cost to consumers
• Advocacy for better professions-based responses to the maldistribution of specialist services
• Support for the development of accessible self-help, mutual support, and other non-professional care agencies
• Promotion of the key roles of carers, particularly to primary care professionals
• Promotion of a broader model of recovery from illness than that associated with the medical notion of 'remission of symptoms'
• Development of novel measures of service quality and mechanisms for collecting such data routinely within health-care services and
• Development of measures of consumer- and carer-based concepts of clinical recovery that can be incorporated in treatment and health-care services research
B. Broader community priorities
• Reduction of stigma through increasing community awareness and the promotion of the experiences of people with depression or anxiety
• Workplace and schools-based education programs
• Development of depression-prevention programs, particularly for young people
• Development of education resources for the wider community concerning common symptoms of depression or anxiety, as well as how to go about accessing appropriate care and
• Initiating response to formal barriers, such as exclusion from life and income protection insurance

Reproduced from McNair BG, Highet NJ, Hickie IB, and Davenport TA (2002) Exploring the perspectives of people whose lives have been affected by depression. *Medical Journal of Australia* 176: s69–s76.

Table 6   Most frequently identified medical and mental disorders by 900 Australian adults

	Major health problems* (% [n])		
All medical and mental disorders	*For all Australians*	*For younger Australians*	*For older Australians*
Cancer	32% (413)	3% (23)	21% (222)
Heart disease and other vascular risks	26% (339)	0	30% (326)
Alcohol or other substance misuse	10% (128)	55% (411)	1% (12)
Diabetes	8% (108)	2% (17)	8% (88)
Infectious diseases (including HIV/AIDS)	6% (78)	8% (58)	0.5% (5)
Asthma	5% (58)	7% (49)	0.3% (3)
Mental health (not specified)	3% (33)	4% (33)	2% (19)
Depression	2% (31)	7% (52)	1% (10)
Anxiety/stress/pressure	2% (31)	3% (21)	1% (6)
Dementia/Alzheimer's disease	0.7% (9)	0	11% (117)
Arthritis	0.7% (9)	0	11% (112)
Gambling	0.3% (5)	0	0
Eating disorders	0.3% (4)	3% (21)	0.1% (1)
Accident/injury	0.2% (3)	3% (20)	0.1% (1)
Suicide	0.1% (1)	0.5% (4)	0
Schizophrenia/psychosis	0.1% (1)	0.5% (4)	0
Other	3% (41)	4% (26)	13% (141)
Total	100% (1292)	100% (739)	100% (1063)

Reproduced from Highet NJ, Hickie IB, and Davenport TA (2002) Monitoring awareness of and attitudes to depression in Australia. *Medical Journal of Australia* 176: s63–s68, with permission.
*Each participant had the opportunity to provide more than one response (ie. *What do you consider to be the major health problem in Australia at present? Are there any other major health problems in Australia?*).

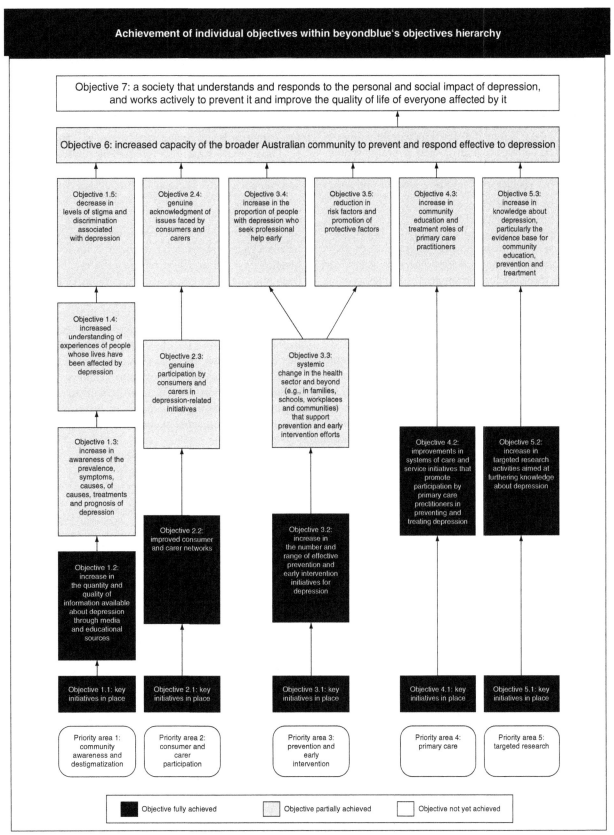

Figure 8   Achievement of individual objectives within beyondblue's objectives hierarchy. Reproduced from Pirkis J, Hickie I, Young L, *et al.* (2005) An evaluation of beyond blue: Australia's National Depression Initiative. *The International Journal of Mental Health Promotion* 7: 35–53 with permission.

and later life (musculoskeletal, cardio- and cerebrovascular, cancer, dementia, and diabetes). Such traditional patterns of organization of services are therefore weakest at that period of life when the need for early and effective intervention for anxiety and depressive disorders is greatest.

In higher-income countries, there has been some recognition of the importance of the adolescent-onset period. This has led to the development of universal primary intervention programs aimed to promote mental health awareness, reduce social, interpersonal, and other known risk factors (including alcohol and other substance misuse and bullying), teach specific cognitive and behavioral skills, and/or enhance other community supports (see Gatehouse Project, 2007; beyondblue Schools Research Initiative, 2007). These have been delivered mainly through school-based settings and more recent projects have attempted to integrate such initiatives into the ongoing early high school curriculum and related school environment. The longer-term value of such programs is not yet evident, but this remains a critical arena for development.

Other clinically based early intervention and indicated prevention programs are now under development internationally (see Headspace, 2008; Headstrong, n.d.). Such programs promote not only new pathways to care for young persons but also earlier engagement through e-health and other primary care health and education systems, provision of effective multidisciplinary care early in the course of illness, long-term professional and self-care packages, reduction of secondary alcohol and other drug use, and return to education, training, and employment as key outcome variables. The effectiveness of e-health-based interventions has been well demonstrated and offers real hope of providing low-cost and accessible interventions to young persons (particularly young men) who do not readily engage with clinical services.

Improving Public Understanding of Anxiety and Depressive Disorders

The lack of provision of effective treatments to persons with anxiety and depression is perceived by health professionals internationally as the major challenge for future health policy and service development. Quite often, however, surveys of those who experience these disorders, and their families and care providers, prioritize the reduction in the consequences of lack of accurate information and overt stigma, as shown in **Table 5**. These negative effects take many forms and extend well beyond the expression of negative personal attitudes to include restrictions of access to health care as well as significant barriers to full participation in employment, education and training, insurance, and other financial systems.

A wide variety of factors have been identified that contribute to these adverse experiences for persons who have these common mental disorders. Some are largely historical and relate to the basic lack of knowledge about the physiological correlates and adverse health and economic consequences of living with untreated forms of anxiety and depression. Others relate to the low priority individuals give to the relative importance of mental health as distinct from physical health problems, as shown in **Table 6**.

These views have underpinned the development of measures of mental health literacy (see Jorm *et al.*, 2006) and supported the implementation of specific regional (see Hickie, 2004), national (Beyondblue, the National Depression Initiative (2008)) and local interventions to increase community awareness, promote positive views of help-seeking, and reinforce accurate knowledge of the benefits of professional or self-care interventions. It has been possible, at least in some better-resourced countries, to develop a comprehensive and integrated approach to increased public awareness, consumer and care provider participation, removal of societal barriers and primary health-care reform (see **Figure 8**). An important part of this movement has been the systematic study of the attitudes and knowledge of different health-care professionals. Consumers of care often report that the most negative attitudes they encounter are expressed by general health and other specialist mental health providers.

Citations

Caspi A and Moffitt TE (2006) Gene-environment interactions in psychiatry: Joining forces with neuroscience. *Nature Reviews Neuroscience* 7: 583–590.

Hall WD, Mant A, Mitchell PB, Rendle VA, Hickie IB, and McManus P (2003) Association between antidepressant prescribing and suicide in Australia, 1992–2000: Trend analysis. *British Medical Journal* 326: 1008–1011.

Hickie I and Scott L (2007) *Understanding Depression.* Sydney, Australia: Educational Health Solutions.

Hickie I, Naismith S, Ward PB, *et al.* (2005) Reduced hippocampal volumes and memory loss in patients with early- and late-onset depression. *British Journal of Psychiatry* 186: 197–202.

Highet NJ, Hickie IB, and Davenport TA (2002) Monitoring awareness of and attitudes to depression in Australia. *Medical Journal of Australia* 176: s63–s68.

Kessler RC, Chiu WT, Demler O, and Walters EE (2005) Prevalence, severity and comorbidity of 12-month DSM-IV disorders in the National Comorbidity Survey Replication. *Archives of General Psychiatry* 62: 617–627.

Lopez AD and Murray CJL (1998) The global burden of disease, 1990–2020. *Nature Medicine* 4: 1241–1243.

Mathers CD and Loncar D (2006) Projections of global mortality and burden of disease from 2002 to 2030. *PLoS Medicine* 3: 2011–2030.

McGorry PD, Hickie IB, Yung AR, *et al.* (2006) Clinical staging of psychiatric disorders: A heuristic framework for choosing earlier, safer and more effective interventions. *Australian and New Zealand Journal of Psychiatry* 40: 616–622.

McNair BG, Highet NJ, Hickie IB, and Davenport TA (2002) Exploring the perspectives of people whose lives have been affected by depression. *Medical Journal of Australia* 176: s69–s76.

Pirkis J, Hickie I, Young L, *et al.* (2005) An evaluation of beyond blue: Australia's National Depression Initiative. *The International Journal of Mental Health Promotion* 7: 35–53.

Rush AJ, Trivedi MH, Wisniewski SR, *et al.* (2006) Bupropion-SR, Setraline, or Venlafaxine-XR after failure of SSRIs for depression. *The New England Journal of Medicine* 354: 1231–1242.

State Government of Victoria Department of Human Services (2001) Current report – Mortality and Morbidity report and DALY worksheets 2001. http://www.health.vic.gov.au/healthstatus/bodvic/bod_current.htm (accessed January 2008).

World Health Organization (2007) Statistical Information System. Ten statistical highlights in global public health. http://www.who.int/whosis/whostat2007_10highlights.pdf (accessed January 2008).

Further Reading

Airan RD, Meltzer LA, Roy M, *et al.* (2007) High-speed imaging reveals neurophysiological links to behaviour in an animal model of depression. *Science* 317(819); 5 July 2007 (10.11126/science/1144400).

Castren E, Voikar V, and Rantamaki T (2007) Role of neurotropic factors in depression. *Current Opinion in Pharmocology* 7: 18–21.

Christensen H, Griffiths KM, and Jorm AF (2004) Delivering interventions for depression by using the internet: Randomised controlled trial. *British Medical Journal* 328: 265.

Hickie I (2004) Treatment guidelines for depression in the Asia Pacific region: A review of current developments. *Australasian Psychiatry* 12 (supplement 1): s33–s37.

Insel TR (2007) Shining light on depression. *Science* 317: 757–758.

Jorm AF, Barney LJ, Christensen H, *et al.* (2006) Research on mental health literacy: What we know and what we still need to know. *Australian and New Zealand Journal of Psychiatry* 40: 3–5.

Kessler RC, Berglund P, Demler O, *et al.* (2005) Lifetime prevalence and age-of-onset distributions of DSM-IV disorders in the National Comorbidity Survey Replication. *Archives of General Psychiatry* 62: 593–602.

Kruijshaar ME, Barendregt J, Vos T, *et al.* (2005) Lifetime prevalence of estimates of major depression: An indirect estimation method and quantification of recall bias. *European Journal of Epidemiology* 20: 103–111.

The Lancet Series on Global Mental Health: Article Collection (2007) http://www.thelancet.com/online/focus/mental_health/collection (accessed January 2008).

Lopez AD, Mathers CD, Ezzati M, Jamison DT and Murray CJL (eds.) (2006) *Global Burden of Disease and Risk Factors.* New York: Oxford University Press.

Mann JJ, Apter A, Bertolote J, *et al.* (2005) Suicide prevention strategies: A systematic review. *Journal of the American Medical Association* 294: 2064–2074.

Patel V, Flisher AJ, Hetrick SE, and McGorry PD (2007) Mental health of young people: A global public-health challenge. *Lancet* 369: 1302–1313.

Pezawas L, Meyer-Lindenberg A, Drabant EM, *et al.* (2005) 5-HTTLPR polymorphism impacts human cingulated-amygdala interactions: A genetic susceptibility mechanism for depression. *Nature Neuroscience* 8: 828–834.

Pirkis J, Hickie I, Young L, *et al.* (2005) An evaluation of beyond blue: Australia's national depression initiative. *The International Journal of Mental Health Promotion* 7: 35–53.

Sanderson K, Andrews G, Correy J, *et al.* (2003) Reducing the burden of affective disorders: Is evidence-based health care affordable? *Journal of Affective Disorders* 77(2): 109–125.

Sartorius N (2001) The economic and social burden of depression. *Journal of Clinical Psychiatry* 62(supplement) 15: 8–11.

Relevant Websites

http://www.beyondblue.org.au – Beyondblue, the National Depression Initiative (accessed January 2008).

http://www.beyondblue.org.au/index.aspx?link_id=4.64 – Beyondblue Schools Research Initiative (accessed January 2008).

http://www.beyondblue.org.au/index.aspx?link_id=94.575 – Beyondblue Postnatal Depression (accessed January 2008).

http://www.rch.org.au/gatehouseproject – Gatehouse Project (accessed January 2008).

http://www.headspace.org.au/default.aspx?page=home – Headspace (accessed January 2008).

http://www.headstrong.ie – Headstrong (accessed January 2008).

http://www.ehub.anu.edu.au/research/moodgym.php – E-hub: e-mental Health Research & Development.

http://www.triplep.net – The Triple P-Positive Parenting Program.

http://www.spheregp.com.au/aboutus.htm – SPHERE: A National Mental Health Project.

Specific Mental Health Disorders: Eating Disorders

S S Delinsky, J Derenne, and A E Becker, Massachusetts General Hospital, Boston, MA, USA

Public Health Significance

Eating disorders comprise a related group of mental disorders characterized by disturbance in dietary patterns, body image, and/or efforts to control weight. Taken together, anorexia nervosa and bulimia nervosa have the highest mortality rate (tied with substance use disorders) of any mental illness (Harris and Barraclough, 1998). Given that these disorders most frequently have their onset in adolescence, this high mortality rate is particularly striking. Premature death in individuals with these disorders is attributable both to suicide – there is a suicide rate of 23 times expected in these disorders (Harris and Barraclough, 1997) – and to medical complications from low weight, poor nutrition, and purging behaviors.

Although eating disorders are considered mental illnesses, their associated behaviors – including restrictive-pattern eating, binge-pattern eating, and purging and other behaviors meant to neutralize the effects of over-eating or to control weight – commonly result in malnu-trition, obesity, and a wide variety of complications that affect nearly every organ system. Individuals with an eating disorder may induce vomiting or misuse laxatives, enemas, diuretics, or stimulants to lose weight. Others restrict eating or exercise compulsively. Those with comorbid insulin-dependent diabetes mellitus have been known to underdose insulin with the intent to lose weight. This is particularly dangerous because it can lead to diabetic ketoacidosis. Chronic purging may cause erosion of dental and gastrointestinal dysfunction (Becker et al., 1999). Metabolic disturbances, such as hypokalemia, may result from chronic vomiting or chronic laxative or diuretic misuse and can contribute to potentially fatal cardiac arrhythmia and renal disease.

Classification

The *Diagnostic and Statistical Manual for Mental Disorders* (DSM)-IV (APA, 1994) consists of three diagnostic cate-gories of eating disorders: Anorexia nervosa (AN), bulimia nervosa (BN), and eating disorder not otherwise speci-fied (EDNOS). The criteria for AN include refusal to maintain adequate body weight (e.g., 85% expected), fear of weight gain, disturbance in how weight/shape are experienced, and amenorrhea. Criteria for BN include objective binge eating and inappropriate compensatory behaviors at least twice weekly for 3 months, plus extreme importance of weight/shape to self-evaluation. If a patient meets criteria for both AN and BN, the diagnosis of AN supersedes the diagnosis of BN. It should be noted, however, that diagnostic criteria, especially 85% expected body weight in AN, are not absolute, and should not be used alone as thresholds for clinical care, especially in children, according to APA (2006) and NICE practice guidelines (Wilson and Shafran, 2005).

EDNOS is the category reserved for eating disorders of clinical severity that do not meet diagnostic criteria for either AN or BN. Although nominally a residual category, EDNOS is the most common eating disorder diagnosis made in most outpatient settings other than those attract-ing highly specialized referrals (Fairburn and Bohn, 2005). Accumulating evidence suggests that EDNOS and AN or BN are indistinguishable on severity of psychopathology and related impairment.

Within EDNOS, binge eating disorder (BED) was pro-posed as a disorder requiring further study in DSM-IV, and uncertainty remains as to whether it constitutes a separate clinical category (see Wilfley et al., 2003). BED is char-acterized by recurrent episodes of binge eating without the compensatory behaviors in BN or other extreme meth-ods of weight control. Night eating syndrome (NES), characterized by wakeful nighttime eating, is a unique combination of eating disorder, sleep disorder, and mood disorder. Various diagnostic criteria for NES have been proposed, and the disorder warrants further research.

Prevalence and Cultural Issues

The majority of individuals with an eating disorder in the United States do not access formal health care for their illness (Hudson et al., 2007). One major reason for this is that up to half of cases presenting in primary care settings are unrecognized by clinicians (Becker et al., 1999). A reluctance to relinquish symptoms that characterize AN and BN, the frequent absence of clinical signs in BN, BED, and EDNOS, and clinician referral patterns (Becker et al., 2003) may contribute to this suboptimal access to care. Even individuals who do access treatment have an unacceptably high rate of continued symptoms (Keel and Mitchell, 1997).

The reported prevalence of eating disorders may under-estimate true prevalence, as both self-report and interview-based ascertainment may miss cases if an individual is unwilling to disclose his or her symptoms. Moreover, dif-ferential access to care may contribute to prolonged dura-tion of illness and elevated prevalence in some populations. Point prevalence of eating disorders in Western Europe and the United States is estimated at 0.3% for anorexia nervosa and 1% for bulimia nervosa in young women. Point preva-lence of BED is at least 1% among all adults (Hoek and van Hoeken, 2003). The incidence of BN appears to have increased over the last half of the twentieth century and data support that incidence of BED may have increased over this time period as well (Hoek and van Hoeken, 2003; Hudson et al., 2007). Fewer data on subsyndromal and atypical eating disorders are available, but lifetime preva-lence of AN together with anorexia-like syndromes is esti-mated at over 3% and of BN together with bulimia-like syndromes is estimated at 8% (CDC, 2006). Moreover, data from the 2005 Youth Behavioral Risk Survey (YRBS) reported by the Centers for Disease Control and Prevention (CDC, 2006) provide some insight as to how commonplace extreme weight-control behaviors are. Female students in the United States who participated in YRBS indicated that within the past month, 6.2% had engaged in self-induced vomiting or laxative abuse to control weight, 8.1% admitted to using diet pills or other products, and 17% fasted for a period of 24 h or more (CDC, 2006).

Female gender is a well-established fixed marker for AN and BN, with at least 90% of cases occurring among females (APA, 1994; Jacobi, 2005). BED is also significantly more prevalent among females, although the gender ratio is not as high (APA, 1994; Jacobi, 2005; Hudson et al., 2007).

Comparison of prevalence estimates of eating disorders across cultures suggests that BN may emerge exclusively in social environments characterized by exposure to so-called Western ideals. In contrast, AN has been reported across diverse social contexts, although the rationale for food refusal is tied to the local cultural context (Keel and Klump, 2003). For example, phenomenological variation in AN between Western and Asian populations is striking (e.g., an absence of fat phobia in the latter; Lee, 2001). Finally, population data have strongly suggested that acculturation, immigration, and modernization contribute to the vulnerability for an eating disorder (Becker *et al.*, 2004).

Within the United States, data vary concerning the relative prevalence of eating disorders among Whites and Blacks. Whereas some large studies suggest they are less common among Blacks, other data suggest that rates of eating disorder symptoms may be quite similar across the major U.S. ethnic groups. In fact, rates of eating disorders may be even greater among Native Americans, Blacks, and Latinos when compared with non-Latino Whites (Crago *et al.*, 1996; Fitzgibbon *et al.*, 1998; Becker and Fay, 2006; Caldwell *et al.*, 2006).

Etiology

Eating disorders have complex, multifactorial etiology, involving the interaction of genes and environment. More than 30 variables have been reported as putative risk factors for the development of eating disorders (Jacobi *et al.*, 2004), including biological, psychological, and sociocultural factors. A taxonomy of risk factor typology and identification methods has been proposed, taking into account timing of risk relative to outcome, study design, and specificity, among other factors (Jacobi *et al.*, 2004). Psycho-developmental risk factors that are common across eating disorders include elevated weight and shape concerns and dieting, early childhood eating and gastrointestinal problems, negative self-evaluation, sexual abuse and other adverse experiences, and general psychiatric morbidity. Factors specific to AN include perfectionism and obsessive-compulsive syndromes. Factors specific to BN include childhood obesity and early onset of puberty. In terms of sociocultural factors, there is strong evidence that social transition (e.g., transitional migration, urbanization, modernization), Western media exposure, and certain peer influences contribute to risk for eating disorders (Becker *et al.*, 2004). Research on biological contributions has focused on genetic factors and neurobiological disturbances (e.g., altered serotonin). Family and twin studies support a strong genetic diathesis to eating disorders, with heritability estimates ranging from 58 to 76% for AN (an estimate similar to that of schizophrenia and higher than most other mental disorders), and 30–83% for BN. Molecular genetic studies have yet to identify well-replicated susceptibility loci, a challenge made more difficult by nosological issues and lack of reliable, valid phenotypes. Vulnerability for the development of an eating disorder may also be related to disturbance in serotonergic activity. As such disturbance seems to persist following recovery, it remains unclear, however, whether such disturbance is a long-term consequence of an eating disorder, rather than a premorbid trait.

Assessment

Multidimensional assessment of eating disorders includes diagnostic interview, medical, nutritional, and family assessments, and self-report questionnaires. Diagnostic interviews can establish past and current eating disorder symptomatology, mental status including suicidality and self-harm, psychiatric comorbidities, including substance abuse, mood, and anxiety disorders, as well as personality disorders. A review should include the patient's height and weight history, restrictive eating patterns, binge eating, purging and compensatory behaviors, and exercise habits. Assessment of body image is essential, although body image disturbance may manifest in different ways across patients. Another important aspect to assess is patient's motivational status, given its influence on course, outcome, and treatment planning. Self-report questionnaires, helpful for ascertaining symptom patterns and progress in treatment, include measures of eating behaviors, dieting, and related beliefs and behaviors, and multidimensional aspects of body image disturbance. Assessment of medical status via full physical examination is strongly recommended, with particular attention to vital signs, physical status, cardiovascular and peripheral vascular function, and dermatological manifestations (APA Workgroup, 2006). Ongoing medical evaluation of changes in weight, cardiovascular indications, and electrolytes may be warranted. Dietary intake and deficiencies may be assessed through self-monitoring (i.e., food records) or interview. While self-monitoring is itself a therapeutic technique, the accuracy of self-reported intake has been challenged, and adherence can be a problem. Family assessment may be important, especially among adolescent patients or patients living with significant others. Family assessment is an opportunity to gather information about family dynamics, especially regarding the topics of food and weight, and also provide psychoeducation to family and significant others.

Course and Outcome

Peak incidence of AN and BN is in adolescence, whereas the onset of BED is typically in late adolescence to the early twenties (APA, 1994). However, clinical experience suggests that eating disorders are becoming common in prepubertal children and middle-aged adults. Patients with eating disorders are often quite conflicted about giving up their symptoms. While most say that they want to be free from disordered eating, many are fearful of gaining weight or finding alternate coping strategies to deal with stress or anxiety. As such, many are reluctant to seek treatment. Patients with AN often come to medical attention more quickly by virtue of low body weight and/ or change in eating and exercise patterns that are often noticed by friends and family. Individuals may protest when clinicians suggest that there is reason for concern; patients will often avoid being weighed or will wear layers of clothing to appear heavier. They may also drink excessive water or carry weights on their bodies to fool providers into thinking that their weight is normal. Similarly, patients struggling with BED may come to attention fairly quickly, particularly if they are overweight. Individuals with BN can be more difficult to detect, as they tend to stay within a relatively normal weight range. In addition, patients struggling with BN are often very reluctant to volunteer their symptoms due to shame. However, when savvy providers identify them, patients with BED and BN are far more likely to accept treatment than are patients diagnosed with AN. This is likely due to the fact that symptoms of binging and purging can be very distressing. Similarly, many individuals are motivated to lose weight for both cosmetic reasons and to avoid long-term health consequences. Those engaged in extreme dietary restriction, on the other hand, tend to take pride in their behaviors and are reluctant to change.

Even with treatment, the natural course of AN tends to be chronic, with symptoms relapsing and remitting several times over the years. However, some patients are able to sustain full recovery after a single episode of illness, sometimes without seeking any formal treatment. Early recovery tends to be more tenuous, with relapse more common in the first 2 years following treatment (Fichter et al., 2006). Relapses tend to be associated with periods of increased psychosocial stress and body image disturbance. Those who recover may continue to experience symptoms. While they may be able to maintain a healthy weight, some continue to observe very rigid behaviors around nutrition and exercise. Others begin binge eating and purging, and some may transition to full-fledged BN (Keel et al., 2005). However, remission rates do improve with time. Poor outcome is strongly associated with chronicity and severity of the eating disorder and mortality also increases over time.

Patients with BN may also have a chronic course, with periods of improvement followed by relapse. Transition to AN is rare, but many continue to engage in binge eating, purging, or compulsive exercise. Again, relapse is common in early remission, but rates of remission increase over time. Often, the frequency of symptoms decreases to a point where diagnostic criteria are no longer met. In a recent long-term follow-up study, 70% of patients no longer met DSM-IV criteria for an eating disorder 12 years after inpatient treatment for BN, 13% met criteria for EDNOS, 10% met criteria for BN, 5% met criteria for AN, and 2% died (Fichter and Quadflieg, 2004). Authors found that the presence of psychiatric comorbidity was the best predictor of outcome in this population.

Lifetime comorbidity with another psychiatric disorder is very common among individuals with an eating disorder, reported as 56% in AN, 95% in BN, and 79% in BED (Husdon et al., 2007).

Treatment

Multidisciplinary team treatment of eating disorders is the standard of care, with coordination among medical, nutritional, and psychiatric treatments. Services range from intensive inpatient programs to residential, partial hospital, day treatment, and varying levels of outpatient care, which may entail general medical treatment, nutritional counseling, individual, group, and family psychotherapy. Level of care should be determined according to a patient's overall physical status, including body mass index and medical stability, as well as psychological symptoms and social circumstances. Hospital-level care is necessary in the context of serious medical complications or seriously impaired psychological function and may also be necessary when there is rapid or persistent decline in intake or weight, inadequate response to lower levels of care, or when psychosocial factors or comorbid illness interfere with effective outpatient management.

Across the eating disorders, psychotherapeutic interventions are the most effective and recommended first-line treatment. Psychopharmacologic treatment can be useful in augmenting psychotherapy for BN and BED but there is inadequate empirical support to recommend specific pharmacologic treatment for the primary symptoms of either AN or EDNOS. In the United States, only one pharmacologic agent has FDA approval for treatment of an eating disorder – fluoxetine for BN – and use of all other agents is considered off-label. The heightened risk for electrocardiographic QT prolongation among individuals with AN and BN requires that clinicians carefully consider risk of QT prolongation prior to initiating certain psychotropic agents in this patient population.

For adult patients with AN, few psychotherapies have been evaluated in randomized control trials and none have demonstrated effectiveness. In contrast to treatment for adults, however, treatment for adolescents with AN has shown promise, and family therapies with this population are recommended (Wilson and Shafran, 2005). Patients may benefit from interventions targeting comorbid anxiety, depression, and obsessive-compulsive symptoms, and psychotherapeutic interventions should comprise the main thrust of the treatment plan. Symptoms of depression and anxiety are exacerbated by the malnutrition that often accompanies eating disorders. Furthermore, individuals with low body weight are more susceptible to troublesome medication side effects (APA Workgroup,

Table 1 Treatment components of cognitive-behavior therapy

Stage 1	• Psychoeducation on cognitive-behavioral model of eating disorders, body weight regulation, consequences of dieting, binge eating, and purging • Establish self-monitoring and weekly weighing • Establish regular pattern of eating and use of alternative behaviors to reduce binge eating and purging
Stage 2	• Reduce/eliminate dieting • Problem-solving skills • Cognitive restructuring, especially of weight and shape concerns
Stage 3	• Relapse prevention

2006), and many patients are reluctant to take medications that could potentially cause weight gain. Typically, slow, monitored, and actively managed weight gain is the most helpful intervention for these individuals. Clinicians should avoid introducing psychotropic agents known to suppress appetite. There are preliminary data to suggest that atypical antipsychotics (risperidone and olanzapine) may have some benefits in ameliorating symptoms of anorexia nervosa.

Cognitive-behavioral therapy (CBT) is the best-established of several empirically supported treatments for BN; numerous randomized controlled trials have shown reliably good outcome, low relapse rates, and superiority to treatment with antidepressants alone. CBT, described in a manual by Fairburn *et al.* (1993), is delineated in **Table 1**. Interpersonal therapy is also an effective treatment for BN. CBT and interpersonal psychotherapy (IPT) have been tested in both individual and group formats in randomized controlled trials and have empirical support (Wilson and Shafran, 2005). Fluoxetine at doses up to 60 mg per day is FDA-approved for the treatment of BN and is the best established pharmacologic agent for treatment of BN (Fluoxetine Bulimia Nervosa Collaborative Study Group, 1992). Combination therapy with both fluoxetine and CBT does seem to provide modest additional benefit (Walsh *et al.*, 1997). Topiramate, an antiepileptic medication, has demonstrated efficacy in reduction of symptoms of BN (Nickel *et al.*, 2005). Other classes of agents have shown efficacy (e.g., some tricyclic antidepressants and some monoamine oxidase inhibitors) but utility is limited by unacceptable side effects. Moreover, bupropion is relatively contraindicated in this population due to increased incidence of seizures in patients who actively binged and purged while taking this medication. CBT – both individual and group – is also the best-established treatment for BED. Topiramate has also been shown effective in the treatment of BED (McElroy *et al.*, 2007) and several pharmacologic agents show promise, although further studies are necessary to establish clear treatment recommendations.

Conclusion

Eating disorders typically have onset in adolescence and young adulthood and are most prevalent among females. Although effective treatments have been developed, access to care for an eating disorder is unacceptably low and eating disorders often follow a chronic course. In addition, they can result in serious medical complications and are associated with high mortality compared with other mental illnesses. Optimal treatment is multidisciplinary and includes medical stability and nutritional counseling in addition to psychotherapeutic and psychopharmacologic interventions.

See also: Specific Mental Health Disorders: Child and Adolescent Mental Disorders.

Citations

American Psychiatric Association (1994) *Diagnostic and Statistical Manual of Mental Disorders*, 4th edn. Washington, DC: American Psychiatric Association.

American Psychiatric Association Work Group on Eating Disorders (2006) Practice Guideline for the Treatment of Patients With Eating Disorders. *American Journal of Psychiatry* 163(supplement).

Becker AE and Fay K (2006) Socio-cultural issues and eating disorders. In: Wonderlich S, de Zwaan M, Steigar H, and Mitchell J (eds.) *Annual Review of Eating Disorders*, pp. 35–63. Chicago, IL: Academy for Eating Disorders

Becker AE, Grinspoon SK, Klibanski A, and Herzog DB (1999) Eating disorders. *New England Journal of Medicine* 340: 1092–1098.

Becker AE, Franko D, Speck A, and Herzog DB (2003) Ethnicity and differential access to care for eating disorder symptoms. *International Journal of Eating Disorders* 33: 205–212.

Becker AE, Keel P, Anderson-Fye EP, and Thomas JJ (2004) Genes (and/) or jeans? Genetic and socio-cultural contributions to risk for eating disorders. *Journal of Addictive Diseases* 23: 81–103.

Caldwell M, et al. (2006) National Institute of Mental Health Workshop on Eating Disorders. Bethesda, MD, 29 June 2006.

Centers for Disease Control and Prevention (2006) *Youth Risk Behavior Surveillance System: Adolescent and School Health*. Atlanta, GA: http://apps.nccd.cdc.gov/YRBSS/index.asp (accessed January 2008).

Crago M, Shisslak CM, and Estes LS (1996) Eating disturbances among American minority groups: A review. *International Journal of Eating Disorders* 19: 239–248.

Fairburn CG and Bohn K (2005) Eating disorder NOS (EDNOS): An example of the troublesome "not otherwise specified" (NOS) category in DSM-IV. *Behaviour Research and Therapy* 43: 691–701.

Fairburn CG, Marcus MD, and Wilson GT (1993) Cognitive behaviour therapy for binge eating and bulimia nervosa: A comprehensive treatment manual. In: Fairburn CG and Wilson GT (eds.) *Binge Eating: Nature, Assessment, and Treatment*, pp. 361–404. New York: Guilford Press

Fichter MM and Quadflieg N (2004) Twelve-year course and outcome of bulimia nervosa. *Psychological Medicine* 34: 1395–1406.

Fichter MM, Quadflieg N, and Hedlund S (2006) Twelve-year course and outcome predictors of anorexia nervosa. *International Journal of Eating Disorders* 39: 87–100.

Fitzgibbon ML, Spring B, Avellone ME, Blackman LR, Pingitore R, and Stolley MR (1998) Correlates of binge eating in Hispanic Black, and White women. *International Journal of Eating Disorders* 24: 43–52.

Fluoxetine Bulimia Nervosa Collaborative Study Group (1992) Fluoxetine in the treatment of bulimia nervosa. A multicenter, placebo-controlled, double-blind trial. *Archives of General Psychiatry* 49: 139–147.

Harris EC and Barraclough B (1997) Suicide as an outcome for mental disorders. A meta-analysis. *British Journal of Psychiatry* 170: 205–228.

Harris EC and Barraclough B (1998) Excess mortality of mental disorder. *British Journal of Psychiatry* 173: 11–53.

Hoek HW and van Hoeken D (2003) Review of the prevalence and incidence of eating disorders. *International Journal of Eating Disorders* 34: 383–396.

Hudson JI, Hiripi E, Pope HG, and Kessler RC (2007) The prevalence and correlates of eating disorders in the national comorbidity survey replication. *Biological Psychiatry* 61: 348–358.

Jacobi C, Hayward C, de Zwaan M, Kraemer HC, and Agras WS (2004) Coming to terms with risk factors for eating disorders: Application of risk terminology and suggestions for a general taxonomy. *Psychological Bulletin* 130: 19–65.

Jacobi C (2005) Psychosocial risk factors for eating disorders. In: Wonderlich S, Mitchell JE, de Zwaan M and Steiger H (eds.) *Eating Disorders: Review Part I*, pp. 59–86. Oxford, UK: Radcliffe Publishing

Keel PK and Klump KL (2003) Are eating disorders culture-bound syndromes? Implications for conceptualizing their etiology. *Psychological Bulletin* 129: 747–769.

Keel PK and Mitchell JE (1997) Outcome in bulimia nervosa. *American Journal of Psychiatry* 154: 313–321.

Keel PK, Dorer DJ, Franko DL, Jackson SC, and Herzog DB (2005) Postremission predictors of relapse in women with eating disorders. *American Journal of Psychiatry* 162: 2263–2268.

Lee S (2001) Fat phobia in anorexia nervosa: Whose obsession is it? In: Nasser M, Katzman M and Gordon R (eds.) *Eating Disorders and Cultures in Transition*, pp. 40–54. London: Routledge

McElroy SL, Hudson JI, Capece KB, Fisher AC, and Rosenthal NR for the Topiramate Binge Eating Disorder Research Group (2007)

Topiramate for the treatment of binge eating disorder associated with obesity: A placebo-controlled study. *Biological Psychiatry* 61: 1039–1048.

Nickel C, Tritt K, Muehlbacher M, *et al.* (2005) Topiramate treatment in bulimia nervosa patients: A randomized, double-blind, placebo-controlled trial. *International Journal of Eating Disorders* 38: 295–300.

Walsh BT, Wilson GT, and Loeb KL (1997) Medication and psychotherapy in the treatment of bulimia nervosa. *American Journal of Psychiatry* 154: 523–531.

Wilfley DE, Wilson GT, and Agras WS (2003) The clinical significance of binge eating disorder. *International Journal of Eating Disorders* 34: S96–S106.

Wilson GT and Shafran R (2005) Eating disorders guidelines from NICE. *Lancet* 365: 79–81.

Further Reading

Fairburn CG, Cooper Z, and Shafran R (2003) Cognitive behaviour therapy for eating disorders: A "transdiagnostic" theory and treatment. *Behavior Research and Therapy* 41: 509–528.

National Institute for Clinical Excellence (2004) *Eating Disorders: Core Interventions in the Treatment and Management of Anorexia Nervosa Bulimia Nervosa, and Related Eating Disorders: Clinical Guideline 9.* London National Institute for Clinical Excellence 2004. http://www. bps.org.uk/downloadfile.cfm?file_uuid=C1173310-7E96-C67F-D396-ADF1B891FSA3text=pdf/.

Shaw H, Ramirez L, Trost A, Randall P, and Stice E (2004) Body image and eating disturbances across ethnic groups: More similarities than differences. *Psychology of Addictive Behaviors* 18: 12–18.

Specific Mental Health Disorders: Mental Disorders Associated with Aging

I Skoog, The Sahlgrenska Academy at the University of Göteborg, Göteborg, Sweden

Dementia

Dementia is strongly associated with increasing age. It is very rare among individuals below the age of 65 years, while the prevalence is more than 50% among individuals above age 90 (**Table 1**). Dementia is a syndrome characterized by a decline in memory and other intellectual functions (i.e., orientation, visuospatial abilities, executive functions, language, and thinking), often accompanied by changes in personality and emotions. The disturbance is a decline from a previous higher level and gives rise to difficulties in everyday life. Around 70 disorders have been associated with a dementia syndrome, the most common being Alzheimer disease (AD) and vascular dementia (VaD). A combination of these disorders (mixed dementia) may be most common. Other psychiatric disorders, such as depression, anxiety, and psychosis, are very common among demented individuals.

Early criteria for dementia were based on the presence of memory dysfunction and disorientation for time and place. The modern concept of dementia emphasizes that dementia is a global decline that affects intellectual functions beyond memory. The most often used definitions of dementia in scientific studies are those released by the American Psychiatric Association; the *Diagnostic and Statistical Manual of Mental Disorders*, 3rd revised version (DSM-III-R; American Psychiatric Association, 1987), and the fourth version (DSM-IV; American Psychiatric Association, 1994), and the classification by the World Health Organization, *International Classification of Diseases* (ICD), 10th version (ICD-10; World Health Organization, 1992). DSM-III-R is most commonly used in epidemiological studies since its criteria were current when several large population studies started in the late 1980s and early 1990s. Both DSM and ICD criteria regard memory disturbance as

Table 1　Prevalence of dementia by age

Age	%
70	2.5
75	5
80	10
85	30
90	40
95	55

mandatory for a diagnosis, but also require the presence of other disturbances of cognitive functions. ICD-10 also requires changes in personality. These diagnostic systems have been questioned because they are based on the symptoms of Alzheimer's disease (AD), where memory disturbance occurs early. Dementia disorders with more circumscribed symptoms, focal signs or an atypical course may therefore not be classified as dementia, e.g., some vascular dementias or frontal lobe dementia. The concept vascular cognitive impairment was introduced to capture the more complex pattern seen in individuals with intellectual disturbances related to cerebrovascular diseases.

Alzheimer's Disease

AD is characterized by an insidious onset with slowly progressive impairments in intellectual functions, typically presenting with memory problems, and changes in personality and emotions. Individuals developing AD, and to some extent VaD, show very mild symptoms regarding memory, executive functions, language, and personality decades before the disease can be diagnosed. These symptoms probably reflect incipient brain pathology. However, at this stage there is a large overlap with normal aging. This dimensional rather than categorical character makes prodromal symptoms of dementia difficult to distinguish from normal aging. The concept of mild cognitive impairment (MCI) was introduced during the early 1990s to capture individuals with prodromal AD. The concept of MCI is uncertain and the prevalence figures vary widely. Besides objective measures of intellectual dysfunction, it also often requires self-reported problems with memory, which means that a large group of elderly persons with intellectual dysfunction will not be classified as MCI. MCI is often divided into three groups based on the symptom pattern, amnestic MCI (only memory impairment), multiple domains slightly impaired, and single non-memory domain impairment. It is reported that 15–20% of patients with MCI develop dementia each year. Other names for this state are age-associated memory impairment (AAMI) and cognitive impairment not dementia (CIND).

The neuropathology of AD includes extensive neuronal loss and deposition of extracellular senile plaques (SP)

and intracellular neurofibrillary tangles (NFT) in the hippocampus and the frontal and temporal cortex, while the motor cortex is spared. The β-amyloid protein is one of the main components of the SP and is also diffusely deposited in the brains of AD patients. Amyloid deposition is often regarded to be central in the pathogenesis of AD, starting a cascade that results in neuronal destruction (the amyloid cascade hypothesis). NFTs are intracytoplasmatic changes, composed of paired helical filaments (PHF), which are proteinaceous filaments twisted around each other in a helical manner. PHFs contain an abnormally hyperphosphorylated form of tau protein. However, extensive brain deposition of β-amyloid and NFTs is often found in normal aging, and in several other brain disorders. Other changes in patients with AD include synaptic loss in the hippocampus and in several cortical regions, and disturbances in the cholinergic, serotonergic, noradrenergic, dopaminergic, glutaminergic, and neuropeptic neurotransmitter systems. Current symptomatic treatment for AD with acetylcholine esterase inhibitors aims to prevent the breakdown of acetylcholine. Lesions in the cerebral microvessels, e.g., amyloid angiopathy and degeneration of the endothelium, are also found in brains of AD patients. Histopathology is often stated to be the gold standard for a diagnosis of AD. Neuropathological criteria for AD are mainly based on age-dependent limits of the amount of SP in the neocortex, although some criteria are based on the pattern of NFT changes. The typical brain changes seen in AD are also found in high proportions of normal elderly, especially among the very old. Several population-based studies report that only about half of individuals who fulfil neuropathological criteria for AD are demented during life. This would mean that all people with AD in their brains do not develop dementia.

Vascular Dementia

VaD is caused by cerebrovascular disorders. Until the 1960s, old age (senile) dementia was considered a result of chronic ischemia secondary to atherosclerosis of cerebral arteries or hardening of the arteries. In 1974, the term multi-infarct dementia was introduced, emphasizing the importance of multiple small or large infarcts, often related to stroke. Other causes of VaD include subcortical white matter lesions (WMLs) and other cerebrovascular diseases.

In epidemiological studies, where brain imaging (CT or MRI) is most often not performed, the diagnosis of VaD is most frequently on history or symptoms of stroke in connection with dementia onset. Stroke-associated dementia is related to small or large brain infarcts. Most cerebral infarcts are caused by thromboembolism from extracranial arteries and the heart. Although this often gives rise to typical focal symptoms (hemiparesis, aphasia), the infarcts are often too small individually to produce a major clinical incident, which means that the diagnosis cannot be made without brain imaging. Therefore, VaD is often underdiagnosed in traditional epidemiological studies. The typical clinical picture is sudden onset, stepwise deterioration, fluctuating course, history of stroke or transitory ischemic attacks, and focal neurological symptoms and signs. However, VaD may also have a gradual onset with a slowly progressive course and without focal signs or infarcts on brain imaging, which makes it difficult to differentiate from AD. The cognitive impairment may have a large variability depending on the site of the lesions, and memory may be relatively preserved.

The importance of subcortical white-matter lesions (WMLs) as a cause of dementia became clear after the advent of brain imaging (CT and MRI) in the 1980s. The neuropathology includes diffuse ischemic demyelination, moderate loss of axons, and incomplete infarctions in subcortical structures of both hemispheres, as well as hyalinization or fibrosis of the small penetrating arteries and arterioles in the white matter. The main hypothesis regarding its pathogenesis is that longstanding hypertension causes lipohyalinosis and narrowing of the lumen of the small perforating arteries and arterioles that nourish the deep WM. The dementia associated with WMLs is probably caused by subcortical–cortical or corticocortical disconnection. WMLs have been associated with a spectrum of clinical pictures. The dementia is supposed to have an insidious onset and a slowly progressive course, which makes it difficult to distinguish from AD. The typical clinical picture includes mild memory problems, psychomotor retardation, urinary incontinence, gait dysfunction, apathy, loss of drive, and emotional blunting. The main risk factors for WMLs are high age and vascular diseases, especially hypertension. WMLs are also common in normal aging and related to mild cognitive symptoms and gait disturbances in otherwise normal elderly.

The main diagnostic problem in dementia is to distinguish AD from VaD. Depending on the criteria used, the proportion of demented individuals diagnosed as AD or VaD may differ considerably. AD may sometimes have a course suggestive of VaD, and VaD may have a course suggestive of AD. AD may be underdiagnosed in persons with cerebral infarcts as neither clinical nor pathological evidence of cerebrovascular disease means that it caused the dementia. However, AD may also be overdiagnosed as many infarctions are clinically silent and infarcts in cases of typical AD may be dismissed as being irrelevant. The common coincidence of AD and VaD is becoming increasingly recognized and may even be the most common form of dementia. This state is often called mixed dementia, in which neither disease alone may be sufficient to cause dementia, but together they may. It was recently reported that concomitant cerebrovascular diseases increase the possibility that individuals with AD pathology will express a dementia syndrome. Pure forms of VaD are probably rare.

Frequency of Dementia

The prevalence of dementia increases with age, from approximately 3% at age 70 to 52% at age 95 (**Table 1**). The figures are uncertain in the very high ages because the number of persons examined in these ages generally has been low. There is an on-going debate whether the prevalence reaches a plateau after the age of 90. Regarding types of dementia, most population studies report that 50–70% of demented individuals have AD and 20–30% VaD, and that the prevalence of AD increases steeply with increasing age, while the prevalence of VaD increases less steeply. One reason may be that silent asymptomatic infarcts become more common with increasing age. In most studies, the prevalence of AD is higher in males than in females among younger old people, and higher among women than among men in the very old. Regarding geographical distribution, the prevalence of dementia is strikingly similar in most parts of the world (although prevalence may be lower in Africa), but there are differences concerning the type of dementia. The prevalence of AD is generally higher in Western European countries and North America, and lower in Asia and Eastern Europe, while the opposite pattern is found for vascular dementia. One explanation for the variation may be that the prevalence and incidence of cerebrovascular disorders differ between countries. More recent prevalence studies from Asia suggest a more similar distribution of AD and VaD to European and North American studies. This may be due to changing diagnostic customs or changes in mortality and morbidity related to cerebrovascular disease.

Also, the incidence of dementia shows an increase with age, although there is a hypothesis that the incidence may decline after the age of 95 years. The relationship between dementia and increasing age has resulted in a debate on whether dementia is an extreme variant of normal aging or different causes of dementia become more common with increasing age.

Risk and Protective Factors

Most studies on risk and protective factors have been published with regard to AD (**Table 2**). Higher age is the most consistent risk factor. Other factors are family history of dementia, Down syndrome, the apoEe4 allele, head trauma, female sex after the age of 80, and vascular risk factors and disorders. Protective factors include higher educational level, use of moderate amounts of red wine, physical exercise, higher leisure time activity, intellectual activities, and larger brain reserve. In observational studies, the use of antihypertensive drugs, anti-inflammatory drugs, statins,

Table 2 Risk factors for dementia

Moderate to strong evidence
- Age
- ApoE e4
- Familial aggregation
- High blood pressure
- Diabetes mellitus
- Antihypertensive drugs (protective)
- Low education
- Leisure-time activity (protective)
- Female sex (after age 85)
- Down syndrome

Some evidence
- Head trauma
- High cholesterol
- Overweight
- Red wine (protective)
- Antiinflammatory drugs (protective)
- Statins (protective)
- Hormone replacement therapy (protective)
- Dietary antioxidants (protective)

estrogens, and dietary antioxidants are reported to decrease risk of dementia and AD. This has not yet been confirmed in placebo-controlled studies. The risk factors suggested for VaD are similar to those in stroke, including advanced age, male sex, hypertension, diabetes mellitus, smoking, and cardiac diseases. VaD is reported to be more common in Finland, the former Soviet Union, and Asian countries than in Western Europe and the United States. Risk factors for dementia in individuals with stroke are similar to those in AD, suggesting that mixed dementia may be common in these cases.

The majority of patients with AD have no obvious family history and are classified as sporadic AD, but there are also rare genetic forms. In these families, the symptoms have an early onset (40–60 years of age). However, sporadic AD is also consistently associated with a family history of dementia. Genetic studies in families with autosomal dominant inheritance for AD, accounting for less than 1% of all AD cases, show that mutations on the genes encoding amyloid precursor protein (APP) on chromosome 21, presenilin-1 on chromosome 14, and presenilin-2 on chromosome 1 segregate with AD. These mutations may elevate the levels of β-amyloid aggregates in the brain. Individuals with Down syndrome (DS) exhibit severe AD neuropathology by age 40. The dominant chromosomal aberration in DS is a trisomy of the long arm of chromosome 21, the site of the APP gene. Alzheimer pathology in DS is probably caused by an overexpression of this gene.

One susceptibility genetic factor, the apolipoprotein E (apoE), has consistently been associated with both familial and sporadic AD. There are three allelic isoforms of the APOE genotype (ε4, ε3, ε2). The ε4 is associated with increased risk for AD and the ε2 with decreased risk. The association is also confirmed in population-based studies,

although it is weaker than in more selected samples and is reduced in the oldest-old. ApoE is a constituent of plasma lipoproteins and is essential in the redistribution of lipids between cells by mediating the uptake of lipoproteins by specific receptors. The apoE ε4 acts as an independent and specific susceptibility gene for AD and several hypotheses exist for its pathogenic role. Presence or absence of the apoE ε4 has been shown to modify the impact of other risk factors, and is also a risk factor for vascular diseases.

AD has recently been associated with vascular risk factors, such as hypertension, coronary heart disease, atrial fibrillation, diabetes mellitus, hypercholesterolemia, and generalized atherosclerosis. Vascular diseases may exacerbate the AD process, or similar mechanisms may be involved in the pathogenesis of both disorders. Those studies reporting an association between hypertension and AD have generally measured blood pressure at least 5–10 years before dementia onset, while studies with shorter follow-ups and cross-sectional studies generally report associations between dementia and low blood pressure. In line with this, it has been reported that blood pressure decreases in the years preceding AD onset and continues to decline during the course of AD. The relationship between declining blood pressure and AD may have several explanations. One possibility is that the declining blood pressure is secondary to the brain lesions seen in AD. Several of the brain regions affected early in AD are regulators of blood pressure. The decline in blood pressure may thus be a very early clinical sign of AD, perhaps even before the cognitive symptoms. Studies showing associations with AD have furthermore generally been based on standardized blood pressure measurements, while studies based on self-report generally do not find associations with AD. One reason for the latter may be that those reporting hypertension may often be on treatment, and a number of epidemiological studies suggest that use of antihypertensive agents decreases the incidence of AD.

Consequences of Dementia

AD is a chronic disorder. During the course of the disease, the patients' functions in daily living inevitably deteriorate. Dementia is the most important cause of dependency in older adults. The burden of care falls mainly on the family, although AD and dementia are also the most important cause of institutionalization in the elderly. Informal family care is particularly important in those parts of the world where health and welfare services and long-term care are less well developed. The caregiver strain is often immense, and related to an increased risk of depression and other mental disorders. In most countries, both in the developed and in the developing world, specialists are few, and primary health care and other services are ill prepared to meet the needs of families for long-term support and care. In 2003, the cost of dementia worldwide was estimated to be almost US $160 billion based on a worldwide prevalence of almost 30 million demented persons. Ninety-two percent of this cost was found in advanced economies, where only about 40% of the demented were found. Due to changing demographics, with a substantial increase in the number of people aged 80 and above, especially in the developing world, the number of people with dementia will increase substantially, to over 130 million, during the next 40 years. Most of this increase will be in the developing world (**Table 3**).

Dementia disorders are the most important predictors of mortality in old age. This is true both for AD and VaD, and VaD has a higher mortality rate than AD. Mortality is also associated with severity of dementia and with cognitive function in nondemented elderly. Although the relative risk of death in dementia is reduced in advanced age, the influence of dementia on survival at high ages is substantial because of its high prevalence. At age 85, population-attributable risk (PAR) for death in AD and VaD was 31% in men and 50% in women.

Depression

A depressive syndrome includes symptoms of depressed mood, tearfulness, diminished pleasure or interest, excessive guilt feelings, low self-esteem, and feelings of worthlessness, hopelessness, pessimism, emotional flatness, poor appetite and weight loss, low energy, or increased fatigue, sleep problems, poor concentration, difficulty making decisions, intellectual problems, withdrawal, psychomotor retardation, reduced talkativeness or agitation, and suicidal ideations.

Elderly people may be predisposed to depression due to age-related structural and biochemical changes, such as underactivity of serotonergic transmission, hypersecretion of cortisol, and low levels of testosterone. This notion is supported by a worldwide report of high suicide rates in the elderly. Furthermore, several risk factors for depression such as bereavement and other psychological losses, loneliness, loss of earlier status in society, vascular and other somatic diseases, and institutionalization become more common with increasing age. With regard to vascular disease, it has been suggested that cerebrovascular diseases, such as stroke and ischemic WMLs are especially important in the etiology of depression in old age. This has led to the concept of vascular depression. However, depression is also a risk factor for myocardial infarction and stroke, and related to worse outcome in these disorders. The association between vascular disease and depression is therefore complicated. On the other hand, some age-related factors may decrease the prevalence of depression in old age. Life stressors might be better tolerated in old age because they are expected, and the wisdom seen in elderly people may also be protective. Old age may also have a positive dimension, with freedom of time, less stressors of work, and less competition.

Frequency of Depression

Most cross-sectional studies report prevalence figures of around 10% for depression, which makes depression an even more common disorder than dementia after age 65. Depression is thus a common cause of disability in the elderly and reduces life satisfaction. Several cross-sectional studies suggest that the prevalence of depressive disorders decreases after age 65. Studies on representative samples that treat the group above age 65 as one entity are, however, heavily weighted towards the age strata 65–75, and the group above age 75 is therefore concealed in these types of studies. Several studies report that depression may have its highest prevalence the 10 years before retirement age (65 years) and its lowest prevalence between age 65 and 75 years, with an increase again after age 75.

Several methodological and confounding factors may act either to increase or decrease the prevalence of depression with age (**Table 4**). First, there is an overlap in symptoms of physical disorders and normal aging and depression (e.g., loss of appetite, tiredness, sleep disturbances), which may

Table 3   Number of people with dementia in different parts of the world (millions)

	2005	2050
Europe	10	19
Asia	18	81
Africa	2	10
North America	4	10
Latin America	3	13
Total	37	133

Based on UN World Population Prospects and a dementia prevalence of 5% age 65–80 and 20% above age 80.

Table 4   Factors that might influence the prevalence of depression and other mental disorders with age

Concomitant physical disorders
Exclusion of institutionalized individuals
Dementia
Manifestation of psychiatric disorders may be different in old age
Criteria for psychiatric disorders are based on younger patient samples
Selective mortality
Birth cohort effects
Misconceptions about normal aging
Differential refusal rates

lead to overdiagnosis of depression. On the other hand, if depressive symptoms are thought to be due to physical disorders or normal aging by the elderly themselves and by their relatives and physicians, the rate of depression may be underestimated. Second, several population studies exclude individuals in institutions, where the prevalence of depressive disorders is high. This has its strongest influence on the prevalence among the oldest old where institutionalization rate is high. Third, most criteria for depression, for example, DSM-IV excludes organic causes of depression such as dementia. As described above, the prevalence of dementia increases dramatically with age. This means that with increasing age, a large proportion of the total population will be removed from the population at risk for depression, giving lower total prevalence of depression in higher ages. Furthermore, even if the demented are not excluded, persons with dementia may underreport these symptoms due to memory problems. Fourth, depression may have other manifestations in the elderly, i.e., other symptom patterns than those in current criteria. This might underestimate the prevalence of depression in the oldest age groups. Instead, depressive symptoms are reported to be more common than the clinical diagnosis, and, in general, the prevalence of depressive symptoms increases with age. However, the symptoms of depression are most often similar in the old and the young. Fifth, the mortality rate is increased in individuals with depression, also in old age. Thus, even if the risk for depression increases with age, the increased mortality may lead to a decreasing prevalence. Sixth, during the twentieth century, a higher prevalence of depression has been reported in later-born generations. Therefore, even if the prevalence is unaffected by age, the cohort effect may give a lower prevalence in the elderly. Seventh, individuals with depression may be more reluctant to participate in studies. If this differential refusal rate is more accentuated in the elderly, it might lead to a lower prevalence of depression in the elderly.

Risk Factors for Depression

Female sex is the most consistent risk factor for depression. The female preponderance is most accentuated in middle life, and the sex difference is supposed to diminish with increasing age. However, depression is generally reported to be more common in women also among the elderly. There are few studies on other risk factors for depression in old age and most are based on retrospective information from cross-sectional data. It is therefore difficult to differentiate between risk factors and consequences of depression. Declining physical health, institutionalization and several medical drugs have been associated with depression. Several physical disorders are related to depression in the elderly including cardiovascular diseases, hypothyroidism, cancer, vitamin deficiencies, Cushing syndrome, anemia, infections, and

lung diseases. Other reported risk factors include previous psychiatric history, family history of depression, bereavement, other life events, personality factors (e.g., locus of control, neuroticism), social factors (social deprivation, loneliness, social support deficits), low education, smoking, and impairments in activities of daily living.

Even if the frequency of depression increases with age, this does not necessarily mean that age as such is a risk factor, as several other proposed risk factors, such as physical disorders, social deprivation, and bereavement, also increase with age. When these other factors are controlled for, age as such may not be an independent risk factor for depression.

Structural brain changes in depression of old age have been reported by several investigators. Theses changes include ventricular enlargement and changes in the caudate nuclei and the putamen. Ischemic white matter lesions and infarcts have also been associated with depression in the elderly. Most studies are, however, hospital-based and may be influenced by selection biases.

Depression and Dementia

High rates of depression have been reported in patients with dementia, with a prevalence of 10–20%. Depressive disorders are generally more common in mild or early dementia. Depression in dementia may be a psychological reaction to the disease, or result from biochemical or structural brain changes. However, a lack of association between dementia and depression has been noted in community studies. Depression may worsen the dementia syndrome and is important to recognize as it is potentially treatable. It has also been suggested that previous depression may be a risk factor for dementia. Furthermore, several studies report that individuals with manifest depression show cognitive decline. This decline is generally of mild degree and not overt dementia.

Consequences of Depression

Among the consequences of depression are social deprivation, loneliness, poor quality of life, increased use of health- and home-care services, increased risk for physical disorders (e.g., stroke, myocardial infarction, cancer), cognitive decline, impairments in activities of daily living, suicide, and an increased nonsuicidal mortality (**Table 5**). Studies on attempted and completed suicides in old age have reported a stronger association with depression, with less alcoholism and fewer personality disorders, than in younger age groups. Furthermore, suicidal attempts in the elderly are often characterized by a greater degree of lethal intent. The depressed elderly have a several-fold increased risk of dying. The causal relationship between depression and the increased risk of dying is not clear.

Table 5   Consequences of depression

Social deprivation and loneliness
Poor quality of life
Impairments in activities of daily living
Increased use of health and home care services
Increased risk for physical disorders
Stroke
Myocardial infarction
Cancer
Cognitive decline
Suicide
Increased nonsuicidal mortality

Untreated depression has consistently been reported to have a poor outcome in the elderly, although it is not clear whether the depressed elderly have worse outcome than younger depressives. Several studies have addressed the question of whether it is possible to identify those with a poor outcome. The findings so far are contradictory.

Despite the high prescription of psychotropic drugs in the elderly, only a minority of those with depression receive specific treatment for their disorder. Most epidemiological studies report that only around 15–20% of individuals diagnosed with depression receive antidepressant therapy. Instead, a high prescription of benzodiazepines in depression has been reported by several investigators. Many elderly may use sedatives for sleep disturbances and anxiolytics for the anxiety accompanying depression, where antidepressants should have been the proper therapy. During recent years, new antidepressants, which are better tolerated by the elderly, have been introduced. At the same time, the prescription of antidepressants has increased in the community. It remains to be elucidated whether these changes have led to a higher treatment rate of depression in the elderly.

Anxiety Disorders

Anxiety disorders include generalized anxiety disorder (GAD), agoraphobia, panic anxiety disorder, obsessive-compulsive disorder (OCD), social phobias, and simple phobias. Studies concerned especially with the epidemiology of anxiety disorders in the elderly are few. The approximate prevalence figures are for social phobia 1%, simple phobia 4%, OCD 0.1–0.8%, panic disorder 0.1%, and generalized anxiety disorder 4%, while the prevalence of agoraphobia varies widely between studies (1.5–8%). For overall anxiety disorder, figures vary widely depending on criteria used, from 3 to 15%. The prevalence of anxiety disorders is reported to decline with age, also after age 65, with the exception of generalized anxiety disorder, which seem to remain stable with age or even increase (if nonhierarchical diagnoses are made; see below

in this section). However, these disorders may occur as primary disorders for the first time in old age. The lower rate of anxiety disorders in the elderly is contradicted by the high consumption of anxiolytic drugs in the elderly. This suggests that anxiety may be an important and underrated problem in this age group. As discussed in relation to depression, the apparent decrease in frequency of anxiety disorders with age may be influenced by birth cohort effects, anxiety-related mortality, cognitive impairment, the exclusion of institutionalized individuals, criteria based on younger and middle-aged persons, anxiety symptoms believed to be caused by physical disorders, and differential refusal to participate in the studies. Another factor may be that the elderly have a different clinical presentation, with less somatic and autonomic symptoms, fewer symptoms, and less avoidance. The requirement that there should be a constriction of normal activities, interference with social or role functioning, and that the individual himself should find the symptoms excessive or unreasonable might also differ by age. Furthermore, anxiety may present differently in the elderly, for example as agitation, irritability, talkativeness, and tension. In most studies, the prevalence of anxiety disorders is higher in women than in men, also among the elderly, but the differences seem to diminish with increasing age.

One important aspect when evaluating frequency of anxiety disorders is whether a hierarchical approach to diagnosis has been made (as in DSM-III and IV and ICD-10 criteria). In such a hierarchy, most anxiety disorders cannot be diagnosed in the presence of concurrent depressive illness. However, anxiety disorders and depression often occur together, also among the elderly, with a reported comorbidity of 75–90%. This has an immense influence on the frequency of anxiety disorders in the population. If comorbidity between depression and anxiety is higher in the elderly, this might explain some of the decrease in frequency of anxiety disorders with age. In fact, the frequency of GAD decreases with age when hierarchical diagnosis is made and increases without a hierarchical system. Another possibility is that individuals with anxiety disorders have an increased risk to develop a depressive disorder, thus shifting their diagnosis from anxiety to depression with increasing age. However, there also seems to be a shift in the opposite direction with increasing age. In the discussion about new criteria, it has been suggested that depression and generalized anxiety should be lumped together as one category. Finally, thresholds for making diagnostic cases seem to be especially important in relation to frequency of anxiety disorders.

Among the consequences of anxiety disorders are an increased mortality rate, increased risk for ischemic heart disease and stroke, and an increased suicide risk. Anxiety disorders seem to be especially common in mild dementia.

Psychosis

The term paraphrenia was previously used to describe psychotic syndromes in the elderly, Currently used terms are late-onset schizophrenia or late-life psychosis, encompassing delusions and visual and auditory hallucinations arising in late life. Compared to early-onset psychosis, late-onset cases have better preserved personality, less affective blunting, less formal thought disorder, more insight and less excess of focal structural brain abnormalities and cognitive dysfunction compared to age-matched controls. The prevalence of psychotic symptoms is high among the demented elderly, ranging from 45 to 50%, while psychotic symptoms and disorders such as schizophrenia are supposed to be rare in the nondemented elderly. Population studies in nondemented elderly are generally based only on self-report and give prevalence figures for psychotic symptoms from 2 to 3% in populations above the age of 65 years. According to currently used criteria, psychotic disorders are even less common, with reported prevalence ranging from 0 to 5%. There are several methodological factors that might explain the low prevalence of psychotic symptoms and syndromes in elderly populations. First, there might be underreporting because the elderly are reluctant to report psychotic symptoms. Recent studies have reported that up to 10% of nondemented elderly above age 85 have psychotic symptoms if information from other sources than self-report (especially close informants) is used in the assessments. Second, individuals with psychotic symptoms are likely to refuse participation in population studies more often than other elderly. Thirdly, as for other psychiatric disorders, diagnostic criteria are developed in young or middle-aged patient samples.

Factors related to late-life psychosis include female sex, previous schizoid and paranoid personality traits, being divorced, living alone, lower education, poor social network and isolation, low social functioning, sensory impairments, especially deafness, and more dependence on community care. Psychosis and psychotic symptoms in elderly populations have been associated with a variety of psychiatric and somatic disorders, such as depression, hypothyroidism, cancer, cerebral tumors, epilepsy, and cerebrovascular disease. Furthermore, many drugs, such as anticholinergics, antiparkinsons, psychostimulants, steroids, and beta-blockers can produce psychotic symptoms in the elderly. Other causes are alcohol and benzodiazepine withdrawal. Studies on the relationship between psychotic symptoms and structural brain changes in the elderly report disparate results. Some studies report a higher ventricle-to-brain ratio, larger third ventricle volume, and volume reductions of the left temporal lobe or superior temporal gyrus. Also, ischemic white matter lesions have been reported in late-onset schizophrenia. Basal ganglia calcifications have also been reported in elderly individuals with psychotic symptoms.

Among the consequences of psychotic symptoms are impairment and disability in daily life, dependence on community care, and cognitive dysfunction. Individuals with late-onset schizophrenia perform significantly worse than age-matched controls on a variety of cognitive tests, although the difference is not as accentuated as for younger age groups. Psychotic symptoms, like most other psychiatric conditions in the elderly, are related to an increased mortality independent of physical disorders. Psychotic symptoms may also be a prodrome of dementia. In Lewy body dementia, early visual hallucinations are even part of the criteria. However, psychotic symptoms frequently accompany dementia disorders and are regarded to be more common late in the course of the disease. The cumulative incidence of hallucinations and delusions for patients with probable Alzheimer's disease is reported to be more than 50% at 4 years.

Alcohol and Drug Abuse

Few epidemiological studies have examined frequency and risk factors for alcohol problems in old age. There is a general decline in alcohol consumption with increasing age, and alcohol problems or abuse are generally believed to be less common among the elderly than in younger populations. One reason may be that alcohol abuse is related to premature mortality. Another reason may be that instruments and diagnostic criteria are developed from younger age groups, and may not be valid at older ages. Birth cohort effects may also influence the results. In epidemiological studies, self-report probably underestimates alcohol problems, due to neglect or early memory problems.

The prevalence of alcohol problems is generally higher in men than in women. Physical and psychiatric disorders, especially dementia and depression, are more common among elderly alcoholics than among other elderly. Increasing age also makes individuals more sensitive to the effect of alcohol to the body. It has been discussed whether late-life alcohol abuse presents differently than alcohol abuse in younger ages, for example, by cognitive dysfunction, falls, self-neglect, incontinence, and malnutrition. Late-onset alcohol abuse may start in connection with bereavement, but may also be an early manifestation of a dementia disorder. Elderly early-onset alcohol abusers are a group who survived into old age, despite the increased mortality in alcohol abusers. Alcohol abuse in the elderly often co-exists with abuse of psychotropic drugs, leading to interactions. There are indications that elderly alcohol abusers who abstain from alcohol may improve in activities of daily living, suggesting a benefit of abstinence.

Multiple medications, drug interactions, and age-related pharmacokinetic and pharmacodynamic changes in the elderly affect drug response and increase the risk for adverse effects, such as delirium and falls. The elderly have a high rate of psychotropic drug use, with figures ranging from 45 to 50% among octogenarians, with lower figures among younger elderly. The highest rates apply to anxiolytic sedatives, mainly benzodiazepines. Women generally have higher rates than men. The extent to which the high use of benzodiazepines reflects drug abuse needs to be elucidated.

See also: Parkinson's Disease.

Citations

American Psychiatric Association (1987) *Diagnostic and Statistical Manual of Mental Disorders: Third Edition Revised*. Washington, DC: American Psychiatric Association.

American Psychiatric Association (1994) *Diagnostic and Statistical Manual of Mental Disorders: Fourth Edition*. Washington, DC: American Psychiatric Association.

World Health Organization (1992) *The ICD-10 Classification of Mental and Behavioural Disorders: Diagnostic Criteria for Research*. Geneva, Switzerland: World Health Organization.

Further Reading

Blazer DG and Hybels CF (2005) Origins of depression in later life. *Psychological Medicine* 35: 1–12.

Blennow K, de Leon MJ, and Zetterberg H (2006) Alzheimer's disease. *Lancet* 368: 387–403.

Farrer LA, Cupples LA, Haines JL, *et al.* (1997) Effects of age, sex, and ethnicity on the association between apolipoprotein E genotype and Alzheimer disease. A meta-analysis. APOE and Alzheimer Disease Meta Analysis Consortium. *Journal of the American Medical Association* 278: 1349–1356.

Johnson I (2000) Alcohol problems in old age: A review of recent epidemiological research. *International Journal of Geriatric Psychiatry* 15: 575–581.

Jorm AF (2000) Does old age reduce the risk of anxiety and depression? A review of epidemiological studies across the adult life span. *Psychological Medicine* 30: 11–22.

Krasucki C, Howard R, and Mann A (1989) The relationship between anxiety disorders and age. *International Journal of Geriatric Psychiatry* 13: 79–99.

Ostling S (2005) Psychotic symptoms in the elderly. *Current Psychosis and Therapeutics Reports* 3: 9–14.

Palsson S and Skoog I (1997) The epidemiology of affective disorders in the elderly: A review. *International Clinical Psychopharmacology* 12 (supplement 2): S3–S13.

Riedel-Heller SG, Busse A, and Angermeyer MC (2006) The state of mental health in old-age across the 'old' European Union – A systematic review. *Acta Psychiatrica Scandinavica* 113: 388–401.

Skoog I (2006) Vascular Dementia. In: Pathy MSJ, Sinclair AJ and Morley JE (eds.) *Principles and Practice of Geriatric Medicine*, 4th edn., pp. 1103–1110Chichester, UK: John Wiley and Sons Ltd.

Skoog I and Blennow K (2001) Alzheimer's disease. In: Hofman A and Mayeux R (eds.) *Investigating Neurological Disease. Epidemiology for Clinical Neurology*, pp. 154–173. Cambridge, UK: Cambridge University Press

Skoog I and Gustafson D (2003) Vascular disorders and Alzheimer's disease. In: Bowler JV and Hachinski V (eds.) *Vascular Cognitive Impairment. Preventable Dementia*, pp. 260–271. Oxford, UK: Oxford University Press

Wimo A, Jonsson L, and Winblad B (2006) An estimate of the worldwide prevalence and direct costs of dementia in 2003. *Dementia and Geriatric Cognitive Disorders* 21: 175–181.

Specific Mental Health Disorders: Personality Disorders

M J Crawford, Imperial College London, London, UK

Personality disorders are a heterogeneous group of conditions which are characterized by relatively stable patterns of interpersonal and intrapsychic functioning that are associated with personal distress and impaired social functioning. People with personality disorder (PD) have an "enduring pattern of inner experience and behavior that deviates markedly from the expectations of the individual's culture" (American Psychiatric Association, 1994: 633–634). These patterns of thinking and behaving are central to a person's sense of self. Indeed, personality disorders can be considered disturbances of the self, of the way a person sees and experiences themselves.

Personality disorders become apparent in childhood and adolescence. In adulthood, they are characterized by long-standing emotional problems and difficulties in relationships with others. Emotional problems may include feelings of anxiety, sadness, and obsessive thoughts that are seen in people with neuroses. However, emotional states among people with PD tend to show greater short-term variation. Some people with PD experience major fluctuations in mood and feelings of emptiness, despair, and suicidal thoughts. Difficulties in relationships with others include weariness of others, a desire to avoid other people, disregard for others' welfare, feeling dependent on others, and fears of rejection by other people.

The diagnosis of personality disorder is controversial and critics have argued that it is simply a means of labeling socially unacceptable behavior (Lewis and

Appleby, 1988). Like 'normal' personality, personality disorders are long lasting and traditional treatments used to manage mental disorders are less effective in reducing mental distress among people with PD. Indeed some people who have been labeled as having a personality disorder complain that they are given this diagnosis as a result of their not responding to treatment for other mental disorders. This concern is supported by surveys of healthcare professionals which have shown that some use the term to refer to people they feel are untreatable. The term has also been used pejoratively to refer to people who are seen as attention-seeking, annoying, and less deserving of care (Lewis and Appleby, 1988). Such views have been challenged by research findings that have demonstrated that many personality-related problems diminish over time (Zanarini *et al.*, 2003) and that psychological treatments can improve the mental health and social functioning of people with these problems.

Classification

Population-based studies indicate that there are aspects of personality called traits that can be reliably measured and are generally stable over time (McGlashan *et al.*, 2005). The most enduring of these traits are extraversion/introversion (the tendency to like or to shun the company of others) and neuroticism (the tendency to worry). However, such characteristics are normally distributed in the population and there are numerous other traits that make a dimensional approach to describing personality in clinical contexts unsatisfactory. As a result, formal systems for classifying personality disorder use operationalized definitions based on clusters of traits associated with different personality types and dichotomize these as being either present or absent according to whether a cut-off point of causing significant personal distress or social problems has been reached.

Types of personality disorder used in the two main systems of classification are illustrated in **Table 1**. Factor analysis of personality traits in community samples suggest that these distinct categories of PD are artificial constructs and a looser system of three broad bands of PD are preferred by some. This system combines personality disorders into three clusters: cluster A (characterized by social distance and eccentricity); cluster B (characterized by flamboyance and emotional instability), and cluster C (characterized by anxiety and a tendency to worry).

An alternative approach to the diagnosis of personality disorder has been suggested by Tyrer and Johnson (1996), based on severity of PD. Abnormal traits that do not cause enduring personal distress are labeled personality difficulty, significant problems associated with disturbance in

Table 1 Systems used to classify personality disorder

DSM IV American Psychiatric Association (1994)	ICD-10 (World Health Organization, 1992)	Clusters
Paranoid Schizoid Schizotypal	Paranoid Schizoid	Cluster A Odd, eccentric, avoid company of others, emotionally detached, suspicious, oversensitive
Borderline Narcissistic Histrionic Antisocial	Emotionally unstable • Impulsive • Borderline Histrionic Dissocial	Cluster B Dramatic, flamboyant, short-tempered, impulsive, fluctuations in mood, difficulties coping with crisis
Anxious Dependent Obsessive-compulsive	Avoidant Dependent Anankastic	Cluster C Worrier, fearful, indecisive, self-conscious, helpless, perfectionist

Source: American Psychiatric Association and World Health Organization (1992) *The ICD-10 classification of Mental and Behavioural Disorers: Criteria for Research*. Geneva, Switzerland: World Health Organization. American Psychiatric Association (1994) *Diagnostic and Statistical Manual of Mental Disorders*, 4th edn. Washington, DC: American Psychiatric Association.

only one cluster are referred to as simple personality disorder, those with disturbance in more than one cluster as having 'diffuse PD', and those with diffuse PD where there is severe disruption, both to the individual and to others, have severe PD.

It seems likely that the current system of classification will be subject to further change, but it does at least have the merit of providing diagnostic labels which relate to patterns of behavior that are familiar to clinicians and have provided a basis for research into the etiology and management of PD.

Prevalence and Outcome

Cross-sectional surveys conducted in Europe and North America indicate that between 5 and 10% of the population have a PD (Coid *et al.*, 2006). The prevalence of PD in resource-poor nations is unknown. Within Western nations, the prevalence of personality disorder tends to be higher in inner-city areas where levels as high as 15% have been reported. Most forms of PD are more prevalent among men, especially antisocial PD, which is five times more common in men than in women. Emotional and interpersonal problems associated with PD mean that the prevalence of personality disorder is generally higher in health-care settings than in the general population. Approximately 15% of people treated by family practitioners and 40% of people treated by mental health services have a PD. Levels of PD are also higher among people in contact with criminal justice services – it is estimated that as many as 80% of people in prison have PD (Singleton *et al.*, 1998).

There have been few long-term follow-up studies of people with PD, but available evidence suggests that psychological and behavioral manifestations of cluster B personality disorders such as impulsivity tend to become less frequent over time (Zanarini *et al.*, 2003). In contrast, personality traits such as suspiciousness, eccentricity, and rigidity that are encountered most frequently among people with cluster A and cluster C PD seem less likely to diminish with advancing age (Seivewright *et al.*, 2002).

Public Health Consequences of Personality Disorder

Much of the research conducted to date has focused on the relationship between personality disorder and mental health-related problems such as depression, suicide, and substance misuse. However, people with PD also have higher rates of physical health problems and premature mortality. The standardized mortality rate for people with PD is estimated to be 184 (95% CI = 140–236). People with PD have higher rates of death from infections and neoplasms as well and suicide and other forms of violent death (Harris and Barraclough, 1998). Levels of social problems such as unemployment are higher, and it is estimated that over one-fifth of homeless people have a PD.

The relationship between PD and other mental disorders is complex, not least because similar problems are experienced by people with mental and personality disorder. For instance, features of cluster A PD have much in common with the prodromal symptoms of schizophrenia and paranoid psychosis, and emotional distress experienced by people with cluster C PD has features that are also seen in those with anxiety neurosis and obsessive-compulsive disorder. Nonetheless, people with personality disorder and especially borderline PD have rates of depression and other mental disorders which are far higher than that among the general population (Zanarini *et al.*, 1998).

Data from psychological autopsy studies indicate that as many as 40% of people who commit suicide have evidence of PD. The relationship between personality disorder and suicide is particularly strong among those with cluster B PDs such as antisocial and borderline PD among whom impulsivity and levels of affective

disturbance are high. Rates of substance misuse are also high among people with PD, especially cluster B PD. This association may be attributable to the difficulties that such people have in coping with intense emotions, for which alcohol and other drugs may provide some temporary relief. However, such drugs may cause disinhibition and this in combination with personality traits such as impulsiveness further increases the risk of suicidal behavior or violence toward others.

Given that impulsivity and disregard for others are the hallmarks of antisocial personality disorder (ASPD), it is not surprising that levels of offending are increased among people with ASPD. It is estimated that, in Britain, one-quarter of violent incidents that result in injury are committed by people with ASPD (Coid *et al.*, 2006); in contrast, hazardous drinking is implicated in over half of all such incidents. One of the traits apparent in some people with ASPD is psychopathy, which is characterized by shallow emotions, a lack of empathy or sense of guilt, and a history of lying, deceit, and criminality. This cluster of personality traits is less prevalent than ASPD, but its association with subsequent violence is far stronger. Attempts to define people who have PD and pose high risks to the public have been made, but past behavior rather than the presence or absence of certain personality traits provides a better guide to the likelihood of future violence in community settings.

Etiology of Personality Disorder

Knowledge of factors that give rise to PD is only partial, but evidence from twin studies suggests that both constitutional and environmental factors are more important. The hereditability of personality disorder is estimated to be 0.6, with narcissistic and anankastic personality disorder having the highest hereditability (Torgersen *et al.*, 2000). Efforts to identify genetic markers for personality disorders have not generated consistent findings, but associations between impulsivity and genes responsible for variations in serotonin receptors have been reported.

High levels of cluster A PD in relatives of people with schizophrenia have led to the suggestion that these may be part of a spectrum of disorders characterized by emotional distance from others, unusual behaviors, and odd beliefs.

More is known about the etiology of borderline PD than that of other groups. As many as two-thirds of people with borderline PD report childhood physical or sexual abuse, and other forms of childhood adversity such as parental mental illness and separation from parents are more frequent than among the general population (Bandelow *et al.*, 2005). These strong associations have led to the view that borderline PD may be the result of deficits in a person's sense of self resulting from disorganized parental relationships. While such risk factors appear to be important in the etiology of personality disorders, they are neither necessary nor sufficient to result in PD.

Intervention

Primary Prevention

Strong links between environmental factors and the development of PD suggest that primary prevention of PD may be possible (Coid, 2003). Such strategies could include whole-population initiatives aimed at improving the family and educational environment of all children or specific interventions aimed at families where children show early indicators of interpersonal problems such as conduct disorder. Few such programs have been evaluated, but emerging evidence suggests that if interventions are delivered early in life they may be effective. For instance, Raine and colleagues (2003) evaluated the impact of a 2-year enrichment program for 3-year-old children on the island of Mauritius. The program combined educational and nutritional interventions with a program of structured physical activity and was delivered over a 2-year period. The team were able to follow up 75 (90%) of 83 children who completed the program and 288 (81%) of 355 matched controls, demonstrating lower levels of personality-related problems and criminal behavior 20 years later. The generalizability of such findings to resource-rich settings have not been explored, but they support the notion that improving the early-childhood environment can impact on adult personality status.

Service Provision

Compared to services for people with mental illness, the development of services for people with PD has been slow. A variety of reasons have been suggested for this. It has been argued that uncertainty about the validity of diagnoses has made it difficult to develop an evidence base for services. Others have pointed to the impact that interpersonal problems associated with PD have on the relationship between therapists and patients. Personality traits such as impulsivity, excessive dependence on others and disregard for others certainly present challenges to health-care professionals working with people with PD. People with PD may also project painful emotions onto health-care workers, especially doctors and others whose position of power and authority may mirror difficult or abusive relationships people experienced at the hands of other authority figures during childhood.

Research among service users who have been given a diagnosis of PD has shown that many feel dissatisfied with the quality of care they receive. In a survey of service users with PD in Britain, a greater proportion believed that they had been harmed, rather than helped by local mental health services (Ramon, 2001).

Table 2 Key features of services for people with PD

Relatively long-term (delivered for over 1 year)
Have consistent boundaries that are made clear to patients at the start of treatment
Help people address social problems
Actively involve the patient in all aspects of treatment
Place an emphasis of interpersonal functioning
Manage expectations so that these are not unrealistic
Anticipate crises and agree on plans to help people manage these when they occur

Despite these problems, specialist services for people with personality disorder have been developed. While the structure and organization of such services varies, there is a good deal of consensus about key features of services for people with PD, which are listed in **Table 2**.

Specific Treatments

A variety of psychosocial interventions have been developed for people with PD, but only a limited number of experimental evaluations have been conducted. Most of the randomized evaluations of interventions for people with personality disorder that have been conducted have focused on people with borderline PD. A systematic review of such studies by Binks and colleagues (2006), concluded that studies have been "too few and too small to allow any definitive statement to be made about their effectiveness."

Some of the earliest studies explored the effectiveness of therapeutic communities. Therapeutic communities aim to facilitate group learning and peer support and place an emphasis on self-efficacy and responsibility. Democratic therapeutic communities do this by flattening the traditional hierarchy that exists between patients and treatment staff and encouraging people to become actively involved in their treatment by involving them in the running of the community. Observational studies comparing the outcome of people with PD who are treated in residential therapeutic communities suggest they are less likely to self-harm and have lower levels of subsequent service utilization that those who are not.

Dialectical behavior therapy is a form of psychotherapy specifically developed for people with borderline PD (Linehan, 1993). It incorporates elements of cognitive therapy and skills training and places specific emphasis on helping patients identify and overcome obstacles to change. Randomized trials of dialectic behavior therapy have demonstrated improved mental health and reduced self-harming behavior among women with borderline PD, including those with comorbid substance misuse.

In recent years, modified forms of psychoanalytical and cognitive therapy have been demonstrated to improve mental health and social function of people with borderline, avoidant, and other personality disorders. In contrast, very little is known about what, if anything, can be done to reduce the likelihood of offending among people with anti-social personality disorder.

Pharmacological interventions have only a limited role in the management of PD. Exceptions to this are low-dose antipsychotic medication that may benefit people with schizotypal personality disorder, and reduce the psychotic-like symptoms that can emerge among people with borderline PD at times of crisis. Antidepressant medication may be of value in treating mood disturbance among people with PD, but response to treatment is generally less marked than among those with depression in the absence of PD. Long-term use of medication in people with cluster B and C PD is not indicated and patients may instead need help in coming off tranquilizers and antidepressants that were started at times of crisis and do not provide long-term benefit.

For patients to benefit from any intervention, they need to be sufficiently motivated to use it. Many people with PD are ambivalent about receiving interventions and a substantial proportion may not want to try to change. Under these circumstances, it has been suggested that a better approach to helping people with PD is to focus on modifying their social circumstances to create a better fit between the person's personality and their environment. Exploratory studies examining the impact of such interventions suggest they can improve patient satisfaction and social functioning (Tyrer *et al.*, 2003). Assessment and support with tackling social problems is an important part of the management of all people with PD.

Conclusion

In summary, personality disorders are important conditions that have negative consequences for the individual and society. While there is only partial understanding of their etiology and debate continues about the most appropriate system for their classification, poor health and social outcomes experienced by people with personality disorder highlight their public health importance. Interpersonal problems inherent in personality disorder mean that providing services for people with these conditions is not straightforward. However, clear links with childhood adversity provide a basis for the development of primary prevention strategies and an evidence base is beginning to emerge that suggests that many forms of personality disorder may be amenable to psychosocial intervention.

See also: Illicit Drug Use and the burden of Disease; Mental Health and Substance abuse; Specific Mental Health Disorders: Child and Adolescent Mental Disorders; Suicide and Self-Directed Violence.

Citations

American Psychiatric Association (1994) *Diagnostic and Statistical Manual of Mental Disorders*, 4th edn. Washington, DC: American Psychiatric Association.

Bandelow B, Krause J, Wedekind D, Broocks A, Hajak G, and Rüther E (2005) Early traumatic events, parental attitudes, family history and birth risk factors in patients with borderline personality disorder and healthy controls. *Psychiatry Research* 134: 169–179.

Binks CA, Fenton M, McCarthy L, Lee T, Adams CE, and Duggan C (2006) Psychological therapies for people with borderline personality disorder. *The Cochrane Database of Systematic Reviews*, Issue 1.

Coid J (2003) Epidemiology, public health and the problem of personality disorder. *British Journal of Psychiatry* 182(supplement 44): s3–s5.

Coid J, Yang M, Tyrer P, Roberts A, and Ullrich S (2006) Prevalence and correlates of personality disorder in Great Britain. *British Journal of Psychiatry* 188: 423–431.

Harris EC and Barraclough B (1998) Excess mortality of mental disorder. *British Journal of Psychiatry* 173: 11–53.

Lewis G and Appleby L (1988) Personality disorder: The patients psychiatrists dislike. *British Journal of Psychiatry* 153: 44–49.

Linehan MM (1993) *Cognitive-Behavioural Treatment for Borderline Personality Disorder*. New York: Guilford.

McGlashan TH, Grilo CM, Sanislow CA, *et al.* (2005) Two-year prevalence and stability of individual dsm-iv criteria for schizotypal, borderline, avoidant, and obsessive-compulsive personality disorders: Toward a hybrid model of axis II disorders. *American Journal of Psychiatry* 162: 883–889.

Raine A, Mellingen K, Liu J, Venables P, and Mednick S (2003) Effects of environmental enrichment at ages 3–5 years on schizotypal personality and antisocial behavior at ages 17 and 23 years. *American Journal of Psychiatry* 160: 1627–1635.

Ramon S, Castillo H, and Morant N (2001) Experiencing personality disorder: A participative research. *International Journal of Social Psychiatry* 47: 1–15.

Seivewright H, Tyrer P, and Johnson T (2002) Change in personality status in neurotic disorders. *The Lancet* 359: 2253–2254.

Singleton N, Meltzer H, and Gatward R (1998) *Psychiatric Morbidity Among Prisoners in England and Wales*. London: Stationary Office.

Torgersen S, Lygren S, Øien PA, *et al.* (2000) A twin study of personality disorders. *Comprehensive Psychiatry* 41: 416–425.

Tyrer P and Johnston T (1996) Establishing the severity of personality disorder. *American Journal of Psychiatry* 153: 1593–1597.

Tyrer P, Sensky T, and Mitchard S (2003) The principles of nidotherapy in the treatment of persistent mental and personality disorders. *Psychotherapy and Psychosomatics* 72: 350–356.

World Health Organization (1992) *The ICD-10 Classification of Mental and Behavioural Disorders: Criteria for Research*. Geneva, Switzerland: World Health Organization.

Zanarini MC, Frankenburg FR, Dubo ED, *et al.* (1998) Axis I comorbidity of borderline personality disorder. *American Journal of Psychiatry* 155: 1733–1739.

Zanarini MC, Frankenburg FR, Hennen J, and Silk K (2003) The longitudinal course of borderline psychopathology: 6-year prospective follow-up of the phenomenology of borderline personality disorder. *American Journal of Psychiatry* 160: 274–283.

Further Reading

Bateman AW and Fonagy P (2004) *Psychotherapy for Borderline Personality Disorder: Mentalization Based Treatment*. Oxford, UK: Oxford University Press.

Holmes J (1999) Psychotherapeutic approaches to the management of severe personality disorder in general psychiatric settings. *CPD Bulletin Psychiatry* 2: 35–41.

Livesley WJ, Jang KL, Jackson DN, and Vernon PA (1993) Genetic and environmental contributions to dimensions of personality disorder. *American Journal of Psychiatry* 150: 1826–1831.

Moran P (1999) *Antisocial Personality Disorder: An Epidemiological Perspective*. London: Gaskell.

Paris J (1996) *Social Factors in the Personality Disorders: A Biopsychosocial Approach to Etiology and Treatment*. New York: Cambridge University Press.

Sampson M, McCubbin R, and Tyrer P (2006) *Personality Disorder and Community Mental Health Teams: A Practitioner's Guide*. Chichester, UK: John Wiley and Sons.

Relevant Websites

http://www.apa.org/topics/topicperson.html – American Psychology Association On-Line (Topic: personality disorders).

http://www.personalitydisorder.org.uk/ – Department of Health, Home Office and Care Service Improvement Partnership. National Personality Disorder website.

Specific Mental Health Disorders: Psychotic Disorders

R Thara and M Taj, Schizophrenia Research Foundation, Chennai, India
S Tirupati, The University of Newcastle, Newcastle, NSW, Australia

Terminology

Psychiatry has always paid great attention to the use of certain terms to denote or describe a particular mental illness or behavior in an attempt to destigmatize and demystify the suffering of people affected by a mental illness. Terms such as madness and insanity, which denoted a mental disorder with severe disturbance of behavior, have fortunately become unusable now. The term psychosis became the officially acceptable term to denote these disorders, qualified by schizophrenic or manic, for example, to identify the individual diagnostic entity. They are also known as severe mental disorders (SMDs) and low-prevalence disorders (LPDs). More recently, the term psychosis has been replaced by the term disorder preceded by the qualifying term (e.g., schizophrenic disorder). The term psychosis has now come to denote a cluster of symptoms rather than a distinct diagnostic entity. The adjective schizophrenic or manic is now used to describe the disorder and not the person suffering from the disorder. We use the term psychotic disorders here to denote a group of mental disorders characterized by a particular set of symptoms, severity of disablement, treatment needs, and public health importance.

History

Psychotic disorders are not new maladies of the emerging modern world. They have been described in ancient texts of various civilizations across the world, some dating back as far as the third millennium BC. It is surprising, in a way, to note the similarities in descriptions of the disorders in the ancient and modern texts. The description "... one who is gluttonous, filthy, walks naked, ... lost his memory and moves about in an uneasy manner..." in the Ayur Veda written in 3500 BC compares with the symptoms described in modern classification systems of psychiatric disorders. A more precise clinical description of psychotic disorders was given by Haslam in 1809 followed by Morel in 1860. It was toward the end of the nineteenth century and early years of the twentieth century that description of what is currently called schizophrenia and its differentiation from what we now know as bipolar disorder were described. Emil Kraepelin of Germany in 1896 and later Eugen Bleuler of Switzerland were accredited with this ground-breaking clinical work. Delineation and description of psychotic disorders underwent many changes during the twentieth century, with major work emerging from the Anglo-American and European schools of thought. It is interesting to note that the clinical classification system currently adopted worldwide, the *Diagnostic and Statistical Manual of Mental Disorders* (DSM) and the *International Classification of Diseases* (ICD), are not far-removed from the seminal works of Krepelin and Bleuer.

Psychotic Disorders

Psychotic disorders are those disorders of mental function and behavior that are severe in nature and cause severe disruption to the individual's functioning capacity and requires active and often long-term medical and psychosocial treatment. They are differentiated from the nonpsychotic or minor mental disorders by the nature of symptoms, morbidity, etiology, treatment, course, and outcome. It is important to note that the so-called minor mental disorders can sometimes cause suffering and disruption to life activities to a level comparable to that caused by psychotic disorders.

Schizophrenia, mood disorders, and paranoid disorder are the commonest forms of psychotic disorders. A fourth group of disorders that have some of the features of the other three but are different in some aspects (etiology, duration, course and outcome, cultural influences) are together classified as 'Other psychotic disorders'. This discussion does not include psychotic disorders caused by known medical conditions such as brain damage or psychotropic substances and some culture-specific syndromes. It focuses on schizophrenia and mood disorders that are the most common and disabling of psychotic disorders.

Symptoms of Psychotic Disorders

The symptoms of a psychotic disorder are manifest in the patient's emotions, perception, thinking, speech, and behavior. Disturbed emotion manifests in the form of excess sadness or happiness. In mood disorders, the patient's thinking and behavior match the mood they are experiencing (e.g., the patient feels worthless, becomes dull and inactive when depressed, is overactive, and indulges in excess spending and social misadventures when manic). Disordered perception takes the form of hallucinations where the person has sensations in the absence of any relevant stimulus and may respond to them as if they were true (e.g., hears voices of people talking to him or her when alone). Thinking disturbance in the form of delusions, which are fixed beliefs, are held even in the presence of definite evidence to the contrary (e.g., a belief that aliens are attacking him or her or that he or she is God). Patients may become mute or their speech rambling and difficult to follow. Their behavior often contravenes the normal behavior expected of the person and can be bizarre or harmful (violent, dirty, and disheveled appearance, silly behavior). Occasionally patients exhibit catatonia, where they may assume peculiar posturing with limbs held rigid for long periods of time. Disturbances in sleep, appetite, and sexual activity are common symptoms. There can be a severe reduction in the patient's interpersonal interactions, emotional life, motivation, and interest in life activities, a drop in academic and work capacity and the ability to take care of oneself. These symptoms are known as negative symptoms. Patients also experience disturbed attention, concentration, memory, and ability to plan and execute day-to-day tasks. Death by suicide occurs in 10–15% of those with psychotic disorders. Patients with psychosis are at a higher risk to commit violent or homicidal crime (Eronen et al., 1996).

Diagnosis

Diagnosis of a psychotic disorder is made mainly through clinical interview with the affected person and observation by a mental health professional with the affected person. Collateral and corroborative information about the person and his or her behavior is sought from relatives, friends, and medical records. Laboratory investigations such as screening for the use of drugs such as amfetamines, blood tests, and neurological investigations such as a CT scan are ordered to identify any medical disorder causing the symptoms of a psychotic disorder (**Tables 1** and **2**).

Diagnosis of schizophrenia is made when a combination of symptoms such as hallucinations, delusions, behavior changes, and negative symptoms predominate. The predominant symptom of a mood disorder is an excess of emotion of depression (depressive disorder) or happiness (manic disorder). Bipolar disorder refers to the condition where both depression and mania occur in the same person at the same time or different points in time. Patients are diagnosed with paranoid disorder when they have only a delusion (e.g., of being persecuted or having a serious disease) but rarely other symptoms.

Epidemiology

The majority of epidemiological studies have produced prevalence estimates in the range of 1.4–4.6/1000 for schizophrenia and 4–5/1000 for bipolar disorder, while it is much higher at 2–5% for major depression. The life-time morbid risk for schizophrenia and bipolar disorder is estimated at 1% and 10–20% for major depression. The annual incidence ranges from 0.017 to 0.054% for

Table 1   Common psychotic disorders

Disorders in which psychosis is a defining feature	Disorders in which psychosis is an associated feature
1. Schizophrenia	1. Mania
2. Substance-induced psychosis	2. Depression
3. Schizophreniform disorder	3. Cognitive disorders
4. Schizoaffective disorder	
5. Delusional disorder	
6. Brief psychotic disorder	
7. Shared psychotic disorder	
8. Psychotic disorder due to a general medical condition	

Table 2   Primary and secondary schizophrenia

Idiopathic/primary	Secondary
1. Schizophrenia	1. Substance-induced psychotic disorders
2. Schizophreniform disorder	2. Psychotic disorders due to a general medical condition
3. Schizoaffective disorder	
4. Delusional disorder	
5. Brief psychotic disorder	
6. Shared psychotic disorder	
7. Bipolar disorders	

schizophrenia and from 0.003 to 0.01% for bipolar disorder. These estimates are unlikely to reflect the true extent of variation that exists in different populations.

Causes

Extensive research has been conducted to identify the causes of the two major psychoses: schizophrenia and mood disorders. Several factors have been put forward to explain their cause. The disorders are probably multifactorial in origin, involving genetic, biological, and environmental factors.

Genes seem to play a rather important role in the causation of schizophrenia. The risk of developing the disorder increases tenfold if a parent or sibling is affected and 40- to 50-fold when an identical twin has the illness (**Figure 1**). Current molecular genetic research has identified several gene loci related to schizophrenia and bipolar disorder but has not yet established a strong and consistent link to the illness. Psychologically stressful experiences throughout life and use of psychotropic substances are also related to the development of psychotic disorders. It is currently being hypothesized that people who develop schizophrenia have a disorder in the development of their brains from the period before birth and/or during the early years of life. These defects could be caused by genetic or environmental factors. Vulnerability is a concept that has helped explain why some individuals and not others develop psychotic disorders, given the same background and environment. This vulnerability could be in the form of a family history of illness or a neurodevelopmental defect. Life stresses or use of psychotropic substances can precipitate an episode of psychosis in a vulnerable individual. It should be noted, however, that a majority of individuals apparently develop psychotic disorders without any identifiable preexisting or precipitating cause.

Abnormalities in the activity of certain areas of the brain such as the temporal and frontal lobes of the cerebrum and changes in neurochemistry have been identified in people with psychosis (**Figure 2** and **3**). For example, increased activity of dopamine, a neurotransmitter that is involved in conducting signals between nerve cells, is implicated as the fundamental defect in schizophrenia. Nothing has yet been concluded about how brain defects are related to the manifestation of and recovery from psychotic disorders.

Treatment and Outcome

A combination of medications and psychological and social interventions provide the best chances of recovery for people with psychotic disorders (**Table 3**). Antipsychotic medications such as clozapine and mood stabilizers such as lithium are used (**Table 4**). Electroconvulsive therapy (ECT) is indicated for a small percentage of severely ill patients, especially those with depression. Psychological interventions include cognitive behavior therapy, social skills training, mental health education, drug abstinence

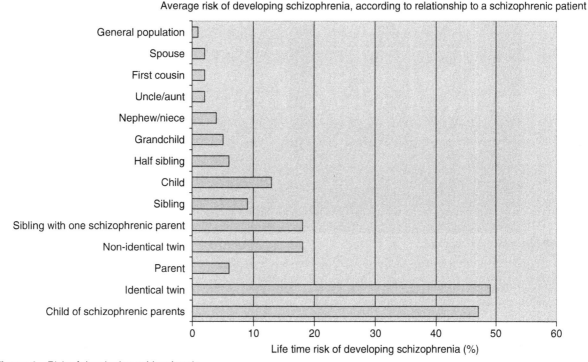

Average risk of developing schizophrenia, according to relationship to a schizophrenic patient

Figure 1   Risk of developing schizophrenia.

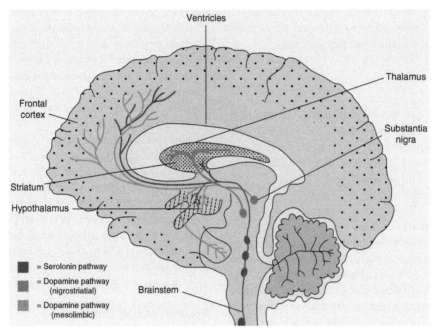

Figure 2   Pathways in the brain affected in psychotic disorders. Source: Target Schizophrenia, ABPI, 2003.

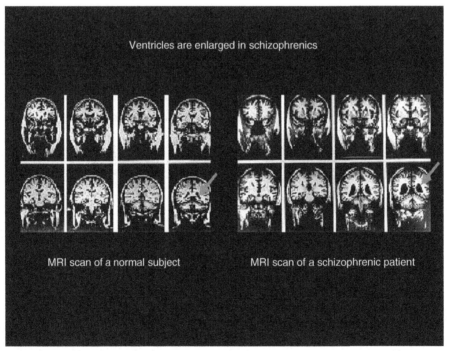

Figure 3   MRI findings in schizophrenia.

programs, stress management, training in independent living skills, and educational and vocational rehabilitation. Social intervention focuses on reducing stigma and supporting patients' reintegration into the mainstream community. It includes public health education programs, empowerment of patients and their caregivers, protection of rights and citizenship, ensuring equal opportunities, encouraging economic independence, social participation, and legal protection. Active and collaborative engagement of the patient, the family, and other caregivers in the treatment process is the recommended practice. Given the social relevance and magnitude of mental illness, an active and informed involvement

Table 3   Factors affecting prognosis of schizophrenia

No.	Good prognosis	Poor prognosis
1.	Acute onset	Insidious onset
2.	Short duration	Long duration
3.	Past psychiatric history absent	Past psychiatric history present
4.	Affective features present	Affective features absent
5.	Clouded sensorium	Sensorium clear
6.	Obsessive features absent	Obsessive features present
7.	Good premorbid functioning	Poor premorbid functioning
8.	Family history of schizophrenia absent	Family history of schizophrenia present
9.	Currently married	Never married
10.	No soft neurological signs	Soft signs present
11.	No structural brain abnormalities	Structural brain abnormalities present

Table 4   Commonly prescribed antipsychotic medications

First-generation or typical antipsychotics (dopamine receptor antagonists)	Low-potency agents
	Chlorpromazine
	Thioridazine
	Moderate-potency agents
	Loxapine
	Trifluoperazine
	High-potency agents
	Fluphenazine
	Thiothixene
	Haloperidol
	Pimozide
Second-generation (atypical antipsychotics)	Clozapine
	Risperidone
	Olanzepine
	Quetiapine
	Ziprasidone
	Aripiprazole
	Sulpiride

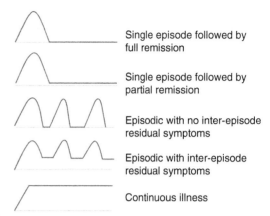

Single episode followed by full remission

Single episode followed by partial remission

Episodic with no inter-episode residual symptoms

Episodic with inter-episode residual symptoms

Continuous illness

Figure 4   Patterns of the course of schizophrenia.

of the legislature, judiciary, and mass media is essential for better outcomes, quality of life, and social reintegration of patients suffering from psychotic disorders.

The course of psychotic disorders varies between individuals. Generally, approximately one-third of patients recover fully after the first episode of illness. A majority experience a course marked by relapses (reemergence of frank symptoms of the disorder) interspersed with periods of varying degrees of recovery or a continuous illness (**Figure 4**).

Public Health and Psychotic Disorders

There is a common perception that psychotic disorders are not of as much public health importance as more prevalent and physically obvious disorders such as infectious diseases, heart disease, and cancer. During the last century, clinical knowledge and the practice of psychiatry and allied disciplines have advanced enormously. Worldwide research has shown that some of the psychotic disorders are no longer so-called low-prevalence disorders. We now know that the disabilities suffered by persons with psychotic disorders are equivalent to those caused by serious medical disorders. The very nature of psychotic disorders, with yet unclear etiology, chronicity with onset often in young age, and lack of a definitive cure tend to create a cumulative public health burden. The widespread lack of public knowledge and misinformation (**Table 5**), the stigma and marginalization faced by people suffering from these disorders, inadequate and inappropriate mental health, and long-term care services place more constraints in the effective management of these disorders. This leads to a substantial unattended public health burden that is often borne by the sufferer and the community.

Morbidity and Mortality

Mortality rates are used as global measures of a population's health status and as indicators for public health efforts and medical treatments. Psychotic disorders often have a fatal outcome. The average life expectancy of patients with schizophrenia is 20% less than that of the community they live in. Approximately 10–20% of people with psychotic disorder die by suicide, while 20–55% make medically serious attempts at suicide. These rates are at least 20 times more than those recorded for the general population.

People with a psychotic disorder suffer from many medical disorders at rates higher than other people. Comorbid medical illnesses have been detected in up to 40% of patients with schizophrenia in the community. The rate is higher among those in a hospital setting. Obesity, type 2 diabetes mellitus, abnormalities in lipid

Table 5   Myths and misconceptions about schizophrenia

Myths	Facts
Schizophrenia is a curse	Schizophrenia is a medical illness
Schizophrenia must be treated by sorcerers and faith healers	Schizophrenia must be treated by qualified medical professionals with medications
Schizophrenia must be treated in places of worship	Practice of religion can have a calming influence on patients and families and religious leaders can often be very effective counselors. However, antipsychotic medicines are required to control symptoms
Schizophrenia is split personality, like Dr. Jekyll and Mr. Hyde	Schizophrenia is not split personality. Jekyll and Hyde is the description of a dissociative state
Patients with schizophrenia are dangerous and should be confined to the house, hospitals, or jails	Most patients with schizophrenia prefer to be left alone and do not harm others unless severely provoked
Patients with schizophrenia are useless and unproductive and a burden on the family	With proper medical treatment, rehabilitation, and a supportive environment, many patients have been able to hold jobs and take care of their homes and families

metabolism, coronary heart disease, hypertension, emphysema, tuberculosis, and cancer occur at higher rates in people with psychotic disorders than the general population. While some of the metabolic abnormalities are associated with treatment with antipsychotic drugs, individuals with schizophrenia are, by nature, said to have a greater tendency to develop these disorders even in the absence of any drug treatment. These medical disorders add to the burden of disease borne by these patients and further reduce their ability to function normally and their quality of life.

Disability and Burden Caused by Psychotic Disorders

The term 'disabled' commonly brings up the picture of a person with impairment in physical function such as vision or mobility. Many fail to recognize that people with mental disorders can suffer disabilities qualitatively and quantitatively similar to those caused by a physical illness. According to the United Nations Standard Rules on the Equalization of Opportunities for Persons with Disabilities, the term disability "summarizes a great number of different functional limitations occurring in any population in any country of the world. People may be disabled by physical, intellectual or sensory impairment, medical conditions or mental illness." The International Classification of Functioning (ICF) developed by the World Health Organization describes and classifies various forms of disability independent of the cause. Psychotic disorders such as schizophrenia have been recognized the world over as conditions that cause major disabilities in several spheres of a person's functioning: self-care, independent living, social activity and social role function, educational and occupational skills, and cognitive capacity.

Psychotic disorders contribute to the overall disease burden, which is generally underestimated. In a major study conducted by the World Bank and the World Health Organization, it was reported that no less than 25% of the total burden of disease in the established market economies was attributable to neuropsychiatric conditions. Measured as a proportion of disability-adjusted life-years (DALY) lost, which is an estimate of healthy years of life lost due to an illness, schizophrenia, bipolar disorder, and major depression together accounted for 10.8% of the total burden of disease in the world. This means that these three disorders together inflict on most communities losses that are comparable to those caused by cancer (15%) and higher than the losses resulting from ischemic heart disease (9%). The study projected depression to rank as the number one cause of disability by the year 2020.

Cost of Psychosis

Psychotic disorders impose considerable cost to the patient, family, and society. Direct costs include cost of mental health services, medicines, and support costs. Indirect costs include loss of productivity of the patients and their carers and the cost of pain and suffering of patient and family. The average costs of psychoses are high even when estimated conservatively. The total cost of schizophrenia alone in the United States in 1990 was estimated at $32.5 billion, followed by affective (mood) disorders at $30.4 billion. Despite the worldwide policy of closing costly-to-run psychiatric hospitals, the cost of psychosis appears to be rising each year. This is worsened by the increasing cost of the new generation of antipsychotic medications that are recommended in place of low-cost medications, with no clearly demonstrated advantages in terms of effectiveness or safety. The cost of psychosis is also borne by the community with varying degrees of willingness and consequence. Absence of welfare support programs and poor public health care in developing countries place the entire cost of patient care on families, resulting in their poverty, marginalization, and downward social drift.

Smit *et al.* (2006) drew attention to some of these issues related to the burden of disease attributable to psychotic disorders and drew up priorities in managing this burden. At the population level, new patients caused a substantial part of the costs. This was a strong argument for strengthening the role of preventive psychiatry in public health, with the aim of reducing incidence, thus avoiding future costs. In particular, reducing the incidence of highly prevalent disorders such as major depression, associated with substantial disability and important economic ramifications, should be a public health priority. Smit *et al.* noted further that the bulk of the costs resulted from production losses; this made employers pertinent stakeholders in mental health promotion. Therefore, thought should be given to the question of how to involve them more actively in health promotion. Adoption of the above-mentioned strategies would need to be supported by more prevention trials and cost-effectiveness studies on the specific disorders. With the costs of mental disorders comparable to those resulting from physical illnesses, there is a need to reconsider how budgets are allocated for research and development in mental illnesses *vis-a-vis* physical illnesses.

Stigma of Psychosis

Stigma is a social phenomenon that places people in a particular social or health status at a disadvantage. WHO defined stigma as a mark of shame, disgrace, or disapproval, which results in an individual being shunned or rejected by others. A diagnostic label such as schizophrenia or mania is often feared and rejected by those who receive it. The need to use psychotropic prescription medications that are often viewed as addicting play a role in creating the stigma. Behavioral deviations in personal hygiene, social skills and communication, homelessness, and unemployment contribute to the stigma faced by people with psychotic disorders. The imbalance in the focus of mass media on disabilities resulting from mental disorders often reinforces stigma.

Stigma has the potential to worsen the course of psychotic disorders. It interferes with the willingness of many people to seek help, which results in a treatment delay, in turn leading to a more severe first manifestation of the illness. It can reduce life opportunities, limit social contacts, reduce self-esteem, and overall reduce quality of life. The central messages of many antistigma campaigns are often positively loaded with statements that mental illnesses are frequent, affect everyone, are treatable, and have a good prognosis if treated. They do not focus on the severe forms of psychosis that the public are often aware of and worried about. The question arises of whether the antistigma campaigns should also cater to psychotic disorders with poorer prognoses and severe disability. Such an approach would bring a more balanced view of mental

disorders and an understanding of patients' suffering. The International Classification of Functioning developed by WHO emphasizes the positive aspects of functioning of people with a health condition such as psychosis. It also turns the focus to the role of environmental factors (community, policies, disability-friendly services) that act as facilitators or barriers to patients' efforts to live as contributing members of the mainstream society. This holistic approach would help the public understand and support people disabled by psychosis so they can attain an optimal level of functioning and improve the quality of their lives.

Inequity of Health Care

There are critical gaps between those who need mental health services and those who receive the services and between optimally effective treatment for psychotic disorders and what many individuals receive in actual practice. Access is a serious problem for people with psychosis. In the U.S., less than 40% of people with severe mental disorders such as schizophrenia received any mental health treatment and a mere 15% received minimally adequate mental health services in a given year. Only 10% of people with bipolar disorder had a consultation with a mental health specialist. Nearly half of people with depression remain untreated. Even those who reach medical services are often not adequately treated in the primary care setting, and there is evidence to suggest that the outcome is worse if treated by the primary physician than when treated by a mental health professional. Given the high rates of morbidity and mortality associated with psychotic disorders, this state of affairs is a major public health concern.

One of the major barriers to narrowing the gap in care is fragmentation of care. This is especially problematic with an illness such as schizophrenia that necessitates a multisystemic interdisciplinary approach. Psychiatrists, nurses, vocational specialists, to name just a few, are integral members of a treatment team. Many services do not have such a team. Finding mental health specialists with the requisite skills and experience to treat psychotic disorders may be lacking, especially in rural areas.

If the gaps in services are as wide in developed countries as reported, it is bound to be worse in economically disadvantaged communities where the national budgetary expenditure on health is grossly inadequate to meet even the minimal needs of people with severe mental disorders. A large percentage of people with psychotic disorders living in developing countries remain untreated for life. Concerns about cost of care, lack of welfare support, medical insurance, cultural models of illness, unawareness, and stigma are among the foremost reasons why people do not seek or receive mental health care in developing countries.

Inequity in mental health care for people with psychotic disorders is influenced by economic status, gender, race, age, education, and geographic distance from services. Women, older persons, ethnic minorities, the economically disadvantaged, and rural populations more often fail to reach treatment and receive less than adequate services. High-prevalence preventable and communicable diseases with definite outcomes take precedence in receiving funding and other support. Parity between coverage for mental health and other health areas is an affordable and effective objective to seek.

Deinstitutionalization and Service Reforms

In the second part of the twentieth century, the development of mental health services in Western Europe was characterized by a dramatic conceptual and structural change: Deinstitutionalization. The focus of care shifted from inpatient care by closing down large and costly mental hospitals to outpatient community care of people with psychotic disorders and other severe mental illnesses. This resulted from several factors, including economic (cost-saving) and social factors (the right of people with severe mental disorders such as psychosis to live in the community). The emergence of effective psychotropic drugs in the 1950s, starting with chlorpromazine, was a further decisive factor contributing to the success of the deinstitutionalization programs.

The deinstitutionalization process led to the development of alternative community mental health services; integration of mental health with other health services; and generic, social, and community services such as accommodation and employment. There was a suspicion that deinstitutionalization might have gone too far. The increase in coercive activities such as compulsory psychiatric treatment, the number of suicides, the increasing number of forensic beds, acute admissions, and bed occupancy indicated a general trend toward reinstitutionalization. On the whole, the European experience made it obvious that a fundamental change in the principles and the organization of mental health care was possible across national borders. At the same time, differences in current mental health-care systems revealed that shared global developments do not necessarily result in comparable patterns of service provision. Reports on mental health-care reforms in several countries suggested that against the background of existing health-care structures as well as economic, social, political, and cultural characteristics, each country has to find its own way in order to accomplish the aims of deinstitutionalization and reintegration of the severely mentally ill into the community. A key task that lies ahead for both mental health service practitioners and researchers is to make sure that progress in mental health services is not lost within the increasing financial crisis of health-care systems.

Consumer and Family Self-Help Movement

The public health importance of self-help groups is in influencing attitudes, health behavior, caring for others, and promoting policy discussion. The emergence of the self-help and support movement initiated by consumers and families has helped to shape the direction and complexion of mental health programs dealing with schizophrenia, depression, and bipolar disorder. Although the origins and philosophy of these organizations differ, they have promoted common and important goals in patient care, protection of rights, and equity of service. Their participation in research and administrative committees has positively influenced the way research or treatment programs are implemented. The consumer and carer forums work toward reducing stigma and discrimination in policies and practices. They focus on recovery and social reintegration and draw attention to the special needs of people with psychotic disorders. The self-help movement has helped bring proper recognition of the individual and the legal rights of people with mental disorders, protecting them from exploitation and social degradation. In addition, families are no longer seen as causing disorders such as schizophrenia or as hindrances to treatment, but rather as valued participating members in the overall therapeutic environment. Organizations such as Rethink (formerly National Schizophrenia Fellowship), the National Alliance of the Mentally Ill (NAMI), Schizophrenics Anonymous, the Depression and Bipolar Support Alliance, and various websites provide information, support, and links to other services for consumers and their families.

Prevention of Psychotic Disorders

Primary prevention of psychotic disorders with undetermined etiology has yet to evolve. Secondary and tertiary prevention of the disorders in the form of intervention during the early phases of the illness and reduction of relapses and deterioration, respectively, are possible. Several studies, particularly in Canada and Australia, have developed guidelines to detect psychotic disorders during the early phases in young people before the frank illness manifests. Although this has raised controversy in terms of labeling people with a mental disorder when they have no frank symptoms of psychosis, evidence has now accrued to show that a full attack of the disorder can be preempted by early intervention methods.

Relapse prevention and minimizing deterioration are the goals of tertiary prevention of psychotic disorders. Mental health education of patients and their caregivers to improve their understanding of the illness and the need for treatment, ensuring adherence to treatment recommendations, education on recognizing early signs of a relapse and proactive management of relapse, assertive follow-up and treatment in the community, minimizing hospitalization, and active multidisciplinary rehabilitation inputs are some of the measures geared toward successful tertiary prevention.

Reducing the Burden of Psychotic Disorders

There are certain principles fundamental to the fulfillment of public health aims for people with psychotic disorders: identifying and providing appropriate help to those disabled by the disorders, gearing services to provide comprehensive and varied programs for short-term and long-term care, integrating services manned by professional and trained service providers, and globally reorienting public health policies and programs toward mental illness and in particular psychotic disorders. Care for patients with psychotic disorders could be improved by using common sense and readily available inexpensive, low-tech, evidence-based practices that reduce relapses and facilitate and maintain recovery. Since public health systems all over the world are invariably faced with resource constraints, establishing priorities, harvesting all resources available within the community rather than depending on public funding alone, and establishing some system of rationing is called for to produce maximum benefit to most people.

First and foremost, measures promoting the well-being of patients with psychotic disorders in the community are awareness, illness education, and reduction of stigma. This is necessary not only at the level of the individual and caregiver, but also at the level of the community. It is important to determine low treatment rates, even in people who have access to primary care medical services, evidence of the need for appropriate skills to identify and treat psychotic disorders in medical professionals in primary care. This can be addressed through training during undergraduate and postgraduate medical education and professional development programs aimed at practicing general practitioners and mental health professionals.

Efficient use of mental health professionals is required so that expert psychiatric care is provided to patients with psychosis. Such professionals are in chronic shortage all over the world, but the situation is worse in developing countries. The general practitioner plays a very crucial role in the pathway to recovery for people with psychotic disorders. While they may not be fully equipped to deal with the problem themselves, adequate support and a shared-care model with mental health professionals could help provide appropriate skilled care. Traditional healers are a common source of medical care in developing societies, especially in rural areas. It is recommended that an active liaison with the healers that includes educating them in identifying patients and referring them to appropriate medical care without prejudice to either system of medical practice be established. Such an approach respects the role of the traditional healer in the community while ensuring evidence-based care for people with psychotic disorders.

The public health burden of psychosis is lessened when the disorders are better treated at low cost, relapses are prevented, and patients live in the community and actively engage in life, fulfilling their family and social roles. Intervention programs that start with early detection and initiation of medical treatment that accompany on-going rehabilitation that focuses on bringing the patient back into mainstream community life are required. The programs need to be geared to the needs of the individual and have relevance to the community and culture. Such programs should provide support for people with psychosis for learning living skills, education, employment, accommodation, and economic independence. Disability support payments, while appropriate to the most disabled, can work as disincentives to engage in productive life and thus increase the burden on society. Public health services alone cannot cater to the diverse needs of people with psychotic disorders. Nongovernmental organizations are now playing an increasingly crucial role in long-term care. Encouraging the role of NGOs in mental health care is an optimal way of utilizing the community's social capital.

The economic cost is probably the most crucial factor that determines the kind of political and policy decisions made that influence care provided for psychotic disorders. The amount of thought, effort, and resource allocation will be determined by how much will be gained by dealing with the problem as a public health issue. Decision makers need to be convinced that treatment of psychotic disorders would lead not only to better public health in general, but also contribute to the economy. There is now clear evidence that providing proper medical care and adequate support for community living cuts the cost of care, and patients brought back into mainstream and gainfully employed contribute to the economy. The increasing importance given to mental health in public health planning in some countries is based on this evidence. This change needs to be continued with the active participation of all stake holders.

See also: Measurement of Psychiatric and Psychological Disorders and Outcomes in Populations; Mental Health Epidemiology (Psychiatric Epidemiology); Mental Health Policy; Women's Mental Health.

Citations

Bleuler E (1911) *Dementia Praecok oder Gruppe der Schizophrenia.* Leipzig, Germany: Deuticke.

Eronen M, Hakola P, and Tiihonen J (1996) Mental disorders and homicidal behavior in Finland. *Archives of Geneneral Psychiatry* 53: 497–501.

Haslan J (1807) *Observations on Madness and Melarcholy,* 2nd edn. London: J. Callow.

Kraepelin E (1896) *Psychiatrie*, 5th edn. Leipzing, Germany: Barth.

Morel BA (1860) *Traites des Maladies Mentales*. Paris, France: Masson.

Smit F, Cuijpers P, Oostenbrink J, Batelaan N, de Graaf R, and Beekman A (2006) Costs of nine common mental disorders: Implications for curative and preventive psychiatry. *Journal of Mental Health Policy and Economics* 9(4): 193–200.

Further Reading

American Psychiatric Association (2000) *Diagnostic and Statistical Manual of Mental Disorders,* 4th edn. Washington DC: American Psychiatric Association.

Andreasen NC and Black DW (2001) *Introductory Textbook of Psychiatry*, 3rd edn. Arlington, VA: American Psychiatric Publishing.

Becker T and Kilian R (2006) Psychiatric services for people with severe mental illness across Western Europe: What can be generalized from current knowledge about differences in provision, costs and outcomes of mental health care? *Acta Psychiatrica Scandinavica* 113 (Supplement 429): 9–16.

Gelder MG, Lopez-Ibor JJ Jr and Andreasen NC (eds.) (2000) *New Oxford Textbook of Psychiatry*. Oxford, UK: Oxford University Press.

Hales RE and Yudofsky SC (eds.) (2003) *Textbook of Clinical Psychiatry*, 4th edn. Washington DC: American Psychiatric Publishing.

Lieberman JA and Murray RM (eds.) (2001) *Comprehensive Care of Schizophrenia*, 1st edn. London: Martin Dunitz.

Murray CJL and Lopez AD (1996) *The Global Burden of Disease.* Boston, MA: Harvard University Press.

Neugebauer R (1999) Mind matters: The importance of mental disorders in public health's 21st century mission. *American Journal of Public Health* 89: 1309–1311.

Sadock BJ and Sadock VA (eds.) (2005) *Kaplan and Sadock's Comprehensive Textbook of Psychiatry,* 8th edn. Philadelphia, PA: Lippincott Williams & Wilkins.

Satcher DS (2000) Executive summary: A report of the surgeon-general on mental health. *Public Health Reports* 115: 89–101.

Stein DJ, Kupfer DJ, and Schatzberg AF (eds.) (2006) *Textbook of Mood Disorders,* 1st edn. Arlington, VA: American Psychiatric Publishing.

Thornicroft G and Tansella M (eds.) (1999) *The Mental Health Matrix: A Manual to Improve Services.* Cambridge, UK: Cambridge University Press.

World Health Organization (1992) *International Classification of Diseases and Related Health Problems (10th Revision).* Geneva, Switzerland: World Health Organization.

World Health Organization (2001) *The World Health Report 2001.* Geneva, Switzerland: World Health Organization.

Relevant Websites

http://www.schizophrenia.com – A non-profit community providing in-depth information, support and education related to schizophrenia.

http://www.bipolar.com.au – Bipolar Disorder website.

http://www.healthcentral.com – Health Central website.

http://www.scarfindia.com – Website of Schizophrenia Foundation, India.

Specific Mental Health Disorders: Trauma and Mental Disorders

D Silove, A Nickerson, and R A Bryant, University of New South Wales, Sydney, NSW, Australia

In recent decades, much attention has been given to the impact of psychological trauma on mental health. Trauma is distinguished from major stresses such as marital separation, financial hardship, and work problems in that it involves a fundamental threat to the life or integrity of individuals or those close to them. The category of posttraumatic stress disorder (PTSD) has tended to dominate the field since its introduction in 1980 into the American Psychiatric Association classification system's third edition of the *Diagnostic and Statistical Manual.* The present article provides an overview of PTSD and its causes, outcomes, and treatment. We will also examine other psychological outcomes of trauma, consider psychological responses to gross human-instigated abuses, and explore issues relevant to a public health response to mass disasters.

Posttraumatic Stress Disorder

Diagnosing PTSD

Four major criteria are applied to diagnose PTSD (DSM-IV; APA, 1994). Criterion A requires exposure to an environmental event that threatens the safety or integrity of the self or someone else. The Diagnostic and Statistical Manual of Mental Disorders, 4th Edition. (DSM-IV) requires that, in addition to the environmental threat, the person responds in a subjective manner with feelings of fear, horror, and/or helplessness. The B criterion involves reliving the traumatic experience in the form of flashbacks or nightmares. The memories are vivid, intrude unbidden into consciousness, and can manifest in multiple sensory modalities. In extreme situations, the survivor may dissociate, that is feel and act as if he or she is detached from the immediate environment and is actually reliving the traumatic experience in the present, albeit in a fragmented and chaotic manner. The re-experiencing phenomena are widely regarded as being the defining features of PTSD, setting the disorder apart from other anxiety and stress-related conditions. In contrast, the remaining two domains of PTSD, avoidance and numbing (Criterion C), and arousal (Criterion D), have features in common with other anxiety disorders, in that they broadly represent defensive responses to extreme fear. Criterion C includes avoidance of thoughts, activities, or places that remind the survivor of the initial trauma. These situations trigger re-experiencing symptoms. Someone who was robbed at a bank not only avoids the specific site where the hold-up occurred, but through conditioning, cues are generalized to include all banks or reminders, for example, advertising on television. In addition, survivors may feel numb in their emotional responses, so that family and friends describe them as being uncharacteristically remote, unresponsive, and unfeeling. Survivors may become socially isolated, preferring their own company to normal interpersonal interactions. The final symptom domain (Criterion D) of PTSD involves psychophysiologic arousal. Symptoms include a rapid heart rate (tachycardia), palpitations, sweating, shakiness, and other somatic experiences. Survivors experience marked startle reactions, insomnia, poor concentration, and difficulties with memory. They can be irritable and are quickly moved to angry outbursts, a response pattern that causes difficulties in family and social interactions.

To make a diagnosis of PTSD, a sufficient number of symptoms from each domain must be present for at least 1 month and the disorder must cause clinically significant distress or impairment in functioning. In its severe form, PTSD can lead to major dysfunction in areas of work, family, and social relationships (**Table 1**).

Triggers and Course of PTSD

A wide range of traumas can lead to PTSD, including accidents, assault, natural disasters, exposure to warfare and other forms of conflict, as well as gross abuses such as

Table 1 Symptoms of PTSD

Re-experiencing symptoms: One or more must be present for diagnosis
- Intrusive memories (including images, thoughts, or perceptions)
- Nightmares
- Flashbacks
- Psychological or physiological distress upon exposure to reminders of traumatic event

Avoidance/numbing symptoms: Three or more must be present for diagnosis
- Avoidance of reminders of the trauma (e.g. people, places, situations)
- Decreased interest in activities
- Feeling detached from others
- Emotional numbing
- Difficulty remembering part of the trauma
- Sense of not having a future

Hyperarousal symptoms: Two or more must be present for diagnosis
- Difficulty sleeping or disturbed sleep
- Increased startle response
- Irritability
- Difficulty concentrating
- Hypervigilance

---

rape, child sexual abuse, torture, and other forms of human-instigated violence. The course of PTSD is somewhat variable. Distress in the acute phase after trauma is common. Persons who have severe PTSD symptoms at this stage together with marked dissociative symptoms qualify for a diagnosis of acute stress disorder (APA, 1994). Nevertheless, in most trauma-affected populations, only a minority go on to develop chronic PTSD. The percentage varies according to the type, severity, and repetitiveness of the trauma. Women and those with a past psychiatric history or with previous exposure to trauma are more vulnerable. Populations exposed to ongoing stresses or danger, for example, people living in dangerous or unsettled refugee camps, tend to experience persistently high rates of PTSD. Nevertheless, following the accidental traumas of everyday life (injuries, motor vehicle accidents, and the like), only a minority of survivors tend to develop chronic PTSD, in the range of 10–15% (McNally et al., 2003). At a population level, the National Comorbidity Study (NCS) conducted in the United States indicated that while 60.7% of men and 51.2% of women are exposed to trauma at some time during their lives, only 8.2% of men and 20.4% of women develop PTSD (Kessler et al., 1995). Survivors of extreme human-instigated trauma such as rape, torture, and exposure to other gross human rights violations tend to have higher rates of PTSD, ranging from 20 to 40% (e.g., Basoglu et al., 1994; de Jong et al., 2001). Hence, except for the most severe forms of trauma, most survivors show high levels of resilience in the posttraumatic phase, recovering from acute feelings of distress.

Predicting those at risk of PTSD based on acute posttraumatic symptoms remains problematic. Emerging evidence indicates that a small group of survivors with very high levels of distress, particularly manifested as repetitive intrusions and heightened arousal, are at great risk of experiencing persisting PTSD (Silove, 2007). The problem remains, however, that another subgroup with intermediate levels of acute symptoms progresses to become full cases of PTSD at a later time. Hence, from a public health perspective, current methods do not allow accurate identification of the whole group at risk of future PTSD, for example, among injury survivors admitted to hospital. Nevertheless, from a service perspective, there is sufficient evidence to warrant identifying the highly symptomatic group in the early posttraumatic phase and to offer them evidence-based interventions that have been shown to prevent the later development of chronic PTSD (McNally et al., 2003).

Causes of PTSD

Although there is ample evidence that PTSD is triggered by life-threatening events, the underlying pathogenesis of the disorder remains unclear. At a biological level, several factors have been implicated, including abnormalities in stress hormone responses mediated via the hypothalamo-pituitary-adrenal axis. Some brain imaging studies have shown that PTSD sufferers have a reduced hippocampal volume, which may be relevant since that brain center is pivotal in contextualizing trauma memories (e.g., Bremner *et al.*, 1997). The amygdala and medial prefrontal cortex have also been implicated, since these centers mediate the learned fear response, mobilizing pathways that activate flight and fight reactions. The prevailing neural network theory of PTSD suggests that there is inadequate regulation of the medial prefrontal cortex of amygdala-generated fear responses, thereby allowing environmental triggers to maintain fear reactions (Rauch *et al.*, 2006). Cognitive theories of PTSD suggest that faulty thought processes or attributions lead to persistence of the learned fear response (Ehlers and Clark, 2000). In other words, expecting catastrophic outcomes perpetuates the PTSD reaction. An evolutionary perspective (Silove, 1998) suggests that the re-experiencing of trauma memories ensures that survivors mobilize defensive responses if exposed to further environmental cues signaling the return of the danger. In some survivors, medial prefrontal mechanisms fail to exert adequate control on this amygdala-mediated normative survival response so that memory rehearsal continues unchecked.

Treatment of PTSD

In Western countries, although many different types of therapy are offered, research has identified two specific domains of treatment (psychotherapy and pharmacotherapy) that are effective for PTSD. All interventions need to be guided by some key principles. These include sensitive engagement with patients in a therapeutic relationship that allays anxiety, promotes trust and dignity, and creates a setting of safety and security. Providing information about the disorder and its causes, and where appropriate, educating the family about the approach to treating the condition are vital. General lifestyle interventions are important, including attention to ongoing stresses, work, family life, leisure activities, and legal and compensation issues where relevant. The specific form of psychotherapy that has most scientific support is cognitive behavioral therapy. The therapy should be provided by trained professionals. In brief, the key interventions include anxiety reduction (relaxation exercises, attention to panic symptoms, for example, by using slow breathing exercises), cognitive restructuring (challenging negative thoughts that perpetuate high levels of anxiety), and exposure therapy where the survivor is guided systematically in imagination through the trauma experience over a number of sessions. Pharmacotherapy involves the use of the newer antidepressants that enhance the action of serotonin and/or norepinephrine. Typical medications

include sertraline, paroxetine, and mirtazapine. In some settings, the older tricyclic antidepressants are used, but close supervision is needed because of potential toxic effects. Other medications such as mood stabilizers, antipsychotics, and sedatives are used, but there is insufficient evidence to recommend these treatments as first-line interventions. All medications can cause side effects and have risks, for example in overdose. The indiscriminate, long-term use of the benzodiazepine tranquilizer class of drugs such as diazepam should be avoided because of dependency, the risk that the dose will be escalated, and withdrawal effects.

Other Psychiatric Disorders Arising from Trauma

PTSD occurs in conjunction with other psychological disorders in over 70% of cases (Kessler *et al.*, 1995). A review of studies has shown that depression is the second most common psychological disorder in survivors of disasters followed by other forms of anxiety (Norris *et al.*, 2002). Other disorders also are common. After the Oklahoma City bombing, 34% of survivors experienced PTSD, 22% depression, 7% panic disorder, 4% generalized anxiety disorder, 9% alcohol use disorder, and 2% drug use disorder; overall, 30% of people had a psychiatric disorder other than PTSD (North *et al.*, 1999). The rates for most of these disorders exceed those in the general population (Brown *et al.*, 2000), indicating that trauma is a significant contributor to the onset of these problems. Traumatic or complicated grief is another response that has only received attention more recently. There is a risk that it will be confused with PTSD since both groups experience intrusive memories. Those with grief, however, have vivid memories of the deceased or missing person, which, although distressing, do not generate a sense of threat in the survivor.

Psychological Responses to Extreme Abuse and Persecution

Survivors of severe abuse such as torture, sexual abuse, and related forms of intentional human violence manifest a range of psychological reactions that are not fully incorporated into the criteria for PTSD. In the past, these reactions were identified according to the cause, for example, the torture or concentration camp syndromes. More recently, more general terms used include complex PTSD or disorders of extreme stress not otherwise specified (referred to but not fully adopted by DSM-IV) and enduring personality change after catastrophic events (EPCACE), a category included for the first time in the International Classification of Diseases Edition 10 (ICD-10). In all these formulations, anger, mistrust, and hostility are prominent, in recognition that these reactions are closely tied to feelings of having one's rights and dignity violated (Silove, 1996). Other features observed include guilt and shame, a tendency to somatic complaints, extreme forms of dissociation, feelings of pervasive isolation and alienation, and unrelenting hopelessness. There are similarities between these descriptions and the criteria for diagnosing borderline personality disorder, a condition linked to early childhood abuse. Further scientific evidence is needed, however, to confirm the specific features (beyond PTSD) that characterize the essential features of these more complex reactions to intentional human abuse.

The following case description illustrates complex PTSD.

An elderly Cambodian refugee who had lived in Australia for 20 years was referred to a trauma treatment service. His family described him as withdrawn, uncommunicative, lost in his own world, irritable and angry at times, and unable to enjoy any aspect of his life. These characteristics had been present for many years but he had become noticeably more depressed and hopeless in recent times. He was interviewed with an interpreter but even so remained monosyllabic through the first few sessions. He did reveal sufficient information to allow PTSD symptoms to be identified and an additional diagnosis of major depression to be made and he was prescribed antidepressants at low dose. He regarded his problem as arising from his karma and he was skeptical that any treatment could work. Over the next 2 months, he appeared to become more trusting of the therapeutic environment. He revealed that during the Pol Pot times (the Khmer Rouge autogenocide of 1975–79), he and his family were subjected to slave labor. He was beaten and tortured on several occasions because he was a member of the professional elite prior to the revolution. On one occasion, he was forced to torture his brother who was accused of being a traitor. He became enraged when he thought of the injustices he had suffered but also felt guilt-stricken and ashamed because of his actions. Psychotherapy focused on dealing with his PTSD symptoms using cognitive-behavioral methods and in addition exploring cautiously and gradually his sense of guilt and shame. He came to realize that he was in a situation of forced choices, that is, he had no control over his actions during his period of captivity. His depression and PTSD symptoms improved and he became more actively engaged in pursuing his Buddhist faith by attending the temple. Improvements overall were modest, however, and the family reported that he never returned fully to his old self preceding the trauma.

Mass Impacts of Trauma

A large proportion of the world's population has been exposed to trauma, particularly taking into account populations experiencing mass violence such as warfare, persecution, and displacement; societies exposed to terrorist attacks; and regions that experience natural disasters such as tsunamis, earthquakes, floods, fires, and hurricanes. Limited resources and professional skills in low- and middle-income countries make it impossible for all survivors to obtain high-quality psychological care. Individual or small group psychological debriefing, where survivors are encouraged to explore their reactions to trauma in the immediate aftermath of disasters, is neither feasible nor effective and can be damaging to those with high levels of arousal. The majority of survivors have the capacity to recover spontaneously and the speed and extent to which that occurs depends largely on the effectiveness of the emergency humanitarian response and the subsequent reconstruction process. The ADAPT model (Adaptation & Development After Persecution and Trauma) (Silove and Steel, 2006) identifies five major psychosocial domains that are threatened by disasters and that, if repaired effectively, support posttraumatic recovery at an individual and population level. These domains or pillars include safety and security; bonds and networks; systems of justice; roles and identities; and institutions and practices that support a sense of meaning and coherence, including culture, religion, and political participation. It is argued that where the aid and reconstruction process assists in rebuilding these psychosocial pillars, survivor populations have a greater capacity to mobilize their own resources to hasten recovery. Conversely, in settings of effective social recovery there should be lower rates of persisting traumatic stress reactions over time. For example, Vietnamese refugees resettled as permanent residents in conditions of security in Australia over 11 years were shown to have low prevalence rates of PTSD, depression, and anxiety (Steel et al., 2002). On arrival in Australia, the Vietnamese were given secure residency status, access to education and work opportunities, and support to sponsor families to join them. They have been free to maintain their culture and to pursue their religious practices. In contrast, other displaced populations exposed to similar traumas in their home countries who continue to live under conditions of insecurity, for example, with temporary protection visas, continue to manifest high levels of PTSD and related mood disturbances (Steel et al., 2006).

It seems likely that aid programs that effectively repair the psychosocial pillars identified by the ADAPT model will achieve the optimal outcomes in terms of population recovery from traumatic stress. From a mental health perspective, this means that the focus moves away from direct psychological debriefing of individual survivors toward what is now referred to as a program of community-wide psychological first aid. The aim is to alleviate acute distress by fostering a calm, safe, and supportive environment, to connect people with family, communities, and support agencies, and to promote self-efficacy, hope, and empowerment in those affected by the trauma. This can be achieved by helping individuals and families to meet their basic needs (food and water, shelter, health care), providing accurate information and practical assistance, helping families to reassemble or stay together, ensuring that people are dealt with in a dignified and nondiscriminating way, giving survivors an active role in planning and implementing the recovery process, and targeting emotional and psychiatric support more accurately to those in special need.

The United Nations Inter-Agency Standing Committee (2007) has developed guidelines to assist humanitarian agencies in planning and implementing psychosocial aid programs in the aftermath of mass trauma. Guidelines are presented in the form of a matrix of action, providing suggested responses for each stage of a disaster. Action sheets offer a step-by-step description of key initiatives. Also listed are available resources, examples of programs from previous emergency situations, and suggestions for interorganizational coordination. Major topic areas include mental health and psychosocial assessments, orientation and training of aid workers, and protecting individuals under threat.

Whereas a population-wide approach is pivotal to an effective mental health response to disasters, a minority of survivors will need direct mental health services because their level of distress is so severe that it prevents them or their families from coping with the demands of the post-traumatic environment. Communities readily identify these persons by their behavioral disturbances (Silove et al., 2004). That heterogeneous group includes people with severe and disabling posttraumatic reactions and others with preexisting mental and neuropsychiatric disorders such as psychosis and epilepsy. If well designed and implemented, community-based emergency mental health clinics can provide critical care to these patients and their families. In developing countries, these clinics can be the forerunner of and shape future service development as the society enters the post-disaster development phase.

Conclusions

Exposure to psychological trauma is extensive around the globe. Most persons and their communities recover from the initial distress that such experiences cause, but a minority continue to suffer a range of psychological problems including PTSD. There is no one intervention that addresses all the needs of survivors and their communities. In settings of mass trauma, particularly in countries with low resources, the emphasis should be on rebuilding the social pillars that assist survivor communities to reestablish their lives and hence achieve psychological equilibrium. Early psychological debriefing for all

survivors is neither necessary nor feasible in settings of large-scale disasters. Nevertheless, there will always be a minority of survivors who manifest severe and disabling traumatic stress reactions and it is vital that they and others with severe psychiatric disorders are identified and provided with best practice interventions to limit chronic disability. Evidence is accruing that cognitive-behavioral therapy adapted to culture and context is the treatment of choice for individuals with established PTSD. All interventions, whether focused on the individual or on whole populations, need to address the challenges of being a survivor struggling to overcome the impact of trauma. Practitioners need to create a context of trust, respect, and safety, encouraging survivors to play an active role in their own recovery.

Citations

American Psychiatric Association (1994) *Diagnostic and Statistical Manual of Mental Disorders*, 4th edn. Washington, DC: American Psychiatric Association.

Basoglu M, Paker M, Paker O, *et al.* (1994) Psychological effects of torture: A comparison of tortured with nontortured political activitists in Turkey. *American Journal of Psychiatry* 151: 76–81.

Bremner JD, Randall P, Vermetten E, *et al.* (1997) Magnetic resonance imaging-based measurement of hippocampal volume in posttraumatic stress disorder related to childhood physical and sexual abuse – A preliminary report. *Biological Psychiatry* 41: 23–32.

Brown ES, Fulton MK, Wilkeson A, and Petty F (2000) The psychiatric sequelae of civilian trauma. *Comprehensive Psychiatry* 41: 19–23.

de Jong JT, Komproe IH, Van Ommeren M, *et al.* (2001) Lifetime events and posttraumatic stress disorder in four postconflict settings. *Journal of the American Medical Association* 286: 555–562.

Ehlers A and Clark DM (2000) A cognitive model of posttraumatic stress disorder. *Behaviour Research and Therapy* 38: 319–345.

Inter-Agency Standing Committee (IASC) (2007) *IASC Guidelines on Mental Health and Psychosocial Support in Emergency Settings*. Geneva, Switzerland: IASC.

Kessler RC, Sonnega A, Hughes M, and Nelson CB (1995) Posttraumatic stress disorder in the National Comorbidity Survey. *Archives of General Psychiatry* 52: 1048–1060.

McNally RJ, Bryant RA, and Ehlers A (2003) Psychological debriefing and its alternatives: A critique of early intervention for trauma survivors. *Psychological Science in the Public Interest* 4: 45–79.

Norris FH, Friedman MJ, Watson PJ, *et al.* (2002) 60 000 disaster victims speak: Part 1. An empirical review of the empirical literature, 1981–2001. *Psychiatry* 65(3): 207–239.

North CS, Nixon SJ, Shariat S, *et al.* (1999) Psychiatric disorders among survivors of the Oklahoma City bombing. *Journal of the American Medical Association* 285: 755–762.

Rauch SL, Shin LM, and Phelps EA (2006) Neurocircuitry models of posttraumatic stress disorder and extinction: Human neuroimaging research – Past, present, and future. *Biological Psychiatry* 60: 376–382.

Silove D (1996) Torture and refugee trauma: Implications for nosology and treatment of posttraumatic syndromes. Mak FL and Nadelson CC (eds.) *International Review of Psychiatry*, vol. 2, pp. 211–232. Washington, DC: American Psychiatric Association

Silove D (1998) Is posttraumatic stress disorder an overlearned survival response? An evolutionary-learning hypothesis. *Psychiatry: Interpersonal and Biological Processes* 61: 181–190.

Silove D (2007) Adaptation, ecosocial safety signals and the trajectory of PTSD. In: Kirwayer LJ, Lemelson R and Barad M (eds.) *Understanding Trauma: Integrating Biological, Clinical and Cultural Perspectives*, pp. 242–258. New York: Cambridge University Press

Silove D and Steel Z (2006) Understanding community psychosocial needs after disasters: Implications for mental health services. *Journal of Postgraduate Medicine* 52: 121–125.

Silove D, Manicavasagar V, Baker K, *et al.* (2004) Indices of social risk among first attenders of an emergency mental health service in post-conflict East Timor: An exploratory investigation. *Australian and New Zealand Journal of Psychiatry* 38: 929–932.

Steel Z, Silove D, Phan T, and Bauman A (2002) Long-term effect of psychological trauma on the mental health of Vietnamese refugees resettled in Australia: A population-based study. *Lancet* 360: 1056–1062.

Steel Z, Silove D, Brooks R, *et al.* (2006) Impact of immigration detention and temporary protection on the mental health of refugees. *British Journal of Psychiatry* 188: 58–64.

Further Reading

Brewin CR, Andrews B, and Valentine JD (2000) Meta-analysis of risk factors for posttraumatic stress disorder in trauma-exposed adults. *Journal of Consulting and Clinical Psychology* 68: 748–766.

Bryant RA and Friedman M (2001) Medication and non-medication treatments of posttraumatic stress disorder. *Current Opinion in Psychiatry* 14: 119–123.

Charney DS, Deutch AY, Krystal JH, Southwick SM, and Davis M (1993) Psychobiologic mechanisms of posttraumatic stress disorder. *Archives of General Psychiatry* 50: 294–305.

Davidson RJ and Foa EB (eds.) (1993) *Posttraumatic Stress Disorder: DSM-IV and Beyond.* Washington, DC: American Psychiatric Press.

Foa EB and Meadows EA (1997) Psychosocial treatments for posttraumatic stress disorder: A critical review. *Annual Review of Psychology* 48: 449–480.

Foa EB, Keane TM, and Friedman MJ (eds.) (2000) *Effective Treatments for Posttraumatic Stress Disorder: Practice Guidelines from the International Society for Traumatic Stress Studies.* New York: Guilford Press.

Litz BT, Gray M, and Bryant RA (2002) Early intervention for trauma: Current status and future directions. *Clinical Psychology: Science and Practice* 9: 112–134.

McNally RJ (2003) *Remembering Trauma.* Cambridge, MA: Belknap Press.

Yehuda R (ed.) (1999) *Risk Factors for Posttraumatic Stress Disorder.* Washington, DC: American Psychiatric Press.

Relevant Websites

http://www.ncptsd.va.gov/ – National Center for PTSD.
http://www.nice.org.uk/ – NICE Treatment Guidelines for PTSD.

Suicide and Self-Directed Violence

D De Leo and K Krysinska, Griffith University, Brisbane, Queensland, Australia

According to the World Health Organization estimates, in the year 2000, suicide (815 000 victims) accounted for almost half of the violence-related deaths worldwide, followed by homicide and war-related fatalities (520 000 and 310 000 victims, respectively). In some countries, the suicide rates have increased by 60% over the last 45 years, and worldwide suicide is among three leading causes of death among adolescents and young adults aged 15–34. With a global rate of 14.5 per 100 000 population, suicide is a major public health problem. In addition to the premature loss of life resulting from a death by suicide and the physical and emotional trauma of suicide attempters, suicide has a serious impact on people who had known the deceased and on society as a whole.

Definition of Suicide

Originally, the word suicide, founded on Latin 'sui' (of oneself) and 'caedes' (killing), was coined by Sir Thomas Browne, a philosopher and a physician, and first appeared in his *Religio Medici* published in 1643. As the conceptualization of suicide has changed over time, a wide range of definitions from a variety of disciplines has been proposed. Durkheim (1897), a sociologist, suggested that suicide constitutes all cases of death directly or indirectly resulting from a positive or negative act of a person who is aware of the consequences of the behavior. Usually there are four elements in the definition of suicide: A suicide has taken place if death occurs, it must be of one's own doing, the agency of suicide can be active or passive, and it implies intentionally ending one's own life. A World Health Organization Working Group recently proposed the definition of suicide as "an act with a fatal outcome which the deceased, knowing or expecting a potentially fatal outcome, has initiated and carried out with the purpose of bringing about wanted changes" (De Leo *et al.*, 2004: 33).

Although the distinction between suicide and attempted suicide seems obvious based upon the outcome of behavior, i.e., a lethal versus nonlethal outcome, not all individuals who die by suicide have intended to die, and not all attempts are failed suicides. The result of such behaviors usually depends on the person's degree of ambivalence ('I want to die, help me to live'), knowledge of lethality of the chosen method and its availability, preparation, and coincidental factors (e.g., rescue). Also, intentions other than wanting to die are frequently involved, including a cry for help, interpersonal communication, or attention seeking. To underscore the fact that many seemingly suicidal behaviors are not directly associated with the intent to die, several terms have been proposed in the literature, including parasuicide, self-injury, and (deliberate) self-harm. As a result of confusion related to the problems in ascertaining the intent behind completed suicides and suicide attempts, the terms fatal suicidal behavior and nonfatal suicidal behavior, considering the physical outcome of the act, have been proposed (De Leo *et al.*, 2004).

Suicidal ideation encompasses phenomena ranging from passive suicidal ideation (e.g., death thoughts and wishes: Life is not worth living or life is a burden) to active suicidal ideation and planning, which might lead to actual suicidal behavior.

Self-mutilation, i.e., direct and deliberate destruction or alteration of body tissue (e.g. skin cutting or burning, head banging, hair pulling) is a relatively common form of self-directed violence; however, its defining feature is a lack of any conscious suicidal intent. Instead, such behaviors might aim at reducing distress and anxiety, communicating anger and self-abhorrence, or coping with dissociation and traumatic memories, and there is general consensus that self-mutilation should not be included in the category of suicidal behaviors.

Epidemiology of Suicidal Behavior

Suicide

Although there is scarcity of data regarding the prevalence of suicide in some parts of the world (including many nations in Africa, Asia, and the Western Pacific), the available epidemiological data show that suicide rates, although quite stable nationally from year to year, differ considerably among countries. Many Eastern European countries report the highest suicide rates in the world, including Lithuania (38.6 per 100 000 in 2005), Belarus (35.1 per 100 000 in 2003), the Russian Federation (34.3 per 100 000 in 2004), and Latvia (24.5 per 100 000 in 2005). High rates have also been reported in other European countries (e.g., 28.1 per 100 000 in Slovenia in 2003, 22.4 per 100 000 in Hungary in 2005, and 20.3 per 100 000 in Finland in 2004), and some Asian countries, including Japan (25.5 per 100 000 in 2003) and the Republic of Korea (25.2 per 100 000 in 2004).

Low suicide rates are found mainly in South American, African, and some Mediterranean countries, for example 5.6 per 100 000 in Italy in 2004, 5.3 in Spain in 2004, and 4.0 per 100 000 in Brazil in 2000. Other countries in Europe, North America, Asia, and the Pacific report moderate suicide rates ranging from 8.1 per 100 000 in

England and Wales in 2005, 10.4 per 100 000 in Australia in 2004 and 10.8 per 100 000 in 2003 in the United States, and 15.9 per 100 000 in Poland in 2004.

The prevalence of suicide differs by age and gender. Suicide rates tend to increase with age, with the global suicide rate among those aged 75 and over (especially for males) being approximately three times higher than the rate among youth under 25 years of age. Between 1970 and 2000, an increase in suicide in young adults aged 19–24 and a decline in suicide rates among the elderly has been observed in a number of countries, especially in the Anglo-Saxon nations, including Australia, Canada, New Zealand, and the United States. Contrary to this, in most Southern European, Latin American, and some Asian countries, suicide rates in old age have presented with less favorable trends and have significantly increased over the last 30 years.

In all nations of the world (except for China) suicide rates are higher in men than in women and, on average, there are three male suicides for every female suicide. The gender ratio of suicide tends to increase with age, up to approximately 12:1 among those over the age of 85. In China, in 2003, the female suicide rates were almost equal to male rates in the urban areas (11.0 per 100 000 vs. 10.9 per 100 000) but exceeded the male rates in rural areas (i.e., 17.4 per 100 000 vs. 15.1 per 100 000).

Attempted Suicide and Suicide Ideation

Fatal and nonfatal suicidal behaviors exhibit opposite tendencies with respect to age: While suicide rates peak in the elderly in most nations, attempted suicide decreases with advancing age virtually everywhere. In the elderly, estimated ratios between attempts and completions vary from 4:1 to 2:1, but in the young they can reach the level of 100–200:1. In contrast to the sex difference in completed suicides, generally there is a higher rate of attempted suicide in women than in men. An international study of nonfatal suicidal behavior in Europe, based upon data on hospital admissions, showed that the attempted suicide rates vary considerably between countries for both gender groups (Schmidtke *et al.*, 2004). For example, the rates of nonfatal suicidal behavior among males ranged from 46 per 100 000 in Spain to 327 per 100 000 in Finland, and from 72 per 100 000 in Spain to 542 per 100 000 in France for females.

Studies based upon the general population indicate that the actual numbers of people engaging in nonfatal suicidal behavior might be even higher, as only a majority of individuals attempting suicide suffer from physical injuries serious enough to seek medical assistance and thus be admitted to hospital. International studies show that between 3% and 5% of individuals in the general population have made a suicide attempt at some time in their life with the ratio of female to male attempters between two and three to one (Weissman *et al.*, 1999). Suicidal ideation is more frequent than attempted or completed suicide and international data indicate that approximately 10–18% of individuals in the general population have ever thought about suicide (Weissman *et al.*, 1999), with the rates declining with increasing age.

Suicide Risk Factors

Suicidal behavior results from complex interactions between a wide range of risk and protective factors encompassing the entire life span of an individual. Characteristics increasing the likelihood of an individual becoming suicidal can be divided into distal and proximal risk factors. The distal risk factors (e.g., psychopathology, genetic and neurochemical factors) are necessary but not sufficient for suicide, and although they form the foundations for suicidal behavior, they may not obviously occur immediately prior to suicide. On the other hand, the proximal risk factors (e.g., negative life events, availability of lethal means) can be considered as triggers or precipitants of suicidal behavior; however, they are neither sufficient nor necessary for suicide to occur. It is the combined action between distal and proximal risk factors that might result in suicidal behavior.

While estimating suicide risk in an individual, one has to be wary of the ecological fallacy, or a logical error in the interpretation of statistical data, in which conclusions about individuals are based upon aggregate statistics collected for the group to which those individuals belong. For example, based upon epidemiological data, it might be incorrectly assumed that a male, a widowed, or an elderly person automatically is at increased risk of suicide. It may also be wrongly assumed, based upon data indicating that the majority of individuals who die by suicide suffer from a mental illness, that all persons who engage in suicidal behavior are mentally ill (one of the common myths about suicide) (**Table 1**).

Demographic Factors

Demographic factors, including gender, age, race, and ethnicity, provide a general indication of those groups in the general population that are at the highest risk of suicide. As indicated in almost all countries, the risk of suicide is greater among males than females, and globally for both genders the suicide risk increases with age.

The prevalence of suicide also varies across racial and ethnic groups. In the United States, the prevalence of suicide among Caucasians is approximately twice that observed in all other races, and American Indian and Alaska Natives have the highest suicide rates of all ethnic groups in the country. In Australia, suicide among Aboriginal and Torres Strait Islander people has increased dramatically

from low rates in the late 1980s to levels substantially higher among young indigenous males than among their nonindigenous counterparts (Hunter and Milroy 2006). For example, in Queensland, where a very accurate Suicide Register is in operation, the global rate of indigenous people is 24.6 per 100 000, which is almost twice as high as the general population rate of 15.0 per 100 000 in 2002–2004. The elevated suicide rates are particularly marked in the younger age groups: In 25- to 34-year-old males (108.0 per 100 000), the suicide rate was almost three times that of the Queensland rate (39.3 per 100 000).

Psychopathology and Psychiatric Hospitalization

A diagnosis of a mental disorder, especially affective disorders, substance-related disorders, and schizophrenia, is one of the strongest risk factors for suicide, with psychiatric comorbidity (e.g., depressive disorder and substance abuse) increasing the risk even further. Studies indicate that between 88% and 99% of suicides (for general population subjects and psychiatric inpatient populations, respectively) have a diagnosis of one psychiatric disorder. However, only a relatively small proportion of individuals with major psychopathology take their own lives, and thus psychiatric disorders alone are not sufficient predictors of suicide; other factors, including the quality and availability of mental health services and effective treatment, and the individual's social support and hopefulness, play a very important role. Periods of psychiatric hospitalization tend to increase the risk of suicide, and after discharge, suicide risk is significantly increased within the first weeks and remains elevated for up to 6 months.

Although persons with practically any mental illness engage in suicidal behaviors more often than individuals in the general population, the diagnoses most frequently related to suicidal behaviors include mood disorders (including major depression and bipolar disorder), schizophrenia and other psychotic disorders, substance-related disorders, personality disorders (especially borderline and antisocial personality disorder), anxiety/somatoform disorders (including posttraumatic stress disorder), and adjustment disorder.

Increased risk of suicidal behavior is related to both depression as a mental disorder and depressive symptoms occurring in the course of other psychiatric illnesses (e. g., schizophrenia, substance abuse, personality disorders) and severe and chronic medical conditions (e.g., cancer, HIV/AIDS). Among patients with affective disorders, suicide risk is higher among inpatients hospitalized following suicidal ideation or attempt, and lower in inpatients admitted for an affective disorder or in depressed outpatients.

There are limited data on suicide risk in people with a diagnosis of bipolar disorder; however, it seems that there is

Table 1   Common risk factors for suicide

Demographic factors	Gender
	Age
	Race and ethnicity
Psychopathology and psychiatric hospitalization	Mood disorders (including major depression and bipolar disorder)
	Schizophrenia and other psychotic disorders
	Substance-related disorders
	Personality disorders (especially borderline and antisocial personality disorder)
	Organic mental disorders
	Anxiety/somatoform disorders (including posttraumatic stress disorder)
	Adjustment disorder
	Psychiatric comorbidity
	Psychiatric hospitalization
	Recent discharge
Previous suicidal behavior and suicidal ideation	History of suicide attempts
	Suicidal ideation
	Self-mutilation
	Aborted suicide attempts
Family history of psychopathology and suicidal behavior	Genetic factors (e.g., genetic predisposition to affective disorders, schizophrenia, alcoholism, deficits in impulsivity control)
	Family history of suicide
Physical illness	Physical illness (e.g., cancer, chronic pulmonary disease, ischemic heart disease, neurological diseases, HIV/AIDS)
	Chronic pain
Life events and coping potential	Negative life events (e.g., relationship problems, family discord, mental and physical health problems, loss of significant other, bereavement, imprisonment, bullying, childhood and adult trauma)
	Low coping potential
Marital status and sexual orientation	Divorced, widowed, separated, single marital status
	Homosexual orientation
Socioeconomic and cultural factors	Low socioeconomic status
	Unemployment
	Religion
	Migration
Neurobiology	Hypoactivity of serotonergic system
	Possible abnormalities in dopaminergic and noradrenergic systems
	Abnormalities in the ventromedial prefrontal cortex
	Hyperactivity of hypothalamic–pituitary–adrenal axis
Psychological factors	Hopelessness
	Aggression and impulsivity
	Lack of reasons for living
	Cognitive rigidity (i.e., dichotomous or all-or-nothing thinking)
	Low ability to solve problems
	Perfectionism
	Psychological pain (i.e., psychache)
Social networks	Social isolation
	Lack of social support
Access to means of suicide	Access to and availability of lethal means of suicide

no substantial difference between suicide risk in unipolar and bipolar major affective disorders. Both are related to elevated risk for fatal and nonfatal suicidal behaviors and between 25 and 50% of people with a diagnosis of bipolar disorder attempt suicide, with up to 20% of individuals in this group dying by suicide. People suffering from bipolar disorder are also at increased risk of premature mortality related to cardiovascular disease and compromised health during the manic phase (e.g., sleep deprivation, malnutrition, and substance abuse).

Between 10 and 15% of patients with a diagnosis of schizophrenia die by suicide, between 18 and 55% make a suicide attempt in their lifetime, and 60–80% experience lingering suicidal thoughts. Individuals with a diagnosis of schizophrenia seem to be at a particularly high risk of suicide in the first 10 years of illness onset, and psychiatric comorbidity (e.g., schizophrenia and depressive disorder or substance abuse) increases the risk of suicide. Patients with schizophrenia are also at extremely high risk of inpatient suicide.

Approximately 2–4% of individuals with an alcohol use disorder die by suicide, and comorbid psychiatric conditions (especially depression and anxiety disorders) significantly increase the risk. The evidence for the association between alcohol abuse and nonfatal suicidal behavior is less consistent, although studies indicate that up to 30% of individuals who attempt suicide cited alcohol addiction as the reason for their attempt. Also, abuse of other substances is related to high incidence of nonfatal and fatal suicidal behavior, although the clinical picture in such cases is often complicated by polysubstance (drug/alcohol) abuse. An increased suicide rate was found in narcotic and opioid addicts, with up to 7% of cocaine abusers and up to 35% of heroin users dying by suicide.

Previous Suicidal Behavior and Suicidal Ideation

A history of a suicide attempt is a major risk factor for both repeated nonfatal suicidal behavior and suicide. Almost one in four suicide attempters makes another nonlethal attempt within 1 year, with the highest risk observed during the first 3–6 months after the initial attempt. Approximately 1% of attempters kill themselves within 1 year after the attempt, and 3–5% (some studies report even higher numbers: up to 13%) over the 5–10 years after the initial attempt (Owens *et al.*, 2002).

Although suicide ideation in the general population is a quite frequent phenomenon, it might lead to a detailed suicide plan resulting in self-harming behavior and suicide. A general population study in the United States showed that suicide ideators with a plan are more likely to attempt suicide than those without a plan, i.e., impulsive suicide attempters (Borges *et al.*, 2006). However, the absence of a suicide plan does not mean the absence of suicide risk; almost half of attempts reported in the study were unplanned – the suicidal behavior occurred without a plan conceived prior to the situation that triggered the suicidal behavior.

The acts of self-mutilation characterized by lack of conscious suicidal intent are usually distinguished from suicidal behaviors; however, individuals who self-mutilate, particularly patients with a diagnosis of borderline personality disorder, might be at increased risk of suicide. Also, individuals with a history of an aborted suicide attempt (i.e., an event without physical injury in which an individual has suicide intent but changes his or her mind before making the attempt) might be at increased risk of actual suicidal behavior. A study on the prevalence of suicidal behavior among psychiatric inpatients showed that there were almost twice as many suicides among patients with aborted attempts as among patients without aborted attempts (Barber *et al.*, 1998).

Family History of Psychopathology and Suicidal Behavior

Different lines of evidence point to the possibility of familial or genetic determinants of suicidal behavior. Clinical and follow-up studies show that individuals with a diagnosis of a mental disorder (especially depression) and a history of suicidal behavior and affective disorder among the first- and second-degree relatives have increased risk of engaging in suicidal behavior themselves. These data are supported by results of twin and adoption studies showing the statistically significant higher incidence of suicide and psychiatric disorder in monozygotic pairs than among dizygotic twins, and among biological relatives of suicides than among the adoptive parents.

Several explanations concerning the familial vulnerability to suicide have been offered. Genetic factors related to suicide may mostly represent a genetic predisposition to psychiatric illness, including affective disorders, schizophrenia, and alcoholism, as well as deficits in impulse control. In addition, the mechanism of social modeling may play an important role: The family member(s) who dies by suicide may serve as a role model(s), pointing to suicide as the best and acceptable solution to life problems.

Physical Illness

Between 30 and 40% of people who die by suicide have a diagnosis of a medical illness, and the number escalates to almost 90% among the elderly victims of suicide. There is documented evidence that cancer, chronic pulmonary disease, ischemic heart disease, neurological diseases (e.g., epilepsy, multiple sclerosis, Huntington's chorea, and stroke), and HIV/AIDS are associated with elevated suicide risk. Also rheumatoid arthritis, diabetes (especially juvenile diabetes), and neoplasms of the cervix and prostate may be related to increased suicide risk.

Medical disorders are associated with suicide in various ways: Some medical disorders may be caused by self-injury or substance abuse stemming from preexisting mental disorders, and a medical disorder and treatment (e.g., medication) may affect brain functioning, leading to personality disorders and mood disturbances. Disfigurement or disability caused by medical illness may result in mood dysregulation, and stigmatized diagnoses may contribute to social isolation and withdrawal. Also, chronic physical pain is a recognized risk factor for suicidal ideation and behavior.

Life Events and Coping Potential

Individuals who attempt or commit suicide experience more stressors and negative life events than individuals in the general population (especially in the month prior to suicide). Among the life stressors most often found in histories of suicidal individuals are relationship problems, family discord, mental and physical health problems, loss of a significant other, bereavement, imprisonment, and work problems (Kõlves *et al.*, 2006). There is a positive correlation between an individual's history of childhood sexual and/or physical abuse and suicidality, and adult traumas (e.g., rape, torture, military combat) may be related to elevated suicide risk.

Life stresses can be important proximal risk factors triggering suicidal ideation and behavior; however, only a minority of individuals faced with life adversities and negative life events become suicidal. Such events must be placed within the context of life-long coping patterns, personality structure, availability of social support and willingness to ask for help, and other distal risk factors, including psychopathology.

Marital Status and Sexual Orientation

There is a strong association between marital status and suicide: Divorced, widowed, and separated persons have the highest suicide rates, while married people have lower suicide rates than never married individuals. Marriage and responsibilities for bringing up children may serve as a protective factor against suicide by reducing social isolation, providing emotional and social stability, and enhancing social integration. Males, especially in the first few months after marital loss or separation, seem to be particularly vulnerable and at increased risk for suicide.

Although completed suicide rates do not appear to be increased among homosexual men and women, there is a greater lifetime prevalence of nonfatal suicidal behavior in these populations, especially among homosexual adolescents and young adults. The factors that may exacerbate the risk of suicidality in these populations include limited sources of support, stress in interpersonal relations, discrimination, abuse of drugs and alcohol, and anxiety about HIV/AIDS.

Socioeconomic and Cultural Factors

Sociological studies have consistently found a correlation between low socioeconomic status and suicide rates, although there are some high-status occupations with increased suicide risk, e.g., dentists, physicians, and veterinarians (Stack, 2000a). Unemployment is often considered as a major risk factor for suicide, especially among men. Studies at both aggregated and individual level indicate that unemployment is directly correlated with suicidality, although the nature of the relationship between those two phenomena has not been fully explained. For example, job loss (and related loss of income and status) or inability to find work over an extended period of time might act as a proximal triggering factor for suicide. Personal

vulnerabilities (including psychopathology) might mediate between the unemployment status and suicidality in a more complex and two-directional way (Stack, 2000).

Religion is an important factor impacting on the prevalence of suicidal behavior. Lower suicide rates have been reported in countries where major religious beliefs include sanctions against suicide, for example countries that are predominantly Muslim or Roman Catholic. At the individual level, religiosity might protect against suicide through the content of religious beliefs (e.g., after-life sanctions against killing oneself); however, its positive correlation with levels of social integration and social support through church attendance and networks with others who share the same beliefs seems to have a stronger impact (Stack, 2000).

The impact of cultural factors on suicide rates can effectively be illustrated by studies on migrants. Such studies have been carried out predominantly in countries with a significant influx of migrants, including the United States, Australia, and Canada. In these countries, suicide rates among diverse migrant groups tend to reflect the rates of their countries of origin; however, a trend of convergence toward the rates of the host country has been observed over time in the United States, the UK, Australia, and Scandinavia. It has also been suggested that the migrant status could increase the risk of suicide in vulnerable individuals (especially those with preexisting psychopathology, people who were forced to leave the country of origin or experienced a downgrading in social status as a result of the move) due to acculturation stress, social isolation, and language barriers (Stack, 2000).

Neurobiology

Research in the area of neurobiology of suicidal behavior has repeatedly shown that suicide attempters and completers have decreased levels of 5-hydroxyindoleacetic acid (a metabolite of serotonin) in the cerebrospinal fluid when compared to depressed subjects and nonclinical controls. Decreased serotonergic function has also been reported in studies using the fenfluramine challenge and observing a decreased prolactin response. The relationship between the hypoactivity of the serotonergic system and suicidality seems to be mediated by lethality of attempts, aggression, and impulsivity (Joiner *et al.*, 2005).

Suicidal individuals show neuroanatomical abnormalities in the ventromedial prefrontal cortex, which may correlate with the neurochemical deficits found in this population, and individuals who made a highly lethal suicidal attempt show decreased prefrontal cortex functioning. Although the results are still inconclusive, it has been suggested that abnormalities in other neurotransmitter systems (i.e., dopaminergic and noradrenergic systems) and hyperactivity of other brain systems, such as the hypothalamic–pituitary–adrenal axis, may be involved in suicidal behavior, and there is also a suggested relationship between low levels of cholesterol and suicidality, although the mechanism of the association remains unclear (Joiner et al., 2005).

Psychological Factors

Psychological characteristics or vulnerabilities of individuals might exacerbate the impact of other risk factors (including psychopathology, negative life events, social factors) and thus increase the risk of suicide. Hopelessness (i.e., a state of negative expectancies concerning oneself and one's future) is one of the strongest predictors for suicidal ideation and behavior, stronger even than depression itself. Studies have established that hopelessness may predict as many as 91–94% of suicides in both outpatient and inpatient populations (Beck et al., 1990). Other psychological and cognitive risk factors for suicide include aggression and impulsivity, lack of reasons for living, cognitive rigidity (i.e., dichotomous or all-or-nothing thinking), poor problem-solving capabilities, and perfectionism (Joiner et al., 2005). Also, the experience of psychological suffering and pain (or psychache) is a strong correlate of elevated suicide risk.

Social Networks

Isolation and lack of social support have been related to many aspects of psychopathology, including ineffective coping with stress and life crises. Suicidal individuals are often described as isolated and alienated from their families and communities, and bereft of emotional and instrumental social support and other resources. This may be due to adverse life circumstances or individuals' inability to maintain satisfactory interpersonal networks. Loneliness may lead to depression and emotional distress or increase their severity, as well as exacerbate the effects of negative stressors. Moreover, isolated and lonely individuals are at higher risk of death when they engage in suicidal behaviors, as the chances of lifesaving intervention by others are severely reduced or nonexistent.

Access to Means of Suicide

Almost all methods used by individuals engaging in suicidal behaviors may lead to death or serious injuries; however, the statistical probability of death as a result of a suicide attempt varies between methods. The choice of means of suicide depends on several factors, including availability of the method, the individual's familiarity with the method, the intent and motivation behind the behavior, the degree of ambivalence, and cultural factors (e.g., gender socialization, symbolic meanings of suicide methods).

The choice of more lethal suicide method by males as compared to females might in part explain the differences in suicide rates among genders. Older individuals (usually characterized by a higher intent to die) tend to choose more lethal methods than their younger counterparts. Also, there are international differences regarding suicide methods used most frequently. For example, in the United States guns are used in approximately two-thirds of all suicides, while hanging is the most frequent method in all other Western nations. In a number of developing countries, pesticide poisoning is the most common cause of suicide mortality; in many areas of China and South East Asia, suicide by pesticide ingestion accounts for 60% of all suicides (Gunnell and Eddleston, 2003).

Protective Factors

Sufficiently strong protective factors can outweigh the impact of risk factors and reduce the risk of suicide. Although this area of study is still in its infancy, several protective factors have been identified. These include family and nonfamily social support, significant and stable relationships (including marriage), children under the age of 18 living at home, physical health, hopefulness, reasons for living, problem-solving and coping skills, cognitive flexibility, plans for the future, constructive use of leisure time, the propensity to seek treatment and maintain it when needed, religiosity, culture and ethnicity, employment, and restricted access to lethal means of suicide.

Prevention of Suicide, Treatment, and Postvention

Suicide is a complex, multidetermined behavior and it would be unrealistic to expect that any single preventive effort could reduce an individual's risk of suicide and the overall suicide mortality rates. In general, the preventive efforts that have been initiated in a number of multidisciplinary settings operate to target risk factors for suicide and to strengthen the protective factors.

Traditionally, there are three levels of prevention with regard to suicide: Universal, selective, and indicated prevention. Universal prevention refers to activities targeted at the general population, including health promotion and education, which may improve the overall emotional and social well-being of individuals, and may target suicide risk factors. Selective prevention refers to interventions aimed at populations identified as being at risk of suicide, while indicated strategies address specific high-risk individuals showing early signs of suicidality. A wide variety of suicide prevention approaches have been developed across the three domains: Treatment of mental disorders and pharmacotherapy, behavioral and relationship approaches, community-based efforts (including suicide prevention centers and school-based interventions), societal approaches including restricting access to suicide means and improved media reporting of suicide, as well as interventions for people bereaved by suicide (i.e., suicide survivors). In 1996, the United Nations issued a document stressing the importance of a guiding policy on suicide prevention: 'Prevention of suicide: Guidelines for the formulation and implementation of national strategies.' Subsequently, in 1999, the WHO launched a worldwide initiative for the prevention of suicide (SUPRE Project).

In some countries, such as Australia, New Zealand, Finland, Norway, Sweden, England, and the United States, comprehensive national suicide prevention strategies have been implemented over the last two decades. Such strategies usually aim at improving detection and treatment of mental disorders (particularly depression) and substance abuse and enhancing access to mental health services. Their goals also include reducing access to lethal means of suicide, improving responsible reporting of suicide in the media, enhancing support for those bereaved by suicide, educating the general public and health-care professionals, and setting up school-based suicide prevention initiatives. Although some components of the strategies may be effective in reducing the risk of suicide, to date there is no evidence for an overall positive impact of the national strategies (with the possible exception of Finland) on countries' rates in the 5 years following their implementation (De Leo and Evans, 2004).

International studies looking at the effectiveness of a range of suicide prevention approaches indicate that restricting access to lethal methods and educational programs for physicians that improve their skills in recognition and treatment of depression reduce suicide rates. More data and more studies are needed to evaluate the effectiveness of other types of interventions, including screening programs, media reporting guidelines, and public education campaigns.

A wide variety of psychosocial treatments for suicidal individuals or patients who have attempted suicide have been developed, including a dialectic and cognitive behavioral approach, a psychodynamic model, problem-solving therapy, multimodal interventions, family interventions, inpatient treatment, and pharmacotherapy (e.g., antidepressants). Unfortunately, despite a large number of studies looking at the effectiveness of such interventions, to date there is only limited evidence regarding recommended treatments for patients at risk of suicidal behavior and its repetition (Hawton et al., 2004). Brief psychological interventions (including problem-solving therapy) and dialectic behavioral therapy for women with a diagnosis of borderline personality disorder seem to be effective treatment options. There is also limited evidence supporting the effectiveness of follow-up and active out-reach (e.g., by home visits or telephone contact) with patients with a history of a suicide attempt who do not attend therapy appointments. Despite many studies, the role of antidepressants in reducing the risk of suicide remains unclear.

Suicide prevention initiatives also include postvention aimed at survivors of suicide, or family members, friends, and other individuals who knew the person who died by suicide and were affected by the death. Although not everyone who experiences loss by suicide requires specialized psychological help, for some it might lead to a serious crisis calling for professional psychotherapy or support from others who have experienced a similar loss. The majority of national suicide prevention strategies aim at enhancing the support available for those bereaved by suicide, and in many Western countries (such as the United States, Western Europe, and Australia) numerous self-help, support, and therapy groups for suicide survivors have been developed.

Conclusions

Although much progress has been made in the field of suicide research and prevention over the decades, many unanswered questions remain on what is really effective in preventing suicide at both the individual and societal levels. Among the greatest challenges is collection of epidemiological data regarding the suicide-related morbidity and mortality around the world and encouraging research in many countries outside the Western (mostly English-speaking) environment. Also, multidisciplinary studies looking at risk and protective factors in suicidal behaviors will allow for further insights into the dynamics of suicidality and should enhance development of innovative and effective prevention strategies.

Citations

Barber ME, Marzuk PM, Leon AC, and Portera L (1998) Aborted suicide attempts: a new classification of suicidal behavior. *American Journal of Psychiatry* 155: 385–389.

Beck AT, Brown G, Berchick RJ, et al. (1990) Relationship between hopelessness and eventual suicide: A replication with psychiatric inpatients. *American Journal of Psychiatry* 147: 190–195.

Borges G, Angst J, Nock MK, et al. (2006) A risk index for 12-month suicide attempts in the National Comorbidity Survey Replication (NCS-R). *Psychological Medicine* 36: 1747–1758.

De Leo D and Evans R (2004) *International Suicide Rates and Prevention Strategies*. Göttingen: Hogrefe & Huber.

De Leo D and Spathononis K (2003) Do psychopharmacological and psychosocial treatments reduce suicide risk in schizophrenia and schizophrenia spectrum disorders? *Archives of Suicide Research* 7: 354–373.

De Leo D, Burgis S, Bertolote JM, et al. (2004) Definitions of suicidal behaviour. In: De Leo D, Bille-Brahe U, Kerkhof ADJF and Schmidtke A (eds.) *Suicidal Behaviour. Theories and Research Findings*, pp. 17–39. Göttingen: Hogrefe & Huber.

Durkheim E (1897) *Le Suicide*. Paris: Felix Alcan. English version (1951) *Suicide*. New York: Free Press.

Gunnell D and Eddleston M (2003) Suicide by intentional ingestion of pesticides: A continuing tragedy in developing countries. *International Journal of Epidemiology* 32: 902–909.

Hawton K, Townsend E, Arensman E, *et al.* (2004) Psychosocial and pharmacological treatments for deliberate self harm. *The Cochrane Library.* Issue 3. Art. No.: CD001764. DOI: 10.1002/14651858. CD001764.

Hunter E and Milroy H (2006) Aboriginal and Torres Strait Islander suicide in context. *Archives of Suicide Research* 10: 141–157.

Joiner TE, Brown JS, and Wingate LRR (2005) The psychology and neurobiology of suicidal behavior. *Annual Review of Psychology* 56: 287–314.

Owens D, Horrocks J, and House A (2002) Fatal and non-fatal repetition of self-harm. *British Journal of Psychiatry* 181: 193–199.

Schmidtke A, Weinacker B, Löhr C, *et al.* (2004) Suicide and suicide attempts in Europe. An overview. In: Schmidtke A, Bille-Brahe U, De Leo D and Kerkhof ADJF (eds.) *Suicidal Behaviour in Europe. Results from the WHO/EURO Multicentre Study on Suicidal Behaviour*, pp. 15–28. Göttingen: Hogrefe & Huber.

United Nations (1996) *Prevention of Suicide: Guidelines for the Formulation and Implementation of National Strategies.* New York: Department of Policy Coordination and Sustainable Development.

Weissman MM, Bland RC, Canino GJ, *et al.* (1999) Prevalence of suicide ideation and suicide attempts in nine countries. *Psychological Medicine* 29: 9–17.

De Leo D, Bille-Brahe U, Kerkhof A, and Schmidtke A (eds.) *Suicidal Behaviour. Theories and Research Findings*. Göttingen: Hogrefe & Huber.

Jacobs DG (ed.) (1999) *The Harvard Medical School Guide to Suicide Assessment and Intervention.* San Francisco, CA: Jossey-Bass Publishers.

Hawton K (ed.) (2005) *Prevention and Treatment of Suicidal Behavior. From science to Practice.* Oxford, UK: Oxford University Press.

Hawton K and Van Heeringen K (eds.) (2000) *The International Handbook of Suicide and Attempted Suicide.* Chichester, UK: Wiley & Sons.

Lester D (ed.) (2001) *Suicide Prevention. Resources for the Millennium.* Philadelphia, PA: Brunner-Routledge.

Maris RW, Berman AL, and Silverman MM (eds.) (2000) *Comprehensive Textbook of Suicidology.* New York: Guilford Press.

Van Heeringen K (ed.) *Understanding Suicidal Behavior. The Suicidal Process, Approach to Research, Treatment and Prevention.* Chichester, UK: Wiley & Sons.

Relevant Websites

http://www.suicidology.org – American Association of Suicidology.

http://www.afsp.org/ – American Foundation for Suicide Prevention.

http://www.griffith.edu.au/school/psy/aisrap/ – Australian Institute for Suicide Research and Prevention.

http://www.crise.ca/eng/index.asp – Centre for Research and Intervention on Suicide and Euthanasia.

http://www.depts.ttu.edu/psy/iasronline – International Academy for Suicide Research.

http://www.med.uio.no/iasp/ – Interventional Association for Suicide Prevention.

http://cebmh.warne.ox.ac.uk/csr/ – University of Oxford Centre for Suicide Research.

http://www.who.int/mental_health/prevention/en/ – World Health Organization Suicide Prevention and Special Programmes.

Further Reading

De Leo D, Bertolote JM, and Lester D (2002) Self-directed violence. In: Krug EG, Dahleberg LL, Mercy JA, Zwi AB and Lozano R (eds.) *World Report on Violence and Health*, pp. 183–212. Geneva, Switzerland: World Health Organization.

Transmissible Spongiform Encephalopathies

E D Belay, Centers for Disease Control and Prevention, Atlanta, GA, USA

Published by Elsevier Inc.

Introduction

Transmissible spongiform encephalopathies (TSEs), also known as prion diseases, are a group of rapidly progressive, uniformly fatal brain degenerative diseases that occur in humans and animals. Neuropathologic characteristics common to most TSEs include neuronal loss, spongiform lesions, astrogliosis, and absence of inflammatory reaction. The presence of protease-resistant prion protein can be demonstrated in the brain and occasionally in other tissues of humans and animals affected by TSEs. Acquired forms of TSEs are characterized by long incubation periods, usually measured in years. Purification of a hydrophobic protein presumed to be the causative agent of TSEs was first reported by Prusiner and colleagues (1982). In 1997, Dr. Stanley Prusiner

was awarded the Nobel Prize for his contribution in the discovery and characterization of the TSE agent.

TSEs in humans include kuru, Creutzfeldt-Jakob disease (CJD), variant CJD, Gerstmann-Sträussler-Scheinker syndrome (GSS), and fatal familial insomnia (FFI) (**Table 1**). Kuru was identified in the 1950s among the Fore tribe of Papua New Guinea and may have affected over 3000 patients, primarily women and children, before virtually disappearing after cessation of the ritualistic cannibalism, which facilitated its transmission (Will *et al.*, 2004). TSEs that occur in animals include scrapie, bovine spongiform encephalopathy (BSE, also called mad cow disease), chronic wasting disease (CWD), transmissible mink encephalopathy (TME), feline spongiform encephalopathy, and ungulate spongiform encephalopathy (**Table 1**). Feline

Table 1   Characteristics of animal and human transmissible spongiform encephalopathies (TSEs)

Type of TSE	Affected host	Year first described or identified	Mode of transmission/disease occurrence	Route of transmission
Sporadic CJD	Humans	1920s	Unknown	None identified
Iatrogenic CJD	Humans	1974[a]	Via pituitary hormones, dura and cornea grafts, neurosurgical equipment	Intramuscular injection, intracerebral, tissue transplantation
Variant CJD	Humans	1996	Consumption of BSE-contaminated cattle products, human blood products	Oral, intravenous
Familial CJD	Humans	1924	Prion protein gene germline mutations	Inherited
Gerstmann-Sträussler-Scheinker syndrome	Humans	1936	Prion protein gene germline mutations	Inherited
Fatal familial insomnia	Humans	1986	Prion protein gene germline mutations, sporadic	Inherited, none identified (sFI)[b]
Kuru	Humans	1950s	Ritualistic cannibalism involving brain tissue ingestion	Oral
Scrapie	Sheep and goats	1700s	Contaminated environment, possibly direct contact	Oral
BSE	Cattle	1986	Contaminated feed	Oral
Chronic wasting disease	Deer, elk, and moose	1967	Contaminated environment, direct animal contact	Oral
Transmissible mink encephalopathy[c]	Mink	1947	Contaminated feed	Oral
Feline spongiform encephalopathy[d]	Domestic and wild cats	1990	BSE-contaminated feed	Oral
Ungulate spongiform encephalopathy[d]	Exotic ruminants (kudu, nyala, etc.)	1986	BSE-contaminated feed	Oral

CJD, Creutzfeldt-Jakob disease; BSE, bovine spongiform encephalopathy.

[a]The first report of iatrogenic CJD was in a recipient of cornea obtained from a CJD decedent; human pituitary growth hormone-associated CJD was first reported in 1985 and dura mater graft-associated CJD in 1987.

[b]Patients with sporadic fatal insomnia (sFI) were reported beginning in 1999; they have clinical and neuropathologic features indistinguishable from that of fatal familial insomnia but lack family history and prion protein gene mutations.

[c]The last known outbreak of transmissible mink encephalopathy occurred in 1981 in Wisconsin.

[d]The known feline and ungulate spongiform encephalopathies are believed to have resulted from BSE transmission.

and ungulate spongiform encephalopathies represent transmission of BSE to domestic cats and zoo animals, respectively. Scrapie in sheep and goats, first reported in the 1700s in Europe, occurs endemically worldwide with the probable exception of Australia and New Zealand. TME has occurred in outbreaks among ranched mink in Canada, Finland, Germany, Russia, and the United States. The last known TME outbreak occurred in 1985 in Wisconsin. TSEs were relatively obscure diseases, but they were catapulted into wider recognition in the 1990s after the emergence of BSE and its presumed transmission to humans attracted much media and public attention.

Causative Agent of TSEs

Several agents had been proposed as possible causative agents of TSEs. Before the 1980s, the most widely implicated agents were 'slow viruses.' However, no viral particles or disease-specific nucleic acids were identified

in association with scrapie transmission in laboratory animals. Replication of the scrapie agent in the absence of nucleic acids and its possible proteinaceous nature were postulated as early as the 1960s by Alper and colleagues, Pattison and Jones, and Griffith. The protein-only hypothesis began to be widely accepted after Prusiner and colleagues purified a hydrophobic protein and demonstrated that the presence of this protein was required for scrapie transmission in laboratory animals. In 1982, Prusiner coined the colloquial term prion to describe this protein by joining the first few letters from the descriptive phrase '*pro*teinaceous *in*fectious' particle. Since then, additional evidence has accumulated indicating that prions may actually be acting alone in causing TSEs. However, some critics of the protein-only hypothesis suggest that nucleic acids undetected by current methods may play a crucial role in the pathogenesis of TSEs.

Prions appear to be composed largely or entirely of a protein designated as PrP^{Sc} and are abnormal conformers of a host-encoded cellular protein designated as PrP^{C}.

PrP^C is a structural component of cell membranes primarily in the brain but also in other tissues of humans and other mammals. Although its function is unknown, it may be involved in supporting neuronal synaptic activity and copper binding and may also interact with other cell-surface proteins to render neuroprotective functions. In humans, PrP^C is encoded by the prion protein gene located on the short arm of chromosome 20.

The fundamental event in the occurrence of TSEs appears to be conversion of the cellular PrP^C into the abnormally folded, pathogenic PrP^{Sc}. This conversion appears to be dictated by the presence of PrP^{Sc} and occurs by a poorly defined posttranslational autocatalytic process, requiring the aid of cofactors such as proteins or nucleic acids. The initial PrP^{Sc} molecule may originate from exogenous sources or within the brain from somatic or germline prion protein gene mutations. Knockout mice devoid of PrP^C do not develop a TSE even after inoculation with infectious prions, indicating that expression of the prion protein gene is a prerequisite for generation and propagation of PrP^{Sc}. Conversion to PrP^{Sc} seems to confer more beta sheet structure and resistance to proteolytic enzymes, conventional disinfectants, and standard sterilization methods. The cellular PrP^C is sensitive to denaturation by these chemical and physical methods, and its structure is primarily composed of alpha helices.

Creutzfeldt-Jakob Disease

CJD, the most common form of TSE in humans, bears the name of two German neurologists who reported patients with rapidly progressive degenerative brain diseases in the early 1920s. Neuropathologic review of Creutzfeldt's initial patient was inconclusive despite having the typical CJD clinical manifestations. In contrast, two of the four patients reported by Jakob had the typical neuropathologic features of CJD (Belay, 1999).

In most patients, CJD is characterized by the onset of dementia, ataxia, or behavioral abnormalities between the ages of 55 and 75 years. As the disease progresses, neurologic dysfunction deteriorates and patients develop speech abnormalities, movement disorders, such as myoclonus and akinetic mutism (Will et al., 2004). Typically, the disease progresses rapidly, and over 50% of the patients die within 6 months and about 80% within 1 year of illness onset. Duration of illness longer than 2 years is extremely rare. A characteristic electroencephalogram (EEG) finding of triphasic, periodic sharp waves can be demonstrated in about 75% of patients. In the appropriate clinical context, elevated cerebrospinal fluid (CSF) levels of 14-3-3 protein may also aid in diagnosing CJD. More recently, abnormal brain magnetic resonance imaging (MRI) findings in the basal ganglia and cortical regions have been reported to be suggestive of a CJD

diagnosis. However, these MRI findings and CSF 14-3-3 protein elevation have been demonstrated in other brain diseases mimicking CJD. A definitive CJD diagnosis requires histopathologic or immunodiagnostic testing of brain tissues obtained at autopsy or biopsy. Histopathologic examination of brain tissue from CJD patients shows the hallmark triad of spongiform lesions, neuronal loss, and astrogliosis. Immunodiagnostic testing, such as immunohistochemistry and Western blot analysis, demonstrates the presence of PrP^{Sc}, confirming a diagnosis of CJD.

CJD occurs in three different forms: a sporadic form with no known environmental source of infection, an iatrogenic form accidentally transmitted via medical interventions, and a familial form associated with prion protein gene mutations. Decades of research have not identified a specific source of infection for sporadic CJD, which accounts for about 85% of patients. Spontaneous generation of PrP^{Sc} was hypothesized as a cause for sporadic CJD, possibly resulting from random somatic mutations or errors during prion protein gene expression. Iatrogenic CJD has resulted from receipt of contaminated cadaveric human pituitary hormones and dura mater and corneal grafts and from exposure to contaminated neurosurgical equipment. In addition, beginning in the mid-1990s, a newly recognized variant form of CJD linked with BSE transmission to humans was reported.

Sporadic CJD can be further subdivided into five different subtypes based on the Western blot characteristics of protease-resistant PrP^{Sc} fragment and the polymorphism at codon 129 of the host prion protein gene (Table 2) (Parchi et al., 1999). The different subtypes correlate with specific clinical and neuropathologic phenotypes. The most common subtype is associated with prion type 1 and the presence of methionine at codon 129 of the prion protein gene.

Bovine Spongiform Encephalopathy

BSE was first recognized in 1986 in the United Kingdom where it caused a large outbreak among cattle (Table 3). Earlier BSE cases were retrospectively identified from 1985, and a modeling study suggested that cases might have occurred since the early 1980s. The number of UK BSE cases increased almost exponentially, peaked during 1992–1993, and markedly declined thereafter. The clinical signs of BSE include unsteady gait with falling, behavioral abnormalities, and abnormal responses to touch and sound. Because of the fearful and aggressive behavior exhibited by some of the earlier BSE-infected cattle, the public media used the term mad cow disease to describe the strange disease affecting many cattle in the UK. This term continues to be used, sometimes erroneously, to describe human TSEs such as CJD.

Table 2   Characteristics of subtypes of sporadic Creutzfeldt-Jakob disease (CJD) and sporadic fatal insomnia (sFI)[a]

Subtype	Number of patients (n = 609)	Percent	Clinicopathologic features
MM1/MV1	352	57.8	Typical CJD clinical and neuropathologic manifestations, typical EEG, rapidly progressive disease
VV2	90	14.8	Commonly ataxia at onset and late dementia, typical EEG rare, short duration, subcortical pathology, plaquelike deposits
MV2	83	13.6	Similar to VV2 but long duration and presence of kuru-type amyloid plaques in cerebellum
MM2	52	8.5	Progressive dementia, typical EEG rare, long duration, cortical pathology, coarse spongiosis
VV1	25	4.1	Usually young age at onset, typical EEG rare, severe pathology in cerebral cortex with relative sparing of cerebellum, faint synaptic prion staining
MM2 (sFI)	7	1.1	Similar to FFI but without prion protein gene mutations

M, methionine; V, valine.
[a]Data used in the table were obtained from the National Prion Disease Pathology Surveillance Center, Cleveland, Ohio.

The original source of the BSE outbreak is unknown. The leading hypotheses include spontaneous occurrence of BSE and scrapie transmission to cattle from feed containing rendered, infected sheep carcasses. The BSE outbreak was greatly amplified by the recycling of the agent through the practice of feeding cattle meat-and-bone meal (MBM), containing rendered cattle carcasses, some of which died of BSE (Wells and Wilesmith, 2004). In the past, cattle feed was rendered using several treatment steps, including prolonged heating in the presence of a hydrocarbon solvent. In the late 1970s and early 1980s, the solvent-extraction steps were omitted, and this may have contributed to the emergence of BSE by allowing infectious prion concentrations to survive the rendering process. Other factors that may have contributed to the emergence of BSE in the United Kingdom include a relatively high rate of endemic scrapie, a high population ratio of sheep to cattle, and the inclusion of MBM at high rates in cattle feed.

In the UK, over 2 million cattle were estimated to have been infected with BSE. Approximately half of these cattle may have been slaughtered for human consumption, potentially exposing millions of UK residents. Beginning in 1988, several protective measures were implemented to prevent further exposure of animals and humans to BSE, including animal feed bans and removal of infectious cattle tissues such as the brain from human food. Infections of additional UK cattle with BSE dramatically declined after implementation of these protective measures.

BSE outside the United Kingdom was first reported in Ireland in 1989 and Portugal and Switzerland in 1990 (**Table 3**). By 2005, the number of countries reporting BSE among native cattle increased to 24; 20 of these were European countries. In most European countries, the BSE outbreak appears to be declining, although some cases continue to occur. The first North American BSE case was reported in 1993 in a cow imported into Canada from the UK. Rendered cohorts of this cow may have been responsi-

Table 3   Number of reported bovine spongiform encephalopathy (BSE) cases and year of first detection by country[a]

Country	Number of BSE cases[b]	Year BSE first detected[c]
Finland	1	2001
Greece	1	2001
Israel	1	2002
United States	2	2005
Austria	4	2001
Liechtenstein	2	1998
Luxembourg	3	1997
Canada	12	1993
Slovenia	8	2001
Denmark	15	1992
Japan	33	2001
Slovakia	23	2001
Czech Republic	26	2001
Poland	55	2002
Netherlands	82	1997
Italy	139	1994
Belgium	133	1997
Germany	415	1992
Switzerland	464	1990
Spain	681	2000
France	984	1991
Portugal	1029	1990
Ireland	1604	1989
United Kingdom	184 533	1986

[a]BSE cases reported to the Office International des Epizooties as of October 5, 2007; data for the UK are as of September 30, 2007.
[b]Because BSE surveillance methods and testing requirements vary by country, the number of reported cases may not be comparable among the different countries.
[c]Year first BSE was detected in imported or domestic cattle.
Source: http//www.oie.int/eng/info/en_esomonde.htm

ble for the 14 BSE cases identified in Canada during 2003–07, including a BSE-positive cow identified in Washington State and traced to a Canadian farm. In the United States, BSE was confirmed in an approximately

12-year-old cow born and raised in Texas and a 10-year-old cow from Alabama. The source of BSE infection in the U.S. cows remains unknown but the Western blot characteristics of the prions seemed to be atypical (H-type), potentially representing a different BSE strain. Other BSE cases with unusual molecular phenotype have also been reported in other countries, including the L-type in Belgium, Italy, and Japan and the H-type in France and Germany.

Because cattle carcasses were included in the production of animal feed, potential BSE transmission to other animals was considered early during the BSE outbreak in the United Kingdom. BSE-like diseases were identified in zoo animals (ungulate spongiform encephalopathy) beginning in the late 1980s and in domestic cats (feline spongiform encephalopathy) beginning in 1990, indicating the potential for the BSE agent to cross the species barrier and spread to other animals. This development led to the reestablishment of CJD surveillance in the UK to monitor the possible transmission of BSE to humans.

Variant Creutzfeldt-Jakob Disease

In 1996, the UK National CJD Surveillance Unit reported a cluster of patients with a TSE having unusual but similar clinicopathologic manifestations (Will *et al.*, 1996). Because the age and clinical and neuropathologic profile for the patients differed from those of classic CJD patients, the term variant CJD (vCJD) was used to describe this emerging TSE in humans. In subsequent years, several laboratory studies showed that the BSE and vCJD agents were indistinguishable, indicating that vCJD was a new disease and that its occurrence represented BSE transmission to humans. As of October 2007, 204 vCJD patients were reported worldwide, including 166 patients from the United Kingdom, 22 from France, 3 from Ireland, 2 each from the Netherlands, Portugal, and Saudi Arabia, and 1 each from Italy and Spain. The worldwide vCJD count includes 5 patients who likely acquired variant CJD during their past residence in the UK but were residents of Canada (1 patient), Ireland (1 patient), Japan (1 patient), and the United States (2 patients) at the time of illness onset.

Clinical and laboratory findings (**Table 4**) distinguish vCJD from the more common, classic CJD. Patients with vCJD have a younger median age at death (28 compared with 68 years), predominantly psychiatric manifestation at onset, delayed appearance of frank neurologic signs, pulvinar sign on MRI, virtual absence of typical EEG findings, and longer illness duration (14 compared with <6 months). All vCJD patients tested to date almost exclusively had methionine homozygosity at the polymorphic codon 129 of the prion protein gene. This homozygosity is present in approximately 35–40% of the general population. The neuropathology in vCJD is distinguished from that of classic CJD by the presence of numerous 'florid plaques' consisting of amyloid deposits surrounded by a halo of spongiform lesions.

In the UK, vCJD transmission has been reported in recipients of blood collected up to 3 years before vCJD onset in the donors (Llewelyn *et al.*, 2004). Because many UK residents have potentially been exposed to BSE, concerns still exist about additional secondary spread of the agent via blood and possibly contaminated surgical instruments.

Human TSEs Associated with Genetic Mutations

One of the intriguing properties of human TSEs is that they can be both inherited and infectious. The inherited

Table 4 Clinical and pathologic characteristics distinguishing variant Creutzfeldt-Jakob disease (vCJD) from classic CJD

Characteristic	Variant CJD	Classic CJD
Median age (range) at death (years)	28 (14–74)	68 (23–97)[a]
Median duration of illness (months)	13–14	4–5
Clinical presentation	Prominent psychiatric/behavioral symptoms, painful sensory symptoms, delayed neurologic signs	Dementia, early neurologic signs
Periodic sharp waves on electroencephalogram	Often absent	Often present
'Pulvinar sign' on magnetic resonance imaging[b]	Present in >75% of cases	Very rare or absent
Presence of 'florid plaques' on neuropathologic sample	Present in great numbers	Rare or absent
Immunohistochemical analysis of brain tissue	Marked accumulation of PrP-res[c]	Variable accumulation
Presence of agent in lymphoid tissue	Readily detected	Not readily detected
Increased glycoform ratio on Western blot analysis of PrP-res	Present	Not present
Genotype at codon 129 of prion protein	Methionine/methionine[d]	Polymorphic

[a]U.S. CJD surveillance data 1979–2001.
[b]Symmetrical high signal in the posterior thalamus relative to that of other deep and cortical gray matter.
[c]Protease-resistant prion protein.
[d]A patient with preclinical vCJD related to bloodborne transmission was heterozygous for methionine and valine.

or genetic forms of TSEs are associated with insertion, deletion, or point mutations of the prion protein gene. At least 24 different point mutations have been described in association with human TSEs, having widely different clinical and neuropathologic manifestations (Kong et al., 2004). Historically, genetic forms of TSEs were classified as familial CJD, GSS, and FFI in part based on their phenotype.

A polymorphism at codon 129 of the human prion protein gene coding either for methionine or valine seems to markedly influence the clinicopathologic phenotype of human TSEs. The most striking example is the phenotype associated with codon 178 mutation which substitutes aspartic acid with asparagine. Patients who have this mutation in combination with methionine on the mutant allele at codon 129 present with the FFI phenotype whereas patients who have valine at codon 129 of the mutant allele present with the familial CJD phenotype.

Familial CJD

Familial CJD patients generally have clinicopathologic phenotype similar to nongenetic forms of CJD. Other family members are commonly affected with the disease because of a dominant inheritance pattern. Familial CJD has been reported among many family clusters from Canada, Europe, Japan, Israel, the United States, and several Latin American countries (Kong et al., 2004). It is most frequently associated with a mutation substituting glutamic acid with lysine at codon 200 of the prion protein gene. This mutation is the most common cause for inherited human TSEs. A majority of family members carrying the mutation eventually die of CJD. The largest familial cluster of codon 200 mutations was reported among Jews of Libyan and Tunisian origin. Fourteen other less frequent mutations associated with familial CJD have been reported from many countries.

Gerstmann-Sträussler-Scheinker Syndrome

The term GSS is used to describe a heterogeneous group of inherited human TSEs characterized by a long illness duration (median about 5 years) and neuropathologic feature of numerous amyloid plaques primarily in the cerebellum. GSS is named after the three physicians who in 1936 reported the disorder in multiple generations of an Austrian family. The disease in this family was later shown to be associated with codon 102 mutation of the prion protein gene and may have been first identified in 1912. At least 13 different prion protein gene mutations in about 56 kindred have been reported in association with the GSS phenotype from Canada, Europe, Japan, Israel, Mexico, and the United States. GSS mutations are associated with a greater degree of variability in disease

phenotype than other inherited TSEs. The most frequent GSS mutation results in leucine for proline substitution at codon 102 and is coupled with methionine at codon 129 of the mutant allele. Patients with this mutation commonly manifest with ataxia, dysarthria, movement disorders, and possibly dementia and akinetic mutism. The illness may last for 6 years in some patients with GSS 102 mutation. An illness duration exceeding 20 years has been reported in other forms of GSS.

Fatal Familial Insomnia

FFI patients have predominant involvement of the thalamus, resulting in severe sleep disturbances, often with intractable insomnia, and autonomic nervous system dysfunction, including abnormalities in temperature regulation, increased heart rate, and hypertension. Pathologic examination of the brain from FFI patients consistently shows preferential involvement of the thalamus with more severe neuronal loss and astrogliosis than seen in other brain regions. Although occasional sporadic fatal insomnia cases with no prion protein gene mutation have been identified, FFI is primarily associated with codon 178 mutation, resulting in the substitution of aspartic acid with asparagine in combination with methionine at codon 129 of the mutant allele. FFI patients have been reported from several European countries, Australia, Canada, Japan, and the United States. The clinical signs and illness duration in FFI patients are influenced by the polymorphism at codon 129 of the nonmutant allele.

Chronic Wasting Disease

CWD is a TSE that affects North American cervids in their natural habitat and captive environment. CWD's known natural hosts are mule deer, white-tailed deer, elk, and moose. It was first identified as a fatal wasting syndrome of captive mule deer in the late 1960s in Colorado and Wyoming research facilities (Williams et al., 2002). It was recognized as a TSE in 1978 and among wild cervids in 1981. CWD can be highly transmissible in affected herds, in some cases reaching a prevalence of over 90% within several years. The mode of transmission among cervids is poorly understood. Transmission is believed to occur by direct animal-to-animal contact or indirect exposure to contaminated feed and water sources.

Surveillance and modeling studies have indicated that CWD may have occurred endemically for decades in a contiguous area in northeastern Colorado and southeastern Wyoming. Since 2000, CWD among free-ranging deer and elk has been increasingly identified in nine additional states and two Canadian provinces (**Figure 1**). CWD has been experimentally transmitted by intracerebral inoculation into other animals, including cattle,

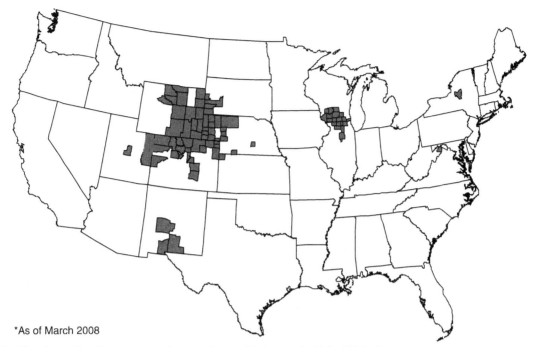

*As of March 2008

Figure 1 Chronic wasting disease among free-ranging cervids by county, United States*.

goats, squirrel monkeys, and laboratory mice. An *in vitro* cell-free experiment demonstrated inefficient conversion of human prion protein by CWD prions. However, no human TSEs with strong evidence of a link with CWD have been identified (Belay *et al.*, 2004).

Citations

Belay ED (1999) Transmissible spongiform encephalopathies in humans. *Annual Review of Microbiology* 53: 283–314.

Belay ED, Maddox RA, Williams ES, Miller MW, Gambetti P, and Schonberger L (2004) Chronic wasting disease and potential transmission to humans. *Emerging Infectious Diseases* 10: 977–984.

Kong Q, Surewicz WK, Peterson RB, *et al.* (2004) Inherited prion diseases. In: Prusiner SB (ed.) *Prion Biology and Diseases*, vol. 14, pp. 673–775Cold Spring Harbor, NY: Cold Spring Harbor Laboratory Press

Llewelyn CA, Hewitt PE, Knight RSG, *et al.* (2004) Possible transmission of variant Creutzfeldt-Jakob disease by blood transfusion. *The Lancet* 363: 417–421.

Parchi P, Giese A, Capellari S, *et al.* (1999) Classification of sporadic Creutzfeldt-Jakob disease based on molecular and phenotypic analysis of 300 subjects. *Annals of Neurology* 46: 224–233.

Prusiner SB (1982) Novel proteinaceous infectious particles cause scrapie. *Science* 216: 136–144.

Wells GAH and Wilesmith JW (2004) Bovine spongiform encephalopathy and related diseases. In: Prusiner SB (ed.) *Prion Biology and Diseases*, vol. 12, pp. 595–628. Cold Spring Harbor, NY: Cold Spring Harbor Laboratory Press.

Will RG, Ironside JW, Zeidlem, *et al.* (1996) A new variant of Creutzfeldt-Jakob disease in the UK. *The Lancet* 347: 921–925.

Will RG, Alper MP, Dormont D, and Schonberger LB (2004) Infectious and sporadic prion diseases. In: Prusiner SB (ed.) *Prion Biology and Diseases*, vol. 13, pp. 629–672. Cold Spring Harbor, NY: Cold Spring Harbor Laboratory Press.

Williams ES, Miller MW, Kreeger TJ, Khan RH, and Thorne ET (2002) Chronic wasting disease of deer and elk: A review with recommendations for management. *Journal of Wildlife Management* 66: 551–563.

Further Reading

Belay ED and Schonberger LB (2005) The public health impact of prion diseases. *Annual Review of Public Health* 26: 191–212.

Collee JG and Bradley R (1997) BSE: a decade on – Part 1. *The Lancet* 349(9052): 636–641.

Collee JG and Bradley R (1997) BSE: a decade on – Part 2. *The Lancet* 349(9053): 715–721.

Knight RS and Will RG (2004) Prion disease. *Journal of Neurology, Neurosurgery, and Psychiatry* 75(Suppl 1): i36–i42.

Prusiner SB (ed.) (2004) *Prion Biology and Diseases*. Cold Spring Harbor, NY: Cold Spring Harbor Laboratory Press.

Relevant Websites

http://www.aphis.usda.gov/newsroom/hot_issues/bse/index.shtml – Animal and Plant Health Inspection Service, U.S. Department of Agriculture.

http://www.defra.gov.uk/animalh/bse/index.html – Bovine Spongiform Encephalopathy (BSE), Department for Environment, Food, and Rural Affairs, Animal Health and Welfare (UK).

http://www.bseinquiry.gov.uk – The BSE Inquiry, Inquiry into BSE and Variant CJD in the UK.

http://www.cjdfoundation.org – Creutzfeldt-Jakob Disease (CJD) Foundation.

http://www.cjdsurveillance.com – National Prion Disease Pathology Surveillance Center.

http://www.cdc.gov/ncidod/dvrd/prions/index.htm – Prion Diseases, Centers for Disease Control and Prevention (CDC).

SECTION 3
PUBLIC HEALTH POLICY AND PRACTICE

Integrated Control of Alcohol

S Casswell, Massey University, Auckland, New Zealand

Alcohol is a major risk factor for burden of disease and injury. Alcohol increases the frequency of injury, both intentional and unintentional, several categories of cancer, neuropsychiatric conditions, and diseases of the cardiovascular system and the liver. Its effects are not confined to the drinker but also result in a significant burden for others. Overall, it is estimated that alcohol contributed to 4% of all disability-adjusted life years lost worldwide in 2002, which means its global impact is comparable to that of tobacco. The lack of adequate data on social costs (Klingemann and Gmel, 2001), particularly to those borne by others, suggests that the total costs may be even higher. Alcohol is a larger net contributor to the global burden of disease and injury than illicit drugs, but there has been no international response aimed at comprehensive and integrated alcohol control.

Other articles in this volume address alcohol policies formulated by governments at national or state level and illustrate a body of research evidence that demonstrates effectiveness. Many such effective policies – for example, random breath testing of drivers, controls on hours of sale via licensing requirements, and early interventions with those experiencing alcohol-related harm – require effective implementation at a local level. Some work has also illustrated the effective impact of community-wide projects focusing on the implementation at the local level of effective government policies.

The development, implementation, and evaluation of effective policies at a local level rely on data gathering of local intelligence, for example, from drunk-driving data or alcohol-related crime, or from operations assessing the willingness of the retail sector to sell to underage patrons, which can help target problem premises or retail outlets for attention. Community groups can also play a useful role in raising local alcohol issues, monitoring local outlets and, if necessary, calling for improvements to policy and legislation or to systems of enforcement to reduce alcohol-related harm.

While the adoption and implementation of effective strategies at the national and local levels are essential to integrated alcohol control, there is also a need for regional and global action, similar to that required for both tobacco and illicit drugs. This article reviews the reasons behind the need for a supranational response, its nature, and some of the factors currently holding back its implementation.

Need for Public Health Policies in Response

A Global Alcohol Industry

As with tobacco, the ownership of alcohol production and the marketing of international and local brands of alcohol is now global business. Alcohol companies that grew in Western Europe and North America through mergers and acquisitions have now gone global. The global consolidation of industry ownership has implications for the public health response to alcohol-related harm. These include the sheer power of these companies, sometimes referred to as transgovernmental corporations (Bendell and Kearins, 2005), to indicate their capacity to act outside national boundaries and constraints. In turn, this capacity allows these corporations to influence international trade agreements, to market their products aggressively to existing and potential consumers, and to engage at all levels with public and private debates on what alcohol control policies are appropriate.

With regard to trade agreements, the alcohol industry has been an active supporter of the liberalization that has both assisted the expansion of the global companies and also challenged effective public health policies at the national level. Alcohol and tobacco have been the subjects of many challenges and not only countries' ability to restrict imports but also their ability to restrict marketing have been reduced as a consequence of the trade agreements (Gould, 2005).

The size and nature of the industry's marketing activity is another spin-off of the globalized industry. The profits available to these corporations and their sophistication as marketers has allowed for effective marketing in mature markets such as Europe and North America, where alcohol companies target products to the cohort of predrinkers (who must be recruited on an ongoing basis to maintain profits), and also to younger cohorts, women, and ethnic groups with below-average patterns of consumption. By 2001, the Council of the European Union noted a disturbing growth in alcohol consumption among children and adolescents. In Western Europe, marketing contributed to shifts away from wine consumption as part of meals toward a more fiesta or intoxication-focused pattern of beer drinking (Gual and Colom, 1997).

Of considerable global public health importance is the use of brand marketing of international alcohol products, and newly acquired local ones, to extend alcohol sales in new markets. The global corporations' primary focus is to reach beyond the mature markets of their country and region of origin to seek emerging markets in other regions: Eastern Europe, Latin America, and Asia. Targeted countries are those with developing economies, growing middle classes, high proportions of young people, and relatively low levels of alcohol consumption, suggesting considerable potential for growth. The rapid increases in consumption of branded products in these emerging markets suggests that the industry's aim of targeted promotion is proving successful.

Also of public health concern is the role and resource of alcohol companies in influencing national alcohol control policies. The largest global companies fund the International Center for Alcohol Policy (ICAP) in Washington, which is engaged in an active program of publication, communication, and lobbying. ICAP has surveyed Health Ministers and other officials developing alcohol policy in countries around the world to identify priority areas for policy development. Its website provides a "comprehensive guide to key issues in alcohol policy development," and its reports are translated into languages widely used in several emerging markets. The Center has released publications that serve to counter public health research by recommending policies that are relatively ineffective or less likely to affect sales (International Center for Alcohol Policies, 2002, 2003, 2004; Stimson et al., 2007). It also advocates a partnership approach between the alcohol industry, governments, and public health groups on alcohol policy and prevention. ICAP's work is complemented by other, less-visible, global associations (such as the Global Alcohol Producers Group) and a growing number of regional and national social aspects organizations, including a number in low- and middle-income countries (Benegal, 2005; Thamarangsi, 2006).

Absence of Effective Policies

In many mature market countries, there are national alcohol policies and laws in place; for example, in regard to the sale of alcohol, driving while intoxicated, and alcohol taxation (which serves a public health goal as well as raising revenue). Shortcomings are often in the operational detail of such policies and laws, including whether the laws and licensing systems are being sufficiently well enforced, and whether sufficient resources are being put behind the most cost-effective policies. Perhaps the weakest area of regulation is that concerned with alcohol advertising and other forms of marketing. In most mature markets, alcohol is heavily advertised. Many countries use a mix of partial restrictions on exposure to alcohol advertisements – in certain media or at certain times – and systems of industry self-regulation in regard

to the content of alcohol advertisements. There is little research or policy on other forms of marketing. For example, there are few studies of integrated marketing of the global alcohol brands that sponsor international sports events and reach loyal and potential drinkers across a range of mature and emerging markets.

Alcohol control often relies too heavily on classroom-based education of young people that seeks to reduce alcohol-related harm. Systematic reviews have consistently shown little or no evidence of effectiveness in terms of either medium- or longer-term behavior change or harm outcomes (Babor et al., 2003; Foxcroft, 2006). However, in part because this approach has face validity and in part because it provides no challenge to vested interests and is actively promoted by industry-funded commentators (International Center for Alcohol Policies, 2004), educational interventions of this kind have been popular. Similarly, there is a focus on public information campaigns and social marketing approaches in some jurisdictions, where, once again, the evidence of effectiveness in reducing alcohol-related harm is lacking.

In emerging markets for alcohol, there is often very little in the way of alcohol policy and regulation, or very little enforcement of such laws as have been passed. Typically, there are very few data on alcohol-related harm on which to base advocacy for government interventions, particularly for restrictive measures to protect public health that may appear contrary to trade principles. The need for assistance with research and data collection, and to share information and technical expertise between countries with regional similarities, has been recognized by the World Health Organization. As in mature markets, there is a danger of over-reliance on less effective strategies, with active promotion of educational approaches despite the lack of a supportive policy environment.

Taxation, including tariffs on imported alcohol products, is often a key policy and a source of government revenue, particularly in countries in which incomes and perhaps economic activity levels are low. For a number of countries, informal illegally produced alcohol or cross-border smuggling may reduce government revenue, and revenue would be increased if governments were able to reduce these nontaxed sources of alcohol. Greater control over alcohol production and distribution would also allow them to increase tax (and therefore price to the consumer). Many emerging markets do not regulate or license the sale of alcohol by bars or stores; alcohol may be sold anywhere. A minimum age at which young people may be sold alcohol may exist in law but often goes unenforced.

It is in this context, that the World Health Organization has been commissioning research and presenting recommendations on effective policies to reduce alcohol-related harm.

Global Governance on Alcohol

NGO Movement in Global Governance

Global governance, as a response to the global nature of the markets and communication networks, requires not just intergovernmental responses, such as those carried out by the UN system (see the section titled 'the UN system' below), but also response from NGOs and voluntary organizations operating at a regional and international level. In response to growing awareness of the contribution alcohol is making to the global burden of disease, a number of NGOs focused on alcohol policy have emerged and a number of health NGOs have demonstrated concern for alcohol policy development. For example, in 2005 the World Medical Association passed a Statement on Reducing the Global Impact of Alcohol on Health and Society, which urged consideration of a Framework Convention on Alcohol Control similar to that of the WHO Framework Convention on Tobacco Control. This was followed in 2006 by a statement from the American Public Health Association, which also urged the adoption by the World Health Organization of a binding international treaty, modeled after the Framework Convention on Tobacco Control.

The World Bank, which in 2000 issued a Note calling for caution in relation to funding of alcohol beverage projects as part of development aid, has more recently in its World Development Report for 2007, *Development and the Next Generation*, emphasized the dangers of alcohol (and tobacco) use by the world's cohort of younger people and called for action via raising taxation, comprehensive bans on advertising and product promotions, age restrictions on sales, and prominent health warnings.

Newly emerging global and regional networks on alcohol policy are monitoring and advocating for action within the U.N. system as well as by national governments. These include the Global Alcohol Policy Alliance, Eurocare, the Asia Pacific Alcohol Policy Alliance, and the Indian Alcohol Policy Alliance.

The UN System

A regional approach to alcohol policy was initially mapped out by Health Ministers in Europe, in consultation with nongovernment organizations. In 1995, a WHO European Charter on Alcohol was adopted, with ten strategies for action. This was followed by an Action Plan, later revised for 2000–07. In 2001, the Health Ministers of WHO Europe countries issued a Declaration on Young People and Alcohol, with policy targets to 2006.

The European Commission also reviewed the policies of its member countries in 1998 and in October 2006 released a European Union Alcohol Harm Reduction Strategy. This strategy had had considerable input from industry representatives and, upon its release, received a more favorable response from industry interests than the NGO sector. Its focus on education as the strategy of choice reflected the lobbying on the part of the industry interests who were pleased to see no specific plan with regard to taxation or product labeling (Anonymous, 2006).

In 2006, following concern raised by public health agencies and community organizations in the Western Pacific Region, the World Health Organization's Western Pacific Regional Office drafted and consulted on a Regional Strategy to Reduce Alcohol-Related Harm that reflects current evidence on effective policy. The Strategy notes that effectiveness will depend on member countries combining as many as possible of the recommended measures, which included: public awareness and health promotion; building capacity among health workers, support for advocacy and community action; regulation of advertising and sponsorship enforced by a government agency; drunk-driving laws with a low blood alcohol concentration (BAC) and frequent random enforcement; collaboration between health and law enforcement on alcohol-related crime and public safety; regulating alcohol sales through a minimum age, restrictions on availability and a licensing system; appropriate enforcement of the above alcohol laws, using taxation based on alcohol content to reduce harmful use, and giving consideration to alcohol harm reduction when participating in trade negotiations.

The Western Pacific Regional Strategy was adopted by the region's Heath Ministers in October 2006. The same month, Health Ministers of WHO's South-East Asian Region adopted a short Resolution endorsing a report on Policy Options for Alcohol Consumption Control as a guide and minimal framework for member states. The report noted research on effective and cost-effective intervention, and its options included taxation and other price controls, regulating alcohol availability, drunk-driving measures, regulation of production and distribution, restrictions on advertising, and community action. It noted the expense and limited effectiveness of mass media moderation campaigns countered by industry advertising. The report also commented on the role of key players, noting that local communities and groups were crucial for effective action and monitoring practices and policies, and there was a more limited role for the industry in ensuring high standards and compliance with regulations (World Health Organization Regional Office for South-East Asia, 2006).

Following evidence of the large contribution that alcohol makes to the burden of injury and disease in all regions of the world, the World Health Organization reviewed current alcohol policies in WHO member countries (World Health Organization, 2004) and sponsored a project to evaluate the most effective and cost-effective alcohol policies to reduce alcohol-related harm (Chisholm *et al.*, 2004, 2006). In 2005, Health Ministers gathered at the 58th

World Health Assembly adopted a report on 'Public health problems caused by harmful use of alcohol' (World Health Organization, 2005). It noted the policy strategies most likely to be effective or ineffective in reducing alcohol-related harm and mandated further work by WHO in this area. In the following year, a resolution supported by more than 40 countries calling for work toward a global strategy on alcohol failed to achieve a consensus and was referred back to the Executive Board for further work.

In addition to the partial progress made to date on regional and global strategy, there have been, as described earlier, calls from NGOs and also in the scientific literature for action more in line with that taken with regard to tobacco, in the form of a binding international agreement – a Framework on Alcohol Control Policy (Room, 2005). There are differences between tobacco and alcohol that militate against such an agreement, the most important of which is probably the much shorter time of widespread use of the two drugs. Whereas tobacco has been widely used only in the last 100 years, alcohol has a much longer history. However, the new situation brought about by vastly increased globalization, resulting in much faster spread of commercial alcohol in contexts without traditional social controls constraining harm, and the size and vulnerability of the world's youth cohort, are factors that are as relevant for alcohol as for tobacco.

There is good evidence of effective policies to reduce alcohol-related harm that may be implemented at the national and local level. An international infrastructure is needed to ensure the appropriate dissemination and adoption of these effective strategies, but such a framework is currently lacking.

See also: Alcohol Consumption: Overview of International Trends; Alcohol: The Burden of Disease; Alcohol—Socio-Economic Impacts (Including Externalities); Alcoholism Treatment; Alcohol Industry; Control and Regulation of Currently Illegal Drugs.

Citations

Anonymous (2006) EU Alcohol Strategy – Is the glass half full or half empty? *The Globe,* Issue 3.

Babor T, Caetano R, Casswell S, *et al.* (2003) Alcohol: *No Ordinary Commodity – Research and Public Policy*. Oxford, UK: Oxford University Press.

Bendell J and Kearins K (2005) The political bottom line: The emerging dimension to corporate responsibility for sustainable development. *Business Strategy and the Environment* 14: 372–383.

Benegal V (2005) India: Alcohol and public health. *The Globe,* Issue 2.

Chisholm D, Rehm J, van Ommeren M, and Monteiro M (2004) Reducing the global burden of hazardous alcohol use: A comparative cost-effectiveness analysis. *Journal of Studies on Alcohol* 65: 782–793.

Chisholm D, Doran C, Shibuya K, and Rehm J (2006) Comparative cost-effectiveness of policy instruments for reducing the global burden of alcohol, tobacco and illicit drug use. *Drug and Alcohol Review* 25: 553–565.

Foxcroft D (2006) Alcohol education: Absence of evidence or evidence of absence. *Addiction* 101: 1057–1058.

Gould E (2005) Trade treaties and alcohol advertising policy. *Journal of Public Health Policy* 26: 359–376.

Gual A and Colom J (1997) Why has alcohol consumption declined in countries of southern Europe. *Addiction* 92(supplement 1): S21–S32.

International Center for Alcohol Policies (2002) *Self-Regulation and Alcohol: A Toolkit for Emerging Markets and the Developing World*. Washington, DC: International Center for Alcohol Policies.

International Center for Alcohol Policies (2003) *International Drinking Guidelines* ICAP Reports 14. Washington, DC: International Center for Alcohol Policies.

International Center for Alcohol Policies (2004) *Alcohol Education and its Effectiveness* ICAP Reports 16. Washington, DC: International Center for Alcohol Policies.

Klingemann H and Gmel G (eds.) (2001) *Mapping the Social Consequences of Alcohol Consumption*. Dordrecht, Austria: Kluwer Academic Publishers.

Room R (2005) Negotiating the place of alcohol in public health: The arguments at the interface. *Addiction* 100: 1396–1397.

Stimson G, Barton A, Grant M, Choquet M, and Garrison P (2007) *Drinking in Context : Patterns Interventions, and Partnerships*. New York: Routledge.

Thamarangsi T (2006) Thailand: Alcohol today. *Addiction* 101: 783–787.

World Health Organization (2004) *Global Status Report on Alcohol*. Geneva, Switzerland: World Health Organization.

World Health Organization (2005) *Public Health Problems Caused by Harmful Use of Alcohol: Report by the Secretariat*. 58th World Health Assembly A58/18. Geneva, Switzerland, WHO.

World Health Organization Regional Office for South-East Asia (2006) *Alcohol Consumption Control – Policy Options in the South-East Asia Region*. http://www.searo.who.int/en/Section1430/Section1439/Section1638/Section2234/Section2272_11902 (accessed 20 October 2007).

Relevant Websites

http://www.apapaonline.org – APAPA, Asia Pacific Alcohol Policy Alliance.

http://www.globalgapa.org/ – Eurocare, European Alcohol Policy Alliance.

http://www.globalgapa.org/ – Global Alcohol Policy Alliance.

http://www.indianalcoholpolicy.org – Indian Alcohol Policy Alliance (IAPA).

http://www.who.int/gb/e/e_wha58.html – World Health Organization, 58th World Health Assembly report Public Health Problems Caused by Harmful Use of Alcohol, A 58, WHA58.26.

http://www.who.int/substance_abuse/en – World Health Organization, Management of Substance Abuse.

http://www.searo.who.int/ – WHO Regional Office for South East Asia, Resolution on Alcohol Consumption Control: Policy Options, Meeting Reports.

http://www.wpro.who.int/ – World Health Organization Regional Office for the Western Pacific, 2006 Resolution adopting Regional Strategy to Reduce Alcohol-Related Harm, Library and Information Sources, Policy Documents, WPR/RC57.R5.

Alcohol Industry

L Hill, The Centre for Social and Health Outcomes Research and Evaluation (SHORE), Massey University, Auckland, New Zealand

Introduction

The quaint history of Stella Artois – 'it all began in the Belgian city of Leuven with a charming house the locals call "Den Horen"... in the year 1466 it was converted to a small brewery ...' – is typical of self-presentation that links global alcohol corporations with local traditions and culture. It is a marketing strategy that perpetuates outdated imagery about breweries, distilleries, and familiar brands. That little brewery is now InBev, the world's largest brewer with around 14% of the global market.

Relatively little research looks at the supply side of alcohol, that is, the dynamics of production, trade, and distribution. (A noteworthy exception was the special issue of the journal *Addiction,* an international project published in 2000; see the section 'Further Reading.') This article reviews the rapid global consolidation of the alcohol industry, based on public information of about 24 of the largest transnational companies. It notes ownership changes, particularly over the last 5 years, and identifies key corporate strategies, including support for free trade agreements.

The Internet is now an important vehicle for the alcohol industry's marketing and communication strategies. Websites target three separate audiences – drinkers, investors, and policy makers. This article draws mainly from corporate websites providing information for shareholders and investors – annual reports, presentations, company policies, media releases – as well as from media commentary and academic analysis. These websites seldom mention government policies on alcohol. The largest corporations now fund separate organizations, at national and global levels, to address the 'social aspects' of alcohol. The strategies of these organizations to influence public opinion and alcohol policies are also identified and discussed.

Global Consolidation of Alcohol Ownership

In 2003 the world's top ten distilling companies produced 306 million 9-liter cases of spirits. Three years later production was dominated by just two companies, who also own much of the world's wine production. In 2005, 60% of the world's commercially brewed beer was produced by global companies, with 44% produced by the largest four. Economies of scale benefit companies with a global footprint, notes SABMiller, the third largest brewer in the world. With consumption stabilizing in industrialized countries, these economies of scale are being achieved through a scramble for position in the emerging markets of Eastern European, Latin America, and Asia.

Brief profiles of the largest alcohol corporations illustrate recent global consolidation.

InBev

In 2004 InBev became the world's largest brewer by volume, and is either the first or second largest brewer in 20 key beer markets. It markets four key global beer brands and over 200 local brands. In December 2006, the company reported a production of 211.6 million hectoliters. Its total revenue from alcohol and nonalcoholic drinks was about US$17 773 million, making 24.2% profit on operations before tax.

InBev was created from the 2004 merger of AmBev, based in Canada and the then second largest brewer worldwide, and Interbrew, the third largest brewer, based in Belgium. AmBev had expanded into Brazil and other Latin American countries, while Interbrew expanded into East Europe, including Poland and Russia. InBev now operates in Korea and in China, where it has 18 breweries in six provinces. It bought the China operations of Lion Nathan, the brewer licensed for InBev brands in Australia, New Zealand, and the Pacific Islands. For the period 2002–04, InBev reported 8–11% returns on investment in its Asia Pacific region.

Anheuser Busch

Anheuser Busch is the second largest brewery, with 11.5% of the world beer market (2005), and 48% of the U.S. market. In 2006 Budweiser and Bud Light were the biggest selling beer brands worldwide and international sales provided a third of the company's income (after alcohol tax) of US$17 717 million.

Anheuser Busch's U.S. operations include malt-based liquor, energy drinks, drinks packaging, and family adventure parks. Its early international operations followed U.S. troop deployments in Korea, Japan, and the Philippines in the 1940s and 1950s. The company boasts '150 years of military support' and a Budweiser Heroes Tour, with draught horses, supported the Iraq war.

In 2004, international beer sales tripled as a result of a growth strategy in Canada, the UK, and China. In Canada Budweiser is brewed under license by the InBev Labatt breweries, in Ireland by the InBev Guinness breweries, and in Italy by Heineken. In Britain, where Budweiser is the top-selling canned or bottled beer in pubs, clubs, and restaurants, the company does its own brewing. In China, Budweiser and Bud Ice sales increased 21.5% in 2002 and by 2003 had achieved nearly half the premium-priced beer market. Anheuser-Busch partly owns 64 breweries, and in 2004 beat SABMiller to buy Harbin, China's fourth largest brewery. China was seen to have great sales potential because "current per-capita consumption levels are only 20% of the levels of many developed countries" (Anheuser-Busch Report, 2006: 15).

Latin America is marked for expansion through local partnerships for similar reasons. Anheuser Busch owns 50% of the leading Mexican brewer Grupo Modelo, which exports its Corona brands to the United States. In 2006 Anheuser-Busch licensed Heineken to brew Budweiser in Panama and also in Russia, the world's fifth-largest beer market.

Anheuser Busch's marketing practices have been at times controversial. Budweiser's cartoon frogs are well recognized by children in the United States. The brand targets different demographic groups through sports – especially major league baseball – music and sponsored concerts, and product placement in films.

Sport is an important strategy internationally. Anheuser Busch has sponsored the U.S. Olympics team since the early 1980s, and now also supports the Chinese Olympics team. It spent US$20 million for Budweiser to be the official beer of the 1996 Olympics in Atlanta, with a further US$100 million spent on related marketing. It paid US$20 million to sponsor World Cup Soccer in 1998, but failed to get the French government to lift its *Loi Evin* (French alcohol policy law) against alcohol company sponsorship of sports. In the United States, it sponsored the 2002 Winter Olympics in Salt Lake City, Utah, a nondrinking Mormon community. Starting in 1996, with a legal challenge, the company pressured the state government into changing a law that allowed advertising for low-alcohol beer only. It was Anheuser Busch that lodged a case against the Utah state government. In 2006 it sponsored the Olympic Winter Games in Italy and the FIFA World Cup Soccer in Germany and will sponsor the 2010 World Cup in South Africa. These sponsorships promote Budweiser to millions of beer drinkers and potential drinkers at matches and through television, by way of official tournament logos, on-field signage, packaging, point-of-sale materials, and advertising campaigns around the globe.

SABMiller

The third largest brewer is SABMiller, with 11.1% of the world market. It operates in 60 markets and produced 176 million hectoliters of lager in 2006, as well as 45 million hectoliters of other beverages. SABMiller was formerly South African Breweries until 2002, when it bought Miller

Brewing Company, the second largest U.S. beer company, with additonal breweries in Central America. Previously, international expansion had been held back by the anti-apartheid boycott but progressed rapidly after 1994. The first purchase was in the Czech Republic. The company is now the largest (or second largest) producer in several Eastern European countries, including Russia. By 2003 it was the largest foreign brewer in China, and operated in seven other Asian countries. In 2005 it doubled its stake in India and with 10 breweries became the second largest brewer there. SABMiller also bought a controlling share in Bavaria, the second largest beer brand in South America. Its 2006 revenue of US $15 307 million was up 19% from the previous year.

SABMiller attributes its global success to experience operating in countries with limited infrastructure. It is the largest brewer in Africa, producing lager and sorghum beer as well as soft drinks (Coca-Cola) and bottling in 20 countries. Sorghum is a grain used to produce traditional African 'cloudy' beer, which was often a source of income for women in poor circumstances. SABMiller played a role in bringing this cottage industry under the licensing system that regulates sales of industrially produced and imported alcohol products in South Africa. SABMiller notes that international brands are often too expensive for many drinkers in developing countries, so it reduces production and transport costs by brewing its brands locally, using local produce and training suppliers as required.

Heineken

Heineken had 7.8% of the world beer market in 2005 yet describes itself as the 'most international brewer.' It owns 115 breweries in more than 65 countries and sells 170 beer brands. Its beer volumes grew 5.3% in 2005 and 13.8% in 2004. In 2006, it sold 111 905 million hectoliters of beer, an increase of 11.8% from the previous year, earning about US$15 749 million.

Heineken is the largest beer brand in Europe, and its Amstel brand is the third largest. Based in the Netherlands, it bought breweries in Germany and Austria, then in Russia, Siberia, Hungary, Poland, and Croatia in the years 2002–03. During that period, it also purchased breweries or increased holdings in Panama, Chile, and Argentina, and formed a partnership with Mexican brewer FEMSA to target the fast-growing Hispanic market in the United States. Heineken also wholesales spirits, wine, and soft drinks in Europe, and produces Budweiser in Italy for Anheuser Busch. In 2004 it formed a 40-brands partnership with Diageo and Namibia Breweries in South Africa and in 2006 consolidated volumes increased by 1.7 million hectoliters, with more than 70% of this increase in Nigeria, Congo, Burundi, Rwanda, and the Democratic Repabulic of the Congo. In 2006 it acquired part-ownership of a Tunisian drinks company and planned a brewery there. In the Middle East, it set up a beer company with

Tempo, the Israeli beer, and increased its minority share-holding of a Lebanese brewery to 79%. In New Zealand, Heineken and Amstel are produced by DB Breweries, which is now owned by two Singapore companies, Fraser and Neave and Asia Pacific Breweries, the latter of which is half-owned by Heineken. In Australia Heineken formed a joint venture with Lion Nathan, DB Breweries' traditional competitor. Through Asia Pacific Breweries' acquisitions in 2006, Heineken now has brewery interests in Vietnam and Laos and has expanded in India. It has fully owned operations in Indonesia and New Caledonia, exporting to Taiwan, Hong Kong, and South Korea, and has a partnership with Kirin in Japan. In China which Heineken describes as the largest beer market in the world it has been buying part-ownership in the largest breweries in several provinces. These will produce Heineken alongside local brands, using local distribution networks and local marketing knowledge.

In 2006 Heineken reported spending 12.6% of revenue on marketing, including films and high-profile football sponsorships. These included the Rugby World Cup in Paris in 2007 (**Figure 1**) – France lifted its ban for international events – and the Rugby World Cup to be held in New Zealand in 2011. By 2008 Heineken anticipates that savings from consolidation of its global operations will enable more money and people to be focused behind 'winning' brands.

Pernod Ricard

This French producer of spirits, champagne, and wine now does nearly 90% of its business outside France,

mainly in Asia and the Americas. In June 2005 it purchased Allied Dolmecq to become the world's second largest spirits and wines company, after Diageo. Its international acquisitions began with Scottish and Irish distilleries, then expanded beyond Europe in the 1980s. The company doubled in size in 2001 when it and Diageo carved up Canadian spirits producer Seagram's. The Allied Dolmecq purchase gave it another nine top international spirits brands, as well as wine interests in Europe, the United States, Argentina, Australia, and New Zealand (Diageo declined an option to purchase half the New Zealand wine industry). Another 25 spirits brands were passed on to Fortune Brands, owner of Jim Beam. This makes Fortune Brands the fourth largest global spirits company, behind Barcardi, a privately owned family company in the Bahamas, which works closely with another family-controlled spirits company, Brown Forman.

With consolidation of these acquisitions, Pernod Ricard's sales (June 2006) were about US$8153 million, with net profit up 32% at about US$1685 million. It spent 17% of revenue on marketing, 70% of which went to 15 'strategic' brands that generated half its 2006 profits. These brands were the focus of new marketing campaigns in 2007.

Constellation Brands

Ownership of wine has also consolidated and globalized. Constellation Brands is now the largest wine maker by volume, alongside Diageo and Pernod Ricard. Acquisitions in California, Australia, and New Zealand put it ahead of E.&J. Gallo, the largest U.S. wine company,

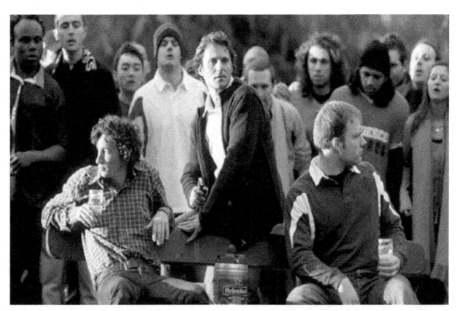

Figure 1   Heineken sponsorship of 2007 Rugby World Cup, with major integrated promotions in rugby-playing countries: 'One world, one cup, one beer'. Television ads – this one of mates watching the match in Paris ('Better get some more') – features the new 5-liter Heineken DraftKeg, now marketed in 54 countries. In 2006 Heineken's EUFA Championship League sponsorship ads showed fans, with keg, watching the games in remote locations in eight countries. From Heineken's website.

and Carlton Fosters, which bought Australia's largest wine company Southcorp in 2005. It has 20% of the U.S. wine market and in 2005 sold 72 million cases of wine worldwide.

Constellation began in the 1950s marketing a cheap, high-alcohol-content dessert wine, then doubled its revenue with wine coolers in the 1980s. A series of acquisitions since the 1990s gives Constellation brands that span the price range. This includes very prestigious vineyards that retain control of production while Constellation focuses on distribution and marketing. In the United States Constellation sells mainly through supermarkets and convenience stores. It also sells spirits brands, including cocktails and mixed drinks, and imported beers, including distribution in 25 states of Corona beer, which is half-owned by Anheuser Busch. Over the past 5 years Constellation's sales grew 16% a year, with sales after alcohol tax of US$4603 million in 2006. In June 2006, Vincor, Canada's leading wine producer and marketer, joined the group.

Diageo

Diageo is the largest alcohol corporation overall, producing leading spirits brands as well as beers and wines. Its 2006 sales after alcohol taxes were about US$14 471 million, up 6% from 2005, and its operating profit was up 18%. Much of this came from international operations (outside the European Union [EU] and the United States), in which volumes were up 14% compared with 6% worldwide, following a 28% increase in marketing expenditure.

Diageo was formed in 1997 from a merger of the Irish and British producers Guinness (including United Distillers) and GrandMet (including International Distillers & Vintners), adding a 60% share of Seagram's in 2001. It operates in 180 countries including emerging markets in Asia, India, the Middle East, Latin America, the Caribbean, and the Pacific. In Africa it is also a leading brewer in 15 countries, with 10 breweries as well as six distilleries. In New Zealand, Diageo's main spirits brands are managed by brewers Lion Nathan (46% owned by Kirin, Japan) and in Australia by its competitor Carlton Fosters – although it recently ran a supermarket price promotion there involving Diageo spirits and Lion Nathan beers.

Diageo's marketing focuses on eight 'global priority' brands, which contributed 59% of total volume sold in 2006. A further 17% of volume came from 30 local priority brands. In 2006 Diageo spent about US$2246 million on marketing its brands.

Global Market Strategies

From annual reports and websites of the top 24 alcohol companies worldwide, a set of industry strategies can be identified. From a shareholder perspective, the first three of these involve corporate ownership, expansion, and consolidation, but they are also a market strategy. The following list outlines industry strategies:

- Global marketing of higher-priced premium brands;
- Targeting emerging markets in growing or recovering economies;
- Buying or part-buying the largest competing local producer, then running international and local brands together;
- Adoption of corporate social responsibility policies.

Political influence is little discussed in annual reports and other public documents, but from what is known about the alcohol industry's lobbying activities, we can add to this list:

- Actively supporting free trade agreements and challenging barriers to competition.

Global alcohol brands are marketed as 'premium' products to bring higher revenue. Production and ownership changes may reflect this. For example, SABMiller's license to produce Heineken in South Africa was terminated because Heineken preferred to profit directly from the growing premium beer sector. In developed countries, regulatory approval of ownership changes may require a brand or two to be shed to avoid an anticompetitive monopoly of a national market – such as seen with the purchases of Seagram's and Allied Dolmecq. Of note is that these companies are consolidating globally, rather than nationally. Profitability comes from owning the most profitable global brands and the most successful local brands in each market, not from owning all brands in any particular market.

Shareholders are told of the economies of scale expected from partnerships and acquisitions in developing countries. There are cost savings in local production of the global brand and distribution through existing customer networks. Relocation of production or other functions also brings cost savings, as with InBev's current 'footprint optimization' program to free up resources for brand building and marketing. A local company can provide cultural knowledge for marketing purposes. For example, the Swedish corporation Vin Spirits now makes puns with Chinese characters in its Absolut vodka advertisements. Buying up or buying into alcohol companies in Eastern Europe, Russia, China, or Brazil gives the global corporation entry into new markets with growing or recovering economies, growing middle classes, and population growth among young adult drinkers. In each market, the strategy is to run premium international brands and popular local brands alongside each other. As SABMiller's 2005 annual report told shareholders (p. 6), "We now have a continuum of businesses from emerging to mature; enabling us to benefit from both value and volume growth.

In many cases, there's also an upward trend towards higher value brands as consumers enter the market at the bottom end and others progress towards the premium end."

What is most striking about this strategy of buying up the local competition is that global alcohol corporations have been doing this out of surplus operating profits. Some report buying a brewery or distillery every few months. The top companies have reported operating profit increases of 7–12% per year in recent years. On a global scale of operation, this provides a great deal of money to be reinvested. Profit itself, as well as the saturation of Western markets, helps drive the need to find new markets and more drinkers.

These strategies ensure business success in the twenty-first century. However, the product is alcohol, not orange juice. The World Health Organization (WHO) reports that alcohol is now the leading risk factor for injury and disease in developing countries with overall low mortality – countries whose growing prosperity and current under-consumption are attracting the alcohol companies.

It is often assumed that investment by global alcohol companies will have positive effects on local economic development and employment, but emerging markets typically lack alcohol policies and appropriate health services. In 2000 the World Bank issued a cautionary statement entitled, *Note on Alcohol Beverages*. Few of its loans now relate to production or consumption of alcohol, and any projects related to alcohol must be consistent with public health issues and social policy concerns. A WHO study of the ambiguous role of alcohol in developing countries shows that alcohol problems increase with development. Yet local politicians often have favorable attitudes toward alcohol, and there is little recognition of negative social and economic effects from increased alcohol consumption (Room and Jernigan, 2000).

Alcohol Globalization and Free Trade Agreements

As alcohol corporations globalize, their interest in policy at the international level necessarily increases. An alcohol industry strategy of active support for free trade agreements is noted from known lobbying activities and media items, as well as from a series of challenges to tariff and nontariff barriers to trade and competition in alcohol. Company size and global consolidation are relevant to resources and influence on these issues, compared to the countervailing views of public health organizations. For example, in 2003 the World Spirits Alliance, representing distillers in mainly industrialized countries, met in Geneva to agree on a unified international trade strategy of open markets. Its position paper on the General Agreement on Trade and Services (GATS) states the industry's priority objectives as significant liberalization,

and where possible, elimination, of tariffs and nontariff barriers, including barriers to distribution and advertising. In mid 2004, World Spirits Alliance representatives from around the world went to Geneva to meet with the World Trade Organization (WTO).

Free trade agreements require governments to progressively eliminate import quotas, tariffs, and regulations to ensure foreign and domestic companies have equal market opportunities. They have opened up markets for global alcohol brands and constrained domestic public health policies in ways that policy makers – and even local alcohol industries – often did not anticipate when the treaties were signed.

In 2000 Grieshaber-Otto and colleagues looked at the impacts of trade treaties on customs and tax policies. For example, the WTO required Japan to allow imports of vodka and other spirits because they were like or substitutable for the traditional drink *shochu*. Alcohol taxes have been challenged and changed under the General Agreement on Trade and Tariffs (GATT), the North American Free Trade Agreement (NAFTA), and WTO Membership, for restricting market access in Canada (including minimum pricing), Denmark, Finland, Chile, and Korea. Tariffs on alcohol imports can be replaced by alcohol excise taxes provided these are evenhanded. In practice, challenges have led to excise taxes being harmonized downward – within the single market of the EU, for example – rather than upward to meet public health costs and goals. The effect of tax reductions on price has resulted in increased consumption. Trade agreements allow governments to temporarily exclude some goods from negotiations. However, in a 2006 report for WHO, Grieshaber and colleagues noted extraordinary difficulty in using 'exceptions' processes under trade agreements to protect public health.

Gould (2005) notes that treaties apply to trade within member countries as well as between countries, and so increasingly constrain domestic policies. Regulation may be considered a barrier to competition or even *de facto* discrimination if it restricts a foreign company from marketing a new product. There have been challenges to Scandinavian policies that specify where different types or strengths of alcoholic drinks can be sold or advertised. In Scandinavia, Canada, and some U.S. states, government monopoly ownership of bottle stores has been challenged under European Treaty, GATT, or NAFTA rules, despite evidence that this reduces alcohol-related harm. Sweden retained most restrictions on alcohol advertising by rewriting the legislation to state clearly that the policy was necessary to achieve public health purposes. France has similarly defended its *Loi Evin* policy restricting alcohol advertising and sport sponsorship against challenges in the French and European courts.

The WTO defines advertising as both goods under GATT and services under GATS. GATS covers the production, distribution, marketing, sale, and delivery of all services unless specifically (and temporarily) excepted. GATS addresses domestic regulation explicitly, requiring it to be no more restrictive than necessary to achieve a specified policy objective. Standards and licensing must not present unnecessary barriers to trade. Although negotiations on GATS have stalled, a growing number of bilateral and regional trade agreements are modeled on it. Some, such as NAFTA, allow companies, not just governments, to challenge noncompliance. Gould (2005) reports that although companies may exaggerate their ability to win such cases, the possibility has had a chilling effect on public health legislation.

It is commonly argued that free trade will improve the availability, choice, and price of products to consumers. Negotiators and decision makers may not have considered the health implications of this with alcohol. Public health groups may be equally unaware of trade issues. Early and ongoing communication between these groups is important. In 2005 and 2007 the inclusion of alcohol and tobacco in the Pacific Islands Countries Trade Agreement (PICTA) was deferred as a result of such efforts by health ministers and nongovernment organizations (NGOs).

The competition principle enshrined in trade treaties is less apparent in the reports and websites of the 24 largest alcohol corporations. More notable are examples of cooperation. Some produce a competitor's brand under license or manage its distribution. Arrangements in new markets may cut across traditional competition in old ones. Mergers that comply with antimonopoly laws have been achieved with the cooperation of competitors. As Pernod Ricard told the media on 31 January 2006, "Our partnership with Fortune Brands will remain an example of cooperation and represents what two groups, otherwise competing, can achieve together when their strategic objectives are complementary."

Global Promotion of Alcohol

Global corporations entering new markets in developing countries have a huge capacity to advertise and promote alcohol products and drinking – in contrast to the limited resources available for health promotion messages. Annual reports usually provide little or no detail on marketing expenditure. However, in 2006 Heineken reported spending 12.6% of net sales on marketing; Diageo, 15.5%; and Pernod Ricard, 17% – that is, about US$1985 million, US$2246 million, and US$3367 million, respectively.

Through a range of marketing strategies, alcohol is linked to desirable middle-class lifestyles, embedded in the enjoyment of sports or music, linked to masculinity, and social success, or to other concepts, aspirations, and cultural traditions specific to a locality or market segment.

As the brand's philosophy on Inbev's website states (cited 4.12.07), "We believe that developing strong brands requires insights into consumer behaviors and motivations. With these insights, we can build powerful connections and, ultimately, enduring bonds with our consumers."

Industry representatives have argued there is little evidence that advertising increases alcohol consumption; its purpose is to increase a brand's share of the market. The statistical studies they refer to are inconclusive when comparing annual advertising expenditure with total consumption, but do show positive effects when data are disaggregated by beverage type, or by age of consumers, or for shorter periods or local markets, to better capture the fluctuations of advertising campaigns. These are studies of saturated markets in industrialized countries, not emerging ones in Latin America or Asia. Annual reports to shareholders express clear expectations that marketing strategies in these new markets will increase consumption of alcohol.

Alcohol companies say their advertising targets adult consumers. There is considerable spillover to younger audiences, however. A large body of research shows that cumulative exposure to alcohol advertisements shapes the perceptions of children and young people, encouraging pro-drinking attitudes and greater consumption. Those who see the most alcohol ads tend to overestimate how much other people drink, and consequently to drink more themselves. Longitudinal research in New Zealand links higher recall of alcohol ads at age 15 to heavier drinking at age 18. Those who responded more positively to alcohol ads at age 18 were heavier drinkers at age 21, reported more alcohol-related aggression, and drank more frequently by age 26 (Casswell et al., 2002). Further research has confirmed the relationship between rising alcohol advertising expenditure and high exposure of children and underage teenagers over a period of policy liberalization and industry self-regulation. In 2004–05, 90% of 5- to 14-year-olds and 91% of 10- to 17-year-olds saw alcohol ads on television at least weekly. Among those who drank, nearly half the heavier drinkers and a third of lighter drinkers said their friends talked about alcohol ads on television and that alcohol ads were among their favorite ads (Huckle and Huakau, 2006).

More than half of all expenditure is now on other forms of alcohol promotion. There is little research on young people's exposure to alcohol messages by way of sponsorships of sports, music, and other events. This is a major marketing strategy for the alcohol industry, as it has been for the tobacco industry. For example, Diageo is paying around US$57 million over ten years for Bundaberg Rum to sponsor rugby union football in Australia. Bundaberg's chairman told *B&T Magazine* "Rugby has achieved record growth in participation, match attendance and TV audiences over the past five years, while Bundy has doubled in size during the period — it's hard to think that is a coincidence."

There is also little research on direct marketing via drinking venues, promotional events, or the new electronic media. The Internet provides a new marketing tool with a global reach. Alcohol corporations often run a separate, highly sophisticated website for each key brand, protected only by a date-of-birth question. The websites are designed to attract niche markets of mainly younger drinkers. They are highly interactive, offering competitions, free software, and music, and branded memorabilia for purchase (**Figure 2**). Some post photos sent in by drinkers. They support other marketing strands by providing news and events calendars for sponsored sports or music, or competitions to win tickets to branded concerts or to 'be a rock star,' and other promotional events. Brand websites also engage in viral marketing by way of emails and text messages to friends.

In 2005, the World Medical Association called for a Framework Convention on Alcohol Control similar to that which had just taken effect for tobacco, and expressed concern about alcohol marketing:

> Alcohol advertising and promotion is rapidly expanding throughout the world and is increasingly sophisticated and carefully targeted, including to youth. It is aimed to attract, influence, and recruit new generations of potential drinkers despite industry codes of self-regulation that are widely ignored and often not enforced (p. 1).

Other NGOs have begun networking internationally to share information about alcohol marketing, trade issues, and effective policies. The Global Alliance on Alcohol Policy has regional networks in India, Asia and the Pacific, and Europe. Members in emerging markets report irresponsible and culturally insensitive promotions that would not be acceptable in the corporation's home country.

Corporate Responsibility

One corporate strategy above has not yet been discussed – corporate social responsibility. This is a public relations strategy. The top alcohol corporations are adopting corporate responsibility policies that reflect the UN Global Compact on labor, environmental, and social issues. This Global Compact arose from public concern about the impacts of global industries, which also led to the 2005 adoption of the Bangkok Charter on Health Promotion in a Globalized World.

Health impacts are a notable omission from both the Global Compact and the policies of alcohol corporations – despite being the key issue in regard to the global marketing of alcohol. Some brand websites give brief mention to health risks and benefits, urging the customer to drink responsibly to reduce the adverse impacts of their product. Just one company, Heineken, has learned from liability cases against the tobacco industry and provides fairly extensive website information on alcohol's adverse effects on health. Lessons from tobacco, as well as threat of regulation, may also have contributed to the UK alcohol industry's voluntary adoption of warning labels to inform drinkers of risks.

Alcohol companies keep the focus on the responsibility of the drinker, not the risk inherent in the product. Most brand websites, and even some ads, now carry 'Drink responsibly' slogans. Some U.S. companies run public service-style advertisements (with brand logos) to encourage responsible drinking, but these are scheduled at times that make them more likely to be seen by parents than by teenagers (Center for Alcohol Marketing and Youth, 2004). SABMiller and Diageo fund responsible drinking campaigns aimed at teenagers and are establishing partnerships on drunk driving with government and nongovernmental agencies in emerging markets. Alcohol company participation in health promotion may send a

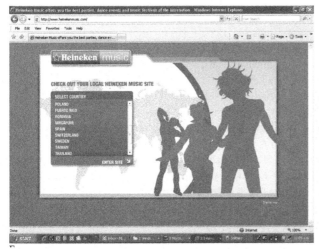
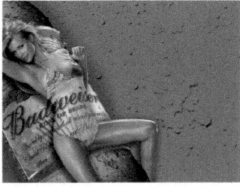

Figure 2   Websites as brand marketing tools: Heineken has music gig guides for each country in which it operates at www.heinekenmusic.com. Anheuser Busch has free 'wallpapers' and other direct marketing downloads at www.budweiser.com.

mixed message, making it less effective. Research shows heavy drinkers ignore responsible drinking messages on ads, favoring those for cut-price bar promotions (Christie *et al.*, 2001). In countries with a high proportion of nondrinkers, campaigns about responsible drinking or not driving while drunk may have the effect of promoting drinking as a new social norm.

In the past two years, the largest alcohol corporations have developed policies on responsibility marketing, although this is not one of the Global Compact's 10 principles. These support national industry codes of standards for alcohol ads but are often less detailed. In its 2003 report Pernod Ricard states that it has actively participated in developing advertising codes as it is "confident that self-discipline is the most effective means of regulating all forms of business communication" (p. 41). Allied Dolmecq urged other alcohol companies to market responsibly to ensure the continuation of industry self-regulation. Since 2003, 39 countries have imposed new and tighter restrictions on the marketing of alcohol, Allied Domecq said in its 2005 Social Report (pp. 5–6); responsible self-disciplined marketing was necessary to avoid a 'regulatory backlash.'

There are frequent reports from public health organizations that alcohol advertising standards are being infringed upon or manipulated by the alcohol, advertising, and media industries. Industry self-regulation is prone to collapse, as happened in Australia (**Figure 3**) and the United States in the 1990s. Studies showing how alcohol ads influence children and young people are based on code-compliant advertisements, not rogue examples.

Industry self-regulation does not limit the many ways in which ads depicting the lifestyles of young adult drinkers are attractive to younger teenagers.

Most importantly, industry self-regulation of alcohol ad content does not, and will not, reduce the exposure of children and young people to the growing volumes of commercial messages promoting alcohol products and a drinking lifestyle. Only legislation – the 'regulatory backlash' – can achieve that.

The alcohol industry argues it has the right to market a legal product, and in the United States commercial speech has a degree of constitutional protection. Yet all industrialized countries have long-standing laws and licensing systems that restrict the sale of alcohol, in recognition of its harmful effects. Policies on alcohol advertising tend to be weaker, and few countries have policy on other forms of marketing. Most restrictions to reduce exposure relate to the broadcast media, and may operate alongside an industry code on the content of ads permitted in other media. The mix of legislation and industry self-regulation in industrialized countries reflects the contested nature of alcohol policy. Saffer and Dave's (2002) comparative research shows, however, that alcohol advertising bans, even partial ones, can reduce alcohol-related harm.

Global Alcohol Commodity Chain

Insights from debates about globalization show the importance of effective policy on alcohol advertising.

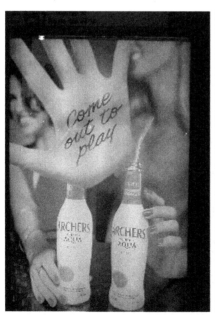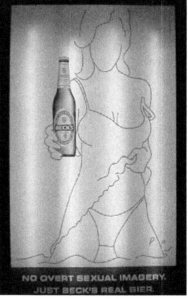

Figure 3 Australia's self-regulatory code for alcohol advertising collapsed in the mid 1990s. A new code was adopted in 1998 but ads continue to infringe the rules. The Archer's ad (Diageo) uses a slogan and other tactics likely to appeal to children. The Becks bus shelter ad (InBev) infringes the rule against linking alcohol with sexual success – she appears to be offering both. From Australian Drug Foundation, Melbourne. See Geoff Munro, A decade of failure: self-regulation of alcohol advertising in Australia, The Globe, 3, 2006. http://www.ias.org.uk/resources/publications/theglobe/globe200603/gl200603_p15.htm

The concept of commodity chains – production networks of multiple firms operating across multiple countries – is used to analyze modern dynamics of power and profit-taking. Globalization takes advantage of cost variations between labor markets, supported by advances in communications and transport. These shape decisions about which links need be owned directly by the corporation. Jernigan (2000) applies this concept to the alcohol industry's networks of local producers, importers, advertisers, and distributors. Exports, distribution agreements, brewing under license, joint ventures, part-ownership, or purchase of local plant or companies are all options in the international expansion of alcohol companies. Commodity chain analysis concludes that to ensure profits accrue to shareholders, corporations should retain direct control over two links in the chain: design/recipe and advertising/marketing. An example of this is the 2006 restructuring of Pernod Ricard into four regional organizations, including subsidiary companies, and four 'brand owner' companies – that is, the separation of local production and logistics from control over global marketing.

As designs/recipes for lager or ethanol are broadly similar, what makes a 'premium' product is partly a marketing strategy targeting the high end of the market. Each brand image is tailored to attract a particular demographic or market segment. In her book, *No Logo*, Klein describes the Absolut vodka brand as a cultural sponge because of the flexibility with which it achieves this. The focus is the iconic bottle shape, filled with whatever symbol or emotion appeals most to the audience targeted by each magazine or other medium in which this award-winning advertising appears.

Commodity chain analysis highlights the importance of advertising and other marketing to a globalized alcohol industry. Policies that restrict brand marketing will affect sales, consumption levels, and global profits. This lies behind the assurances of responsible marketing and lobbying to retain industry self-regulation.

Social Aspects Organizations

A responsible face for the industry as a whole is presented by social aspects organizations. These are collaboratively funded by the large corporations to represent their noncompetitive interests. They have a strong focus on responsible drinking, and corporate websites cite support for these organizations as evidence of responsibility. A key function, however, is to influence policy and public opinion.

The International Center for Alcohol Policy in Washington operates at the global level, publishing reports on policy issues and offering advice to developing countries. The European Forum for Responsible Drinking (The Amsterdam Group, until 2006) plays the same role in Europe, and similar national organizations operate in most industrialized countries – for example, the Portman Group in Britain and the Century Council in the United States (**Figure 4**). Other industry bodies may represent beer, wine, or spirits producers, so it is not always apparent to the public that these responsible-sounding organizations represent the interests of 'Big Alcohol.'

The advocacy organization Eurocare (2002) identifies five viewpoints promoted by social aspects organizations:

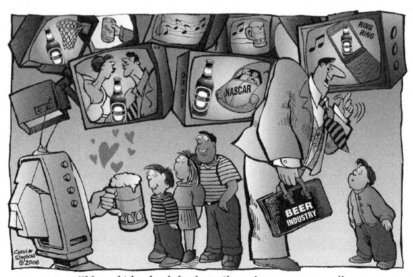

"Now, kids, don't look until you're twenty-one."

Figure 4   An e-postcard from the Get Serious campaign for effective alcohol policies in the United States. Source: Join Together, a program of the Boston School of Public Health, www.jointogether.com.

1. Individuals' patterns of drinking, rather than volume of alcohol consumption, is the best basis for alcohol policy.
2. Responsible drinking can be learned, so education should be the cornerstone of alcohol policy.
3. Alcohol, despite its potential for abuse, confers a net benefit to society.
4. Marketing should be self-regulated by the alcohol industry itself.
5. Social aspects organizations or other industry representatives should have an equal place at the policy table.

The first three views are not consistent with research evidence. Social aspects organizations support policies that are not effective in reducing alcohol-related harm, such as the youth education and designated driver programs for which they generously provide funding. These policy positions are promoted by directly lobbying policy makers, by discrediting evidence and funding alternative research, and by seeking to work in partnership with public health agencies and NGOs.

Partnership is a core value for community-based public health organizations. However, Eurocare has issued a public health 'warning' about partnerships with the alcohol industry and its social aspects organizations, as they result in weak policies being adopted and less effective use of public resources. In Australia, a partnership relationship with industry to promote responsible drinking led an advocacy group to change its previous position on alcopops (flavored alcoholic beverages) and support the appeal of an alcohol company against the licensing authority's decision to prohibit distribution of its alcoholic milk product, Moo Joose. Attendance at industry conferences has been used to imply endorsement of industry positions. Meetings to debate issues have later been used as evidence that industry participation in policy development is legitimate.

Eurocare's warning concludes with recommendations for relations with the alcohol industry. Governments should base policies on independent research and the public interest, recognizing that social aspects organizations are not impartial. NGOs play an important advocacy role on alcohol policy but for this role to be effective, they should maintain their independence from the industry and its organizations. The editors of the leading journal on alcohol, *Addiction,* have made similar recommendations to ensure the integrity of alcohol research (Edwards and Savva, 2001). In their view, any relationship with the industry, particularly funding, should be at arm's length, entered into with care, and made public.

These rules of engagement are consistent with the European health ministers' Declaration on Alcohol and Young People in 2001: "Public health policies concerning alcohol need to be formulated by public health interests, without interference from commercial interests" (p. 1).

Conclusion

The recent rapid global consolidation of the alcohol industry in the hands of relatively few large corporations has implications for public health. This is particularly so for developing countries now targeted as emerging markets for alcohol. Such countries typically have few alcohol policies or health services in place and governments may lack awareness of potential negative social and economic consequences of increased consumption.

Brand marketing is a feature of globalized companies. Economies of scale confer an unprecedented capacity to market alcohol and promote drinking – and this is a matter that requires policy attention. Company size and consolidation also mean increased resources for influencing policy to align with the interests of industry rather than of public health.

A globalized alcohol industry requires a globalized public health response. As policy makers and public health organizations formulate policies to reduce alcohol-related harm in communities, they need to be aware of industry strategies at both national and global levels. Effective responses will include international policy statements and precautionary trading principles agreed to by governments, supported by information sharing and collaboration between public health networks in industrialized and developing countries.

See also: Alcohol Consumption: Overview of International Trends; Alcohol: The Burden of Disease; Alcohol—Socio-Economic Impacts (Including Externalities); Alcoholism Treatment; Socio-Cultural Context of Substance Use/Abuse (Alcohol/Drugs/Tobacco); Regulation of Drugs and Drug Use: Public Health and Law Enforcement.

Citations

B & T (2005) Bundy sinks $30m into Australian rugby. http://www.bandt.com.au/news/sf/oc03865f.asp
Casswell S, Pledger M, and Pratap S (2002) Trajectories of drinking from 18 to 26 years: Identification and prediction. *Addiction* 97: 1427–1437.
Center on Alcohol Marketing and Youth (2003) Drops in the bucket: Alcohol industry 'responsibility' advertising on television in 2001. Washington DC: Georgetown University. www.camy.org.
Christie J, Fisher D, Kozup JC, Smith S, Burton S, and Creye EH (2001) The effects or bar-sponsored alcohol beverage promotions across binge and non-binge drinken. *Journal of Public Policy and Marketing* 20: 240–253.
Edwards G and Savva S (2001) ILSI Europe, the drinks industry, and a conflict of interest undeclared. *Addiction* 96(2): 197–202.
Eurocare (2002) The beverage alcohol industry's social aspects organizations: A public health warning. www.eurocare.org See also commentary in *Addiction* 99: 1375–1381.
Gould E (2005) Trade treaties and alcohol advertising policy. *Journal of Public Health Policy* 26(3): 359–376.
Grieshaber-Otto J, Sinclair S, and Schacter N (2000) Impacts of international trade, services and investment treaties on alcohol regulation. *Addiction* 95 (Supplement 4): S491–S504.

Grieshaber-Otto JN, Schacter N, and Sinclair S (2006) Dangerous Cocktail: International trade treaties, alcohol policy, public health. Cedar Isle Research. Report for the World Health Organization.

Huckle T and Huakau J (2006) Exposure and response of young people to marketing of alcohol in New Zealand. Auckland, New Zealand: The SHORE Centre.

Jernigan DH (2000) Applying commodity chain analysis to changing modes of alcohol supply in a developing country. *Addiction* 95 (Supplement 4): S465–S575.

Klein N (2001) No logo. London: Flamingo.

Room R and Jernigan D (2000) The ambiguous role of alcohol in economic and social development. *Addiction* 95 (Supplement 4): S523–S535.

Saffer H and Dave D (2002) Alcohol consumption and alcohol advertising bans. *Applied Economics* 34(11): 1325–1334.

World Bank Group (2000) Note on alcohol beverages. 14 March.

World Health Organization (2005) Bangkok charter for health promotion in a globalised world. Proceedings of the 6th Global Conference on Health Promotion, Bangkok, Thailand, August. http://www.who.int/healthpromotion/conferences/6gchp/bangkok_charter/en.

World Medical Association (2005) Statement on reducing the global impact of alcohol on health and society. Resolution of WMA Annual Assembly, Santiago, Chile. 14 October.

Casswell S and Maxwell A (2005) Regulation of alcohol marketing: A global view. *Journal of Public Health Policy* 26: 343–358.

Center for Alcohol Marketing and Youth (2004) Clicking with kids: Alcohol marketing and youth on the Internet. Washington, DC: CAMY March www.camy.org.

Hill L and Casswell S (2004) Alcohol advertising and sponsorship: Commercial freedom or control in the public interest? In: Heather N and Stockwell T (eds.) *The Essential Handbook on Treatment and Prevention of Alcohol Problems.* Chicester, UK: John Wiley & Sons.

Holder HD (ed) (2000) Special issue: The supply side Initiative International collaboration to study the alcohol supply. *Addiction* 95(Sup. 4).

Jernigan DH (1997) *Thirsting for Markets.* San Rafael: Marin Institute.

Jernigan DH and Mosher JF (eds) (2005) Special section: Global Alcohol marketing and youth-public health perspectives. *Journal of Public Health Policy* 26(3): 287–376.

Marshall M (2003) Market highs: Alcohol, drugs and the global economy in Oceania. In: Lockwood V (ed.) *Globalization and Culture Change in the Pacific Islands.* New Jersey: Prentice-Hall.

Room R, Jernigan D, Carlini-Marlatt B, *et al.* (2002) Alcohol in developing countries: A public health approach. Helsinki, Finland: Finnish Foundation for Alcohol Studies/World Health Organization.

Riley L and Marshall M (1999) *Alcohol and Public Health in 8 developing Countries.* Geneva, Switzerland: World Health Organization.

Further Reading

Babor T, Caetano R, Casswell S, *et al.* (2003) Regulating alcohol promotion. *In: Alcohol: No;Public Policy*, pp. 173–188. Oxford: Oxford University Press/World Health Organization.

Caetano R and Laranjeira R (2005) A 'perfect storm' in developing countries: Economic growth and the alcohol industry. *Addiction* 101: 149–152.

Relevant Websites

http://www.policyalternatives.ca – Canadian Centre for Policy Alternatives (CCPA).

http://camy.org – Center on Alcohol Marketing and Youth.

http://www.eurocare.org – Eurocare.

http://www.globalgapa.org – Global Alcohol Policy Alliance (GAPA).

Control and Regulation of Currently Illegal Drugs

J A Buxton, University of British Columbia, Vancouver, BC, Canada
M Haden, Vancouver Coastal Health, Vancouver, BC, Canada
R G Mathias, University of British Columbia, Vancouver, BC, Canada

Introduction

Worldwide debate continues regarding the best way to control the use of psychoactive substances. The distinction between currently legal and illegal drugs is not based on any analysis of the benefits of the drug or the best way to maximize the positive aspects and reduce harms. There is an increasing recognition that criminal justice tools, in isolation, are ineffective to manage the criminal, health, and social problems associated with illegal drug use (Bertram *et al.*, 1996). Evidence suggests that drug prohibition not only fails to address the problems, but also produces significant negative health and societal impacts. To address the problems created by drug prohibition the concept of a regulated market for all currently illegal drugs is being developed. This concept has grown out of the harm-reduction movement in which services are provided to active drug users without requiring abstinence (Health Officers Council of British Columbia [BC], 2005) Regulated market models are based on both public health and human rights principles that recognize psychoactive drug use as being a choice made by many people around the world.

Context of Use and Size of the Issue

Psychoactive drugs are used by many species and have been used by humans for as long as history has been recorded. Psychoactive drugs alter brain function, resulting in temporary changes in mood, perception, and behavior. These drugs may be used recreationally to intentionally alter one's consciousness, as entheogens

(Ruck *et al.*, 1979) for ritual or spiritual purposes, or as medication. Psychoactive substance use occurs along a spectrum from beneficial use, to nonproblematic use, through to problematic or harmful use, when use becomes habitual despite negative health impacts. Physical dependence may develop in some classes of drugs.

The *2006 World Drug Report* estimates that 200 million people, or 5% of the global population age 15–64 years have used currently illicit drugs as defined by the United Nations (UN) at least once in the last 12 months (UN Office on Drugs and Crime, 2006). This rate of drug use supports the concept that the majority of users are not addicted. Persons who use drugs do so because of perceived benefits in terms of the drug's desirable effects whether they are mental, physical, social, or spiritual. When addiction does develop, the reasons for it are a complex interaction of biological, psychological, social, spiritual, and environmental factors. In response to this complexity, a public health model has much to offer in the structuring of pragmatic responses (Tucker *et al.*, 1999).

Harms from drugs come from a variety of causes, which include toxicity (e.g., liver cirrhosis), overdose, addiction, and behavioral (e.g., drinking and driving) issues. Some drugs have minimal adverse behavior changes and few toxic effects, such as marijuana (Kalant *et al.*, 1999). Other drugs are highly toxic or are associated with undesirable behaviors such as crystal methamphetamine. An evidence-based approach to the control of drugs must recognize the benefits while minimizing the harms. Responding to both the harms and benefits of drugs will require drug-specific approaches rather than a one-size-fits-all approach.

History

Drug laws have been a common feature of human culture throughout history. Alcohol was prohibited under Islamic law and banned by the Koran more than a thousand years ago. Tobacco smokers returning from the Americas to Spain in the sixteenth century were subjected to torture, and in Russia Czar Michael Federovitch executed anyone on whom tobacco was found.

The United States antidrug legislation began in the late nineteenth century when smoking opium was banned in opium dens in San Francisco in 1875. The law was reported to have been a response to moral panic based on the fear that women, young girls, and young men were induced to visit the Chinese opium dens and were ruined morally and otherwise. These laws affected the use and distribution of opium by Chinese immigrants but not the use of laudanum, a combination of opium and alcohol used by Caucasian Americans. The laws were racist in both origin and intent.

In the United States the Harrison Narcotics Act was passed in 1914. This act required sellers of cocaine and opiates to have a license (usually only given to Caucasian people). It was originally intended to act as a revenue-tracking mechanism requiring a paper trail between doctors, drugstores, and patients. In 1920, the Supreme Court upheld, as a violation of the Harrison Act, that if a physician provided prescription narcotics for an addict, s/he was liable to prosecution. The Controlled Substances Act in 1970 replaced the Harrison Narcotics Act as the primary drug law in the United States. Drugs were classified according to their medicinal use, potential for abuse, and their likelihood of producing dependence.

The UN Single Convention on Narcotic Drugs was introduced in 1961, and this established the current system of global drug prohibition. It considered that addiction to narcotic drugs constituted a significant evil for the individual and economic danger to society. U.S. President Richard Nixon's War on Drugs began in 1969. Countries throughout the world have accepted drug prohibition because of the enormous pressure from the U.S. government, which continues to lead the War on Drugs and has found drug prohibition useful for its own purposes (Levine, 2002). The UN Convention Against Illicit Traffic in Narcotic Drugs and Psychotropic Substances was adopted in 1988, which further entrenched the prohibitionist framework.

The United States has the highest prison population rate in the world (Walmsley, 2003). According to the U.S. Justice Department, "while the number of offenders in each major offence category increased (from 1995 to 2003), the number of persons incarcerated for a drug offense accounted for the largest percentage of total growth (49%)" (Harrison and Beck, 2005b: 10).

There are many parallels between drug prohibition and alcohol prohibition. Despite the prohibition of alcohol going into effect in 1920, alcohol was readily available in most of the United States. Beer drinking was reduced, but consumption of stronger, hard liquor increased. When alcohol use was outlawed, it gave rise to gang warfare and spurred the formation of some of the most well-known criminals. The end of prohibition in 1933 led to an immediate decrease in murders and robberies.

Public Health and Social Harms of Prohibition

Tobacco and alcohol are currently legal drugs in most countries and have been branded and advertised. The long history of the commercialism of these two legal drugs has intentionally increased consumption of these drugs, both of which have significant potential for harm. Their widespread use results in greater morbidity, mortality, and overall economic costs than illegal drugs (World Health Organization [WHO], 2003; Rehm *et al.*, 2006).

Therefore, an evidence-based model with the goal of reducing health and social harms from psychoactive substances should also include tobacco (Borland, 2003; Callard *et al.*, 2005) and alcohol (Babor *et al.*, 2003) as they are currently underregulated substances. If tobacco and alcohol were regulated according to public health principles, there would be significant changes to the current system. For example, unbranded tobacco could be sold in plain, inconvenient packaging with ingredient labeling and dominant warning labels. The concentration of nicotine could be slowly reduced to achieve specific public health goals. Pricing and taxation of alcohol could be more strategic with the goal of reducing harms.

Prohibition is defined as a law, order, or decree that forbids something. Drug prohibition criminalizes the production, possession, sales, and – in some countries – the consumption of drugs. It aims to reduce demand by disrupting drug production, supply, and distribution, and to identify consumers of illegal drugs by using law enforcement resources to prosecute and punish them. Prohibition reduces demand and consumption only if the producers, consumers, and sellers of drugs respect the law.

Many of the harms typically attributed to illegal drug consumption are due not to the drugs *per se*, but to the *prohibition* of them. Drug prohibition creates a robust black market, which makes concentrated, sometimes toxic drugs widely available and produces many health and social pathologies, including:

- Increased transmission of HIV
- Corruption of police, civic, and elected officials
- Violence
- Crime
- Destabilization of governments
- Destabilization of world markets
- Criminalization of youth
- Creation and support for organized crime groups
- Disrespect for the law.

Consequently, there is inconsistency between the declared motives of the law enforcement agencies to reduce crime and the laws themselves. This is beginning to change; in the United States, law enforcement officials are starting to challenge drug prohibition (Law Enforcement Against Prohibition, 2007).

Evidence suggests that drug prohibition is ineffective, as the amount of drug use in societies fluctuates independently of the severity of enforcement measures (MacCoun and Reuter, 2001; Nolin 2002). The continued arrest, prosecution, and incarceration of people violating the drug laws have failed to reduce the chronic, societal problem of drug abuse and its public and economic costs. Despite the increasing amounts of money being spent on prohibition, drugs have become more accessible, cheaper, and more potent through the illegal drug trade in the United States and Europe (UN Office on Drugs and Crime, 2006).

A public health approach to the individual and societal problems associated with substance use stresses the need to shift resources into research, education, prevention, and treatment as an alternative to the continued use of criminal sanctions (Geller, 1997; Tucker *et al.*, 1999; King County Bar Association, 2005). Public and population health tools can be used to examine the social determinants of health, which include the economic and social conditions that interact to influence the health of individuals and communities. Over the last century, the improvements in the health of individuals in developed countries have not been shared equally among all members of society. Illicit drug use and addiction are associated with marginalized and disadvantaged populations. To further improve the health of the population, we must reduce the health inequities between social groups (Wilkinson, 1997) and improve the social determinants of health among the most vulnerable groups.

Seeing drug use as a health issue, and not a criminal issue, allows policy makers to explore a wide range of public health tools to manage the problems in a more effective way. The social determinants of health require a focus on policies, organizations, and social structure (Sanders, 2006). The formation of the Commission on the Social Determinants of Health by the WHO in 2005 recognizes that there needs to be greater focus on these upstream determinants (Marmot, 2005).

Unintended Consequences of Prohibition

Crime and violence

The unintended consequences of prohibition have considerably negative criminal, health, and social impacts. The vast majority of the negative impacts to society stems from black market culture (e.g., organized crime and dealer disputes). Prohibition leads to wealth transfer to criminals and thus corruption. It encourages the development of a robust black market, some of which may be managed by highly cohesive, large, organized criminal groups, with spillover into seemingly legitimate businesses (Robinson, 1999; Office of the Auditor General of Canada, 2001; Sher and Marsden, 2003). The use of criminal funds to corrupt public officials, both elected and appointed, is all too common. Violence can occur because people in the drug 'industry' have wealth in highly portable forms (i.e., drugs and cash), which make them obvious targets for theft or robbery. Miron (2004) observes that violence occurs as a form of dispute resolution among people who cannot use legal channels because their disputes are occurring in an illegal industry.

The United States has more people per capita in jail than any other country, and 55% of federal prisoners are there due to drug crimes (Harrison and Beck, 2005b). However, the United States has more drug use per capita than most European countries (Hibell *et al.*, 2003). Miron found a strong correlation between the violent crime and homicide rates with drug law enforcement. He suggests eliminating drug prohibition would likely cut the homicide rate in the United States by 25–75% (Miron, 2004).

Overdose

Heroin overdose risk is directly related to its strength and purity (Brugal *et al.*, 2002; Buxton, 2005). To conceal drugs, suppliers will produce and ship the drug in the most concentrated forms (Thornton, 1998). Due to the illegal production and distribution of drugs the user is unaware of the purity and strength of the purported drug, and ignorant of other active constituents, adulterants, and diluents contained in the substance they purchase. Consequently, prohibition increases uncertainty about the product quality.

Emphasis on supply reduction and police crackdowns can result in unsafe injection practices as users inject hastily without 'tasting' their drugs to avoid police detection and therefore increase the risk of overdose. Police may force users 'underground' and away from health and other support services (Canty *et al.*, 2005).

Drug price

Prohibition may reduce the price of drugs. Although prohibition may raise supply costs as production and distribution is by illegal means, drug suppliers do not pay income or social security taxes, nor do they need to obey minimum wage laws or other labor regulations. As a result, prohibition does not appear to raise the price of drugs or reduce consumption as much as is commonly thought (Thornton, 1991).

Ethnic and racial disparities

The use and effects of drug use are not evenly distributed among different ethnic groups. Vulnerable populations have experienced the overall negative impact of drug abuse and drug prohibition more severely than the general population (Clifford, 1992). Cocaine and crack in particular affect low-income neighborhoods (Reinarman and Levine, 1997). There are disproportionate arrests and incarcerations of ethnic minorities (King County Bar Association, 2005). In the United States, African-Americans constitute 12.1% of the population (U.S. Census Bureau, 2000) but represent 47.3% of all state inmates for drug offences and 74% of all those sentenced to prison for drug possession (Harrison and Beck, 2005b). Among males aged 25–29 years, 12.6% of African-Americans are in prison or jail compared to 3.6% of Hispanics and about 1.75% of Caucasians (Harrison and Beck, 2005a). Most are poor people of color imprisoned for possessing an illicit drug or 'intending' to sell small amounts (Reinarman and Levine, 1997; Levine, 2002).

Youth involvement

An inability to enforce drug laws results in the engagement of youth with the drug culture and high-school-aged youth become a popular conduit through which drugs are distributed. It is difficult to persuade a youth who is making hundreds of dollars in an evening that he should work at a minimum-wage job. This directly contradicts the 'protect the children' arguments from those who argue for prohibition.

Harm Reduction: Philosophy and Current Initiatives

The concept of a regulated market for currently illegal drugs began with the concept of harm reduction, which is slowly becoming the accepted model of treatment in many countries around the globe (Levine, 2002). Although the harm-reduction movement stresses the freedom of individuals' and users' rights, its main incentive is to improve the population's health (Tammi and Hurme, 2007). Harm reduction is a philosophical, ethical, and pragmatic approach. It focuses on the harms resulting from substance use rather than the substance use itself. Therefore the aim is to keep people safe and minimize death, disease, and injury associated with higher risk behaviors. It does not insist on abstinence, but involves a range of nonjudgmental strategies aimed at enhancing the knowledge skills, resources, and supports for individuals, their families, and communities to be safer and healthier (Tucker *et al.*, 1999; Denning, 2000). Tammi and Hurme reflect that:

> drug use is a normal action that inevitably occurs in modern society, and therefore users should be treated fairly as sovereign citizens and their possible problems should be tackled pragmatically and on the basis of scientific knowledge. (2007: 86)

Levine and Reinarman (2004) suggest that harm reduction in effect, though not always in intent, pushes drug policies from the more punitive forms of drug prohibition toward the more tolerant and regulated forms. The Harm Reduction Model of Controlled Drug Availability proposed by Burrows states that:

> drug policy should: have realistic goals; take into account the different patterns and types of harms caused by specific drugs; be shown to be effective or changed; separate arguments about the consequences of drug use from arguments about morals; be developed in the light of the costs of control as well as the benefits; ensure that the harms caused by the control regimes themselves do not outweigh the harms prevented by them; and recognise the existence of multiple goals, but ensure that contradictory goals are minimised. (2005: 8–9)

Harm-reduction initiatives such as needle or syringe exchange programs and methadone maintenance treatment, despite being initially controversial, are now generally accepted in many countries. Even the UN agencies that supervise worldwide drug prohibition recognize the public health benefits of harm-reduction services within current drug prohibition regimes (Levine and Reinarman, 2004). However, more recent initiatives such as supervised injection/consumption sites, heroin prescription, and distribution of crack pipes and other paraphernalia to facilitate safer crack use, have received less support and have been actively opposed by some political and enforcement agencies. The City of Vancouver, British Columbia has been largely successful in the implementation of new harm-reduction programs which were initially controversial but are now accepted and supported. It is useful to examine these programs as they begin to fundamentally challenge the utility of drug prohibition.

City of Vancouver 'four-pillar' approach and supervised injection facility

The City of Vancouver is typical of the harm-reduction movement by adopting a 'four-pillar' approach (MacPherson, 2001). This policy integrates four pillars: prevention, treatment, harm reduction, and enforcement. Each pillar should not be considered an isolated pillar, as the name implies. The Vancouver Police Department was a partner in the establishment of the Vancouver supervised injection site; the first site of its kind in North America. As the supervised injection facility (SIF) does not provide drugs on prescription, all users would enter the facility in possession of illegal drugs. This forced unprecedented discussions and cooperation between the Vancouver Police Department and health service providers. The police recognized the importance of the SIF as a harm-reduction initiative for public health benefits – such as reducing transmission of infectious diseases and overdose deaths – rather than a means to reduce criminal activity.

The SIF has been found to be effective in improving public order (Kerr et al., 2006), and increases in both safer injecting practices and reduced syringe sharing have been observed (Kerr et al., 2005). This service has increased use of detoxification programs and other addiction treatments (Wood et al., 2006). Despite these and other positive evaluations being published in peer review literature, the SIF has been subject to nonevidence-based political pressures (McKnight, 2007).

Prescription heroin

The usefulness of opiates for controlling pain is well accepted worldwide. Hence there are regulations around opiate production, manufacture, and use that recognize the benefits and try to reduce potential harms. Prescription heroin trials were introduced in Switzerland in 1994 and in the Netherlands in 1998. Co-prescription of heroin was found to be cost effective compared to methadone alone (Dijkgraaf et al., 2005), and individuals in this study showed improvements in mental and physical health (Rehm et al., 2001). A randomized controlled trial of prescription heroin is currently underway in Canada, known as the North America Opiate Medication Initiative (NAOMI) in Vancouver and Montreal, the results of which will be available in 2008.

If prescribed heroin were available, drug dealers would be unable to sell this drug to opiate dependent users who would obtain the drug more cheaply on prescription. With no dealers to apprehend, police could focus their limited resources on more serious criminals. Property crime, formerly committed by users to obtain money to purchase drugs, would be reduced dramatically. The head of the British Association of Chief Police Officers suggested heroin should be prescribed to long-term addicts to prevent them from committing crimes to feed their habits (Bennetto, 2007). However, providing users with drugs would require additional funding, to distinguish recreational users from dependent individuals.

Netherlands 'coffee shops'

The cannabis policies of the Netherlands are a regulated form of *de facto* drug legalization for consumers. Coffee shops are heavily controlled business establishments where adults can purchase small quantities of soft drugs for personal use in the form of joints, pastry, drinks, and packages. Cannabis and other 'soft' drugs are available only in small quantities. Advertising is not allowed and there is a limit on individual transactions (5 grams) and maximum stock (500 grams). Although sales appear to be completely legal, the importation and commercial production of cannabis is illegal in the Netherlands. Hence, the coffee shops are supplied by illegal importers and growers. In spite of the open availability of cannabis, the Netherlands have a lower rate of cannabis use with an average 3% regular use (17% lifetime) (Trimbos Institute, 2002), compared to U.S. 5.4% recurring use (36.9% lifetime) (U.S. Department of Health and Human Services Substance Abuse and Mental Health Services Adminstration, 2002). This addresses the fear that open availability always leads to increased consumption. Consumption patterns are influenced by many forces in society including the drug-using culture, which is very difficult to influence in the prohibitionist model.

The success of the Netherlands less punative cannabis policy has contributed to the spread of *de facto* and formal cannabis decriminalization in Spain, Switzerland, Portugal, Germany, and the UK (Reinarman et al., 2004).

Compassion clubs

Medical cannabis dispensaries, also called compassion clubs, supply cannabis for therapeutic use on recommendation from a licensed health-care practitioner through Canada's Medical Marijuana Access Division established in 1999. Although communities, law enforcement, and criminal courts across Canada have shown support and tolerance for medical marijuana the legal supply of cannabis remains problematic and Canadian dispensaries are currently operating without a license (Capler and Lucas, 2006). It has been observed that allowing medical cannabis use does not increase use in the general population (Gorman, 2007).

Many industrial countries have developed policies or practices that challenge global drug prohibition. These range from official nonenforcement of cannabis laws to state-sanctioned SIFs and heroin prescription programs made possible through exemptions from the prohibition-based legal framework and not through fundamental changes of that framework (King County Bar Association, 2005). These steps are all slowly and incrementally leading to a fundamental reconsideration of drug prohibition.

Alternate Models of Drug Control

The Development of a Regulated Market Concept

It is slowly becoming recognized that harm-reduction programs are insufficient. They still exist within a prohibitionist framework, which is responsible for the creation of many of the problems that harm reduction attempts to alleviate (Health Officers Council of BC, 2005). Therefore, the debate is shifting toward development of the concept of a regulated market for all psychoactive drugs (Nolin, 2002; Health Officers Council of BC, 2005; Transform Drug Policy Foundation, 2006) including what are considered the most dangerous drugs, the smokable and injectable stimulants (Haden, 2008).

A regulated market model should be based on public health and human rights principles, which could interact to address the benefits and the problems produced by drugs and the problems produced by drug prohibition. Decriminalization or just withdrawing the legal sanctions is insufficient, as this would allow the black market to thrive. A model of regulated access needs to be developed to apply evidence-based, cost-effective models of use.

Unlike some debates regarding control of illegal drugs, there is not a strict dichotomy between prohibition and legalization (Haden, 2002). Examining the range of options through the enforcement lens leads to the observation of three models of community-based drug law enforcement (Canty et al., 2005). At one end is the prohibitionist model in which police are totally dedicated to supply reduction; next is the modified supply reduction model, in which police see supply reduction as their overriding goal but acknowledge the legitimacy of harm-reduction work and try not to undermine it; and, finally, market regulation, in which police are committed to harm minimization and

recognize that supply reduction is just one of a range of methods to reduce drug-related harms.

Some prohibitionists mistakenly perceive legalization as being the same as a free, uncontrolled market and that addictive psychoactive substances might be available as branded and commercial products without controls and regulations. In fact, a public-health-based regulated market could produce a more controlled market than currently exists under prohibition. For example, prohibition actively engages our youth, who then often sell to each other with no age or other controls. The Monitoring the Future report documents the high level of perceived availability of currently illegal drugs. For example, for grade 12 students in the United States, 84.9% report marijuana is 'fairly easy' or 'very easy' to obtain, 46.5% report the same for cocaine, and 52.9% report the same for amfetamines (Johnston et al., 2006).

A regulated market would acknowledge that heroin, cocaine, Ecstasy, and marijuana have very different pharmacological and behavioral effects. The mode and frequency of administration may vary, and be subject to drug availability. The potential for different drugs to cause dependence and acute and chronic harms also varies widely. A regulated market would need to match the appropriate regulatory options with specific administrative and social controls for each classification of drugs. These options would be based on a benefit to harm ratio for each substance.

King County Bar Association

In 2001, a group of lawyers within the King County Bar Association in Seattle, Washington, put forward four principles to guide reform of drug control policies and practices. These principles stated that public policy should result in no more harm than the drug use itself, and it should address the underlying causes and resultant harms of drug abuse rather than discouraging drug use through criminal sanctions. It should also recognize citizens' individual liberties and the efficient use of scarce public resources (King County Bar Association Drug Policy Project, 2001).

The King County Bar Association proposed a new legal framework intended to render illegal markets of psychoactive substances unprofitable, to restrict access by young persons, and to provide health care to persons with chemical dependency and addiction. They suggest that such a framework would serve to reduce crime, improve public order, enhance public health, protect children, and use scarce public resources better than current drug policies (King County Bar Association, 2005). This framework would begin to develop the foundational principles of a new post-prohibition model.

Public Health Approaches to Drug Regulation

Haden examined ways in which drugs should be regulated (Haden, 2004). Some of the approaches or mechanisms that would be considered in a public health approach include:

Age of purchaser. There are currently restrictions to access of alcohol and tobacco based on age, but there is no control of the age when illegal drugs can be purchased. Drug dealers today do not ask their customers for age identification.

Degree of intoxication of purchaser. In Canada, the sale of alcohol is restricted based on the degree of intoxication of the purchaser. Sellers can refuse to sell to a customer whom they perceive to be engaging in high-risk, substance-using behavior.

Volume rationing. Quantities would be limited to a certain amount deemed appropriate for personal consumption.

Proof of dependence prior to purchase. Initially sales could be limited to those with addiction concerns.

Proof of 'need' to purchase. Beyond those drugs on which people are dependent, other drugs such as LSD and MDMA (Ecstasy), which have been shown to have potential psychotherapeutic benefits when used in controlled therapeutic environments, could be used with registered and trained psychiatrists and psychologists. Need can also be defined as a cultural/spiritual need, as peyote and ayahuasca (Tupper, in press) have been used by aboriginal groups in sacred traditions for centuries.

Required training for purchasers. Training programs could provide information to drug users about addiction, treatment services, and other public health issues, such as sexually transmitted diseases and bloodborne illnesses. The programs could provide the knowledge and skills aimed at discouraging drug use, reducing the amount of drug use, and reducing the harm of drug use.

Registrations of purchasers. This would allow the purchasers to be tracked for 'engagement' and health education.

Licensing of users. Like licenses for new motor vehicle drivers that restrict where and when they drive and whom they are permitted to drive with, these licenses would control time, place, and associations for new substance users. This would be a graduated program with demonstrated responsible, nonharmful drug use. The license could be given demerit points or be suspended based on infractions, such as providing substances to nonlicensed users, driving under the influence, or public intoxication. The licenses could also specify different levels of access to various substances based on levels of training and experience. People in some professions, such as airplane pilots or taxi drivers, could be restricted from obtaining licenses to purchase long-acting drugs that impair motor skills.

Proof of residency with purchase. Some societies have gone through a process of developing culturally specific social controlling mechanisms that form over time a certain amount of relatively healthy, unproblematic relationships with substances. 'Drug tourists' who have not been integrated into this culture may behave in problematic ways that do not adhere to the local restraining social practices. Therefore, purchasers may be restricted to residents of a country, state/province, city, or neighborhood.

Limitations in allowed locations for use. Alcohol is often restricted from public consumption and some public locations do not allow tobacco consumption. Locations for substance use could vary based on the potential for harm. Options of locations include supervised injection rooms for injected drugs, supervised consumption rooms for the smoking of heroin and cocaine, and home use for drugs with less potential for harm.

Administration of test prior to purchase. A short test could be administered at the distribution point to demonstrate to the staff that the purchaser has the required knowledge of safe use of the substance, which is likely to minimize harm.

Tracking of consumption habits. Registered purchasers would have the volume and frequency of purchasing tracked. This could be used to instigate health interventions by health professionals who could register their concerns with the user and offer assistance if a problem is identified. The tracking may be a deterrent to use, as well as a possible increase in price of the substance once the user has passed a certain volume threshold.

Required membership in a group prior to purchase. Drug users can belong to advocacy or union groups that would act similarly to existing professional regulatory bodies that provide practice guidelines for their members. If the user acts outside of the norms of the discipline, the group can intervene or ultimately refuse membership. The norms are enforced through a variety of peer processes and education.

Shared responsibility between the provider and the consumer. Sellers could be partially responsible for the behaviors of the consumers. To that end, the sellers would monitor the environment where the drug is used and restrict sales based on the behavior of the consumers. Proprietors could be held responsible through fines or license revocations for automobile accidents or other socially destructive incidents for a specified period of time after the drug is consumed. The consumer would not be absolved of responsibility but a balance would be established in which the consumer and seller were both liable.

Maximum allowable limit for the consumer. A previously negotiated, maximum allowable limit for each individual could be implemented or the consumer could be allowed to put a 'stop purchase' order on themselves for a fixed period of time.

Order/delivery delay times. A delay of hours or days between time of order and product delivery may serve to reduce the incidence of out-of-control sequential use patterns.

Regulatory controls can also be targeted at sales/distribution outlets. The amount per package, formulation, and concentration of product can be specified. Examples include:

- Licensing of outlets, that is, municipalities can specify where outlets exist, hours of operation, and appearance.
- Warning posters and handout information can be available to consumers.
- A pharmacy specialist may be required to be on-site to provide information to consumers.
- Clean needles or new smoking equipment can be provided with purchase.
- Adjunctive services (i.e., withdrawal services, medical, or nursing care) may be required to be available either on-site or nearby.

Corporate restrictions include:

- Price can be controlled to initially eliminate the black market and then to generate a revenue stream for government.
- Profit controls can ensure that health and social issues always have priority over the need for corporations to maximize profitability.
- Sales can be restricted to government-run outlets only.
- Taxation levels can be specified by government.
- A percentage of the taxation can be allocated to prevention and treatment programs.
- There can be a ban of public trading of stocks for companies who sell these products.
- Advertising and sponsorship of events can be prohibited, as the intended outcome of promotion is increased consumption.

Product and packaging restrictions include:

- The design of the package can be specified. The use of color, logos, and images can be controlled.
- Governments can be responsible for all packaging.
- Warning and ingredient labels can be mandatory.
- Branding must be prohibited as allowing branding is the beginning of a process that inevitably leads to advertising, which encourages consumption. Governments would therefore have to be responsible for the packaging and sales of these products.

The Medical Health Officers Council of British Columbia proposed a policy framework for a comprehensive approach to psychoactive substances. With the overall goal to minimize harms from use, policies and programs are associated with all psychoactive substances and a realization of the benefits for individuals, families, communities, and society. The policy is based on rational and respectful discussion, and includes involving those directly affected, being explicit when policies and strategies are made without supporting evidence and encouraging pilot research (when evidence is lacking) with careful evaluation (Health Officers Council of BC, 2005).

Prohibitionist drug policy has not evolved in response to evaluation, but rather is a response to historical, moral, and political influences (Transform Drug Policy Foundation, 2006). The concept of regulated market should be explored as an evidence-based model that has the goal of reducing health and social harms from currently illegal drugs.

Critics

Critics of legalization, who assume that this means free market access, warn that the legalization of a 'soft drug' (e.g., cannabis) in an area may lead to increased sales of harder drugs (e.g., heroin). They propose that problems associated with illegal heroin use (e.g., fatalities, muggings, burglaries, use of infected needles) would rise in the area, possibly leading the authorities to conclude that the full legalization of cannabis would exacerbate the situation.

The experience of the Netherlands is significant as they have shown that openly selling a drug does not lead to societal collapse. In fact, *de facto* legalization of cannabis for consumers has been used as a tactic to separate 'soft' and 'hard' drug markets and has not lead to high rates of cannabis use. That legal sanctions are not usually correlated with consumption rates was observed in 11 American states and several jurisdictions in Australia where decrimalization and subsequent recriminalization of cannabis neither increased nor decreased consumption rates (Single *et al*, 2000).

Market Regulation: Controlling Drugs Not Legalization

A regulated market could be implemented to substantially reduce the illegal drug business and most of the crime, violence, and corruption associated with it (Levine and Reinarman, 2004). A regulated market with a public health and human rights orientation would also seek to substitute milder and weaker drugs and make them available in safer preparations to reduce the demand for more dangerous substances. Also, there would need to be comprehensive education about risks and benefits of the different modes of administration. An evidence-based model is needed which explores how increased availability of weaker oral solutions of some drugs can reduce the demand for more dangerous substances.

Legalizing and regulating drug production and supply would lead to a dramatic decrease in crime at all levels, as legally regulated supplies of heroin and cocaine to active addicts do not necessitate fundraising offending and would therefore have the potential to reduce property-associated crime (Transform Drug Policy Foundation, 2006).

Despite many benefits of regulating drug markets, there will be a minority of users who continue to use irresponsibly and suffer harms, and some will die as a direct result of their use. Regulation will remove the health and social problems associated with drug prohibition and the criminal markets, which encourage out-of-control use patterns. A regulated market would allow the creation of consumption facilities, which are supervised and therefore create spaces where harmful, drug-using behaviors can be directly influenced to actually reduce harm.

When drugs are purchased in the underground market they may be cut with other substances or sold under different guises to increase profit or user addiction potential. The purity and constituents are unknown. A regulated market would control for both concentration and purity of drugs.

When our society is able to move forward on the creation of a regulated market, policy makers would need to anticipate a brief period when there may be more experimentation of drugs. This can be controlled by making changes incrementally and slowly and evaluating the effects of each change. We would therefore be able to create a regulated market for all currently illegal drugs that is evidence based and actually reduces the harms created by both drugs and drug prohibition.

See also: Primary Prevention Strategies for Illicit Drug Use; Illicit Drug Trends Globally; Illicit Drug Use and the burden of Disease.

Citations

Babor T, Caetano R, Casswell S, et al. (2003) *Alcohol: No Ordinary Commodity, Research and Public Policy.* Oxford, UK: Oxford University Press.

Bennetto J (2007) Police chief calls for heroin to be available on the NHS. London: *The Independent.*

Bertram E, Blachman M, Sharpe K, and Andreas P (1996) *Drug War Politics: The Price of Denial.* Berkley, CA: University of California Press.

Borland R (2003) A strategy for controlling the market of tobacco product: A regulated market model. *Tobacco Control* 12: 372–382.

Brugal TM, Barrio G, Fuente LDL, Regidor E, Royuela L, and Suelves JM (2002) Factors associated with non-fatal heroin overdose: Assessing the effect of frequency and route of heroin administration. *Addiction* 97: 319.

Burrows D (2005) Towards a regulated market for illicit drugs: Effects of the harm reduction model of control drug availability. *International Journal of Drug Policy* 16: 8–9.

Buxton J (2005) Vancouver drug use epidemiology: Vancouver site report for the Canadian Community Epidemiology Network on Drug Use (CCENDU). Vancouver, BC.

Callard C, Thompson D, and Collishaw N (2005) Transforming the tobacco market: Why the supply of cigarettes should be transferred from for profit corportations to non-profit enterprises with a public health mandate. *Tobacco Control* 14: 278–283.

Canty C, Sutton A, and James S (2005) Strategies for community-based drug law enforcement: From prohibition to harm reduction. In: Stockwell T, Gruenewald PJ, Toumbourou JW, and Loxley W (eds.) *Preventing Harmful Substance Use: The Evidence Base for Policy and Practice,* pp. 225–236. London: Wiley.

Capler R and Lucas P (2006) Guidelines for the community-based distribution of medical cannabis, British Columbia Compassion Club Society and the Vancouver Island Compassion Club Society Vancouver, BC: Compassion Club Sociey.

Clifford PR (1992) Drug use, drug prohibition and minority communities. *Journal of Primary Prevention* 12(4): 297–310.

Denning P (2000) *Practicing Harm Reduction Psychotherapy: An Alternative Approach to Addiction.* New York: Guilford Press.

Dijkgraaf MGW, Zanden BPvd, Borgie CAJMd, Blanken P, Ree JMv, and Brink Wvd (2005) Cost utility analysis of co-prescribed heroin compared with methadone maintenance treatment in heroin addicts in two randomised trials. *British Medical Journal* 330: 1297.

Geller A (1997) Comprenhensive treatment programs. In: Lowinson JH, Ruiz P, Millman RB, and Langrod JG (eds.) *Substance Abuse: A Comprehensive Textbook,* 3rd edn., pp. 425–429. Baltimore, MD: Williams and Wilkins.

Gorman DM (2007) Do medical cannabis laws encourage cannabis use? *International Journal of Drug Policy* 18: 160–167.

Haden M (2002) Illicit IV drugs: A public health approach. *Canadian Journal of Public Health* 93: 431–434.

Haden M (2004) Regulation of illegal drugs: An exploration of public health tools. *International Journal of Drug Policy* 15: 225–230.

Haden M (2008) Controlling illegal stimulants: a regulated market model. *Harm Reduction Journal* 5: 1.

Harrison PM and Beck AJ (2005a) *Bureau of Justice Statistics, Prison and Jail Inmates at Midyear 2004.* Washington, DC: U.S. Dept of Justice.

Harrison PM and Beck AJ (2005b) *Bureau of Justice Statistics, Prisoners in 2004.* Washington, DC: U.S. Dept of Justice.

Health Officers Council of British Columbia (2005) *A Public Health Approach to Drug Control in Canada.* Victoria, BC: Health Officers Council of British Columbia.

Hibell B, Andersson B, Bjarnason T, et al. (2004) The ESPAD report 2003: Alcohol and other drug use among students in 35 European countries, Swedish Council for Information on Alcohol and Other Drugs, the Pompidou Group at the Council of Europe. Printed in Sweden by Modintryckoffset AB, Stockholm, November 2004.

Johnston LD, O'Malley PM, Bachman JG, and Schulenberg JE (2006) Monitoring the future: National results on adolescent drug use, overview of key findings, U.S. Department of Health and Human Services. Bethesda, MD: National Institute on Drug Abuse.

Kalant H, Corrigall W, Hall W, and Smart R (1999) *The Health Effects of Cannabis.* Toronto, ON: Addiction Research Foundation, Centre for Addiction and Mental Health.

King County Bar Association Drug Policy Project (2001) Is it time to end the war on drugs: An examination of current law and practice in drug abuse prevention, drug addiction treatment, and the use of criminal sanctions, King County Bar Association, Board of Trustees. Seattle, WA: King County Bar Association.

King County Bar Association Drug Policy Project (2005) *Parameters of a New Legal Framework for Psychoactive Substance Control.* Seattle, WA: King County Bar Association.

Law Enforcement Against Prohibition (LEAP) (2007) http://www.leap.cc (accessed February 2008).

Levine HG (2002) The secret of worldwide drug prohibition. The varieties and uses of drug prohibition. *Independent Review* 7: 165–180.

MacPherson D (2001) A framework for action: A four pillar approach to drug problems in Vancouver. Vancouver, BC: City of Vancouver.

Marmot M (2005) Social determinants of health inequalities. *The Lancet* 365: 1099–1104.

McKnight P (2007) It isn't balanced when opinion runs as fact. *Vancouver Sun* Saturday May 12, 2007.

Nolin PC (2002) *Cannabis: Our Position for a Canadian Public Policy.* Ottawa, ON: Senate Committee, Government of Canada.

Rehm J, Baliunas D, Brochu S, et al. (2006) *The Costs of Substance Abuse in Canada 2002.* Ottawa, ON: Canadian Centre on Substance Abuse.

Rehm J, Gschwend P, Steffen T, Gutzwiller F, Dobler-Mikola A, and Uchtenhagen A (2001) Feasibility, safety, and efficacy of injectable heroin prescription for refractroy opioid addicts: A follow-up study. *The Lancet* 358: 1417–1420.

Reinarman C, Cohen P, and Kaal HL (2004) The limited relevance of drug policy: Cannabis in Amsterdam and San Francisco. *American Journal of Public Health* 94: 836–842.

Reinarman C and Levine HG (1997) The crack attack: Politics and media in the crack scare. In: Rienarman C and Levine HG (eds.) *Crack in America: Demon Drugs and Social Justice,* pp. 15–81. Berkeley, CA: University of California Press

Robinson J (1999) *The Merger: How Organized Crime Is Taking Over Canada and the World*. Toronto, ON: McClelland and Stewart.

Ruck C, Bigwood J, Staples D, Ott J, and Wasson RG (1979) Entheogens. *Journal of Psychedelic Drugs* 11: 145–146.

Sanders D (2006) A global perspective on health promotion and the social determinants of health. *Health Promotion Journal of Australia* 17: 165–167.

Sher J and Marsden W (2003) *The Road to Hell: How the Biker Gangs Are Conquering Canada*. Toronto, ON: Random House of Canada.

Single E, Christie P, and Ali R (2000) The impact of cannabis decriminalisation in Australia and the United States. *Journal of Public Health Policy* 21: 157–167.

Tammi T and Hurme T (2007) How the harm reduction movement contrasts itself against punitive prohibiton. *International Journal of Drug Policy* 18: 84–87.

Thornton M (1991) *The Economics of Prohibition*. Salt Lake City: University of Utah Press.

Thornton M (1998) The potentency of illegal drugs. *Journal of Drug Issues* 28: 725–740.

Transform Drug Policy Foundation (2006) After the war on drugs: Options for control. London: Transform Drug Policy Foundation.

Trimbos Institute (2002) *Report to the EMCDDA by the Reitox National Focal Point, The Netherlands Drug Situation 2002, European Monitoring Centre for Drugs and Drug Addiction, November, 2002*. Utrecht, the Netherlands: Trimbos Institute.

Tucker JA, Donovan DM, and Marlatt GA (1999) *Changing Addictive Behavior: Bridging Clinical and Public Health Strategies*. New York: Guilford Press.

Tupper KW (in press) The globalization of ayahuasca: Harm reduction or benefit maximization? *International Journal of Drug Policy*.

UN Office on Drugs and Crime (2006) *2006 World Drug Report*. Geneva, Switzerland: UN Office on Drugs and Crime.

U.S. Census Bureau (2000) Census 2000 redistricting data (PL94–171) summary file for states, population by race and Hispanic or Latino origin for the United States, Department of Commerce. Washington, DC: U.S. Census Bureau.

U.S. Department of Health Human Services Substance Abuse and Mental Health Services Adminstration (2002) National household survey on drug abuse: Volume I. Summary of national findings, Washington, DC. Washington, D.C: U.S. Department of Health and Human Services Substance Abuse and Mental Health Services Adminstration.

Walmsley R (2003) *World Prison Population List*. 5th edn. London: Home Office Research, Development and Statistics Directorate.

Wilkinson RG (1997) Socioeconomic determinants of health: Health inequalities: Relative or absolute material standards. *British Medical Journal* 314(7080): 519.

Wood E, Tyndall MW, Montaner JS, and Kerr T (2006) Summary of findings from the evaluation of a pilot medically supervised safer injecting facility. *Canadian Medical Association Journal* 175(11): 1399–1404.

Wood E, Tyndall MW, Zhang R, *et al.* (2006) Attendance at supervised injecting facilities and use of detox services. *New England Journal of Medicine* 354: 2512–2514.

World Health Organization (2003) *The World Health Report*. Geneva, Switzerland: WHO.

Primary Prevention Strategies for Illicit Drug Use

F Faggiano, Avogadro University, Novara, Italy
F Vigna-Taglianti, Piedmont Centre for Drug Addiction Epidemiology, Grugliasco, Italy

Background

Substance misuse, including tobacco and alcohol, is currently the predominant health burden in developed countries, accounting for 20% of all deaths and 22% of potential years of life lost (Single, 2000). In the European Community smoking alone accounted annually for 520 000 deaths (Peto, 2006).

Apart from impact on mortality, substance misuse has a considerable effect on personal safety, mental health, and social well-being. A comprehensive evaluation of the annual social costs of drugs carried out in Australia at the end of the past decade estimated that losses equivalent to 5.6% of the gross domestic product are attributable to social harm caused by alcohol, tobacco (including passive smoking), and illicit drugs (Collins, 2002).

This article provides an outline of the programs, interventions, and policies shown to be effective in the primary prevention of the use of tobacco and illegal drugs, and of misuse of alcohol. This overview does not consider other kinds of preventive strategies, such as harm reduction or others generally called 'secondary prevention' or those aimed at smoking, alcohol, or drugs cessation.

Drug Addiction versus Drug Use

Drug addiction is commonly described both medically and socially as a chronic, relapsing disease, characterized by the effects of the prolonged use of the drug itself and by the behavioral disorder caused by its compulsive seeking (Leshner, 1997). This condition is shared by alcohol and illicit drugs as well as by tobacco.

Drug users are commonly divided into "sensation seekers" and those who "use drugs as a way to deal with life's problems or with dysphoric mood" (Leshner, 1999). Not all users become addicted. Once established, however, addiction "is often an uncontrollable compulsion to seek and use drugs" (Leshner, 1999). Experimental use affects mainly adolescents, who "use drugs simply for the pleasant feelings or the euphoria that drugs can produce, or to feel accepted by their peers" (Leshner, 1999). Since the neurological or psychological factors affecting the risk of addiction are not known, "even occasional drug use can inadvertently lead to addiction" (Leshner, 1997; Leshner, 1999). The natural history of addiction has been written in terms of a gateway theory or stepping-stone hypothesis, in that involvement in drug use may follow culturally determined steps from one substance to another. Hard liquors and tobacco, for example, are viewed as intermediate between beer/wine and marijuana, whereas marijuana may be a stepping stone to other illicit drugs (Kandel, 1975; Fergusson, 2000).

Apart from those related to addiction, drug use can lead to a wide range of health and social problems, such as traffic accidents and occupational injuries for alcohol consumption, violence, and child abuse. For this reason, primary interventions should be aimed to reduce first use, as well as to prevent the transition from experimental use to addiction.

Primary Prevention

Although the conceptual definition of drug addiction was settled many years ago, the factors linking first or recreational use with addiction have not been clearly explained. Yet many years of research have resulted in the identification of a long list of factors influencing the probability to become addicted (Hawkins, 1992). The list is so comprehensive, ranging from genetic to educational factors, from parental relationship to national legislation, that a single intervention cannot tackle all the identified factors; moreover, because of the multifactorial essence of addiction, interventions should be generally aimed to increase protective factors rather than to tackle risk factors (Hawkins, 1992).

The age of onset of substance use is critical for the choice of intervention. In the Health Behavior in School-aged Children (HBSC) survey, the mean age at onset of tobacco use is 12.1 for boys and 12.8 for girls (European HBSC countries), and 11.5 and 12.3 in the United States (Currie, 2004). The same figures for the onset of drinking alcohol are 12.3 for boys and 12.9 for girls (European HBSC countries), and 11.8 and 13.2 in the United States (Currie, 2004). Adolescents who begin smoking at younger ages are more likely to become regular smokers and less likely to quit (Tyas, 1998). The same applies to drug use: those who initiate drug use at an earlier age are at greatest risk for later drug misuse (Hawkins, 1992). Results from the North American National Longitudinal Alcohol Epidemiologic Survey (Grant, 1997) showed that the life-time alcohol dependence rate of those who initiate alcohol use by age 14 is four times as high as those who start by age 20; the odds of dependence decreases by 14% with each additional year of delayed initiation.

These data suggest that although the main aim of prevention is to avoid use, the delay of initiation can be also considered a positive outcome.

An Attempt to Classify Preventive Interventions

The European Council approved in 2004 the EU drug strategy for 2005–2012 (Council of the European Union, 2004). Two main policy fields are addressed to tackle the drugs problem at the international and national level: supply reduction and demand reduction. Although the strategy is aimed at the control of illegal drugs, it serves as an example of a global strategy – including transnational law enforcement cooperation, treatment service supply, and prevention programs – that is relevant also to tobacco and alcohol.

Primary prevention of substance use may be classified as:

- universal prevention, targeted to the general population as well as to specific unselected populations (school, family, community);
- selective prevention, targeted to subsets of the population identified as having a higher risk of drug use than average;
- indicated prevention, which targets those who have already taken drugs and are considered to be at risk of becoming addicted.

Methods

This article is based on secondary publications, such as systematic reviews, reports of international agencies, and guidelines of preventive practice. The Cochrane Library (Issue 1/2007) and the Medline database have been searched for systematic reviews on the effectiveness of tobacco, alcohol, and illicit drugs prevention programs. The websites of the major international agencies involved in the control of such risk factors have been explored in order to find reports on effectiveness evaluations; National Institute for Clinical Excellence (NICE), Centers for Disease Control and Prevention (CDC), European Union, World Health Organization (WHO), Scottish Intercollegiate Guidelines Network (SIGN), National Institute on Drug Abuse (NIDA), and European Monitoring Centre for Drugs and Drug Addiction (EMCDDA) websites have been visited and useful reports have been downloaded and examined.

For a limited set of items for which no secondary publications were available, a bibliographic search has been performed in Medline, without temporal limitation, using specific search terms, and looking for randomized controlled trials (RCTs) of interventions on individuals, on groups (group or cluster RCT), and nonexperimental studies for interventions provided at the population level.

Universal Prevention

Mass Media Campaigns

Mass media interventions generally consist of brief, recurring messages, disseminated through broadcast, Internet, and print media, to inform and motivate individuals to remain tobacco free (Hopkins, 2001), abstain from excessive alcohol use, and avoid using illicit drugs.

Evidence on tobacco

A Cochrane systematic review published in 1998, included six controlled trials evaluating the effectiveness of mass media campaigns for preventing smoking uptake in young people (Sowden, 1998). Since only two of these studies were associated with reductions in smoking prevalence, the conclusions of the author were that "there is some evidence that media campaigns can be effective, but overall the evidence is not strong." The effective campaigns were guided by theoretical concepts about how behaviors are acquired; the first was based on provocative messages, and the second was based on the social learning theory approach (Bandura, 1977). Both campaigns were intensive, a characteristic of effective campaigns already known (Flay, 1987).

A more recent systematic review included 14 controlled studies evaluating the effectiveness of mass media campaigns (Hopkins, 2001) in preventing smoking onset in young people, 12 of them reporting a quantitative evaluation of effect. In 13 out of 14 studies, the mass media campaign was a component of a larger strategy, including contests or school-based interventions, community education programs, and tax increase of tobacco products. Among the five studies reporting results as differences in prevalence, with follow-up periods ranging from 2 to 5 years, the median absolute reduction was 2.4%. Among the six studies reporting results as odds ratios (ORs), two did not find an effect and the median OR for the four remaining was 0.60. A single study evaluated a campaign in addition to a school based program showing a reduction of 11% in the prevalence of smoking. The authors concluded that a strong scientific evidence exists that mass media campaigns are effective in reducing tobacco use prevalence in adolescents when combined with other interventions.

The bulk of evidence comes from North America, but there are some European studies confirming these results. For example, an evaluation of an anti-tobacco multimedia campaign in Norway found that nonsmoking youth in the intervention counties were less likely to take up smoking than youth in control counties (Farrelly, 2003). In general, mass media campaigns appear to have raised awareness, improved attitudes about tobacco use, and/or reduced prevalence and consumption among youth, though it is difficult to ascertain the degree to which the effect is attributable to the campaigns specifically, particularly when they are part of comprehensive programs (Farrelly, 2003). Mass media campaigns are most likely to succeed if designed according to social marketing theory, with sufficiently large, sustained campaigns, and appropriately targeted messages based on empirical evidence for the intended population (Lantz, 2000).

Mass media campaigns, sustaining attention and legitimatizing and reinforcing community actions, can also help to maintain tobacco control as a priority issue in the public health agenda (Bala, 2004; Wilde, 1993).

Based on recent evidence, the WHO Europe states that "multimedia campaigns can be used to increase awareness" while making use of all of the effective options available (Gilbert, 2003).

Evidence on alcohol

A recent WHO review (Hawks, 2002) summarized the results of different reviews on the effectiveness of mass-media interventions for reducing alcohol use and misuse. Media-based campaigns that are pursued in conjunction with complementary and reciprocal community actions seem to be more effective than media campaigns alone in changing both attitudes toward alcohol and use itself (Boots, 2001, Casswell, 1990). Media campaigns have been shown to be effective in raising the general level of awareness with regard to alcohol and of lending support to policy initiatives in this area. However, their effectiveness in precipitating changes to individual using behavior is less clearly demonstrated (Proctor, 2001; Casswell, 1990; Makkai, 1991), even in recent studies (Flynn, 2006).

In the case of alcohol (and in some countries, tobacco also), concurrent and frequent broadcasting of advertisements for these substances represents a frustrating, if not hostile influence, and the consequence may be to weaken if not nullify the effects of health messages (Slater, 1996; Wallack, 1984, 1983; Aitken, 1989). This is clearly shown in many studies: the advertising of alcohol products, particularly beer, especially when associated with sporting values has been found to influence the perceptions and future drinking intentions of underage viewers, particularly males (Grube, 1992; Connolly, 1994; Slater, 1996). Alcohol advertising during very early adolescence can influence both beer drinking and drinking intentions in the short term. Children at extremely high levels of overall advertising exposure were found to be subsequently 50% more likely to drink and 36% more likely to intend to drink as those at low levels (Collins, 2007). Moreover, despite restrictions on the advertising of alcohol to underage audiences, studies have shown such audiences to be aware of alcohol advertisements. The positive perception of these advertisements is associated with intention to drink and heavy drinking at a later stage. This trend is more apparent for males than females (Connolly, 1994; Aitken, 1988; Hill,

2001). To confirm the influence of advertising, studies evaluating the effect of bans on the broadcast advertising of alcohol showed that these measures are associated with lower per capita consumption and fewer motor vehicle accidents (Saffer, 1991). Cross-national analyses comparing different levels of advertising restrictions showed lower levels of alcohol consumption and alcohol-related harm in countries with stricter regulatory mechanisms – although there may be other (confounding) factors that account for some of this variability (Hill, 2001).

Exposure to promotional items appears to have an influence on drinking habits: in a cross sectional survey, one-fifth of students reported owning at least one alcohol promotional item, and these students were three times more likely to have tried alcohol and 50% more likely to report current alcohol use than students without such items (Hurtz, 2007).

From another point of view, there is strong evidence that mass media campaigns against alcohol and driving are effective in reducing alcohol-related crashes. A review (Elder, 2004) focused on the campaigns for reducing drinking and driving and alcohol-involved crashes showed that the campaigns were effective in reducing alcohol-related crashes, with a median decrease in crashes across all studies and all levels of crash severity of 13%, and a median decrease in injury-producing crashes of 10%. The studies evaluating the rate of intoxicated drivers showed a 158% net decrease (−37% intervention group; +121% control group). No clear difference on the effectiveness of campaigns that used legal deterrence messages and those that used social and health consequences messages were shown.

A more recent systematic review including 11 studies confirmed Elder's results: mass media campaigns reduced crashes resulting in injury by 10% (Tay, 2005). Moreover mass media campaigns resulted in large savings in medical costs, property damage, and productivity. There were no significant differences in outcomes among message types emphasizing legal, social, or health consequences of drunk-driving.

Evidence on illicit drugs

Few papers have reviewed the effectiveness of mass media campaigns against illicit drugs. An extensive recent review failed to identify papers producing quantitative data (Hawks, 2002), and this is a recognized gap in the research in the field (Proctor, 2001).

On the other hand, the very recent results of the evaluation of the American National Youth Anti-drug Media Campaign, planned by the Office of National Drug Control Policy (ONDCP) and funded in 1997 by the U.S. Congress with US$1 billion, raises concern. The main objective of the campaign was to "educate and enable America's youth to reject illegal drugs as well as alcohol and tobacco"; however, alcohol and tobacco were omitted from the main focus of the campaign, and this attracted

comments from several critics (Proctor, 2001). The centerpiece of the campaign, which focused mainly on minimizing illegal drug use (particularly marijuana and inhalants) among young adolescents who have not yet become 'regular' users of illegal substances, consisted of televised anti-drug public service announcements (PSAs).

The evaluation of the effectiveness of the campaign was committed by ONDCP to an external research corporation, who conducted a separate evaluation of the campaign (Orwin, 2006). A longitudinal panel study on children's and parents' exposure and response to the campaign has been carried out, using a national probability sample. Data collection was conducted by means of audio computer-assisted self-interview, allowing privacy, over four rounds (1999–2004), each about one year apart from the next round in nine waves of interviews. The evaluation aimed to assess whether the exposure to the campaign affected the self-reported knowledge, attitudes, beliefs, and drug use among exposed youth. Because the campaign was addressed to youth nationwide, an experimental design was inapplicable; therefore, the evaluation has been carried out by linking variations in self-reported exposure to the campaign messages with outcomes that the campaign intended to bring about (Orwin, 2006). The effects of the exposure to the campaign on the outcomes have been measured and detected within individuals over time, after controlling for factors that could have influenced outcomes.

This study shows disappointing results. It provides no evidence that the campaign had a positive effect in relation to teen drug use, and shows some indications of a negative impact. Some intermediate outcomes, such as parents talking with children about drugs, and doing fun activities with their children, showed positive results. However, other intermediate outcomes, such as parents' monitoring of their children's behaviors, were not shown to be affected by the campaign.

Preliminary findings from the evaluation were reported in 2002: the past month use of marijuana appeared significantly increased by 2.5% among 14–18 years (Orwin, 2006). Following these results, in 2002, ONDCP modified the campaign, enlarging the concentration of anti-marijuana messages, in order to strengthen the power of the campaign to achieve positive results. However, even if no increase in marijuana use was detected in the second phase of the campaign, the post-2002 results yielded no evidence of positive impacts and some evidence of negative and unintended consequences in relation to marijuana use. Specifically, exposure to advertisements during the redirected campaign was associated with statistically significantly higher rates of marijuana use initiation among youth who were prior nonusers (2000 to 2004 change 2.1%). Most parents and youth recalled exposure to the campaign messages, thus the failure of the campaign cannot be attributed to a lack of recognition of the messages themselves. Preliminary results from research trying to explain the counterintuitive effect of the ONDCP campaign have pointed out that socially oriented factors, such as peer influence and normative belief, are more likely to account for the unintended effects rather than psychological or cognitive explanations (Jacobsohn, 2007). The author suggests that the most persuasive message of the campaign was the unintended meta-message on the high prevalence of peer use of marijuana contained in the advertisements. This possibly resulted in a "boomerang effect" on youth perceptions, thus leading to an increase in marijuana use.

The risk of increasing the perceived prevalence of use, shared by any anti-drug campaign (Perkins, 1986), raises concerns about the capacity of mass media campaigns to influence teen drug attitudes and behaviors, and in general questions concerning the understanding of the factors that are most salient to teens' decision making about drugs (GAO, 2006). Moreover it suggests that it is most important to evaluate thoroughly the effectiveness of any campaign prior to widespread implementation.

Policy Interventions: Price and Availability of Selling Products

One of the fundamental principles of economics is that when the price of goods rises, demand falls. Price elasticity is the extent to which demand falls in response to a price increase (Gilbert, 2003).

Evidence on tobacco

Price increase of tobacco products is considered one of the most productive and cost-effective means for reducing the demand for tobacco (Chaloupka, 2000).

Several reviews have showed that a price increase of 10% results in a decrease of 2.5% to 5% in cigarette consumption (Townsend, 1996; Gilbert, 2003; Lantz, 2000; Hopkins 2001). It has been estimated that such a 10% price increase could result in 600 000 to 1.8 million prevented deaths in the World Bank European and central Asian region, at a cost of US$3 to US$78 per disability-adjusted life year (DALY) (Ranson, 2002). This intervention is estimated to be the one with the highest cost-effectiveness value. These estimates can be considered as minimum, since they are based on the short-run response of smokers to price increases. In fact, several studies have estimated that the demand for tobacco could be reduced twice as much in the long-run as in the short-run., on condition that increases are repeated over time.

A recent systematic review found that in seven out of eight studies, increases in the price of tobacco products decrease both the overall prevalence of use and the quantity consumed (Hopkins, 2001). According to this extensive review, as well as to the one of the Europe Health Evidence Network, the effect of price increases is expected to be higher among young people, women, and lower social strata (Hopkins, 2001; Gilbert, 2003).

In countries where consumption has actually fallen in response to price increases, taxes account for 65% to 80% of the price of a pack of cigarettes (Gilbert, 2003). It has been estimated that price increases may also contribute to the effectiveness of tobacco control programs, especially when a portion of the tobacco tax revenues are allocated to anti-tobacco interventions (Gilbert, 2003; Chaloupka, 2000).

An important policy intervention with the aim of preventing use of tobacco among adolescents is the restriction of sales to minors. A Cochrane review recently concluded that legislation alone is not sufficient to prevent sales to minors (Stead, 2005). Simply giving information to retailers about the law is not effective (DiFranza, 1992, 1996). Both enforcement and community policies, if including a variety of strategies, can improve compliance by retailers (Altman, 1999). Enforcement, or warnings of it, generally had an positive effect on retailer behavior, but checking must occur frequently, more than six times a year (Jason, 1996). The penalty for infringement may also be important, although there is little direct evidence of the relative deterrent effect of different penalties. Revoking of a license to sell tobacco can be more effective, if the licensing itself is strictly monitored (Chapman, 1994). However, the effect of these measures can be counterproductive if community attitudes are not supportive. For example, retailer interventions may not work if neighboring districts have discordant policies (Landrine, 1994). Both retailers' compliance and density of vendors are very important in light of the effectiveness of the measure (Rigotti, 1997; Levy, 2000, 2001); a study in Erie County in the United States (Cummings, 1995; Cummings, 2003) suggests that the threshold for compliance must be greater than 80% for the measure to be effective. Moreover, although the potential for enforcement of sales laws to reduce underage smoking may be limited, a recent cost-effectiveness analysis suggests that even if it can only reduce youth tobacco use by 5% it is likely to be as cost-effective as other prevention activities (DiFranza, 2001).

Evidence on alcohol

An extended review published in 2002 (Chaloupka, 2002) targeted the price sensitivity of alcohol consumption; it was carried out mainly using data from studies taking advantage of the substantial variation in alcohol prices across the United States due to the differences in excise tax rates on alcoholic beverages. This review was focused on youths and young adults, because of the frequency of motor vehicle accidents from alcohol use, the high prevalence of misuse and dependence in the age group 20–39, and the fact that drinking behaviors in adolescence is linked with alcohol misuse in late life. Among the four studies included in the review, especially targeted to the youth ages 16 to 21, the results are consistent: the price of alcohol, generally resulting from variation in taxes, reduced the number of frequent and fairly frequent young drinkers and, to a lower extent, the fraction of infrequent drinkers (Chaloupka, 2002). Two studies included in the review analyzed the effect of price increases of alcoholic beverages on motor vehicle fatalities due to drinking and driving: both studies concluded that, based on the variation of prices across the United States, increased prices are able to reduce accidents from drinking and driving (Chaloupka, 2002). The authors of the review concluded that price increase can be considered one of the most cost-effective interventions to control alcohol consumption and related risks.

Five studies examining the health effects of alcohol were included in the review: four of them concluded that price increases are able to reduce mortality rates of causes directly linked to alcohol, such as liver cirrhosis, and those indirectly linked to alcohol, such as traffic fatalities, as well as the incidence of gonorrhea (Chaloupka, 2002). It has been estimated that an increase of $1 of the price of distilled spirits can reduce the rates of cirrhosis mortality by about 5.4–10.8%, and that an increase by 10% of the prices of alcoholic drinks can reduce the cirrhosis mortality by 8.3–12.8%.

Although these conclusions came from experiences limited to North America, some European evidence appears to confirm them: in Switzerland, following a reduction of prices for spirits, an increase of consumption has been noticed, during a period of generally declining consumption of alcohol (Heeb, 2003). An analysis of the relationship between prices of alcoholic beverages and consumption during 1984 and 1994, carried out in Sweden, showed a net tendency toward reduction of consumption as a response of price increase (Gruenewald, 2006).

Evidence on illicit drugs

The analysis of the role of price policies on the frequency of consumption is obviously not applicable for illicit drugs. Nevertheless control policies could affect the availability of substances in the illegal market, and criminalization policies could determine the career of users and consequently the prevalence of use. No reviews have been traced on this topic by our literature search, only a few research reports. A study comparing prevalence and career of use of illegal drugs in a city characterized by an informal tolerance toward cannabis, that is, Amsterdam, with those of San Francisco, which has a punitive prohibition law, has been recently published (Reinarman, 2004). The authors concluded that no evidence supports claims that criminalization, or decriminalization, are able to reduce prevalence of drug use. The ineffectiveness of punitive drug policies are described in other, less formal, studies, showing that in the 'tolerant' Netherlands the prevalence of cannabis users is lower than in the UK or

Germany (Korf, 2002) and that countries with weaker enforcement of prohibition laws do not encounter an increase of prevalence of use (MacCoun, 2001).

Smoking and Alcohol-Free Workplaces

Evidence on tobacco

Many countries have established regulations to ban or restrict the consumption of tobacco in enclosed public places (health centers, workplaces, educational institutions, sports centers, social centers, waiting rooms, restaurants, shops, and public transport) to promote smoking cessation and protect nonsmokers from exposure to environmental tobacco smoke (ETS).

Totally smoke-free workplaces are associated with reductions in prevalence of smoking of 3.8% and 3.1 fewer cigarettes smoked per day per continuing smoker. Combination of both those effects yields a mean reduction of 1.3 cigarettes per day per employee, which corresponds to a relative reduction of 29%. To achieve similar results through taxation would require an increase in the price of cigarettes of 73% (Fichtenberg, 2002).

Different no-smoking policies can be implemented: some may include a total ban on smoking, or restrictions with signs warning and clearly marked areas specifically for smokers with separate ventilation. Comprehensive no-smoking interventions in public places usually include educational campaigns for employees, visitors, and managers, posting of signs about the policy, health advice, and smoking cessation counseling for employees.

In 2000a Cochrane systematic review (Serra, 2000), which summarized results of 11 studies carried out in hospitals, workplaces, shops, barbershops, supermarkets, elevators, and cafeterias, concluded that the most effective interventions were those in which institutions developed, resourced, and supported comprehensive programs to achieve compliance with a policy decision to ban smoking. Strategies that includes education, dissemination of information, training for managers, and support in quitting for individual smokers showed the highest rate of success (Becker, 1989; Stillman, 1990). Commitment from management and communication with those affected by bans appeared to be an important part of the successful interventions.

Recently, the introduction of a comprehensive smoke free legislation, covering all indoor workplaces in the Republic of Ireland offered a natural experiment for identifying effects of this law, because the ban was introduced in the Republic but not in Northern Ireland (Allwright, 2004). In the evaluation study, the smoking ban led to a clear reduction in self-reported exposure to ETS in and outside work: in nonsmokers salivary cotinine concentration dropped by 80% and respiratory symptoms declined by 16.7% (Allwright, 2005).

Similar results were found in a previous U.S. study: in 1998, California statewide legislation prohibited tobacco smoking in bars and taverns. It was possible to evaluate the relationship between ETS exposure and respiratory symptoms, sensory irritation symptoms, and pulmonary function in bartenders. After the smoking ban, the self-reported ETS exposure at work significantly decreased from a median of 28 to 2 hours for week. Of those symptomatic at baseline, 59% no longer had symptoms at follow-up. Of those bartenders who at baseline reported sensory irritation symptoms, 78% had resolution of symptoms (Eisner, 1998).

A new law in Italy, introduced in the beginning of 2005, banned smoking from work and public places. The impact evaluation carried out by the Ministry of Health (Ministero della Salute, 2006) showed very high levels of compliance and acceptance of the ban both in public and in workplaces, besides a reduction in prevalence and an increase in sales of smoking cessation drugs. An evaluation at a regional level estimated that during the year after the introduction of the law, hospital admissions for first episode of myocardial infarctions decreased by 11% (Barone-Adesi, 2006).

Evidence on alcohol

Alcohol misuse not only affects work performance in general, but also results in higher rates of absenteeism, accidents, illness, and mortality, with all their related costs.

Most countries have restrictions on alcohol consumption; these can vary from complete bans or partial restrictions to voluntary or local agreements. In general, among countries involved in WHO Global Status Report Alcohol Policy 2004, alcohol consumption in official settings is strictly controlled, with around 50% of them having total bans (WHO, 2004).

Besides alcohol restrictions, there is a long tradition of programs to address the problem of substance misuse by workers. A series of evaluation studies has indicated that the workplace programs succeeded in restoring substantial proportions of employees with alcohol problems to effective performance (McAllister, 1993; Walsh, 1992; Blum, 1995). A workplace prevention training program for stress management has been shown to reduce problem drinking from 20 to 11% and missing work because of a hangover from 16% to 6% (Bennett, 2004).

School-Based Prevention

Schools are appropriate settings for illicit drug use prevention programs for three reasons: first, four out of five tobacco smokers begin before adulthood. Second, schools offer the most systematic and efficient way of reaching a large number of young persons every year. Third, schools can adopt and enforce a broad spectrum of educational policies (United Nations, 2003). Most substance

prevention programs, therefore, are school-based. According to Nancy Tobler's (Tobler, 1986) systematic review on tobacco, alcohol, and drugs prevention, prevention programs can be divided into those founded on (1) knowledge-only interventions, in which description of the effects of drug use sets out to build negative attitudes toward drugs and hence decrease their use; (2) affective-only (e.g. self-esteem or self-awareness building) interventions, based on the assumption that psychological factors place people at risk of use; (3) peer-based interventions, namely refusal skills and social life skills programs, the former focused on resistance skills or peer role models and the latter on inter-personal or intra-personal skills, both founded on the assumption that peer pressure can lead to drug use; (4) knowledge plus affective interventions, in which knowledge is combined with affective education to provide values and build decision-making patterns; or (5) alternative approaches (activities and competence), such as interventions encouraging alternative activities to drug use or those aimed at enforcing control abilities.

Evidence on tobacco

In 2004, a Cochrane review summarizing the results of the studies on the effectiveness of school-based programs for tobacco prevention was published (Thomas, 2004). Due to the differences in approaches between the studies, the review did not produce a quantitative summary of the evidence. However, the review pointed out that rigorous studies evaluating programs based on information are lacking, and there is little positive available evidence to support this approach. On the contrary, school programs incorporating social influence models are effective in reducing smoking behavior in the short term. Among studies with long-term follow-up, the Life Skills Training studies showed a 25% reduction in cigarette smoking at the 12th grade (Botvin, 1990; Botvin, 1995), and the TNT project showed a 30% reduction of smoking initiations and a 60% reduction of weekly use across the two-year junior high to senior high school period (Sussman, 1993). However, the Hutchinson Smoking Prevention Project, a large high-quality study, failed to find an effect of a social influence intervention program on smoking behavior, either at school-leaving or later follow-up (Peterson, 2000).

The review underlined also that there is not enough evidence to clarify whether interventions combining social competence with social influence are more effective than pure social influence interventions; moreover, studies evaluating social influence interventions delivered in conjunction with wider, multimodal initiatives reached conflicting results on the prevalence of smoking.

Another important conclusion of this review was that since "cost is an important factor in planning school-based programs, those planning services will need to determine whether these costs are justified in the light of the existing evidence." The Hutchinson Smoking Prevention Project, for example, delivered 65 classroom sessions to each group of students, requiring investment in teacher-training, and employing time usually dedicated to other academic activities. Therefore, according to the current status of the evidence, the cost/benefit ratio of engaging such programs remains unclear.

Evidence on alcohol

In 2002, the Cochrane Library published a systematic review summarizing the evidence of effectiveness of primary prevention interventions for alcohol misuse in young people (Foxcroft, 2002; Foxcroft 2003). Regarding studies evaluating a school-based component, the review concluded that the Strengthening Families Program (Spoth, 2001a, 2001b), an intervention involving both the families and the school, is effective over the long term for the primary prevention of alcohol misuse. The number needed to treat (NNT) over four years is nine, which means that for every nine individuals who receive the intervention, there will be one fewer student using alcohol, using alcohol without permission, or having drunkenness episodes four years later. Moreover, according to the review, culturally focused skills training (Schinke, 2000) is potentially effective in the long term, with a NNT of 17, whereas evidence supporting the effectiveness of the Life Skills Training program is less convincing (Botvin, 1995).

Evidence on illicit drugs

Many studies have evaluated the efficacy of illicit drug use prevention programs implemented in the school setting, and several reviews have summarized their results (Bangert-Drowns, 1988; Cuijpers, 2002; Ennett, 1994; Hansen, 1992; Kroger, 1994; McBride, 2003; Mellanby, 2000; White, 1997; Tobler, 1997; White, 1998; Tobler, 2000; Skara, 2003). In 2005, the Cochrane Library published the first systematic review (Faggiano, 2005) taking into account all the characteristics of the programs, the quality of the studies, and classifying the programs according to Tobler's scheme.

The Cochrane review revealed differences in the efficacy of the prevention programs (classified into knowledge, skills, and affective-focused). Skills-focused programs showed a positive effect on both mediating variables (drug knowledge, decision making, self-esteem, and peer pressure resistance) and final outcomes, compared to usual curricula, with a 20% lower use of marijuana in the intervention groups at the post test and a 55% lower use of hard drugs. From the meta-analysis on marijuana use, based on four randomized control trials (RCTs) involving 7287 students, the number needed to treat (NNT) was 33, meaning that one out of every 33 students (20% of the new initiators) receiving the intervention will abstain from drug use because of it. Knowledge focused programs were more effective in improving drug knowledge than the usual curricula, but were not more effective than

skills-based programs and less effective than affective programs. Their effects on drug use were comparable to the usual curricula and the other two types of programs, not different from resistance training programs, and less effective than normative education programs. Affective-focused programs were effective in improving decision-making skills and drug knowledge compared to both usual curricula and knowledge-focused interventions, but no evidence of effectiveness was shown for the prevention of drug use. Programs administered by peers appeared to be more effective than programs administered by teachers. However, no difference was shown for peers compared to external educators.

Parental Interventions

Evidence on tobacco

A recent Cochrane review summarized the results of the effectiveness of family-based programs for preventing smoking by children and adolescents (Thomas, 2007). The review was based on 19 RCT studies, some of which were of low quality. Excluding the low-quality studies, the authors found that family interventions may prevent adolescent smoking. Four of the nine studies that tested a family intervention, such as printed activity guides, parenting tip sheets, child newsletters, incentives, or more complex ones such as Strengthening Families Program and Family-School partnership, against a control group had significant positive effects (Jackson, 2006; Josendal, 1998; Spoth, 2004; Storr, 2002) at short- and long-term follow-up. However, four RCTs found no differences and one found negative results. Only one of the five RCTs that tested a family intervention against a school intervention detected significant positive effect (Spoth, 2004). None of the remaining comparisons (family-plus-school versus school, family tobacco versus family nontobacco, parent plus-teens versus teens for general risk reductions) detected evidence of significant intervention effects. Across all the included studies, the number of sessions was not related to positive outcomes, but the extent of implementer training and the fidelity of implementation appeared to be higher in the studies with positive outcomes.

Evidence on alcohol

The Cochrane systematic review (Foxcroft, 2002, 2003) on effectiveness of primary prevention intervention for alcohol misuse in young people found the Strengthening Families Program, involving both the families and the school, to be effective over the long term (Spoth, 2001a, 2001b). The same review, evaluating the Project Northland, a school-based intervention associated with strong parental and community involvement, showed significant effects on drinking behavior while the intervention was ongoing but not afterwards, and no effects at four years follow-up.

Evidence on illicit drugs

The Cochrane review on interventions delivered in non-school settings (Gates, 2006) found evidence of effectiveness (vs. no intervention group) only for the three family interventions (Focus on Families, Iowa Strengthening Families Program, and Preparing for the Drug-Free Years) (Catalano, 1997; Spoth, 2004). Calculated results showed at six years follow-up an advantageous effect of the Iowa Strengthening Families Program on self-reported lifetime cannabis use $(RR = 0.55, 95\%CI: 0.32–0.95)$ and on self-reported past-year cannabis use $(RR = 0.44, 95\% CI: 0.20–0.96)$.

Community Interventions

Community interventions also need to be considered by policy makers because the potential benefit goes beyond youth. If community interventions can have a significant impact on important youth substance misuse outcomes while having an impact also on other groups within a community, then ultimately there may be an economy of scale. Instead of different interventions for different groups, a single community intervention that covers all the groups may be more cost-effective.

Evidence on tobacco

The Cochrane review on community interventions for preventing smoking in young people (Sowden, 2003) stated that "there is limited support for the effectiveness of community interventions in helping prevent the uptake of smoking in young people." Seventeen controlled trial studies were included in the review. Two out of twelve evaluations comparing community-wide interventions with no intervention reported differences in smoking prevalence between the intervention and control groups (Perry, 1994; Vartiainen, 1998); both studies were part of larger community-wide cardiovascular disease prevention programs. A third study comparing two similar interventions with standard health education did not find consistent results (Piper, 2000). Of the four studies comparing community-wide interventions with school-based interventions (Biglan, 2000; Sussman, 1998; Gordon, 1997; Schinke, 2000), only one showed a statistically significant effect on smoking prevalence (Biglan, 2000). However, when samples of expired air carbon monoxide were taken into account, differences between groups disappeared. A study evaluating a community-wide intervention including a school-based component and one without, did not show differences in smoking rates between the two groups (Kaufman, 1994). However, in the follow-up survey, smoking prevalence was decreased in both groups. A study evaluating a community-wide intervention with

a mass media component and a control with only the media component (Pentz, 1989) showed an effect on smoking rates in the intervention group.

Most of the programs included in this review mentioned some kind of theoretical basis. Three of the studies that reported reductions in smoking prevalence between intervention and control groups were based on Social Learning Theory and one referred to the social influences approach. These studies also reported significant changes in mediating variables after the intervention (negative attitudes, perceived positive consequences, intention to smoke in the future).

Evidence on alcohol

Community-based prevention programs focus on changing the environment in which a person consumes alcohol rather than the behavior of the individual drinker (Treno, 2002). The Cochrane systematic review (Foxcroft, 2002; Foxcroft, 2003) on effectiveness of primary prevention intervention for alcohol misuse in young people pointed out the value of community interventions on youth alcohol misuse. Three large-scale community-based interventions were included in the review. The first one (Holder, 1997) demonstrated a 10% annual reduction in alcohol-related crashes among all drivers (not specifically youth) across three communities, and a greater reduction in the number of retail outlets selling alcohol to apparent underage buyers in the intervention communities (-30%) than in the control communities (-12%) in the first year of follow-up. The second large community trial included was the Communities Mobilizing for Change on Alcohol program (Wagenaar, 2000), which reported no clear statistically significant effects apart from a statistically significant effect on arrests for drinking and driving among 18–20-year-old youth. The third trial was Project Northland (Perry, 1996) with a predominantly school-based intervention associated with strong parental and community involvement, which found significant effects of the intervention on drinking behavior while the intervention was ongoing, but not afterward, and no effects at four-years follow-up.

Evidence on illicit drugs

A recent Cochrane systematic review (Gates, 2006) summarized the evidence concerning the interventions intended to prevent or reduce use of drugs by young people delivered in nonschool settings. Although 17 studies were included, the authors underline that many studies had methodological drawbacks, especially high levels of loss to follow-up, so that no firm conclusions can be drawn. One study of motivational interviewing (McCambridge, 2004) suggested that this intervention was beneficial on cannabis use. Three family interventions (Focus on Families, Iowa Strengthening Families Program, and Preparing for the Drug-Free Years) (Catalano, 1997;

Spoth, 2004) suggested that they may be beneficial in preventing cannabis use. The studies on multicomponent community interventions did not find any strong effect on drug use outcomes (Perry, 2003; Flay, 2004; Biglan, 2000; Schinke 2000), and the two studies of education and skills training (Lindenberg, 2002; Palinkas, 1996) did not find any differences between the intervention and control groups.

Selective Interventions for Vulnerable Groups

A comprehensive review on the effectiveness of interventions to reduce substance misuse among vulnerable and disadvantaged young people was recently published by the UK National Centre for Drug Prevention (Jones, 2006). From the recommendations of the review, we summarize in the following paragraphs only evidence statements classified as "A: likely to be applicable across a broad range of settings and populations" or "B: likely to be applicable across a broad range of settings and populations, assuming appropriately adapted."

Multicomponent Community-Based Interventions

Multicomponent community-based approaches are more effective for high-risk youth at preventing, delaying, or reducing drug use than school and community projects alone. Compared with low-risk youth, this population may respond more favorably to comprehensive interventions targeting alcohol, cannabis, tobacco, and generic substance use (Streke, 2004).

Multicomponent interventions including a component delivered at school combined with community components can be effective in reducing substance use in the short-term (LoSciuto, 1999); however, there is inconsistent evidence about their effectiveness in the long-term, with studies either indicating no change or a reduction in patterns of alcohol use (Roe, 2005; Harmon, 1995; Eddy, 2003). A study found that they are not effective in producing long-term changes in willingness or intent to use substances; they have no effects on family functioning or absences and suspensions from school, and they increase negative behaviors (Hostetler, 1997).

A multicomponent intervention offered in addition to usual school prevention services may produce an immediate decrease in problem behaviors and a long-term decrease in association with deviant peers and involvement in criminal activity (Eddy, 2000, 2003).

As regards young people with a substance-using family member (i.e., parent, sibling, or carer), multicomponent interventions targeting parental drug use and parenting practices in combination with drug treatment have no effect on children's drug use in the short-, medium or long-term compared to treatment only (Catalano, 1999, 2002). No effect is shown on children's behavioral outcomes or school and family factors (Catalano, 1999, 2002), but the interventions can improve parental outcomes in terms of problem-solving, parenting practices, and depression, although there are few intervention effects on family factors such as bonding and conflict (Catalano, 1999, 2002; Whiteside-Mansell, 1999), and they may help drug-using parents stabilize or reduce their own use in the short to medium term (Catalano, 1999; Magura, 1999; Whiteside-Mansell, 1999).

Community-Based Interventions

Behavioral skills programs, information focused programs, recreational focused programs, and affective programs targeting high-risk youth have no effect on illicit drugs, alcohol, and tobacco use and mental health outcomes both in the short and long term (Hermann, 2002; Husler, 2005a, 2005b; Sambrano, 2005; Springer, 2002a, 2002b).

There is insufficient evidence to determine whether family, educational, or multicomponent community interventions *per se* are effective in reducing drug use behavior in vulnerable or disadvantaged young people (Gates, 2006).

Interventions incorporating cultural values are no more effective in reducing substance misuse than interventions that do not (Bledsoe, 2002; Yuen, 2005).

Drug prevention programs targeting populations of mixed ethnicities which incorporate refusal skills training are more effective in reducing substance misuse among high risk youth as well as other behavioral outcomes related to substance use than programs that do not (Bledsoe, 2002).

Support groups combined with peer mentor training delivered to young people with substance-using parents or other family members can increase negative attitudes to substance use and can be effective at improving intervention-targeted outcomes such as emotion-focused coping and self-esteem in the short to medium term (Horn, 1998; Short, 1995).

Self-administered drug education programs for pregnant adolescents do not impact on substance use behaviors in the medium term and improve substance-related knowledge but no effect are shown on attitudes to substance use (Sarvela, 1993).

School-Based Interventions

There is evidence to suggest that school-based Life Skills Training (LST) or generic life skills, on their own or in combination with other approaches, are not effective in reducing substance misuse in the long term on high-risk youth. When delivered as a stand alone intervention, Life

Skills Training or generic life skills may produce medium, but not short- or long-term, reductions in substance use (Griffin, 2003; Smith, 2004; Vicary, 2004), and the effect on substance use may be strongest in girls (Smith, 2004). In combination with other approaches, including parent workshops, staff training, or mentoring, they have no effects on substance use outcomes in the short-, medium or long-term (Brown, 2005; Demers, 2000; Forman, 1990; Losciuto, 1996; Palinkas, 1996; Rentschler, 1997; Richards-Colocino, 1996). However, delivering generic life skills with family components can produce both immediate and medium-term reductions in alcohol use and frequency of use, but only immediate effects on the frequency of cannabis use (DeWit, 1998, 2000). Curricula addressing other risky behaviors (violence, sexual activity) have no direct final or medium term effects on substance use outcomes (Farrell, 2003; Donnelly, 2001).

There is inconsistent evidence about the effectiveness of life skills approaches at changing attitudes and knowledge relating to substance misuse: Life Skills Training can produce long-term decreases in young people's association with substance-using peers (Gottfredson, 1996). These approaches do not show long-term effects of generic life skills with family and diversionary components on intentions to use substances, although with the addition of either mentoring or outreach with generic skills training may produce short- and medium term decreases in favorable attitudes toward substance use (DeWit, 1998, 2000; Rentschler, 1997). Specialized teacher training, in the context of a skills development approach, has no long-term effects on substance use norms (O'Donnell, 1995).

There is evidence to suggest that some school-based educational/skills interventions can improve young peoples' educational skills and positive behaviors, as well as parents' family-based care giving; specialized teacher training, in the context of a cognitive skills development approach, may be associated with long-term improvements in educational skills and other classroom behaviors (O'Donnell, 1995). Life skills curricula with parental, mentoring, and/or social support components can produce both short- and long-term increases in mood, anxiety, community engagement, positive school-based outcomes, and family bonding (DeWit, 1998, 2000; Forman, 1990; LoSciuto, 1996). However, a weakly implemented LST program may be associated with long-term iatrogenic effects, and decreases in positive school-based outcomes (Gottfredson, 1996).

Brief, single substance interventions can be more effective at producing short-term reductions in alcohol use than interventions targeting multiple substances (including alcohol) (Werch, 2005).

There is inconsistent evidence about the effectiveness of school-based counseling and therapy on behavioral and social functioning in young people. However, there is some evidence that school-based social work schemes may produce long-term decreases in reported thefts and truanting (Bagley, 1998).

Family-Based Interventions

Family case management interventions can increase positive parenting skills in families with young children considered at risk (Baydar, 2003).

There is some evidence that family-based interventions may be effective in producing long-term reductions in substance use, except for tobacco and alcohol. The Adolescent Transitions Program produces long-term increases in overall substance use abstention (although tobacco smoking may increase) (Dishion, 2002, 1995; Poulin, 2001). The Family Check Up intervention reduces long-term substance use (Dishion, 2003). The Preparing for the Drug Free Years program reduces alcohol and cannabis initiation at long-term follow-up but increases tobacco smoking and alcohol consumption (Park, 2000).

Family-based interventions can be effective in producing long-term improvements in parenting skills: for example, the early intervention Healthy Start Program was found to have no effects on child developmental status, perceived parental competence, parents' stress levels or mother-child interaction in the medium term, or on use of physical assault as discipline and child developmental status in the long-term, but the intervention might produce improvements in nonviolent discipline in the long-term (Duggan, 1999).

Preparing for the Drug Free Years may lead to long-term improvements in parenting skills and family responses to substance use but not family conflict or adolescent refusal skills (Kosterman, 1997, 2001; Spoth, 1998; Park, 2000).

Nonprogrammed multicomponent family based approaches may increase some parenting skills and parental self-efficacy and self-esteem in the long-term but have no effects on parenting stress (Miller-Heyl, 1998). Programmed multicomponent family based approaches, such as the Family Check Up, can produce long-term increases in parental monitoring of child activities (Dishion, 2003).

There is no consistent evidence on the effects of home visitations interventions for families with substance-using members: in the long-term there is no difference in substance use between children with drug-using mothers who receive home visitation at birth and those who do not (Olds, 1998). Adolescents who receive home visitation as infants do not have improved outcomes of dysfunctional behaviors; although stops by police may be higher, there are fewer arrests and convictions in the long-term among children who receive home visitation at birth compared to those who do not (Olds, 1998). Home visitation does not produce long-term increases in the number of mothers who are drug free compared to no visits, and there are no effects of home visitation on parenting stress or child abuse potential compared to no visits (Black, 1994; Nair, 2003).

Employment-Skills Programs

There is evidence to suggest that comprehensive employment programs (including outreach and admissions, basic education, vocational training, residential living, health care and education, counseling, and job placement assistance) for high-risk youth are not effective in reducing substance use in the long-term, but they can have long-term positive effects on participation in employment and training and arrest and conviction rates, and reduce the amount of time spent in jail (Schochet, 2001).

Counseling

There is insufficient evidence to determine whether individual counseling is effective in reducing substance use in the long-term in young people with multiple vulnerabilities. Motivational interviewing with video feedback has no effect upon delinquent, home, or school behaviors and decreased perception of control over the consequences of individual actions (Knopes, 2004).

Indicated Interventions

As for selective interventions, in the following paragraphs we summarize evidence statements on the effectiveness of interventions to reduce substance misuse among young people who reported substance use, but not substance dependence, according to the review published by the UK National Centre for Drug Prevention (Jones, 2006).

Brief Intervention or Motivational Interviewing

Motivational interviewing and brief intervention can have short-term effects on the use of cigarettes, alcohol, and cannabis and on attitudes and intentions to use (Tait, 2003; McCambridge, 2004; Oliansky, 1997; Aubrey 1998), but there is no evidence of medium-term impact on the use of cigarettes, alcohol, or cannabis (McCambridge, 2005).

Brief intervention enhanced with additional support may have a positive impact on attendance at community treatment agencies and psychological well-being compared to usual hospital treatment (Tait, 2004).

Family Therapy

Family therapy (in particular when it is multidimensional) is reported to be more effective at reducing substance use than other types of group therapy interventions (Austin, 2005; Liddle, 2001, 2004; Joanning, 1992);

however, these interventions are no more effective in improving school or family-related factors compared to educational or group therapy approaches in the immediate or medium term (Liddle, 2001, 2004; Joanning, 1992).

Brief family therapy interventions are more effective than group therapy in producing immediate reductions in cannabis use (Santisteban, 2003) and overall substance use (Lewis, 1990).

Counseling or Therapy Sessions for Adolescents

There is insufficient evidence to determine whether counseling and behavior therapy interventions targeting young substance users are effective in reducing substance use.

Other Interventions

There is some evidence that skills training for parents of young substance users is effective in producing immediate reductions in cannabis use among young substance users compared to no intervention (McGillicuddy, 2001); moreover, these interventions can produce an immediate improvement in parent coping but not other measures of parent and family functioning (McGillicuddy, 2001).

Conclusions

The evidence presented in this overview is weak in some types of interventions but other interventions are supported by relatively robust scientific studies of effectiveness: examples include mass media campaigns for tobacco use, bans and restrictions for tobacco and alcohol use, school programs based on the comprehensive social influence approach, and family programs for selected populations. Interventions known to not be effective include knowledge-based school programs and employment skills programs.

In general the availability of data on effectiveness of interventions is far from satisfactory. Many interventions supplied at a population level, such as mass media campaigns against drugs other than tobacco and alcohol, have little evidence of impact, and no evidence is available on the interaction among market advertising, preventions campaigns, and programs at the community level. In general, very few studies have tried to estimate which are the active components of the multicomponent interventions.

One possible reason for this weakness is that the classical evaluation study design, the randomized controlled trial, is seldom applicable to the assessment of the effectiveness of such interventions, because they are supplied at a population level. For interventions supplied at a group level the group RCT has been recently developed

(Murray, 2004), but for interventions supplied at a population level, when the "unexposed" population cannot be easily identified, only before and after design can be proposed (Spasoff, 1999). In the future these study designs will be more developed methodologically and this will help the conduction of evaluations of prevention interventions (Spasoff, 1999). A second possible weakness is the lack of systematic reviews in many fields of primary prevention. However, in our view, the evidence collected so far is sufficient on which to base a number of effective public health policies.

See also: Alcoholism Treatment; Illicit Drug Trends Globally; Illicit Drug Use and the burden of Disease.

Citations

Aitken PP (1989) Alcohol advertising in developing countries. *British Journal of Addiction* 84: 1443–1445.

Aitken PP, Eadie DR, Leathar DS, McNeill RE, and Scott AC (1988) Television advertisements for alcoholic drinks do reinforce underage drinking. *British Journal of Addiction* 83: 1399–1419.

Altman DG, Wheelis AY, McFarlane M, Lee H, and Fortmann SP (1999) The relationship between tobacco access and use among adolescents: A four community study. *Social Science and Medicine* 48: 759–775.

Allwright S (2004) Republic of Ireland's indoor workplace smoking ban. *British Journal of General Practice* 54(508): 811–812.

Allwright S, Paul G, Greiner B, et al. (2005) Legislation for smoke-free workplaces and health of bar workers in Ireland: Before and after study. *British Medical Journal* 331: 1117.

Aubrey LL (1998) Motivational interviewing with adolescents presenting for outpatient substance abuse treatment. *Dissertation Abstracts International: Section B: The Sciences Engineering* 59(3-B)B.

Austin AM, Macgowan MJ, and Wagner EF (2005) Effective family-based interventions for adolescents with substance use problems: a systematic review. *Research Social Work Practice* 67–83.

Bala M, Strzeszynski L, and Hey K (2004) Mass media interventions for smoking cessation in adults. *Cochrane Database of Systematic Reviews* Issue 2.

Bandura A (1977) *Social Learning Theory*. Eaglewood Cliffs, NJ: Prentice-Hall.

Bagley C and Pritchard C (1998) The reduction of problem behaviours and school exclusion in at-risk youth: an experimental study of school social work with cost-benefit analyses. *Child and Family Social Work* 3(4): 219–226.

Bangert-Drowns RL (1988) The effects of school-based substance abuse education. *Journal of Drug Education* 18: 243–264.

Barone-Adesi F, Vizzini L, Merletti F, and Richiardi L (2006) Short-term effects of Italian smoking regulation on rates of hospital admission for acute myocardial infarction. *European Heart Journal* 27: 2468–2472.

Baydar N, Reid MJ, and Webster-Stratton C (2003) The role of mental health factors and program engagement in the effectiveness of a preventive parenting program for Head Start mothers. *Child Development* 74(5): 1433–1453.

Becker DM, Conner HF, Waranch HR, Stillman F, Pennington L, Lees PSJ, and Oski F (1989) The impact of a total ban on smoking in the Johns Hopkins Children's Center. *Journal of the American Medical Association* 262: 799–802.

Bennett JB, Patterson CR, Reynolds GS, Wiitala WL, and Lehman WE (2004) Team awareness, problem drinking, and drinking climate: workplace social health promotion in a policy context. *American Journal of Health Promotion* 19: 103–113.

Biglan A, Ary DV, Smolkowski K, Duncan T, and Black C (2000) A randomised controlled trial of a community intervention to prevent adolescent tobacco use. *Tobacco Control* 9(1): 24–32.

Black MM, Nair P, Kight C, et al. (1994) Parenting and early development among children of drug-abusing women: effects of home intervention. *Pediatrics* 94(4:Pt:1): t-8.

Bledsoe KL (2003) Effectiveness of drug prevention programs designed for adolescents of color: A meta-analysis. *Dissertation Abstracts International: Section B: The Sciences and Engineering* 63(9-B)B.

Blum TC and Roman PM (1995) Cost-Effectiveness and Preventive Implications of Employee Assistance Programs. Rockville, MD: Substance Abuse and Mental Health Services Administration Publication RP0907.

Boots K and Midford R (2001) mass media marketing and Advocacy to Reduce Alcohol-Related Harm. In: Heathers N, Peters TJ and Stockwell T (eds.) *International Handbook of Alcohol Dependence and Problems*, pp. 805–882. Chichester: John Wiley and Sons.

Botvin GJ, Baker E, Dusenbury L, Tortu S, and Botvin EM (1990) Preventing adolescent drug abuse through a multimodal cognitive-behavioral approach: results of a 3-year study. *Journal of Consulting Clinical Psychology* 58(4): 437–446.

Botvin GJ, Baker E, and Dusenbury L (1995) Long-Term follow-up results of a randomized drug abuse prevention trial. *Journal of the American Medical Association* 273: 1106–1112.

Brown EC, Catalano RF, Fleming CB, et al. (2005) Adolescent substance use outcomes in the Raising Healthy Children project: a two-part latent growth curve analysis. *Journal of Consulting Clinical Psychology* 73(4): 699–710.

Casswell S, Ransom R, and Gilmore L (1990) Evaluation of a mass-media campaign for the primary prevention of alcohol-related problems. *Health Promotion International* 5(1): 9–17.

Catalano RF, Gainey RR, Fleming CB, et al. (1999) An experimental intervention with families of substance abusers: one-year follow-up of the focus on families project. *Addiction* 94(2): 241–254.

Catalano RF, Haggerty KP, Gainey RR, and Hoppe MJ (1997) Reducing parental risk factors for children's substance misuse: preliminary outcomes with opiate-addicted parents. *Substance Use and Misuse* 32(6): 699–721.

Catalano RF, Haggerty KP, Fleming CB, Brewer DD, and Gainey RR (2002) Children of substance-abusing parents: Current findings from the Focus on Families project. In: McMahon RJ and Peters RD (eds.) *The effects of parental dysfunction on children*, pp. 179–204. New York: Kluwer Academic/Plenum Publishers.

Chaloupka FJ and Warner JE (2000) The economics of smoking. In: Culyer AJ and Newhouse (eds.) *Handbook of Health Economics*, pp. 1539–1627. New York: Elsevier.

Chaloupka FJ, Grossman M, and Saffer H (2002) The effects of price on alcohol consumption and alcohol-related problems. *Alcohol Research and Health* 26–34.

Chapman S, King M, Andrews B, McKay E, Markham P, and Woodward S (1994) Effects of publicity and a warning letter on illegal cigarette sales to minors. *Australian Journal of Public Health* 18: 39–42.

Collins DJ and Lapsley HM (2002) Counting the cost: estimates of the social costs of drug abuse in Australia in 1998–9 National Drug Strategy Monograph Series No. 49. Canberra: Commonwealth Department of Health and Ageing.

Collins RL, Ellickson PL, McCaffrey D, and Hambarsoomians K (2007) Early adolescent exposure to alcohol advertising and its relationship to underage drinking. *Journal of Adolescent Health* 40 (6): 527–534.

Commission of the European Communities (2007) *Green Paper: Towards a Europe Free from Tobacco Smoke: Policy Options at EU Level*. Brussels: CEC.

Connolly GM, Casswell S, Zhang J, and Silva PA (1994) Alcohol in the mass media and drinking by adolescents: A longitudinal study. *Addiction* 89: 1255–1263.

Council of the European Union (2004) *EU Drugs Strategy (2005–2012)*. Brussels: EEU.

Cuijpers P (2002) Effective ingredients of school-based drug prevention programs. A systematic review. *Addictive Disorders* 27: 1009–1023.

Cummings KM, Hyland A, Perla J, and Giovino GA (2003) Is the prevalence of youth smoking affected by efforts to increase retailer compliance with a minors' access law? *Nicotine and Tobacco Research* 5(4): 465–471.

Cummings KM, Hyland A, Saunders-Martin T, Perla J, Coppola PR, and Pechacek TF (1988) Evaluation of an enforcement program to reduce tobacco sales to minors. *American Journal of Public Health* 88: 932–936.

Currie C, Roberts C, Morgan A, Smith R, Settertobulte W, Samdal O, Barnekow and Rasmussen VB (eds.) (2004) *Young people's health in context – Health Behaviour in School-aged Children (HBSC) study: international report from the 2001/2002 survey.* Copenhagen: WHO, Health Policy for Children and Adolescents; No. 4.

Demers J, French DC, and Moore D (2000) The preliminary evaluation of a program to help educators address the substance use/prevention needs of special students. *Journal of Alcohol and Drug Education* 46(1): 14–26.

DeWit DJ, Ellis K, Rye BJ, et al. (1998) Evaluations of "Opening Doors". Addiction Research Foundation, Toronto. A drug prevention program for at-risk youth: Three reports. ARF Research Document Series No. 143.

DeWit DJ, Steep B, Silverman G, et al. (2000) Evaluating an in-school drug prevention program for at-risk youth. *Alberta Journal of Educational Research* 46(2): 117–133.

DiFranza JR and Brown LJ (1992) The Tobacco Institute's "It's the Law" campaign: Has it halted illegal sales of tobacco to children? *American Journal of Public Health* 82: 1271–1273.

DiFranza JR, Savageau JA, and Aisquith BF (1996) Youth access to tobacco: the effects of age, gender, vending machine locks, and "It's the Law" programs. *American Journal of Public Health* 86: 221–224.

DiFranza JR, Peck RM, Radecki TE, and Savageau JA (2001) What is the potential cost-effectiveness of enforcing a prohibition on the sale of tobacco to minors? *Preventive Medicine* 32: 168–174.

Dishion TJ and Andrews DW (1995) Preventing escalation in problem behaviors with high-risk young adolescents: immediate and 1-year outcomes. *Journal of Consulting Clinical Psychology* 63 (4): 538–548.

Dishion TJ, Kavanagh K, Schneiger A, et al. (2002) Preventing early adolescent substance use: a family-centered strategy for the public middle school. *Prevention Science* 3(3): 191–201.

Dishion TJ, Nelson SE, and Kavanagh K (2003) The Family Check-Up with high-risk young adolescents: Preventing early-onset substance use by parent monitoring. *Behavior Therapy* 34(4): 553–571.

Donnelly J, Ferraro H, and Eadie C (2001) Effects of a health and relationship education program on drug behaviors. *North American Journal of Psychology* 3(3): 453–462.

Duggan AK, McFarlane EC, Windham AM, et al. (1999) Evaluation of Hawaii's Healthy Start Program. *Future of Children* 9(1): 66–90.

Eddy JM, Reid JB, Stoolmiller M, et al. (2003) Outcomes during middle school for an elementary school-based preventive intervention for conduct problems: Follow-up results from a randomized trial. *Behavior Therapy* 34(4): 535–552.

Eddy JM, Reid JB, and Fetrow RA (2000) An elementary school-based prevention program targeting modifiable antecedents of youth delinquency and violence: Linking the Interests of Families and Teachers (LIFT). *Journal of Emotional Behavioral Disorders* 8(3): 176.

Eisner MD, Smith AK, and Blanc PD (1998) Bartenders' Respiratory Health After Establishment of Smoke Free Bars and Taverns. *Journal of the American Medical Association* 280: 1909–1914.

Elder RW, Shults RA, Sleet DA, Nichols JL, Thompson RS, and Rajab W (2004) Effectiveness of mass media campaigns for reducing drinking and driving and alcohol-involved crashes: A systematic review. *American Journal of Preventive Medicine* 27(1): 57–65.

Ennett ST, Tobler NS, Ringwalt CL, and Flewelling RL (1994) How effective is drug abuse resistance education? A meta-analysis of project DARE outcome evaluations. *American Journal of Public Health* 84: 1394–1401.

Faggiano F, Vigna-Taglianti F, Versino E, Zambon A, Borraccino A, and Lemma P (2005) "School-based prevention for illicit drugs' use" *Cochrane Database of Systematic Reviews* Issue 2.

Farrell AD, Meyer AL, Sullivan TN, et al. (2003) Evaluation of the Responding in Peaceful and Positive Ways (RIPP) seventh grade violence prevention curriculum. *Journal of Child and Family Studies* 101–120.

Farrelly MC, Niederdeppe J, and Yarsevich J (2003) Youth tobacco prevention mass media campaigns: past, present, and future directions. *Tobacco Control* 12(S1): I35–I47.

Fergusson DM and Horwood LJ (2000) Does cannabis use encourage other forms of illicit drug use? *Addiction* 95(4): 505–520.

Fichtenberg CM and Glantz SA (2002) Effect of smoke-free workplaces on smoking behaviour: systematic review. *British Medical Journal* 325: 188.

Flay BR (1987) Selling the smokeless society: fifty-six evaluated mass media programs and campaigns worldwide. Washington: American Public Health Association.

Flay BR, Graumlich S, Segawa E, Burns JL, and Holliday MY for the Aban Aya Investigators (2004) Effects of 2 prevention programs on highrisk behaviors among African-American youth: a randomized trial. *Archives of Pediatriatric and Adolescent Medicine* 158(4): 377–384.

Flynn BS, Worden JK, Bunn JY, Dorwaldt AL, Dana GS, and Callas PW (2006) Mass media and community interventions to reduce alcohol use by early adolescents. *Journal of Studies on Alcohol* 67(1): 66–74.

Forman SG, Linney JA, and Brondino MJ (1990) Effects of coping skills training on adolescents at risk for substance use. *Psychology of Addictive Behaviors* 4(2): 67–76.

Foxcroft DR, Ireland D, Lister-Sharp DJ, Lowe G, and Breen R (2002) Primary prevention for alcohol misuse in young people. *Cochrane Database of Systematic Reviews* Issue 3.

Foxcroft DR, Ireland D, Lister-Sharp DJ, Lowe G, and Breen R (2003) Long-term primary prevention for alcohol misuse in young people: a systematic review. *Addiction* 98: 397–411.

GAO, United States Government Accountability Office (2006) Report to the Subcommittee on Transportation, Treasury, the Judiciary, Housing and Urban Development, and Related Agencies, Committee on Appropriations, U.S. Senate, Washington, D.C.: ONDCP Media Campaign – Contractor's National Evaluation Did Not Find That the Youth Anti-Drug Media Campaign Was Effective in Reducing Youth Drug Use. http://www.gao.gov/cgi-bin/getrpt?GAO-06–818 (accessed February 2008).

Gates S, McCambridge J, Smith LA, et al. (2006) Interventions for prevention of drug use by young people delivered in non-school settings. *Cochrane Database of Systematic Reviews* Issue 1.

Gilbert A and Cornuz J (2003) Which are the most effective and cost-effective interventions for tobacco control? WHO Regional Office for Europe's Health Evidence Network (HEN). http://www.euro.who.int/document/e82993.pdf (accessed February 2008).

Gordon I, Whitear B, and Guthrie D (1997) Stopping them starting: evaluation of a community-based project to discourage teenage smoking in Cardiff. *Health Education Journal* 46: 42–50.

Gottfredson DC, Gottfredson GD, and Skroban S (1996) A multimodel school-based prevention demonstration. *Journal of Adolescent Research* 11(1): 115.

Grant BF and Dawson DA (1997) Age at onset of alcohol use and its association with DSM-IV alcohol abuse and dependence results from the National Longitudinal Alcohol Epidemiologic Survey. *Journal of Substance Abuse* 9: 103–110.

Griffin KW, Botvin GJ, Nichols TR, et al. (2003) Effectiveness of a universal drug abuse prevention approach for youth at high risk for substance use initiation. *Preventive Medicine* 36(1): 1–7.

Grube JW and Wallack L (1992) *The Effects of Television Beer Advertising on Children.* Berkeley, CA: Prevention Research Center.

Gruenewald PJ, Ponicki WR, Holder HD, and Romelsjo A (2006) Alcohol Prices, Beverage Quality, and the Demand for Alcohol: Quality Substitutions and Price Elasticities. *Alcoholism: Clinical and Experimental Research* 30: 96–105.

Hansen WB (1992) School-based substance abuse prevention: a review of the state of the art in curriculum, 1980–1990. *Health Education Research* 7(3): 403–430.

Harmon MA (1996) Reducing Drug Use among Pregnant and Parenting Teens: A Program Evaluation and Theoretical Examination. Dissertation Abstracts International (56): Feb, 3319-Feb, 3320.

Hawks D, Scott K, McBride N, Jones P, and Stockwell T (2002) Prevention of Psychoactive Substance Use: A Selected Review of

What Works in the Area of Prevention. Geneva: World Health Organization.

Hawkins JD, Catalano RF, and Miller JY (1992) Risk and protective factors for alcohol and other drug problems in adolescence and early adulthood: implications for substance abuse prevention. *Psychological Bulletin* 112: 64–105.

Heeb J-L, Gmel G, Zurbrügg C, Kuo M, and Rehm J (2003) Changes in alcohol consumption following a reduction in the price of spirits: a natural experiment in Switzerland. *Addiction* 98: 1433–1446.

Hermann J, Sambrano S, Springer JF, et al. (2002) The national cross-site evaluation of high-risk youth programs: findings on designing and implementing effective prevention programs for youth at high risk. *ERIC Monograph Series.* no. ED477134.

Hill L and Caswell S (2001) Alcohol advertising and sponsorship: commercial freedom or control in the public interest? In: Heathers N, Peters T and Stockwell T (eds.) *International Handbook of Alcohol Dependence and Problems*, pp. 823–846. Chichester: John Wiley and Sons.

Holder HD (1997) A community prevention trial to reduce alcohol-involved trauma. *Addiction* 92.

Hopkins DP, Briss PA, Ricard CJ, et al. (2001) Reviews of Evidence Regarding Interventions to Reduce Tobacco Use and Exposure to Environmental Tobacco Smoke. *American Journal of Preventive Medicine* 20(2S): 16–66.

Horn KA (1998) Examination of a cumulative strategies model for drug abuse prevention: Risk factor reduction in high risk children. *Dissertation Abstracts International Section A: Humanities and Social Sciences* 58(12-A)A.

Hostetler M, Fisher K, and Project CARE (1997) substance abuse prevention program for high-risk youth: A longitudinal evaluation of program effectiveness. *Journal of Community Psychology* 25(5): 419.

Hurtz SQ, Henriksen L, Wang Y, Feighery EC, and Fortmann SP (2007) The relationship between exposure to alcohol advertising in stores, owning alcohol promotional items, and adolescent alcohol use. *Alcohol and Alcoholism* 42(2): 143–149.

Husler G, Werlen E, and Rehm J (2005a) The Action Plan–a new instrument to collect data on interventions in secondary prevention in adolescents. *Substance Use and Misuse* 40(6): 761–777.

Husler G, Werlen E, and Blakeney R (2005b) Effects of a national indicated preventive intervention program. *Journal of Community Psychology* 33(6): 725.

Jackson C and Dickinson D (2006) Enabling parents who smoke to prevent their children from initiating smoking. Results from a 3-year intervention evaluation. *Archives of Pediatriatric and Adolescent Medicine* 160: 56–62.

Jacobsohn L (2007) Explaining the Boomerang Effect of the National Youth Anti-Drug Media Campaign. 15th annual meeting Society for Prevention Research. Washington, 30 May 2007.

Jason L, Billows W, Schnopp Wyatt D, and King C (1996) Reducing the illegal sales of cigarettes to minors: analysis of alternative enforcement schedules. *Journal of Applied Behavioral Analysis* 29: 333–344.

Joanning H (1992) Treating Adolescent Drug Abuse: A Comparison of Family Systems Therapy, Group Therapy, and Family Drug Education. *Journal of Marital and Family Therapy* 18(4): 345–356.

Jones L, Sumnall, Witty K, Wareing M, McVeigh J, and Bellis MA (2006) A review of community-based interventions to reduce substance misuse among vulnerable and disadvantaged young people. National Collaborating Centre for Drug Prevention, Centre for Public Health, Liverpool John Moores University.

Josendal O, Aaro LE, and Bergh I (1998) Effects of a school-based smoking prevention program among subgroups of adolescents. *Health Education Research* 13: 215–224.

Kandel D (1975) Stages in adolescent involvement in drug use. *Science* 190: 912–914.

Kaufman JS, Jason LA, Sawlski LM, and Halpert JA (1994) A comprehensive multi-media program to prevent smoking among Black students. *Journal of Drug Education* 24: 95–108.

Knopes DR (2004) Motivating change in high-risk adolescents: An intervention focus on the deviant friendship process. *Dissertation Abstracts International: Section B: The Sciences and Engineering* 65(2-B)B.

Korf DJ (2002) Dutch coffee shops and trends in cannbis use. *Addictive Behaviors* 27: 851–866.

Kosterman R, Hawkins JD, Haggerty KP, et al. (2001) Preparing for the drug free years: session-specific effects of a universal parent-training intervention with rural families. *Journal of Drug Education* 31(1): 47–68.

Kosterman R, Hawkins JD, Spoth R, et al. (1997) Effects of a preventive parent-training intervention on observed family interactions: Proximal outcomes from preparing for the drug free years. *Journal of Community Psychology* 25(4): 352.

Kroger CB (1994) A review of the effectiveness of health education and health promotion. Utrecht: IUPHE-International Union for Health Promotion and Education.

Landrine H, Klonoff EA, and Fritz JM (1994) Preventing cigarette sales to minors: The need for contextual, sociocultural analysis. *Preventive Medicine* 23: 322–327.

Lantz PM, et al. (2000) Investing in youth tobacco control: a review of smoking prevention and control strategies. *Tobacco Control* 9(1): 47–63.

Leshner AI (1997) Drug abuse and addiction treatment research: the next generation. *Archives of General Psychology* 54: 691–694.

Leshner AI (1999) Science-based views of drug addiction and its treatment. *Journal of the American Medical Association* 282: 1314–1316.

Levy DT and Friend KB (2000) A simulation model of tobacco youth access policies. *Journal of Health Politics, Policy, and Law* 25: 1023–1050.

Levy DT, Friend K, Holder H, and Carmona M (2001) Effect of policies directed at youth access to smoking: results from the SimSmoke computer simulation model. *Tobacco Control* 10: 108–116.

Lewis RA, Piercy FP, Sprenkle DH, et al. (1990) Family-based interventions for helping drug-abusing adolescents. *Journal of Adolescent Research* 5(1): 95.

Liddle HA, Dakof GA, Parker K, et al. (2001) Multidimensional family therapy for adolescent drug abuse: results of a randomized clinical trial. *American Journal of Drug and Alcohol Abuse* 27(4): 651–688.

Liddle HA, Rowe CL, Dakof GA, et al. (2004) Early intervention for adolescent substance abuse: pretreatment to posttreatment outcomes of a randomized clinical trial comparing multidimensional family therapy and peer group treatment. *Journal of Psychoactive Drugs* 36(1): 49–63.

Lindenberg CS, Solorzano RM, Bear D, Strickland O, Galvis C, and Pittman K (2002) Reducing substance use and risky sexual behavior among young, low-income, Mexican-American women: comparison of two interventions. *Applied Nursing Research* 16(3): 137–148.

LoSciuto L, Rajala AK, Townsend TN, et al. (1996) An outcome evaluation of Across Ages: An intergenerational mentoring approach to drug prevention. *Journal of Adolescent Research* 11(1): 129.

LoSciuto L, Hilbert SM, Fox MM, et al. (1999) A two-year evaluation of the Woodrock Youth Development Project. *Journal of Early Adolescence* 19(4): 488–507.

MacCoun R and Reuter P (2001) Evaluating alternative cannabis regimes. *British Journal of Psychiatry* 178: 123–128.

Magura S, Laudet A, Kang SY, et al. (1999) Effectiveness of comprehensive services for crack-dependent mothers with newborns and young children. *Journal of Psychoactive Drugs* 31(4): 321–338.

Makkai T, Moore R, and McAllister I (1991) Health education campaigns and drug use: The 'drug offensive' in Australia. *Health Education Research* 6(1): 65–76.

McAllister PO (1993) An evaluation of counseling for employer-referred problem drinkers. *Health Bulletin* 51: 285–294.

McBride N (2003) A systematic review of school drug education. *Health Education Research* 18: 729–742.

McCambridge J and Strang J (2004) The efficacy of single-session motivational interviewing in reducing drug consumption and perceptions of drug-related risk and harm among young people: results from a multi-site cluster randomized trial. *Addiction* 99(1): 39–52.

McCambridge J and Strang J (2005) Deterioration over time in effect of Motivational Interviewing in reducing drug consumption and related risk among young people. *Addiction* 100(4): 470–478.

McGillicuddy NB, Rychtarik RG, Duquette JA, *et al.* (2001) Development of a skill training program for parents of substance-abusing adolescents. *Journal of Substance Abuse Treatment* 20(1): 59–68.

Mellanby AR, Rees JB, and Tripp JH (2000) Peer-led and adult-led school health education: a critical review of available comparative research. *Health Education Research* 15: 533–545.

Miller-Heyl J, MacPhee D, and Fritz JJ (1998) DARE to be you: A family-support, early prevention program. *Journal of Primary Prevention* 18(3): 257–285.

Ministero della Salute-Centro Nazionale per la Prevenzione e il Controllo delle Malattie (2006) Il rapporto sull'impatto della legge 16 gennaio 2003, n. 3 art. 51 "tutela della salute dei non fumatori" Roma. http://www.ccm.ministerosalute.it/resources/static/primopiano/255/conferenzaFumo.pdf (accessed February 2008).

Murray DM, Varnell SP, and Blitstein JL (2004) Design and analysis of Group-randomized trials: a review of recent methodological developments. *American Journal of Public Health* 94: 423–432.

Nair P, Schuler ME, Black MM, *et al.* (2003) Cumulative environmental risk in substance abusing women: early intervention, parenting stress, child abuse potential and child development. *Child Abuse and Neglect* 27: 997–1017.

O'Donnell J, Hawkins JD, Catalano RF, *et al.* (1995) Preventing school failure, drug use, and delinquency among low-income children: long-term intervention in elementary schools. *American Journal of Orthopsychiatry* 65(1): 87–100.

Olds D, Henderson CR, Cole R, *et al.* (1998) Long-term effects of nurse home visitation on children's criminal and antisocial behaviour: 15-year follow-up of a randomized controlled trial. *Journal of the American Medical Association* 280(14): 1238–1244.

Oliansky DM, Wildenhaus KJ, Manlove K, *et al.* (1997) Effectiveness of brief interventions in reducing substance use among at-risk primary care patients in three community-based clinics. *Substance Abuse* 18 (3): 95–103.

Orwin R, Cadell D, Chu A, *et al.* (2006) *Evaluation of the National Youth Anti-Drug Media Campaign: 2004 Report of Findings Executive Summary*. Rockville, MD: Westat.

Palinkas LA, Atkins CJ, Miller C, *et al.* (1996) Social skills training for drug prevention in high-risk female adolescents. *Preventive Medicine* 25(6): 692–701.

Park J, Kosterman R, Hawkins J, *et al.* (2000) Effects of the 'Preparing for the Drug Free Years' curriculum on growth in alcohol use and risk for alcohol use in early adolescence. *Prevention Science* 1(3): 125–38.

Pentz MA, Dwyer JH, Mackinnon DP, Flay BR, Hansen WB, Wang EY, and Johnson CA (1989) A multicommunity trial for primary prevention of adolescent drug abuse. Effects on drug use prevalence. *Journal of the American Medical Association* 261: 3259–3266.

Perkins HW and Berkowitz AD (1986) Perceiving the community norms of alcohol use among students: some research implications for campus alcohol education programming. *International Journal of Addiction* 21: 961–976.

Perry CL, Kelder SH, and Klepp K (1994) Community-wide cardiovascular disease prevention in young people: long-term outcomes of the Class of 1989 Study. *European Journal of Public Health* 4: 188–194.

Perry CL, Williams CL, Veblen-Mortenson S, Toomey TL, *et al.* (1996) Project Northland: outcomes of a community-wide alcohol use prevention program during early adolescence. *American Journal of Public Health* 86: 956–965.

Perry CL, Komro KA, Veblen-Mortensen S, Bosma LM, Farbakhsh K, Munson KA, *et al.* (2003) A randomized controlled trial of the middle and junior hig school DARE and DARE plus programs. *Archives of Pediatrics and Adolescent Medicine* 157(2): 178–184.

Peterson AV Jr, Kealey KA, Mann SL, Marek PM, and Sarason IG (2000) Hutchinson Smoking Prevention Project: Long-Term Randomized Trial in School-Based Tobacco Use Prevention-Results on Smoking. *Journal of the Nationall Cancer Institute* 92: 1979–1991.

Peto R, Lopez AD, Boreham J, and Thun M (2006) *Mortality from Smoking in Developed Countries 1950–2000.* 2nd ed. http://www.deathsfromsmoking.net (accessed February 2008).

Piper DL, Moberg DP, and King MJ (2000) The Healthy for Life Project: behavioral outcomes. *Journal of Primary Prevention* 21: 47–73.

Poulin F, Dishion TJ, and Burraston B (2001) Three-year iatrogenic effects associated with aggregating high-risk adolescents in

preventive interventions. *Applied Developmental Science* 5(4): 214–224.

Proctor D and Babor TF (2001) Drug wars in the post-Gutenberg galaxy: Mass media as the next battleground. *Addiction* 96: 377–381.

Reinarman C, Cohen PDA, and Kaal HL PhD (2004) The Limited Relevance of Drug Policy: Cannabis in Amsterdam and in San Francisco. *American Journal of Public Health* 94: 836–842.

Ranson MK, Jha P, Chaloupka FJ, and Nguyen SN (2002) Global and regional estimates of the effectiveness and cost-effectiveness of price increases and other tobacco control policies. *Nicotine and Tobacco Research* 4: 311–319.

Rentschler DM (1997) A longitudinal study to determine the long-term effects of prevention and intervention substance abuse strategies on at-risk fourth grade students and their families. *Dissertation Abstracts International Section A: Humanities Social Sciences* 57(8-A)A.

Richards-Colocino N, McKenzie P, and Newton RR (1996) Project Success: Comprehensive intervention services for middle school high-risk youth. *Journal of Adolescent Research* 11(1): 163.

Rigotti NA, DiFranza JR, Chang Y, Tisdale T, Kemp B, Singer DE (1997) The effect of enforcing tobacco-sales laws on adolescents' access to tobacco and smoking behaviour. *New England Journal of Medicine* 337: 1044–1051.

Roe S and Becker J (2005) Drug Prevention with Vulnerable Young People: A Review. *Drugs: Education, Prevention, and Policy* 12(2): 85–99.

Saffer H (1991) Alcohol advertising bans and alcohol abuse: An international perspective. *Journal of Health Economics* 10(1): 65–79.

Sambrano S, Springer JF, Sale E, *et al.* (2005) Understanding prevention effectiveness in real-world settings: the National Cross-Site Evaluation of high risk youth programs. *American Journal of Drug and Alcohol Abuse* 31(3): 491–513.

Santisteban DA, Coatsworth JD, Perez-Vidal A, *et al.* (2003) Efficacy of brief strategic family therapy in modifying Hispanic adolescent behavior problems and substance use. *Journal of Family Psychology* 17(1): 121–133.

Sarvela PD and Ford TD (1993) An evaluation of a substance abuse education program for Mississippi delta pregnant adolescents. *Journal of School Health* 63(3): 147–152.

Schinke SP, Tepavac L, and Cole KC (2000) Preventing substance use among native American youth: three-year results. *Addictive Behavior* 25(3): 387–397.

Schochet PZ, Burghardt J, and Glazerman S (2001) National Job Corps Study: The Impacts of Job Corps on Participants' Employment and Related Outcomes {and} Methodological Appendixes on the Impact Analysis. Princeton, NJ: Mathematical Policy Research.

Serra C, Cabezas C, Bonfill X, and Pladevall-Vila M (2000) Interventions for preventing tobacco smoking in public places. *Cochrane Database of Systematic Reviews* Issue 3.

Short JL, Roosa MW, Sandler IN, *et al.* (1995) Evaluation of a preventive intervention for a self-selected subpopulation of children. *American Journal of Community Psychology* 23(2): 223–247.

Single E, Rehm J, Robson L, and Truong MV (2000) The relative risks and etiologic fractions of different causes of death and disease attributable to alcohol, tobacco and illicit drug use in Canada. *Canadian Medical Association Journal* 162: 1669–1675.

Skara S and Sussman S (2003) A review of 25 long-term adolescent tobacco and other drug use prevention program evaluations. *Preventive Medicine* 37: 451–474.

Slater MD, Rouner D, Murphy K, Beauvais F, Van Leuven J, and Domenech Rodriguez M (1996) Male adolescents' reactions to TV beer advertisements: The effects of sports content and programming context. *Journal of Studies on Alcohol* 57: 425–433.

Smith EA, Swisher JD, Vicary JR, *et al.* (2004) Evaluation of life skills training and infused-life skills training in a rural setting: outcomes at two years. *Journal of Alcohol and Drug Education* 48(1): 51–70.

Sowden AJ and Arblaster L (1998) Mass media interventions for preventing smoking in young people. *Cochrane Database of Systematic Reviews* Issue 4.

Sowden A and Stead L (2003) Community interventions for preventing smoking in young people. *Cochrane Database of Systematic Reviews* Issue 1.

Spasoff RA (1999) *Epidemiologic Methods for Health Policy.* New York: Oxford University Press.

Spoth R, Redmond C, Shin C, et al. (1998) Risk moderation of parent and child outcomes in a preventive intervention: a test and replication. American Journal of Orthopsychiatry 68(4): 565–579.

Spoth R, Redmond C, Trudeau L, and Shin C (2001a) Longitudinal substance initiation outcomes for a universal preventive intervention combining family and school programs. Psychology of Addictive Behavior 16: 129–134.

Spoth R, Redmond C, and Shin C (2001b) Randomized trial of brief family interventions for general populations adolescent substance use outcomes 4 years following baseline. Journal of Consulting Clinical Psychology 69: 1–15.

Spoth R, Redmond C, Shin C, and Azevedo K (2004) Brief family intervention effects on adolescent substance initiation: school-level growth curve analyses 6 years following baseline. Journal of Consulting Clinical Psychology 72(3): 535–542.

Springer JF, Sambrano S, Sale E, et al. (2002a) The National Cross-Site Evaluation of High-Risk Youth Programs. Preventing Substance Abuse: Major Findings from the National Cross-Site Evaluation of High-Risk Youth Programs. ERIC Monograph Series.

Springer JF, Sambrano S, Sale E, et al. (2002b) The National Cross-Site Evaluation of High-Risk Youth Programs: Making Prevention Effective for Adolescent Boys and Girls: Gender Differences in Substance Use and Prevention. ERIC Monograph Series.

Stead LF and Lancaster T (2005) Interventions for preventing tobacco sales to minors. Cochrane Database of Systematic Reviews Issue 1.

Stillman FA, Becker DM, Swank RT, Hantula D, Moses H, Glantz S, and Waranch R (1990) Ending smoking at the Johns Hopkins Medical Institutions: an evaluation of smoking prevalence and indoor air pollution. Journal of the American Medical Association 264(12): 1565–1569.

Storr CL, Ialongo NS, Kellam SG, and Anthony JC (2002) A randomized controlled trial of two primary school intervention strategies to prevent early onset tobacco smoking. Drug and Alcohol Dependency 66(1): 51–60.

Streke AV (2004) Meta-analysis of adolescent community-based drug prevention programs. Dissertation Abstracts International 65Dec, 2388-Dec, 238A.

Sussman S, Dent CW, Stacy AW, Hodgson CS, Burton D, and Flay BR (1993) Project Towards No Tobacco Use: implementation, process and post-test knowledge evaluation. Health and Education Research 8: 109–123.

Sussman S, Dent CW, Stacy AW, and Craig S (1998) One-year outcomes of Project Towards No Drug Abuse. Preventive Medicine 27: 632–642.

Tait RJ and Hulse GK (2003) A systematic review of the effectiveness of brief interventions with substance using adolescents by type of drug (DARE structured abstract). Drug Alcohol Review 22: 337–346.

Tait RJ, Hulse GK, and Robertson SI (2004) Effectiveness of a brief-intervention and continuity of care in enhancing attendance for treatment by adolescent substance users. Drug and Alcohol Dependency 74(3): 289–296.

Tay R (2005) Mass media campaigns reduce the incidence of drinking and driving. Evidence-based Healthcare Public Health 9(1): 26–29.

Thomas R (2004) School-based programs for preventing smoking. Cochrane Database of Systematic Reviews Issue 2.

Thomas RE, Baker P, and Lorenzetti D (2007) Family-based programs for preventing smoking by children and adolescents. Cochrane Database of Systematic Reviews Issue 1.

Tobler NS (1986) Meta-Analysis of 143 Adolescent Drug Prevention Programs: Quantitative Outcome Results of Program Participants Compared to a Control or Comparison Group. Journal of Drug Issues 16(4): 537–567.

Tobler NS and Stratton HH (1997) Effectiveness of school-based drug prevention programs: a meta-analysis of the research. Journal of Primary Prevention 18(1): 71–128.

Tobler NS, Roona MR, Ochshorn PM, Diana G, Streke AV, and Stackpole KM (2000) School-based adolescent drug prevention programs: 1998 meta-analysis. Journal of Primary Prevention 20(4): 275–336.

Townsend J (1996) Price and consumption of tobacco. British Medical Bulletin 52: 132–142.

Treno AJ and Lee JP (2002) Approaching alcohol problems through local environmental interventions. Alcohol Research and Health 26(1): 35–40.

Tyas SL and Pederson LL (1998) Psychosocial factors related to adolescent smoking: a critical review of the literature. Tobacco Control 7: 409–420.

United Nations Office for Drug Control and Crime Prevention (2003) School-Based Drug Education: A Guide for Practitioners and the Wider Community. New York: UN.

Vartiainen E, Paavola M, McAlister A, and Puska P (1998) Fifteen-year follow-up of smoking prevention effects in the North Karelia Youth Project. American Journal of Public Health 88: 81–85.

Vicary JR, Henry KL, Bechtel LJ, et al. (2004) Life skills training effects for high and low risk Rural Junior High School Females. Journal of Primary Prevention 25(4): 399–416.

Wagenaar AC, Gehan JP, Jones-Webb R, Toomey TL, and Forster JL (2000) Communities mobilizing for change on alcohol outcomes from a randomized community trial. Journal of Studies on Alcohol 61: 85–94.

Walsh DC, Hingson RW, Merrigan DM, et al. (1992) A randomized trial of alternative treatments for problem-drinking employees: Study design, major findings, and lessons for worksite research. Journal of Employee Assistance Research 1: 112–147.

Wallack L (1984) Television programming, advertising, and the prevention of alcohol-related problems. In: Gerstein DR (ed.) Towards the Prevention of Alcohol Problems. Government, Business, and Community Action: 79–169. Washington: National Academy Press.

Wallack LM (1983) Mass media campaigns in a hostile environment: Advertising as anti-health education. Journal of Alcohol and Drug Education 28: 51–63.

Werch CE, Moore MM, DiClemente CC, et al. (2005) Single vs. multiple drug prevention: is more always better?: a pilot study. Substance Use and Misuse 40(8): 1085–1101.

White D and Pitts M (1998) Educating young people about drugs: A systematic review. Addiction 93(10): 1475–1487.

White D and Pitts M (1997) Health promotion with young people for the prevention of substance misuse. London: Health Education Authority.

Whiteside-Mansell L, Crone CC, and Conners NA (1999) The development and evaluation of an alcohol and drug prevention and treatment program for women and children. The AR-CARES program. Journal of Substance Abuse Treatment 16(3): 265–275.

Whilde GJ (1993) Effects of mass-media communications on health and safety habits: an overview of issues and evidence. Addiction 88: 983–996.

WHO, Regional Office for Europe (2002) Why Smoking in the Workplace Matters: An Employer's Guide. A publication of the WHO European Partnership Project to Reduce Tobacco Dependence.

WHO (2004) Global status report on alcohol. World Health Organization, Department of Mental Health and Substance Abuse Geneva.

Yuen RK (2005) The effectiveness of culturally tailored interventions: A meta-analytic review. Dissertation Abstracts International 2005: Section B: The Sciences and Engineering 65(8-B)B.

Relevant Websites

http://www.cdc.gov – Centers for Disease Control and Prevention.
http://www.cochrane.org – The Cochrane Collaboration.
http://ec.europa.eu – European Commission.
http://www.consilium.europa.eu – Council of the European Union.
http://www.deathsfromsmoking.net – Deathfromsmoking.net.
http://www.emcdda.europa.eu – European Monitoring Centre for Drugs and Drug Addiction.
http://www.hbsc.org – Health Behaviour in School-aged Children, WHO Collaborative Cross-national Study.
http://www.cancer.gov – National Cancer Institute, U.S. National Institutes of Health.
http://www.drugpreventionevidence.info – National Collaborating Center Drug Prevention.

http://www.nice.org.uk – National Institute for Health and Clinical Excellence.

http://niaaa.census.gov – National Institute on Alcohol Abuse and Alcoholism, National Epidemiologic Survey on Alcohol and Related Conditions.

http://www.nida.nih.gov – National Institute on Drug Abuse, National Institutes of Health.

http://www.mediacampaign.org/ – National Youth Anti-Drug Media Campaign.

http://www.whitehousedrugpolicy.gov – Office of National Drug Control Policy.

http://www.lifeskillstraining.com – LifeSkills Training.

http://www.sign.ac.uk – Scottish Intercollegiate Guidelines Network.

http://www.strengtheningfamilies.org – Strengtheningfamilies.org.

http://www.strengtheningfamiliesprogram.org – Strengthening Families Program.

http://www.unicri.it – United Nations Interregional Crime and Justice Research Institute.

http://www.unodc.org – United Nations Office on Drugs and Crime.

http://www.gao.gov – U.S. Government Accountability Office.

http://www.who.int – World Health Organization.

http://www.euro.who.int – World Health Organization Regional Office for Europe.

Effective Alcohol Policy

H D Holder, Prevention Research Center, Pacific Institute for Research and Evaluation, Berkeley, CA, USA

Alcohol use and abuse represents a significant public health issue across the world. Heavy drinking over a period of time in the life of an individual contributes to the alcohol-related burden of disease. Alcohol contributes to social, health, and safety problems in two ways, that is, drinking can have acute or immediate and chronic or long-term consequences. First, alcohol is a psycho-active drug which affects one's ability to carry out complex tasks and/or to make socially appropriate or safe decisions, especially in a stressful situation. For example, an automobile driver who has been drinking, even one drink of alcohol, has a reduced ability to operate the vehicle. The more drinks consumed on the average the greater the driver's impairment. Second, alcohol, consumed regularly in high amounts, can have a direct harmful effect on the body. The most obvious threat is the liver which must process alcohol for the body and where long-term drinking substantially increases the risk of liver cirrhosis, or fatty liver, and thus shortens the life of a heavy drinker. Many other diseases also have a substantial association with extended heavy drinking. Both domains of risk are important challenges for public health.

Alcohol policy can be defined broadly as any public health effort to reduce alcohol problems by altering the social, economic, and physical environment that affects alcohol markets and manufacturing, production, promotion, distribution, sales, or consumption. Alcohol dependence for some individuals can create special demands for interventions and treatment. However, the majority of alcohol-related problems are associated not with the small minority of addicted or dependent persons but rather with those who occasionally drink to excess, or in ways or contexts where risk is increased. This article discusses policies that affect alcohol and our knowledge of relative effectiveness in promoting public health.

Policies and Evidence of Effectiveness

Because alcohol is a legal product in most countries, the regulation of these products through policies has often been part of a public health approach to both limiting the damage associated with alcohol and increasing tax revenues in industrialized countries. Government policies can in some cases actually determine the retail price of beverages, the opening hours or days for retail sales, the number and location of retail outlets, how the alcohol can be advertised and promoted, and restrictions on who may purchase alcohol. Restricting alcohol availability through law has been a key policy in many parts of the world. All policy occurs within an individual society and reflects the unique attitudes and values of that society, and so the potential effectiveness of any policy relates directly to public acceptability and compliance with these policies. The following general policies have been utilized in public health efforts to reduce alcohol-related harm.

Retail Price

The consumption of alcohol, like that of any retail product, is related to purchase price; the higher the price set for alcohol, the lower the consumption. Because alcohol consumption is influenced by price, the retail price of alcohol can have a direct effect on the level of alcohol consumption and related problems. Econometric studies suggest that raising the price of alcohol as a part of public health policy could reduce a number of public health problems related to alcohol use. Cirrhosis mortality has been shown to be responsive to price as locations with higher alcohol taxes have fewer such deaths. Furthermore, alcohol tax increases have the potential to reduce the rate of fatal car accidents involving alcohol. For example, it is estimated that a 10% increase in the price of alcoholic beverages in the United States could reduce the probability of drinking and driving by about 7% for men and 8% for women, with even larger reductions among those 21 years and under. One example of increasing retail price as a part of policy occurred in the Northern Territory of Australia under a 'Living with Alcohol Program' which increased the cost of standard drinks by five cents in 1992, followed by other problem reduction strategies in 1996 including lowering the legal blood alcohol content (BAC) limit and a special levy on case wine (Stockwell *et al.*, 2001). Over these first four years, there were statistically significant reductions in acute conditions such as road deaths (34.5%) and other mortality (23.4%) as well as traffic crashes requiring hospitalization (28.3%). Several studies have examined the impact of the price of alcoholic beverages on homicides and other crimes, including rape, robbery, assaults, motor vehicle thefts, domestic violence, and child abuse. See the section titled 'Further reading' for these studies.

Minimum Drinking Age of Alcohol Purchase

Setting a higher minimum legal drinking age to reduce alcohol consumption among youth is also an important public policy. There are legal ages of alcohol purchase in many countries but most often they are ignored or not enforced. One example of a national policy to reduce youth drinking using minimum age occurred in the United States in the 1980s with a 21 minimum purchase or drinking age for all alcoholic beverages. Studies uniformly show that increasing the minimum drinking age significantly decreases self-reported drinking by young people, the number of fatal traffic crashes, and the number of arrests for 'driving under the influence' of alcohol. Studies using data from all 50 states and the District of Columbia for the years 1982 through 1997 concluded that the enactment of the uniform age 21 minimum drinking age law was responsible for a 19% net decrease in fatal crashes involving young drinking drivers after controlling for driving exposure, beer consumption, enactment of zero tolerance laws, and other relevant changes in the laws during that time period. Studies in Canada report findings similar to those in the United States concerning youth drinking and alcohol problems.

The most extensive summary of international research on the effects of minimum drinking age is that of Wagenaar and Toomey (2002) who analyzed all identified published studies from any country from 1960 to 1999 and found that a majority of studies reported that a higher legal drinking age was associated with reduced alcohol consumption among youth, whereas only a few found that a higher drinking age had little or no effect on adolescent drinking. Of the published studies that

assessed the effects of changes in the legal minimum drinking age on incidents of drunk driving and traffic crashes, for example, fatal crashes, drunk-driving crashes, or self-reported driving-after-drinking, a clear majority found that raising the drinking age reduced crashes and associated problems and that lowering the minimum age raised the crash rate.

Even with higher minimum drinking age laws, young people can and do purchase alcohol. Such sales result from low and inconsistent levels of enforcement of laws prohibiting underage alcohol sales, especially when there is little community support. Even moderate increases in enforcement can reduce sales of alcohol to minors by as much as 35% to 40%, especially when combined with media and other community and policy activities.

Number and Densities of Alcohol Outlets

Alcohol outlets in every community are sources of alcohol. Their geographical concentration in neighborhoods and communities can either enhance or delay alcohol access. Gruenewald and colleagues (1993), using a time-series cross-sectional analysis of alcohol consumption and density of alcohol outlets over 50 U.S. states, found that a 10% reduction in the density of alcohol outlets would reduce consumption of spirits by from 1% to 3% and consumption of wine by 4% across all ages. Similar findings have been reported in other countries. A recent study by Treno, Grube, and Martin (2003) found that although outlet density did not directly affect either youth driving after drinking or youth riding with drinking drivers, density did interact with the driver licensing status of the youth on both behaviors. Thus, higher density was positively related to drinking and driving among licensed youth drivers and negatively related to riding with drinking drivers among youth who did not have driver's licenses. This is the first solid evidence of a relationship between alcohol outlet densities and drinking-related risky behavior by youth. See 'Further reading' for a summary of alcohol outlet density and policy research.

Hours and Days of Retail Sale

The length of time during a week when alcohol can be consumed and/or purchased has a demonstrated relationship with alcohol-involved harm. Reducing the days and times of alcohol sales restricts the opportunities for alcohol purchasing and can reduce heavy consumption, and is a common policy strategy for reducing drinking-related problems, although the trend in recent years has been to liberalize such restrictions in many countries. One policy change in Western Australia permitted 'Extended Trading Permits' which enabled longer opening hours. It was found that these extended hours significantly increased monthly assault rates for those hotels with the permits, due to greater sales of high-alcohol-content beer, wine, and spirits. In the 1980s Sweden re-instituted Saturday closings for liquor and wine sales in retail monopolies' stores. As a result, as studies showed, Saturday sales had increased rates of domestic violence and public drunkenness. A recent Swedish study found a net 3% increase in alcohol sales in a new test of Saturday openings of liquor and wine stores, compared with other stores that were not opened on Saturday. A study of an isolated Aboriginal community (Tennant's Creek) in Australia evaluated the effects of banning take-away sales of alcohol on Thursdays, limiting take-away sales to the hours of noon to 9 p.m. on other days, and closing bars until noon on Thursday and Friday. This policy produced a 19.4% decrease in drinking over a 2-year period, and a reduction in arrests, hospital admissions, and women's refuge admissions. In one of the few studies focusing on youth, it was found that temporary bans on the sales of alcohol from midnight Friday through 10 a.m. Monday because of federal elections reduced cross-border drinking in Mexico by young Americans. A local policy in Diadema, Brazil, limited opening hours for alcohol sales and produced a significant decrease in murders. Thus, from a policy perspective, restricting hours and specific days of sale can have considerable impact on acute alcohol problems such as traffic crashes, violence, and heavy drinking.

Government Alcohol Retail Monopolies

One alcohol policy is for the government to operate a retail monopoly for the sale of alcohol. Such monopolies exist in several countries including Iceland, India, Norway, Sweden, Finland, Canada, and the United States. The evidence is quite strong that these government retail systems result in lower rates of alcohol consumption and alcohol-related problems. (See the recent study on youth drinking and harm by Miller *et al.* (2006) associated with the existence of retail monopolies.) Furthermore, the elimination of such monopolies does typically increase total alcohol consumption and alcohol-involved problems; for example, in the United States, those states with retail monopolies have lower numbers of alcohol outlets. A summary of seven time-series analyses of six U.S. states and New Zealand found a consistent increase in total consumption when government-owned or community-trust-operated off-premise outlets were replaced with privately owned outlets (Wagenaar and Holder, 1996). Typically, the networks of stores in these government-operated systems are sparse rather than dense, and the open hours are limited. Elimination of a private profit interest also typically facilitates the enforcement of rules against selling to minors or the already intoxicated and eliminates or reduces alcohol promotion.

Responsible Beverage Service or Sales

In general, responsible beverage service or sales (RBS) involves the creation of clear policies, for example, making a public statement that the establishment does not wish to serve intoxicated persons, or requiring clerks and servers to check identification for all customers appearing to be under the legal alcohol purchase age. RBS also means training staff, for example, teaching clerks and servers how to recognize intoxicated patrons, teaching them effective approaches to intervention, and instructing them in the detection of false age identification. RBS can be implemented at both on-license establishments, which sell alcohol for consumption on site, and off-license establishments which sell alcohol for consumption elsewhere. The serving staff in bars, pubs, and restaurants who encounter heavily intoxicated patrons often frequently continue to serve them alcohol. It has been estimated that obviously intoxicated persons are served alcohol over 60% of the time when they attempt to purchase. As a result, RBS involves efforts to decrease service to intoxicated patrons. Studies of RBS have demonstrated that server training is most effective when coupled with changes in the serving policy and practices of a bar or restaurant. RBS has been found to reduce the number of intoxicated patrons leaving a bar and to reduce the number of car crashes. RBS training has also been associated with an increase in self-reported checking of age identification by servers, a behavior that can continue among trained servers for as long as four years.

There is increasing recognition of the need to focus on house rules and management support for RBS, as well as regular enforcement by police and licensing authorities. Many RBS programs include training managers in the implementation of standard house policies, or use a 'risk assessment' approach to policy development (Saltz, 1997). A typical policy checklist for assessing risks covers the following topics: providing positive incentives for avoiding intoxication (e.g., food, cheaper prices for low or no-alcohol drinks), avoiding incentives for intoxication (e.g., specials on low-cost drinks), policies to minimize harm (e.g., increasing safe transportation options), and policies to minimize intoxication (e.g., slowing then refusing service to intoxicated patrons). An increased emphasis on alcohol serving policies often shows a dramatic impact on reducing bar, pub, or restaurant service to intoxicated individuals. The findings suggest that RBS training, if supported by actual changes in the serving policies of licensed establishments and reinforced by means of enforcement, can reduce heavy consumption and high-risk drinking.

Alcohol Promotion and Advertising Restrictions

Restrictions and outright bans on alcohol promotion and commercial advertising have been employed as part of public health policy. The evidence of the effects of advertising bans has been mixed, but recent research suggests that limits on point-of-purchase advertising and promotion could have specific effects on youth drinking. Saffer (2002) completed a review of published international research literature on the potential effects of alcohol advertising on consumption and in particular the effects on youth drinking. He concluded that the results of his review suggest that alcohol advertising does increase consumption, but that a general alcohol advertising ban alone is insufficient to limit all forms of promotion and a comprehensive ban was needed. On the other hand, Nelson (2003), using a panel of 45 U.S. states for the period 1982–1997, studied the effect of several restrictive alcohol regulations, including advertising bans for billboards, bans of price advertising, state monopoly control of retail stores, and changes in the minimum legal drinking age. He concluded that "bans of advertising do not reduce total alcohol consumption, which partly reflects substitution effects." Saffer and Dhaval (2003) concluded, following an analysis of national alcohol consumption related to total advertising expenditures across the world, that alcohol advertising bans decrease alcohol consumption. Their findings indicated that one more advertising ban on beer and wine or on spirits would reduce consumption by about 5%, and that one more ban on all alcohol advertising in a media would reduce consumption by about 8%.

Promotion of alcohol and its effect on youth drinking has been a significant public health issue. Studies have examined the relationship between exposure to different forms of alcohol advertising and subsequent drinking among adolescents. It was found that for 12-year-old children exposure to in-store beer displays predicted drinking onset by age 14. Similar research concluded that exposure to magazines with alcohol advertisements and to beer concession stands at sports or music events for 12-year-olds predicted frequency of drinking at age 14. Snyder and colleagues (2006) found that youth who saw more alcohol advertisements on average drank more (each additional advertisement seen increased the number of drinks consumed by 1%). These researchers found that restrictions on point-of-purchase price advertising at liquor stores reduced the probability of drinking and driving among all drinkers and that when price advertising is permitted, prices may be expected to fall, thereby leading to increases in overall consumption. They found that drinkers who lived in locations with policies permitting grocery stores to sell beer and wine had a significantly higher probability of drinking and driving, and concluded that advertising and availability of alcohol promotes drinking.

Drinking and Driving Policies

Policies that discourage drinking and driving can reduce alcohol-related crashes and the injury and death that result from it. Strategies for reducing alcohol-related traffic crashes include increased and highly visible law enforcement, for example, sobriety checkpoints and random breath testing, and the level of legal blood alcohol concentration at which a driver is considered legally drunk or impaired.

Random breath testing

Random breath testing, or RBT, involves extensive and continuous random stops of drivers who are required to take a breath test to establish their blood alcohol concentration (BAC). Studies of RBT in Australia, Canada, and Great Britain show that it can reduce traffic crashes. Shults and colleagues (2001) reviewed 23 studies of RBT and intensive enforcement and found a median decline of 22% (range 13% to 36%) in fatal crashes, with slightly lower decreases for non-injury and other accidents. Sobriety checkpoints, a limited version of RBT, are often implemented in individual U.S. states under proscribed circumstances often involving prenotification about when and where they will be implemented. Even under these restricted circumstances there is some evidence that such selective enforcement can reduce drinking and driving.

Lowering BAC limits

BAC limits are public laws that legally define drunk driving using a BAC at or above a prescribed level for the whole population (e.g., from 0.08 to as low as 0.02). Jonah *et al.* (2000) reviewed the evidence internationally for the impact of lower BAC laws, which outside of the United States involve BAC limits down to 0.05 or, in the case of Sweden, to 0.02, and found that consistently lower BAC limits produced positive results for all drivers, but especially for younger drivers.

Zero-tolerance laws for youth

Zero-tolerance laws set lower specific BAC limits for young drivers and commonly invoke penalties such as automatic license revocation. An analysis of the effect of zero-tolerance laws in the first 12 U.S. states enacting them found a 20% relative reduction in the proportion of single vehicle nighttime (SVN) fatal crashes among drivers under 21, compared with nearby states that did not pass zero-tolerance laws. A study of all 50 U.S. states and the District of Columbia found a net decrease of 24% in the number of young drivers with low BACs as a result of the implementation of zero-tolerance laws.

Administrative license suspensions

Under administrative license suspensions or revocations for drinking and driving, licensing authorities can suspend licenses more quickly and closer in time to the actual offense without a court hearing. That administrative license suspension dramatically affects alcohol-related traffic accidents has been consistently positive in international studies.

The threat of loss of license has been shown to be very effective in deterring drinkers from getting into their automobile and driving.

Graduated licensing

Graduated licenses establish unique driving restrictions for young and novice drivers, for example, restricting night-time driving and prohibiting driving with other adolescents. A graduated licensing program in Connecticut (USA) led to a 14% net reduction in crash involvement among the youngest drivers. Similarly, in New Zealand, a 23% reduction in car crash injuries among novice drivers was found after implementation of a graduated licensing system.

In general, the most substantial evidence of effectiveness in reducing alcohol-involved traffic problems exists for RBT, lower BAC laws including special limits for young drivers, and administrative removal of driver's licenses. These enforcement strategies have even greater potency when coupled with strategies to reduce the impairment level of drinkers leaving public drinking venues, with increases in and enforcement of the minimum drinking age, and with increased community support for drinking and driving enforcement.

Community Alcohol Policy Interventions

Policies can be implemented at the community level. Local public policy can be reflected in any established process, priority, or structure that is purposefully sustained over time in the community. At the local level, policy makers can establish the priorities for community action to reduce risky behavior involving alcohol, which in turn can reduce the number of alcohol-involved problems. Possible local alcohol policies can include making a priority of drinking and driving enforcement by the local police; mandating server training for bars, pubs, and restaurants; setting a written policy for responsible alcoholic beverage service by a retail licensed establishment; or allocating enforcement resources to prevent alcohol sales to underage persons. Local alcohol policy, at whatever level it is implemented, is an environmental or structural response to drinking problems. Following are three examples from international community prevention projects that illustrate how local alcohol policy has been used successfully.

Communities Mobilizing for Change on Alcohol

A community intervention program called 'Communities mobilizing for change on alcohol,' or CMCA, was designed to bring about change in policies regarding access to alcohol by those under 21 years of age in communities in the United States. Through numerous contacts with groups and organizations that might be able to affect policies, practices, and norms for minors' access

to alcohol, a strategy team was created in each community to lead efforts to bring about change. Local news was used to bring public attention to issues involving drinking by children and youth. The local policy teams implemented quite a variety of activities to reduce alcohol access. These included steps to get alcohol merchants not to sell to young people, to increase enforcement of laws regarding underage sales, to instigate changes in community events to make alcohol less readily available to young people, and to prevent underage drinking parties at hotels. They provided information to parents, and encouraged alternative punishments for youth who violated drinking laws. Specific policy activities varied across communities. Communities involved in CMCA had lower levels of sales of alcohol to minors in their retail outlets and had marginally lower sales to minors at bars and restaurants compared with control communities. Phone surveys of 18- to 20-year-olds indicated that they were less likely to try to buy alcohol and less likely to provide alcohol to others. Arrests of 18- to 20-year-olds for driving under the influence of alcohol declined significantly more in CMCA communities than in control communities (Wagenaar *et al.*, 2000).

The STAD (Stockholm Prevents Alcohol and Drug Problems) Project

The STAD alcohol policy project, conducted in downtown Stockholm, was designed to reduce alcohol and drug problems in this area of Stockholm County. The effort comprised three elements: an emphasis on reducing the sales of beer to underage young people in food shops, an intervention with primary care physicians to increase their discussions with patients about harmful drinking, and a RBS program that followed the content of other RBS programs described in this article. The local effort achieved a modest effect on sales of medium-strength beer to youth. The RBS component achieved a reduction in sales to obviously intoxicated persons from 5% (pre-intervention) to 47% (post-intervention). As a result of manager and staff training and policy development in alcohol establishments, findings indicated, using interrupted time-series analyses, a decrease in violent crime in the area served (Wallin *et al.*, 2003).

The Community Trials Project

The community trials project in the United States, a local alcohol policy project, tested a five-component three-community intervention to reduce alcohol-related harm among people of all ages. It sought to reduce acute injury and harm related to alcohol, that is, drunk-driving injuries and fatalities and injuries and deaths related to violence, drowning, burns, and falls. The effects of the program were evaluated by comparing three communities that received the intervention with matched-comparisons communities. Overall, off-premise outlets in experimental communities were half as likely to sell alcohol to minors as were the comparison sites. This was the joint result of special training of clerks and managers to conduct age identification checks, the development of effective off-premise outlet policies, and, especially, the threat of enforcement on sales to minors. Moreover, the drinking and driving component produced increased enforcement of drinking and driving laws and a significant reduction in alcohol-involved traffic crashes overall. Comparing experimental and control communities, it was found that the policy intervention produced significant reductions in nighttime injury crashes (10% lower in experimental than in comparison communities) and in crashes in which the driver was found by police to 'have been drinking' (6%). Assault injuries observed in hospital emergency departments declined by 43% in the intervention communities versus the comparison communities, and hospitalized assault injuries related to drinking declined by 2%. There was a 49% decline in reports of driving after 'having had too much to drink' and 51% in self-reports of driving when 'over the legal limit.' There was a significant reduction in problematic alcohol use: average drinks per occasion declined by 6% and the variance in drinking patterns (an indirect measure of heavy drinking) declined by 21% (Holder *et al.*, 2000).

Summary of Substance Abuse Prevention Effectiveness

Public decision makers who have the difficult task to reduce alcohol use and alcohol-related problems are faced with many complex and competing forces. Decisions about which prevention strategies to actually implement (or provide funds for) at a local, state, or national level are usually a compromise between political values and scientific evidence. This article has sought to provide a summary of the international evidence on the effectiveness of potential alternative alcohol policy strategies across countries and communities. The greater the generalizability of the findings internationally, the greater confidence one can have that any one policy strategy works in diverse settings and cultures.

Policy strategies that have been shown to be consistently effective over time and in two or more countries or cultural settings include the following:

- Retail price of alcohol
- Minimum age for drinking or purchase of alcohol
- Density of alcohol outlets
- Drinking/driving deterrence especially via regular and highly visible enforcement such as RBT

- Hours and days of alcohol sales
- RBS – alcohol serving and sales policies and training
- Lower BAC limits for driving.

This article has emphasized the importance of evidence of effectiveness as a critical condition for any public health policy concerning alcohol. However, in a time of restricted resources for prevention, the cost of a public policy relative to its demonstrated (or potential) effectiveness should be increasingly considered in the modern approach to substance abuse prevention. For example, a particular policy or strategy may be shown to be effective in a number of controlled studies, but, compared with an alternative policy or strategy, its potential to yield desired effects must be considered in terms of its cost to design, implement, and sustain. These are additional standards that alcohol policy in all countries should meet in the future.

One specific guide for decision makers in selecting cost-effective public policies in reducing alcohol harm is provided by the World Health Organization (see the section titled 'Relevant Website'). The analyses include taxation or retail price, RBT, a comprehensive ban on alcohol advertising, and brief intervention, as well as various combinations of these strategies. The research on which these recommendations are based can be found in the section, 'Further Reading.'

Based on the research evidence, policy recommendations are best matched with the cultural, economic, and policy situation of the country. The following can provide further guidance in considering potential effectiveness as well as cost:

- Less developed alcohol policy. For countries or communities in which there is no tradition of alcohol policy, the most directly effective policy is to increase the retail price of alcohol, usually through increased excise or direct alcohol sales taxes, if allowed by law. This is a low-cost policy and can increase government revenue while reducing alcohol problems. Such a policy is often opposed by producers and sellers of alcohol and can stimulate illegal alcohol production and smuggling.
- Moderately developed alcohol policy. For countries that have already implemented taxes on alcohol but wish to further reduce alcohol problems, adding restrictions on hours and days of sale as well as reducing the density and concentration of alcohol outlets is recommended. These two policies can be established at low cost but, to be effective, must be supported by sufficient government enforcement to ensure compliance. Some of this cost could be offset by licensing fees paid by alcohol outlets and by alcohol tax revenues. Retail outlets that sell alcohol will oppose such restrictions and will press for maximum hours and days of sale.
- More developed alcohol policy. For countries that have already implemented more comprehensive alcohol

policies involving retail price and restrictions on sales of alcohol, adding RBS and consistent enforcement will further reduce heavy drinking at bars, pubs, restaurants, and clubs. RBT and low BAC limits for driving will reduce traffic crashes involving alcohol, and lower minimum drinking or purchase ages supported by enforcement will reduce youth drinking, especially high-risk drinking. These more targeted policies have additional associated costs for enforcement and training, and require the support of citizens to implement and sustain.

This article has identified those public policies that have scientific evidence of effectiveness in reducing population-level alcohol problems. All of the policies for which effectiveness has been shown require a context that includes active implementation. This often requires regular police enforcement. It is also likely, based on the new research showing the impact of marketing, that regulation to reduce exposure, particularly of young people, to all forms of marketing could prove effective. In practice, the mix of policies that can actually be implemented reflects what is politically and economically possible within any country.

See also: Alcohol Consumption: Overview of International Trends; Alcoholism Treatment; Alcohol Industry.

Citations

Gruenewald PJ, Ponicki WR, and Holder HD (1993) The relationship of outlet densities to alcohol consumption: A time series cross-sectional analysis. *Alcoholism: Clinical and Experimental Research* 17: 38–47.

Holder HD, Gruenewald PJ, Ponicki WR, et al. (2000) Effect of community-based interventions on high-risk drinking and alcohol-related injuries. *Journal of the American Medical Association* 284: 2341–2347.

Jonah B, Mann R, Macdonald S, Stoduto G, Bondy S, and Shaikh A (2000) The effects of lowering legal blood alcohol limits: A review. In: *Proceedings of the 15th International Conference on Alcohol, Drugs and Traffic Safety*. Stockholm, Sweden: Ekom press.

Miller T, Snowden C, Birckmayer J, and Hendrie D (2006) Retail alcohol monopolies, underage drinking, and youth impaired driving deaths. *Accident Analysis and Prevention* 38: 1162–1167.

Nelson J (2003) Advertising bans, monopoly, and alcohol demand: Testing for substitution effects using state panel data. *Review of Industrial Organization* 22: 1–25.

Saffer H (2002) Alcohol advertising and youth. *Journal of Studies on Alcohol* Supplement 14: 173–181.

Saffer H and Dhaval D (2003) Alcohol consumption and alcohol advertising bans. *Applied Economics* 34: 1325–1334.

Saltz RF (1997) Prevention where alcohol is sold and consumed: Server intervention and responsible beverage service. In: Plant M, Single E and Stockwell T (eds.) *Alcohol: Minimising the Harm*, pp. 72–84. London: Free Association Books.

Shults RA, Elder RW, Sleet DA, et al. the Task Force on Community Preventive Services(2001) Review of evidence regarding interventions to reduce alcohol-impaired driving. *American Journal of Preventive Medicine* 31: 66–88.

Snyder L, Milici F, Slater M, Sun H, and Strizhakova Y (2006) Effects of alcohol advertising exposure on drinking among youth. *Archives of Pediatric and Adolescent Medicine* 160: 18–24.

Stockwell T, Chikritzhs T, Hendrie D, et al. (2001) The public health and safety benefits of the Northern Territory's Living with Alcohol programme. *Drug and Alcohol Review* 20: 167–180.

Treno AJ, Grube JW, and Martin SE (2003) Alcohol availability as a predictor of youth drinking and driving: A hierarchical analysis of survey and archival data. *Alcoholism: Clinical and Experimental Research* 27: 835–840.

Wagenaar AC and Holder HD (1996) The scientific process works: Seven replications now show significant wine sales increases after privatization. *Journal of Studies on Alcohol* 57: 575–576.

Wagenaar AC, Murray DM, and Toomey TL (2000) Communities mobilizing for change on alcohol (CMCA): Effects of a randomized trial on arrests and traffic crashes. *Addiction* 95: 209–217.

Wagenaar AC and Toomey TL (2002) Effects of minimum drinking age laws: Review and analyses of the literature from 1960 to 2000. *Journal of Studies on Alcohol.* Supplement 14: 206–225.

Wallin E, Norström T, and Andréasson S (2003) Alcohol prevention targeting licensed premises: A study of effects on violence. *Journal of Studies on Alcohol* 64: 270–277.

Further Reading

Babor T, Caetano R, Casswell S, et al. (2003) *Alcohol: No Ordinary Commodity: Research and Public Policy.* New York: Oxford University Press.

Chisholm D, Rehm J, Van Ommeren M, and Monteiro M (2004) Reducing the global burden of hazardous alcohol use: A comparative cost-effectiveness analysis. *Journal of Studies on Alcohol* 65: 782–793.

Cook PJ and Moore MJ (2002) The economics of alcohol abuse and alcohol-control policies. *Health Affairs* 21: 120–133.

Edwards G, Anderson P, Babor TF, et al. (1994) *Alcohol Policy and the Public Good.* Oxford, UK: Oxford University Press.

Holder HD (1998) *Alcohol and the Community: A Systems Approach to Prevention.* Cambridge, UK: Cambridge University Press.

Relevant Website

http://www.who.int/choice/interventions/rf_alcohol/en/index.html – World Health Organization (WHO).

Happiness, Health & Altruism

S G Post, Case Western Reserve University, Cleveland, OH, USA

Public health focuses in large part on contagion, pollutants, violence, and innumerable other sources – both natural and human – of illness, disability, and premature death; yet it also focuses on the emotional, relational, behavioral, and environmental aspects of well-being that contribute to individual and public flourishing. While public health most obviously concerns the amelioration of disease and dysfunction, primary prevention will often involve efforts to enhance human well-being (i.e., happiness), often through pro-social and altruistic (other-regarding) behaviors.

In both the European Union and the United States, self-reported happiness has been flat over the last 50 years, or has even slightly declined since 1936, despite each generation having more material wealth than did the preceding one; depression and anxiety rates have risen dramatically even when corrected for lower detection and reporting in the past. While those whose basic material needs are met are happier than those who struggle in poverty, once basic needs are met, increased material prosperity does not bring increased happiness. This is in part because people tend to assess their level of relative prosperity by making comparisons with those who have more, and thus always perceive themselves as wanting (Easterbrook, 2003). In addition, financial capital does not equate with social capital. Americans today, while better off materially than their forebears, now report having only two very close friends, whereas 20 years ago they had three. This loss of 'social capital,' which occurs despite material prosperity, has been described in terms of 'bowling alone' (Putnam, 2001). Psychologist Dan Kindlon (2001) addresses the problem of 'affluenza' in his nationwide survey of American teens, discovering that high levels of depression and anxiety are associated with low engagement in positive helping behaviors, loss of meaning, and material as well as emotional overindulgence by parents. The United States, despite its relative wealth per capita, ranks 23rd among nations in the first-ever 'world map of happiness,' (http://www.physorg.com/news73321785.html) which is based on self-reported life satisfaction.

Feeling Well by Doing Good

In response to the above problematic issues, researchers have begun to focus on the benefits to the agent of altruistic or 'other-regarding' behavior in the domains of families, neighborhood, and society. Rowe and Kahn (1998) point to the public health benefits of volunteerism for older adults. They point out that older adults for the most part agree with these two statements: 'Life is not worth living if one cannot contribute to the well-being of others'; 'Older people who no longer work should contribute through community service' (p. 178). They also point out that less than one-third of all older men and women work as volunteers, and those who do spend on average a bit less than 2 h per week. Midlarsky (1991) posed five reasons for benefits to older adults who engage in altruistic behavior: enhanced social integration; distraction from the agent's own problems; enhanced meaningfulness; increased perception of self-efficacy and competence; improved mood or more physically active lifestyle.

The idea of encouraging positive prosocial behavior as a means to well-being and health is not a new idea. For example, the transition in the 1820s in the United States and England from the maltreatment of mentally ill individuals – usually bound in shackles and physically abused – to 'moral treatment' was based not only on treating the insane with kindness and sympathy, but also on occupying their time with helping behaviors in the community and cultivating the love of nature. This evidently was quite successful, giving rise to the sweeping grounds of the Connecticut Retreat for the Insane (founded in 1822) in Hartford, now known as the Institute of Living; McLean Hospital in Belmont, Massachusetts; and several other sister institutions in eastern cities in the United States. Residents would do everything from milking cows and harvesting gardens to washing the dishes and sewing gifts for the needy (Clouette and Deslandes, 1997). Another example of the therapeutic use of altruism can be found in the 12 Steps of Alcoholics Anonymous. Step 12 requires the recovering alcoholic to help other persons with alcoholism. The framework is one of paradox. The recovering individual who helps others with this disease is to do so freely and with no expectation of reward:

> And then he discovers that by the divine paradox of this kind of giving he has found his own reward, whether his brother has yet received anything or not. (Alcoholics Anonymous, 1952: 109)

The AA member finds 'no joy greater than in a Twelfth Step job well done' (1952: 110). Those experienced with recovering alcoholics will widely attest as to how important such individuals feel that helping others is with regard to their own continued recovery, however much such helping behavior is in effect an AA recruitment activity.

To cite a more controversial instance of disinhibited altruism in relation to well-being, psychiatrist Mark Galanter, based on two decades of research, concluded that young people – often from middle-class or affluent families – who joined demanding new religious movements in the 1970s and 1980s had in general a somewhat more significant history of substance abuse than the general population, and were relatively socially isolated. In joining such groups, they reported relief from anxiety, meaninglessness, and depression through being members of communities requiring self-sacrifice and service, however much they may have been subject to authoritative manipulation and misplaced utopian idealism. Disillusionment and attrition after a year or two was the norm, but many still felt that they had discovered a more satisfying way of living (Galanter, 1999).

Most healthy people, however, are not so altruistically inhibited, at least in self-reported sentiment. The U.S. National Opinion Research Center's (NORC) landmark survey, the General Social Survey (GSS), has been administered across a U.S. national sample 24 times since 1972. Its 2002 administration, with support from the Fetzer Institute, included an item developed by epidemiologist Lynn G. Underwood regarding unselfish love: 'I feel a selfless caring for others.' Based on sample methods of the U.S. population that enjoy the highest level of confidence across a highly diversified sample pool, the following results were found with regard to the above question: many times a day (9.8); every day (13.2); most days (20.3); some days (24.0); once in a while (22.3); never or almost never (10.4) (Fetzer Institute, 2002).

There is a caveat – when caring for others is overwhelming and itself a cause of stress, the agent experiences negative health consequences, as is well-documented in caregivers of persons with dementia (Kiecolt-Glaser *et al.*, 2003). However, rather than harping on 'the burden of care,' as is characteristic of the gerontological literature, it needs to be stated that giving to others under ordinary circumstances seems to have significant benefits for the agent. A relevant study (Schwartz *et al.*, 2003) points to health benefits in generous behavior, but with the important proviso that there are adverse health consequences associated with being overly taxed.

Mental Health

Well-being consists of feeling hopeful, happy, and good about oneself, as well as energetic and connected to others. An early study compared retirees over age 65 who volunteered with those who did not (Hunter and Linn, 1980). Volunteers scored significantly higher in life satisfaction and will to live, and had fewer symptoms of depression, anxiety, and somatization. Because there were no differences in demographic and other background variables

between the groups, the researchers concluded that volunteer activity helped explain these mental health benefits. The nonvolunteers did spend more days in the hospital and were taking more medications, which may have prevented them from volunteering. However, the mental health benefits persisted after controlling for disability.

The mental health benefits of volunteerism include reduction in depressive symptoms (Musick and Wilson, 2003; Musick *et al.*, 1999), happiness, and enhanced well-being. Schwartz *et al.* (2003) focused on a stratified random sample of 2016 members of the Presbyterian church located throughout the United States. The study's purpose was to investigate whether altruistic social behaviors such as helping others were associated with better physical and mental health. Mailed questionnaires evaluated giving and receiving help, prayer activities, positive and negative religious coping, and self-reported physical and mental health. Multivariate regression analysis revealed no association between giving or receiving help and physical functioning, although the sample was skewed toward high physical functioning. After adjusting for age, gender, stressful life events, income, general health, religious coping, and asking God for healing, both helping others and receiving help were associated with mental health (i.e., anxiety and depression). Giving help was more significantly associated with better mental health than was receiving help. The authors concluded that:

> helping others is associated with higher levels of mental health, above and beyond the benefits of receiving help and other known psychospiritual, stress, and demographic factors. (2003: 782)

The authors add that feeling overwhelmed by others' demands had a stronger negative relationship with mental health than helping others had a positive one.

Physical Health

A review of existing studies indicates that research on the effect of kindness and volunteerism on health may have begun inadvertently in 1956, when a team of researchers from Cornell University School of Medicine in the United States began following 427 married women with children under the hypothesis that housewives with more children would be under greater stress and die earlier than women with few children (Moen *et al.*, 1993). Surprisingly, they found that numbers of children, education, class, and work status did not affect longevity. After following these women for 30 years, however, it was found that 52% of those who did not belong to a volunteer organization had experienced a major illness, compared to 36% who did belong. While a potential confounding factor is that people who volunteer may start out in better physical health, this would not greatly diminish the study's implications.

Oman of the University of California at Berkeley is one of the leading researchers in this field. Oman and colleagues (1999) focused on 2025 community-dwelling residents of Marin County, California, who were first examined in 1990–91. All respondents were 55 or older at this baseline examination; 95% were non-Hispanic white, 58% were female, and a majority had annual incomes above $15 000. Residents were classified as practicing 'high volunteerism' if they were involved in two or more helping organizations, and as practicing 'moderate volunteerism' if they were involved in one. The number of hours invested in helping behavior was also measured, although this was not as predictive as the number of organizations. Physical health status was assessed on the basis of reported medical diagnoses, as well as such factors as 'tiring easily' and self-perceived overall health. After controlling for age, gender, number of chronic conditions, physical mobility, exercise, self-rated general health, health habits (smoking), social support (marital status, religious attendance), and psychological status (depressive symptoms), those who volunteered for two or more organizations had a highly significant 44% lower mortality rate.

On a cross-cultural level, Krause and colleagues (1999) at the University of Michigan studied a sample of 2153 older adults in Japan, examining the relationships between religion, providing help to others, and health. They found that those who provided more assistance to others were significantly more likely to indicate that their physical health was better.

Brown *et al.* (2003) report on a 5-year study involving 423 older couples. Each couple was asked what type of practical support they provided for friends or relatives, if they could count on help from others when needed, and what type of emotional support they gave each other. A total of 134 people died over the 5 years. After adjusting for a variety of factors – including age, gender, and physical and emotional health – the researchers found an association between reduced risk of dying and giving help, but no association between receiving help and reduced death risk. Brown concluded that those who provided no instrumental or emotional support to others were more than twice as likely to die in the 5 years as people who helped spouses, friends, relatives, and neighbors. Despite concerns that the longevity effects might be due to a healthier individual's greater ability to provide help, the results remained the same after the researchers controlled for functional health, health satisfaction, health behaviors, age, income, education level, and other possible confounders. The researchers concluded:

> If giving, rather than receiving, promotes longevity, then interventions that are currently designed to help people feel supported may need to be redesigned so that the emphasis is on what people do to help others. (Brown *et al.*, 2003: 326)

The benefits of altruism may not be limited to older adults; the differences in health outcomes between helpers and nonhelpers is more difficult to detect in younger age groups, however, where health is not affected by susceptibilities associated with aging. Ironson and colleagues (2002) at the University of Miami compared the characteristics of long-term survivors with AIDS ($n = 79$) with an HIV-positive comparison group equivalent (based on CD4 count) that had been diagnosed for a relatively shorter time ($n = 200$). These investigators found that survivors were significantly more likely to be spiritual or religious. The effect of spirituality/religiousness on survival, however, was mediated by 'helping others with HIV.' Thus, helping others (altruism) accounted for a significant part of the relationship between spirituality/religiousness and long-term survival in this study.

Explanatory Models

Altruism results in deeper and more positive social integration, distraction from personal problems and the anxiety of self-preoccupation, enhanced meaning and purpose as related to well-being, a more active lifestyle that counters cultural pressures toward isolated passivity, and the presence of positive emotions such as kindness that displace harmful negative emotional states. It is entirely quite plausible, then, to assert that altruism enhances happiness and health.

The idea that human beings are inclined toward helpful pro-social and altruistic behavior seems incontrovertible, and it is highly plausible that the inhibition of such behavior and related emotions would be unhealthy. What conceptual models would help explain the connection between altruism and health? Three closely interwoven models can be suggested: evolutionary biology, physiological advantages, and positive emotion.

First, the association between a kind, generous way of life and health prolongevity can be interpreted in light of evolutionary psychology. Group selection theory suggests a powerfully adaptive connection between widely diffuse altruism within groups and group survival. Altruistic behavior within groups confers a competitive advantage against other groups that would be selected for (Sober and Wilson, 1998).

Second, this association can be interpreted in the context of reduced stress. The 'fight-or-flight' response, with its well-documented physiological cascade, is adaptive in the face of perceived danger. If the threat continues for an extended period, however, the immune and cardiovascular systems are adversely impacted, weakening the body's defense and making it more susceptible to abnormal internal cellular processes involved in malignant degeneration (Sternberg, 2001). Altruistic emotions can gain dominance over anxiety and fear, turning off the fight-or-flight response. Immediate and unspecified physiological changes may occur as a result of volunteering and helping others, leading to the 'helper's high' (Luks, 1988). Two-thirds of helpers report a distinct physical sensation associated with helping; about half report that they experienced a 'high' feeling, while 43% felt stronger and more energetic, 28% felt warm, 22% felt calmer and less depressed, 21% experienced greater self-worth, and 13% experienced fewer aches and pains.

Third, this association can be understood in light of the salutary aspects of positive emotions. Norman B. Anderson (2003) of the American Psychological Association highlights six dimensions of health:

- biology (biological well-being)
- thoughts and actions (psychological and behavioral well-being)
- environment and relationships (environmental and social well-being)
- personal achievement and equality (economic well-being)
- faith and meaning (existential, religious, spiritual well-being)
- emotions (emotional well-being).

According to the Anderson model, positive emotions (kindness, other-regarding love, compassion, etc.) enhance health by virtue of pushing aside negative ones. Anderson draws on a wealth of studies to conclude that 'the big three' negative emotions are 'sadness/depression, fear/anxiety, and anger/hostility' (2003: 243). It is difficult to be angry, resentful, or fearful when one is showing unselfish love toward another person. These findings suggest possible mechanisms through which chronic unforgiving responses (grudges) may erode health, whereas forgiving responses may enhance it (Witvliet *et al.*, 2001).

Conclusions

There is a strong association between the well-being, happiness, health, and longevity of people who are emotionally kind and compassionate in their charitable helping activities – as long as they are not overwhelmed, and here world view may come into play. Of course, this is a population generalization that provides no guarantees for the individual.

Proverbs 11:25 reads: 'a generous man will prosper, he who refreshes others will himself be refreshed.' Plato, too, suggested that virtue is its own reward. The purported link between helping behavior and happiness is at the core of Dickens's story of Ebenezer Scrooge, for with each new expression of kindness Scrooge became more buoyant, until finally he was among the happiest and most generous men in all of England. He surely felt a great deal happier

with life the more generous he became, following the pattern of the 'helper's high' (Luks, 1988).

The freedom from a solipsistic life in which one relates to others only insofar as they contribute to one's own agendas, as well as a general freedom from the narrow concerns of the self, bring us internal benefits, as all significant spiritual and moral traditions prescribe. Here, epidemiology of health, happiness, and altruism can enter a fruitful dialogue.

Citations

Alcoholics Anonymous (1952) *Twelve Steps and Twelve Traditions*. New York: Alcoholics Anonymous.

Anderson NB (2003) *Emotional Longevity: What Really Determines How Long You Live*. New York: Viking.

Brown S, Nesse RM, Vonokur AD, and Smith DM (2003) Providing social support may be more beneficial than receiving it: Results from a prospective study of mortality. *Psychological Science* 14(4): 320–327.

Clouette B and Deslandes P (1997) The Hartford retreat for the insane: An early example of the use of "moral treatment" in America. *Connecticut Medicine: The Journal of the Connecticut State Medical Society* 61(9): 521–527.

Easterbrook G (2003) *The Progress Paradox: How Life Gets Better While People Feel Worse*. New York: Random House.

Fetzer Institute/National Institute on Aging Working Group (2002) *Multidimensional Measurement of Religiousness/Spirituality for Use in Health Research*. Kalamazoo, MI: Fetzer Institute.

Galanter M (1999) *Cults: Faith, Healing, and Coercion,* 2nd edn. New York: Oxford University Press.

Hunter KI and Linn MW (1980) Psychosocial differences between elderly volunteers and non-volunteers. *International Journal of Aging and Human Development* 12(3): 205–213.

Ironson G, Solomon GF, and Balbin EG (2002) Spirituality and religiousness are associated with long survival, health behaviors, less distress, and lower cortisol in people living with HIV/AIDS. *Annals of Behavioral Medicine* 24: 34–40.

Kiecolt-Glaser JK, Preacher KJ, MacCallum RC, Malarkey WB, and Glaser R (2003) Chronic stress and age-related increases in the proinflammatory cytokine interleukin-6. *Proceedings of the National Academy of Sciences* 100: 9090–9095.

Kindlon D (2001) *Too Much of a Good Thing: Raising Children of Character in an Indulgent Age*. New York: Hyperion.

Krause N, Ingersoll-Dayton B, Liang J, and Sugisawa H (1999) Religion, social support, and health among the Japanese elderly. *Journal of Health and Social Behavior* 40: 405–421.

Luks A (1988) Helper's high: Volunteering makes people feel good, physically and emotionally. *Psychology Today* October: 34–42.

Midlarsky E (1991) Helping as coping. *Prosocial Behavior: Review of Personality and Social Psychology* 12: 238–264.

Moen P, Dempster-McCain D, and Williams RM (1993) Successful aging. *American Journal of Sociology* 97: 1612–1632.

Musick MA and Wilson J (2003) Volunteering and depression: The role of psychological and social resources in different age groups. *Social Science and Medicine* 56(2): 259–269.

Oman D, Thoresen CE, and McMahon K (1999) Volunteerism and mortality among the community-dwelling elderly. *Journal of Health Psychology* 4: 301–316.

Putnam RD (2001) *Bowling Alone: The Collapse and Revival of American Culture*. New York: Simon & Schuster.

Rowe JW and Kahn RL (1998) *Successful Aging*. New York: Pantheon.

Schwartz C, Meisenhelder JB, Ma Y, and Reed G (2003) Altruistic social interest behaviors are associated with better mental health. *Psychosomatic Medicine* 65: 778–785.

Sober E and Wilson DS (1998) *Unto Others: The Evolution of Unselfish Behavior*. Cambridge, MA: Harvard University Press.

Sternberg EM (2001) *The Balance Within: The Science Connecting Health and Emotions*. New York: W.W. Freeman.

Witvliet CV, Ludwig TE, and Kelly LVL (2001) Granting forgiveness or harboring grudges: Implications for emotion, physiology and health. *Psychological Science* 12(2): 117–123.

Further Reading

Berkman LS and Syme L (1970) Social networks, host resistance, and mortality: A nine-year follow-up study of Alameda county residents. *American Journal of Epidemiology* 109(2): 186–204.

Justice B (1987) *Who Gets Sick: Thinking Through Health.* Houston, TX: Peak Press.

Keyes LM and Haidt JH (eds.) (2003) *Flourishing: Positive Psychology and the Life Well-Lived.* Washington, DC: American Psychological Association Press.

Peterson C and Seligman MEP (eds.) (2004) *Character Strengths and Virtues: A Handbook and Classification.* New York: Oxford University Press.

Post SG (ed.) (2007) *Altruism and Health: An Empirical Approach.* New York: Oxford University Press.

Post SG, Underwood LG, Schloss JR, and Hurlbut WB (eds.) (2002) *Altruism and Altruistic Love: Science, Philosophy and Religion in Dialogue.* New York: Oxford University Press.

Health-Related Stigma and Discrimination

R L Barrett, Stanford University, Stanford, CA, USA

Introduction

Stigma was originally a Greek term for a permanent mark that branded a person as a criminal, traitor, or slave. In recent decades, stigma has referred to the process of negative discrimination against people for having certain physical, behavioral, or social attributes. Many health conditions are socially stigmatized in certain societies. Where present, stigma and discrimination can have a significant impact upon the epidemiology, course, and control of human diseases. For this reason, it is important to better understand the biosocial dynamics of disease discrimination and address it as a public health problem.

From Deviance to Discrimination

It was not until the late 1950s that social discrimination became a major topic of study in public health and the social sciences. Before then, research had been focused upon deviance from socially established norms – undesired personal attributes that contrasted with cultural beliefs about how people should appear and act under a given set of circumstances. Deviance was considered pathological by definition, a social disease whose underlying cause and ultimate cure had yet to be discovered. Numerous studies focused upon causal factors such as poverty, education, family structure, and heredity. Yet few studies considered the other side of the equation: How and why societies become intolerant to certain human differences.

The emphasis on deviance as pathology began to change in the decades following World War II, influenced by revelations of the Holocaust, an emerging Civil Rights Movement in the United States and Europe, and numerous independence struggles throughout the world. Within this historical context, attention shifted from discredited to discreditor, focusing on the processes by which negative labels are constructed and assigned to particular human attributes, in particular sociocultural contexts. Tracing its intellectual roots to thinkers such as Marx and Manheim, this social constructivist movement sought to understand the ways in which these categories are constructed into objective realities and internalized into unconscious norms. In this manner, the study of social deviance gave way to the study of social discrimination.

Howard Becker (1963) and Ernest Goffman (1963) were early proponents of this constructivist approach to discrimination. Becker focused on the lines of toleration for behavioral attributes that marked certain people as social outsiders. Becker observed what he called the moral career of the discredited, in which people who were beyond the point of societal reintegration would amplify their differences in order to gain acceptance into a smaller out-group having similar attributes. Becker also identified moral entrepreneurs, people who wield power within a society by defining the categories of normal and abnormal. In similar studies, health professionals were seen as imputational specialists with the power to define and adjudicate matters of health and illness (Friedson, 1979). Under these circumstances, deviance could no longer be seen as a simple fact. It was the result of exchanges between the discredited, their discreditors, and the people who defined their terms of interaction.

Although innovative, Becker nevertheless worked with the same terminology as the deviance researchers before him. By contrast, Goffman chose to relabel the entire phenomenon as stigma. Whereas the original Greek term referred to a permanent physical mark, Goffman redefined this mark as the social disgrace itself. Goffman's definition is commonly used in studies of health-related discrimination today. He also developed the notion of master status, a physical, behavioral, or tribal attribute that eclipses all other aspects of a person's identity. A master status becomes objectified when both attribute and disgrace merge into a single unquestionable reality. This objectification occurs within the minds of the discredited as well, insofar as they have long been socialized to have the same prejudices as their discreditors.

At the community level, Goffman described how courtesy stigma – sanctions against normals for their association with the stigmatized – perpetuates social discrimination, even among those who were sympathetic to their situation. Moreover, the discredited perpetuate their own stigmata even as they attempt to disavow their condition. These disavowal mechanisms included: (1) covering – the concealment of the mark; (2) passing – techniques to minimize the tension of social interactions; and, (3) sheltering – segregation from protective environments. Although these disavowal techniques provide short-term palliation for stigmatization, they often do so at the cost of reinforcing underlying social prejudices.

Stigma and Infectious Diseases

In addition to its personal consequences, health-related stigma can impede the prevention and control of infectious diseases. This can occur with stigmatized diseases when people actively conceal their condition to avoid social sanctions. Even with an accurate understanding of disease contagion, people may not want to risk the consequences of unemployment and ostracism for themselves and their families. Concealment strategies are therefore common among people with stigmatized infections, and many are disinclined to seek early testing as a consequence. For these undetected cases, the opportunities for transmission increase exponentially according to the number of susceptible contacts, their contacts, and so forth. In this manner, stigma can perpetuate the spread of infectious diseases.

Avoidance of testing is especially common in countries where the treatment of certain diseases is not well integrated with primary health services. In India, for example, people often avoid being seen in the vicinity of a leprosy treatment worker lest they be publicly branded as having the disease. In addition, the segregation of treatment services can result in a segregation of knowledge. Without proper training, primary health providers may miss the early signs of a disease and fail to make appropriate referrals in a timely manner (Barrett, 2005).

The stigma of AIDS presents similar challenges for early detection as well as efforts to prevent behaviors

having a high risk for disease transmission. For instance, advocating condom use can be seen as accusatory in some societies, or it may raise the suspicion that the person requesting a condom already has a sexually transmitted disease. Suspicions notwithstanding, it may not be socially feasible to advocate for safer sexual exchanges if there are significant power differences between partners due to other forms of discrimination. In a study of HIV prevention among single women in Uganda, the subjects described how their diminished social and economic status prevented them from insisting upon safer sexual exchanges, despite having accurate knowledge of disease transmission and easy access to condoms (McGrath *et al.*, 1993).

Social stigma can also impede patient adherence to disease treatment regimens. People may travel much further for treatment to avoid social detection. These circumstances tend to reduce the frequency and quality of patient–provider communications. Reduced communications increase the possibility of nonadherence, especially when the prescribed regimen is lengthy, requires behavior changes, or is subject to side effects. If, in addition to the disease stigma, the patient also belongs to a historically discriminated social group, they may be distrustful of their providers if the latter do not share the same background.

In the event of a major infectious disease outbreak, the stigma of infection can slow the ability of public health providers to control the spread of infection in a population. This is especially the case for surveillance–containment, or ring vaccination programs, in which providers rely upon cases to provide them with complete, accurate, and timely information about their contacts. When people are reticent to provide this information, contact tracing may not keep pace with the spread of the disease – a failure in the so-called race to trace in epidemic control. Under these circumstances, providers are not able to establish a sufficient ring of immunity around cases and contacts. They must resort instead to more expensive and difficult mass vaccination programs.

Finally, social discrimination can lead to an unequal or inappropriate distribution of public health resources, which may in turn result in avoidable disease morbidity and mortality. For example, an historical analysis of institutional responses to epidemics in North America found that medical authorities affected the social and geographic distribution of diseases such as cholera and polio, by distinguishing between innocent and guilty victims according to socioeconomic status (Risse, 1988). As a result, many public health initiatives for improving urban environments neglected poor neighborhoods that were hardest hit by these diseases, thereby exacerbating health differences between socioeconomic groups and developing reservoirs that would eventually pose risks to affluent and poor communities alike. These same processes have been attributed to many re-emerging infectious diseases of the late twentieth century, for which the borders between rich and poor countries have been more permeable to pathogens than the resources with which to control them (Farmer, 1996).

Stigma and Chronic Health Conditions

There are several ways that social stigma can significantly affect the severity and course of chronic noninfectious diseases. First, the negative attribution of degenerative diseases can influence their symptomatic experience. Studies of chronic pain patients found that the absence of physical signs compromised the social legitimacy of their condition, which, in turn, was associated with the severity and quality of their pain (Good, 1992). In this manner, the stigma of an illegitimate illness can create a perpetual cycle of feedback between social and physical suffering.

Second, the psychological impact of stigma and discrimination can be expressed through physical problems. For example, some socially marginalized communities in China describe physical problems in similar terms to that of their social alienation (Kleinman, 1992). Under these circumstances, it may as difficult for health providers to distinguish between emotional and physical problems as it is for the patients themselves. These kinds of examples have been described as nocebo phenomena (Hahn, 1997). Just as pharmacologically neutral placebos can mitigate psychosomatic suffering in a variety of physical and psychological conditions, so too can professional and community practices act as nocebos to worsen psychosomatic experiences. There is evidence that the quality of the physician–patient relationship can act as a placebo or nocebo to affect the symptomatic course of conditions ranging from asthma to heart disease (Hahn, 1997).

Some studies have shown correlations between social discrimination and the trajectory of chronic degenerative conditions. For example, a small but significant association has been found between the emotional tensions of racial discrimination and increased incidence of high blood pressure among African-Americans (Dressler, 1993). Insofar as discrimination is related to segregation, this association is further supported by the longitudinal study of over 1000 people born in Alameda, California, in which measures of social isolation were shown to correlate with suicide, diabetes, heart disease, and significantly lower overall life expectancies (McGuire and Raleigh, 1986).

It should also be noted that social stigma can significantly diminish the economic status of the discredited, thereby increasing their risk for diseases strongly associated with poverty. A person who has been socially and economically ostracized due to one health condition could be at greater risk for other diseases due to poor living conditions, undernutrition, and psychological stress. By this process, the stigma need not be health-related for it to play a role in all manner of health conditions. For all these reasons, stigma itself is a public health problem.

Theories of Etiology and Prevention

A public health approach to stigma and discrimination entails an understanding of its etiological factors and potential areas for prevention. Similar to past studies of deviance as pathology, some theories explain that certain health conditions are universally stigmatized because of their intrinsic biological characteristics. Accordingly, one can predict that conditions associated with physical deformation, contagiousness, incurability, and high mortality will result in a proportional degree of negative attribution, independent of cultural and historical conditions. These associations suggest that negative social attitudes constitute an adaptive human response to potentially dangerous diseases.

Other more constructivist theories counter that there is considerable variation in public attitudes toward some of the most commonly stigmatized diseases, and that this variation is often independent of biological factors. Leprosy, for example, is not a universally stigmatized disease. Cross-cultural studies of social attitudes toward leprosy show significant differences between societies and historical periods (Gussow, 1989). Even the most negative attitudes toward leprosy defy the fact that it is a mildly contagious and easily treated disease. This then leads to the question of why the disease would be stigmatized within certain social and temporal contexts more than others.

There are several alternative theories to explain sociohistorical variation in health-related stigma and discrimination. A common set of theories emphasizes the aggravating effects of ignorance on discrimination; these theories typically describe an inverse relationship between the degree of accurate medical knowledge about a given health condition and social attitudes toward the people who have it. Examples may include relatively new infections such as HIV/AIDS, rare neurological conditions such as Huntington's chorea or Machado-Joseph disease (Boutte, 1987). They may also include psychiatric conditions such as depression and schizophrenia, for which the causes are as poorly understood as their means for effective treatment.

Other theories predict discrimination against physical and mental disabilities, even when the conditions themselves are commonly known. In these cases, unfamiliarity with the challenges and capacities of the disabled creates tensions during social interaction. In a well-known study conducted by Robert Murphy (1988), a disabled anthropologist, one community of recently paralyzed people describes these tensions and the social ambiguity with which they are associated. Murphy argues that many social categories are linked to basic physical acts such as sex and ambulation. When a person is unable to perform such acts as expected, then he or she falls between social categories and becomes stigmatized as a consequence.

Building on Goffman's (1963) description of courtesy stigma, another theory states that certain health conditions become socially discredited because of a perceived association with other discredited behaviors or membership in marginalized racial, ethnic, or gender groups. A related theory in social psychology states that these dual associations are a coping mechanism for reducing the perceived susceptibility to an unwanted condition. By associating a disease or other tragedy with another human group and somehow blaming its members for the tragedy, the discriminating group constructs a just world in which they can more easily deny their vulnerability to random misfortune.

Finally, health professionals can inadvertently stigmatize particular conditions even as they attempt to assist their patient populations. Although sometimes unavoidable, isolation procedures can exacerbate community fears and create a sense of alienation among patients. Health prevention campaigns and fundraisers may highlight the worst aspects of certain diseases in order to maximize behavioral changes and financial support, but they also risk distorting community perceptions and attitudes. Further research is needed to determine how best to balance these competing interests, as well as the causes, consequences, and means for preventing health-related discrimination.

See also: Stigma of Mental illness.

Citations

Barrett RL (2005) Self-mortification and the stigma of leprosy in northern India. *Medical Anthropology Quarterly* 19(2): 216–230.

Becker HS (1963) *Outsiders: Studies in the Sociology of Deviance*. New York: Macmillan.

Boutte MI (1987) 'The stumbling disease:' A case study of stigma among Azorean-Portugese. *Social Science and Medicine* 24(3): 209–217.

Dressler WW (1993) Health in the African American community: Accounting for health inequalities. *Medical Anthropology Quarterly* 7(4): 325–335.

Farmer P (1996) Social inequalities and emerging infectious diseases. *Emerging Infectious Diseases* 2(4): 259–269.

Friedson E (1979) *Profession of Medicine: A Study of the Sociology of Applied Knowledge*. New York: Dodd Mead & Co.

Goffman E (1963) *Stigma: Notes on the Management of Spoiled Identity*. Engelwood Cliffs, NJ: Prentice Hall.

Good BJ (1992) The body in pain: The making of a world of chronic pain. In: Good BJ (ed.) *Pain as Human Experience: An Anthropological Perspective*, pp. 29–48. Berkeley, CA: University of California Press.

Gussow Z (1989) *Leprosy, Racism, and Public Health: Social Policy in Chronic Disease Control*. Boulder, CO: Westview Press.

Hahn RA (1997) The nocebo phenomenon: Concept, evidence, and implications for public health. *Preventative Medicine* 26: 607–611.

Kleinman A (1992) Pain and resistance: The delegitimation and relegitimation of local worlds. In: Good BJ (ed.) *Pain as Human Experience: An Anthropological Perspective*, pp. 169–197. Berkeley, CA: University of California Press

McGrath JW, Rwabukwali CB, Schumann DA, *et al.* (1993) Anthropology and AIDS: The cultural context of sexual risk behavior among urban Baganda women in Kampala Uganda. *Social Science and Medicine* 36(4): 429–439.

McGuire MT and Raleigh MJ (1986) Behavioral and physiological correlates of ostracism. *Ethology and Sociobiology* 39(187): 187–200.

Murphy RF, Scheer J, Murphy Y, and Mack R (1988) Physical disability and social liminality: A study in the rituals of adversity. *Social Science and Medicine* 26(2): 235–242.

Risse GB (1988) Epidemics and history: Ecological perspectives and social responses. In: Fee E and Fox D (eds.) *AIDS: The Burdens of History*, pp. 33–66. Berkeley, CA: University of California Press

Further Reading

Ablon J (1981) Stigmatized health conditions. *Social Science and Medicine* 15B: 5–9.

Ainlay SC, Coleman LM, and Becker G (eds.) (1986) *The Dilemma of Difference: A Multidisciplinary View of Stigma*. New York: Plenum.

Allport GW (1954) *The Nature of Prejudice*. Reading, UK: Addison-Wesley.

Becker G (1981) Coping with stigma: Lifelong adaptation of deaf people. *Social Science and Medicine* 15B: 21–24.

Cohen L (1998) *No Aging in India: Alzheimer's, the Bad Family, and Other Modern Things*. Berkeley, CA: University of California Press.

Farmer P (1992) *AIDS and Accusation: Haiti and the Geography of Blame*. Berkeley, CA: University of California Press.

Inhorn M (1986) Genital herpes: An ethnographic inquiry into being discreditable in American society. *Medical Anthropology Quarterly* 17: 59–63.

Jones EE, Scott RA, and Markus H (1984) *Social Stigma: The Psychology of Marked Relationships*. New York: WH Freeman and Co.

Major B and O'Brien LT (2005) The social psychology of stigma. *Annual Review of Psychology* 56: 393–421.

Pfohl S (1985) *Images of Deviance and Social Control*. New York: McGraw Hill.

Pfuhl EH and Henry S (1993) *The Deviance Process*. New York: Aldine de Gruyter.

Rubel AJ and Garro LC (1992) Social and cultural factors in the successful control of tuberculosis. *Public Health Reports* 107(6): 626–635.

Sontag S (1977) *Illness as Metaphor*. New York: Vintage Books.

Volinn IJ (1983) Health professionals as stigmatizers and destigmatizers of diseases: Alcoholism and leprosy as examples. *Social Science and Medicine* 17(7): 385–393.

Waxler N (1981) Learning to be a leper: A case study in the social construction of illness. In: Mishler EG (ed.) *Social Contexts of Health, Illness, and Patient Care*, pp. 169–194. Cambridge, UK: Cambridge University Press

Illicit Drug Trends Globally

P Griffiths and M Meacham, EMCDDA, Lisbon, Portugal
R McKetin, University of New South Wales, Sydney, Australia

Introduction: From American Disease to Global Epidemic

When David Musto penned his influential history of narcotic control in 1973, *The American Disease* would have seemed an appropriate title. Throughout the twentieth century, drug use in America had regularly been an issue of concern, and by the 1970s, it had become one of the key U.S. domestic policy issues. In reality, the use of psychoactive substances by humans is virtually universal. In many parts of the world indigenous people were continuing to use psychoactive substances, including those controlled under the United Nations (UN) drug control conventions, in much the same way as they had for centuries. But this kind of drug consumption remained largely unrecognized or simply ignored at a global level. Similarly, in some parts of Europe drug use among the artistic and fashionable elite had existed since the beginning of the nineteenth century, and postwar Europe to some extent mirrored the American association of drug use with a growing youth and counterculture. However, in the 1970s, it appeared that drug use was predominantly a problem of the developed world, and in only a handful of nations was it becoming recognized as an important public health issue.

To a large extent, this condition has changed, and drug use has now become recognized as a global problem. While a debate still exists that sets drug consumers in the affluent developed world against drug producers in poorer developing countries, this paradigm is increasingly being replaced with a discourse that acknowledges a shared responsibility for the illicit drug problem. There are a number of reasons for this paradigm shift. First, drug consumption in many developing countries is now considerable. Second, the development of new patterns of synthetic drug use, along with technological developments that allow cannabis to be intensively produced, mean that significant drug production is now occurring in developed countries. Finally, governments in many developing and transitional countries have recognized the potential costs of drug problems and their links to other pressing social concerns, such as crime, community safety, AIDSinfection, corruption, and general political instability.

As drug use has become recognized as a widespread problem, there has been a gradual change in how it is being tackled. If any moment can be said to mark the recognition of the drug problem as a common global responsibility, it was the 1998 UN General Assembly Special Session (UNGASS) on the world drug problem. The UNGASS was accompanied by a 10-year action plan to reduce drug use, and more importantly, it also committed signatories in the accompanying Declaration on Guiding Principles of Drug Demand Reduction. This declaration outlined the need to balance drug interdiction efforts with initiatives to reduce the demand for illicit drugs, and the need for these initiatives to be based on a comprehensive and regular assessment of the illicit drug situation.

Looking to the future, drug use problems are likely to be increasingly associated with the developing rather than developed world because of the combined impact of globalization, urbanization, and that a far greater proportion of those in the developing world are young – the predominant risk group for drug use. Moreover, because drug problems have a tendency to coalesce with and exacerbate other health and social ills, the developing world may disproportionately pay the public health and social cost of future drug epidemics.

Monitoring Illicit Drug Trends

Measuring Illicit Drug Use

A number of problems hamper any discussions of illicit drug trends at the global level. A large part of uncovering the public health aspect of illicit drug trends involves appreciation of the nuances regarding which substances are classified as drugs, what constitutes drug use, and when drug use becomes drug 'abuse' or problematic. Drug use encompasses a complex set of behaviors that are usually found at low prevalence and tend to be stigmatized and well hidden. This presents the researcher with a number of practical, methodological, and even ethical challenges, a review of which can be found in *Epidemiology of Drug Abuse,* edited by Zili Sloboda (2005). For practical and methodological reasons, monitoring the extent of drug use is typically restricted to simple behavioral measures of drug use within a temporal reference period. Currently the most common measures used for monitoring purposes are lifetime prevalence, past-year prevalence, past-month prevalence and, if available, the number of days the drug was used in the past month. Although it is theoretically possible with this sort of approach to also look at combined use of different substances, in practice this can be quite difficult. Growing recognition of this issue has led to a greater interest in adapting current approaches to be more sensitive to multi- or poly-drug use (for more on multidrug use, see under the section titled 'Concluding remarks').

From a public health perspective, it is not only the use of drugs *per se* that is of interest, but the identification of drug users that would meet a clinical definition of drug 'abuse' or 'dependence,' who disproportionately account for drug consumption and drug-related harm. Both the DSM-IV (*Diagnostic and Statistical Manual of Mental Disorders*) and ICD-10 (*International Classification of Diseases*) have diagnostic criteria that are useful at the individual, or clinical, level in assessing dependence on drugs. Clinical assessment of drug dependence is usually not feasible within the context of routine drug-monitoring systems, necessitating the use of behavioral proxies of problem drug use, such as daily drug use or other high-risk drug-using behaviors (e.g., injecting drug use) (**Figure 1**).

Even defining which psychoactive substances fall under the general heading of illicit drug use can be problematic. Illicit drugs are scheduled by the UN and national governments according to their perceived degree of harm and other considerations. However, not all drugs that are prohibited at a national level necessarily fall under international control. *Khat*, for example, is currently prohibited in some countries but freely available elsewhere, and in its natural plant form it is not subject to international control.

Drug problems can also occur through the misuse of diverted medicines intended for therapeutic or pharmaceutical purposes, or by imbibing household or industrial products that contain psychoactive chemicals. The innovative nature of the contemporary synthetic drug market also lends itself to discovery of new psychoactive substances that do not fall under current UN international drug control conventions.

Classification of drug types is a further concern when monitoring global illicit drug trends. Some countries still classify drugs as being narcotics or psychotropics, according to whether they fall under the 1961 UN Single Convention on Narcotic Drugs (including cocaine, heroin, and cannabis), or the later conventions on psychotropic substances, which cover a range of synthetic drugs. Contemporary classification of illicit drugs is more specific, and there have been significant efforts to harmonize the reporting of illicit drug trends along globally recognized drug classification systems. The most problematic area in terms of drug classification is the nomenclature used to describe various types of synthetic drugs, where drug market conditions can preclude monitoring specific substances (e.g., pills containing a combination of illicit psychoactive ingredients).

Global, Regional, and National Drug Monitoring Mechanisms

Historically, the engine driving drug monitoring was the need to assess the effectiveness of supply reduction measures and the adherence of UN member states to the drug control conventions; however, public health concerns have increasingly risen in prominence. At the international level an outcome of this transition can be seen in the range of bodies with an interest in collecting data on drug use: the UN Office on Drugs and Crime (UNODC), which acts as a secretariat for the Commission on Narcotic Drugs (CND);

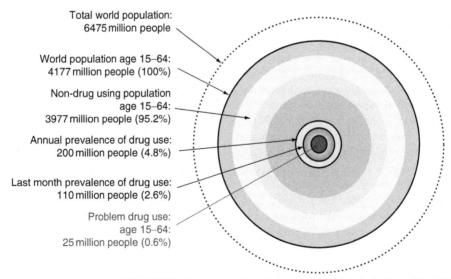

Total world population:
6475 million people

World population age 15–64:
4177 million people (100%)

Non-drug using population age 15–64:
3977 million people (95.2%)

Annual prevalence of drug use:
200 million people (4.8%)

Last month prevalence of drug use:
110 million people (2.6%)

Problem drug use:
age 15–64:
25 million people (0.6%)

Figure 1   Illegal drug use at the global level (2005/2006). In percent of population age 15–64. Adapted from World Drug Report (2006). United Nations Office on Drugs and Crime (2006a) *World Drug Report 2006. Volume 1: Analysis*. Vienna, Austria: UNODC.

the International Narcotics Control Board (INCB), which acts as the guardian of the drug control conventions; as well as the World Health Organization (WHO) and the UNAIDS program.

At the regional level, the Inter-American Drug Abuse Control Commission (CICAD) plays an important role in monitoring drug use in the Americas through a multi-evaluation mechanism. The European Monitoring Centre for Drugs and Drug Addiction (EMCDDA), a decentralized agency of the European Union, takes on the sole task of collecting data and reporting on drug use in Europe, using some of the epidemiological approaches developed by the Pompidou Group of the Council of Europe. Regional reporting is often structured around epidemiological working groups or supports regional political initiatives that exist in many parts of the world. Currently the most active initiative is the ACCORD network (ASEAN and China Cooperative Operations in Response to Dangerous Drugs) in Southeast Asia. Through its Global Assessment Programme (GAP), the UNODC is supporting the developments of regional reporting systems elsewhere (mainly Africa and Central Asia).

A number of national systems are also fundamental to note, namely the National Institute on Drug Abuse (NIDA) in the United States, which supports scientific research and dissemination of information, as well as data collection and training in various parts of the world through its international program. The U.S. Community Epidemiological Working Group (CEWG) has been particularly groundbreaking and influential, with its approach imitated and adopted elsewhere, including by the aforementioned Pompidou Group. The Canadian Centre on Substance Abuse provides information and advice through similar methods of data collection and dissemination. Australia has also invested considerable resources in developing national sentinel monitoring systems, such as the Illicit Drug Reporting System, which supports more comprehensive national data collection activities. In South Africa, SACENDU (South African Community Epidemiological Network on Drug Abuse) is probably the best example of a long-standing and successful monitoring program in the developing world. A good overview of data collection approaches and the bodies working in these areas can be found in the 2002 and 2003 double issues of the international *Bulletin on Narcotics*.

Indicators of Illicit Drug Use Used in Monitoring Systems

In one version of an old fable, a king wishing to test his wisest sages sends them into a dark room containing an elephant. Each sage subsequently describes the animal according to the part of its body he had encountered,

comparing this feature to the observation of some other object, such as a wall or a tree. None of their descriptions in isolation provided an adequate depiction of the animal and all could be said to be in some respects both accurate and misleading. However, taken collectively the accounts did allow the king, who was unaware of the animal's identity, to draw a picture of the complete creature.

In many respects this fable provides a good analogy for the approach taken in describing patterns and trends in drug use. A range of data sources usually referred to as indicators is available, all of which are deficient in some respects and require careful interpretation, but when taken together nonetheless provide an image of the phenomenon. By using a variety of indicators, none of which is sufficient on its own, in combination they can provide a more accurate picture of drug use in a given population and allow changes over time to be identified. Certain methods are often more appropriate than others for measuring specific types of drug use, depending on general prevalence in the population, degree of hidden use and stigmatization, and cost effectiveness.

The main indicators used to monitor illicit drug use can be found in the UN Annual Reports Questionnaire (ARQ) and through many of the regional and national reporting mechanisms listed at the end of this article. These indicators are also explicitly listed in the Lisbon Consensus, an agreement among international and regional bodies on the core components of a drug monitoring system.

An important distinction between illicit drug epidemiology and approaches to other public health topics is the prohibited nature of illicit drug use. For this reason, monitoring illicit drug use is driven by both concern about drug control (interdiction efforts against production, trafficking, and use) and public health issues (treating drug dependence and preventing HIV transmission through injecting drug use). As such, much of the data available on illicit drug trends stem from law enforcement efforts to control illicit drugs (e.g., arrests for drug use and drug seizure data) as well as its consequences (e.g., demand for drug treatment).

Obtaining a comprehensive picture of the illicit drug situation involves thoughtful and cautious examination of these various illicit drug indicators. Some of the more commonly used indicators of illicit drug use, and their limitations, are outlined here.

Interdiction statistics

For supply-related drug interdiction efforts, intelligence and law enforcement authorities monitor trends on drug seizures and arrests for drug-related offences, as well as market price and purity information. Methodological approaches vary, as does the quality of the information available, with data on price and purity being generally poor or unavailable. Because reporting on the number and quantity of illicit drugs seized is obligatory for countries who are signatories to the UN drug control conventions, this data set is generally relativity robust at the international level. Nonetheless, seizure data are problematic to interpret because they are heavily influenced by large-volume seizures, most of which relate to drugs in transit rather than being reflective of local drug consumption trends. The UNODC and the U.S. Drug Enforcement Agency (DEA) also report on opium and cocaine crop production, based on ground and satellite surveys. Estimating the overall production of cannabis or synthetic drugs is extremely difficult, and consequently, the global production figures reported by the UN should be regarded as 'best estimates' rather than precise figures.

School surveys

The most comprehensive and comparable global data set on illicit drug use arises from school surveys on drug use, which are inexpensive and easy to conduct. These surveys are particularly useful because they target adolescents, who are a high-risk group for drug use. At the global level, questions on cannabis use are included in the WHO survey on Health Behavior in School-aged Children (HBSC). In the United States, the Monitoring the Future annual survey of eighth-, tenth-, and twelfth-graders represents one of the most developed and largest survey exercises, running since 1975. Other notable school survey data sources include CICAD, which has prioritized school surveys on drug use in Latin America, and adopted a common methodological approach across countries to facilitate intraregional comparisons. And in Europe, the ESPAD study group (European School Survey Project on Alcohol and other Drugs) reports on drug use among 15- to 16-year-olds in over 30 countries every 4 years.

Problems of bias related to nonresponses and dishonest responses can be a difficulty for any survey, but they present a particular challenge when surveying illicit drug use. Techniques have been developed to ensure confidence in anonymity to improve the honesty and accuracy of responses. However, school surveys face additional problems: in many countries, the children most at risk of using drugs do not attend school for various reasons, while in the developing world, education is often not universal, or is limited to the early years of schooling. Therefore, generalizations from the results of school surveys to the wider population of young people need to be made with some caution.

School-aged children are not the only special target population selected for assessing drug use levels: surveys of military conscripts have been conducted in some countries, while at-risk groups such as out-of-school youth, the homeless, and sex workers have also been targeted for surveys.

Household surveys

Less commonly available for the developing world, but a mainstay for reporting on drug use in North America, Australia, and Europe, are national household surveys on the health habits of the general population, like the U.S. National Survey on Drug Use and Health (NSDUH). Such surveys are costly and methodologically complex, but they include numerous approaches developed to reduce reporting biases, such as the use of computer-aided interviewing. Despite these state-of-the-art methods, general population surveys are generally regarded as inadequate for measuring stigmatized and infrequent drug use behaviors (e.g., injecting drug use), which are disproportionately found in marginalized communities. For this reason a number of statistical techniques (e.g., capture-recapture and benchmark-multiplier methods) have been developed that try to extrapolate from known data sources to estimate the unknown, or hidden, proportion of drug users. Nevertheless, well-conducted household surveys are useful for examining the relative prevalence of illicit drugs, and they can provide time-series data on more commonly used drugs, which is important for evaluating trends and compensating for other data limitations.

Health-care services and criminal justice indicators

In addition to techniques to estimate the prevalence of drug use, drug information systems also report on people who are identified as having a drug problem through their contact with health-care services or the criminal justice system. In the United States, approaches in this area include drug testing among arrestees (Arrestee Drug Abuse Monitoring, or ADAM) and reported drug use among medical emergency patients (Drug Abuse Warning Network, or DAWN). More common is the practice of monitoring the characteristics of people seeking drug treatment, which provides a convenient tool for analyzing global drug trends. The Treatment Demand Indicator is one of the key epidemiological measures adopted by the EMCDDA, while similar treatment-demand monitoring systems have been established in a number of non-European countries. Clearly, information on the characteristics of those seeking help for drug problems is influenced by the availability of drug treatment services and factors such as court-mandated treatment. Nonetheless, this type of data is useful in monitoring problematic drug use and shifts in treatment demand. Other key indicators include monitoring drug-related deaths (by acute poisoning) and levels of infectious disease (principally HIV and hepatitis C) among injecting drug users. Finally, data from *ad hoc* research studies and more qualitative information from interviews with researchers, health-care providers, and social workers – and drug users themselves – all contribute to the global information base on drug use trends.

A Global Overview of Illicit Drug Use

The quality and type of information available on illicit drug use varies greatly between geographic regions, in part because illicit drug data collection activities tend to receive greater funding in developed countries. For this reason, some parts of the world base their understanding of the illicit drug situation on sophisticated and standardized reporting methods, while others rely almost solely on drug arrest and seizure data or on the opinion of available experts. It is possible to describe the overall illicit drug situation quite comprehensively in North America, Europe, and Australia, while in South America and parts of Southeast Asia only limited data exist, which are often localized and more difficult to compare. In Africa, with the exception of South Africa, data are extremely limited, with only a few rapid assessments and some *ad hoc* surveys in Northern Africa and a few Middle Eastern countries. Similar deficits exist in much of Central Asia, where again only sporadic information sets are available. This paucity of data is reflected in the submission rates for the ARQs, which are provided to the UN to prepare the annual global drug situation report for the CND: only around 110 of the 193 UN member states submit data through the ARQ.

Despite the information deficits it is possible to draw a rough picture of the global drug problem and to identify some significant trends and developments. The reader should be aware that drug use is a dynamic phenomenon and reporting tends to be based on data that are often slow to compile (for more contemporary data sources that can be accessed, see the section titled 'Relevant Websites'). In particular, the *World Drug Report*, which is published each year by the UNODC, provides the best global overview on many aspects of the drug problem. However, this report is very general and the inadequacies of some of the data sources used are not always apparent. For this reason, the reader should refer to local drug monitoring systems to gain insight into drug use trends within any particular country or region.

According to the *World Drug Report 2006* (UN, 2006a), the global consumption of illicit drugs continues unabated. An estimated 5% of the world's population had used an illicit drug in the past year, while drug production and trafficking was estimated to be a US$320 billion industry. Most of this drug use was sporadic: only about half of those who had used drugs in the past year, or 2.7% of the global adult population, had used drugs in the last month. Those with serious problems were a far smaller number, with an estimated 25 million drug addicts or problem drug users worldwide, or 0.6% of the global population aged 15–64. In nearly all regions of the world, drug users are disproportionately young and male, though in some regions there are concerns of a narrowing gender gap or evidence of an aging population of drug users (**Table 1**).

Cannabis

Cannabis is by far the most widely used, produced, and trafficked illicit drug in the world. An estimated 162 million people worldwide use cannabis, and the drug is grown in at least 176 countries. Cannabis resin (hashish) is primarily produced in Morocco and in a few other countries, with Europe as the world's main resin consumer. Herbal cannabis production is practically impossible to monitor, but is particularly intensively cultivated in the Americas. The widespread availability of this drug is a likely factor in its ubiquitous high prevalence in comparison to other illicit drugs. Any limitation on the drug's cultivation by climate, land space, or crop detection has been circumvented by the development of indoor hydroponic cultivation. High prevalence of cannabis use can be found in Australia and New Zealand, North America, and West and Central Europe, where annual prevalence estimates range from around 7 to 15%. Cannabis use is

Table 1   Extent of drug use (annual prevalence) estimates 2004/05 (or latest year possible)[a]

		Amfetamine-type stimulants				
	Cannabis	Amfetamines	Ecstasy	Cocaine	Opiate (including heroin)	Heroin
(million people)	158.8	24.9	8.6	14.3	15.6	11.1
in % of global population age 15–64	3.8%	0.6%	0.2%	0.3%	0.4%	0.3%

[a]Annual prevalence is a measure of the number/percentage of people who have consumed an illicit drug at least once in the 12-month period preceding the assessment.
From United Nations Office on Drugs and Crime (2006a) *World Drug Report 2006. Volume 1: Analysis, p. 34.* Vienna: United Nations Office on Drugs and Crime.

undoubtedly prevalent in many other parts of the world, but the absence of comprehensive prevalence surveys in many developing nations makes it difficult to verify the extent of use. For example, cannabis is the main drug used throughout most of Africa and the Pacific Islands. It is also widely used in Asia, but its use is this region is overshadowed by problems with opiates and methamfetamine.

Cocaine

While cannabis is the most widely used illicit drug, historically two other products that are based on illicit crop production have been the predominant drugs associated with severe health and social problems. Cocaine, produced from the leaves of the coca bush, and heroin, derived from opium poppies, both remain responsible for some of the world's most damaging drug problems. While chewing of unprocessed coca leaves was a common traditional habit in many Andean indigenous communities, nearly all modern coca cultivation goes toward production of cocaine. Most of the estimated 910 metric tons of cocaine produced each year comes from Colombia (50%), and to a lesser extent Peru (32%), and Bolivia (15%). In line with the production of cocaine in this region, around two-thirds of the estimated 13.4 million users worldwide live in the Americas. Although the United States is the country most associated with cocaine use problems and particularly crack cocaine abuse (a concentrated and smokable form of the drug), cocaine consumption in the United States appears to have stabilized. This country still reports the world's highest annual prevalence figure for the adult population (2.8%), although Spain and the UK in Europe as well as Canada now report levels of use approaching those in the United States (2.7%, 2.4%, and 2.3%, respectively).

Opiates

The use of heroin and other opiates remains a major public health concern, largely because of their potential to bring about dependence, but also because they are often injected, creating a population susceptible to infection by blood-borne viruses (i.e., hepatitis B and C, HIV). UN estimates suggest that there are almost 16 million opiate users worldwide, 11.3 million of whom are heroin users. Opium production is currently concentrated in Afghanistan, which is thought to be responsible for 89% of global opium production (estimated at 4620 metric tons in 2005). Opium is still produced in parts of Southeast Asia, but opium poppy cultivation has declined significantly over the past decade, and within that region is now mainly limited to Myanmar. Opium poppy cultivation has also been noted in South and Central America (Colombia, Mexico, Peru, and Venezuela) and other Asian countries (Laos PDR, Pakistan, Thailand, and Vietnam).

Declines in the cultivation of opium in Southeast Asia could be argued to underlie recent declines in opioid use in parts of Southeast Asia and Australia. However, heroin use continues to be a significant concern in China and Vietnam, while opium remains the major illicit drug of abuse in Myanmar. In Europe, there is a stable overall trend in heroin consumption, while heroin use in North America also appears to have stabilized. The picture is different in the Russian Federation and the former Soviet republics and Central Asia. In 2004, the annual prevalence of heroin use was estimated at 2.0% for the adult population, and high prevalence was also found in the Ukraine (0.8%), Kyrgyzstan (2.3%), Kazakhstan (1.3%), and Tajikistan (1.0%). Of particular concern, heroin injecting appears to be the main vector for the HIV epidemics in Russia, Central Asia, and the Baltic states. The world's highest prevalence for heroin use is from Iran (estimated annual prevalence of 2.8% in 1999). Relatively high prevalence rates have also been reported by Pakistan (0.8%) and Afghanistan (1.4%).

Heroin use is comparatively lower in Latin America, and there appears to be little use in the Pacific Islands. Despite a dearth of prevalence data in Africa, there have been anecdotal reports of heroin use along drug-trafficking routes that extend from East Africa across the continent, evidence of use in Nigeria (estimated prevalence of 0.6% in 1999), and a growing demand for heroin treatment in South Africa. In contrast to the seemingly low prevalence of heroin use in mainland Africa, the island country of Mauritius has a long-standing heroin use problem, with an estimated annual prevalence of 2.0%.

Synthetic Drugs

Although plant-based substances remain an important part of the global drug problem, a clear trend since the early 1990s has been increased availability and use of a range of synthetically produced drugs, most notably amfetamine-type stimulants (ATS). An estimated 24 million people use ATS each year, often with devastating health and social consequences. The category of ATS includes methamfetamine, amfetamine, ecstasy (3,4-methylenedioxymethamfetamine, or MDMA), and ecstasy-related drugs (e.g., 3,4-methylenedioxamfetamine (MDA), 3,4-methylenedioxy-N-ethylamfetamine (MDEA)). Methamfetamine and ecstasy currently demand the most attention of all the drugs within this class, and of these synthetic stimulants, methamfetamine has a higher dependence liability and is associated with far greater harm. Amfetamine, the less potent analogue of methamfetamine, sometimes found in controlled medicines, has been superseded by methamfetamine in most parts of the world, while ecstasy derivatives are usually inadvertently produced in an attempt to manufacture ecstasy, rather than being intended for a designated market. Other synthetic drugs, such as gamma-hydroxybutyrate (GHB or GBH) have become popular among niche drug markets, although they represent a growing concern for some countries. Here we restrict our attention to the most widely used synthetic drugs in the current global illicit drug market: methamfetamine and ecstasy.

Methamfetamine

The global rise in methamfetamine use and related problems since the late 1990s has disproportionately impacted the Asia Pacific region and North America. Southeast Asia, in particular, is a global hub for the production and trafficking of methamfetamine, accounting for 58% of global methamfetamine seized in 2004. Significant production of the drug also occurs in North America. As with all synthetic drugs, methamfetamine production is not restricted to any particular location, as this is limited only by the availability of precursor chemicals (sometimes found in cold and flu medicines) and the capacity to manufacture the drugs undetected. Areas of the globe most affected by methamfetamine use are those proximal to major manufacturing regions. Smoking crystalline methamfetamine (*shabu*, or ice) has been a historical trend in the Pacific islands of Japan, Hawaii, and the Philippines, while this pattern of drug use is also apparent in Brunei, Darussalam, Indonesia, and Malaysia (UNODC, 2006b). A more contemporary trend is the large-scale production of methamfetamine pills called *ya ba* in the Shan State of Myanmar, which have also been used in epidemic proportions in neighboring Thailand. The production and use of combination ATS pills, many of which also contain methamfetamine, has become a broader issue affecting countries within the sub-Mekong region (Laos, Vietnam, and Thailand) (UNODC, 2006c).

Outside of Southeast and East Asia, methamfetamine has also become a significant problem in both New Zealand and Australia, with additional concerns due to use by injection. In North America, crystalline methamfetamine use is expanding eastward from the West Coast, particularly through rural areas, while increases in methamfetamine use have recently affected Vancouver, Canada. A sharp rise in treatment demand for the drug has also been reported in South Africa (Parry *et al.*, 2004). Significant use of this drug in Europe is limited to the Czech and Slovak republics, where a localized problem has existed since the mid-1980s. Other parts of Europe have a long history of amfetamine use, including in the United Kingdom and Scandinavia and surrounding Nordic countries, although amfetamine use has fallen dramatically in the UK, being superseded by cocaine and ecstasy use, a trend apparent across Europe as a whole.

Ecstasy

A more fashionable synthetic drug trend is the rapidly growing popularity of ecstasy (MDMA). The recreational use of ecstasy can be traced back to the 1970s in the United States, but it was only in the mid-1980s that the drug became popular, first in Europe, and subsequently on a worldwide scale. Unlike many other drug use patterns, ecstasy is predominantly associated with recreational drug use among integrated young adults, very few of whom report substantial problems from their drug use or seek drug treatment. A relatively low number of deaths have been reported from ecstasy use. For example, in 2005, 77 deaths were identified in Europe as being ecstasy-related – in comparison with 8000 deaths per year attributed to opiate overdose.

Europe remains the global center of ecstasy production, with laboratories based predominantly in the Netherlands and Belgium, although increasingly the relative importance of Europe is declining as production increases elsewhere, particularly in North America and East and Southeast Asia. Levels of ecstasy use have been relatively stable in Europe (annual prevalence estimates range from 0.5–2.5%), although there has been a continuing upward trend in some countries. Despite rising in the 1990s, ecstasy trends in North America also appear to have stabilized, with annual prevalence estimates of around 1.0%. In contrast, Australia has experienced a sustained increase in the prevalence of ecstasy use since the late 1990s, and the annual prevalence is now 3.4% among adults. Several countries in East and Southeast Asia are also seeing increases in ecstasy use, albeit at lower levels.

Concluding Remarks

In this article, we have summarized the main approaches to monitoring the illicit drug problem, noted some of the more important conceptual and methodological difficulties in this area, and provided a simple overview of the global illicit drug situation. By necessity, our brush strokes are broad, but it is hoped that they are sufficient to provide a basic understanding of illicit drug trends, related data collection methods, and more importantly, direct the reader to further information on illicit drug monitoring.

There are a number of important issues that were not covered in the current article, but require due attention. An issue of paramount importance is the association between injecting drug use and HIV infection. In many parts of the world injecting drug use is a major cause of the continuing HIV/AIDS epidemic, with alarmingly high HIV prevalence rates among injecting drug users in Asia, South America, and Eastern Europe.

An increasingly acknowledged issue in the illicit drug arena is the high level of comorbidity between drug use and other mental health disorders, such as depression and psychotic disorders. In particular, there is a growing emphasis on the development of treatment approaches that address both drug use and mental health problems.

Also worth noting are patterns of multi- or poly-substance use, including the combined use and interaction with substances that are legal in most countries, such as alcohol and tobacco. From a policy and public health pers-pective, many countries are now developing responses that target substance consumption in general, rather than the use of specific substances.

In recognition of changing illicit drug trends associated with globalization, further development of data collection and treatment capacity is needed in developing nations. Within these countries, there is typically little informa-tion from which to assess potentially growing drug pro-blems. Adherence to internationally recognized ethnical standards in monitoring illicit drug trends is also a global imperative, while dedicated global efforts are required to sustain a balance between understanding both the demand and the supply aspects of illicit drug trends.

See also: Illicit Drug Use and the burden of Disease; Mental Health and Physical Health (Including HIV/AIDS); Mental Health and Substance abuse; Regulation of Drugs and Drug Use: Public Health and Law Enforcement.

Citations

Parry C, Myers B, and Plüddemann A (2004) Drug policy for methamphetamine use urgently needed. *South African Medical Journal* 94: 964–965.

Sloboda Z (ed.) (2005) *Epidemiology of Drug Abuse.* New York: Springer.

United Nations Office on Drugs and Crime (2006a) *World Drug Report 2006. Volume 1: Analysis.* Vienna, Austria: UNODC.

United Nations Office on Drugs and Crime (2006b) East Asia and the Pacific 2005 Regional Profile. Bangkok, Thailand: UNODC, Regional Centre for East Asia and the Pacific.

United Nations Office on Drugs and Crime (2006c) Patterns and trends of amphetamine-type stimulants (ATS) and other drugs of abuse in East Asia and the Pacific 2005. Bangkok, Thailand: UNODC, Regional Centre for East Asia and the Pacific.

Further Reading

European Monitoring Centre for Drugs Drug Addiction (EMCDDA). *Modelling Drug Use: Methods to Quantify and Understand Hidden Processes.* Lisbon, Portugal: EMCDDA.

Hartnoll R (2004) *Drugs and Drug Dependence: Linking Research, Policy and Practice. Lessons Learned, Challenges Ahead.* Strasbourg, France: Council of Europe.

Musto D (1973) *The American Disease: Origins of Narcotic Control.* New Haven, CT: Yale University Press.

United Nations and General AssemblySpecial, Session (UNGASS) (1998) United Nations General Assembly Special Session: Declaration on guiding principles of drug demand reduction. http://www.un.org/ga/20special/demand.htm (accessed September 2007).

United Nations (1961) Single convention on narcotic drugs, 1961, as amended by the 1972 protocol amending the single convention on narcotic drugs, 1961. http://www.unodc.org/pdf/convention_1961_en.pdf (accessed September 2007).

United Nations (1971) Convention on psychotropic substances, 1971. http://www.unodc.org/pdf/convention_1971_en.pdf (accessed September 2007).

United Nations (1988) Convention against the illicit traffic in narcotic drugs and psychotropic substances, 1988. http://www.unodc.org/pdf/convention_1988_en.pdf (accessed September 2007).

United Nations Office of Drugs, Crime (UNODC) (2002) *Bulletin on Narcotics: The Science of Drug Abuse Epidemiology* vol. 54). Vienna, Austria: UNODCnos. 1 and 2.

United Nations Office of Drugs and Crime (2003) *Bulletin on Narcotics: The Practice of Drug Abuse Epidemiology* vol. 55, nos. 1 and 2. Vienna: UNODC.

Relevant Websites

http://www.aihw.gov.au/drugs/datacubes/index.cfm – Alcohol and Other Drug Treatment Services National Minimum Data Set (AODTS-NMDS).

http://www.ojp.usdoj.gov/nij/adam – Arrestee Drug Abuse Monitoring (ADAM).

http://www.aseansec.org/645.htm – ASEAN and China Cooperative Operations in Response to Dangerous Drugs (ACCORD).

http://www.adin.com.au – Australian Drug Information Network (ADIN).

http://www.ccsa.ca – Canadian Centre on Substance Abuse (CCSA).

http://www.drugabuse.gov/about/organization/CEWG/CEWGHome.html – Community Epidemiological Working Group (CEWG).

http://www.dawninfo.samhsa.gov – Drug Abuse Warning Network (DAWN).

http://www.aic.gov.au/research/duma – Drug Use Monitoring in Australia (DUMA).

http://www.emcdda.europa.eu/?nnodeid=25328 – EMCDDA Drug Profiles.

http://www.emcdda.europa.eu – European Monitoring Centre for Drugs and Drug Addiction (EMCDDA).

http://www.espad.org – European School Survey Project on Alcohol and Other Drugs (ESPAD).

http://www.hbsc.org – Health Behavior in School-Age Children Survey (HBSC).

http://www.ndp.govt.nz/publications/illicitdrugmonitoringsystem.html – Illicit Drug Monitoring System (IDMS).

http://ndarc.med.unsw.edu.au – Illicit Drug Reporting System (IDRS) and the Ecstasy and Related Drugs Reporting System (EDRS).

http://www.incb.org – International Narcotics Control Board (INCB).

http://www.cicad.oas.org – Inter-American Drug Abuse Control Commission (CICAD).

http://www.monitoringthefuture.org – Monitoring the Future.

http://www.aihw.gov.au – National Drug Strategy Household Survey (NDSHS).

http://www.drugabuse.gov – National Institute of Drug Abuse (NIDA).

http://www.oas.samhsa.gov/nhsda.htm – National Survey on Drug Abuse and Health (NSDUH).

http://www.sahealthinfo.org/admodule/sacendu.htm – South African Community Epidemiological Network on Drug Abuse (SACENDU).

http://www.samhsa.gov – Substance Abuse and Mental Health Services Administration (SAMHSA).

http://www.unodc.org – United Nations Office on Drugs and Crime (UNODC).

http://www.unodc.org/unodc/en/cnd_questionnaire_arq.html – UNODC Annual Reports Questionnaire.

http://www.unodc.org/unodc/en/drug_demand_gap.html – UNDOC Global Assessment Programme on Drug Abuse.

http://www.unodc.org/unodc/en/drug_demand_gap_datacollection.html#core – UNDOC Lisbon Consensus.

http://www.unaids.org – United Nations Program on HIV/AIDS (UNAIDS).

http://www.who.int – World Health Organization (WHO).

Mental Health Policy

R Jenkins, Institute of Psychiatry, London, UK

Why Do We Need Mental Health Policy?

Burden

Mental disorders are common everywhere in the world and contribute to disability, mortality, loss of economic productivity, and poverty (Murray and Lopez, 1996; Mathers and Loncar, 2006). Across the globe, in both developed and developing countries, mental ill health affects 10–15% of people at any one time, and more in high-risk populations. Mental ill health accounts for 14% of the total global burden of disease (World Health Organization, 2005). Conflict, increasing numbers of refugees, the impact of HIV/AIDS, and nutritional deficiencies contribute further to the burden of mental ill health of those living in poor countries (World Health Organization, 2001a).

Poverty and Education

Poverty and mental health are intertwined and the association reflects causality in both directions: Poverty worsens mental ill health and mental ill health makes poor people poorer. Therefore, the effective provision of mental health services should form an integral part of national poverty reduction as well as general health strategies (Gureje and Jenkins, 2007).

Impact on Children

Parental illness contributes to intellectual and emotional consequences for the next generation.

Impact on Physical Health

The presence of untreated mental disorders also influences the success of prevention and treatment programs for physical illness such as malaria, cholera, HIV/AIDS, tuberculosis, leprosy, and other infectious diseases.

Mental Ill Health can be Addressed

Most cases of mental ill health are amenable to cost-effective interventions, whether preventive, therapeutic, or rehabilitative, and can be managed in the community (Institute of Medicine, 2001).

Challenge of Limited Resources

Delivery of these interventions in resource-poor settings poses significant challenges for health systems, communities, and individuals. Many of the difficulties in delivering effective mental health services reflect generic problems within the health system. Specialist services are limited, and few primary health workers have received adequate training in mental health.

Evolving More Effective and Accessible Services

Most countries in the world are undergoing mental health reform to a greater or lesser extent; the precise nature of those reforms and the current situation in each country are variable. However, the common goal is to achieve comprehensive, local, needs-led, evidence-based, and sustainable care that is in as unrestricted an environment as is compatible with the health and safety of the affected individual, family, and public, tailored to the local context and resources. Many Western countries, and much of Eastern Europe have extensive custodial and institutional care, resulting in impaired health and social outcomes compared to active treatment and rehabilitation in community settings. On the other hand, many low- and middle-income countries have very little or no institutional care, but they often also lack adequate access to treatment and rehabilitation in the community. Many countries are also contemplating reform of the legislative framework so that it can support appropriate care in flexible settings, with appropriate attention to human rights.

Both these movements require reform of other areas and, if the public health burden of mental illness is to be tackled effectively, it is necessary for governments to adopt a strategic approach that encompasses all the necessary components (Jenkins *et al.*, 1998). Most countries focus their policy efforts on the specialist services, but this ignores the problem that the overall mental health-care system is extremely complex, comprising many different agencies that inevitably interact with people with mental illness. The interfaces and patient flows through the system also need to be carefully considered as a blockage in one part of the system will have inevitable consequences for the rest of the system. For example, it is very difficult to resettle people with severe mental illness in the community if stigma surrounding people with mental illness is not tackled through public education and education in schools. Similarly, it is impossible for relatively scarce specialists to focus on those with the greatest need if they are constantly deluged by many referrals of less ill people from primary care. Systems need to be developed so that the most highly trained professionals focus on the most difficult cases, while the front-line health workers address the bulk of mental disorder, in order to achieve access to care for all who need it.

Summary

It is important to support governments to adopt mental health policies and to integrate mental health policy into public health policy and general social policy because mental disorder causes a heavy burden for societies, impedes the development of other health and development targets, contributes to poverty, differentially affects the poor, and because mental health itself is of intrinsic value, as is physical health (Jenkins, 2003).

What Is a Mental Health Policy?

A mental health policy is a written statement of intent by the government on mental health issues and mental health services. Health policy at the national level will identify the range of health, morbidity, disability, and mortality issues it intends to tackle, the relevant settings covered by the policy, the overall framework for implementing policy in the relevant settings, including, for example, health services, social services, the education sector, the workplace, and the criminal justice sector. The policy may set desired goals and will set a framework for planning at local level. The policy document addresses the issues in mental health which require multidisciplinary and intersectoral collaboration at all levels of human development as well as socioeconomic development (World Health Organization, 2001b).

How Can Policy Impact on the Mental Health of Populations?

Policy, or a mission statement, is required at national and local levels to set broad goals for mental health and the means of achieving those goals. A written National Mental Health Policy is important because it informs the Health Sector Policy Framework, which in turn informs the National Development and Planning Policies.

The policy document can bring all mental health issues into sharp focus and act as an advocacy tool for equitable resource allocation at individual, family, community, national, and international levels.

The policy document can assist in the national allocation of both human and nonhuman resources such as mental health personnel, financing, and supplies and equipment. National mental health policy helps government include mental health into the health and social sector plans so it is not marginalized. It informs the process of mental health legislation. It is a key pillar for the development of national mental health program of action and mental health service delivery in an integrated decentralized manner (including coprogramming with programs for HIV, malaria, other infectious diseases, reproductive health, and child health). A policy is capable of bringing mental health priorities to the same level as physical health and social well-being and of addressing issues of stigmatization, not just within the general population but also within policy makers and professionals. It can help raise awareness in other government departments.

Mental health policy must be integrated with the overall national health policy, including the general health sector reform strategy, package of essential health interventions, essential medicine kit, health information systems, curricula for all health workers, and country-level work on global burden of disease. The policy must form part of government policy; budgetary and public expenditure processes contribute to the national poverty reduction strategy and involve ministries of finance, education, social welfare, domestic affairs/criminal justice, and employment (Jenkins et al., 2002).

The Need for Locally Tailored Solutions

Mental health policy will need to take into account the contextual factors, the epidemiology (range, severity, frequency, and duration) of disorders, their accompanying social disability, their mortality, and the relationship to sociodemographic variables, including geographic variation. Epidemiology is fundamental to the overall goals of mental health policy. A few countries are embarking on a specific rolling program of detailed national mental health surveys (e.g., Jenkins and Melzer, 2003) and WHO is coordinating a world mental health survey program in a variety of participating countries (Ustun and Kessler, 2002).

Cultural and religious issues are also very important. They influence the value placed by society on mental health, the presentation of symptoms, illness behavior, access to services, pathways through care, the way individuals and families manage illness, the way the community responds to illness, the degree of acceptance and support experienced on the one hand, and the degree of stigma and discrimination, on the other hand, experienced by the person with mental illness. Each country has a unique context, culture, resources, and existing service structures and each will require its own mental health strategy containing locally tailored solutions (Jenkins et al., 2004; Jenkins, 2007).

Common Policy Aims

While each country has special needs, problems, resource constraints, and challenges, there are nevertheless some consistent areas that national policy needs to address (Jenkins *et al.*, 2002). The overall goals of public policy on mental health generally include some or all of the following:

- To promote mental health;
- To prevent mental and neurological disorders;
- To improve the health and social functioning of people with mental illness;
- To deliver appropriate services for early detection, care, treatment, and rehabilitation;
- To reduce the premature mortality of people with mental disorders;
- To reduce stigma;
- To protect the human rights and dignity of people with mental illness;
- To promote the psychological aspects of general health care;
- To engage in appropriate development of human resources;
- To develop a program of research to support the above aims.

Common Policy Components

The components of an effective mental health policy include:

1. National components:
    - The construction of a national strategy to promote mental health, reduce morbidity, and reduce mortality;
    - The establishment of policy links with other government departments including home affairs, criminal justice, education, housing, and finance;
    - The enaction of specific mental health legislation to set the overall philosophy of the approach to care of people with mental disorders, together with precise provision for assessment and treatment without consent under certain defined conditions in the interests of the individual and the public, with regard to safeguarding human rights;
    - Financing, to remove perverse incentives, to ensure sustainable local financing, and develop funding streams for disseminating good practice models. In all countries, especially poor ones, finance is a major limiting factor and prioritization of services will be necessary. A basic package should include the provision of medicines for patients at primary care level with psychosis, epilepsy, and severe depression; the ability to refer very ill patients

for hospital admission; primary care workers supported by specialists in the community; mental health promotion in the community, and intersectoral linkages;
    - Implementation plans and a system of accountability and governance.
2. Supportive infrastructure components:
    - A human resources strategy;
    - A consumer involvement strategy;
    - A research and development strategy;
    - A mental health information strategy (which should include context, needs, inputs, processes, and outcomes; information systems provide an essential resource for clinicians, managers, planners, and policy makers and allows the audit cycle to proceed; users and care providers also require relevant information, and the general public requires information for public accountability);
3. Service components:
    - Primary care and specialist care, with the links between the two;
    - Good practice guidelines;
    - Liaison with NGOs, police, prisons, and the social sector;
    - Dialogue with traditional healers;
    - Mental health promotion in schools, workplaces, and the community;
    - Addressing needs of refugees and internally displaced people;
    - Disaster preparedness.

The Construction of a National Strategy

The first step in getting mental health into national policy is to identify and engage key agencies and stakeholders in the overall process so that there is shared ownership of the vision and its implementation. The next step is to undertake a detailed situation appraisal to obtain a good understanding of the context, needs, demands, current policy, service inputs, processes, and outcomes; this is best done in collaboration with key sectors and stakeholders. The third activity is to develop an overall mission statement, set goals and targets, including detailed recommendations on structures to support integrated coordination, liaison, and implementation. The fourth step is to develop strategic plans and implementation frameworks with those agencies that take the local situation into account and that specifically tackle local issues, constraints, and disincentives. The fifth and final step is to review progress regularly using a variety of outcome measures and to fine-tune strategy and implementation.

The policy document should be developed in a democratic and equitable manner with all the stakeholders involved at all stages of its development as well as its implementation.

Policy Partnerships Outside the Health Sector

Education

Inadequate education contributes to social exclusion because of the increased subsequent difficulties in finding work and in participating fully in other social roles. People with poor educational attainment are overrepresented in prisons and in specialized hospitals; they are overrepresented in prisoners with psychological disorder.

Besides their primary educational role, schools are important settings for mental health promotion in order to teach children important life skills aimed at reducing acute and chronic social stresses and enhancing social supports, all of which have a direct influence on mental health.

Policy needs to ensure that the general health education program, which is likely to have already established good links to schools, the media, and health-care workers, now develop and include education of the community on mental health and mental illness, life skills and coping strategies, and responsible community attitudes to people with a mental or physical disability.

The curriculum needs to include education on mental health as part of its health and social skills element and to develop the higher education appropriate for the country's needs, including generic courses, vocational qualifications, distance learning, and occupational standards.

Children often receive too little policy attention. Specific learning difficulties, including dyslexia in schools, lead to educational failure, dropping out of school, and unemployment, as well as overrepresentation in prisons. It is therefore important for policy to address specific learning difficulties in schools. Provision of spectacles to schoolchildren increases performance, and reduces dropout rates and entry into child labor and child prostitution.

Children Not in a Home Setting

Large numbers of children across the world are looked after in orphanages and children's homes, which often contain children who have been abused and neglected, children whose home life has broken down, children with developmental delay and retardation, speech delay, seizures, severe hyperactivity and aggression, chronic physical illness, and disability. It should be an important policy imperative to ensure adequate mental and physical health promotion and care to children not in their home setting and to prevent their subsequent overrepresentation in prisons.

Police

To be effective, mental health policy needs to provide a framework for health staff and police to cooperate to ensure that people with mental illness who come into contact with the police receive speedy assessment and treatment. Police may be helpful in bringing acutely disturbed patients to the attention of the health service. However, it is not acceptable for people with mental illness to spend long periods in a police cell. There needs to be liaison, leadership, and agreement at a senior level between the ministry responsible for the police and the Ministry of Health. This needs to provide a framework for liaison between primary care teams, outpatient clinics or outreach teams, and the police. Education and the establishment of agreed procedures for police officers are important.

Prisons

Mental illness is very common in prisons, and in some Western countries suicide is very high among prisoners. We need systems to prevent and treat anxiety and depression in prison, ensure people with psychosis are treated in hospital rather than prison, prevent suicide and suicide attempts, and tackle dyslexia and educational failure in prisoners.

Mental health policy needs to address the principles and mechanisms of diversion of mentally disordered offenders from the criminal justice system into the health-care system and the implications of this for specialist services. Offenders with less severe mental disorders will need to receive treatment while in prison, and therefore liaison with and education of prison staff on depression and management of suicide risk is important.

Employment

Work, unemployment, and specific conditions at work have been shown to have a considerable influence on mental health and mental illness and utilization of mental health services. Rates of illness are higher in the unemployed than in the working population. There is evidence from longitudinal studies that both unemployment, actual redundancy itself, and the threat of redundancy causes mental illness, although it is also true that people who are already ill are more likely to become either voluntarily or involuntarily unemployed.

Workplaces are also a key environment for mental health promotion as well as physical health promotion. Employers bear the cost of the consequences of untreated mental illness in terms of sickness absence, labor turnover, accidents, and poor performance. Employers should therefore be encouraged to include mental health in their workplace health policies, as well as drugs, alcohol, and HIV/AIDS.

Ministries covering employment, trade, and industry therefore need to consider environmental conditions at work; access to employment for all, including sheltered employment for those who need it; opportunities for employment rehabilitation; the introduction of workplace mental health policies, and the provision of occupational health for the workforce in order to support a successful economy and to make an appropriate contribution to the prevention of discrimination against people with mental illness.

Housing and Overcrowding

Crowding has been conceptualized as two distinct but interrelated concepts: Excess stimulation and lack of privacy. Culture defines what is perceived as excessive demands and responses, with differences not only between cultures and countries but also between generations. There is a strong relationship between internal housing density and psychological symptoms in women experiencing very low as well as high levels of density.

Children seem more vulnerable to the effects of crowding than adults, and there is a relationship between large family size and delinquency, low verbal IQ, and poor reading skills.

Homelessness is generally associated with much higher levels of both severe mental illness and depression and anxiety.

Urban–Rural Differences

There is a consistent tendency across different counties for rates of mental illness to be higher in urban than rural areas, although not all studies find differences. In adults in the UK, urban areas have higher rates of psychiatric morbidity, alcohol dependence, and drug dependence than rural areas, with semi-rural areas in between. Most of the factors differentiating urban from rural areas include higher rates of acute life events and chronic social stresses, less social support, and more mobility in urban areas. In addition, there is a tendency for people with severe mental illness to drift to the cities, where they are overrepresented among the homeless, those living in shanty towns, and other marginalized groups.

Therefore, ministries responsible for the environment and housing will need to consider the impact of its planning decisions on the mental as well as the physical health of the population and to consider the needs for sheltered housing for people with severe mental illness if they cannot live with their families.

Another key urban–rural issue is the fact that in low-income countries, and indeed often in richer ones, most psychiatrists and psychiatric beds are in the large cities, greatly limiting access to specialist care for those in rural areas, and where those from rural areas do manage to access urban services, the large distances involved exacerbate institutionalization and difficulty in rehabilitating the patient back home. These issues are addressed further in the section titled 'Key Service Provision Issues.'

Key Cross-Cutting Issues

Human Resource Development

Countries need a sustainable human resources strategy to carry out the implementation of policy and the delivery of services. Low-income countries will have difficulty in meeting all their training requirements for health- and social-care professionals. They will therefore need a sustainable plan for production and continuing development both at home and elsewhere, of primary and secondary care staff.

User Involvement

The views of service users and care providers will be particularly important, as they will be directly affected by the strategy and will have personal experience of the problems in the current system (e.g., Mirza *et al.*, 2006). They will also be able to comment on those aspects of the current mental health system that are working well. User involvement is one of the great innovations in mental health and provides a framework for placing people who use mental health services at the center of decisions and activities that affect them. It is important to extend the principle of user involvement from users of specialist services to users of primary care services and also to the other sectors besides health that are key for mental health such as schools, universities, prisons, and institutional care of children and the elderly. User involvement is not simply an add-on to existing ways of doing things. Neither is it simply a process of consultation by those in power or authority. Rather it presents a challenge to everyone involved in mental health to reflect and rethink on how traditionally excluded people and groups can be empowered and included in society. People with mental illness, their care providers, and the community are the customers of mental health services. Their involvement can greatly improve the planning and delivery of services since they can spot gaps and problems as well as comment on what is working well. Government pump priming of a national mental health NGO can be a cost-effective way of encouraging progress.

Research and Development

All countries need to establish a sustainable research and development strategy to support its policy development and implementation program. Epidemiology and mental health economics are particularly important contributors to policy and planning. Poor countries cannot meet all their research needs and will have to rely largely on research produced elsewhere; however, there are some crucial questions that can only be answered by local research and this should be planned for.

Policy makers need both qualitative and quantitative information. Qualitative information is just as important as quantitative information and indeed quantitative information will frequently not be available. Policy makers therefore have the task of obtaining qualitative and quantitative evidence from a variety of sources – including research, audit, routine data, user and professional groups, and the general public – and of integrating very disparate bits of evidence, knowledge, experience, and values into a reasonably cohesive whole.

Policy makers need both broad and narrow information on which to base their decisions. Evidence covering contextual issues, needs, service inputs, human resources, service processes and health, and social and economic outcomes is required for policy making. Broad information helps inform decisions such as how much money should be spent overall and how it should be divided between promotion, prevention, treatment, and rehabilitation services. It also helps decide the balances that should be sought between public and private health care, generalist and specialist health care, and mental health care and social care. Finally, it helps determine the importance of public policy on mental health. In contrast, narrow information helps inform decisions on specific treatment options and interventions (Jenkins *et al.*, 2007).

There are rarely any studies available on which to base broad information decision-making; useful information that can be shared between countries is urgently needed. The systematic review is the narrow information instrument of choice to guide decision making that has proved very useful. However, the quality of the systematic review is entirely dependent on the quality and quantity of the existing investigations on which it is based, and high-quality investigations aimed at issues relevant to the proposed policy are not always available, especially in middle- and low-income countries. Only a very restricted set of policy questions have been addressed by systematic review and as soon as one looks beyond the specific to broader health care and the interplay of health care, welfare, criminal justice, education, and environmental policies, experimental trials become difficult or impossible. Given these circumstances, there are a number of steps we can take to improve mental health policy making.

A fundamental tenet of the evidence-based approach is that strong evidence of effectiveness should be established before a practice is adopted. It has generally been assumed that where possible strong evidence comes from randomized controlled evaluations. However, the RCT approach does not always lend itself to key problems, and other approaches also have much to offer and are also valid. Arguably, therefore, government policies should, wherever possible, be subject to the principle of being evidence based.

Health Management Information Systems

Good information is essential within countries to ensure effective planning, budgeting, and documentation of outcomes of resource expenditure. It is therefore important to collect routine data for mental health on:

- Population needs;
- Primary care consultation rates;
- Primary care treatments and outcomes;
- Referrals to specialist care;
- Specialist treatment and outcomes;
- Suicide rates.

Such data can be collected by a combination of household surveys, mortality records, and routine consultation data at primary and secondary care levels.

In addition, more detailed information on country context, needs, resources, provision, and outcome can be collated and compared between countries (e.g., Jenkins, 2004a; Jenkins *et al.*, 2004, 2007).

Legislation

Each country needs a legal framework that balances the need and desire of professionals to treat people when they are unable to consent with the need for legal protection of the individual's rights and regulation of the circumstances in which involuntary detention and treatment can take place. Governments should also develop legislation on disability, antidiscrimination, and welfare benefits.

Addressing Stigma Within a Policy Framework

In developing mental health policy, it is important to include consideration of stigma about mental health issues and mental illness. As well as the impact on the individual with mental illness, stigma results in a lack of attention from ministers and the public, which then results in a lack of resources and morale, decaying institutions, lack of leadership, inadequate information systems, inadequate legislation, and inadequate attention to key public health committees. By resulting in social exclusion of people with mental illness, stigma is detrimental not just to people with mental illness, but also to the health of society as a whole. All too often, our services are departure points for exclusion when they should be stepping stones for social inclusion. The development of civil society, greater local democracy, and local institutional frameworks for the expression of the plurality of views in mental health provides the impetus for more transparency in the creation and evaluation of policy options. As the policy process becomes more open and local, it may gain greater legitimacy for particular policies. As the agenda of public action in mental health increasingly includes the issues of citizenship and human rights, mental health becomes part of the wider human development agenda.

Policy Partnerships Within the Health Sector

Partnerships with Generic Health Policy

Mental health policy needs to be linked to generic health policy. It is particularly important that any general public health strategy address mental as well as physical health so that national mortality indicators include death from suicide and relevant measures of morbidity due to mental illness, and health impact assessments must explicitly include mental health. Some of the generic health policy issues that will impact on mental health include primary care funding, training and incentive arrangements, and government generic health targets.

An effective policy will see mental health included in generic health reforms such as development of health information systems, because it is important to develop the facilities and instruments for routine monitoring of needs, inputs, processes, and outcomes for planning purposes, hospital optimization programs, quality standards, basic training standards, and accreditation procedures.

Governments need to ensure that all relevant agencies are aware of the importance of mental health for the population, that they are aware of the influence that their activities can have on mental health and that appropriate coordination between relevant agencies takes place. This coordination is often in place for action on alcohol and drugs and for AIDS programs but is as yet rarely in place for mental health programs despite mental illness forming the greater burden across the population.

Partnerships with Other Health Programs on Communicable and Noncommunicable Disease

There is a need for a partnership rather than a competition for resources between those working on noncommunicable diseases and infectious diseases. For example, mental health promotion is essential in schools if we are to reduce the risk of AIDS from unprotected sex and drugs and support girls in being assertive and confident in ensuring their sexual health and safety, and if we are to address the lack of acceptance of condoms in the male culture. It is much more efficient if such mental health promotion in schools is carried out collaboratively between the HIV, substance abuse, and mental health teams rather than as separate initiatives.

Partnership with Traditional Healers

Traditional healers are very common across the world (1 per 50 population in sub-Saharan Africa) and will remain a key deliverer of health care for large proportions of the population for many decades if not centuries. Their practice is variable and there is no doubt that some traditional practice is very harmful, but it is also likely that some of the herbal medicines used have helpful psychoactive properties and that some interventions give important psychosocial support to individuals, families, and communities. Rather than seeking to destroy traditional healing, it is more productive to research their provision and outcomes, seek dialogue with the aim of eliminating frankly harmful practices, and engage in joint training using diagnostic algorithms to encourage referral of difficult or chronic cases.

Integration with Primary Care

Primary health care has been defined by the World Health Organization as:

> essential health care made accessible to individuals and families in the community, by means acceptable to them, through their full participation and at a cost that the community and the country can afford. It forms an integrated part of the country's health care system, of which it is the nucleus, and of the overall social and economic development of the country (WHO, 1978).

The rationale for primary care arises from comparison of the prevalence and burden of severe mental illness and the common mental disorders, with the relative availability of specialist services. For example, in the national psychiatric morbidity surveys of Great Britain of 1994 and 2000, 16% of the adult population were suffering from a common mental disorder such as depression and anxiety and 0.5% from psychosis, with one psychiatrist per 50 000 in 1994 and approaching one per 10 000–20 000 population in 2005. Therefore no country, however rich, can afford anything approaching sufficient specialist personnel to see and care for everyone with a mental disorder.

Whatever the country, whether rich or poor, mental disorder is so common that most people with mental disorders will need to be seen and cared for by members of a primary health-care unit. It is therefore essential that both mental health policy and general health sector reforms aim to strengthen the basic and continuing training of primary health-care personnel in assessment, diagnosis, management, and criteria for referral of people to secondary care. This is as essential in the developed world as it is in low-income countries.

In richer countries, people with severe mental illness may be cared for by specialist services, with some shared care with primary care for long-term support. In poorer countries, there may often only be capacity for a small number of people with psychosis to be cared for in specialist care and most will need to be assessed, diagnosed, and treated in primary care, with support from specialist services.

We know from epidemiological studies that there is a high prevalence of common mental disorders in the general population and these may also be severe, disabling, and of long duration. This high prevalence in all countries means that not even rich countries can afford sufficient specialists to look after everyone with a mental disorder.

Because of their high socioeconomic costs, it is not tenable to argue that the burden of common mental disorders should be ignored. These costs arise from the repeated primary care consultations, and if patients remain untreated, absence due to sickness, labor turnover, reduced productivity, and the impact on families and children. Primary care therefore needs to play a central role in overall mental health care in rich countries as well as in poor countries. In addition to the logistical necessity of primary care, primary care has particular advantages in that it allows attention to both physical health and social needs, it allows continuity of care, it is often preferred by consumers, it is often more accessible than specialist care, and studies have shown it is possible to achieve good clinical and social outcomes.

In the development of policy on primary care of mental illness, it is important to examine the existing primary care system, its staffing, its system of basic and continuing training for each of the professional groups involved, and the existing system of information collection from primary care. Some key questions remain:

- Is the lead professional in the team a doctor or a medical assistant or a nurse, and what are their respective roles? For example, in some countries health workers with months rather than years of training are in the front line, dealing with screening and case finding, assessment and treatment. In Pakistan, the first tier are health-care workers, usually married women with grown children, who receive a short training, and the second tier is the primary care doctor. In the UK, the first tier is usually the primary care doctor, although this is now changing in some areas to allow nurses to conduct initial triages. A few still work alone but most work in groups and employ a number of primary care nurses. They also collaborate with a community nursing structure of district nurses and health visitors.
- What does the basic training for each tier and professional in the primary care unit consist of and how much if any mental health is included? For example, in Iran and Pakistan, the village health-care workers receive a few months training in selected priority topics so that they can screen, assess, diagnose, and treat. In Zanzibar,

there is a 4-year basic training for all nurses and the fourth year is devoted to mental health.
- What continuing training is available for each tier? In Zanzibar, there are education coordinators whose task is to organize and deliver continuing training for all the staff in the primary health-care units. This continuing training is regular, consisting of several weekends a year for which the primary care staff receive transport allowances and incentive payments to attend.
- What quality monitoring exists in primary care? In Iran, health psychologists perform a quality monitoring role for the village health workers, and visit every month to support, supervise, and check on the quality of the work. Systems for information collection in primary care are needed for adequate planning. This can be effective without involving expensive technology. For example, in Iran, health workers routinely collect and display annual data on prevalence and outcome of priority disorders.
- How proactive should primary care be? Should it mostly concentrate on active consulters or should it take a broader population perspective and seek to find and treat common disabling conditions? Primary care capacity for outreach is important. Transport is necessary for outreach from secondary care to primary care and from primary care to the community. It may need to be subsidized, be appropriate to the terrain, and preferably not be shared with other specialties with different working patterns.

In countries where there is a low psychiatrist-to-population ratio, specialists must support primary care to assess and manage all but the most severe cases. Specialists need to spend a major proportion of their time as a supportive consultant advisor (e.g., supervision, teaching, local planning, service development, and researching key local issues) for the service as a whole rather than purely as a hands-on clinician if they are to have maximum impact on the population for which they are responsible and if specialist nurses and primary care teams are to be adequately supported. However, in practice, it is difficult to achieve this when psychiatrists tend largely to be trained for their clinical role rather than for their leadership role in service development, intersectoral partnerships, support and supervision to primary care, etc., and where psychiatrist's remuneration is often dependent on the clinical role.

The integration of primary and secondary care is assisted by communication, including regular meetings to discuss criteria for referral, discharge letters, shared care procedures, need for medicines, information transfer, training, good practice guidelines, and research, and by agreeing to prescribing policies and ensuring supply of essential medicines.

Logistical consideration of the availability of the specialist services relative to primary care and to the population epidemiology of disorders is essential in order to plan the precise framework for specialist support to primary care.

In low-income countries, there is often only one psychiatrist per million population and in a few countries this is as low as one psychiatrist per five or six million.

Integration of Mental Health with District-Level and Provincial-Level Health Care

However rich a country may be, specialist mental health staff will nonetheless be in relatively short supply and therefore policy is needed to ensure their efficient deployment. In low-income countries, specialist services are usually in extremely short supply, and it is important to use them to best effect. Often the distribution of specialists is not equitable relative to the population, with most concentrated in the main cities for a variety of reasons, including the availability of private practice, the availability of academic links and posts, and the availability of schools and other facilities for families. For example, in Tanzania over half the country's psychiatrists live and work in Dar es Salaam. A similar situation exists in Australia and many other countries. Attention therefore needs to be given to the construction of attractive posts that offer exciting and interesting work, are suitable for people with families, but which nonetheless meet the overall service needs of the country. During specialist training and continuing professional development, attention will also need to be paid to the wide range of skills required by specialists responsible for service delivery for large populations, which may range from 500 000 to 5 000 000. Indeed Malawi has only one psychiatrist for its 13 million population. Clearly, service leadership, intersectoral liaison, support from the regional level to the district services, and capacity building at the district level to support and supervise primary care will be crucial components of the leadership role, as well as advocacy and construction of annual operational plans and budgets within the health sector.

The availability of specialist doctors, psychologists, and nurses is even less than it appears because of the time devoted to private practice in order to supplement the basic salary. Apart from availability for direct clinical work, it is also important to consider availability for audit, planning, service development, and essential research. It is therefore important for countries, when determining salary structures, to consider the opportunity costs of losing a significant proportion of a highly trained specialist's time not just from clinical work, important though it is, but also from the strategic planning and service development function, which is also essential.

There is growing concern that relatively rich countries are increasing their relative proportions of specialists per head of population, not so much by training greater numbers of specialists, but rather by recruiting trained specialists from low-income countries who can ill afford to lose them. It is crucial that governments agree on international guidelines to prohibit active poaching from low- and middle-income countries, and to give adequate recompense to governments in low- and middle-income countries for the loss of their health-care workers, both for their training and for the opportunity costs of losing such people often at a relatively senior stage in their careers.

Policy on Planning and Resourcing Specialist Services

To achieve good outcomes, people with severe mental illness should be cared for as close to home as is compatible with health and safety of the individual and the safety of the public, in an environment that is the least restrictive possible, with due regard to their rights as human beings and respect for their dignity, religion, and culture. The precise service structure and configuration needs to be determined in the context of local needs, culture, and resources, and in the West may include a small flexible mixture of acute inpatient beds, halfway houses, respite houses, outpatient clinics, occupational rehabilitation, day care, employment, and social activities aimed at promoting each individual's self-determination and personal responsibility. In low-income countries, resource constraints greatly limit the extent of specialist provision, which may be limited to district level outpatient clinics, and very small numbers of inpatient beds in the provincial hospitals (e.g., 20 beds per 5 000 000 population). Some countries with a colonial history have inherited a large national mental hospital, which is usually being downsized and converted to other uses such as training. Attention needs to be paid to the appropriate siting of inpatient beds so that relatives can visit frequently. Apart from maintaining emotional links with the family, in poor countries, relatives are relied on to make significant contributions to the patient's diet and patients may become significantly malnourished without such input. Where the only beds available are hundreds of miles away, it is all too easy for family ties to be disrupted, contributing to long-term institutionalization.

Before planning future service developments, it is crucial to assess the existing specialist services, their distribution relative to the population, their balance, and their current pattern of use. Where large asylums exist, they tend to be in poor repair, with inadequate resources for maintaining the fabric of the building, staffing, treatment, and rehabilitation. Policy needs to consider the future of such asylums, which research has shown encourage institutionalization and the accumulation of significant social handicap. There is an inevitable tension between putting resources into developing a range of local services in each locality, however defined, and continuing to put adequate resources into the asylum until it can close. In essence, it is necessary to provide double running costs for a period of time. In practice, most governments do not budget for double running costs and this leads in many countries to the existence of mental hospitals, which are in a far worse state of repair than the general hospitals, with worse staffing, training, and worse morale, and even too few resources to give the patient an adequate diet. It is therefore essential for policy to address the mechanics and time scale, resourcing of the transition period, and to build in adequate monitoring of progress.

In some countries, most acute admissions are to general beds in general hospitals where the patients are cared for by general nurses. If this is the case, policy needs to consider how far the quality of care can be improved by additional training for the general nurses.

Key Service Provision Issues

Supply of Essential Medicines and Therapies

It is important to assess the needs for essential medicines and basic psychosocial interventions; even though there is a significant cost attached to ensuring adequate availability of medicines and psychological treatments. Nonetheless if there is adequate availability of treatments in primary care, then the number of inpatient beds needed in the new community-oriented system will be much smaller than that originally provided in the asylums. In some countries, senior policy makers do not recognize that mental illness is a real illness or that it can be treated, or that not to do so incurs considerable financial and social costs to the country. This attitude leads to inadequate provision for essential medicines in the medication budget.

Basic psychosocial interventions include general support, cognitive behavior therapy, marital therapy, psychological education, and relapse prevention. Occupational therapy is especially important. All inpatients should be in an appropriate rehabilitation and activity program every day.

Where countries cannot afford a wide variety of different specialists, it is not uncommon for one professional to fulfill a variety of roles. For example, the psychiatric nurse may take on the role of occupational therapist or social worker. If this is the case, then policy needs to consider how far the basic training of psychiatric nurses should take into account and support this situation by incorporating modules on occupational therapy and social work.

Standards of Care

Where patients are cared for in places other than their own homes, it is essential to have some system of quality assurance to ensure that some basic standards are met. For example, it is reasonable to expect an adequate diet, adequate spacing of meals, hygienic cooking facilities,

and hygienic washing and toilet facilities, with appropriate privacy and freedom from sexual harassment for women. It would not be realistic to expect low-income countries to be able to afford the kinds of inspection that richer countries can deploy, but it is reasonable to expect that psychiatric hospitals be regularly visited by senior politicians, policy makers, and influential lay people so that the conditions in the hospital are clearly known and visible.

Good practice guidelines are helpful educational tools for ensuring that best practice is routine and may be useful in inpatient, outpatient, and community settings. All referred patients will need routine assessment of the physical, psychological, and social needs and a care plan to meet those needs (e.g., Jenkins, 2004b).

Provision for Women

Women, by virtue of their increased exposure to acute life events, chronic social stresses, lower social status and income, and smaller social networks, are often particularly vulnerable to common mental disorders. There is also a small group of disorders specific to women, disorders associated with menstruation, pregnancy, and childbirth. Governments will therefore need to consider access to education, training, and health care for women as well as the influence of other government policies on these issues. Liaison between government departments on policies to improve family cohesiveness, for example, mechanisms such as taxation and welfare benefits in place to support families, reduce family breakdown, and reduce the burden on women as they struggle to raise their children will impact on mental health. In some countries, mental illness is a sufficient reason for divorce, and such premature divorces will often leave a parent without financial support, to the detriment of both the mother and the child. It is therefore important to make available marital support and therapy. This is an activity that can often be usefully delivered by a nongovernmental organization.

Provision for Children

Children are a nation's most precious resource, yet services for children and adolescents are often the least developed and supported. Children's cognitive and emotional development is greatly influenced by the mental health of their parents, especially the mother, and particularly when the mother is the main carer. In addition to the general rates of adult illness, women experience higher rates of illness around the time of childbirth. If untreated, these disorders can severely affect the mother's relationship with her children, thus damaging the child's cognitive and emotional development. Particular childhood disorders that need to be considered include emotional and conduct disorders, epilepsy, mental retardation, cerebral malaria, and specific learning problems such as dyslexia.

It is important to develop facilities for sick postnatal mothers to be cared for with their babies, and older children with their mothers. All children with epilepsy should receive adequate medication (often in very short supply in low-income countries) and school teachers should receive training in detecting and managing dyslexia, which is a significant contributor to conduct disorders and depression in children and to antisocial behavior in adult life.

Cognitive Disability

Children and adults with cognitive disabilities should be able, encouraged, and supported to lead as normal a life as possible. Children with cognitive disabilities, as well as those with special educational needs, often also have social, physical, and psychological needs. This means that close liaison between the ministries of health and education is important. Policy makers will need good estimates of the prevalence of cognitive disabilities, and an appreciation of the possibilities for prevention of some cases, for example in areas where iodine deficiency is a significant cause, such as Cambodia. Many children with cognitive disabilities also have specific neurological problems such as cerebral palsy and epilepsy, and essential medicines are needed to ensure that the cognitive deficit is not aggravated by these associated conditions.

The psychiatric services need to plan how they can deliver an assessment and management service to children with cognitive disabilities and their care providers. There also needs to be an orientation to the needs of children and adults with cognitive disabilities and their families in primary health care. This may be supported by the use of good practice guidelines on assessment and management of cognitive disabilities. Depending on the availability of resources, consideration needs to be given to the training of child psychologists, speech therapists, and special teachers and to the incorporation of cognitive disability into basic, specialist, and continuing training.

Public Health Measures

Reduction of Suicide and Homicide by Mentally Ill People

Government health policies usually implicitly, or sometimes explicitly, aim to protect, promote, and improve health and to reduce premature avoidable mortality. Premature death from suicide is a significant cause of mortality around the globe; official suicides alone form the tenth leading cause of death in the world, equivalent in magnitude to deaths from road traffic accidents or to deaths from malaria. A number of countries are now

developing national suicide prevention policies (United Nations, 1996; Anderson and Jenkins, 2008).

Psychiatric homicide prevention programs will include improved training in risk assessment, improved coordination, continuity of care, and communication between care providers and improved provision of support for those in greatest need, particularly the provision of 24-h nursing care for people in whom a lesser degree of support is insufficient.

Reduction in Mortality from Physical Illness in Mentally Ill People

People with severe mental illness tend to have a higher mortality than the general population from cardiovascular disease, respiratory disease, and malignancy. It is therefore extremely important to ensure adequate physical health care and health promotion to people with mental illness, particularly those being looked after by the hospital. In tropical countries this may include particular public health attention to the quality of the water supply and sanitation to reduce the risk of cholera, for example. In cold countries, this will include particular attention to housing.

Preparedness for Disasters

No country can afford to ignore the possibility of disasters, whether instigated by humans or natural. More than 50 countries have experienced conflict in the last 20 years. Conflicts are much more common in poor countries, and 15 of the 20 poorest countries of the world have had a major conflict in the last 15 years. Nearly all low-income countries are next to a country that has experienced war and therefore frequently carry the burden of caring for refugees. Women and children are particularly vulnerable to war, frequently being witness to or forced participants in murder, victims of rape, victims of infection with AIDS, rejection, abduction of child soldiers, with the subsequent difficulty rehabilitating them.

Psychosocial issues are often neglected in postconflict situations even though the presence of psychosocial disorders contributes to low compliance with vaccination, nutrition, oral rehydration, antibiotics, and risky sexual behavior, and hence to the high morbidity and mortality from preventable and treatable infectious disease.

Sometimes the sheer volume of refugees and their movements make practical arrangements very difficult. For example, in Macedonia during the Kosovo crisis, there were over 250 000 refugees and large transfers at short notice between camps as new refugees arrived, making psychosocial work very difficult during the initial phase. In Kashmir, the affected population was extremely widely dispersed through vast mountain areas and did not want to abandon their homes to be centralized into camps. Therefore, primary care is crucial in disaster management, and the central importance of involving primary care teams in the management of the medium- and long-term psychological consequences of a disaster has long been argued. In any disaster affecting large numbers of people, there will be preexisting disorders, the severity of which have been exacerbated by the disaster, and there will be new disorders caused by the disaster. Thus, the whole range of mental disorders (psychosis, common mental disorders, childhood disorders, dementia, substance abuse) as well as common neurological problems such as epilepsy need to be addressed, not just PTSD. Disasters often uncover or highlight preexisting public deficiencies and problems, such as the lack of a preexisting strong primary care and public health system; consequently, much of the postdisaster task is in fact the construction of what should have been in place before the disaster, namely the establishment of a strong primary care system, supported by decentralized district specialist services, and mechanisms for intersectoral liaison. Experience indicates over and over again that countries beset by disaster then undergo a second disaster, which is the lack of coordination by the multiple agencies who respond to disasters. Coordination is crucial, and all assisting agencies must liaise closely with the WHO country office and government ministries who have the overall lead responsibility (see Inter-agency Standing Committee, 2007).

Implementation of Policy

Implementation is even more challenging than strategy formulation, and particular attention needs to be paid to:

- Communications: Public relations on strategy, cascading information within organizations, organizing feedback, and alliance-building between key partners;
- Resources: Accessing key budgets, securing capital, ensuring revenue flows, maximizing the use of generic budgets, sponsorship, and aid;
- Staff: Planning the development of the human resource, training for changing service configurations, basic and continuing education for mental health staff, training generic staff such as primary care and teachers, communicating with staff, engaging professional bodies and educational institutions;
- Embedding the strategy: Engaging generic organizations, managers, politicians;
- disseminating good practice;
- Implementing an R & D strategy: Including evaluation, learning from mistakes, and successes and fine-tuning of strategy, quality assurance, accreditation, and inspection;

- Addressing stigma: There is a need to address high-level stigma within government surrounding mental health so that mental health policy is well integrated with general health policy and so that de-institutionalization is seen as an important step toward achieving better health and social outcomes for people with mental illness, but not as an opportunity to save money on the costs of health care;
- Political will: Political will at national level is essential to support mental health in public policy and must include a high profile for mental health within the ministry of health, liaison with other ministries and a cabinet committee for mental health; political will at international level will foster debate in the international media and international cooperation.

An important component of the way forward includes building capacity for policy development, health monitoring, research architecture, for innovation, development, and empowering leadership. This means creative use of attachments and secondments during training and career development. It is important to know much more about national and local epidemiology and to build capacity in local epidemiology.

The Facilitating Role of International Agencies in Stimulating Policy Development

In 2001, WHO devoted both its annual health day and its annual health report to mental health, which called on countries to develop mental health policies. In the same year, the Institute of Medicine, in Washington, launched a scientific report on neurological, psychiatric, and developmental disorders in low-income countries, which called for immediate strategic action to reduce the burden of brain disorders (Institute of Medicine, 2001). The EC plays an important role both in Europe and elsewhere and has recently produced a public health framework for mental health. At national level, various governments, national NGOs, professional bodies, and the media have played important roles in prioritizing mental health in their countries.

Conclusions

All countries have a mixture of developed and developing features, and we can learn from each other. Large-scale applications are dangerous and we need locally tailored solutions. We need to build capacity for strategic policy work, tackle stigma, enhance human rights, consumer involvement, individual assessment of needs and individually tailored care plans, evidence of interventions, public relations, and evaluation of outcomes. Psychiatrists have a key role to play in influencing their governments to increase the priority afforded to mental health, develop well-tailored mental health policies, and support their implementation and fine-tuning. It is therefore essential that every country create a strategic mental health policy that is well integrated, both with its general public policies and its overall health policy at ministerial, regional, and local levels and that covers the three broad tasks:

1. Community action to promote mental health;
2. Primary care of mental disorders for prevention and prompt and efficient treatment of common mental health disorders;
3. Specialist services (as local as is affordable) to support those patients in greatest need and to support and sustain expertise in primary care.

Mental health in a population depends on much more than the policies of the health and social services, and is influenced by policies on housing, employment, taxation, and issues such as the availability of alcohol. Policy is likely to work best if it is integrated as far as possible with existing systems for education, human resources, organizing feedback, and alliance building between key partners.

It needs to be accompanied by a strategic implementation program, a timetable for action, and substantial political will. It is essential to access key budgets, secure capital, ensure revenue flows, maximize the use of generic budgets as well as specific budgets, and obtain sponsorship and aid. Mental illness is stigmatized and suffers from lack of resources everywhere. Giving it its own budget gives it status and visibility.

The best of plans will remain on the shelf unless a powerful strategic mechanism is devised for their implementation with direct senior official and ministerial accountability. The implementation strategy needs to address all levels of action, at the national, regional, and local level, including the specialist sector, primary care sector, and the community.

See also: Mental Health Promotion; Mental Health Resources and Services.

Citations

Anderson M and Jenkins R (2008) National suicide prevention strategies across the world. In: Waserman D and Waserman C (eds.) *Oxford Textbook of Suicidology: The Five Continents Perspective*. Oxford, UK: Oxford University Press.
Gureje O and Jenkins R (2007) Mental health and development: Re-emphasising the link. *The Lancet* 369: 447–449.
Inter-agency Standing Committee (2007) *Guidelines on Mental Health and Psychosocial Support in Emergency Settings*. Geneva, Switzerland: Inter-agency Standing Committee.
Institute of Medicine (2001) *Neurological, Psychiatric and Developmental Disorders. Meeting the Challenge in the Developing world*. Washington, DC: National Academy Press.
Jenkins R (2001) World Health Day 2001 – Minding the world's mental health. *Social Psychiatry and Epidemiology* 36: 165–168.
Jenkins R (2003) Supporting governments to adopt mental health policies. *World Psychiatry* 2: 14–19.
Jenkins R (ed.) (2004a) International Project on Mental Health Policy and Services. Phase 1: Instruments and Country Profiles. *International Review of Psychiatry* 16(1–2): 1–176.
Jenkins R (ed.) (2004b) *WHO Guide to Mental and Neurological Health in Primary Care*. London: Royal Society of Medicine Press.
Jenkins R (2007) Health research and policy. In: Bhui K and Bhugra D (eds.) *Culture and Mental Health: A Comprehensive Textbook*, pp. 70–86. London: Hodder Arnold
Jenkins R and Meltzer H (2003) A decade of national surveys of psychiatric epidemiology in Great Britain 1990–2000. *International Review of Psychiatry* 15(1–2): 19–28.
Jenkins R, McCulloch A, and Parker C (1998) *Supporting Governments and Policy Makers on Mental Health Policy*. Geneva, Switzerland: World Health Organization.
Jenkins R, McCulloch A, Friedli L, and Parker C (2002) *Developing a National Mental Health Policy: Maudsley Monograph 43*. Hove, UK: Psychology Press, Taylor and Francis.
Jenkins R, Gulbinat W, Manderscheid R, et al. (2004) The mental health country profile: Background, design and use of a systematic method of appraisal. The International Consortium on Mental Health Policy and Services: Objectives, design and project implementation. *International Review of Psychiatry* 16: 31–47.
Jenkins R, McDaid D, Brugha T, Cutler P, and Hayward R (2007) The evidence base in mental health policy. In: Knapp M, McDaid D, Mossialou E and Thornicroft G (eds.) *Mental Health Policy and Practice Across Europe*, pp. 100–125. Maidenhead, UK: Open University Press.
Mathers CD and Loncar D (2006) Projections of global mortality and burden of disease from 2002 to 1030. *PLoS Medicine* 3: e442.
Mizra I, Hassan R, Chaudrey H, and Jenkins R (2006) Eliciting explanatory models of common mental disorders using the Short Explanatory Model Interview (SEMI) Urdu Adaption – a pilot study. *Journal of Pakistan Medical Association* 56: 461–462.
Murray C and Lopez AD (1996) *The Global Burden of Disease – A Comprehensive Assessment of Mortality and Disability from Diseases, Injuries and Risk Factors in 1990 and Projected to 2020*. Cambridge, MA: Harvard University Press.
United Nations (1996) *Prevention of Suicide: Guidelines for the Formulation and Implementation of National Strategies*. New York: United Nations.
Ustun TB and Kessler RC (2002) Global burden of depressive disorders: The issue of duration. *British Journal of Psychiatry* 181: 181–183.
World Health Organization (1978) *Report and Declaration from the World Health Organization*. Alma Ata, USSR, Geneva: World Health Organization.
World Health Organization (2001a) *The World Health Report 2001. Mental Health: New Understanding, New Hope*. Geneva, Switzerland: World Health Organization.
World Health Organization (2001b) *Mental Health Policy Project – Policy and Service Guidance*. Geneva, Switzerland: World Health Organization.
World Health Organization (2005) *The World Health Report 2005*. Geneva, Switzerland: World Health Organization.

Further Reading

World Health Organization (2005) *Mental health Policy and Service Guidance Package*. Geneva, Switzerland: WHO.
World Health Organization (2005) *Mental Health Policy, Plans and Programmes* (updated version) (2005). Geneva, Switzerland: WHO

World Health Organization (2005) *Child and Adolescent Mental Health Policies and Plans*. Geneva, Switzerland: WHO.

World Health Organization (2005) *Improving Access and Use of Psychotropic Medicines*. Geneva, Switzerland: WHO.

World Health Organization (2005) *Planning and Budgeting to Deliver Services for Mental Health* (2003).

Relevant Websites

http://www.who.int/mental_health/evidence/atlas – World Health Organization, Project Atlas: Resources for Mental Health.

http://www.who.int/mental_health/emergencies/en/ – World Health Organization, Mental Health and Psychosocial Support in Emergencies.

http://www.who.int/entity/mediacentre/factsheets/ – World Health Organization, Fact Sheets.

http://www.who.int/mental_health/policy/en – World Health Organization, Mental health Improvements for Nations Development: The WHO MIND Project.

http://www.who.int/mental_health/policy/legislation/policy/en/ – World Health Organization, Mental health, human rights and legislation.

http://www.world-mental-neurological-health.net

Mental Health Promotion

H Herrman and R Moodie, University of Melbourne, Melbourne, VIC, Australia
S Saxena, World Health Organization, Geneva, Switzerland

Introduction

Mental health promotion is an area of study and practice integral to the new public health and health promotion. The recognition of mental health within public health is nonetheless a recent development in many parts of the world. Mental health theory and practice have a long history of separation from physical health theory and practice. The change to a more integrated approach relates to greater public awareness of mental health and evidence of its importance to overall health and social and economic development.

Like health promotion, mental health promotion involves actions that (1) support people to adopt and maintain healthy ways of life and (2) create living conditions and environments that allow or foster health. Actions such as advocacy, policy and project development, legislative and regulatory reform, communications, and research and evaluation are relevant in countries at all stages of economic development. Mental health promotion relates to the whole population of a locality or country, often through vulnerable subgroups and particular settings. It focuses on maintenance and growth of positive mental health. The Ottawa Charter for Health Promotion provides a foundation for health promotion strategies that can be applied usefully to the promotion of mental health (see Lahtinen *et al.*, 2005). It considers the individual, social, and environmental factors that influence health. It places emphasis on the control of health by people in their everyday settings in the context of healthy policy and supportive environments. The Charter's five strategies are building healthy public policies, creating supportive environments, strengthening community action, developing personal skills, and reorienting health services.

Mental health promotion refers to improving the mental health of everybody in the community, including those with no experience of mental illness as well as those who live with illness and disability. Activities designed to promote other aspects of health, to reduce risk behaviors such as tobacco, alcohol, and drug misuse and unsafe sex, or to alleviate social and economic problems such as crime and intimate partner violence, will often promote mental health. Suicide prevention programs in countries or districts will also typically include interventions that promote mental health. Conversely, the promotion of mental health will usually have additional effects on health, productivity, and on social and economic conditions. The evaluation of outcomes can be designed to take these wider changes into account, although such an integrated view has been rare in the past.

Awareness of the importance of mental health has grown through advocacy for prevention and treatment of mental illnesses. Reports on the global burden of disease, the release of the World Health Organization's World Health Report in 2001, 'Mental Health: New Understanding, New Hope,' and the release of national reports on mental health since 1990 have resulted in a significant increase in awareness and action to improve the outcomes for people affected by mental illnesses or at risk of becoming ill. Even so, this attention in itself results in a restricted view of the public health approach to improving mental health. As with all other components of health, illness claims the attention of the community and policy makers. Indeed the term mental health is commonly understood as referring to mental illnesses and their prevention and treatment. The stigma attached to people living with mental illness encourages this vague use of terms and concepts in a way that is similar to but generally more pronounced than for illnesses of other types. As noted by Norman Sartorius in 1998 and in several of his other publications, this creates confusion about the meaning and value of mental health, and lowers the chance of its promotion becoming a high priority for public policy or action. Mental health is a positive set of attributes, in a person or community, which can be enhanced or compromised by environmental and social conditions.

Mental Health Promotion Across Cultures

Mental health has been described in an extensive literature in terms of a positive emotion (affect) such as feelings of happiness, a personality trait that includes the psychological resources of self-esteem and mastery, and as resilience, or the capacity to cope with adversity. Each of these models contributes to understanding what is meant by mental health. Research has aided the understanding, although much of the accessible evidence is recorded in the English language and generated in high-income countries. Progress in generating the evidence for mental health promotion depends on defining, measuring, and recording mental health in all parts of the world (see Kovess-Masfety *et al.*, in Herrman *et al.*, 2005).

Mental health is defined by WHO as "a state of well-being in which the individual realizes his or her own abilities, can cope with the normal stresses of life, can work productively and fruitfully, and is able to contribute to his or her community" (as quoted in Herrman *et al.*, 2005: 2). The term positive mental health is sometimes used to emphasize the value of mental health as a personal and community resource. This core concept of mental health is consistent with its wide and varied interpretation across cultures.

Positive mental health contributes to personal well-being, quality of life and effective functioning, and also contributes to society's effective functioning and the economy. It describes a personal characteristic as well as a community characteristic. Geoffrey Rose (1992) used the mental health attributes of populations to exemplify his restatement of the ancient view that healthiness is a characteristic of a whole population and not simply of its individual members. He went on to note that just as the mildest subclinical degree of depression is associated with

impaired functioning of individuals, so surely the average mood of a population must influence its collective or societal functioning. Yet the measurement of population mental health and the study of its determinants are still relatively neglected.

Concepts fundamental to public health, as distilled by key thinkers such as Marmot, Wilkinson, Syme, and Rose, are also fundamental to the improvement of mental health. For example, health and illness are determined by multiple factors, health and illness exist on a continuum, and personal and environmental influences on health and disease may be studied and changed and the effects evaluated. Yet these ideas are foreign to mental health for many professionals and nonprofessionals whose views are shaped by the image of asylum care for people living with apparently incurable mental illnesses. Furthermore, the promotion of mental health is sometimes seen as far removed from the problems of the real world and even as diverting resources from the treatment and rehabilitation of people affected by mental illness. As a result, the opportunities for improving mental health in a community are not fully realized. Activities that can improve mental health include the promotion of health, the prevention of illness and disability, and the treatment and rehabilitation of those affected. As in public health overall, these are different from one another, even though the actions and outcomes overlap. They are all required and are complementary to one another (Sartorius, 1998) (**Figure 1**).

Although the attributes defining mental health may be universal, their expression differs individually, culturally, and in relation to different contexts. An understanding of a particular community's concepts of mental health is a

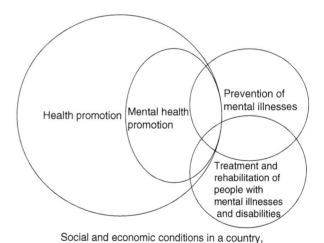

Social and economic conditions in a country, locality or population

Figure 1 Notional diagram of the relationships between mental health promotion, prevention, and treatment of mental illnesses and the new public health or health promotion.

prerequisite to engaging in mental health promotion (see Sturgeon and Orley, in Herrman *et al.*, 2005). Sensitivity to the factors valued by different cultures will increase the relevance and success of potential interventions. Understanding the effects of discrimination on the lives of women in patriarchal societies or people living with HIV/AIDS, for instance, will make a major contribution to developing relevant intervention programs. It is equally important to be aware that a culture-specific approach to understanding and improving mental health may be unhelpful if it ignores the variations within most cultures today and fails to consider individual differences. The beliefs and actions of people and groups need to be understood in their political, economic, and social contexts.

Determinants of Mental Health

Mental health and mental illnesses are determined by interacting social, psychological, and biological factors. This is similar to the mechanism of multiple interactions understood to determine health and illness in general. Ideas about the social determinants of mental health and mental illness have evolved to reach the current understanding that gene expression can be influenced by external agents and may be shaped by social experience (see Anthony, in Herrman *et al.*, 2005). Studies with animal models are demonstrating the mechanisms by which social experience influences the developing brain. For instance, the closeness of maternal care in laboratory mice has molecular consequences that modify the brain. Other studies are illustrating, conversely, how the brain can process social information, for example how unique molecules influence memory of social events (see Insel, in Herrman *et al.*, 2005). A life-course approach helps in understanding social variations in health and mental health.

Research designs need to take into account these systemic interactions rather than rely only on risk factor epidemiology, by which is meant a selectively narrow focus on individual-level characteristics and behaviors. Eminent critics such as Claus Bahne Bahnson in the 1970s had earlier advocated for more research using designs that avoid old controversies about the relative significance of biological or sociological or other factors, but instead consider a larger matrix integrating the several levels or types of determinants (see Anthony, in Herrman *et al.*, 2005).

Social Disadvantage: Poverty, Gender Disadvantage, and Indigenous Populations

In the developed and developing world, poor mental health and common mental disorders are associated with indicators of poverty, including low levels of education. The association may be explained by such factors as the experience of insecurity and hopelessness, rapid social change, and the risks of violence and physical ill health (Patel and Kleinman, 2003). Most evidence of this association relates to the prevalence of mental disorders. When mental health is understood in positive terms, the need becomes apparent for studies using positive as well as negative indicators of mental health, as well as documenting the process of health-promoting interventions.

Mental, social, and behavioral health problems can interact to intensify each other's effects on behavior and health. The authors of the influential volume *World Mental Health* (Desjarlais *et al.*, 1995) define this idea clearly. They marshal the evidence to state that substance abuse, violence, and abuses of women and children on the one hand, and health problems such as heart disease, depression, and anxiety on the other, are more prevalent and more difficult to cope with in conditions of high unemployment, low income, limited education, stressful work conditions, gender discrimination, unhealthy lifestyle, and human rights violations.

Human Rights

Respect for and protection of civil, political, economic, social, and cultural rights is fundamental to mental health promotion in a community. Good mental health does not coexist with abuse of fundamental human rights. The Bill of Rights and other United Nations (UN) human rights instruments reflect a set of universally accepted values and principles of equality and freedom from discrimination, and the right of all people to participate in decision-making processes. The related legal obligations on governments can assist vulnerable and marginalized groups to gain influence over matters that affect their health. These UN instruments also serve to guide countries in the design, implementation, monitoring, and evaluation of mental health policies, laws, and programs. They provide additional protection to vulnerable groups, including women and children in many settings, who are marginalized and discriminated against and at high risk for poor mental health and mental disorders. As human rights have civil, cultural, economic, political, and social dimensions, they provide a mechanism to consider mental health across the wide range of mental health determinants. They also underscore the need for action and involvement of a wide range of sectors in mental health promotion (see Drew *et al.*, in Herrman *et al.*, 2005).

Case study: Mental health and psychosocial support in emergency settings: The Inter-Agency Standing Committee guidelines

The Inter-Agency Standing Committee (IASC) is formed by the heads of a broad range of UN and non-UN humanitarian agencies. It is the primary mechanism for interagency decisions in response to complex emergencies and natural disasters. In 2005 in the aftermath of the Asian tsunami, an IASC Task Force on Mental Health and Psychosocial Support (MHPSS) in Emergency Settings was established to develop intersectoral guidelines. The guidelines are a foundational reference and guide for policy leaders, agencies, and practitioners worldwide. The *Guidelines* emphasize the need for protection and human rights standards, including the application of a human rights framework through MHPSS, and the need to identify, monitor, prevent, and respond to protection threats through social and legal protection.

Human rights violations are pervasive in most emergencies. Many of the defining features of emergencies – displacement, breakdown in family and social structures, lack of humanitarian access, erosion of traditional value systems, a culture of violence, weak governance, absence of accountability and a lack of access to health services – entail violations of human rights. In emergency situations, an intimate relationship exists between the promotion of mental health and psychosocial well-being and the protection and promotion of human rights:

• Advocating for the use of human rights standards such as the rights to health, education or freedom from discrimination contributes to the creation of a protective environment and supports social protection and legal protection. Using international human rights standards promotes accountability and the introduction of measures to end discrimination, ill treatment, or violence. Taking steps to promote and protect human rights will reduce the risks to those affected by the emergency.

• At the same time, humanitarian assistance helps people to realize numerous rights and can reduce human rights violations. Enabling at-risk groups, for example, to access housing or water and sanitation increases their chances of being included in food distributions, improves their health, and reduces their risks of discrimination and abuse. Providing psychosocial support, including life skills and livelihoods support, to women and girls may reduce their risk of having to adopt survival strategies such as prostitution that expose them to additional risks of human rights violations.

The IASC guidelines are designed for use by all humanitarian actors, including community-based organizations, government authorities, UN organizations, nongovernmental organizations, and donors operating in emergency settings at local, national, and international levels. Implementation requires extensive collaboration. The active participation at every stage of communities and local authorities is essential for successful, coordinated action, the enhancement of local capacities, and sustainability. Action sheets in the guidelines outline social supports relevant to the core humanitarian domains, such as disaster management, human rights, protection,

general health, education, water and sanitation, food security and nutrition, shelter, camp management, community development and mass communication. Mental health professionals seldom work in these domains, but are encouraged to use this document to advocate with communities and colleagues from other disciplines to ensure that appropriate action is taken to address the social risk factors that affect mental health and psychosocial well-being.

Social Capital

Lomas (1998) notes that the way we organize society, the extent to which we encourage social interaction, and the degree to which we trust and associate with each other are probably the most important determinants of health. Putnam used the term social capital in 1995 to refer to features of social organization such as those that facilitate coordination and cooperation for mutual benefit (Putnam, 1995). While Putnam and other scholars note the potential ill effects as well as benefits of social cohesion, research in recent years has demonstrated links between social capital and economic and community development. Higher social capital may protect individuals from social isolation, lower crime levels, improve schooling and education, enhance community life, and improve work outcomes. The relationships between social capital, health, and mental health, and the potential of mental health promotion to enhance social capital are now subject to active investigation (Sartorius, 2003), although related themes have a long history of study. In 1897, Durkheim proposed that weak social controls and the disruption of local community organization were factors producing increased rates of suicide (Durkheim, 1897). In 1942, Shaw and McKay linked crime to similar factors (Shaw and McKay, 1942). The study of the links between levels of social cohesion and antisocial and suicidal behavior continues, as reported by the Organization for Economic Cooperation and Development (OECD) in 2001 (OECD, 2001). Much work remains to be done in accounting for the mechanisms underlying the health–community link and the interrelations between social capital and mental health.

Social capital is a population attribute, not an individual status or perception, and the concept has helped to redirect research on the social determinants of health and mental health. Population health measures are usually considered as the aggregate of the individual characteristics in the population. Anthony (in Herrman *et al.*, 2005) illuminates how the perspective of networks of individuals interacting with environments, as offered by the concept of social capital, has the potential to explain a series of collective outcomes additional to those explained by research based on individual health outcomes.

Physical Health

Physical health and mental health are closely associated through various mechanisms (see Jane-Llopis and Mittelmark, 2005). Physical ill health has adverse effects on mental health, just as poor mental health contributes to poor physical health. For example, malnourishment in infants can increase the risks of cognitive and motor deficits, and heart disease and cancer can increase the risk of depression. Depression is an acknowledged risk factor for heart disease, and the mechanisms are now being studied. Poor social support, or a perception of this, and certain types of adverse working conditions are detrimental to both physical health (e.g., cardiovascular morbidity) and mental health (e.g., depression). People living with HIV/AIDS and their families frequently experience stigma and discrimination as well as depression and other mental illnesses. Persistent pain is linked with depression, anxiety, and disability.

Mental and physical health and functioning influence each other over time by various pathways (see WHO, 2001), interacting with the social and environmental influences on health. The first pathway is directly through physiological systems, such as neuroendocrine and immune functioning. The second pathway is through health behavior. The term health behavior covers a range of activities, such as eating sensibly, getting regular exercise and adequate sleep, avoiding smoking, engaging in safe sexual practices, wearing safety belts in vehicles, and adhering to medical therapies. The physiological and behavioral pathways interact with one another and with the social environment: Health behavior can affect physiology (for example, smoking and sedentary lifestyle lower immune functioning) and physiological functioning can influence health behavior (for example, tiredness contributes to accidents). In an integrated and evidence-based model of health, mental health (including emotions and thought patterns) emerges as an important determinant of overall health (WHO, 2001).

Mental Health Promotion and the Prevention and Treatment of Illnesses

Promotion and prevention are necessarily related and overlapping activities. Promotion is concerned with the determinants of health and prevention focuses on the causes of disease. Although the starting points are different, and the range of actions and those primarily responsible for them are also different, the activities and outcomes overlap with each other. The evidence for prevention of mental disorders (see WHO, 2004; Hosman and Jane-Llopis in IUHPE, 2000 noted below) contributes to the evidence base for promoting mental health.

Table 1   The actors in mental health promotion

Progress in mental health promotion depends on the work of several groups of people:
1. Local communities aware of the value of mental health
2. Those working in health and non-health sectors of government, business, and other nongovernmental organizations whose decisions affect mental health in ways that they may not fully realize
3. Mental health professionals who need to endorse and assist the promotion of mental health while continuing to deliver and advocate for services for people living with mental illnesses
4. Those working to develop policies and programs in countries with low, medium, and high levels of income and resources
5. Those concerned with guidelines for international action

Beyond that, evidence for the effectiveness of mental health promotion is gained through evaluation of public health actions and social policies in various sectors and in different countries and settings (Herrman *et al.*, 2005). The actions that promote mental health will often have as an important outcome the prevention of mental disorders. The evidence is that mental health promotion is also effective in the prevention of a whole range of behavior-related diseases and risks, as described above. It can help, for instance, in the prevention of smoking or of unprotected sex and hence of AIDS or teenage pregnancy (Orley and Weisen, 1998).

Mental health promotion actions are often social and political: Implementing interventions in schools, influencing housing and working conditions, working to reduce stigma and discrimination of various types, and developing policy initiatives to reduce violence are examples. The changes occur through decisions taken by politicians, educators, and members of nongovernmental organizations. Health practitioners are important as advocates and as aids to introducing policies that promote mental health (**Table 1**).

Evidence for Mental Health Promotion

Several authoritative sources summarize the evidence available for mental health promotion interventions. The landmark review from Mrazek and Haggerty in 1994 (Mrazek and Haggerty, 1994) describes a consensus on clusters of known risk and protective factors for mental health, as well as evidence that interventions can reduce identified risk factors and enhance known protective factors. The International Union for Health Promotion and Education (IUHPE) endorses the idea that mental health promotion programs work and that there are a number of evidence-based programs to inform mental health promotion practice (IUHPE, 2000; McQueen and Jones, 2007). Accumulating evidence demonstrates the feasibility of implementing effective mental health promotion programs across a range of population groups and settings (see Hosman and Jane-Llopis, 2005; Jane-Llopis *et al.*, 2005). A major task is to promote the application of existing evidence into good practice on the ground.

The published evidence comes mainly from high-income countries. Evidence is least available from places that have the greatest need, including low-income countries and populations affected by conflicts. A challenge now is to evaluate programs and practices in these settings and populations. This may include evaluation of programs and practices based on existing evidence, or initiating research and evaluation of practices and programs established in low-resource settings. Large-scale intervention trials are needed in a range of settings. Another challenge is to monitor the mental health effects of interventions in fields other than mental health. Patel and colleagues in South Asia (Patel *et al.*, 2004) demonstrate, for example, that maternal mental health is a critical and previously ignored factor in the association between social adversity and childhood failure to thrive in poor countries, an enormous problem in these countries. Interventions for preventing and treating postnatal depression as well as nutrition and social programs may be required, designed by members of the community according to the circumstances. Evaluation will require a variety of approaches and study designs, using qualitative and quantitative methods and indicators of process and outcome (Barry and McQueen, in Herrman *et al.*, 2005). Violence prevention is now seen as a major element of HIV prevention and as these programs expand it will be sensible to measure their mental health outcomes.

Empowerment is the process by which groups in a community who have been traditionally disadvantaged in ways that compromise their health can overcome these barriers and can exercise all the rights that are due to them with a view to leading a full and equal life in the best of health. The empowerment of women, violence prevention in the community, and microcredit schemes for the alleviation of debt are examples of empowerment programs that have had a mental health impact (see Patel *et al.*, in Herrman *et al.*, 2005). The evidence for the effects of these programs on mental health is so far little documented. Doing so will strengthen the evidence base in order to inform practice and policy globally.

The evidence base is important to several groups for different reasons, as described by Nutbeam in relation to health promotion more broadly (see IUHPE, 2000). Researchers will have a primary concern with the quality of the evidence, its methodological rigor, and its contribution to knowledge. Policy makers are likely to be concerned with the need to justify the allocation of resources and demonstrate added value. Practitioners need to have confidence in the likely success of implementing interventions, and the people who are to benefit need to see that both the program and the process of its introduction are participatory and relevant to them. Mental health promotion considers mental health in positive rather than in negative terms. This shift requires further work in establishing positive indicators of mental health outcomes (Zubrick and Kovess-Masfety, in Herrman *et al.*, 2005). It also requires a focus on research methods that will document the process as well as the outcomes of promoting positive mental health and identify the necessary conditions for successful implementation.

The systematic study of program implementation has been relatively neglected. A continuum of approaches is needed ranging from randomized controlled trials (RCTs) to qualitative process-oriented methods such as narrative analyses, interviews, surveys, and ethnographic studies. Collections of this kind of data will advance knowledge on best practice in real settings. The development of user-friendly and accessible information systems and databases is required for both practitioners and policy makers.

These systems would respond to the urgent need to identify effective programs that are transferable and sustainable in settings such as schools and communities. Examples are the application of programs based on community development and empowerment methods, such as mutual support for mothers and for widows and school-based programs for young people (Barry and McQueen, 2005). These have been shown to be highly effective, low-cost, replicable programs successfully implemented and sustained by nonprofessional community members in disadvantaged community settings. The principle of prudence recognizes that we can never know enough to act with certainty (see Mittelmark *et al.*, in Herrman *et al.*, 2005). Despite uncertainties and gaps in the evidence, we know enough about the links between mental health behavior and social experience to apply and evaluate locally appropriate policy and practice interventions to promote mental health (Herrman *et al.*, 2005: XIX).

Effective programs for universal, selective, and indicated prevention of conduct disorders, depression, anxiety disorders, eating disorders, substance use-related disorders, and psychotic disorders are summarized in a WHO publication on prevention of mental disorders (WHO, 2004). Reducing the risk of aggressive behavior and conduct disorders, for instance, focuses on improving the social competence and pro-social behavior of children, parents, teachers, and peers. Malleable risk factors include mothers' smoking during pregnancy, substance abuse among parents, child abuse, early substance use, deviant peer relationships, and poor and socially disorganized neighborhoods with high levels of crime. The onset of depression and its recurrence is influenced by a wide range of malleable risk and protective factors at different stages of life from infancy, including depression-specific factors such as parental depression, and generic risk factors such as child abuse and neglect, stressful life events, and bullying at school, and protective factors such as a sense of mastery, self-esteem, and social support. Effective prevention of depression therefore needs multiple actions at several levels. Prevention is possible for several forms of developmental and intellectual disabilities (for example, cretinism due to iodine deficiency) and disorders due to brain injury, although neglected in much of the world (Sartorius and Henderson, 1992). Suicide prevention programs rely on a range of social and health service interventions in any country or district, including interventions that improve treatment of depression, provide continuing care for people living with psychotic disorders, reduce harmful use of substances or control access to the means of suicide, and that promote mental health in the population in other ways. The proof that an intervention or a program is effective in preventing suicide is difficult and complicated, as suicide is a rare event (even though a leading cause of death in young people in several parts of the world) with determinants at several levels.

The effectiveness of exemplary mental health promotion programs and policies is summarized in recent publications (Hosman and Jane-Llopis, in Herrman et al., 2005; Jane-Llopis et al., 2005). In addition, research demonstrates that mental health can be affected by non-health policies and practices, for example in housing, education, and child care (see Petticrew et al., in Herrman et al., 2005) (**Table 2**). This work emphasizes the need to assess the effectiveness of policy and practice interventions in diverse health and non-health areas. It also demonstrates the effectiveness of a wide range of programs and interventions for enhancing the mental health of populations. These include:

- early childhood interventions;
- economic and social empowerment of women;
- social support to old-age populations;

- programs targeted at vulnerable groups such as minorities, indigenous people, migrants, and people affected by conflicts and disasters;
- mental health promotion activities in schools;
- mental health interventions at work;
- housing policies;
- violence prevention programs;
- community development programs (Herrman et al., 2005).

Improving the mental health of individuals and communities is a primary goal for some of these interventions, for example policies and programs that improve parenting skills and those that encourage schools to prevent bullying. Mental health is enhanced as a side benefit in other interventions that are mainly intended to achieve something else, for example policies and resources that ensure girls in a developing country attend school and programs to improve public housing. This distinction helps in recognizing the shared and primary responsibilities in countries and communities. Monitoring the effect on mental health of public policies relating to such things as housing and education is becoming feasible (Petticrew et al., in Herrman et al., 2005). Mental health programs in a country or locality can advocate for this, and help to ensure that findings are translated into action. Other groups will need to do the work, however, and ensure that policies and practices are shaped by the findings.

A Public Health Framework for Mental Health Promotion

Mental health promotion is expected to improve overall health, quality of life, and social functioning. Interventions designed to promote mental health, with a focus on the major determinants in vulnerable population groups, and

Table 2 Cost–outcome domains for the economic analysis of mental health promotion

	Level 1: Individuals (e.g., school children and workers)	Level 2: Groups (e.g., households and communities)	Level 3: Population (e.g., regions and countries)
Resource inputs	Health-seeking time	Program implementation	Policy development and implementation
	Health and social care	Household support	
	Lifestyle changes (e.g., exercise)		
Process indicators	Change in attitudes or behavior	Change in attitudes or behavior	Change in attitudes or behavior
Health outcomes	Functioning and quality of life	Family burden	Summary measures (e.g., DALYs)
	Mortality (e.g., suicide)	Violence	
Social and economic benefits	Self-esteem	Social capital/cohesion	Social inclusion
	Workforce participation	Reduced unemployment	Productivity gains
			Reduced health-care costs

From Petticrew M, Chisholm D Thomson H, and Jane-Llopis E (2005) Evidence: The way forward. In: Herrman H, Saxena S, and Moodie R (eds.) *Promoting Mental Health: Concepts, Emerging Evidence, Practice*, pp. 203–214. Geneva: World Health Organization.

through complex interactions including intermediate outcomes at individual, organizational, and societal levels, can result in a number of long-term benefits. In addition to improved mental health, the benefits can include lower rates of some mental illnesses, improved physical health, better educational performance, greater productivity of workers, improved relationships within families, and safer communities. The actions likely to be feasible and effective can be planned and monitored within a public health framework.

The first step in planning the activities of mental health promotion in any community or country is gathering local evidence and opinion about the main problems and potential gains, and the social and personal influences on mental health. A public health framework can help the process of assessing needs, developing partnerships, and planning actions and their evaluation. A framework includes the locally identified determinants of mental health, the population groups and areas and settings that have high priority for action, and a description of the anticipated benefits. In the case of the framework shown as an example in **Figure 2** (VicHealth, 2005), the three identified determinants of mental health are social inclusion, freedom from discrimination and violence, and economic participation.

Success in promoting mental health relies on the development of partnerships between a range of agencies in the public, private, and nongovernmental sectors. Common interests need to be identified. The focus on health rather than illness can help in doing this, as well as avoid the perception of competing for resources with the health services sector, already poorly resourced in most of the world.

Research, government policy making, and practice tend to take place in systems or organizations that have little involvement with each other. Effective mental health promotion interventions in a population require integrated activity across these so-called silos: Long-term planning, investment, and evaluation are required. Long-term gains are generally not attractive to governments with immediate concerns in other areas. Effective advocacy and communication with decision makers must be developed. International collaborations can assist advocacy for mental health promotion activity in low-income as well as high-income countries and the sharing of information and expertise (Walker *et al.*, in Herrman *et al.*, 2005).

Policy and Practice

Mental health promotion strategies need support from the community and the government. As collective action, the success of the strategies depends on shared values as much as on the quality of scientific evidence. In some communities, the practices and ways of life

maintain mental health even though mental health may not be identified as such. In other communities, people need to be convinced – as by the results of large-scale intervention trials – that making an effort to improve mental health is realistic and worthwhile (Sartorius, 1998; Herrman *et al.*, 2005: XIX). A government's work to develop mental health promotion strategies involves its social development policies as well as its health and mental health policies. It can use the public health framework at this level, with three main ingredients: A concept of mental health, strategies to guide mental health promotion, and a model for planning and evaluation.

Community Development and Mental Health Promotion

Community development aims to develop the social, economic, environmental, and cultural well-being of communities with a focus on marginalized people. Solutions to community problems are developed by local people, based on local knowledge and priorities. Work done in rural areas of India exemplifies some aspects of the relationship between community development and promotion of mental health, even where the objectives of the program may not include a specific focus on mental health. For example, a large primary health-care program in rural Indian villages directly targeting poverty, inequality, and gender discrimination has led indirectly to significant gains in mental health and well-being (Arole *et al.*, in Herrman *et al.*, 2005). As the interventions succeeded, the people realized the advantages of working together and they became open to approaching other issues affecting the village such as health needs and caste discrimination. An approach that is aware of the needs, interests, and responsibilities of men and women and that focuses on reducing the vulnerability and increasing the participation of women is the likely basis of the success of community development in these villages and the associated improvement in mental health (**Figure 3**).

Intersectoral Linkage and Community Change in Mental Health Promotion

Mental health can be improved through the collective action of society. Improving mental health requires policies and programs in government and business sectors including education, labor, justice, transport, environment, housing, and welfare, as well as specific activities in the health field relating to the prevention and treatment of ill health. Policy makers are now recognizing that emphasis is best placed on adding programs that sharpen the capacity of systems, such as primary

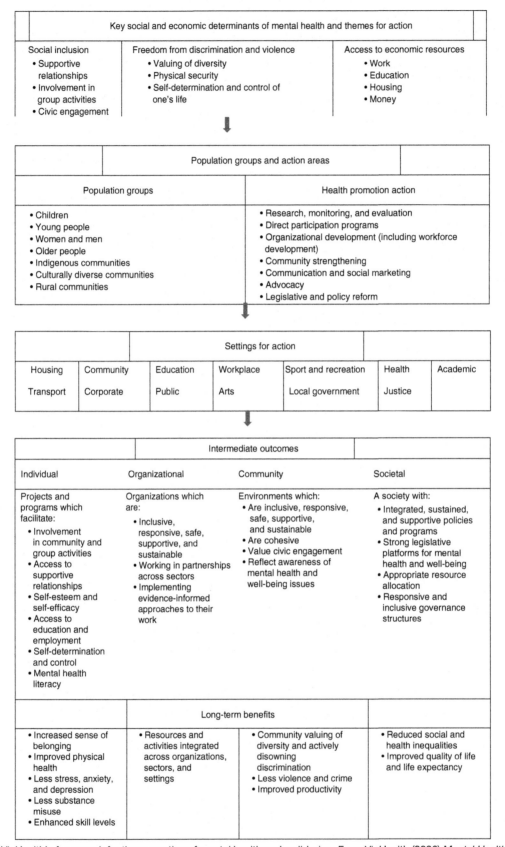

Figure 2 VicHealth's framework for the promotion of mental health and well-being. From VicHealth (2006) *Mental Health Promotion Framework 2005–2007*. www.vichealth.vic.gov.au (accessed October 2007).

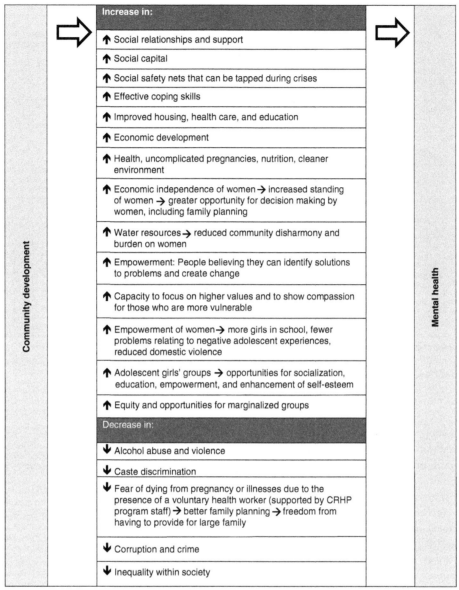

Figure 3 The relationship between community development and mental health in rural villages in India. From Arole R, Fuller B, and Deutschmann P (2005) Community development as a strategy for promoting mental health: Lessons from rural India. In: Herrman H, Saxena S, and Moodie R (eds.) *Promoting Mental Health: Concepts, Emerging Evidence, Practice*, pp. 243–251. Geneva: World Health Organization.

health-care systems and school systems, to be more health-enhancing. Investigating the sustainability of mental health promotion actions is therefore less about the technological aspects of programs and more about programs as change processes within organizations or communities. Programs are opportunities to recalibrate systems to higher or better levels of functioning. Evaluation also includes a more systematic analysis of the context within which programs are provided and factors within that context (such as preexisting attitudes and relationships) that could predict why some programs fade over time while others succeed and grow (see

Hawe *et al.*, in Herrman *et al.*, 2005; Rowling and Taylor, in Herrman *et al.*, 2005) (**Figure 4**).

Conclusions

Mental health is everybody's business. Those who can do something to promote mental health and who have something to gain include individuals, families, communities, health professionals, commercial and not-for-profit organizations, and decision makers in governments at all levels. International organizations can ensure that countries at

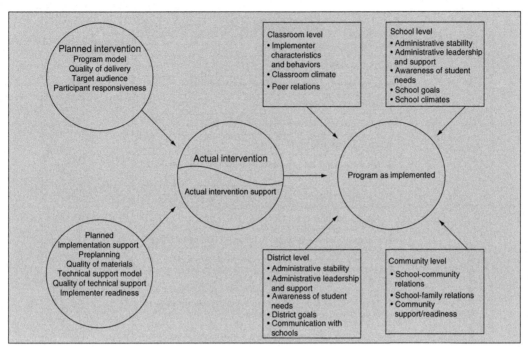

Figure 4   A model for implementing school-based programs. From Barry M, Domitrovich C, and Lara MA (2005). The implementation of mental health promotion programmes. In: Jane-Llopis E and Mittelmark M (eds.) (2005) *What Works in Mental Health Promotion. Special Issue. Promotion and Education*. 42(supplement 2): 30–36.

all stages of economic development are aware of the importance of mental health for human, community, and economic development and of the possibilities and evidence for intervening to improve and monitor the mental health of the population. A wide range of health and non-health decisions made by organizations and governments at local and national levels affect mental health. Mental health promotion ultimately depends on activities at the local level supported by local people and partnerships.

See also: Mental Health and Substance abuse; Mental Health Epidemiology (Psychiatric Epidemiology); Mental Health Policy; Mental Health Resources and Services; Historical Views of Mental Illness; Specific Mental Health Disorders: Child and Adolescent Mental Disorders; Stigma of Mental illness; Women's Mental Health.

Citations

Anthony J (2005) Social determinants of mental health and mental disorders. In: Herrman H, Saxena S and Moodie R (eds.) *Promoting Mental Health: Concepts, Emerging Evidence, Practice*, pp. 120–131. Geneva, Switzerland: World Health Organization.

Arole R, Fuller B, and Duetschmann P (2005) Community development as a strategy for promoting mental health: Lessons from rural India. In: Herrman H, Saxena S and Moodie R (eds.) *Promoting Mental Health: Concepts, Emerging Evidence, Practice*, pp. 243–251. Geneva, Switzerland: World Health Organization.

Barry MM and McQueen DV (2005) The nature of evidence and its use in mental health promotion. In: Herrman H, Saxena S and Moodie R (eds.) *Promoting Mental Health: Concepts, Emerging Evidence, Practice*, pp. 108–120. Geneva, Switzerland: World Health Organization.

Barry M, Domitrovich C, and Lara MA (2005) The implementation of mental. health promotion programmes. In: Jane-Llopis E and Mittelmark M (eds.) *What Works in Mental Health Promotion. Special Issue. Promotion and Education* 42(supplement 2): 30–36.

Drew N, Funk M, Pathare S, and Swartz L (2005) Mental health and human rights. In: Herrman H, Saxena S and Moodie R (eds.) *Promoting Mental Health: Concepts, Emerging Evidence, Practice*, pp. 89–108. Geneva, Switzerland: World Health Organization.

Durkheim E (1897, 1951) *Suicide: A Study in Sociology*. Spaulding JA and Simpson G (trans.). New York: The Free Press.

Hawe P, Ghali L, and Riley T (2005) Developing sustainable programs: Theory and practice. In: Herrman H, Saxena S and Moodie R (eds.) *Promoting Mental Health: Concepts, Emerging Evidence, Practice*, pp. 252–263. Geneva, Switzerland: World Health Organization.

Hosman CMH and Jane-Llopis E (2005) The evidence of effective interventions for mental health promotion. In: Herrman H, Saxena S and Moodie R (eds.) *Promoting Mental Health: Concepts, Emerging Evidence, Practice*, pp. 169–189. Geneva, Switzerland: World Health Organization.

Insel T (2005) Promoting mental health: Lessons from brain research. In: Herrman H, Saxena S and Moodie R (eds.) *Promoting Mental Health: Concepts, Emerging Evidence, Practice*, pp. 2–13. Geneva, Switzerland: World Health Organization.

Jane-Llopis E, Barry M, Hosman C, and Patel V (2005) Mental health promotion works: A review. In: Jane-Llopis E and Mittelmark M (eds.) *What Works in Mental Health Promotion. Special Issue. Promotion and Education* 42(supplement 2): 9–25.

Kovess-Masfety V, Murray M, and Gureje O (2005) Evolution of our understanding of positive mental health. In: Herrman H, Saxena S and Moodie R (eds.) *Promoting Mental Health: Concepts, Emerging Evidence, Practice*, pp. 35–46. Geneva, Switzerland: WHO.

Lahtinen E, Joubert N, Raeburn J, and Jenkins R (2005) In: Herrman H, Saxena S and Moodie R (eds.) *Promoting Mental Health: Concepts, Emerging Evidence, Practice*, pp. 226–242. Geneva, Switzerland: World Health Organization.

Lomas J (1998) Social capital and health – Implications for public health and epidemiology. *Social Science and Medicine* 47(9): 1181–1188.

McQueen D and Jones C (eds.) (2007) *Global Perspectives on Health Promotion Effectiveness*. New York: Springer.

Mrazek P and Haggerty RJ (eds.) (1994) *Reducing Risks of Mental Disorder: Frontiers for Preventive Intervention Research*. Washington, DC: National Academies Press.

OECD (2001) *The Well-Being of Nations. The Role of Human and Social Capital. Education and Skills*. Paris: Organisation for Economic Co-operation and Development Centre for Educational Research and Innovation.

Orley J and Weisen RB (1998) Mental health promotion. *The International Journal of Mental Health Promotion* 1: 1–4.

Patel V and Kleinman A (2003) Poverty and common mental disorders in developing countries. *Bulletin of the World Health Organization* 81: 609–615.

Patel V, Rahman A, Jacob KS, and Hughes M (2004) Effect of maternal mental health on infant growth in low income countries: New evidence from South Asia. *British Medical Journal* 328(7443): 820–823.

Patel V, Swartz L, and Cohen A (2005) The evidence for mental health promotion in developing countries. In: Herrman H, Saxena S and Moodie R (eds.) *Promoting Mental Health: Concepts, Emerging Evidence, Practice*, pp. 189–202. Geneva, Switzerland: World Health Organization.

Petticrew M, Chisholm D, Thomson H, and Jane-Llopis E (2005) Evidence: The way forward. In: Herrman H, Saxena S and Moodie R (eds.) *Promoting Mental Health: Concepts, Emerging Evidence, Practice*, pp. 203–214. Geneva, Switzerland: World Health Organization.

Putnam R (1995) Bowling alone: America's declining social capital. *Journal of Democracy* 6(1): 65–78.

Rowling L and Taylor A (2005) Intersectoral approaches to promoting mental health. In: Herrman H, Saxena S and Moodie R (eds.) *Promoting Mental Health: Concepts, Emerging Evidence, Practice*, pp. 264–283. Geneva, Switzerland: World Health Organization.

Sartorius N (2003) Social capital and mental health. *Current Opinion in Psychiatry* 16(supplement 2): S101–S105.

Sartorius N and Henderson S (1992) The neglect of prevention in psychiatry. *Australian and New Zealand Journal of Psychiatry* 26: 550–553.

Shaw C and McKay H (1942) *Juvenile Delinquency and Urban Areas*. Chicago, IL: University of Chicago Press.

Sturgeon S and Orley J (2005) Concepts of mental health across the world. In: Herrman H, Saxena S and Moodie R (eds.) *Promoting Mental Health: Concepts, Emerging Evidence, Practice*, pp. 59–70. Geneva, Switzerland: World Health Organization.

Walker L, Verins I, Moodie R, and Webster K (2005) Responding to the social and economic determinants of mental health: a conceptual framework for action. In: Herrman H, Saxena S and Moodie R (eds.) *Promoting Mental Health: Concepts, Emerging Evidence, Practice*, pp. 89–108. Geneva, Switzerland: World Health Organization.

Zubrick SR and Kovess-Masfety V (2005) Indicators of mental health. In: Herrman H, Saxena S and Moodie R (eds.) *Promoting Mental Health: Concepts, Emerging Evidence, Practice*, pp. 148–169. Geneva, Switzerland: World Health Organization.

Further Reading

Albee GW and Gullotta TP (1997) *Primary Prevention Works*. Thousand Oaks: Sage Publications.

Desjarlais R, Eisenberg L, Good B, and Kleinman A (1995) *World Mental Health: Problems and Priorities in Low-Income Countries*. New York: Oxford University Press.

Herrman H, Saxena S and Moodie R (eds.) (2005) *Promoting Mental Health: Concepts, Emerging Evidence, Practice. A Report from the World Health Organization Department of Mental Health and Substance Abuse in Collaboration with the Victorian Health Promotion Foundation (VicHealth) and The University of Melbourne*. Geneva, Switzerland: World Health Organization.

Hosman C (2001) Evidence of effectiveness in mental health promotion. In: Lavikainen J, Lahtinen E and Lehtinen V (eds.) *Proceedings of the European Conference on Promotion of Mental Health and Social Inclusion*. Ministry of Social Affairs and Health (Report 3). Helsinki, Finland: Edita.

Institute of Medicine (2001) *Health and Behavior: The Interplay of Biological, Behavioral, and Societal Influences*. Washington, DC: National Academies Press.

IUHPE (2000) The Evidence of Health Promotion Effectiveness: Shaping Public Health in a New Europe, 2nd edn. Brussels, Belgium: International Union for Health Promotion and Education.

Jane-Llopis E and Mittelmark M (eds.) (2005) *What Works in Mental Health Promotion. Special Issue. Promotion and Education*. 42(supplement 2): 9–45.

Jenkins R and Ustun TB (eds.) (1998) *Preventing Mental Illness: Mental Health Promotion in Primary Care*, pp. 141–153. Chichester, UK: John Wiley.

Keys CL and Haidt J (eds.) (2003) *Flourishing: Positive Psychology and the Life Well-Lived*. Washington, DC: American Psychological Association.

Lahtinen E, Lehtinen V, Riikonen E and Ahonen J (eds.) (1999) *Framework for Promoting Mental Health in Europe*. Helsinki, Finland: National Research and Development Centre for Welfare and Health (STAKES).

Rose G (1992) *The Strategy of Preventive Medicine*. Oxford, UK: Oxford University Press.

Sartorius N (1998) Universal strategies for the prevention of mental illness and the promotion of mental health. In: Jenkins R and Ustun TB (eds.) *Preventing Mental Illness: Mental Health Promotion in Primary Care*, pp. 61–67. Chichester, UK: John Wiley.

Tudor K (1996) *Mental Health Promotion: Paradigms and Practice*. London: Routledge.

VicHealth (2006) *Mental Health Promotion Framework 2005–2007*. www.vichealth.vic.gov.au (accessed October 2007).

World Health Organization (2001) *Mental Health: New Understanding, New Hope. The World Health Report*. Geneva, Switzerland: World Health Organization.

World Health Organization (2004) *Evidence for Prevention of Mental Disorders: Effective Interventionsand Policy Options*. Summary Report. Geneva, Switzerland: World Health Organization.

Relevant Websites

http://www.cartercenter.org – The Carter Center.
http://www.cliffordbeersfoundation.co.uk/ – The Clifford Beers Foundation.
http://www.internethealthlibrary.com/Professional-Associations/ healtheducationauthority.htm – The Health Education Authority.
http://www.humanitarianinfo.org/iasc – Inter-Agency Standing Committee.
http://www.med.uio.no/iasp – International Association for Suicide Prevention.
http://www.iuhpe.org – International Union of Health Promotion and Education (IHPE).
http://www.mentality.org.uk – Mentality.
http://www.stakes.fi/english/#text – National Research and Education Centre for Welfare and Health (STAKES), Finland.
http://www.sdcmh.org.uk – Scottish Development Centre for Mental Health.
http://www.vichealth.gov.au – Victorian Health Promotion Foundation (VicHealth).
http://www.wfmh.org/ – World Federation for Mental Health.
http://www.who.int/en – World Health Organization.

Mental Health Resources and Services

S Saxena, World Health Organization, Geneva, Switzerland
P Sharan, All India Institute of Medical Sciences, New Delhi, India

Introduction

Although substantial information is available on the burden that mental and behavioral disorders place on society, until recently, very little was known about the resources available in different countries to alleviate these problems. Most of the available information on mental health resources was related to a few high-income countries. Furthermore, because available studies had used different units of measurement, the information that was accessible was not comparable across different countries or over time. In 2000, the World Health Organization launched Project Atlas to address this gap. The objectives of this project include the collection, compilation, and dissemination of relevant information about mental health resources in different countries.

Burden of Mental Disorders

According to World Health Report for 2001, approximately 450 million people alive today have mental or neurological disorders or suffer from psychosocial problems, such as those related to alcohol and drug abuse. It is estimated that neuropsychiatric disorders account for 14% of the global burden of disease (WHO, 2004a; Prince et al., 2007). Currently, major depression ranks fourth in the ten leading causes of the global burden of diseases. If projections are correct, within the next 20 years, it will become the second leading cause of global disease burden. While neuropsychiatric disorders account for 27.2% of disability-adjusted life years (DALYs) lost in high-income countries (World Bank, 2004) in comparison to 8.6% in low-income countries (WHO, 2004b), in terms of actual caseload, three-fourths of those affected by neuropsychiatric disorders live in developing countries.

It is now obvious that the social and economic burden of mental illness is enormous. In addition, mental illnesses impose the burden of human suffering and stigma, discrimination and humiliation on the affected people and their families.

Public Health Approach to Mental Health

The importance of mental health has been recognized by WHO since its origin and is reflected by the definition of health in the WHO Constitution as "not merely the absence of disease or infirmity," but rather "a state of complete physical, mental and social well-being" (United Nations, 2006: 186). Mental health is as important as physical health to the overall well-being of individuals, societies, and countries. Yet only a small minority of people suffering from a mental or behavioral disorder are receiving treatment. The World Mental Health Surveys (Demyttenaere et al., 2004) in 14 countries in the Americas, Europe, the Middle East, Africa, and Asia that covered six less developed and eight developed countries showed that even for serious disorders that were associated with substantial role disability, almost two-fifths of cases in developed countries and four-fifths in less developed countries received no treatment in the 12 months before the interview.

Advances in neuroscience and behavioral medicine have shown that, like many physical illnesses, mental and behavioral disorders are the result of a complex interaction between biological, psychological, and social factors. While there is still much to be learned, we already have the knowledge and power to reduce the burden of mental and behavioral disorders worldwide. Effective psychiatric care provision, indeed, is not a matter of sophisticated technologies, but rather a matter of equitable and rational organization of human resources. The World Mental Health Survey (Demyttenaere et al., 2004) showed that due to the high prevalence of mild and subthreshold cases, the number of those who received treatment for mild disorders far exceeded the number of untreated serious cases in every country. It suggested that reallocation of treatment resources could substantially decrease the problem of unmet need for treatment. As the ultimate stewards of any health system, governments must take the responsibility for ensuring that appropriate mental health policies are developed and implemented.

Mental Health at the International Level

Some of the important statements of international bodies like the United Nations including its specialized agency – the World Health Organization, the World Psychiatric Association, and the World Federation for Mental Health are detailed in the following paragraphs.

The United Nations resolution on the right of everyone to the enjoyment of the highest attainable standard of physical and mental health adopted in 2003 states that the enjoyment of the highest attainable standard of physical and mental health is a human right, and that such right derives from the inherent dignity of the human person.

The United Nations mental health principles for protection of persons with mental illness and the improvement of mental health care addresses issues such as the right to consent to treatment, protection of minors, standards of care, resources for mental health facilities, etc.

The United Nations standard rules on equalization of opportunities for persons with disability is an ambitious set of practical principles aimed at the equal exercise of rights by individuals with disabilities, of which a portion of individuals with mental disorders constitute a subgroup. It covers preconditions for equal participation (awareness raising, medical care, rehabilitation, and support services), target areas (e.g., accessibility, employment, family life and personal integrity, culture, religion, etc.), and guidelines on how the standard rules can be implemented and monitored. The rules have been strengthened by the United Nations Convention on the Rights of Persons with Disabilities (UN, 2006). The convention does not establish any new rights but rather emphasizes and consolidates the existing rights and freedoms of persons with disabilities and the international commitments of States. It defines disability as an element of human diversity and praises the contributions of persons with disabilities to society. It prohibits obstacles to the participation and promotes the active inclusion of persons with disabilities in society. The long-term goal of this Convention is to change the way the public perceives persons with disabilities, thus ultimately changing society as a whole.

The World Health Organization recognizes that mental health problems are of major importance to all societies and to all age groups and are significant contributors to the burden of disease and loss of quality of life. It is working toward a greater understanding of the mental health issues among policy makers and other partners to facilitate effective development of policies and programs to strengthen and protect mental health (WHO, 2002).

The World Psychiatric Association's ethical guidelines on psychiatric practice (Hawaii Declaration in 1977, its amendment in Vienna in 1983, and the Madrid Declaration of 1996) prohibit abuse and treatment against a patient's will unless such treatment is necessary for the welfare and safety of the patient and others. It emphasizes information and advice to the patient or caregiver on details of management, confidentiality, and the ethics of research.

The World Federation for Mental Health Declaration of Human Rights and Mental Health, first adopted in 1989, mentions that the diagnosis of mental illness by a mental health practitioner should be in accordance with accepted medical, psychological, scientific, and ethical standards. It states that the fundamental rights of mentally or emotionally ill or distressed persons shall be the same as those of all other citizens (e.g., right to coercion-free, dignified, humane, and qualified treatment; right to privacy and confidentiality; right to protection from physical or psychological abuse; right to adequate information about clinical status, etc.). The Declaration also mentions that all mentally ill persons have the right to be treated under the same professional and ethical standards as other ill persons.

Current State of Mental Health Resources in the World

Project Atlas was launched by WHO in 2000 in an attempt to map mental health resources in the world (Saxena *et al.*, 2002). The analyses of the global and regional data collected in 2001 were compiled and presented in the publication *Atlas: Mental Health Resources in the World* (WHO, 2001b), and individual country profiles and some further analyses were presented in *Atlas: Country Profiles of Mental Health Resources in the World, 2001* (WHO, 2001a). Atlas 2005 was a part of the second set of publications from the project and it presented country profiles and detailed analyses of global and regional data (WHO, 2005; Saxena *et al.*, 2006).

Information for this project was obtained from the focal points for mental health in the Ministries of Health in each WHO Member State, Associate Member, and Area through WHO Regional Offices (Saraceno and Saxena, 2002). Also, for Atlas 2005, comprehensive literature searches on epidemiological data pertaining to mental health and mental health services and resources (focusing on low- and middle-income countries) were conducted. Information was also obtained from documents received from countries, travel reports submitted by WHO staff, feedback from experts and member associations of the World Psychiatric Association, and data available with WHO regional offices (WHO, 2005; Saxena *et al.*, 2006).

Any comparison of data collected in the years 2001 (Atlas 2001) and 2004 (Atlas 2005) would benefit from the understanding that some of the changes involve relatively few countries reporting changes in status, and that this may reflect reporting error or unreliability rather than genuine trends. It should also be remembered that the denominator for the two data sets (years 2001 and 2004) is often different because many countries responded to questions in 2004 that they had been unable to answer previously.

National Policies and Legislation on Mental Health

Governments, as the ultimate stewards of mental health, have to assume the responsibility for the complex activities required to improve mental health services and care. Mental health policy, programs, and legislation are necessary steps for significant and sustained action.

Mental Health Policy

Mental health policy is a specifically written document of the government or Ministry of Health containing the goals for improving the mental health situation of the country, the priorities among those goals, and the main directions for attaining them. It may include the following components: Advocacy for mental health goals, promotion of mental well-being, prevention of mental disorders, treatment of mental disorders, and rehabilitation to help mentally ill individuals achieve optimum social and psychological functioning.

Only 62.1% of countries, accounting for 68.3% of the world population, have a mental health policy. In the African Region, approximately half of the countries do not have a mental health policy. A mental health policy is present in 51%, 70%, 68%, and 70% of countries of the low-income, lower-middle-income, upper-middle-income, and high-income countries, respectively. Mental health policies of most countries that have them cover most of the broad domains such as treatment (98.1%), prevention (95.3%), rehabilitation (93.4%), promotion (91.4%), and advocacy (80.4%). Policies in some countries also addressed other components such as intersectoral collaboration, social assistance, human resource development, and improvement of facilities for the underserved (e.g., Maoris in New Zealand).

Many developed countries such as the Scandinavian countries, the United Kingdom, Australia, and New Zealand have comprehensive national mental health policies. Some countries without a national mental health policy may still have good mental health services, e.g., some European countries do not have a stated policy but have well-developed action plans, and others such as the United States have a policy at the state or provincial level rather than the national level. On the other hand, it is possible that a country with a mental health policy may not have implemented its policy completely (**Table 1**).

National Mental Health Program

A national mental health program is a national plan of action that includes the broad and specific lines of action required to give effect to the policy. It helps to prioritize mental health issues in a country, sets time frames, and provides for budgetary support. Most countries with national mental health programs have emphasized deinstitutionalization, community-based care, and intersectoral collaboration. At times these programs also lend support to other specific populations (e.g., children and adolescents, the elderly, refugees, indigenous people); specific conditions (e.g., depression, suicide, HIV-related mental disorders) or specific issues such as domestic violence.

Seventy percent of countries, accounting for 91% of the world population, have a national mental health program. In the European Region, only 52.9% of countries have a program. In keeping with this, only 59.1% of high-income countries have specified their national mental health programs. On one hand, the low figures can be explained by the fact that many of these countries have laid down plans in various sectors of mental health (rather than a unified plan) or have plans at the state or provincial

Table 1   National policies and legislation on mental health and substance misuse

WHO regions	Mental health policy (n = 190) (%)	Mental health program (n = 191) (%)	Mental health legislation (n = 173) (%)	Disability benefits (n = 189) (%)	Therapeutic drug policy (n = 187) (%)
WHO regions					
Africa	50.0	76.1	79.5	45.5	93.5
Americas	72.7	76.5	75.0	90.9	90.9
Eastern Mediterranean	72.7	90.9	57.1	85.7	95.2
Europe	70.6	52.9	91.8	100	81.6
South-East Asia	54.5	72.7	63.6	81.8	100
Western Pacific	48.1	63.0	76.0	65.4	85.2
World	62.1	69.6	78.0	77.8	89.3
Income group of countries[a]					
Low	50.8	70.5	74	55.2	93.4
Lower middle	69.1	72.2	69.2	87	98.2
Upper middle	65.7	77.8	81.3	80	93.9
High	70.5	59.1	92.7	100	61.9

[a]Four of the responding countries classified according to WHO Regions could not be classified according to the World Bank income categories. From World Bank (2004) http://www.worldbank.org (accessed January 2008). Washington, DC: World Bank Group.

level (rather than at a national level); on the other hand, they point to the relative neglect of mental health in otherwise well-resourced countries. It is essential to revise programs as needs and management issues change over time. Nearly 11% of the programs date from before 1980 and it is unlikely therefore that deinstitutionalization and use of the newer psychotropic drugs would figure prominently in them.

Countries such as Norway and the Netherlands have well-defined programs. Importantly, some countries with limited resources such as Chile, Egypt, Jordan, India, Mexico, and the Philippines also have established programs. In the African Region, Niger has recently developed a program, Ghana updated its program in 2000, and Zambia is in the process of developing one.

Mental Health Legislation

Mental health legislation provides for the protection of the basic human and civil rights of people with mental disorders and deals with treatment facilities, personnel, professional training, and service structure. Some countries such as Cuba, Hungary, Iceland, and Spain include mental health legislation within their laws on general health.

Seventy-eight percent of countries, accounting for 69.1% of the world population, have specific mental health legislation. In the Eastern Mediterranean Region, only 57.1% of countries have laws in the field of mental health, compared with 97.8% of countries in the European Region. There is a large disparity between countries in different income groups, with 93% of high-income countries having specific mental health legislation, and 69% and 74% of lower-middle-income and low-income countries having such legislation.

Earlier legislation tried to isolate dangerous mentally disordered patients from the community, but more recently the focus has shifted toward ensuring consistency with international human rights obligations. This suggests that legislation needs to be updated and revised on a regular basis to make it comprehensive and in line with international norms. Scotland provides an example of a process where consumers, service providers, and policy makers were actively involved in revising legislation. Many other countries such as Jordan, Niger, Uganda, the UK, Zambia, etc., are also in the process of revising existing legislation. On the other hand, almost one-sixth of countries have mental health legislation that dates from before 1960, when the majority of the current effective methods for treating mental disorders were not available and focus on human rights was deficient.

Policy on Disability Benefits

Disability benefits are benefits that accrue to persons with illnesses that reduce their capacity to function as a legal right (from public funds). While disability benefits for physical illnesses exist in most countries, disability benefits for mental illnesses do not. Even when they do, they are often inadequate, difficult to obtain, and those affected are often unaware that they exist.

Some disability benefit is provided in 77.8% of countries that account for 93% of the world's population. While provisions for disability benefits exist in only 45.5% and 65.4% of countries in the African and South-East Asian Regions, respectively, such provisions have been made in all countries in the European Region. Categorization of countries by World Bank (2004) income groups revealed that only 55.2% of countries in the low-income group provide disability benefits for mental illness, compared with nearly five-sixths of countries in middle-income groups and all countries in the high-income group.

Countries such as Austria, France, Germany, Spain, the UK, the United States, have well-developed (and rigorously implemented) legislation on disability benefits. In many countries, provision of disability benefit is limited to small one-time monetary help, paid leave for a specified duration, or early retirement with a pension. Also, the disbursement of disability benefits is often restricted to specific groups (e.g., those with severe chronic mental disorders, employed personnel) or by procedural difficulties (lack of uniform assessment procedures).

Policy on Therapeutic Drugs

A therapeutic drug policy is a document endorsed by the Ministry of Health or the government to ensure accessibility and availability of essential therapeutic drugs. The essential list of drugs is usually adapted from the WHO Model List of Essential Drugs. The therapeutic drug policy often specifies the number and types of drugs to be made available to health workers at each level of the health service according to the functions of the workers and the conditions they are required to treat. A country may specify an essential list of drugs even in the absence of a therapeutic drug policy.

Almost 90% of countries report the existence of a therapeutic drug policy or essential list of drugs. More than four-fifths of countries in all WHO regions, including all countries in the South-East Asia Region, have a therapeutic drug policy/essential list of drugs. While, more than 90% of low- and middle-income countries have a therapeutic drug policy/essential list of drugs, only 61% of high-income countries have them. This is probably related to the fact that therapeutic medications are governed by independent/other (nonfederal) agencies in these countries; nonetheless, it could lead to inequities in the provision of therapeutic medication to their populations. Two-thirds of the policies or essential lists of drugs were formulated after 1990. Antidepressants such as serotonin-specific reuptake inhibitors (SSRIs) and atypical antipsychotics are also included in the list of essential drugs in some countries.

Overall, there was a slight increase in number of countries with mental health policy, mental health legislation, and therapeutic drug policy/essential drug list between the two rounds of data collection (2001 and 2004). The trend for legislation was more pronounced in the African (8.4%) and American (7.1%) regions. More countries were providing disability benefits; the change in this regard was most marked in the Eastern Mediterranean Region (10.7%) and the lower middle-income (9.5%) countries.

Budgetary Issues

A specified budget for mental health denotes the regular allocation within a country's budget for actions directed at achievement of mental health objectives, e.g., implementation of mental health policies or programs or the establishment of psychiatric care facilities. Many countries do not make a specific allocation for mental health in their national budgets, but make such allocations at the provincial or state level. In other countries, where mental health is a part of the primary health-care system, it is difficult to ascertain the specific budget for mental health care.

In spite of the importance of a separate mental health budget within the total health budget, 30.8% of countries reported not having a specified budget for mental health care. In the Regions of Africa and the Western Pacific, such a budget is present in 62.2% and 59.3% of countries, respectively. On the other hand, 78.1% of countries in the American Region have a specified budget for mental health care.

One hundred and one countries provided information on the actual budget for mental health. One-fifth of these countries, covering a population of more than 1 billion, spend less than 1% of the total health budget on mental health. In the Regions of Africa and South-East Asia, 70.0% and 50.0% of countries, respectively, spend less than 1% of their health budget on mental health care. In contrast, more than 61.5% of countries in the European Region spend more than 5% of their health budget on mental health care. Categorization of countries according to World Bank (2004) income groups showed that 29.2% of low-income countries versus 0.7% of high-income countries spend less than 1% of their budget on mental health care.

Examination of the percentage of the mental health budget out of the total health budget versus the gross domestic product (GDP) for countries shows that countries that have higher GDP tend to earmark higher percentages of their total health budget for mental health.

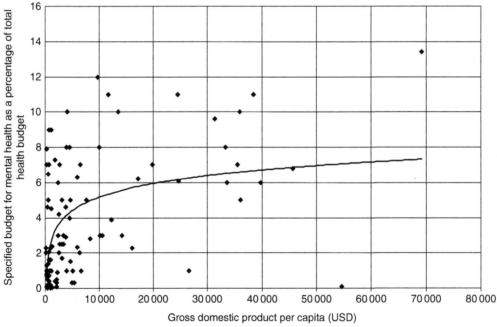

Figure 1 Specified mental health budget as a proportion of total health budget by GDP per capita ($n = 101$). Logarithmic trendline: $y = 1.1041\ln(x) - 4.9884$, $R2 = 0.2507$. Saxena S, Sharan P, Garrido Cumbrera M, and Saraceno B (2006) World Health Organization's Mental Health Atlas – 2005: Implications for policy development. *World Psychiatry* 5: 179–184.

Table 2   Budget and financing for mental health care

WHO regions	Specified budget for mental health (n = 185) (%)	Most common method of financing mental health care countries (n = 180) (%)				
		Out-of-pocket payment	Tax-based	Social insurance	Private insurance	External grants
WHO regions						
Africa	62.2	38.6	54.5	0	4.5	2.3
Americas	78.1	12.9	74.2	6.5	3.2	3.2
Eastern Mediterranean	71.4	15.8	68.4	5.3	0	10.5
Europe	70.0	0	55.1	44.9	0	0
South-East Asia	90.0	30.0	70.0	0	0	0
Western Pacific	59.3	18.5	70.4	3.7	0	7.4
World	69.2	17.8	62.8	14.4	1.7	3.3
Income group of countries[a]						
Low	70.2	42.9	50.0	0	3.6	3.6
Lower middle	63.6	16.0	72.0	8.0	0	4.0
Upper middle	77.1	0	63.6	30.3	0	6.1
High	74.4	0	64.9	32.4	2.7	0

[a]Four of the responding countries classified according to WHO Regions could not be classified according to the World Bank income categories. From World Bank (2004) http://www.worldbank.org (accessed January 2008). Washington, DC: World Bank Group.

A logarithmic trend line (**Figure 1**) confirms this relationship. This illustrates the double disadvantage suffered by mental health in low-income countries; they have, even proportionally, a lower mental health budget. It is obvious that mental health is one of the most neglected areas of health in poor countries. Even considering the limitations of the current data, it is obvious that countries spending less than 1% of their total health budget on mental health care need to substantially increase it (**Table 2**).

Methods of Financing

Since mental health financing is a relatively new area of investigation, most countries do not have the information required to provide accurate data on this index. The ratings provided are at best approximations, because this project only sought information ranked by order of importance of each source of financing.

The dominant methods of financing mental health in countries are out-of-pocket payment (17.8%), tax-based funding (62.8%), social insurance (everyone above a certain income level is required to contribute a fixed percentage of their income to a government-administered health insurance fund, which pays for part or all of the consumer's mental health services; 14.4%), private insurance (1.7%), and external grants to countries by other countries or international organizations (3.3%). Across all WHO Regions, tax-based financing is the dominant method of financing mental health care in one-half to three-quarters of countries. Out-of-pocket payment is the dominant method of financing in 38.6%

and 30% of countries in the African and South-East Asia Regions, respectively. In the European Region, social insurance is the primary method of financing in 44.9% of countries.

Categorization of countries according to World Bank (2004) income groups showed that tax-based care is the primary method of financing mental health in countries of all income groups. Out-of-pocket payment is the primary method of financing in 42.9% of low-income countries, while social insurance is the primary method of financing in 32.4% and 30.3% of high-income and upper-middle-income countries, respectively.

Out-of-pocket payment is unsatisfactory because severe mental disorders can lead to heavy financial expenditure. Mental health care should preferably be financed through taxes or social insurance, as private health insurance is also inequitable because it favors the more affluent sections of society and is often more restrictive in the coverage of mental illness than in the coverage of somatic illness.

A comparison of data between 2001 and 2004 showed that 23.3% more countries in South-East Asia Region reported that they had a specific budget for mental health. There was a decrease in emphasis on out-of-pocket payment (5.4% and 10.8%, respectively) and an increase in emphasis on tax-based systems (7.5% and 7.8%, respectively) in the American and Eastern Mediterranean Regions, while in the Western Pacific Region there was an increase in emphasis on out-of-pocket payment (11.2%) and social insurance (5.7%). In terms of income groups of countries, a decrease in emphasis on social insurance (8.9%) and an increase in emphasis on private insurance (8.0%) were observed in lower-middle-income countries; and a decrease in emphasis on social insurance (8.3%) occurred in high-income countries.

Resources for Mental Health Services

Mental Health Beds

The term psychiatric bed denotes a bed maintained for continuous use by patients with mental disorders. These beds are located in public and private psychiatric hospitals, general hospitals, hospitals for special groups of the population such as the elderly and children, military hospitals, long-term rehabilitation centers, etc. Though inpatient facilities are essential for managing patients with acute mental disorders, efforts should be made to reduce beds in stand-alone psychiatric hospitals and increase beds in general hospitals and long-term community rehabilitation centers. Some regions within countries such as Italy have completely eliminated asylum-like psychiatric hospitals.

The median number of psychiatric beds in the world per 10 000 population is 1.69 (mean, 4.36; standard deviation, 5.47). The median figure per 10 000 population varies from 0.33 in the South-East Asia Region and 0.34 in African Region to 8.00 in the European Region. The median figure per 10 000 population in low-income countries is 0.68 in comparison to 8.94 in high-income countries.

More than two-thirds of psychiatric beds in the world are located in mental hospitals, while only about one-fifth are found in general hospitals. More than four-fifths of beds in the Eastern Mediterranean, South-East Asia, and American Regions are in mental hospitals. The Western Pacific Region has the highest proportion of psychiatric beds in general hospitals (34.5%). On the other hand, only about 10% of beds in South-East Asia, American, and Eastern Mediterranean regions are in the general hospital setting. More than three-fourths of beds in low- and middle-income countries and approximately 55% of beds in high-income countries are located in mental hospitals.

In 40.5% of countries, covering 44.7% of the population, there is less than one psychiatric bed per 10 000 population. In the South-East Asia and African Regions, 94.9% and 82.9% of the population, respectively, has access to less than one bed per 10 000 population. On the other hand, in the European Region only 25.7% of the population has access to less than five psychiatric beds per 10 000 population. Nearly five-sixths of low-income countries, covering 96% of the world population, have less than one psychiatric bed per 10 000 population. In high-income countries, only roughly 10% of the population has access to fewer than five psychiatric beds per 10 000 population.

A comparison of data between 2001 and 2004 showed that there was a decrease in the median number of beds in regions that had high bed-to-population ratios, i.e.,

American (a decrease of 0.9 per 10 000 population) and European (a decrease of 0.7 per 10 000 population) Regions, and an increase in regions with intermediate bed-to-population ratio, i.e., in the Eastern Mediterranean (an increase of 0.24 per 10 000 population) and Western Pacific (an increase of 0.08 per 10 000 population) Regions. No change was observed in regions with low bed-to-population ratio, i.e., in the African and South-East Asian Regions. A decrease in number of beds was noted in high-income countries (a decrease of 1.20 per 10 000 population), an increase in middle-income countries, particularly upper-middle-income countries (an increase of 2.30 per 10 000 population), and no change was observed for low-income countries. There was a decrease in proportion of mental hospital beds (denominator: all psychiatric beds) in the African (5%), European (7%), and Western Pacific (9.2%) Regions and low-income countries (11.7%). A general trend toward an increase (3.9%) in the proportion of general hospital beds to total beds was observed; this was relatively marked for the African (8.6%), European (11.7%), and Western Pacific (11.8%) Regions (**Table 3**).

Human Resources

Inputs from mental health professionals are required in patient care, policy advice, administration, and for training other personnel.

The median number of mental health professionals per 100 000 population in the world is quite low (psychiatrists, 1.2; psychiatric nurses, 2; psychologists working in mental health, 0.6; social workers in mental health, 0.4), even though some countries may have overreported the number of psychiatric nurses, psychologists, and social workers in mental health fields (by mistakenly including general nurses working in the mental health field, and psychologists and social workers employed in general health and related sectors such as education).

Psychiatrists

The term psychiatrist denotes a medical doctor who has had at least 2 years of postgraduate training in psychiatry at a recognized teaching institution. The median number of psychiatrists per 100 000 population varies from 0.04 in the African Region to 9.80 in the European Region. In actual numbers, this amounts to approximately 1800 psychiatrists for 702 million people in the African Region compared to more than 89 000 psychiatrists for 879 million people in the European Region. The median figure for low-income countries is 0.05 per 100 000 population and that for high-income countries is 10.5 per 100 000 population.

In 47.6% of countries, covering 46.5% of the world's population, there is less than one psychiatrist per 100 000 population. All countries in the South-East Asia Region and 89.1% of countries in the African Region have fewer than one psychiatrist per 100 000 population.

Table 3   Distribution of psychiatric beds per 10 000 population

	Psychiatric beds per 10 000 population in each category of countries (n = 185) (%)			
	0–1	1.01–5	5.01–10	>10
WHO regions				
Africa	78.3	17.4	4.3	–
Americas	29.0	29.0	16.1	25.8
Eastern Mediterranean	50.0	40.9	9.1	–
Europe	–	25.5	49.0	25.5
South-East Asia	75.0	25.0	–	–
Western Pacific	48.1	37.0	7.4	7.4
World	40.5	27.6	19.5	12.4
Income group of countries[a]				
Low	84.5	12.1	3.4	–
Lower middle	34.6	44.2	19.2	1.9
Upper middle	12.1	27.3	30.3	30.3
High	2.6	28.9	36.8	31.6

[a]Four of the responding countries classified according to WHO Regions could not be classified according to the World Bank income categories. From World Bank (2004) http://www.worldbank.org (accessed January 2008). Washington, DC: World Bank Group.

Five-sixths (87.9%) of low-income countries have fewer than one psychiatrist per 100 000 population. Even when available, most psychiatrists are based in large cities and large populations living in rural areas have no access to them (**Table 4**).

Psychiatric nurses

The term psychiatric nurse denotes a graduate of a recognized, university-level nursing school with a specialization in mental health. Psychiatric nurses are registered with the local nursing board (or equivalent) and work in a mental health-care setting. The median number of psychiatric nurses per 100 000 population varies from 0.1 in the South-East Asia Region to 24.8 in the European Region; and 0.16 in low-income countries to 32.95 in high-income countries. More than three-fourths of countries in the South-East Asia Region and in low-income countries have access to fewer than one psychiatric nurse per 100 000 population. In many developed and in some developing countries such as Botswana, Fiji, Ghana, Jamaica, and Tanzania, community psychiatric nurses contribute significantly to mental health care.

Psychologists working in mental health

The term psychologist working in mental health denotes a graduate from a recognized, university-level school of psychology with a specialization in clinical psychology. These psychologists are registered with the local board of psychologists (or equivalent) and work in a mental health setting.

The median number of psychologists per 100 000 population varies from 0.03 in the South-East Asia and Western Pacific Region to 3.10 in the European Region, and from 0.04

in low-income countries to 14.0 in high-income countries. There is fewer than one psychologist per 100 000 population in 61.6% of countries, accounting for 66.0% of the world's population. Ninety percent or more of the population in South-East Asian and African Regions and of low-income countries have access to fewer than one psychologist per 100 000 population.

Social workers working in mental health

The term social worker working in mental health denotes a graduate from a recognized, university-level school of social work, registered with the local board of social workers (or equivalent) and working in a mental health setting.

The median number of social workers working in mental health per 100 000 population varies from 0.04 in the South-East Asian Region to 1.5 in the European Region, and from 0.04 in low-income countries to 15.7 in high-income countries. In 64% of countries, accounting for three-fourths of the world's population, there is fewer than one social worker per 100 000 population. In the African and Eastern Mediterranean Regions, more than 85% of the countries have access to fewer than one social worker per 100 000 population. Nearly 92.7% of low-income countries are served by fewer than one social worker per 100 000 population, while 38.7% of high-income countries are served by approximately ten social workers per 100 000 population.

A comparison of data between 2001 and 2004 showed that there was an increase in the number of mental health professionals in the world. The greatest increase was noted for psychologists engaged in mental health care (increase in median: 0.2 per 100 000 population, greater improvement occured in American and European

Table 4   Median number of mental health professionals per 100 000 population

	Psychiatrists (n = 187)	Psychiatric nurses (n = 176)	Psychologists (n = 177)	Social workers (n = 168)
WHO regions				
Africa	0.04	0.20	0.05	0.05
Americas	2.00	2.60	2.80	1.00
Eastern Mediterranean	0.95	1.25	0.60	0.40
Europe	9.80	24.8	3.10	1.50
South-East Asia	0.20	0.10	0.03	0.04
Western Pacific[b]	0.32	0.50	0.03	0.05
World	1.20	2.00	0.60	0.40
Income group of countries[a]				
Low	0.05	0.16	0.04	0.04
Lower middle	1.05	1.05	0.60	0.28
Upper middle	2.70	5.35	1.80	1.50
High	10.50	32.95	14.0	15.70

[a]Four of the responding countries classified according to WHO Regions could not be classified according to the World Bank income categories. From World Bank (2004) http://www.worldbank.org (accessed January 2008). Washington, DC: World Bank Group.
[b]The median numbers for the Western Pacific Region are 0 as a number of the smaller countries do not have these professionals.

Regions and upper middle-income group countries), and social workers engaged in mental health care (increase in median: 0.1 per 100 000 population, greater improvement occured in the European Region). When the median number of psychiatrists per 100 000 population was compared, it was seen that an increase had occurred in the European Regions (0.8) and in high-income countries (1.5). The South-East Asia Region showed a decrease in the number of psychiatrists (by approximately 40%) and psychiatric nurses (by roughly 60%). A decrease (roughly 20%) in the number of psychiatric nurses was reported in the Eastern Mediterranean Region. Availability of more accurate figures as well as the flight of professionals to more affluent countries could be reasons for this trend.

There was a decrease (5.1%) in the number of countries with fewer than one psychiatrist per 100 000 population. This trend was more pronounced in the African and American Regions and in middle-income countries. Also, there was a decrease (6.7%) in the number of countries with fewer than one psychologist per 100 000 population. This trend was supported by figures for the American, European, and Eastern Mediterranean Regions and in low-income and upper-middle-income countries. Similarly, fewer (9.7%) countries in the Eastern Mediterranean Region reported having fewer than one social worker per 100 000 population.

Primary and Community Care

Primary Care

Mental health in primary care can be defined as the provision of basic preventive and curative mental health at the first level of the health-care system. In many countries, a nonspecialist who can refer complex cases to a more specialized mental health professional provides such care. Most mental disorders can be managed effectively at the primary care level if adequate resources are made available. Shifting mental health care to primary level also helps to reduce stigma, improves early detection and treatment, leads to cost efficiency and savings, and partly offsets limitations of mental health resources through the use of community resources (WHO, 2001a).

Mental health facilities at the primary level are reported to be present in 87.3% of countries that cover 96.5% of the world's population. They are available in more than 77% of countries in the Eastern Mediterranean and Western Pacific Regions and in approximately 95% of countries in the Americas and European Region. Across income groups, they are present in 76.3% of low-income countries and 97.4% of high-income countries. However, in reality, the population coverage is lower, as primary care services are not evenly distributed.

Treatment facilities for severe mental disorders in primary care settings were reported to be available in only 61.5% of countries in the world, covering 52.8% of the population. Such facilities are available in only 44.4% of countries in the South-East Asia Region. Across countries of different income groups, such facilities are available in 55.2% of low-income countries, 44.4% of lower-middle-income countries, and 86.8% of high-income countries. Treatment facilities for severe mental disorders in primary care settings across different countries also vary greatly. Most countries provide only follow-up care to the severely mentally ill in primary health-care facilities.

Mental health-care facilities in primary care are an integral part of the system in countries such as Australia,

Table 5   Primary and community care for mental health

	Mental health in primary care (n = 189) (%)	Facilities for SMD[a] in primary care (n = 187) (%)	Training, primary care personnel (n = 186) (%)	Essential[b] psychotropics in primary care (n = 192) (%)	Community care for mental health (n = 185) (%)
WHO regions					
Africa	82.6	60.9	58.7	67.4	56.5
Americas	93.9	62.5	27.3	62.9	75.0
Eastern Mediterranean	81.8	63.6	81.8	50.0	68.2
Europe	96.1	68.6	68.8	62.7	79.2
South-East Asia	80.0	44.4	90.0	63.6	50.0
Western Pacific	77.8	51.9	55.6	81.5	66.7
World	87.3	61.5	59.7	65.1	68.1
Income group of countries[c]					
Low	76.3	55.2	60.3	52.5	51.7
Lower middle	87.0	44.4	61.1	68.5	51.9
Upper middle	100	72.7	55.9	81.3	90.9
High	97.4	86.8	66.7	83.3	97.4

[a]Severe mental disorder.
[b]Phenytoin, amitriptyline, and chlorpromazine.
[c]Four of the responding countries classified according to WHO Regions could not be classified according to the World Bank income categories.
From World Bank (2004) http://www.worldbank.org (accessed January 2008). Washington, DC: World Bank Group.

Austria, Italy, the Netherlands, the UK, and the United States. Integration of mental health into primary care has been found to be useful in countries such as Barbados, Cambodia, China, India, Iran, Jamaica, Nepal, and Zimbabwe (**Table 5**).

Training of primary care personnel

Training of primary care personnel involves the provision of essential knowledge and skills in identification, prevention, and care of mental disorders. Approximately 59% of countries have some training facilities for primary care personnel in the field of mental health. Whereas 90% of countries of the South-East Asia Region have such facilities, the same are available in only 41.9% of countries in the American Region. Many high-income countries of the European and American Regions provide regular training programs for doctors, nurses, and social workers working at primary care level. Some other countries such as Cambodia, Pakistan, Botswana, and Lesotho have also developed training facilities for primary care professionals.

Therapeutic psychotropic medication

Project Atlas sought information on the availability in primary care, the most common basic strength, and the cost of a specific list of drugs. Among antiepileptics, phenobarbital is available in 93% and phenytoin in 77% of

countries. Amitriptyline, an antidepressant, is available in 86.4% of countries. Among antipsychotics, chlorpromazine is available in 91.4% and haloperidol in 91.8% of countries. Lithium, a mood stabilizer, is available in 65.4% of countries. Carbamazepine and sodium valproate, which are antiepileptics with mood-stabilizing properties are available in 91.4% and 67.4% of countries, respectively. Anti-Parkinson drugs are available in fewer countries, with levodopa, carbidopa, and biperiden being available in only 61.9%, 51.1%, and 43.5% of countries, respectively. Almost two-thirds of countries report that they make the three essential drugs: Amitriptyline (an antidepressant), chlorpromazine (an antipsychotic), and phenytoin (an antiepileptic) available in primary care. However, in many countries these drugs are either not available at all primary care centers or are not available at all times.

Community Care

Community mental health care includes provision of crisis support, protected housing, and sheltered employment in addition to management of disorders to address the multiple needs of individuals. Community-based services can lead to early intervention and limit the stigma of treatment. They can improve functional outcomes and quality of life of individuals with chronic mental disorders, and are cost-effective and respectful of human rights.

Community care facilities exist in only 68.1% of countries, covering 83.3% of the world population.

In the African, Eastern Mediterranean, and South-East Asian Regions, such facilities are present in roughly half the countries. Across different income groups, community mental health facilities are present in 51.7% of the low-income and in 97.4% of the high-income countries. Countries such as Australia, Canada, Finland, Norway, the UK, and the United States, among others, have well-established community care facilities. Some Latin American countries have undertaken innovative services that provide useful demonstration experiences, for example in Argentina, Brazil, and Nicaragua. Other countries such as Barbados, Ghana, and Qatar have also developed some community care facilities. Services of traditional healers are being used as part of community care in many countries such as Cambodia, Guinea, Niger, Nigeria, and Senegal.

A comparison of 2001 and 2004 data showed that more countries (13.6%) in the Eastern Mediterranean Region had made treatment for severe mental disorders available in primary care. However, a 15.5% reduction was noted in the number of countries that made the three essential psychotropic drugs (amitriptyline, chlorpromazine, and phenytoin) available in primary care. This is mainly reflective of the fact that some countries, particularly in the European Region, added newer psychotropics to their essential list of drugs.

Monitoring Mental Health Systems

Monitoring is necessary to assess the effectiveness of mental health prevention and treatment programs and to identify its deficits. Indicators for monitoring should include data on clients of mental health services, quality of the services rendered, and general measures of the mental health of communities.

Mental Health Reporting Systems

Annual reporting systems cover health and health services functions and utilization of allocated funds. Annual mental health reporting systems exist in 75.7% of countries. They are reported to be present in 100% and 87.5% of countries, respectively, of South-East Asian and European Regions versus only 57.8% of countries in the African Region. Only 62.1% of low-income countries have an annual mental health reporting system compared with 86.1% of high-income countries. A comparison of data between 2001 and 2004 showed that a greater number of countries in the African (5.5%), American (8.1%), and South-East Asian (10%) Regions and the lower-middle-income group (9.3%) reported the presence of mental health reporting systems.

Programs for Special Populations

Programs for special populations are programs that address the mental health concerns (including social integration) of the most vulnerable and disorder-prone groups of the population. Programs for indigenous people are present in 14.8%, for minority groups in 16.5%, for refugees in 26.2%, for disaster-affected populations in 37.7%, for elderly persons in 50.5%, and for children in 62.4% of countries.

With 42.6% of its population made up of children (below 14 years), the African Region has programs for children in only 37% of countries, compared to 77.6% of countries in the European Region, where children account for 19.1% of the total population. Whereas 86.8% of high-income countries have a program for children, only 34.5% of low-income countries have one.

Programs for the elderly exist in 15.6% of countries in the African Region, in comparison to 77.4% of countries in the Region of the Americas. Such programs are present in 89.5% of high-income countries but in only 17.9% of low-income countries.

A comparison of data between 2001 and 2004 showed that there was an increase in services for children and the elderly in countries of the American (9.9% and 9.7%, respectively) and Western Pacific (7.7% and 11.5%, respectively) Regions. Similarly, services for children and the elderly increased in the lower-middle-income (13.3% and 5.6%, respectively) and upper-middle-income (7% and 9.6%, respectively) countries (**Table 6**).

Table 6   Distribution of mental health programs for children, adolescents, and the elderly

	Children and adolescents (n = 186) (%)	Elderly (n = 184) (%)
WHO regions		
Africa	37.0	15.6
Americas	81.3	77.4
Eastern Mediterranean	72.7	54.5
Europe	77.6	63.3
South-East Asia	54.5	54.5
Western Pacific	50.0	50.0
World	62.4	50.5
Income group of countries[a]		
Low	34.5	17.9
Lower middle	73.6	50.9
Upper middle	72.7	66.7
High	86.8	89.5

[a]Four of the responding countries classified according to WHO Regions could not be classified according to the World Bank income categories. From World Bank (2004) http://www.world bank.org (accessed January 2008). Washington, DC: World Bank Group.

Current Emphases in Psychiatric Care

Human Rights

The persisting question is how to balance the civil rights of mentally ill individuals against the limitations on their freedom required by society and contemporary healing techniques. Violation of human rights can be perpetrated both by neglecting patients through carelessness and by forcing them into restraining or even violent care systems. To prevent abuses, there is an urgent need to improve the quality of mental health care, to strengthen the management of institutions, and to closely monitor the rights of the mentally ill.

People with mental disorders are entitled to the enjoyment and protection of their fundamental human rights. The fundamental human rights obligations covered in the three instruments that make up what is known as the International Bill of Rights (the Universal Declaration of Human Rights, the International Covenant on Civil and Political Rights, and the International Covenant on Economic, Social, and Cultural Rights) include the protection against discrimination; the right to health including the right to access rehabilitation services; the right to dignity; the right to community integration; the right to reasonable accommodation; the right to liberty and security of person; and the need for affirmative action to protect the rights of persons with disabilities, which includes persons with mental disorders; and protection against torture, cruel, inhuman, or degrading treatment.

Deinstitutionalization and Care in the Community

Deinstitutionalization is a complex process in which reduction of beds in stand-alone mental hospitals is associated with implementation of a network of community alternatives that can avoid the institutionalization of individuals with mental illness. Neither closure of mental hospitals without provision of extramural alternatives (which can lead to homelessness and transinstitutionalization in prisons, nursing homes, etc.), nor creation of extramural alternatives without restriction on admission to mental hospitals (adding new services eventually recruits new patients but leaves the mental hospital unaffected) is optimal. In many European countries (e.g., Italy, Denmark, Finland, Spain, Sweden, and the United Kingdom) and the United States, a substantial shift from a hospital-based to a community-based system has already taken place.

The deinstitutionalization process has also begun in some Latin American countries, for example Brazil, based on the policy guidelines of the Caracas Declaration. The principles set forth in this declaration refer to the need to develop psychiatric care that is closely linked to primary care and within the framework of the local health system. Deinstitutionalization has also been started in countries such as Burkina Faso, Croatia, Czech Republic, Jamaica, Iran, and Lithuania.

Integration with General and Primary Health Care

Many patients with psychological problems seek treatment from general health services. Studies conducted by WHO in many countries have shown that between 10% and 20% of primary care patients meet diagnostic criteria for psychiatric conditions (Harding *et al.*, 1980). The WHO advocates that mental health care should be decentralized and integrated into primary health care, with the necessary tasks carried out as far as possible by general health workers rather than specialists in mental health. Equipping primary health-care workers to deal with mental health problems avoids wasted effort and cost. Importantly, the responsibility for mental health is not an extra burden for primary health-care services; on the contrary, it increases their effectiveness. Experiences in China, India, and African countries show that adequate training of primary health-care workers to early recognition and management of psychological disorders can reduce institutionalization and improve clients' mental health.

Consumer and Family Involvement

The involvement of consumers and family is closely related to community-based management. Communities, families, and consumers can be included in the development and decision making of policies, programs, and services. This should lead to services becoming better tailored to people's needs. Consumer and family associations have emerged as a major force in creating reciprocal social networks between mentally ill persons. Consumer and family movements have a long and important tradition in the United States and Europe, and recently similar movements have emerged in Latin America, Asia, and Western Pacific Regions. As a positive and promising example, in recent years, the Brazilian Ministry of Health gave impressive support to consumers and family organizations, which are now actively influencing the mental health policy, advocating for their rights and taking part in decision making in service organizations.

Conclusions and Future Directions

It is clear that mental disorders cause considerable burden on individuals, families, and societies and are of immense public health importance. Yet, they are underrecognized, undertreated, and underprioritized the world over, even though effective management options are available and psychiatric care provision does not require sophisticated technologies. In addition, the rights of mentally ill people (which includes the right to access to care) are often trampled upon.

Project Atlas, launched by WHO in 2000 in an attempt to map mental health resources in the world, has presented a worrisome picture. Global mental health resources continue to remain low and are grossly inadequate to respond to the high level of need. Regional imbalances and differences across income groups of countries persist. These data emphasize the urgent need to enhance resources devoted to mental health, especially in low- and middle-income countries. WHO has argued for a substantial enhancement in resources invested in mental health (WHO, 2003).

The ten recommendations of the *World Health Report 2001* (WHO, 2001c) remain as valid today as when they were made:

1. Provide treatment in primary care.
2. Make psychotropic drugs available.
3. Give care in the community.
4. Educate the public.
5. Involve communities, families, and consumers.
6. Establish national policies, programs, and legislation.
7. Develop human resources.
8. Link with other sectors.
9. Monitor community mental health.
10. Support more research.

These recommendations can be adapted by every country according to its needs and its resources.

Fortunately, the importance of mental health and rights issues is beginning to be recognized and international and national bodies have started advocating for effective, equitable, and rights-based mental health services. The world is also witnessing a welcome trend toward integration of mental health into primary health care, deinstitutionalization, community care, and involvement of communities, families, and consumers in the development of policies, programs, and services.

See also: Mental Health and Substance abuse; Mental Health Policy; Mental Health Promotion; Stigma of Mental illness; Women's Mental Health.

Citations

Demyttenaere K, Bruffaerts R, Posada-Villa J, *et al.* (2004) Prevalence, severity, and unmet need for treatment of mental disorders in the World Health Organization World Mental Health Surveys. *Journal of American Medical Association* 291: 2581–2590.

Harding TW, Arango MV, Baltzar J, *et al.* (1980) Mental disorders in primary health care: A study of their frequency and diagnosis in four developing countries. *Psychological Medicine* 10: 231–241.

Prince M, Patel V, Saxena S, *et al.* (2007) No health without mental health. *Lancet* 370: 859–877.

Saraceno B and Saxena S (2002) Mental health resources in the world: Results from Project Atlas of the WHO. *World Psychiatry* 1: 40–44.

Saxena S, Maulik PK, O'Connell K, and Saraceno B (2002) Mental health care in primary community settings: Result from WHO's Project Atlas. *International Journal of Social Psychiatry* 48: 83–85.

Saxena S, Sharan P, Garrido Cumbrera M, and Saraceno B (2006) World Health Organization's Mental Health Atlas – 2005: Implications for policy development. *World Psychiatry* 5: 179–184.

United Nations (2006) *Convention on the Rights of Persons with Disabilities*. http://www.un.org/esa/socdev/enable/documents/tccconve.pdf (accessed January 2008). New York: United Nations.

World Bank (2004) *The World Bank*. http://www.worldbank.org (accessed January 2008). Washington, DC: World Bank Group.

World Health Organization (2001a) *Atlas: Country Profiles on Mental Health Resources*. Geneva, Switzerland: World Health Organization.

World Health Organization (2001b) *Atlas: Mental Health Resources in the World 2001*. Geneva, Switzerland: World Health Organization.

World Health Organization (2001c) *The World Health Report 2001: Mental Health: New Understanding, New Hope*. Geneva, Switzerland: World Health Organization.

World Health Organization (2002) *Strengthening Mental Health*, EB109. R8. Geneva, Switzerland: World Health Organization.

World Health Organization (2003) *Investing in Mental Health*. Geneva, Switzerland: World Health Organization.

World Health Organization (2004a) *The World Health Report 2004: Changing History*. Geneva, Switzerland: World Health Organization.

World Health Organization (2004b) *Revised Global Burden of Disease (GBD) 2002 Estimates*. http://www.who.int/healthinfo/bodgbd2002revised/en/index.html (accessed January 2008).

World Health Organization (2005) *Mental Health Atlas 2005*. Geneva, Switzerland: World Health Organization.

Futher Reading

Department of Health Human Services (1999) *Mental Health: A Report of the Surgeon General*. Pittsburgh, PA: Department of Health and Human Services, United States Public Health Service.

Ustun TB and Sartorius N (eds.) (1995) *Mental Illness in General Health Care*. Chichester, UK: John Wiley and Sons.

World Health Organization (2005) *WHO Resource Book on Mental Health, Human Rights and Legislation*. Geneva, Switzerland: World Health Organization.

Relevant Website

http://www.who.int/globalatlas/default.asp – Mental Health Atlas.

Historical Views of Mental Illness

D Pilgrim, University of Central Lancashire, Preston, Lancashire, UK

Comprehensive histories of mental illness can be found in Shorter (1998), Stone (1997), and Hunter and MacAlpine (1963). This article draws from these and other specific sources but starts with some cautions about reading the past from the present.

Reading the Past from the Present: Three Main Starting Points

For the past 40 years psychiatric knowledge has been contentious. For this reason any historical reading of mental illness requires some declaration about a philosophical stance toward that body of knowledge. Broadly three starting points can be described.

'Medical naturalism' starts from the premise that current medical terminology describing mental abnormality is valid and has global and transhistorical applicability. Diagnoses such as 'schizophrenia' or 'depression' are taken to be labels for naturally occurring phenomena embodied in their sufferers. Here the object (mental illness) is assumed to precede the subject (those using the term). Mental illness is assumed to exist 'out there' and to be independent of its observers or diagnosticians. In other words the factual status of mental illness is deemed to be nonproblematic. The codifications used by mainstream psychiatry, and found in the two main current nosologies of the American Psychiatric Association's *Diagnostic and Statistical Manual* (DSM) and the World Health Organization's *International Classification of Diseases* (ICD), reflect medical naturalism.

'Radical constructivism' inverts the first position and assumes instead that subject precedes object. Here the emphasis is on how diagnoses are context-specific human products. They are deemed to be socially negotiated outcomes that reflect the cognitive preferences and vested interests of the negotiators (in this case in modern times the psychiatric profession being the most important, but not only, group). In this view mental illness does not exist as a natural free-standing entity but is a by-product of psychiatric activity. The oft-quoted campaign of the dissident psychiatrist Thomas Szasz to deem mental illness to be a myth reflects this position (Szasz, 1961), although he treats physical illness as nonproblematic, which is not the case with other constructivists.

'Critical realism' is a bridge between the two positions, in that reality is deemed to precede the subject but is represented by shifting subjective or intersubjective activity. The latter needs to be critically evaluated in order to identify interests operating (thus it supports the radical constructivist position to an extent). But critical realists concede the reality of some sort about mental abnormality (supporting to some extent the medical naturalists). Mental illness is not dismissed as being merely a by-product of professional activity but it is criticized for its poor conceptual validity. Critical realists emphasize that knowledge claims in human or social science are not the same as in natural science, as they are context specific to time and place (partly but not wholly agreeing with the constructivists).

Madness and Misery before Psychiatry

In line with this author's starting point of critical realism, it is reasonably safe to argue that from antiquity to the present, all societies have described people in their midst who are notably miserable or whose conduct is idiosyncratic and not readily intelligible to others. As Rosen (1968) notes, in antiquity madness was associated stereotypically with aimless wandering and violence. The modern English use of the term 'to be mad' reflects this conflation of lunacy and fury and the ancient stereotypes remain with us.

But once we get beyond these very broad generalizations and stereotypes, detailed accounts suggest that psychological deviance is described and judged in a very context-specific way. Moreover, cross-cultural comparisons tell us that cultures vary in the number of words used to describe internal states. For example, some cultures have no word for 'depression,' even though the latter medical term has now entered the vernacular in Anglophone societies (Pilgrim and Bentall, 1999).

Another difficulty in making clear transhistorical statements about mental illness relates to contested attributions about dysfunction. For example, ancient philosophers were ambivalent about the value of madness. Currently it is simply disvalued in medically codified dysfunctional states, such as 'schizophrenia' or 'bipolar disorder.' But Socrates considered that madness and sanity had equal value. For him, positive aspects of mad rapture included prophesying (a 'manic art'), mystical initiations and rituals, poetic inspiration, and the madness of lovers (Screech, 1985).

As Leuder and Thomas (2000) point out, an irony of Socrates being idealized as the epitome of rational thought as a founder of philosophy is that he freely admitted to experiencing what are now called 'command hallucinations' (then called his 'daemon'). Pythagoras, another founding father of philosophy, also heard voices. So, too, did Mohammed, Joan of Arc, and Luther.

And Jesus and the Buddha could both be accused of being deluded and of operating grandiose certainty about the meaning of life. Thus, if we succumb to retrospective psychiatric diagnosis, many religious and philosophical leaders of the past might be described as being 'mentally ill,' yet they now enjoy hypercredibility.

The medicine of antiquity began to systematize mental abnormality based upon single symptoms (such as sadness, excitement, confusion, and memory loss). This single-symptom approach was adopted by Roman medicine in the system of Galen – a view that operated in the main in Western medicine until the eighteenth century, overlain by religious assumptions in the Judeo-Christian view about sin as the source of insanity.

Mental Illness and Psychiatry

The single-symptom approach adopted by Galen began to be superseded in the eighteenth century in Britain and France. The Scottish physician Cullen suggested a classificatory system which he called the 'neuroses.' This very wide notion, which today would subsume most mental disorders, contained the etiological premise that madness and misery reflected damage to the nervous system. He argued that the healthy person had adequate levels of nervous energy (*vis nervosa*), which, when diseased, would be depleted. Cullen also suggested syndromes within this broad description of energy shortage.

By the middle of the nineteenth century, Cullen's overarching notion of 'the neuroses' was revised by Feuchterleben, who argued that the psychoses should be seen as a separate category because of symptom severity. However, the notion of 'severe' or 'serious' mental illness remains problematic, as some neurotic patients may be more socially disabled than some psychotic patients. Likewise the notion of 'insight' does not consistently distinguish the two broad groups of patients.

In late eighteenth-century France, de Sauvages offered a general classification of diseases of ten broad categories, the eighth of which was 'insanity.' Just prior to the French Revolution, Pinel, following the strictures of Hippocrates, on close observation, began the modern trend of basing the classification of mental illness on groups of symptoms and suspending etiological speculation or assertion. For example, Hippocrates opposed the common assumption, of his time, of mental abnormality being seated in the heart and diaphragm or *phren* (hence later English terms such as 'schizophrenia,' 'frenzy,' and 'frantic'). He argued that with no direct evidence of causation, this assumption should be dropped in favor of simply observing and recording the patient's speech and action.

Pinel delineated categories such as mania with delirium, mania without delirium, melancholia, confusion, and idiocy. This focus on group categories, which individual patients were then fitted into, was continued by Esquirol in France, who added the notion of 'monomania' or 'partial insanity.' This included both isolated delusions and more recent descriptions of obsessive-compulsive disorder. Neither Pinel nor Esquirol included the neuroses (mild sadness and anxiety) in their incipient psychiatric nosologies because these were deemed to be the responsibility of physicians, not alienists. In other words, from the outset psychiatry focused on madness and left neurotic misery to others; in recent times the latter has been mainly dealt with by primary care physicians.

Subsequently, German alienists also began to categorize. For example, Kahlbaum argued that psychological dysfunction could be observed in patients about their judgment ('paranoia'), their moods ('dysthymia'), or their will ('diastrephia'). This empiricist approach to classification started by Pinel, Esquirol, and Kahlbaum found its most noteworthy champion in Kraepelin.

Kraepelin (1883) set the scene for the main paradigm in modern Western psychiatry, which was characterized by three main features:

- The mental illnesses were considered to be separate, naturally occurring categories (hence the epistemological position of 'medical naturalism' noted earlier).
- These illnesses were considered to be a function of degeneracy; they were inherited conditions, with a predicable deteriorating course. To signify this assumption about predictable deterioration, Kraepelin used the term 'dementia praecox.' He argued that cases of the latter could be divided into three types: catatonia; paranoia; and hebephrenia (a term he took from Hecker). Later (1908) the term 'dementia praecox' was to be re-labeled 'schizophrenia' by Bleuler.
- Kraepelin held the view that all symptoms of mental illness were caused by diseases of the brain or nervous system. Even Freud, Kraepelin's contemporary, who emphasized psychological determinism, considered that all mental illness would eventually be explicable in physical terms. Thus if Kraepelin was a biodeterminist, Freud was a hoped-for-biodeterminist. Similarly, when Krafft-Ebing first used the term 'psychopathology,' he made it clear that all psychiatric symptoms implied underlying neural endopathology (Krafft-Ebing, 1875).

As Kraupl-Taylor (1966) noted when discussing the work of German psychopathologists in the late nineteenth century, the problem they were already encountering was that signs were only implied and still not proven (even post-mortem) for the great bulk of patients with psychiatric symptoms. The gap between symptoms and demonstrable neurological signs continues to dog the credibility of psychiatry today.

This Victorian *zeitgeist* then framed the modern psychiatric view of mental illness, with its emphasis on naturalism, hereditarianism, and biodeterminism. This epistemological position was also a political one for the developing profession, as it justified full medical control of the asylum system. The Victorian *zeitgeist* was manifested in a scientific and political ideology based upon the paradoxical blend of positivism and eugenics. This blend was commonplace in the intellectual circles of Western societies in the late nineteenth century, and it was to guarantee the controversial status of psychiatric knowledge in the twentieth century.

The Controversial Legacy of Mental Illness

By 1900, "psychiatry looked on itself with uncritical matter-of-factness as natural scientific enlightenment, as a flight against demonologic and other social superstitions and for the rights of the mentally ill..." (Doerner, 1970: 292). The seminal work of Kraepelin epitomized this scientific self-confidence and lack of collective professional self-doubt. It distilled the logic of his empiricist medical predecessors in France and Germany in the nineteenth century and it came to dominate Western psychiatry in the twentieth century.

The recent status of the neo-Kraepelinian orthodoxy (expressed in the DSM and ICD classificatory systems) has been summarized as follows:

> ...if there is one central intellectual reality at the end of the twentieth century, it is that the biological approach to psychiatry – treating mental illness as a genetically influenced disorder of brain chemistry – has been a smashing success.   (Shorter, 1998: vii)

This confirms that the lack of self-doubt, recorded by Doerner above, was as true at the end of the twentieth century as it was at the beginning.

But all was not completely well. By 1960 some psychiatrists restated the problem about the symptom–sign gap for confident classification (Stengel, 1960). After all, the term 'mental illness' reflects a lack of confident commitment to knowledge claims about mental 'disease' derived from proven endopathological states. The subsequent two decades then became dominated by the Szaszian critique of 'the myth of mental illness" (Szasz, 1961). The controversies of more recent decades have centered on the three main features of Kraepelin's legacy.

The first relates to the refusal of many mental health professionals (including some psychiatrists) to concede naturalism and its purported categories of mental illness and to favor instead dynamic wholism, biographical uniqueness, and continua rather than categories. The seminal major protagonist in this regard was Meyer, who developed his 'psychobiological approach' prior to the Second World War. Meyerian psychiatry was the basis of the later development of the 'biopsychosocial model,' which offers a holistic alternative to the dominant 'biomedical model.'

The biopsychosocial model is indebted to Meyer's work and that of the biologist Weiss in the 1920s and his student von Bertalanffy, who developed General Systems Theory in the 1950s (Pilgrim, 2002). Meyer conceded the role of broad inherited psychological tendencies but saw mental illnesses as reactions to peculiar biographical circumstances. His main question of interest was not "What is this patient's diagnosis?" but "Why is this particular patient presenting with these particular symptoms at this time in his or her life?" This sort of question undermines the 'lumping' tendency found in the Kraepelinian tradition, which fits patients, Procrustean-style, into preformed professionally preferred categories. Meyerian psychiatry also gave confidence to social psychiatry, an interdisciplinary project, which conceded the conceptual problems of functional mental illness but got on with studying social determinants of madness and misery (Pilgrim and Rogers, 2005).

But a great sustaining advantage of Kraepelin's system for the medical profession was that it generated a checklist approach to diagnosis and it created diagnostic-related groups. In this way, demands for medical services could be predicated on mapping the frequency of first cases (incidence) and accumulated cases (prevalence). However, psychiatric epidemiology was weak from the outset. Whereas strong medical epidemiology was based on mapping and correlating cases and causes, the cause of mental illness was strictly unknown (and still is for the major functional groups).

Apart from the Meyerian viewpoint challenging the categorical view, psychoanalysis also offered an alternative. However, psychoanalysts have been inconsistent in their opposition. Freud certainly considered that we are all ill to some extent (emphasizing a dimensional rather than categorical view). At the same time, other analysts accepted a categorical approach to classification willingly or rejected it out of hand as pseudo-science. What the psychodynamic view more significantly introduced was a challenge to the eugenic orthodoxy of asylum psychiatry in relation to the 'shellshock' problem of the First World War. The officers and gentlemen and the working-class volunteers breaking down with predictable regularity in the trenches were 'England's finest blood,' thus contradicting that orthodoxy.

Turning to the second feature of the Kraepelinian legacy, the English eugenic roots in the work of Galton and subsequent psychologists Spearman and Pearson found its most notorious expression in German psychiatry, during the Nazi period, in the work of Rudin and Kallmann (Meyer, 1988; Marshall, 1990). This genetic methodology, developed in inter-War Munich and based on twin studies, became the basis for respectable post-War psychiatric genetics promulgated by their English collaborator Slater. It is still a commonly held view in psychiatry that the psychoses are overwhelmingly genetically determined, reflecting a strong intellectual inertia, dating back to the eugenic roots of the profession in Nazi Germany and the Victorian England of Galton.

The third assumption about biodeterminism also resonates strongly today in relation to treatment preferences and etiological assumptions in psychiatry. Mental illness is treated overwhelmingly by using biological methods (medication, electro-shock, and a residue of psychosurgery). The dominant etiological theories in psychiatry reflect biodeterminism. However, the latter is no longer crudely hereditarian because it also emphasizes neuro-developmental effects. Such congenital and childhood insults remind us that biology cannot be conflated narrowly with heredity. This has opened up a space to argue that psychosis is a function of early trauma interacting with genetic predisposition, rather than it simply being the latter.

These three aspects of neo-Kraepelinian psychiatry have been the focus of criticism both within psychiatry from 'anti-psychiatry' and 'critical psychiatry,' as well as from disaffected service users (the mental health service users' movement). These critics have tended to emphasize constructivist and critical realist arguments when opposing medical naturalism. Such criticisms inevitably remain alive in a branch of medicine which, as was noted earlier, overwhelmingly deals with symptoms not signs.

Finally, a historical review of mental illness allows us to see some repeated patterns. For example, Galen's emphasis on single symptoms has its advocates today in clinical psychologists who reject diagnosis and favor working instead with presenting problems. Socrates' view that madness is an ambiguous state that holds personal and social strengths as well as weaknesses can be found in voice hearers sharing their different experiences. It is also evident in people with a diagnosis of psychosis pointing up its extra-ordinary subjective features and their special insights on life.

The reticence of Hippocrates to leap into etiological speculation is mirrored now in the DSM system, which, since 1980, has rejected etiology in favor of symptom checklists. Prior to that, DSM conceded both biological and psychodynamic etiological factors in its diagnostic listings. But this Hippocratic and Kraepelinian tradition *ipso facto* fails to deliver certainty about etiology and conceptual validity. As a result, the orthodox satisfaction with symptom checklists continues to attract criticisms of the concept of mental illness both inside and outside of the psychiatric profession.

See also: Mental Health Policy; Mental Health Resources and Services; Specific Mental Health Disorders: Child and Adolescent Mental Disorders; Stigma of Mental illness; Women's Mental Health.

Citations

Doerner K (1970) *Madmen and the Bourgeoisie*. Oxford, UK: Blackwell.
Hunter R and MacAlpine I (1963) *Three Hundred Years of Psychiatry 1535–1860*. London: Oxford University Press.
Kraepelin E (1883) *Compendium der Psychiatrie*. Leipzig: Abel.
Krafft-Ebing RF von (1875) *Ein Lehrbuch der Gerichtilichen Psychopathologie mit Berucksichtigung der Gesetzgebung von Osterreich, Deutschland und Frankreich*. Stuttgard: Enke.
Kraupl-Taylor L (1966) *Psychopathology*. London: Butterworth.
Leuder I and Thomas P (2000) *Voices of Reason, Voices of Insanity*. London: Bruner/Routledge.
Marshall R (1990) The genetics of schizophrenia: Axiom or hypothesis? In: Bentall RP (ed.) *Reconstructing Schizophrenia*. London: Routledge.
Meyer JE (1988) The fate of the mentally ill in Germany during the Third Reich. *Psychological Medicine* 18: 575–581.
Pilgrim D (2002) The biopsychosocial model in Anglo-American psychiatry: Past, present and future? *Journal of Mental Health* 11(6): 585–594.
Pilgrim D and Bentall RP (1999) The medicalisation of misery: A critical realist analysis of the concept of depression. *Journal of Mental Health* 8(3): 261–274.
Pilgrim D and Rogers A (2005) The troubled relationship between psychiatry and sociology. *International Journal of Social Psychiatry* 51(3): 228–241.
Rosen G (1968) *Madness in Society*. New York: Harper.
Screech MA (1985) Good madness in Christendom. In: Bynum WF, Porter R and Shepherd M (eds.) *The Anatomy of Madness: Essays in the History of Psychiatry* Volume I. London: Tavistock.
Shorter E (1998) *History of Psychiatry: From the Era of the Asylum to the Age of Prozac*. New York: Wiley.
Stengel E (1960) A comparative study of psychiatric classifications. *Proceedings of the Royal Society of Medicine* 53: 123.
Stone MH (1997) *Healing the Sick Mind: A History of Psychiatry from Antiquity to the Present*. New York: Norton.
Szasz TS (1961) The uses of naming and the origin of the myth of mental illness. *American Psychologist* 16: 59–65.

Regulation of Drugs and Drug Use: Public Health and Law Enforcement

C L Fry, Monash University, Frankston, VIC, Australia
S Cvetkovski, Turning Point Alcohol and Drug Centre Inc., Fitzroy, VIC, Australia

Introduction

Drug use has developed historically as part of wider social practices. Drug-related harms, including harms to health and social order, need to be understood in a sociocultural context, as do the regulatory frameworks that have developed to control drug demand, supply, and use. Contemporary drug policy reflects an uneasy balance between public health and law enforcement responses. This dichotomy creates avoidable complications and unintended consequences for associated regulatory practices. Balanced approaches to drug control and regulation should consider a number of central issues, including the role of science and evidence, ethics, public opinion, and the socioeconomic and political context.

Historical Overview

The Role of Drug Use in Context

The use of naturally occurring psychoactive substances predates modern history, with evidence of tobacco, cannabis, alcohol, opium, coca, psilocybin, and peyote occupying important cultural, spiritual, medicinal, and economic roles in ancient societies. Historically, the distribution and use of psychoactive substances was not State regulated in the manner that is seen today, although in some countries taxes on psychoactive substances provided a significant source of government funding which predated income taxation systems.

Indian opium was imported into the UK as early as 1606 by trade ships chartered by Elizabeth I. In the seventeenth and eighteenth centuries, hemp cropping for rope and sail manufacture was widespread in the North American colonies. In many countries, opium, morphine, and cocaine were used widely in a range of home remedies and tonics. Since the advent of modern toxicology in the early nineteenth century, the manufacture of new drugs for medicinal and other purposes has steadily increased the available range of psychoactive drugs.

Responses to Drug Use

It is beyond the scope of this article to fully discuss the antecedents of the regulatory legal approach to the control of drug supply and use (for a detailed history refer to Courtwright, 2001; MacCoun and Reuter, 2001; Davenport-Hines, 2004). Some of the key events and social changes are overviewed here to illustrate the shift toward progressively inclusive drug regulation and control by the State, together with harsher penalties for drug use, supply, and manufacture.

A number of important socioeconomic and political developments influenced the development of international drug control conventions and treaties and related jurisdictional laws. The Opium Wars of 1839–42 and 1856–80 were the result of clashes involving international politics, commercial interests, and moral opinion on drugs. The conflicts followed the persistent supply of opium to China by the Dutch, Portuguese, English, and British India despite the 1729 ban on importation and the 1799 prohibition of importation, cultivation, and use.

A key post-industrial revolution theme that developed as populations became more mobile was a sense of moral panic about drug use. This legitimized prejudice against the lower socioeconomic classes and minority immigrant groups, their drugs of preference, and perceived racial and cultural difference. In some countries during the nineteenth century gold rush era, this was first evident in relation to Chinese immigrants and their use of opium, culminating in fears about social order and laws banning opium smoking directed at the Chinese opium dens (Goode and Ben-Yehuda, 1994).

State concerns about the prevention of drug-related health harms can be traced in England back to the 1868 Pharmacy Act, involving the first regulation of drugs. This was prompted by accidental and intentional drug poisonings and the recreational use of opium and chloral hydrate by the working classes. Initial concerns around the need for regulation of the patent medicine industry via State legislation paved the way for the early foundations of an international drug control system.

The 1912 Hague Opium Convention focused on reduced production, distribution, and consumption of opiates; restricted use for legitimate medical purposes; and domestic legislation to prevent narcotics abuse. Since then drug control measures have become progressively more inclusive and more punitive (for a description of development of international conventions on drugs, see Courtwright, 2001; MacCoun and Reuter, 2001; Davenport-Hines, 2004).

Another important development was the rise of the Temperance Movement in the UK and United States, leading to prohibition in those and other countries. Prohibition became a popular vehicle for social control in the context of industrial expansion, urbanization, increased population, immigration, and associated social order problems. Prohibition initially focused on alcohol but later extended to opium and other drugs, taking a punitive moral stance toward drug use and users. This laid the foundations for the medical-disease model of addiction in which drug use was seen as a marker of individual deficit and lack of agency, thus requiring the paternalism of both law enforcement and public health responses (Berridge, 1980).

Although the pursuit of altered consciousness through drug use has been a constant in human history, the shifting public and State view on the permissibility of this owes a debt to the emphasis during the seventeenth and eighteenth century Enlightenment on reason and rationality as the underpinnings of the perfect society.

Current Situation: Drug Use and Harms

Drug use practices and the associated harms, both individual and social, continue to be shaped by changing sociocultural, economic, and political norms. Although it is difficult to find comparable data across nations, the available estimates show that tobacco and alcohol use is prevalent in most populations, and accordingly is responsible for the majority of drug-related mortality and morbidity compared with illicit drugs.

Worldwide there are an estimated 2 billion people who consume alcoholic beverages and 1.3 billion people who currently smoke cigarettes or use other tobacco products (Shafey *et al.*, 2003; World Health Organization, 2004). Alcohol-related harms largely occur in developed countries, but these harms are increasing in some developing countries as a result of commercial interests establishing alcohol beverage markets. Globally, there are around 76 million people with a diagnosable alcohol use disorder. Alcohol use is estimated to cause "around 20–30% of esophageal cancer, liver cancer, cirrhosis of the liver, homicides, epileptic seizures, and motor vehicle accidents world wide" (World Health Organization, 2004: 1).

Tobacco use is also a major cause of morbidity and mortality in developed nations, and as with alcohol, it is a growing problem in developing countries where increasing affluence is associated with increased use and associated health harms. There were an estimated 4.9 million premature deaths worldwide in the year 2000 from smoking. By 2020 the global burden is expected to exceed 9 million deaths annually, with 7 million of these occurring in economically developing countries (Shafey, 2003: 7).

The annual global prevalence of illicit drug use has been estimated to be 200 million people between 15–64

years of age (5% of the world population), with around 25 million people (0.6% of the world population) having problematic drug use (United Nations Office of Drugs and Crime, 2006). The most prevalent illicit drug is cannabis, followed by amfetamine-type stimulants (amfetamines and ecstasy), cocaine, and opiates. Illicit drug use has been greatest in developed countries, although here, too, the pattern has been shifting. The demand for treatment for problematic amfetamine-type stimulants use, for example, is highest in Asia, followed by Oceania, North America, Europe, and Africa (United Nations Office of Drugs and Crime, 2006: 9).

Contemporary Drug Policy – Public Health or Law Enforcement?

A key historical development is the dichotomization of drug use and harms into primarily a public health and social issue or a law enforcement and criminal justice issue (largely coinciding with the 'legal' and 'illegal' classification of substances). This dichotomy is reflected in the relative emphasis of regulatory strategies. A particular jurisdiction's policy will be determined by the relative importance placed on the nexus of 'drugs and crime' compared with the relationship between drug use and dependence or addiction.

Prohibitionist policy frameworks for the use of certain drugs have led to most jurisdictions giving public health strategies fewer resources and a role subordinate to law enforcement. Critics have pointed out that the emphasis on law enforcement has made it difficult for public health interventions to effectively operate, and that there are unintended negative consequences of policies that have stressed law enforcement (Kerr *et al.*, 2005).

Range of Current Legal Responses

There is a general expectation that the State will bear responsibility for implementing systems of control and sanction in order to prevent and punish individuals whose behavior transgresses accepted rules and standards. Today there is a range of drug use and related behaviors that are considered criminal offences in law and law enforcement. These behaviors are subject to a variety of punitive measures (ranging from community service to the death penalty) or to civil regulatory actions and other sanctions (e.g., civil commitment, court-ordered treatment, and diversion-to-treatment programs, or compulsory drug treatment to avoid loss of social assistance, welfare benefits, or child custody).

The most common types of criminal offence are for the use, possession, trafficking, and manufacture of drugs of dependence. However, supply control and regulatory measures have in recent times extended to the diversion and nonmedical use of prescription pharmaceuticals, diversion from legitimate commerce of precursor chemicals (e.g., methamphetamine manufacture), the regulation of alcohol and public smoking, and, most recently, counterfeit drugs and Internet trafficking (see *Monitoring the Future Survey*; Makkai and McAllister, 1998; EUROPHEN, 2004).

A powerful factor motivating public expectations around the regulation of illicit drugs is the perceived relationship between drugs and crime. Politically, the regulation of drugs through legal mechanisms has been made possible through the characterization of certain drug use (and drug users by association) as immoral and a threat to social order. As noted, this developed historically in relation to the State's desire to control minority immigrant and other groups viewed as problematic. However, the enshrinement of this control in binding international legal frameworks has positioned drug use as a behavior for which legal control and sanctioning is viewed as a justified response. Implicit in this justification is the contested assumption of a causal link between drug use and crime, and a belief that drug use can be reduced or even eliminated through supply reduction means.

There has been a long tradition of research into possible links between drug use, dependence, and crime, leading to the development of various theoretical models (e.g., see Makkai, 2002 for a discussion of models of enslavement, criminality, escalation, psychopharmacology, economic compulsive, and systemic violence). However, although the evidence consistently shows that people who use illicit drugs have a significantly higher than average crime rate and are more likely to have been arrested, no direct causal relationship has been identified (Lipton and Johnson, 1998; Deitch *et al.*, 2000; Stevens *et al.*, 2003). Current research into the drugs and crime issue engages with transdisciplinary assessment of inequalities in environmental factors such as poverty, education, and unemployment to further an understanding of the relationship.

The Addition of a Range of Public Health Responses

Broad public health discussion on the relationship between drugs and dependence or addiction has focused on the presence or absence of personal responsibility. There are various disease models under the umbrella of addiction that view drug users as powerless to address their addiction. In this context, it is argued that drug user responsibility is limited, since autonomy or agency is affected by a pathology or defect leading to addiction (from psychosocial factors to genetic predispositions) (see Kellehear and Cvetkovski, 2004). Given this lack of autonomy, it is argued, appropriate regulatory strategies should be adopted – that is, the relative emphasis of

strategies should be based on public health rather than law enforcement responses.

However, arguments that minimize responsibility for drug use owing to addiction can be challenged as they are based on a small group of problematic drug users and do not represent the patterns of drug use by most people. Further, those who support abstinence and prohibition counter the argument about lack of autonomy due to addiction by insisting that it is the individual's responsibility to avoid drugs in the first place.

Within the public health and law enforcement spectrum, there is a range of intervention strategies that are possible. Various types of legal and law enforcement strategies have been applied, such as legalization, supply reduction, border and domestic interdiction, street saturation policing, cautioning, and court and police diversion of offenders. In public health, harm reduction and minimization strategies can take the form of various kinds of demand reduction – such as primary, secondary, and tertiary prevention plus or minus health promotion – or use human rights approaches and strategies for drug law reform.

Different jurisdictions vary in their place on the spectrum between public health harm reduction and minimization or law enforcement approaches. The differential application and operation of strategies such as needle and syringe programs (NSP), supervised injecting facilities (SIF), and law enforcement reflect this orientation. Paradoxically, it is not possible to predict the use of particular interventions from the prevalence of drug-related harms or even the available evidence of efficacy. For example, although NSPs have operated for more than two decades in Australia and Europe, with widespread acceptance of evidence demonstrating their effectiveness in preventing human immunodeficiency virus (HIV) and hepatitis C virus (HCV) transmission, they are still prohibited in many American states and have been only recent additions in parts of Asia and other developing countries where HIV and HCV are most established. Differential outcomes are also evident across jurisdictions attempting to implement SIF trials, and even within certain countries (e.g., in Australia establishment of a SIF trial in Sydney and failed attempts in Melbourne and Canberra).

Finally, there are examples of mixed approaches in which law enforcement innovations are defined by some as key components of the harm reduction and minimization response (e.g., community policing, drug courts, court diversion to treatment schemes, decriminalization of possession, cannabis normalization and nonenforcement policy, drug and driving programs).

Opponents of a primary emphasis on law enforcement responses have pointed out that international drug control mechanisms are failing on a number of fronts and produce unintended consequences. The direct and indirect costs include a lack of success in reduction of illicit market supply of heroin, cocaine, methamphetamine, and cannabis;

the additional negative social impact of law enforcement approaches; the deemphasis on drug-related harms such as HCV and HIV/AIDS; the lack of evidence regarding the efficacy of law enforcement policies and programs in reducing drug use and associated health and social problems; and the undermining of the operation of existing public health interventions – for example, riskier drug use to avoid police detection and non-uptake of NSP services (see Kerr *et al.*, 2005; Rhodes *et al.*, 2005). The important idea that laws, as they are written and enforced, shape the risk environment for drug users is attracting growing acceptance (Burris *et al.*, 2004).

Issues for Debate

Drugs use and the harms associated with their use, together with the regulatory frameworks designed to address them, are closely linked to the socioeconomic and political contexts; therefore, consideration of context is important in addressing contemporary drug use and related harm. Irrespective of one's views on the different approaches, regulation is the foundation of both public health and law enforcement. The relative emphasis on public health or law enforcement approaches, although important, should not detract from the discussion of their broader context. Issues such as the unequal social, economic, and political power of competing groups, the State as the site of competition between different strategies to regulate and protect citizens from drug use and its harms, the function of science and the status of evidence, and ethical questions related to these dimensions must all be considered.

The different jurisdictional outcomes in debates about supervised injecting facilities (SIFs) provide a good example of the crucial role of context. The relative socioeconomic and political power exerted by opposition groups in some jurisdictions has prevented trials from going ahead. These groups used a variety of strategies, from engaging in media debates to lobbying for legislation. Both those for and against SIFs engaged with the available scientific evidence, by critiquing and rejecting it or by interpreting it in ways that supported their positions. In this context, drug users were marginalized and their participation in the development of policies that affected them was directly minimized. Ethical issues, such as how we are to understand the relationship between drug use and dependence, individual autonomy, and rights, were difficult to discuss when debates circulated around the simple dichotomy of drug users as addicted and lacking autonomy or as criminal and autonomous.

Even where regulatory interventions such as SIFs (which are seen as politically progressive by supporters) have been successfully implemented, there is the possibility that rather than displacing more punitive measures, such policy shifts may actually incorporate these in the overall governance of drug users, drug use, and the associated harms. For example, in relation to SIFs, Fischer and colleagues (2004) note that "little attention has been given to their implications as a substantial shift from the punitive repression of injection drug use (IDU) to the government of drug use as a form of regulated risk consumption and sociospatial ordering under the guises of public health" (p. 357). The unintended end point may be more punitive targeting of drug users who refuse to submit to new rules and regulations with harsher measures than originally in place (e.g., saturation policing around new SIFs).

The example of SIFs demonstrates how drug use regulation is influenced by the socioeconomic and political context and can lead to the entrenchment of a simplistic public health versus law enforcement dichotomy. Public debates are influenced by powerful lobby groups. Choices can be dominated by strategic and technical details or by simplistic moral and punitive responses. Specific strategic regulatory responses are important, both public health and law enforcement responses, but they must be considered within the wider social, economic, and political context to achieve a better understanding of their negative and positive consequences.

Conclusion

The State regulation and control of drugs, legal and otherwise, shifts according to current sociocultural and political determinants. At different points in history, most known psychoactive substances have been freely available and unregulated. Historically, public health, in addition to law enforcement, has played a role in the justification of drug control – from the earliest application of epidemiologic methods to illustrate the prevalence of drug use and associated mortality and morbidity in the population to the regulatory frameworks (legislative and taxation) governing the manufacture, distribution, and sale of pharmaceuticals to controls of the licit drugs of highest consumption, tobacco and alcohol.

Many countries have pragmatic drug control policies that sit within increasingly strict prohibition regimes (e.g., cannabis normalization, diamorphine prescription, supervised drug consumption facilities). However, taking a long-term view, there is nothing inevitable or permanent about prohibitionist drug regulation and control, nor are public health approaches to the regulation of drug use and harms stable and guaranteed. Beyond strict prohibition, drug law reformists currently advocate for a sophisticated view of drug regulation that encompasses a range of prohibitory, prescription, and regulatory drug control regimes. Another important theme gaining momentum in the debate about drugs and legal issues is the consideration of the international human rights legal framework as a means of achieving a balanced approach to drug policy through an emphasis on human dignity, enforceable limits on State actions, remedies for mistreatment, and State public health obligations.

The fluidity of the place of drugs in society poses a challenge for public health to be flexible and creative in working for the right balance of harm reduction and law enforcement approaches to drug use. Achieving this may require a better understanding of drug use and the related ethical, health, and legal issues in their sociocultural, economic, and political context. It may also necessitate further thinking about disputes regarding the use of science and evidence, as well as definitions of the relationship between drug use and dependence and individual autonomy and rights.

See also: Illicit Drug Trends Globally; Control and Regulation of Currently Illegal Drugs.

Citations

Berridge V (1980) The making of the Rolleston Report, 1908–1926. *Journal of Drug Issues* 7: 28.

Burris S, Blankenship KM, Donoghoe M, *et al.* (2004) Addressing the ''risk environment'' for injecting drug users: The mysterious case of the missing cop. *The Milbank Quarterly* 82: 125–156.

Courtwright DT (2001) *Forces of Habit: Drugs and the Making of the Modern World.* Cambridge, MA: Harvard University Press.

Davenport-Hines RPT (2004) *The Pursuit of Oblivion: A Global History of Narcotics.* New York: W.W. Norton & Company Inc.

Deitch D, Koutsenok I, and Ruiz A (2000) The Relationship Between Crime and Drugs: What We Have Learned in Recent Decades. *Journal of Psychoactive Drugs* 32: 391–397.

European Public Health Ethics Network (EUROPHEN) (2004) Attitudes to government intervention in public health issues: Overview of findings of qualitative research across Europe. C12507. Sheffield: University of Sheffield. http://www.shef.ac.uk/scharr/sections/ph/research/genetics_ethics/research/europhen/about.html/

Fischer B, Turnbull S, Poland B, and Haydon E (2004) Drug use, risk and urban order: examining supervised injection sites (SISs) as 'governmentality.' *International Journal of Drug Policy* 15: 357–365.

Goode E and Ben-Yehuda N (1994) *Moral Panics: The Social Construction of Deviance.* Cambridge, MA: Blackwell.

Kellehear A and Cvetkovski S (2004) Grand theories of drug use. In: Hamilton M, King T and Ritter A (eds.) *Drug Use in Australia: Preventing Harm,* 2nd edn., pp. 53–63. Melbourne, Australia: Oxford University Press in association with Turning Point Alcohol & Drug Centre.

Kerr T, Small W, and Wood E (2005) The public health and social impacts of drug market enforcement: a review of the evidence. *International Journal of Drug Policy* 493: 1–11.

Lipton DS and Johnson BD (1998) Smack, crack, and score: Two decades of NIDA-funded drugs and crime research at NDRI 1974–1994. *Substance Use and Misuse* 33: 1779–1815.

MacCoun RJ and Reuter P (2001) *Drug War Heresies: Learning from Other Vices, Times and Places.* Cambridge, UK: Cambridge University Press.

Makkai T (2002) Illicit drugs and crime. In: Graycar A and Grabosky P (eds.) *The Cambridge Handbook of Australian Criminology,* pp. 110–125. Cambridge, UK: Cambridge University Press.

Makkai T and McAllister I (1998) *Public Opinion Towards Drug Policies in Australia: 1985–95.* Canberra, Australia: Commonwealth of Australia. http://www.health.gov.au/internet/wcms/Publishing.nsf/Content/health-pubhlth-publicat-document-opinions-cnt.htm (accessed August 2007).

Monitoring the Future Survey, Institute for Social Research, University of Michigan. http://www.monitoringthefuture.org (accessed July 2007).

Rhodes T, Singer M, Bourgois P, Friedman SR, and Strathdee SA (2005) The social and structural production of HIV risk among injecting drug users. *Social Science and Medicine* 61: 1026–1044.

Shafey O, Dolwick S and Guindon GE (eds.) (2003) *Tobacco Control Country Profiles.* 2nd edn. Atlanta, GA: American Cancer Society, Inc., World Health Organization, and International Union Against Cancer.

Stevens A, Berto D, Kerschl V, *et al.* (2003) *Summary Literature Review: The International Literature on Drugs, Crime and Treatment.* Canterbury, UK: University of Kent.

United Nations Office of Drugs and Crime (2006) *World Drug Report. Volume 1: Analysis.* http://www.unodc.org/pdf/WDR_2006/wdr2006_volume1.pdf (accessed August 2007).

World Health Organization (2004) *Global Status Report on Alcohol 2004.* Geneva, Switzerland: WHO, Department of Mental Health and Substance Abuse.

Further Reading

Booth M (1996) *Opium: A History.* London: Simon & Schuster.

Goode E (1989) *Drugs in American Society,* 3rd edn. New York: McGraw-Hill.

Hamilton M, King T and Ritter A (eds.) (2004) *Drug Use in Australia: Preventing Harm.* 2nd edn. Melbourne, Australia: Oxford University Press in association with Turning Point Alcohol & Drug Centre.

Maher L and Dixon D (1999) Policing and public health: Law enforcement and harm minimisation in a street-level drug market. *British Journal of Criminology* 39: 488–511.

Musto DF (1999) *The American Disease: Origins of Narcotic Control,* 3rd edn. New York: Oxford University Press.

Musto DF (ed.) (2002) *Drugs in America: A Documentary History.* New York: New York University Press.

Relevant Websites

http://www.aic.gov.au – The Australian Institute of Criminology.

http://www.internationaldrugpolicy.net – The Beckley Foundation Drug Policy Programme.

http://www.drugpolicy.org – The Drug Policy Alliance.

http://www.erowid.org – Erowid.

http://www.emcdda.eu.int – European Monitoring Centre for Drugs and Drug Addiction.

http://www.shef.ac.uk/scharr/sections/ph/research/genetics_ethics/research/europhen – European Public Health Ethics Network.

http://www.harmreduction.org – Harm Reduction Coalition.

http://www.kcl.ac.uk/icpr – The Institute for Criminal Policy Research.

http://www.ihra.net – International Harm Reduction Association.

http://www.monitoringthefuture.org – *Monitoring the Future Survey,* Institute for Social Research, University of Michigan.

http://www.drugabuse.gov/l – The National Institute on Drug Abuse.

http://www.whitehousedrugpolicy.gov – Office of National Drug Control Policy.

http://www.rand.org – RAND Drug Policy Research Center.

http://www.release.org.uk – Release Drugs, the Law and Human Rights.

http://www.druglibrary.org – Schaffer Library of Drug Policy.

http://www.unodc.org – United Nations Office on Drugs and Crime.

http://www.who.int/en – World Health Organization.

Stigma of Mental Illness

L H Yang and S H Cho, Columbia University, New York, NY, USA
A Kleinman, Harvard University, Cambridge, MA, USA

Introduction

Stigma is a pervasive social force that has powerful consequences for those who are stigmatized and for society itself. Stigma acts to decrease life opportunities among those that it affects by reducing social contacts, housing options, and employment opportunities. Further, stigma causes affected individuals to underutilize health care in order to avoid becoming stigmatized. As a result, larger society is adversely affected. Society becomes burdened by the costs of those who neglect adequate treatment and whose illness conditions worsen due to fear of stigma. Further, society suffers from the spread of infectious diseases (such as AIDS) that remain untreated due to the threat of stigma. Finally, society is adversely impacted by the loss of productive citizens and a further loss of fundamental human rights by the stigmatized.

Instead of being confined to a strict definition, stigma has been understood primarily through the ideas of several leading theorists. These ideas have ranged from conceptions that focus on individuals to those that examine society to explain how stigma works. The concept of stigma has included internal psychological processes within the person, interpersonal social processes between individuals and groups, and large-scale processes on the level of culture and politics.

Stigma is closely associated with concepts such as discrimination and racism. However, some important distinctions exist. While stigma has traditionally been applied to either behavioral or physical deviance, discrimination has been applied much more generally to social characteristics such as race, gender, and socioeconomic status. Further, while stigma has typically been applied to individual traits, discrimination usually has been applied to group characteristics. Lastly, discrimination has tended to focus responsibility on those doing the discriminating. Stigma, in contrast, has focused more attention on the stigmatized person him- or herself. Researchers are currently examining the limits of each concept both theoretically and empirically to determine how these closely related processes complement or contradict one another.

Definitions of Stigma

Because thinking regarding this concept has changed over time, definitions of stigma have also been adapted as theorists and researchers have modified their views toward what this concept should encompass. As a result, although most definitions of stigma share common features, particular definitions of stigma may emphasize one or more dimensions as central. Further, because stigma has been studied from various disciplinary perspectives (e.g., sociology, psychology, or anthropology), a particular theory may also emphasize the theoretical orientation or the discipline of that particular investigator.

Sociologist Irving Goffman's book written in 1963, *Notes on the Management of a Spoiled Identity,* is widely viewed as the first essential social and behavioral science formulation of stigma. Goffman defines stigma as "an attribute that is deeply discrediting" and proposes that the stigmatized person is reduced "from a whole and usual person to a tainted, discounted one" (Goffman, 1963: 3). While Goffman's definition implies that stigma takes place because of some characteristic that an individual possesses, he also emphasizes the importance of how others interpret the stigma by describing stigma as "a special kind of relationship between an attribute and a stereotype" (Goffman, 1963: 4). Here an attribute could be a physical blemish or functional impairment, or a psychological trait. From Goffman's perspective, stigma occurs when a person is characterized by society (i.e., the meanings that others attach to the stigmatized attribute) in a way that differs from the characteristics that person actually possesses.

The next definition of stigma, proposed by social psychologists (Jones *et al.,* 1984), uses the term mark to describe how society identifies a deviant condition that initiates the stigmatizing process. The mark, which is seen as central to who the person is, then discredits the stigmatized person by defining the person as flawed, spoiled, contaminated, or undesirable (e.g., similar to the process of branding a slave in ancient times). This perspective emphasizes how the mark and its associated negative meanings engulf how the person is seen by other members of society and accordingly emphasizes stigma as being located within the person who is stigmatized.

Similarly, a definition of stigma proposed by another group of social psychologists (Crocker *et al.,* 1998) defines stigma as taking place when an objective characteristic of the individual leads to a negatively valued social identity. For example, someone who walks with a limp may be discredited by the term cripple. However, this perspective also emphasizes that the negative attribute is interpreted within the social context of the stigmatized individual. These authors thus incorporate the social context in defining whether and how a stigmatized attribute devalues an individual. That is to say, a person with epilepsy may be discredited by having uncontrollable seizures that powerfully alter behavior or because within a certain cultural context, the seizures are attributable to supernatural factors.

A separate psychological perspective approaches stigma from the viewpoint of evolutionary psychology (Kurzban and Leary, 2001). Evolutionary psychology is based on the principle of natural selection, which is defined as a process by which the organisms best adapted to their environment tend to survive and transmit their genetic characteristics to succeeding generations. According to this view, natural selection favors the survival of those species who adapt to or overcome obstacles posed to them over time by evolution. To aid in this adaptation, distinct information-processing structures exist within the mind to solve specific problems encountered in the social domain. These cognitive structures motivate the individual to avoid interactions with certain categories of people that would lessen that individual's likelihood of eventual survival. The first category resulting from these cognitive structures is that of a poor social exchange partner: individuals are avoided who may cheat in a social exchange and who provide little in terms of social benefit. The second category is that of outgroup exploitation: Individuals are excluded from gaining the benefits of group membership and instead are targeted for exploitation as an inferior group. The third category consists of parasite avoidance: Individuals who are viewed as likely to carry contagious diseases are avoided. Stigma results from the categorization of people into these groups by adaptive cognitive mechanisms: By classifying people into such categories, the stigmatizing individual thus increases his or her probability of survival.

In addition to the aforementioned conceptualizations, one sociological framework has focused on how a combination of societal forces result in stigmatized individuals being excluded from everyday life (Link and Phelan, 2001). Rather than emphasizing one or two primary components to define stigma, Link and Phelan view stigma as a broader concept that connects together six interrelated components. The first component, labeling, consists of when people distinguish a human difference as important and give it a label. An example might be after an individual hears voices and talks to him- or herself, he or she is then labeled as having mental illness. The second component, stereotyping, takes place when beliefs of a cultural group connect labeled individuals to negative characteristics. For example, people with mental illness might be seen as being very dangerous. The third component, cognitive separation, takes place when labeled persons are seen as so different from normal people that a complete separation of us (normals) from them (deviants) is achieved. The fourth component, emotional reactions, includes the emotional responses to stigma felt by both stigmatizers (e.g., fear) and the people who are stigmatized (e.g., shame). The fifth component, status loss and discrimination, results when labeled individuals feel themselves to be less valued than other members of society and are treated unfairly (i.e., discriminated against) by others. Link and Phelan describe discrimination as primarily occurring either when one person treats another person unfairly or when practices of larger institutions or laws disadvantage stigmatized groups. Lastly is the idea that the entire stigma process depends on one group possessing the power (either social, economic, or political) to actually make these stigma components harmful to those who are stigmatized. That is, the group who stigmatizes must be higher in status than the group who is stigmatized in order for the negative effects of stigma to occur.

From these multiple definitions, we can thus trace how stigma has evolved from a conceptualization involving a stigmatizing attribute and cognitive stereotyping processes to a more complex formulation incorporating evolutionary forces, social factors, and political processes. The manifold domains of stigma continue to be refined as researchers further identify the empirical processes by which stigma works.

Categorical Versus Dimensional Definitions of Stigma

As definitions of stigma have incorporated a wider array of processes, there has been a shift in defining stigma according to dimensions as opposed to categories (or typologies; see **Table 1**). Two stigma frameworks emphasize categories of stigma, or classifications of the different manifestations that stigma may take (Goffman, 1963; Kurzban and Leary, 2001). Like the evolutionary framework described earlier, Goffman (1963) separates stigma into three types. The first type, physical deformities, indicates abominations of the body. The second, blemishes of character, includes characteristics (e.g., having served a jail sentence) that impugn the person's moral integrity. The last category, tribal stigma of race, nation, and religion, encompasses stigmas that can be inherited and equally affect all family members. Using this classification, a particular stigma (e.g., attached to being an alcoholic) could be categorized as belonging to one of these three types (e.g., a blemish of character).

Later definitions emphasize dimensions of stigma – attributes or components of stigma that could apply singly or in combination in a matter of degree to any given stigma. The stigma framework proposed by Jones *et al.* (1984) is particularly known for its proposed six dimensions of stigma. The first dimension, concealability, indicates how detectable the stigmatized characteristic is to others. The second, course, describes whether the

Table 1   Categories and dimensions of stigma

Source	Typologies of stigma	Dimensions of stigma

Goffman, 1963	1. Physical deformities
	2. Blemishes of character
	3. Tribal stigma of race/nation/religion
		1. Visibility
		  a. Discreditable
		  b. Discredited
		2. Obtrusiveness

Jones et al., 1984	None	1. Concealability 2. Course 3. Disruptiveness 4. Aesthetics 5. Origin 6. Peril
Kurzban and Leary, 2001	1. Poor social exchange partner 2. Outgroup exploitation 3. Parasite avoidance	None

Link and Phelan 2001	None	1. Distinguishing and labeling differences
		2. Associating differences with negative attributes
		3. Separating 'us' from 'them'
		4. Emotional responses
		5. Status loss and discrimination
		  a. Individual discrimination
		  b. Structural discrimination
		  c. Status loss
		  d. Internalized processes
		6. The dependence of stigma on power

Corrigan et al. (2004)		1. Structural discrimination
		  a. Intentional
		  b. Unintentional

stigmatizing condition is reversible over time. The third dimension, disruptiveness, indicates the extent to which a stigmatizing trait strains interpersonal interactions. The dimension of aesthetics reflects concerns about the extent to which a stigmatizing characteristic elicits an instinctive reaction of disgust. The fifth, origin, refers to how the condition came into being, with an emphasis on how perceived responsibility for the condition greatly influences others' reactions. The last dimension, peril, refers to feelings of danger that the stigmatized trait induces in others. Other theories of stigma that identify dimensional aspects similarly organize stigma into characteristics that vary in degree rather than assigning them into fixed categories. For example, utilizing Link and Phelan's (2001) dimensional definition, a person encountering a stigmatizing event (e.g., being hospitalized in a psychiatric unit) may undergo labeling more or less strongly, may encounter negative stereotyping and separation of us from them that is more or less complete, etc. A stigma may vary on these dimensions in accordance with the nature of the stigma, the individual's particular circumstance, and the sociocultural context. Although stigma dimensions can hypothetically function independently, in reality they are often intertwined and exert influence upon one another. For example, utilizing Jones et al.'s framework, stigmas that are genetic in nature (origin) may tend to be relatively inflexible to future change (course).

How a stigma varies on different dimensions can be seen to give rise to the stigma classification systems. For example, Goffman's typologies of physical deformities and blemishes of character are likely to differ in concealability (a stigma dimension). These differences in concealability (i.e., blemishes of character tend to be concealable while physical deformities are not) may in great part determine why these two types of stigmas are viewed as categorically different. One advantage to definitions of stigma that emphasize its dimensional aspects is that they provide a more nuanced view of what the salient aspects of stigma consist of. Further, considering the dimensions of stigma provides a set of attributes that may illustrate how that stigma affects the individual.

Models of How Stigma is Experienced by the Individual

We next describe the most prominent models of how stigma is seen to affect the individual. Reviewing such models is essential to conceptualizing how stigma works. Like the definitions of stigma, models of how stigma exerts its negative effects on individuals have developed from processes that primarily focus on individuals to models that incorporate the larger social and political context. Further, although many of these models focus on mental illness stigma specifically, they can be used to illustrate how the stigma process works more generally.

Goffman's Model of Stigma

Goffman (1963) describes stigma as a process where the person is socialized into a new stigmatized identity. This process begins with a stigmatized person learning society's view of the stigma and what it might be like to have a particular stigma. The person then adopts a stigmatized role by gradually identifying with the stigmatized status. For example, a person with mental illness (whose stigma is viewed as not being visible) thus passes from a normal status when diagnosed with mental illness to the status of a person who is potentially discreditable (if others find out about the illness). If others discover the person's condition, he or she will pass onto a discredited status. In this view, stigma occurs as the person assumes a new identity that is socially constructed.

Social Psychological Models of Stigma

Following Goffman, Jones *et al.* (1984) utilize a social psychological perspective to examine the role of the individual in response to stigma. Jones *et al.* conceptualize stigma as mainly working through cognitive processes of assigning individuals into categories. Stigma takes place when the mark (the stigmatizing attribute) links the identified person to undesirable characteristics (i.e., stereotypes). The negative meanings conveyed by these stereotypes then lead to discrediting of the stigmatized individual. Disruption in the community member's emotions, cognitions, and behaviors then occurs when interacting with the stigmatized person.

From another social psychological perspective, Crocker *et al.* (1998) expanded stigma to include how people maintain their self-esteem through cognitive coping strategies. They also incorporate how social identities are constructed through cognitive processes and how the social context is instrumental in shaping one's identity. A key addition of this formulation is that both stigmatizers and the stigmatized individual may internalize a negative stereotype that in turn has harmful effects. For example, among stigmatizers, negative stereotyping of stigmatized groups occurs automatically and often outside of the stigmatizer's awareness. An example of internalized stigma that occurs among stigmatized individuals is that of stereotype threat. Individuals labeled with stigma encounter situations when specific negative stereotypes about a group are known by the stigmatized individual. The threat provided by this stereotype to a person's self-esteem then negatively impacts the individual's performance in that situation. For example, a female student who is asked to take a math test (and is aware of the stereotype that females tend to perform more poorly than males on tests of arithmetic ability) will tend to perform worse on the test than a male student due to this threat to self-esteem.

At the heart of Crocker *et al.*'s formulation is that stigma threatens the stigmatized individual's self-worth. Stigmatized individuals then select among several possible cognitive coping strategies to avoid threats to self-esteem. For example, the female student in the above situation may psychologically disengage her self-esteem from her ability to do math. Stigma thus may impact the individual by working through psychological well-being (including life satisfaction, self-esteem, and depression) and school achievement.

From another social psychological perspective, Major and O'Brien (2005; **Figure 1**) organize stigma within an identity threat model that integrates how people assess and cope with stigma-related stress. When an individual possesses a devalued social identity, he or she encounters situations that threaten one's identity. In such situations, the individual first appraises environmental threats to his or her well-being. Appraisal is influenced by three factors: (1) immediate situational cues (how much a situation conveys the risk of being devalued); (2) collective

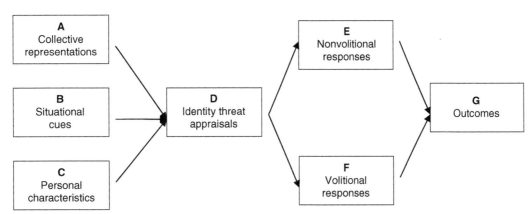

Figure 1 An identity-threat model of stigma. Reprinted with permission from the Annual Review of Psychology, Volume 56 © 2005 by Annual Reviews www.annualreviews.org.

representations (knowledge of cultural stereotypes that shape a situation's meaning), and (3) personal characteristics of the individual (e.g., how sensitive that individual might be to stigma). Identity threat occurs when an individual appraises the stigma present in the situation as being harmful to one's social identity and as surpassing one's ability to cope with this stress. An individual may then respond to this stigma-induced stress in two ways: (1) through an involuntary stress response (e.g., anxiety) and (2) a voluntary coping response. Voluntary coping responses consist of cognitive strategies that reduce threat to the self in reaction to stressful events. For example, a stigmatized individual may attribute a negative outcome (e.g., not getting a job promotion) to discrimination (e.g., racial hiring preferences) rather than to one's own efforts or abilities at work. Stress due to identity threat then affects individuals through impacts on self-esteem, academic achievement, and health.

Other social psychologists have added emotional and behavioral aspects of stigma to its cognitive aspects. The cognitive, affective, and behavioral components of stigma are represented as stereotypes, prejudice, and discrimination. Stereotypes are cognitive representations that describe individuals as having characteristics that are inaccurate or exaggerated. An example might be people with mental illness being seen as unable to care for themselves. Prejudice in turn refers to a negative emotional reaction toward a stigmatized person. For example, a person might feel fearful toward someone who has mental illness. Discrimination then refers to negative behaviors enacted toward a stigmatized person. An example might be an employer not hiring someone with mental illness. These three components are seen as causally related to one another. Endorsement of negative stereotypes may thus lead to prejudice and subsequent discrimination. The perceived controllability of the stigmatized person's condition is central to this process. For example, if others view the stigma to be controllable, this will greatly influence how they will feel about (e.g., anger) and then behave toward (e.g., seek to punish) the stigmatized person.

Watson and River (2005) present a model of personal response to mental illness stigma that parallels the stereotyping – prejudice – discrimination model. The first step of self-stigma takes place when stigmatized individuals are aware of the negative images about their group (self-stereotyping). The second step occurs when stigmatized individuals agree with and apply the stereotype to the self. This leads to negative emotional reactions such as low self-esteem (self-prejudice). The final step results in behavioral responses by the individual (such as not pursuing work) which limits life opportunities (self-discrimination).

Watson and River further propose a two-part model to explain the personal response of individuals to stigma (**Figure 2**). An individual first appraises whether an instance of stigma encountered in a specific situation is

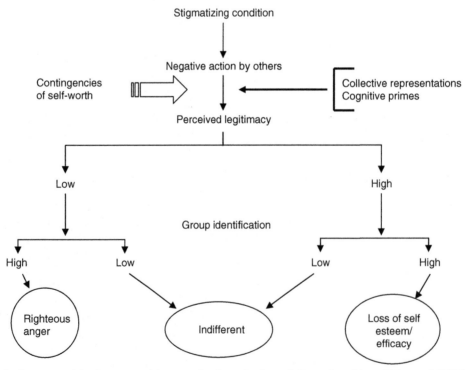

Figure 2 A path diagram explains the personal response to stigma by the self. Reproduced from Kleinman A (2006) *What Really Matters: Living a Moral Life Amidst Uncertainty and Danger*. New York: Oxford University Press.

legitimate or illegitimate. Appraisal is determined through collective representations (which consist of cultural stereotypes and perceived social statuses), which are activated by cognitive primes (information emerging from the situation). After appraisal occurs, whether an individual highly identifies with the broader stigmatized group will determine personal reactions. For example, an individual who perceives stigma based on nationality as illegitimate and who closely identifies as a person from a particular national group will respond with righteous anger and an increase in self-esteem.

Sociological Models of Stigma

In comparison, models based on sociological theory have used labeling theory to describe stigma. This concept, based on symbolic interactionism, proposes that the meaning and value of interpersonal actions are socially constructed. That is, the meaning of deviant behavior is continuously interpreted by how that behavior is described by language and symbols. Social responses to behaviors are shaped by shared cultural descriptions of what the behavior means. For example, a person who hears voices and talks aloud to himself is commonly described as someone who has mental illness, and that his behavior is erratic and unpredictable. The potential dangerousness of such a person is symbolized by how psychiatric patients are locked away and secluded during inpatient treatment. How a person comes to view oneself then arises from perceptions of how others view and respond to him or her. When these self-conceptions become fixed, individuals become socialized into a specific role. These roles are accompanied with behaviors that the individual then is expected to fulfill.

Scheff (1966; **Figure 3(a)**) proposed a labeling theory where deviant labels lead to changed perceptions and social opportunities for an individual. Mental illness stereotypes (i.e., identifying what is considered crazy) are learned as part of socialization and engaging in everyday life. When deviant behaviors repeatedly violate social rules, this may be perceived by others as a sign of mental illness, or a characteristic of the person. Once labeled as mental illness, a patient role may emerge as a master status that dominates other statuses due to its highly discrediting nature. Responses from others (such as rejection from social networks) then limit the person to the role of someone who is mentally ill and block attempts to return to normal social roles. Individuals labeled with mental illness may further conform to their altered roles, which results in future symptomatic behavior. Scheff proposed that labeling was one of the most important factors in continued psychiatric symptoms.

Link *et al.* (1989; **Figure 3(b)**) proposed a Modified Labeling Theory that stated that mental illness labeling and stigma placed people at risk for negative outcomes that may worsen already existing mental disorders. Link *et al.* proposed that all members of a society internalize notions of what it means to be labeled with mental illness. They emphasized two components of these internalized conceptions. These components consist of the degree that all members of society believe that people with mental illness will be devalued (i.e., lose status) and discriminated against (e.g., be denied life opportunities such as employment). Labeling occurs through contact with treatment. At this point, beliefs about how the community will treat a person with mental illness now become personally relevant. Labeled individuals may then respond to perceived future rejection in one of three ways: (1) secrecy or concealing one's treatment history, (2) withdrawal or restricting social contact to people who accept one's condition, and (3) education or changing others' views to ward off negative attitudes. Negative consequences may result from the individual's response to stigma. For example, while a response such as withdrawal may protect patients from some harmful aspects of stigma, it may also limit life chances by reducing opportunities for social contact. These negative impacts on self-esteem, social contacts, and employment opportunities are then seen to increase vulnerability to future episodes of mental disorders.

Models of Stigma That Utilize Perspectives from Society

Another model describes mental illness from the perspective of society that includes an analysis of economic, political, and historical factors (Corrigan *et al.*, 2004; **Figure 4**). Such a framework is important in understanding how stigma may be generated by larger forces in society. Corrigan *et al.* describe two types of structural discrimination. The first, intentional institutional discrimination, occurs when policies of institutions intentionally restrict the rights of people with mental illness. Here the decision-making group of an institution intentionally implements policies to reduce a particular group's opportunities. For example, government legislatures may craft laws that restrict people with mental illness from voting. The second type of structural discrimination takes place when policies limit the rights of people with mental illness in unintentional ways. For example, insurance companies within the United States do not insure mental illness at the same level as physical illnesses because they judge that it would be too expensive. This decision is not specifically intended to discriminate against people with mental illness. However, such a decision results in fewer financial resources being devoted to treating people with mental disorders. What is key in both types of structural discrimination is that people with mental illness are negatively affected by discriminatory policies that take place on broader levels of society.

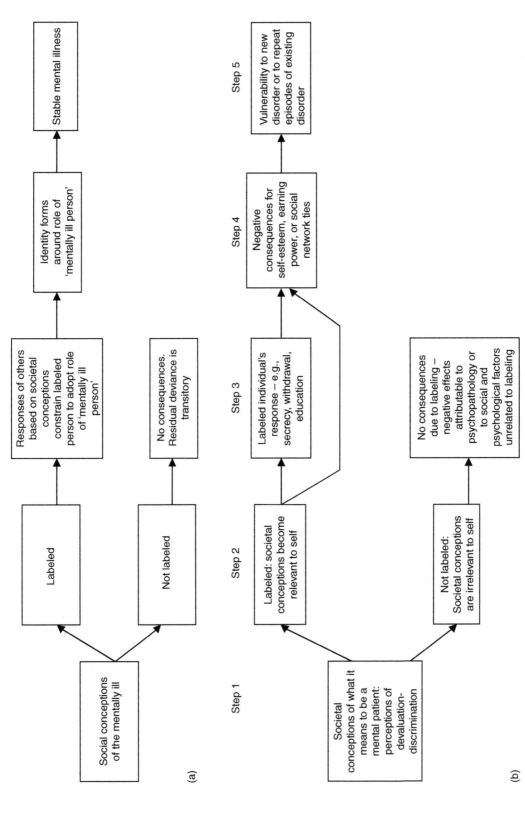

Figure 3 Diagrammatic representation of Scheff's Labeling Model (a) and the Modified Labeling Approach (b). Reproduced from Link BG, Cullen FT, Struning EL, Shrout PD, and Dohrenwend BP (1989) A modified labeling theory approach in the area of mental disorders: An empirical assessment. *American Sociological Review* 54: 100–123.

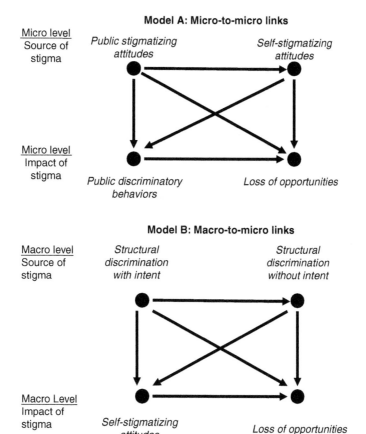

Figure 4 Macro and micro levels of analysis in mental illness stigma and discrimination. Reproduced from Corrigan PW, Markowitz FE, and Watson AC (2004) Structural levels of mental illness stigma and discrimination. *Schizophrenia Bulletin* 30: 481–491.

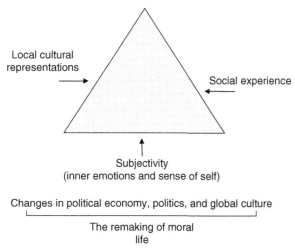

Figure 5 Triangle illustrating the intersection of cultural meanings, social experience and subjectivity. Reproduced from Kleinman A (2006) *What Really Matters: Living a Moral Life Amidst Uncertainty and Danger*. New York: Oxford University Press. By permission of OUP, Inc.

One other perspective, proposed in regards to HIV/AIDS, identifies stigma in a broader framework of power and as central to reproducing means of social control within a society (Parker and Aggleton, 2003). These authors draw from philosophers and sociologists who propose that forms of social control are embedded in each society's formalized way of knowing and perceiving the world. Because these means of social control are seen as natural and accepted, the ability of stigmatized individuals and groups to resist marginalization is limited. These authors argue that stigma is utilized by identifiable actors within social groups who use such social control to legitimate their dominant positions in society.

One final anthropological perspective proposes that stigma is embedded in what is most at stake for sufferers and their social world (Yang *et al.*, 2007; **Figure 5**). What matters most in a local world is determined by the interaction of cultural meanings, social experience, and subjectivity (inner emotions and sense of self). Thus, people within particular social worlds find certain things to greatly matter, such as status, money, life chances, health, good fortune, a job, or relationships. Stigma is felt most powerfully by people in their social contexts by threatening the life domains that matter most to them. For example, in Chinese cultural groups, the effects of stigma are not limited to the individual but are felt most acutely on the family's ability to continue the family lineage. Since both the stigmatized and stigmatizers struggle with the daily activities that make social life matter, understanding what is most valued enables us to understand how stigma shapes the behaviors of both groups. This perspective also enables us to identify the family, health and social service providers, and even the stigmatized persons as potential sources of stigma.

Summarizing the Models of Stigma

In tracing through the above models, we can observe the different mechanisms by which stigma has been seen to affect individuals and groups. Although these models emphasize different components as key to the stigma process (e.g., one highlights the effect of internalized stereotypes, while another emphasizes societal processes), these models can be seen to complement rather than contradict one another. These models also provide valuable perspectives by which to intervene with the negative effects of stigma.

How Stigma Affects Health and Recovery from Illness

Stigma not only negatively impacts a person's social status, but it also detrimentally affects both psychological and physical health. The above models illustrate possible mechanisms by which stigma causes its negative effects. A great deal of research has also demonstrated the harmful effects of stigma on health and recovery, especially among the stigmatized conditions of mental illness and HIV/AIDS.

Both mental illness and HIV/AIDS have been identified by public attitude surveys across cultures as being among the most stigmatized of conditions. The label of mental illness evokes a great deal of negative and fearful reactions. In public attitude surveys, the label of mental illness is commonly linked to adjectives such as dependent and helpless, on the one hand, and dangerous, different, and unpredictable, on the other. AIDS-related stigma differs from mental illness but also is quite negative. Because the primary routes of transmission for HIV – sexual intercourse and sharing of infected needles – are perceived as voluntary behaviors, people infected with HIV are seen to be responsible for their condition. A great amount of stigma is also attached to HIV/AIDS because: (1) it is perceived as contagious, (2) its course is seen to be unalterable, and (3) the illness is apparent to others in its advanced stages. What the two conditions have in common is that the stereotype of dangerousness appears to underlie much of the public's willingness to reject these stigmatized individuals.

These negative stereotypes toward people with mental illness and HIV/AIDS have several harmful effects. First of all, stigma acts as a critical barrier to effective treatment for persons with mental illness and HIV/AIDS. Among mental illnesses, stigma causes two negative effects in regards to treatment: (1) many people with mental illness never pursue treatment or (2) others begin but fail to adhere to prescribed treatment. For example, in a representative national study conducted in the U.S., less than 40% of respondents with mental illness in the past year received ongoing treatment (Kessler *et al.*, 2001). Similarly, fears of AIDS stigma may prevent people at risk for HIV from being tested and seeking assistance for reducing risk of contracting the illness. For example, in China over 90% of the estimated 1 million people who are HIV-positive have not yet been tested for HIV because of the intense fear of stigma (Jing, 2006).

The negative stereotypes associated with mental illness and HIV/AIDS also lead to the devaluation and rejection of people with these conditions. On the individual level, such stigmatized persons face direct discrimination. In one survey of community outpatients with mental illness in the U.S., 42% of respondents reported having been shunned at least sometimes when others learned of their psychiatric treatment (Dickerson *et al.*, 2002). Similarly, people with AIDS have reported suffering from individual discrimination such as being fired from their jobs, evicted from their homes, and denied services. A second form of devaluation occurs through structural discrimination when institutional practices lead to unequal opportunities for stigmatized groups. One prominent example for those with mental illness includes unequal treatment by health insurers toward psychiatric as opposed to physical illnesses. A third form of devaluation takes place through stigmatized individuals themselves, once they have adopted the belief that they will be discriminated against after receiving a stigmatizing label. Once stigma becomes internalized, the patient's manner of coping with stigma (e.g., through withdrawal or secrecy) can result in negative outcomes.

As a result of these processes, stigma has been linked with many negative outcomes for both people with mental illness and HIV/AIDS. The negative psychological effects of stigma among people with mental illness include low self-esteem, depressive symptoms, and less psychological integration with the community. Other harmful effects include constricted social networks, avoidance of non-family members, and noncompliance with treatment programs. Similarly, people with AIDS have been reported to suffer from social isolation, self-blame, increased psychological distress, and self-destructive behaviors. Stigma also limits life opportunities of members of both groups through income loss, increased time of unemployment, and limited access to housing and medical care. The evidence thus overwhelmingly indicates that stigma denies people from both of these stigmatized groups access to important means of recovery. The stigma process also initiates stressors such as rejection and discrimination that make rehabilitation from these chronic illnesses even more difficult to achieve.

Intervening with Stigma: Anti-Stigma Campaigns

Because of stigma's numerous negative effects, intervening with stigma has become a critically important area of research. Further, stigma interventions benefit society by promoting stigmatized individuals' opportunities for recovery and enabling them to become productive citizens. The above models of how stigma works have greatly shaped existing interventions to reduce stigma. Because of the prominent place that negative stereotypes have in the formation of stigma, many anti-stigma campaigns have sought to decrease stigma by changing public attitudes toward stigmatized groups.

In recent years, there have been several anti-stigma campaigns as well as public and private research to reduce stigma. The European Federation of Associations of Families of People with Mental Illness's (EUFAMI) anti-stigma campaign, Zerostigma, began in October 2005, seeking to replace fear with facts about mental illness. Zerostigma works with various health-care organizations, volunteers, and media across Europe to increase knowledge about stigma for those who suffer from mental illness. One of EUFAMI's major contributions to anti-stigma is directing the government's money to be used more efficiently. Another way EUFAMI helps reduce stigma is by evaluating and promoting new research.

Changing Minds is another anti-stigma campaign funded by the United Kingdom Royal College of Psychiatrists. Launched in 1998, this program targets community members ranging from health-care professionals to the general public. They use print and video media to relay an anti-stigma message to others. Another anti-stigma campaign is taking place in over 20 countries with the World Psychiatric Association's Open the Doors campaign in 1996. This program specifically targets the stigma associated with schizophrenia. Further, novel interventions have been developed to address the perspectives of specific community groups, including medical professionals, journalists, school children, law enforcement officials, employers and church leaders. Regarding HIV/AIDS, the Ford Foundation funded the HIV/AIDS Anti-Stigma Initiative by involving community-based organizations in the U.S. to increase awareness and to decrease stigma. This campaign also produces research for those who are stigmatized and for the disease itself.

It should be noted, however, that most public education campaigns have occurred in Western countries (such as Germany and the United Kingdom). Also, the positive effects on public conceptions of mental illness due to such programs have been described as modest in impact. Much research has yet to be done to determine what the content of programs should be to most effectively reduce stigma and what form such programs should take to maximize positive attitude change among the general community (Thornicroft, 2006).

The above campaigns and clinical research on stigma intervention have used one of three common approaches: protest, education, and contact.

Protest

By means of protest, a person or a group objects to negative ideas, images, and attitudes about a stigmatized group. Protesting is an active way to reduce offensive and demeaning representations of stigmatized groups in the media. By decreasing stigmatizing images in the media, protesters believe they can reduce stereotypes and stigmatization. For example, a group called Stigma Busters responds to negative media portrayals of people with mental illness in the United States by using actions ranging from letters of concern to protests such as boycotting. While such actions can lessen certain stigmatizing images and behavior, it does not change the public's stigmatizing attitudes. In fact, protest merely suppresses the targeted negative ideas. Research has shown that when people are forced to suppress negative stereotypes, they become more sensitized to such stereotypes. This in turn may lead to unwanted thoughts about the initial stigmatized group. Additionally, those who suppress stigmatizing ideas and attitudes learn less accurate information about the stigmatized group during educational programs (Corrigan and Penn, 1999).

Education

Education seeks to challenge inaccurate ideas with factual information through the media (such as public announcements, lectures, books, and movies). For example, one form of education might be to expose the public to productive works of people with mental illness. Education is not only useful for the general public, but also for those who are stigmatized. Education gives people who are stigmatized alternate strategies to cope with feelings of difference and shame. Education yields positive results in improving conceptions toward people with mental illness. For example, one study demonstrated that after education, participants showed more willingness to believe that people with psychiatric problems benefit from medical treatment and psychotherapy (Corrigan and Penn, 1999). Another study, conducted in rural Pakistan, showed that educating children through a school-based intervention program improved attitudes toward people with mental illness not just among the children but also positively changed the attitudes of the people who they came into contact with (their parents, friends, and neighbors; see **Figure 6**; Rahman *et al.*, 1998).

The Elimination of Barriers Initiative (EBI), developed by The Center for Mental Health Services, is a large-scale

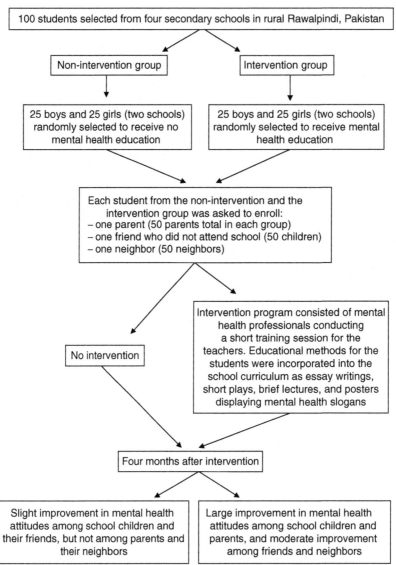

Figure 6 In-depth examination of an educational anti-stigma intervention.

campaign based in the United States that educates the public about inaccurate stereotypes of mental illness. This campaign combats stigma through town meetings, radio, television, and printed announcements, and has reached approximately 150 million people. While EBI is an example of broad-based intervention based on education, it is uncertain whether those who hold stigmatizing views (rather than those who are already aware of and affected by the stigma) were actually exposed to the message and had their views influenced by it.

Contact

The final strategy of contact is accomplished by having personal contact with someone from the stigmatized group. For example, while many people with mental illness work and live among us, they are stigmatized as being unable to work and function normally. Contact gives those who stigmatize an opportunity to engage in a mutual and informal conversation with members of a stigmatized group. These conversations in conjunction with education have led to decreases in stereotyping and stigma among potential stigmatizers. Contact increases acceptance and positive attitudes by exposing community members to people of stigmatized groups who are functioning normally. One study found greater improvements in attitudes after intervention through contact when compared with education alone (Corrigan *et al.*, 2002). It appears that collaborative interaction with a stigmatized person who moderately disconfirms a preexisting stereotype is the most effective form of personal contact.

While each of the three interventions has its specific purpose, these strategies can also be combined. For example, education about a stigmatized group is often combined with the strategies of protest or contact. While contact yields the best results among the three strategies, it is unknown whether stigma is truly decreased or merely suppressed. It is also unclear whether education has an enduring impact on stigma and whether factual information alone is sufficient to bring about change in attitudes. Further, it is not certain whether increasing positive attitudes toward stigmatized persons actually decreases discriminatory behavior toward such individuals. Lastly, stigma's most harmful effects vary by culture, and stigma intervention should be targeted toward areas that most severely limit a group's integration into society. In sum, many areas remain unexplored in regards to stigma intervention, and diminishing the impact of stigma may ultimately depend equally upon policy-makers crafting legislation that combats structural discrimination and more easily allows stigmatized persons to integrate into society. Advancing the study of stigma will better enable researchers and other public health experts to identify those areas most in need of government intervention, to reduce the suffering of stigmatized individuals, and to decrease the burden in the societies to which they belong.

See also: Health-Related Stigma and Discrimination; Historical Views of Mental Illness.

Citations

Corrigan PW, Markowitz FE, and Watson AC (2004) Structural levels of mental illness stigma and discrimination. *Schizophrenia Bulletin* 30: 481–491.

Corrigan PW and Penn DL (1999) Lessons from social psychology on discrediting psychiatric stigma. *American Psychologist* 54(9): 765–776.

Corrigan PW, River PR, Lundin RK, *et al.* (2001) Three strategies for changing attributions about severe mental illness. *Schizophrenia Bulletin* 27(2): 187–195.

Corrigan PW, Rowan D, Green A, *et al.* (2002) Challenging two mental illness stigmas: Personal responsibility and dangerousness. *Schizophrenia Bulletin* 28: 293–310.

Crocker J, Major B, and Steele C (1998) Social stigma. In: Fiske S, Gilbert D and Lindzey G (eds.) *Handbook of Social Psychology*, pp. 504–553. Boston, MA: McGraw-Hill.

Dickenson FB, Sommerville J, Origoni AE, Ringel NB, and Parente F (2002) Experiences of stigma among outpatients with schizophrenia. *Schizophrenia Bulletin* 28: 143–155.

Goffman E (1963) *Stigma: Notes on the Management of Spoiled Identity.* New York: Prentice Hall.

Jing J (2006) Fear and stigma: An exploratory study of AIDS patient narrations in China. In: Kaufman J, Kleinman A and Saich T (eds.) *AIDS and Social Policy in China.* Cambridge, MA: Harvard University Press.

Jones EE, Farina A, Hastorf AH, *et al.* (1984) *Social Stigma: The Psychology of Marked Relationships.* New York: Freeman.

Kessler RC, Berglund PA, Bruce ML, *et al.* (2001) The prevalence and correlates of untreated serious mental illness. *Health Services Research* 36: 987–1007.

Kleinman A (2006) *What Really Matters: Living a Moral Life Amidst Uncertainty and Danger.* New York: Oxford University Press.

Kurzban R and Leary MR (2001) Evolutionary origins of stigmatization: The functions of social exclusion. *Psychological Bulletin* 127(2): 187–208.

Link BG, Cullen FT, Struning EL, Shrout PE, and Dohrenwend BP (1989) A modified labeling theory approach in the area of mental disorders: An empirical assessment. *American Sociological Review* 54: 100–123.

Link BG and Phelan JC (2001) Conceptualizing stigma. *Annual Review of Sociology* 27: 363–385.

Major B and O'Brien LT (2005) The social psychology of stigma. *Annual Review of Psychology* 56: 393–421.

Parker P and Aggleton P (2003) HIV and AIDS-related stigma and discrimination: A conceptual framework and implications for action. *Social Science and Medicine* 57: 13–24.

Rahman N, Mubbashar M, Gater R, and Goldberg D (1998) Randomised trial impact of school mental-health programme in rural rawalpindi, Pakistan. *Lancet* 352: 1022–1026.

Scheff TJ (1966) *Being Mentally Ill: A Sociology Theory.* Chicago, IL: Aldine.

Thornicroft G (2006) *Shunned: Discrimination Against People with Mental Illness.* New York: Oxford University Press.

Watson AC and River LP (2005) A social-cognitive model of personal responses to stigma. In: Corrigan PW (ed.) *On the Stigma of Mental Illness: Practical Strategies for Research and Social Change,* 1st edn. Washington DC: American Psychological Association.

Yang LH, Kleinman A, Link BG, *et al.* (2007) Culture and stigma: Adding mood experience to stigma theory. *Social Science and Medicine* 64(7): 1524–1535.

Further Reading

Corrigan PW (2004) How stigma interferes with mental health care. *American Psychologist* 59(7): 614–625.

Corrigan PW and Gelb B (2006) Three programs that use mass approaches to challenge the stigma of mental illness. *Psychiatric Services* 57(3): 393–398.

Herek GM (1999) AIDS and stigma. *American Behavioral Scientist* 42(7): 1106–1116.

Keusch GT, Wilentz J, and Kleinman A (2006) Stigma and global health: Developing a research agenda. *The Lancet* 367: 525–539.

Lee S, Lee MTY, Chiu MYL, and Kleinman A (2005) Experience of social stigma by people with schizophrenia in Hong Kong. *British Journal of Psychiatry* 186: 153–157.

Link BG, Yang LH, Phelan JC, and Collins PY (2004) Measuring mental illness stigma. *Schizophrenia Bulletin* 30(3): 511–541.

Markowitz FE (2005) Sociological models of mental illness stigma: Progress and prospects. In: Corrigan PW (ed.) *On the Stigma of Mental Illness: Practical Strategies for Research and Social Change,* pp. 129–144. Washington DC: American Psychological Association.

Mead GH (1934) *Mind, Self and Society.* Chicago, IL: University of Chicago Press.

Phelan JC (2005) Geneticization of deviant behavior and consequences for stigma: The case of mental illness. *Journal of Health and Social Behavior* 46: 307–322.

Phelan JC, Link BG, and Meyer J (in press) Stigma and discrimination: one animal or two? *Social Science and Medicine.*

Yang LH and Kleinman A (in press) Face and the embodiment of stigma in China: The cases of schizophrenia and AIDS. *Social Science and Medicine.*

Relevant Websites

http://www.repsych.ac.uk/campaigns/changingminds.aspx – Changing Minds, an anti-stigma campaign against mental illness, which is funded by the United Kingdom Royal College of Psychiatrists.

http://www.eufami.org – The European Federation of Associations of Families of People with Mental Illness.

http://www.hivaidsstigma.org – Ford Foundation's HIV/AIDS Anti-Stigma Initiative.

http://www.stigmaconference.nih.gov – National Institutes of Health Stigma Conference, 2001.

http://www.openthedoors.com – World Psychiatric Association's international effort to combat the stigma of schizophrenia.

Stress and (Public) Health

U Lundberg, Stockholm University, Stockholm, Sweden

The Concept of Stress

In daily life, the concept of 'stress' is frequently used without a precise definition. However, a common meaning of stress is a condition characterized by, for example, a high work pace, complex problem solving, time pressures, or conflicts between different demands, that is, a condition in which one feels that the demands exceed what one can manage.

In scientific research, the concept of 'stress' is not only used both as a stimulus and as a response but also as an interaction between the individual and the environment. Responses to stress involve psychological, behavioral, and bodily components. Stress responses can be induced not only by psychological and psychosocial factors but also by physical (noise, heat, cold, vibration) and biological conditions (exhaustion, infections). Human and animal responses to stress have developed during evolution and contributed to adaptation to various environmental conditions. In animals, the evolutionary principles are still very important. In humans today, however, evolution is not supposed to determine life or death; humans try to protect individuals with major handicaps or chronic diseases in order to give all individuals a chance to spread their genes. It has taken millions of years for the present physiological stress systems to evolve. From a human historical perspective, it is obvious that past environmental conditions quite different from the present ones have formed these response patterns. During the last ten thousand years, human living conditions have undergone dramatic changes, which have accelerated in speed in the recent centuries. The increase in the world population, migration, farming, and technological developments are just a few examples of this. From an evolutionary perspective, this is a very short period in which evolution provides no significant influence on the functioning of human bodily systems. Considering that relatively small adjustments of the human body and biological functions through natural selection or mutations would take thousands of years, from a biological perspective, human beings today are very much the same as they were a hundred thousand years ago.

In order to describe under which conditions stress responses may arise, a number of models have been proposed. All of these models have received empirical support in terms of relations to biological markers of stress, for example, stress hormone secretion, but also in terms of prediction of stress-related health outcomes, such as cardiovascular disorders.

According to one model, psychological stress is caused by an imbalance between perceived environmental demands and the individual's perceived resources to cope with these demands. This means that individual differences in coping abilities and in their interpretation of the situation will determine their stress responses. Based on these appraisal models of stress, not only overstimulation in terms of, for example, a heavy workload or time pressure, but also lack of stimulation can induce imbalance and stress. Understimulation may occur when individuals are unable to use their education, skills, abilities, resources, and experiences. Examples of individuals who may be suffering from this kind of stress are those who are unemployed, retired, on sick-leave, and those who have simple, repetitive, and monotonous work tasks.

Another model of stress, the Cognitive Activation Theory of Stress (CATS), has also been influential. According to the CATS model, stress is defined as 'a negative expectancy outcome.' Stress will occur in a threatening or demanding situation when individuals expect that their actions are not likely to eliminate the threat or help in coping with situational demands. In other words, if one believes that any action will lead to failure, 'hopelessness' would be experienced whereas if one expects that there is no causal relation between one's actions and outcome, feelings of 'helplessness' would be experienced. In so doing, stress will be reduced only when actions and threats are linked by an individual's expectancy of a positive response outcome, that is, successful coping.

A third and very well-known model of stress is the Demand-Control Model, which has been used frequently during the last three decades to describe stress in the work environment. According to this model, high demands combined with lack of influence and control will cause high job strain. High demands combined with a high level of control and influence, however, would contribute to an active and stimulating work situation. Lack of social support has been added as a third factor contributing to stress. Social support involves instrumental and emotional help and appreciation from colleagues and managers. The Demand-Control Model was initially developed to identify stress in industrial work and has been found very useful to predict elevated health risks among workers. In some modern work situations, characterized by information handling and informal work conditions, work stress is likely to be induced in a more complex way. In such jobs, the worker has to define the work tasks and set qualitative and quantitative limits for work performance.

Siegrist (2002) developed a more recent occupational stress model, which is known as the Effort-Reward Imbalance (ERI) model. This model is relevant for identifying stress in the modern work environment. According to this model, the employee has formed a contract with the employer, in which both parties have certain expectations. The employee is expected to carry out a specific work task, and the employer is expected to compensate the employee by some kind of reward. The reward is usually monetary but it could also involve career opportunities, appreciation by colleagues and managers, and occupational status. Stress is induced when this contract is broken and the employee's effort is not adequately rewarded. Characteristics of the employee can also contribute to additional health risks. For example, overcommitted individuals will put increasing effort into their work in order to make sure that they fulfill all possible expectations than those who are not overly committed.

Health Problems in Modern Society

In the beginning of the twentieth century, infectious diseases such as pneumonia, diphtheria, and epidemics were common reasons for death. However, in the industrialized countries today, there has been a shift in the causes of death to diseases with a more complex background, such as cardiovascular disorders and cancer. Myocardial infarctions, stroke, and other cardiovascular diseases cause the death of almost 50% of the population, and various forms of cancer cause the death of about a third of the population. In less developed countries, such as in several countries in Africa, infectious diseases such as acquired immunodeficiency syndrome (AIDS), malaria, diphtheria, and pneumonia are still common causes of death. In these countries, women as well as their infants are also at risk of dying during childbirth.

However, the major health problems affecting the working population in the industrialized countries today are nonfatal disorders with a complex and multifactorial etiology, where stress seems to play an important role. Although these disorders cause absenteeism from work, illness, and an enormous economic societal burden, they may not necessarily increase mortality. For instance, women generally report more health problems than men, but women usually live longer.

In Europe, America, Australia, and in many countries in Asia, musculoskeletal disorders, such as neck, shoulder, and back pain, and various mental illnesses, such as chronic fatigue, burnout syndromes, depression, memory impairment, and sleeping problems, are dominating health problems. In addition, behavioral disorders such as drug addictions (alcohol, narcotics) and eating disorders (obesity, bulimia, anorexia) are important public health problems. Among other frequently reported health problems are headaches, gastrointestinal disorders (e.g., irritable bowel syndrome), infections, and type 2 diabetes.

Socioeconomic Status and Health

A typical feature of these disorders is that social, psychological, and behavioral factors interact with exposure to different physical and social environments (Sapolsky, 1998). Considerable health differentials can be found between as well as within countries since health is closely linked to social position, education, income, and income distribution. The mechanisms behind these relationships have been investigated and discussed extensively, but are not yet fully understood (Marmot, 2004).

The association between socioeconomic status (SES) and health exists in all parts of the world (Östlin, 2004). Individuals with higher education, income, and occupational status are almost always healthier and living longer than individuals with lower education, income, and occupational status. In economically poor countries, lack of medical care, inadequate nutrition, polluted water, substandard housing, and poor sanitary conditions are important explanations for these health differentials, but in affluent societies other factors linked to SES, such as relative deprivation, life style behaviors (smoking, alcohol, unhealthy food, lack of exercise, violence, etc.), work conditions, and access to social networks are likely to be more important (Adler *et al.*, 1999). Indeed, understanding the developmental pathways of these various stress-related factors in various communities worldwide could lead to a better understanding of the link between SES and health.

In a recent review summarizing findings on social position and the physiological mediators of the SES–health relationship in different species, Sapolsky (2005) concluded that stress-induced health problems related to social position depend on the stability of the social hierarchy. In relatively stable social hierarchies such as among humans, rats, and mice, where subordinates are exposed to social stressors and low availability of social support, low social rank gives rise to a particular psychophysiological profile. An association based on a reverse causal order is unlikely. Based on his review, psychophysiological profiles of single animals do not predict their subsequent ranks in social groups. In social groups where dominance has to be repeatedly and physically defended (e.g., among male chimpanzees), high social status is associated with elevated physiological arousal and increased risk for adverse health.

Since humans may belong to a number of different hierarchies, social position or rank is more difficult to determine than in animals. For example, an individual in a low-status job or with a low level of education may be a top player in the local football team or receive a lot of prestige as a musician or as a performing artist.

In addition, early-experienced SES has been linked to health over time. Parents' SES seems to influence their children's health status during childhood as well as adulthood. Thus, describing the physiological mechanisms linking SES to health can be expected to be more complex in humans than in animals. Measures of social position, income, education, and rank in social hierarchies may also differ. Nevertheless, the SES–health associations are very consistent in humans (Marmot, 2004).

Bodily Responses to Stress

Mental stress causes bodily reactions. By signals from the cortex, other centra in the brain, such as thalamus, hypothalamus, and hippocampus, are influenced and, in turn, send signals via nerves, hormones, and/or the immune system to other centra and, eventually, to all parts of the body. These bodily responses include the cardiovascular, the immune, and the gastrointestinal systems, the muscles, sleep, and healing processes, to name only a few. Via feedback mechanisms, the brain is informed about these bodily responses and thus regulates various systems in order to keep, for example, an adequate heart rate or blood pressure. However, under certain conditions, such as under chronic stress, these regulatory mechanisms might fail and initiate vicious circle processes through which inadequate or exaggerated responses will contribute to negative health outcomes. For example, an increase in heart rate due to stress may enhance the individual's perception of stress and thus induce an additional increase in heart rate, as well as other biological changes. Two neuroendocrine systems are of particular importance in coping with stressful conditions: the sympathetic adrenal medullary system (SAM) and the hypothalamic pituitary adrenocortical (HPA) axis.

The SAM system is activated by sympathetic nerve stimulation from the hypothalamus. It stimulates the adrenal medulla to secrete the two catecholamines epinephrine and norepinephrine into the blood stream. Elevated epinephrine levels in the blood will increase heart rate, cause vasodilation of the arteries in the muscles and the brain, and stimulate lipolysis, that is, the release of energy in terms of glucose and lipids into the blood. Norepinephrine is also a transmitter substance in the sympathetic nervous system. During activation of this system, norepinephrine will be released into the blood from sympathetic nerve endings. It is important to mention that it also has an important role in controlling blood pressure homeostasis by vasoconstriction of the blood vessels. During stress, vasoconstriction of the blood vessels will cause a redistribution of blood from the gastrointestinal system and the skin to the muscles and the brain, as well as contribute to an increased supply of energy and oxygen to the cells. This will happen in less than a minute after stress exposure, and this energy mobilization will increase the individual's possibilities to survive by

fight and flight in a threatening situation. Both, epinephrine and norepinephrine can be measured in blood and in urine.

The HPA axis is also activated by signals from the cortex. By means of the hypothalamus and hippocampal formation, the pituitary is affected by hormonal signals (corticotropin releasing factor, CRF) and responds by increasing the secretion of ACTH (adrenocorticotropin hormone). Through the blood stream, ACTH will stimulate the adrenal cortex to secrete cortisol. It takes about 30 min after exposure to a stressful situation for the cortisol level to reach its peak. Cortisol affects the metabolism in the cells and has an important role in controlling the immune system (antiinflammatory effects). Moreover, this system prepares the organism for sustained stress exposure. Cortisol can be measured in blood, urine, and saliva.

In an acute stress situation, for example, in response to a sudden physical threat, the elevated levels of stress hormones will start a series of bodily responses. There is an increase in heart rate and blood pressure and a rapid release of energy from the liver in terms of glucose and lipids into the blood stream, metabolic activity is attenuated (decreased salivary production and gastrointestinal activity), reproductive activity is reduced (decreased secretion of sex hormones), and some of the immune functions are activated during an acute stress response. In addition, pain sensitivity is reduced, pupils are dilated, concentration will narrow in on the immediate threat (tunnel vision), and certain memory systems will be strengthened. As a result, more energy to the muscles and the brain will increase physical and mental capacity. Reduced pain sensitivity will make the individual capable to continue to fight or run, even in the case of tissue damage, and increased coagulation will reduce bleeding. By remembering under which circumstances the threat appeared, the individual will also have a better chance to avoid similar threats in the future. In conclusion, this well-orchestrated series of actions in various systems will increase the individual's mental and physical resources to cope with an acute physical threat, but it is less adequate or may even be harmful during mentally induced stress. In addition, the responses to chronic or long-term stress may be quite different, and sometimes even the opposite series of actions can occur. Chronic stress may cause increased pain sensitivity and impaired immune and memory functions. During chronic stress, activity in the HPA axis is particularly important.

Stress as a Health-Promoting or Health-Damaging Factor

In modern society, exposure to mental and psychosocial stress is probably more common than exposure to physical threats. Under conditions of psychological stress, an increase in heart rate, blood pressure, and blood lipid levels may be more harmful than protective. For example, it has been reported that psychological strain contributes to cardiovascular disorders. In addition, psychosocial stress conditions in terms of economic difficulties, relational problems, unemployment or threat of unemployment, unsatisfactory working conditions, to name a few, are usually more long-lasting than physical threats or demands. In response to physically exhausting work, it is possible to take a break in order to rest and recover, whereas psychosocial problems exist steadily over time and may influence the individual continuously. Today, just as psychological stress exposure is more common than physical threats, individuals are more likely to experience long-term or chronic stress induced by psychosocial conditions rather than by physical demands or threats.

In ancient times, it is likely that acute threats to survival, induced by confrontations with dangerous animals, human enemies, hunting, extreme weather conditions, and so forth, were the dominating sources of stress. Between these acute stress episodes and moments with sufficient access to food, it is possible that individuals had more time to sleep, rest, and recover. Lack of artificial light also made it necessary to be inactive or sleep during a large part of the day. Although human beings are rather resistant and can survive under long-term stressful conditions, there is likely to be an upper limit for each individual beyond which stress-related symptoms start to appear. For long-term health and survival, an adequate balance is necessary between energy mobilization and rest and recovery. As pointed out by Sapolsky (1998), animals living in their natural habitats, such as zebras on the savannah, are unlikely to develop stress-related disorders. He explains that animals do not spend time on rumination after a stressful event by thinking about what could have happened if they had not escaped from a lion or another predator. Animals are also less likely to anticipate and become stressed by possible future threats. As a consequence, after an acute stressful event, animals will unwind rapidly and change from catabolic (energy mobilization) to anabolic processes, such as eating, digesting, healing, mating, and sleeping.

In order to describe when stress responses are health protective versus health damaging, McEwen (1998) and others have proposed the Allostatic Load Model. Allostasis refers to bodily responses necessary for adjustment, protection, and survival. An adequate economic and healthy response to acute stress exposure means a rapid activation of the allostatic systems in order to cope with the stressor and, at the end of the stress exposure, a rapid return to baseline in order to be able to rest and recover. According to the Allostatic Load Model, health problems may be caused by too frequent activation of the allostatic systems or by an inability to shut off these responses. Also an inadequate (blunted) response, due to dysregulation or exhaustion of a system, may cause health problems because an inability to mobilize resources by one system may cause compensatory overactivation of other systems.

Sympathetic arousal is considered to reflect an active 'defense reaction' (fight-or-flight), whereas activation of the HPA axis is representing a 'defeat reaction.' In species living in relatively stable social hierarchies, subordination has been linked to activation of the HPA axis (secretion of cortisol or hydrocortisone in primates and corticosterone in rodents) (Sapolsky, 2005). It has been suggested that the HPA axis is influenced by social position even in humans, where the SAM system is involved, too (Cohen *et al.*, 2006). Such findings, however, are not consistent (Kristenson *et al.*, 2004).

In conclusion, the physiological stress systems have evolved due to their protective role in human and animal development. These systems are also necessary for survival today, but as indicated above, the threats and demands of modern society can be quite different from conditions that faced our ancestors. The mobilization of energy induced by the bodily responses to stress will enhance resources for 'fight or flight,' but is less adequate in situations requiring mental problem solving or an ability to deal with conflicting information, to name only a few.

Stress-Related Disorders

Sympathetic activation involves elevated blood pressure and heart rate, and increased cholesterol levels. Sustained sympathetic activation is considered to contribute to coronary heart disease. Dysregulation or hyperactivity of the HPA axis contributes to a number of health problems, such as coronary heart disease, type 2 diabetes, reduced immune function, and memory impairment.

An association between stress and coronary heart disease has been demonstrated in a number of studies. In the 1970s, men characterized by the stress-related type A behavioral pattern, that is, time urgency, impatience, hostility, and competitiveness, were found to be at significantly greater risk of developing a myocardial infarction compared to their more relaxed type B counterparts, independent of other physical risk factors such as hypertension, blood lipid levels, cigarette smoking, and diabetes. Type A individuals have also been found to respond to stress with more elevated stress hormones and cardiovascular responses. Work stress as measured by the Demand-Control Model or the Effort-Reward Imbalance Model has also been linked to cardiovascular illness in prospective studies (Siegrist, 2002).

The mechanisms linking psychosocial stress and behavior to cardiovascular disorders, such as myocardial infarction, have been investigated extensively. The following series of events has been suggested:

1. Psychosocial stress will cause an increase in blood pressure and heart rate, as well as a release of energy in terms of glucose and free fatty acids into the blood stream.

2. Frequent or chronic elevation of the blood pressure will contribute to structural changes in the arteries, for example in the coronaries supplying blood to the heart itself (myocardium).

3. High blood pressure will lead to thicker and stiffer walls of the blood vessels and a smaller diameter (lumen) will reduce the blood flow, which will, due to higher vascular resistance, increase the blood pressure even more.

4. A high heart rate and elevated blood pressure may cause damage to the inner walls (endothelium) of the blood vessels, particularly where a vessel branches off.

5. Fatty acids will be built into the walls at these places on the blood vessels and form foam cells in the intima (atherosclerosis).

6. The high level of blood lipids during stress will enhance the atherosclerotic process.

7. A narrowing of the coronary arteries due to thicker walls and atherosclerosis will reduce the blood to the myocardium. The individual will feel pain (angina) when exposed to physical and mental effort requiring more energy and oxygen to the heart.

8. Blood clotting (coagulation) increases during stress and will in combination with atherosclerosis further increase the risk of a myocardial infarction, that is, a complete obstruction of the blood flow to parts of the heart muscle.

9. Furthermore, atherosclerotic arteries have been found to respond paradoxically to stressful demands by vasoconstriction rather than by vasodilation (Harris and Matthews, 2004).

Behavioral factors influenced by stress, such as unhealthy food habits (fast food, lack of vegetables and fruit), sedentary behavior, cigarette smoking, and alcohol abuse, will contribute to cardiovascular risk and to the metabolic syndrome (see below).

Early stress exposure and responsivity to stress may determine the function of the stress systems later in life as illustrated in animal studies (Adler et al., 1999). It has also been found that elevated blood pressure reactivity at the age of 20 may predict increased risk of hypertension 20 years later.

High cortisol levels cause an accumulation of fat in the central parts of the body, due to the high density of cortisol receptors on the fat cells. In addition, cortisol contributes to a decrease in the secretion of anabolic hormones, such as sex and growth hormones, which reduces muscle mass in men and contributes to fat distribution from hips and buttocks to the abdominal region (visceral fat) in women. This visceral fat is rich in energy, and free fatty acids are readily released into the blood. In heavy physical work this resource supports the muscles with energy, but in response to psychosocial stress the same release of lipids into the blood increases the atherosclerotic process. Patients suffering from Cushing's syndrome, a condition caused

by very high cortisol levels, demonstrate all these effects in a dramatic way. However, similar but less extreme effects can be seen in individuals exposed to long-term stress. By reducing cortisol levels, some of these processes can be reversed. It has also been suggested that cortisol mediates the effect of the intra-uterine environment on adult circulatory disease, but the evidence is contradictory.

Overactivity of the HPA axis causes insulin resistance and thus contributes to type 2 diabetes. The body responds with increased insulin secretion, which may not be enough to compensate for this effect. Consequently, the cells' uptake of glucose from the blood will be reduced and they will lack energy. The combination of high blood pressure, high lipid levels, and abdominal fat is commonly referred to as the metabolic syndrome (Grundy et al., 2005), which is linked to cardiovascular disease as well as to type 2 diabetes. Life style factors such as cigarette smoking, a high-fat diet, and sedentary behaviors are also associated with this syndrome.

An additional consequence of long-term stress and chronic overactivity of the HPA axis is impairment of the immune system, with increased risk of infections and delayed healing processes. Cohen (2005) has performed a series of controlled experiments in order to demonstrate how susceptibility to the common cold increases with the amount of chronic psychosocial stress in a dose–response fashion, and that this association is mediated by impaired immune functions. It has also been shown that chronic stress and depression contribute to a more rapid deterioration of the immune system of HIV patients, reducing the time before AIDS develops. Social support seems to have the opposite effect. It not only increases the time before AIDS develops but also reduces the risk of viral infection irrespective of stress level (Cohen, 2005).

Cortisol serves as a reliable marker of HPA activity in humans. Measurements from saliva, in particular, have several advantages as they reflect plasma levels and contain free (active) cortisol where the concentration is unrelated to saliva flow. Another benefit is that samples can be stored at room temperature for up to three weeks. Saliva samples are also easy to collect without interfering with the participants' normal environment or causing any pain or discomfort. The cortisol-awakening response and the difference between morning and evening levels seem to be of particular importance. Chronic stress and depression have been found to be associated with a flatter diurnal curve, attenuated responses to stress, and elevated baseline levels. High SES and psychological well-being seem to reduce HPA activity (Ryff et al., 2004), but the results are inconsistent. Specific conditions such as burnout syndromes and posttraumatic stress disorders have been found to be associated with suppressed cortisol levels.

The role of stress in gastrointestinal disorders such as irritable bowel syndrome and ulcers has been discussed for a long time. When a bacterium, Helicobacter pylori, was found to be responsible for the development of stomach ulcers, the role of stress in this disorder was questioned. However, most do not develop ulcers despite the fact that they have this bacterium, and some individuals develop ulcers without *Helicobacter pylori*. According to Sapolsky (1998), the gastrointestinal system (saliva production, stomach function, and intestinal activity) is not prepared to digest food after a period of stress because the mucous membrane in the stomach is thinner. The release of hydrochloric acid in response to food intake is therefore likely to damage the inner walls of the stomach and give the helicobacter a chance to invade the stomach wall.

Memory impairment (episodic memory) is also caused by high cortisol levels due to a breakdown of the dendrite connections between the neurons of the hippocampal formation in the brain. By reducing cortisol levels, these connections are reestablished and memory functions can be restored.

Despite considerable improvements of the physical work environment such as less heavy lifting and better ergonomic conditions, musculoskeletal disorders (MSD) remain a major health problem and constitute one of the most important reasons for long-term sick leave from work. In addition, neck, shoulder, and back pain are common not only in heavy physical work but also in jobs requiring very little physical strength but which may be psychologically stressful, such as work at a computer and light assembly work. This indicates that other factors, such as mental and psychosocial stress, are likely to play an important role in these disorders, a notion that is supported by epidemiological studies showing that work stress may predict MSD. In order to explain how long-term but low muscular activity may develop into muscular pain problems, a number of different models have been proposed (Lundberg and Melin, 2002). One of these models, the Cinderella Hypothesis, is based on an orderly recruitment of motor units in the trapezius muscle, covering the neck, shoulders and upper part of the back, in response to increased muscular force. At low levels of force, motor units with low thresholds are activated first and remain activated until complete relaxation of the muscle. Under long-term and low levels of muscle activity, these motor units may become exhausted and various degenerative processes may start that eventually lead to pain conditions. Recently, it has been demonstrated that mental stress may activate the same motor units as physical demands and, consequently, it may keep these low-threshold motor units active even in the absence of biomechanical work. As mental and psychosocial stress can be long-lasting, this may be an important factor for the development of muscle pain in psychologically stressful but physically light work. Additional reasons for the development of muscle pain due to psychological stress are the lack of time for healing of damaged muscle fibers

that are constantly active and the lack of adequate signals of fatigue when very little muscular capacity is used. Under such conditions, the individual may continue to work until a chronic pain syndrome develops, without any awareness of motor unit exhaustion.

Muscle pain associated with psychological factors at the workplace can be explained by a blocking of pauses in muscle activity unrelated to the actual biomechanical work being performed. This will reduce restitution and contribute to sustained activity in low-threshold motor units. This is consistent with data showing that women unable to relax during breaks at work, and women with few 'EMG-gaps,' were more likely to develop pain syndromes (trapezius myalgia) during their first year in a new job involving repetitive tasks than their counterparts in the workplace (Veiersted *et al.*, 1993).

Additional explanatory models for stress-induced muscle pain are based on the following:

- the effects of stress-induced hyperventilation on blood pH-levels (alkalosis) leading to muscle tension and increased sensitivity to stress hormones;
- the interaction between nerves and stretching of blood vessels in the muscle, contributing to the secretion of substances increasing pain sensitivity;
- stress-induced dysfunction of the muscle spindles regulating muscle force and coordination of movements, which may start a vicious circle of successively increased muscle tension and an accumulation of pain-inducing substances.

Because the responses to stress are part of a dynamic process, single measures showing high or low levels of stress hormones are usually not sufficient to identify health risks. Chronic stress seems to change the regulation of various physiological processes rather than causing high or low activity in specific systems. This could happen due to excessive and/or long-term stress hormone secretion, combined with high or low regulation of receptor sensitivity.

Whereas some disorders, such as hypertension, atherosclerosis, hyperlipidemia, and diabetes, can be diagnosed reliably by medical examinations and laboratory tests, a large number of disorders, termed as subjective health complaints or medically unexplained symptoms, cannot be objectively confirmed. Muscular pains, stomach discomfort, headaches, and various psychological problems (depression, chronic fatigue, burnout syndrome, sleep problems) can only be measured by self-reports. Similarly, in medical examinations of these disorders, the physician has to make the diagnosis on the basis of the patient's subjective reports. These disorders usually have a multifactorial etiology and represent the most common reasons for absence due to sickness from work. Stress is assumed to play an important role in the development of subjective health complaints.

Gender Differences in Stress-Related Health

Women generally report more health problems, seek more medical care, and use more medication than men. Yet women usually live longer, which may seem like a health paradox. It is important to mention that gender differences in longevity vary between countries. The most pronounced gender difference, of about 13 years, is seen in Russia. In other European countries and in North America, the corresponding gender differences vary between four and eight years. In poor countries, where women are at great risk of dying during childbirth, there are smaller or no gender differences in longevity, and in some countries, men may even live longer than women. The 'health paradox' in most countries may be due to other reasons than the nonfatal health problems affecting people in daily life.

In industrialized countries in Europe and North America, men's shorter life span is due to a number of factors, such as life style, work conditions, risk behaviors, and biological factors, many of which are stress-related. Women usually eat healthier food, exercise more, and less often drink excessive amounts of alcohol. Cigarette smoking has, until recently, been more common among men than among women, and continues to be the case in many countries. However, in Europe and North America smoking has decreased among men and increased (or remained common) among women, which is reflected in an increasing incidence of death from lung cancer among women. On the other hand, men are still dying from lung cancer and cardiovascular disorders due to decades of cigarette smoking. With regard to work conditions, men are more often exposed to hazardous conditions at the job whereas fatal accidents at work are rather unusual among women. In addition, men more often expose themselves to various risks and neglect to use protective means or follow proper safety instructions for dangerous equipment, not only at work but also in traffic. As a consequence, men die more often than women due to accidents, particularly in car and motorcycle accidents. Men also commit suicide more often than women, although suicide attempts are more common among women. Compared with men, women also seem to be more attentive to minor symptoms. Combined with seeking medical care and the more frequent use of medication, this may protect women from more serious diseases. However, another important explanation for why men die earlier than women is gender differences in age when cardiovascular diseases appear. Although women die of myocardial infarctions, strokes, or other cardiovascular disorders about as often as do men, they seem to be somewhat protected before menopause. Specifically, before the age of 50, myocardial infarctions are 3–4 times more common among men than women. After menopause, when women's estrogen production ceases, their risk of cardiovascular diseases increases and,

consequently, they often contract and die due to cardiovascular diseases when they are older than do men.

With regard to gender differences in nonfatal health problems, a number of factors are likely to contribute, such as biological factors, violence, and work conditions. From a stress perspective, gender differences in type of job and work tasks, as well as in total workload, may be of importance for health. Women and men often have different types of jobs and even when they have the same job they often do different tasks. For example, as physicians, women are often working within emotionally demanding specialties, such as geriatrics and psychiatry, where patients remain for long periods of time because they recover slowly or not at all, whereas men work within surgery and cardiology, where treatment usually is more efficient and rapid and the long-term emotional load therefore is likely to be less pronounced.

Women more often than men are performing repetitive tasks, which are associated with lack of unwinding after work and with health problems such as upper extremity disorders. As lack of rest and recovery seems to be an important health risk, these findings seem relevant for gender differences in health. Occupations dominated by women are also often characterized by low control and lack of autonomy, which according to the Demand-Control Model are likely to induce job strain and health problems.

With regard to total workload, unpaid work from household duties and child care may in some cases contribute to work overload and lack of opportunities for rest and recovery, a situation which is more common for women than for men. Despite women's equal participation in the paid work force, women still carry the primary responsibility for child care and other unpaid duties at home. Consequently, the total workload (sum of paid and unpaid work) of full-time-employed women is greater than that of men, particularly in families with children. Women's employment *per se* is generally associated with positive health consequences, but there may be a limit at which the combined load from paid and unpaid work responsibilities becomes a health problem. For example, in a recent study comparing paid and unpaid workload in matched groups of full-time-employed men and women, it was found that more women than men had a total workload exceeding 80 hours per week and that women reported more conflicts between paid and unpaid work. Also in these matched groups, women reported significantly more symptoms than men. In recent years, the prevalence of stress-related health problems has increased dramatically in many industrialized countries and the gender differences have become even more pronounced.

In order to compare stress and work conditions in men and women, several studies have been performed on full-time-employed and highly educated women and men matched for age, occupation, education, and number of children (Lundberg, 2002). Measurements of stress levels during and after work show that there are no pronounced gender differences during work. However, men generally unwind rapidly at the end of the work day, whereas women's physiological stress levels remain high for hours after work. Both women and men report a peak total workload between 35 and 40 years of age. As would be expected, the number of children at home was found to be of considerable importance for the total workload in terms of hours per week. In families with no children at home, the total workload was about the same, that is, a little more than 60 hours per week. However, in families with three or more children, women's total workload was almost 90 hours and men's total workload was about 70 hours. The conflict between demands increased and the control over household work decreased with an increase in number of children at home.

In families with small children at home, the number of extra hours in paid work (overtime) has been associated with elevated epinephrine levels during weekends in women but not in men. Moreover, women who regularly work more than 50 hours per week were found to have twice as high cortisol levels in the morning during the weekend compared with women working fewer hours. In a study of 600 000 male and 400 000 female workers it was found that overtime at work (10 hours or more per week) was associated with elevated risk of myocardial infarction during a one year follow-up for women but not for men. However, in a study of telework among women and men, it was found that men had significantly higher epinephrine levels than women in the evening after working from the home but not when working at the office, indicating that men continued to work in the evening when working from the home.

The influence of mental stress on women's muscular tension seems to be enhanced in repetitive physical work. Jobs combining mental and physical demands, for example, data entry and assembly work, which are often held by women, may in turn form a particular risk for the development of neck and shoulder disorders. Although biomechanical factors and mental stress seem to contribute to muscle tension in both men and women, lack of influence over the work–rest balance, repetitive work tasks, and unpaid work responsibilities may contribute to keep women's stress levels and muscle tension elevated off the job as well. Furthermore, women generally report more sleeping problems than men. As sleep is the most important form of rest, where many important anabolic processes are activated, lack of sleep may contribute to the allostatic load in women.

Research indicates that the stress of employed women is determined by an interaction between conditions at work and conditions at home, whereas men respond more selectively to the specific stress situations at work. Men's stress levels seem to be determined by their actual stress exposure at work, which means that they are better able to relax compared with women when they come home in the evening and during weekends. The most stress-inducing factors may consist of the anticipation of future commitments and events. This is consistent with the fact that stress from paid and unpaid work interacts more for women than for men and that women's occupational stress may not always be seen in terms of elevated physiological stress levels at work, but may just as well be reflected in elevated physiological arousal at home. Indeed, total workload, role conflicts, responsibilities, and family issues influence women's life and stress responses in a complex way.

In conclusion, the different roles occupied by men and women are likely to have negative as well as positive health consequences. Work overload and role conflicts are assumed to add to the 'wear and tear' of the organism according to the Allostatic Load Model. However, occupying different roles may also increase social and economic status and serve as a buffer against stress-related ill health. Yet, one role may also 'spill over' into other roles. Therefore, public health efforts to improve health gaps between men and women need to incorporate both family and work life.

Positive Health

There are considerable individual differences in sensitivity to stress exposure. Although an overwhelming amount of research has been focused on psychosocial factors contributing to ill health, some studies have been performed in order to investigate factors contributing to good health and protection against stress. Social support and high social status are examples of factors known to protect against stress-related disorders.

Ryff et al. (2004) have identified six factors contributing to 'positive health' or 'psychological well-being': self-acceptance, positive relations with others, autonomy, environmental mastery, personal growth, and purpose in life. These factors are measured by the Ryff Psychological Well-Being Scale. High scores on this scale are associated with physical and mental health, longevity, and a buffer against stressful life events. As mentioned above, psychological well-being has also been linked to biological markers.

Sense of coherence (SOC) is another concept used to describe factors contributing to good health. Conceptually, it includes perceptions of the environment as structured, predictable, and understandable. A well-known instrument measuring dimensions of manageability, meaningfulness, and comprehensibility has been developed for measuring SOC. In recent studies, it has been shown that women with high SOC have lower systolic blood pressure, better lipid profiles, and lower allostatic load.

Conclusions

Stress is a major health problem in most industrialized countries today. Part of the population seems to suffer from stress induced by work overload, time pressures, and too much responsibility, whereas another part of the population is suffering from stress induced by unemployment, economic problems, and understimulation. Whatever the underlying cause, stress influences various bodily functions that are at times health protective and at others health damaging. Short-term stress exposure is usually not a health risk, whereas long-term stress exposure, even on a low level, may contribute to symptoms by influencing various bodily organs and functions. Stress may also influence health indirectly by various risk behaviors such as unhealthy food habits, lack of physical exercise, cigarette smoking, drug abuse, accidents, and suicide.

By definition, stress means activation of physiological systems and mobilization of energy, that is, a catabolic response, which in the long run has to be balanced by anabolic processes. The human body is rather robust and may be activated rather frequently, intensely, and for long periods of time without health problems. However, sooner or later, these processes have to be replaced by anabolic processes, such as digestion, healing, rest, and reproduction. The long-term balance between catabolic and anabolic processes becomes critical for health. Research indicates that women and individuals in low-status positions are at particular risk of stress-related disorders. Today, it is possible that lack of relaxation is an even more important health problem than the absolute level of mental and physical stress exposure.

Acknowledgments

This article has been prepared with support from the Swedish Research Council and the Swedish Council for Working Life and Social Research.

See also: Happiness, Health & Altruism; Health Behavior and Risk Factors; Mental Health Etiology: Social Determinants; Mental Health and Physical Health (Including HIV/AIDS); Mental Health: Morbidity and Impact.

Citations

Adler NE, Marmot M, McEwen B, and Stewart J (eds.) (1999) Socioeconomic status and health in industrial nations: Social, psychological and biological pathways. *Annals of the New York Academy of Science* Volume 896.
Cohen S (2005) The Pittsburgh common cold studies: Psychosocial predictors of susceptibility to respiratory infectious illness. *International Journal of Behavioral Medicine* 12: 123–131.
Cohen S, Doyle WJ, and Baum A (2006) Socioeconomic status is associated with stress hormones. *Psychosomatic Medicine* 68: 414–420.
Grundy SM (2005) Diagnosis and management of the metabolic syndrome. *Circulation* 112: 285–290.
Harris KF and Matthews KA (2004) Interactions between autonomic nervous system activity and endothelial function: A model for the development of cardiovascular disease. *Psychosomatic Medicine* 66: 153–164.
Kristenson M, Eriksen HR, Sluiter JK, Starke D, and Ursin H (2004) Psychobiological mechanisms of socioeconomic differences in health. *Social Science and Medicine* 58: 1511–1522.
Lundberg U (2002) Psychophysiology of work: Stress, gender, endocrine response and work-related upper extremity disorders. *American Journal of Industrial Medicine* Suppl. 2, 383–392.
Lundberg U and Melin B (2002) Stress in the development of musculoskeletal pain. In: Linton S (ed.) *Avenues for the Prevention of Chronic Musculoskeletal Pain and Disability*, pp. 165–179. Amsterdam: Elsevier Science.
Marmot M (2004) *Status Syndrome: How Our Position on the Social Gradient Affects Longevity and Health.* London: Bloomsbury Publishing.
McEwen BS (1998) Stress adaptation and disease: Allostasis and allostatic load. *New England Journal of Medicine* 338: 171–179.
Östlin P (2004) *Priorities for Research to Take Forward the Health Equity Policy Agenda. Report from the WHO Task Force on Health System Research Priorities for Equity in Health.* Geneva, Switzerland: WHO.
Ryff C, Singer B, and Dienberg Love G (2004) Positive health: Connecting well-being with biology. *Philosophical Transactions of the Royal Society of London* 359: 1383–1394.
Sapolsky R (1998) *Why Zebras Don't Get Ulcers: An Updated Guide to Stress, Stress-Related Disease and Coping.* New York: W H Freeman.
Sapolsky R (2005) The influence of social hierarchy on primate health. *Science* 308: 648–652.
Siegrist J (2002) Effort-reward imbalance at work and health. In: Perrew P and Ganster D (eds.) *Research in Occupational Stress and Well Being, Vol. 2: Historical and Current Perspectives on Stress and Health*, pp. 261–291. New York: Elsevier.
Veiersted KB, Westgaard RH, and Andersen P (1993) Electromyographic evaluation of muscular work pattern as a predictor of trapezius myalgia. *Scandinavian Journal of Work and Environmental Health* 19: 284–290.

Further Reading

Blechman EA and Brownell KD (eds.) (2000) *Behavioral Medicine and Women: A Comprehensive Handbook.* New York and London: Guilford Press.
Frankenhaeuser M, Lundberg U, and Chesney M (eds.) (1991) *Women, Work and Health: Stress and Opportunities.* New York: Plenum Press.
Karasek RA and Theorell T (1990) *Healthy Work: Stress, Productivity, and the Reconstruction of Working Life.* New York: Basic Books.
Kawachi I and Kennedy BP (2002) *The Health of Nations: Why Inequality is Harmful to your Health.* New York: The New Press.
Kolk A, Bekker M, and van Vliet K (eds.) (1999) *Advances in Women and Health Research: Toward Gender-Sensitive Strategies.* Tilburg The Netherlands: Tilburg University Press.
McEwen BS and Lasley EN (2002) *The End of Stress as We Know It.* Washington DC: Joseph Henry Press.
Marmot M (2004) *Status Syndrome: How Our Position on the Social Gradient Affects Longevity and Health.* London: Bloomsbury Publishing.
Wamala S and Lynch J (eds.) (2002) *Gender and Social Inequalities in Health.* Stockholm, Sweden: Studentlitteratur.
Yehuda R and McEwen B (eds.) (2004) Biobehavioral stress response: Protective and damaging effects. *Annals of the New York Academy of Science* Volume 1032.

Women's Mental Health

P S Chandra and V N G P Raghunandan, National Institute of Mental Health and Neuro Sciences, Bangalore, India
V A S Krishna, Washington University School of Medicine, St. Louis, MO, USA

Introduction

It is now widely understood that women's well-being is multifactorial and is not only determined by biological factors and reproduction, but also by the effects of poverty, nutrition, stress, war, migration, and illness. Approaching mental health problems from a female perspective and mainstreaming it requires a broad framework of health for women that addresses mental health throughout the life cycle and in domains of both physical and mental health. First, we present evidence demonstrating that women disproportionately suffer from certain mental disorders and are more frequently subject to social issues that lead to mental illness and psychosocial distress. Subsequently, the article will deal with the nature and types of mental disorders in women; factors contributing to vulnerability; and specific issues such as poverty, migration, HIV, war, natural disasters, and pregnancy-related psychiatric problems. It will also describe landmark studies that have been conducted in the area and report interventions that have been attempted with a public health perspective.

Sex Differences and Mental Disorders

Which Mental Disorders Are More Common in Women?

Mental disorders affect women and men differently: some disorders are more common in women and some express themselves with different symptoms. Researchers are only now beginning to tease apart the contribution of various biological and psychosocial factors to mental health and mental disorders in both women and men.

The disability-adjusted life year data recently tabulated by the World Bank reflect these differences. Depressive disorders account for close to 30% of the disability from neuropsychiatric disorders among women, but only 12.6% of that among men. Conversely, alcohol and drug dependence accounts for 31% of neuropsychiatric disability among men, but accounts for only 7% of the disability among women. These patterns for depression and general psychological distress and substance-abuse disorders are consistently documented in many quantitative studies carried out in societies throughout the world (Murray and Lopez, 1996). **Table 1** describes the sex differences in prevalence of various psychiatric disorders.

Clinical Profile of Various Mental Disorders in Women

Depression

Epidemiological and clinical studies have consistently documented that depression across different cultures is about twice as common in women as in men. Research shows that before adolescence and late in life, females and males experience depression at about the same frequency. Because the gender difference in depression is not seen until after puberty and decreases after menopause, scientists hypothesize that hormonal factors are involved in women's greater vulnerability. In addition, the changing psychological status and role of women in society following puberty may place them in a vulnerable position in times of stress.

The manifestation of depression also tends to be different in women. They very often present with medically unexplained symptoms including vague aches and pains. Though severity has been reported to be similar in both genders, depression in women has been found to be associated with increased functional impairment and rates of suicide attempts are higher than in men. Women also tend to have onset of depression at an earlier age and often become symptomatic in mid-adolescence, while depression in men usually begins in their twenties. Longitudinal studies have shown that women develop more recurrent depression and the individual episodes last longer. Comorbid medical disorders such as thyroid problems, migraine, and rheumatologic disorders are particularly common. In addition, depression in women frequently coexists with other psychiatric disorders, particularly panic disorder and simple phobia. Other psychiatric conditions such as eating disorders and personality disorders are often associated with depression in women and add to functional impairment and diagnostic problems.

Anxiety disorders

Anxiety disorders include generalized anxiety disorder, panic disorder, phobias, and posttraumatic stress disorder (PTSD), with women outnumbering men for each of these illness categories. Women not only have a higher risk of developing posttraumatic stress disorders, but they are also more likely to develop long-term PTSD than males, with higher rates of co-occurring medical and psychiatric problems.

Table 1   Lifetime prevalence of DSM III psychiatric disorders by gender

Psychiatric disorder	ECA[a]		NCS[b]	
	Men (%)	Women (%)	Men (%)	Women (%)
Prevalence of any disorder	36	30	48	50
Schizophrenic disorders	1.2	1.7	–	–
Affective disorders	2.3	5.0	17.5	24.9
Major depression	2.6	7.0	12.9	20
Alcohol abuse and/or dependence	23.8	4.6	19.6	7.5
Drug abuse and/or dependence	7.7	4.8	11.6	4.8
Panic disorder	0.99	2.1	3	6.2
Agoraphobia	3.18	7.86	1	1.6
Social phobia	2.53	2.91	11	13
Obsessive compulsive disorder	2	3	1	2.6
Somatization disorder	0.02	0.23	–	–
Antisocial personality	4.5	0.8	–	–

[a]Data from Robins LN and Regier DA (1991) *Psychiatric Disorders in America: The Epidemiologic Catchment Area Study.* New York: The Free Press.
[b]Data from Kessler RC, Berglund PA, Demler O, *et al.* (2005) Lifetime prevalence and age-of-onset distributions of DSM-IV disorders in the National Comorbidity Survey Replication (NCS-R) *Archives of General Psychiatry* 62(6): 593–602.

Schizophrenia

Schizophrenia is the most chronic and disabling of the mental disorders, affecting about 1% of women and men worldwide. The illness typically appears earlier in men, usually in their late teens or early twenties, while women are generally affected in their twenties or early thirties. Thus, schizophrenia starts later in women compared to men, with a second peak in the menopausal period. The later age of onset confers some protection to women as they are usually better socialized and have a better clinical outcome.

Though the disease is reportedly less severe in women, they may have more depressive symptoms, paranoia, and auditory hallucinations than men and tend to respond better to typical antipsychotic medications. A significant proportion of women experience increased symptoms during the postpartum period and may also have significant problems in bonding with the child. Despite the better clinical outcome, women with schizophrenia often have to face higher stigma and face major problems in assimilating with the mainstream. In addition, they are prone to abuse – both physical and sexual – which puts them at further risk for physical and mental health problems. Additional problems that women with serious mental illness face include problems related to parenting, sexuality, and being more prone to drug side effects such as extrapyramidal symptoms, endocrine side effects, and osteoporosis.

Dementias: Alzheimer's Disease

The main risk factor for developing Alzheimer's disease (AD) is increased age. Studies have shown that while the number of new cases of AD is similar in older adult women and men, the total number of existing cases is somewhat higher in women. Possible explanations include that AD may progress more slowly in women than in men, that women with AD may survive longer than men with AD, and that men, in general, do not live as long as women and die of other causes before AD has a chance to develop.

Caregivers of a person with AD are usually family members – often wives and daughters. The chronic stress often associated with the care-giving role can contribute to mental health problems; indeed, caregivers are much more likely to suffer from depression than the average person. Since women in general are at greater risk for depression than men, female caregivers of people with AD may be particularly vulnerable to depression.

Suicide

Although men are four times more likely than women to die by suicide, women report attempting suicide about two to three times as often as men. Self-inflicted injury, including suicide, ranks ninth out of the ten leading causes of disease burden for females worldwide. A recent study on causes of maternal mortality in the first year after childbirth in the UK reported suicide as being the most common reason for death among women within 1 year of childbirth.

Substance Use

Several studies have reported a marked difference in rates of all substance use, with men outnumbering women. However, complications related to substance use such as alcoholic liver disease, neurological problems including cognitive deficits, and sexual and reproductive consequences of substance use in women lead to substantial disability.

What Are the Factors That Contribute to Increased Vulnerability in Women to Mental Health Problems?

Life Stress and Mental Health Problems in Women

Serious adverse life events are clearly implicated in the onset of depression (**Table 2**). Most work investigating the relationship of stressful life events and major depression has largely or exclusively employed samples of women and few studies have examined sex differences with regard to stress and depression. However, initial research in this area

Table 2 Factors that contribute to increased vulnerability among women

Life stresses
Sexual abuse and coercion
Intimate partner violence
Economic determinants: poverty
Migration
War
Natural disasters
Reproductive health: menstrual cycle, pregnancy, and
  menopause
Hormonal and endocrine factors
Gender disadvantage and discrimination
Medical conditions
Self-esteem and body image issues

has demonstrated that women are three times more likely than men to experience depression in response to stressful events. Brown and Harris were among the first to systematically describe the relationship of life stress to depression and subsequent research has confirmed the role of stress in women's mental health.

One of the first research studies to look at the role of social factors in depression in women was published by George Brown and Tirril Harris in 1978 (Brown and Harris, 1978). This study, conducted in inner city London, delineated three important sets of factors in the causation and manifestation of depression among women. The factors included vulnerability factors (lack of a confiding and intimate relationship, three children under the age of 14 at home, and loss of the mother before the age of 11), provoking factors (stressful life events), and symptom formation factors (past history of depression, severe life event after the onset of depression, and any past loss). The study was among the first that described a conceptual and interactive model for the social and personal causes of depression in women.

Sexual Abuse and Sexual Coercion

Trauma experienced by women such as childhood sexual abuse, adult sexual assault, and intimate partner violence also have been consistently linked to higher rates of depression in women, as well as to other psychiatric conditions (e.g., posttraumatic stress disorder, eating disorders) and physical illnesses. Features of abuse that determine the nature and severity of mental health problems include the duration of exposure to abuse, use of force, and relationship to the perpetrator. In addition, cognitive styles such as low self-esteem and even related appraisals also have an important impact on how women cope with abusive and traumatic life situations. In the context of sexual assault, characteristics such as degree and nature of physical force and perceived fear of death or injury significantly affect psychological outcome.

Intimate Partner Violence

Depression is also highly prevalent among women who experience male partner violence, which is often repetitive and concealed. Depression and posttraumatic stress disorder, which have substantial comorbidity, are the most prevalent mental health sequelae of intimate partner violence. Depression in women experiencing intimate partner violence has also been associated with other life stressors that often accompany domestic violence, such as younger age at marriage, childhood abuse, daily stressors, many children, coercive sex with an intimate partner, and negative life events. While some women might have chronic depression that is exacerbated by the stress of a violent relationship, there is also evidence that first episodes of depression can be triggered by such violence. Though most research focuses on physical and sexual abuse, the impact of psychological abuse on mental health is also evident. Most of the data point to the association of substance use (particularly alcohol use) in women experiencing intimate partner violence. Substance use has also been found to be a sequel to the experience of violence among women. A postulated explanation of substance use as an outcome of intimate partner violence is through posttraumatic stress disorder. Women with posttraumatic stress disorder might use drugs or alcohol to calm or cope with the specific groups of symptoms associated with posttraumatic stress disorder: Intrusion, avoidance, and hyperarousal. Women can also begin to abuse substances through their relationships with men or from wanting to escape the reality of intimate partner violence. It is important to address and understand these complex relations between intimate partner violence, mental health, and behavior to make an accurate diagnosis and intervene in substance abuse problems. In addition to mental health problems, women who experience violence use medical and emergency services more often and are known to present to primary care with unexplained somatic symptoms.

Poverty

Poverty among women has been steadily increasing and it has been linked to mental health problems among women. This association was observed more than two decades ago by Brown and Harris (1978), and this link has been established in recent studies. Affective disorders are common among both men and women living in poverty and it has been observed that more women live in poverty than men. Poverty among women increases their risk for exposure to traumatic life experiences such as physical and sexual victimization. These experiences at times serve as barriers to accessing mental health services. In addition, women in poverty find it difficult to access health care because of lack of insurance and transportation and inflexible jobs.

Mental health problems, when untreated, can lead to severe disabilities for women in poverty. In addition, mental health problems, specifically depression, have been reported to contribute to significant economic burden in women living in poverty (Patel *et al.*, 2007).

Migration

Migration involves uprooting oneself fully or partially from the familiar, traditional community and relocating in a foreign land. Immigration can be planned and voluntary for better prospects in life or it can be unplanned, unanticipated, and forced, as in the case of civic unrest, armed conflict, and violation of human rights. Migration always calls for making adaptations, as people traverse several interpersonal, cultural, language, ecological, and geographic boundaries. The sociocultural differences and scarcity of resources could lead to feelings of fear, isolation, alienation, and helplessness in migrants. Migration as such may not affect the mental health of the immigrants, but the process of migration and adaptation can cause increased stress and vulnerability to mental health problems. For instance, evidence from South Asian immigrant women in Canada suggests that these women are specifically at risk for mental health problems because of the rigid gender roles in the South Asian community that make smooth integration into the adopted country a challenge. Likewise, South Asian women residing in the UK were more likely to report anxiety and depressive symptoms compared to their male counterparts. Loss of social support, low social status, constraints in finances, and accessing health services were major stressors for immigrant women in Canada (Ahmad *et al.*, 2004). Research studies conducted on divergent ethnic and racial immigrant groups residing in Europe found that complicated grief and posttraumatic stress disorder were noted to be common psychiatric problems among refugees and asylum seekers.

War

Wars are known to cause immense human suffering in several ways. War results in a shortage of food, water, fuel, and electricity that are basic requirements of every human being. During war, many civilians are exposed to traumatic experiences such as shooting and shelling and also seeing dead and wounded people, witnessing and experiencing violence, and injuries to self and others. Experiences of separation and displacement from relatives and forced migrations are very common. In addition to loss of valuable human resources, war results in damage of infrastructure and depletion of natural resources. There is substantial evidence on the mental health consequences of war for individuals. High rates of posttraumatic stress disorder as well as depressive and anxiety

disorders were documented even among civilians. Studies documented inconsistent but high prevalence rates of PTSD among women affected by war. In addition, the aftermath or the postwar sociopolitical conditions are likely to contribute to mental health problems in women. For instance, life in Afghanistan has been disrupted for the past 20 years because of social and political disturbances. The war had extraordinary health outcomes for Afghan women, and women in Afghanistan have been found to have significantly poorer mental health compared to men (Cardozo, 2005).

Natural Disasters

Natural disasters are out of human control but the consequences of natural disasters overlap with the consequences of war or combat. In both contexts, there is human suffering caused by damage to life, personal property, and infrastructure. Families are displaced and victims lose shelter. This is complicated further by immense shortages of food and drinking water. Several medical and psychological problems among the victims are major offshoots of natural disasters. A summary of research studies conducted between 1981 and 2004 in both developing and developed nations yielded consistent results with regard to the psychological consequences of disasters on women. PTSD and major depressive and anxiety disorders were the common mental health consequences. The gender of the victims predicted several post-disaster outcomes in many of these studies; consistently, women were more likely to be affected than men. For PTSD alone, the rates for women exceeded those for men by a ratio of 2:1. In a few studies, being married was found to be a risk factor because the severity of husbands' symptoms predicted the severity of wives' symptoms more than vice versa (**Figure 1**).

Clinical Interface of Women's Mental Health with Reproductive Health and Medical Disorders

Psychiatric Disorders in Relation to Pregnancy and the Postpartum Period

Studies on psychiatric disorders among pregnant women in community-derived samples have shown lifetime depression risk estimates between 10% and 25%, while studies that screened obstetric patients at random for depressive symptoms found that up to 20% of patients met criteria for a diagnosis of a depressive episode. Risk factors for depression during pregnancy include young age, low education, a large number of children, a history of child abuse, a personal or family history of mood disorder, and stressors such as marital dysfunction.

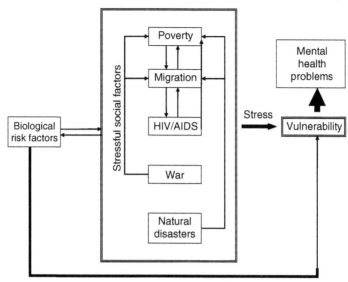

Figure 1   Hypothetical model demonstrating the interaction between biological and social factors leading to mental health problems among women.

Marcus *et al.* (2003) found that one in five pregnant women experience depression, but few seek treatment. The stigma of having depression during pregnancy may prevent women from seeking active treatment because they may feel guilty for suffering during what is supposed to be a happy period. The impact of untreated depression during pregnancy is known to have negative effects on both mother and child.

Major consequences of untreated maternal depression

In the mother
Mothers with depression may suffer from impaired social function, emotional withdrawal, and excessive concern regarding their future ability to parent. They are less likely to regularly attend obstetrical visits or have regular ultrasounds and show lack of initiative and motivation to seek help, and experience a negative perception regarding any potential benefit of obstetric services. Mothers suffering from depression are also more likely to smoke or use alcohol and have lower-than-normal weight gain throughout pregnancy because of diminished appetite. Severe depression also carries the risk of self-injurious, psychotic, impulsive, and harmful behaviors. Untreated depression may have associated obstetric complications such as spontaneous abortion, bleeding during gestation, and spontaneous early labor.

In the child
Untreated maternal depression has also been associated with low birth weight in babies, babies small for their gestational age, preterm deliveries, perinatal and birth complications, admission to a neonatal care unit, and neonatal growth retardation. Neurobehavioral effects include

reduced attachment, reduced mother–child bonding, and delays in offsprings' cognitive and emotional development. Lower language achievements and long-term behavioral problems may also be seen in some children whose mothers suffered from depression.

Postpartum psychiatric disorders
Postpartum psychiatric disorders are unarguably one of the most complex groups of disorders that encompass human experience. The joy of having a baby coupled with distress caused by impaired mental health can render the experience particularly traumatic to the mother, infant, and family. History taking in overburdened emergency maternity wards usually does not allow for details about the mother's psychiatric history, let alone her current emotional status. In addition, short hospital stays and lack of follow-up make early recognition of emotional disorders difficult. The consequences of undiagnosed and hence untreated puerperal disorders can have negative consequences both on the mother and the developing infant. Psychiatric disorders in the postpartum period include depression, anxiety-related disorders such as panic disorder and obsessive compulsive disorders, mother–infant bonding disorders and the relatively less common group of severe mental illness. In addition, women with preexisting psychiatric problems may also have worsening of symptoms in the postpartum period.

Epidemiology
Epidemiological surveys by Kendell *et al.* (1987) and Terp *et al.* (1999) have established the incidence of postpartum psychosis as somewhat less than 1/1000 deliveries. Postpartum depression affects approximately 10–15% of all mothers in the developed world, while slightly higher

Table 3   Prevalence rates for postpartum depression across various sites

Country/(state)	Percentage (%)
India/(Goa)	23
China	11.2
Japan	17
Arabia	15.8
Zimbabwe	16
South Africa	34.7
Australia	14–17
Western population[a]	10–15[a]

[a]Data from meta analysis: O'Hara MW and Swain AM (1996) Rates and risk of postpartum depression: A meta-analysis. *International Review of Psychiatry* 8: 37–54.

rates have been reported from India (Patel, 2002) and South Africa. **Table 3** gives the prevalence rates based on studies done in several countries around the world.

The presence of depression in the last trimester of pregnancy is a strong predictor of postpartum depression. The preference for male children, deeply rooted in some societies, coupled with the limited control a woman has over her reproductive health may make pregnancy a stressful experience for some women. Local cultural factors are also pertinent in shaping maternal socioaffective well-being. For example, in rural China, mother-in-law conflict was reported in nearly one-third of young women who attempted suicide, as reported by Pearson (2002). Similar data on the role of mothers-in-law in domestic violence in pregnancy are available from different cultures such as Hong Kong, India, Korea, and Japan.

Severe mental illness in the postpartum period

Psychoses in the postpartum period have been classified as organic psychosis, schizophrenia, mania, or acute psychosis. Several studies report a relationship between puerperal psychosis and bipolar disorders. Some of the common clinical features of psychosis in the postpartum include a polymorphic presentation, perplexity, confusion, emotional lability, and psychotic ideas related to the infant. In addition, preexisting severe mental illness can also worsen in the postpartum period. Severe mental illness after childbirth may raise several psychosocial issues, particularly related to safety of the mother and the infant. The Confidential Enquiry into Maternal Deaths 1997–1999, carried out in the UK, reported that psychiatric disorder, and suicide in particular, was the leading cause of maternal death in the first year after childbirth. The study has highlighted the need for routine assessment of preexisting and recent-onset psychiatric disorder in obstetric settings. It also emphasized the need for specialized clinical services for mothers with severe mental illness.

Table 4   Risk factors for postpartum depression

Low marital age
Low education
Marital discord and violence
Inadequate social support
Low socioeconomic status
Past depression
Personality vulnerability
Life events during pregnancy or near delivery
Complicated delivery
Adverse in-law relationship

Depression

The presentation of this group of disorders can be heterogeneous. Mothers with chronic dysthymia, prepartum depression continuing into the puerperium, depression associated with recent adversity, and bipolar depression all fall into this common heading. Postnatal depression can have untoward effects on infant development, and depression may lead to reduced interaction and irritability misdirected at the child.

One of the most popular and widely used screening tools used for detection of postpartum depression is the Edinburgh Postnatal Depression Scale (EPDS) (**Table 5**) originally designed by Cox *et al.* (1987). This scale is available in several languages around the world. A high score on this ten-item self-rating questionnaire needs to be followed by an interview clarifying the symptoms of depression and comorbid psychiatric disorders. In addition to detecting depression, it is also important to explore the wider context, including the mother's life history, personality, and circumstances; the course of the pregnancy, including parturition and the puerperium; and relationships with the spouse, other children, family of origin and, especially, the infant. In addition to diagnosing depression and other disorders, one must identify vulnerability factors and the availability of support (**Table 4**).

Treatment and prevention of maternal mental disorders

Several studies have assessed the efficacy of different forms of treatment and prevention of postpartum depression. These include interpersonal psychotherapy, home visits by nurses, prenatal and postnatal classes, debriefing visits, and continuity of care models. A recent meta-analysis on the efficacy of psychosocial interventions in preventing postpartum depression has reported that interventions that target at-risk women, are individually based, and are done in the postpartum period rather than during pregnancy appear to show more benefit. Interpersonal psychotherapy has also been used in the treatment of postpartum depression with some efficacy.

Acute treatment of bipolar illness and psychosis is usually with psychotropic drugs including mood stabilizers. However, knowledge regarding the safety of

Table 5 Edinburgh Postnatal Depression Scale (EPDS)

1. I have been able to laugh and look at the funny side of things.
   As much as I always could.
   Not quite so much now.
   Definitely not so much now.
   Not at all.
2. I have looked forward with enjoyment to things.
   As much as I always did.
   Rather less than I used to.
   Definitely not so much now.
   Not at all.
3. I have blamed myself unnecessarily when things went wrong.
   Yes, most of the time.
   Yes, some of the time.
   Not very often.
   No, never.
4. I have been anxious or worried for no reason.
   No, not at all.
   Hardly ever.
   Yes, sometimes.
   Yes, very often.
5. I have felt scared or panicky for no very good reason.
   Yes, quite a lot.
   Yes, sometimes.
   Not very often.
   No, never.
6. Things have been getting on top of me.
   Yes, most of the time I have not been able to cope at all.
   Yes, sometimes I have not been coping as well as usual.
   No, most of the time I have coped quite well.
   No, I have been coping as well as ever.
7. I have been so unhappy that I have had difficulty sleeping.
   Yes, most of the time.
   Yes, some of the time.
   Not very often.
   No, never.
8. I have felt sad or miserable.
   Yes, most of the time.
   Yes, quite often.
   Not very often.
   No, never.
9. I have been so unhappy that I have been crying.
   Yes, most of the time.
   Yes, quite often.
   Not very often.
   No, never.
10. The thought of harming myself has occurred to me.
   Yes, quite often.
   Sometimes.
   Hardly ever.
   No, never.

Cox JL, Holden JM, and Sagovsky R (1987) Detection of postnatal depression: Development of the 10-item Edinburgh Postnatal Depression Scale. *British Journal of Psychiatry* 150: 782–786.

antipsychotics and mood stabilizers in pregnancy and lactation is needed and second-generation antipsychotics may be safer. Lithium and other mood stabilizers are useful in treatment of bipolar disorders provided they are used with monitoring and also following discussions with the mother and the family. Antidepressants are indicated for moderate to severe depression, especially when biological functions are impaired or there is prominent suicidal ideation. Inpatient care may be indicated in more severe cases and requires specialized nursing and psychiatric care.

Postpartum psychosis has a recurrence rate of at least one in five pregnancies and mothers with a past history of puerperal or nonpuerperal psychosis have an enhanced risk. There is some evidence that prophylaxis, given immediately after delivery, reduces this risk.

Mother–infant bonding disorders that can occur as a consequence of psychiatric problems or infant-related issues are treated depending on the cause. Play therapy and baby massage under supervision or done in a graduated manner are often quite effective.

Menstrual Cycle and Menopause

Mild mood changes in relation to the premenstrual phase have been reported commonly; however, significant mental health problems have been reported in 3–5% of women. This usually occurs in the form of late luteal phase dysphoric disorders, which are mainly characterized by mood changes that significantly impair social, personal, and occupational functioning.

Mental health problems in menopause may be attributable to a combination of factors including hormonal, cognitive, and life-stage-related causes. Psychosocial factors including exit events such as illness or death of spouse, retirement, and loneliness may contribute significantly to mental health in the postmenopausal stage.

While the emphasis of the Women's Health Initiative (WHI) was more on the role of estrogen and progesterone on osteoporosis, breast cancer, and cardiovascular disease, the study also generated a large amount of data relevant to mental health. The WHIMS (Women's Health Initiative Memory Study) found a lack of evidence for the role of hormone therapy (estrogen alone or estrogen and progesterone) in protection against dementia among older women. The study also has important findings in the area of quality of life and lifestyle issues related to physical health, alcohol use, trauma, and panic disorders in older women. The study included Caucasian, African-American, and Asian women, was conducted in the U.S., and has important implications in the care of women over 65 years of age.

Reproductive Health Problems and Women's Mental Health

Infertility, female sterilization, and reproductive tract complaints have all been related to poor mental health in women. Infertility and the newer reproductive technologies are often fraught with uncertainties, leading to depression. Infertility in cultures where fertility and having children often determine the status of women has important implications for mental health. Vaginal discharge – both pathological (resulting from infections) and nonpathological – is often associated with symptoms of depression and anxiety. Women with somatic complaints and depression are known to present to clinics with a presenting complaint of vaginal discharge and need to be screened for mental health problems.

A recent study from West Africa (Coleman *et al.*, 2006), explored associations between depression and reproductive health conditions in 565 rural African women of reproductive age. The weighted prevalence of depression in the community was 10%, but more importantly, being depressed was significantly associated with widowhood or divorce, infertility, and severe menstrual pain.

Malignancies and Impact on Mental Health

Cancer of the cervix and breast cancer are the commonest cancers among women (the former in the developing world) and have several mental health implications. Mental health influences help seeking, early detection, and participation in cancer screening programs. Subsequent to diagnosis, depressive disorders are common and may influence coping methods used in handling the illness. Studies done on women with breast cancer have emphasized the role of coping not only in the context of mental health but also in the progression of the disease.

HIV/AIDS

The efficacy of antiretroviral drugs has resulted in the decline in the incidence of AIDS cases in developed parts of the world but the proportion of women living with AIDS in resource-poor countries has been increasing steadily. Feelings of shame, guilt, fears related to stigma, death, and dying, concerns associated with childbearing and transmission of HIV to children are common sources of stress among women with HIV/AIDS. HIV-infected women face higher stigma and lesser social support than men. A high incidence of depressive symptoms and anxiety disorders among women with HIV has been found in recent studies. HIV-infected women were found to be four times more likely to report current major depressive disorder and report anxiety symptoms compared to HIV-seronegative women. In the current context of antiretroviral treatment being available to a growing number of HIV-infected women even in the developing world, the recent literature has reported that depressive symptoms among women with HIV could lead to poor antiretroviral treatment utilization and adherence (Cook *et al.*, 2002). Early detection and treatment of mental health problems in HIV-infected women therefore may have an impact on help-seeking behaviors and medication compliance. In addition, psychosocial factors such as poor socioeconomic conditions, race, and ethnicity are also likely to be associated with mental health problems among women infected with HIV. For instance, HIV-infected women in the United States are disproportionately African-American or Latina and often live in poverty, and are as a result vulnerable to several social disadvantages. Understanding the psychological response to AIDS among women and the psychosocial context in which AIDS occurs is vital to prevent mental health problems and improve adherence to treatment.

Medical Disorders and Impact on Mental Health

Several medical conditions, especially endocrinological diseases (such as thyroid and parathyroid disorders) and collagen vascular disorders occur more commonly in women. These can cause mental health problems in two ways, one resulting from direct neuropsychiatric effects and the other a consequence of the disability caused by these conditions. Pain and somatic symptoms in medical disorders can be worsened because of coexisting mood disorders, which are commoner among women.

Interventions

Primary Prevention

Health policies that incorporate mental health into public health and address women's needs and concerns in different life stages can be developed in numerous ways. Health promotion through public health initiatives related to education, men's attitudes toward women, gender discrimination, violence, safety, substance abuse, prenatal care, and regular health assessments of older women will help in preventing several mental health problems. Health policies must also face the challenge of formulating ethical but culturally sensitive responses to practices that are damaging to the emotional and physical health of women and girls (such as female circumcision, female infanticide, gender-specific abortion, and feeding practices that discriminate against girl children).

Secondary Prevention

Integrated health programs that address and handle the stigma of major mental illness, consequences of sexual or domestic violence, the consequences of gender discrimination, and the stress of poverty are an important part of public health. One of the more troubling mental health consequences of the general health status of communities is the effect on mothers of high infant and child mortality rates and high HIV infection rates affecting multiple family members across generations. Communication between health workers, physicians, and women patients (and often men as well) needs to be emphasized to facilitate disclosure of mental health issues by women to facilitate early detection. Training of nonmental health professionals in the use of simple screening tools to detect mental health problems such as the use of the General Health questionnaire or the EPDS (see the section titled 'Depression') will strengthen early detection efforts in primary care. Training and enhancing the competence of primary care physicians, mental health professionals, and health workers to detect and treat the consequences of domestic violence, sexual abuse, and psychological distress can also play an important role. Helplines for women in distress and suicide helplines have been shown to be effective for women in early and accessible help seeking in the community. Women in most communities will need services near their homes and without causing inconvenience to child care and family.

Tertiary Prevention

Skilled clinicians as well as broader multidisciplinary programs in the community with links to hospitals are necessary to address the more distressing and difficult needs of women with serious psychiatric problems. These services should also be available in other medical centers such as those dealing with oncology or HIV infection and in obstetric and gynecology clinics.

Although the social roots of many of these problems mean that they cannot be managed only with medical interventions, there is a need to strengthen the potential role of the health-care system. In addition, there should be increased consumer participation by women in formulating health-care policies and programs.

Conclusion

Women's mental health needs to be considered in the context of the interaction of physical, reproductive, and biological factors with social, political, and economic issues at stake. The multiple roles played by women such as childbearing and child rearing, running the family, caring for sick relatives, and, in an increasing proportion of families, earning income are likely to lead to considerable stress. The reproductive roles of women, such as their expected role of bearing children, the consequences of infertility, and the failure to produce a male child in some cultures are examples of mechanisms that make women vulnerable to suffering from mental disorders. In addition, biological factors may play a major role, particularly in reproductive life events such as pregnancy, the postpartum period, and menopause as well as in the clinical manifestations of various mental health problems.

Public health and social policies aimed at improving the social status of women are needed along with those targeting the entire spectrum of women's health needs.

Efforts to improve and enhance social and mental health services and programs aimed at increasing the competence of professionals are also required.

See also: Mental Health Policy; Mental Health Promotion; Mental Health Resources and Services; Specific Mental Health Disorders: Trauma and Mental Disorders; Stigma of Mental illness.

Citations

Ahmad F, Shik A, Vanza R, et al. (2004) Voices of South Asian women. *Immigration and Mental Health* 40: 113–129.

Brown GW and Harris T (1978) *Social Origins of Depression. A Study of Psychiatric Disorder in Women.* London: Tavistock.

Cardozo BL (2005) Mental health of women in postwar Afghanistan. *Journal of Women's Health* 14: 285–293.

Coleman R, Morison L, Paine K, Powell RA, and Walraven G (2006) Women's reproductive health and depression: A community survey in the Gambia West Africa. *Social Psychiatry and Psychiatric Epidemiology* 41(9): 720–727.

Cook JA, Cohen MH, Burke J, et al. (2002) Effects of depressive symptoms and mental health quality of life on use of highly active antiretroviral therapy among HIV-seropositive women. *Journal of Acquired Immune Deficiency Syndrome* 30: 401–409.

Cox JL, Holden JM, and Sagovsky R (1987) Detection of postnatal depression: Development of the 10-item Edinburgh Postnatal Depression Scale. *British Journal of Psychiatry* 150: 782–786.

Kendell RE, Chalmers JC, and Platz C (1987) Epidemiology of puerperal psychoses. *British Journal of Psychiatry* 150: 662–673.

Kessler RC, Berglund PA, Demler O, et al. (2005) Lifetime prevalence and age-of-onset distributions of DSM-IV disorders in the National Comorbidity Survey Replication (NCS-R). *Archives of General Psychiatry* 62(6): 593–602.

Marcus SM, Flynn HA, Blow FC, et al. (2003) Depressive symptoms among pregnant women screened in obstetrics settings. *Journal of Women's Health (Larchmont)* 12: 373–380.

Murray CJL and Lopez AD (eds.) (1996) *The Global Burden of Disease and Injury Series, vol. 1: A Comprehensive Assessment of Mortality and Disability from Diseases, Injuries, and Risk Factors in 1990 and Projected to 2020.* Cambridge MA: Harvard School of Public Health.

O'Hara MW and Swain AM (1996) Rates and risk of postpartum depression: A meta-analysis. *International Review of Psychiatry* 8: 37–54.

Patel V, Rodrigues M, and DeSouza N (2002) Gender, poverty, and postnatal depression: A study of mothers in Goa India. *American Journal of Psychiatry* 159: 43–47.

Patel V, Chisholm D, Kirkwood BR, and Mabey D (2007) Prioritizing health problems in women in developing countries: Comparing the financial burden of reproductive tract infections, anaemia and depressive disorders in a community survey in India. *Tropical Medicine and International Health* 12(1): 130–139.

Pearson V (2002) Attempted suicide among young rural women in the People's Republic of China: Possibilities for prevention. *Suicide and Life-Threatening Behavior* 32: 359–369.

Robins LN and Regier DA (1991) *Psychiatric Disorders in America: The Epidemiologic Catchment Area Study.* New York: The Free Press.

Terp IM and Mortensen PB (1999) Post-partum psychoses: Clinical diagnoses and relative risk of admission after parturition. *British Journal of Psychiatry* 172: 521–526.

Further Reading

Benjamin L, Hankin L, and Abramson Y (2001) Development of gender differences in depression: an elaborated cognitive vulnerability-transactional stress theory. *Psychological Bulletin* 127: 773–796.

Carta MG, Bernal M, Hardoy MC, *et al.* (2005) Migration and mental health in Europe (The State of the Mental Health in Europe Working Group: Appendix I): Review. *Clinical Practice and Epidemiology in Mental Health* 1: 13.

Fischback RL and Herbert B (1997) Domestic violence and mental health: Correlates and conundrums within and across cultures. *Social Science and Medicine* 45: 1161–1170.

Judith L, Lindsey W, Rhonda S, *et al.* (2006) PRISM (Program of Resources Information and Support for Mothers): A community-randomized trial to reduce depression and improve women's physical health six months after birth. *BioMed Central Public Health* 6: 37.

Kornstein SG and Clayton AH (eds.) (2003) *Women's Mental Health: A Comprehensive Textbook.* New York: Guilford Press.

Mazure CM, Keita GP, and Blehar MG (2002) *Summit on Women and Depression: Proceedings and Recommendations.* Washington DC: American Psychological Association.

Miranda J and Green B (1999) The need for mental health services research focusing on poor young women. *The Journal of Mental Health Policy and Economics* 2: 73–80.

Oates M (2003) Perinatal psychiatric disorders – A leading cause of maternal morbidity and mortality. *British Medical Bulletin* 67: 219–229.

Patel V, Araya R, de Lima A, *et al.* (1999) Women, poverty and common mental disorders in four restructuring societies. *Social Science and Medicine* 49: 1461–1471.

Rehaman A, Iqbal Z, Bum J, *et al.* (2004) Impact of maternal depression on infant nutritional status and illness: A cohort study. *Archives of General Psychiatry* 61(9): 946.

Watson M, Homewood J, Havilland J, *et al.* (2005) Influence of psychological response on breast cancer survival: 10-year follow-up of a population-based cohort. *European Journal of Cancer* 41(12): 1710–1714.

Relevant Websites

http://www.cdc.gov/hiv/ – Center for Disease Control and Prevention: HIV/AIDS.

http://www.who.int/mental_health/resources/gender/en/ – Gender and Women's Mental Health, World Health Organization.

http://www.womensmentalhealth.org/ – Massachusetts General Hospital Center for Women's Mental Health.

http://www.ncptsd.va.gov/ncmain/index.jsp – National Center for Posttraumatic Stress Disorder, United States Department of Veterans Affairs.

http://www.whi.org/ – Women's Health Initiative.

http://www.who.int/mental_health/media/en/67.pdf – Women's Mental Health: An evidence-based review, World Health Organization.

Subject Index

Notes

The index is arranged in set-out style with a maximum of three levels of heading. Major discussion of a subject is indicated by bold page numbers. Page numbers suffixed by T and F refer to Tables and Figures respectively. vs. indicates a comparison.

A

Abacavir
    AIDS dementia complex 212
Aboriginal peoples *see* Indigenous peoples
Abscess(es)
    bacterial, HIV patients 217
Absence seizures 292–293
Abulia, AIDS dementia complex 210
Abuse
    alcohol *see* Alcohol use/misuse
    children *see* Child abuse
    drugs *see* Drug abuse/misuse
    extreme, psychological responses 354
    partner *see* Partner abuse
    substance *see* Substance abuse/misuse
Acamprosate, alcohol use disorders 140
Accidental deaths 124
Acellular pertussis (aP) vaccine
    inactivated polio vaccine combination 276–277
Acetaminophen (paracetamol)
    migraine 231–232
Acetylsalicylic acid (ASA) *see* Aspirin (acetylsalicylic acid)
Acoustic admittance 198
Acoustic impedance measurement 198
Acoustic neuroma (vestibular schwannoma) 200, 201
Acoustic (stapedial) reflex 195–196
    acoustic impedance testing 198–199
Acoustics 196
Acquired immune deficiency syndrome (AIDS) *see* HIV/AIDS
Actigraphy, sleep disorders 299
Activity, ICF definition 173*t*
Acute anterior poliomyelitis *see* Polio
Acute flaccid paralysis (AFP)
    surveillance 273
Acute Stress Disorder 353
Acute stroke unit (ASU) 173
    average length of stay calculations 162
    mobile stroke team *vs.* 173
Adaptation & Development After Persecution and Trauma (ADAPT) model 355
ADAPT model (Adaptation & Development After Persecution and Trauma) 355
Adolescents/adolescent health
    anxiety/anxiety disorders 324
    anxiety disorders 120
    mental health 119
        comorbidity 120
        costs on society 120
        promotion 307
        see also Child and adolescent mental disorders
    mood disorders 316–317
    risk behavior 305
    tobacco use *see* Tobacco consumption/use
Adolescent Transitions Program, substance misuse prevention 407
Adrenocorticotropin hormone (ACTH)
    stress 498
Adult onset diabetes mellitus *see* Type 2 diabetes mellitus
Adverse Childhood Experience (ACE) studies 39, 41*f*
Advocacy
    mental health promotion 454
AESOP (Aetiology and Ethnicity in Schizophrenia and Other Psychoses) study 115
Aetiology and Ethnicity in Schizophrenia and Other Psychoses (AESOP) study 115
Africa
    alcohol consumption 6*f*, 7*f*
    mental health services, treatment gap 89*t*
    onchocerciasis control programs 149
Age-associated memory impairment (AAMI) *see* Mild cognitive impairment (MCI)
Age-related macular degeneration 148
Aging/age-related changes
    cognitive disorders *see* Cognitive disorders, aging-related
    mental disorders **330–338**

Agoraphobia, elderly 336
AIDS *see* HIV/AIDS
AIDS dementia *see* AIDS dementia complex (ADC)
AIDS dementia complex (ADC) 210
    behavioral symptoms 210
    CD4 counts 210, 211
    cognitive manifestations 210
    development 210
    diagnosis 211
    differential diagnosis 210–211
    laboratory evaluation 211
    memory difficulties 210
    motor symptoms 210
    neuroimaging 212, 213*f*
    psychomotor slowing 210
    staging system 210–211, 211*t*
    subacute dementia 210
    treatment 212
    viral loads 211
Alcohol, definition 126
Alcohol consumption
    biochemical effects 12
    brain tumor risks 158
    burden of disease **12–28**
        age at death 24*t*, 27
        disability-adjusted life years 23*t*, 26*t*, 27
        global 17, 18, 19*t*
        risk factors 12
        years of life lost 23*t*
    category definitions 16*t*
    characteristics 5, 5*t*, 21*t*
    cognitive decline 181
    dimensions 2
    diseases associated 13, 14*t*, 15*t*, 17, 19*t*
    elderly 337
        prevalence 337
    health/social consequences 12
    injuries associated 13, 14*t*, 15*t*, 19*t*
    measurement 6, 14
        adult per capita 14, 16, 21*f*
        Global Alcohol Database, WHO *see* Global Alcohol Database, WHO
        models 12, 13*f*
    mortality 6, 22*t*
        age at death 24*t*
        premature 22*t*
    prevalence 16
    trends, international **2–11**
        Global Alcohol Database *see* Global Alcohol Database, WHO
        methodological issues 2
        see also Alcohol use/misuse
Alcohol dependence 12
Alcohol dependence syndrome (ADS) 137–138
Alcohol Harm Reduction Strategy, European Union 376
Alcoholics Anonymous 141–142
    efficacy 142
    Twelve Step Facilitation 142, 421
Alcohol-induced mood disorder 138
Alcohol-induced psychotic disorder 138
Alcohol industry **378–388**
    advertising 399–400
    corporate responsibility 384
    free-trade agreements 382
    global consolidation 378
    global promotion 383, 385*f*, 386*f*
        commodity chain 385
        market strategies 381
    social aspects organizations 386
    sport sponsorship 379
Alcohol policy/control **414–420**
    advertising restrictions 416
    community interventions 418

Campylobacter pyloridis see Helicobacter pylori
Canada
  alcohol consumption 5, 6–8, 7*f*
  drug policy, City of Vancouver 'four-pillar' harm reduction
    approach 391
Cancer
  depression comorbidity 87–88, 89*f*
  diet in *see* Diet-cancer relationship
  etiology
    tobacco association 132
  personality and 83
  psychological issues 82
Canine rabies
  control 284–285
  presentation 285, 285*f*, 286*f*
  transmission 283, 284–285
  vaccination 284–285
Cannabis dependence syndrome 59
Cannabis use
  adverse health effects 58
  global trends 433, 433*t*
  morbidity 59
  mortality 58
  prevalence 57, 58*t*
  sociocultural influences 129–130, 132
Capgras syndrome 179
CAPN3 gene 253–254
Carbamazepine (CBZ) 294
  side effects 294
  teratogenicity 294
Cardiomyopathy type 1F 255
Cardiomyopathy type 1G (CMD1G) 255
Cardiovascular disease (CVD)
  absolute 5-year development risk 168–169, 170*f*
  behavioral factors 500
  depression association 82
  psychological attributes associated 82
  risk factors
    menopause 502
    stress 498–499, 499–500
Caregivers
  Alzheimer's disease 506
  mental disorders 124
Care in the community 473
Carers *see* Caregivers
Caribbean
  alcohol consumption 8
Carnitine palmitoyl transferase (CPT) deficiency 223
Cartesian dualism *see* Mind-body dualism
Case-control studies
  mental health epidemiology 69, 101
  observational epidemiology *see* Observational epidemiology
Cataplexy, narcolepsy-related 300
Cataracts
  public health prevention strategies 146
    blindness 146
Catechol O-methyltransferase (COMT) 268
Cattle
  bovine spongiform encephalopathy 367
Cellular telephones, brain tumor risk 156
  exposure misclassification 156
Censuses
  mental health epidemiology 69
Centers for Disease Control and Prevention (CDC), US
  epilepsy-related initiatives 296
Central auditory nervous system 195
Central nervous system (CNS), HIV infiltration 80
Central nervous system cancers
  definition 151
  incidence 152*t*
Central nervous system tuberculosis (CNSTB)
  HIV/AIDS associated 206
    clinical features 206
    diagnosis 206
    extrameningeal lesions 206
Central nervous system tumors 151
Central pontine myelinolysis (CPM) 188
Cerebral blood flow (CBF), traumatic brain injury 183–184, 184*f*
Cerebral insult, cognitive disorders 177
Cerebral perfusion pressure (CPP), traumatic brain injury
  183–184, 187

Cerebral stroke *see* Stroke
Cerebral toxoplasmosis 204
  clinical features 205
  diagnosis 205
  HIV-related 204
    induction-dose therapy 205–206
  treatment 205
Cerebrospinal fluid (CSF)
  AIDS dementia complex 211–212
  bacterial meningitis 217–218
  corticosteroid therapy 221
  examination, multiple sclerosis diagnosis 243
  HIV/AIDS 211–212
    central nervous system tuberculosis 206
    cerebral cryptococcosis 215
    progressive multifocal leukoencephalopathy 207–208
Cerebrovascular disease (CeVD) **161–176**
  incidence 161
  pathology 161
  prevalence 161
  risk factors 167
Cervical cancer
  mental health 512
Cervids, chronic wasting disease 370
Changing Minds, anti-stigma campaign 493
Child abuse **32–43**
  definition 32–33, 34*t*
  epidemiology 34
  evaluation 41
  incidence studies 35, 41*f*
  interventions 41
    service delivery 41
  investigation 41
  physical consequences 38, 39*f*
  prevention 42
  psychological consequences 38, 39
  risk factors 35*f*
  sexual *see* Child sexual abuse (CSA)
  typologies 33, 34*t*
Child and adolescent mental disorders **303–310**, 304*t*
  comorbidity 120
  costs on society 120
  disability-adjusted life years 303–304
  economic implications 304
  etiology 303
  impairment 303
  interventions 307, 307*t*, 308
  longitudinal studies 304
  morbidity 119
  parental burden of care 303
  prevalence 303, 305*t*
  prevention 307
  protective factors 303, 306*t*
  public health policy response 308
    future development 308
    standards 308*t*
  public health significance 303
  risk behavior association 305
  risk factors 303, 306*t*
  stigma 306
Childhood brain tumors (CBT)
  maternal cured meat consumption 155
  maternal infection, pregnancy 157
  parental smoking 158
Child maltreatment *see* Child abuse
Child neglect
  definition 33, 34*t*
  see also Child abuse
Child protective services (CPS), USA 41–42
Children/children's health
  anxiety disorders 316
  media health impact *see* Media coverage/campaigns
  mental health policy 440, 446
  mental health promotion 307
  mental health resources 465, 472*t*
  mental illness *see* Child and adolescent mental disorders
  parental educational attainment and *see* Educational attainment
  social gradients health impact *see* Social gradients
  violence, exposure/witness to *see* Violence
Child sexual abuse (CSA)
  definition 33, 34*t*

Printed in the United States
By Bookmasters